Recurrent Pregnancy Loss

Online Contents

1. A comprehensive up to date guide on diagnostic protocols and research-based therapies in Recurrent Pregnancy Loss.
2. Includes 3 free videos and case analysis.
3. Appendix 2-guidelines for further reading.

Video Contents

Chapter 54: Hysteroscopic Evacuation of the Uterus

Video 1: Hysteroscopic evacuation of a missed miscarriage at 6 weeks

Video 2: 9 weeks missed miscarriage with a gestational sac in anterior wall with fetus and an anembryonic gestational sac in posterior wall

Video 3: Ultrasound guided hysteroscopic evacuation of the uterus

**Kindly refer to the video,
Appendix 2-guidelines for further reading
by scanning the QR code**

Recurrent Pregnancy Loss

Fourth Edition

Editors

Mala Arora
FRCOG (UK) FICOG DA (UK) D Obst (Ireland)
Director, Noble IVF Center
Faridabad, Haryana
Senior Consultant, Fortis La Femme, New Delhi, India
Founder Director, Indian Recurrent Pregnancy Loss Foundation (IRPLF)
Vice Chairperson, International Society of Recurrent Pregnancy Loss (ISRPL)
Editor-in-Chief, International Journal of Recurrent Pregnancy Loss (IJRPL)
Past Chairperson, Indian College of Obstetricians and Gynaecologists (ICOG)
Past Vice President, Federation of Obstetric and Gynaecological Societies of India (FOGSI)

Asher Bashiri MD
Full Professor
Director, Recurrent Pregnancy Loss (RPL) Prevention Clinic and Maternity C Ward
Soroka University Medical Center
Department of Obstetrics and Gynecology
Faculty of Health Sciences
Ben-Gurion University of the Negev, Beer -Sheva, Israel
President World Congress Recurrent Pregnancy Loss (WCRPL)
President International Society Recurrent Pregnancy Loss (ISRPL)

Neelanjana Mukhopadhaya MBBS DGO MMed FICOG FRCOG
Consultant in Gynecology
Department of Obstetrics and Gynecology
Bedfordshire Hospitals, UK
Honorary Senior Lecturer, University College Hospital, London
Member, EBCOG Standing Committee on Examinations
Past Chair, Part 1 MRCOG at the Royal College of Obstetricians and Gynaecologists

Co-Editor

BS Susheela Rani MBBS MD (Obs & Gyne) PGDMLE (Medical Law & Ethics) FICOG
Director and Consultant
Manjushree Speciality Hospital
Consultant, Sparsh Hospital, Infantry Road
President of Bangalore Society of Obstetrics and Gynaecology 2008–2009
Chairperson, BSOG PG Forum from 2000–2021
Secretary, IMS, Bangalore Chapter

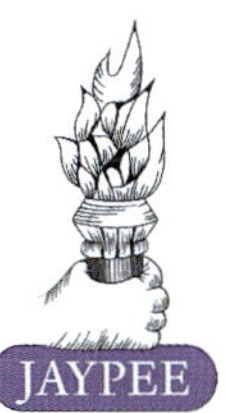

JAYPEE BROTHERS MEDICAL PUBLISHERS
The Health Sciences Publisher
New Delhi | London

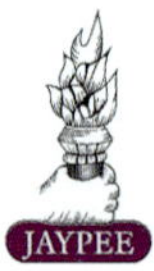

Jaypee Brothers Medical Publishers (P) Ltd

Headquarters
Jaypee Brothers Medical Publishers (P) Ltd
EMCA House, 23/23-B
Ansari Road, Daryaganj
New Delhi 110 002, India
Landline: +91-11-23272143, +91-11-23272703
+91-11-23282021, +91-11-23245672
Email: jaypee@jaypeebrothers.com

Corporate Office
Jaypee Brothers Medical Publishers (P) Ltd
4838/24, Ansari Road, Daryaganj
New Delhi 110 002, India
Phone: +91-11-43574357
Fax: +91-11-43574314
Email: jaypee@jaypeebrothers.com

Overseas Office
JP Medical Ltd
83 Victoria Street, London
SW1H 0HW (UK)
Phone: +44 20 3170 8910
Fax: +44 (0)20 3008 6180
Email: info@jpmedpub.com

Website: www.jaypeebrothers.com
Website: www.jaypeedigital.com

Inquiries for bulk sales may be solicited at: jaypee@jaypeebrothers.com

Recurrent Pregnancy Loss

First Edition: 2003

Second Edition: 2007

Third Edition: 2019

Fourth Edition: **2025**

ISBN: 978-93-6616-946-0

Printed at: Samrat Offset Pvt. Ltd.

Dedication

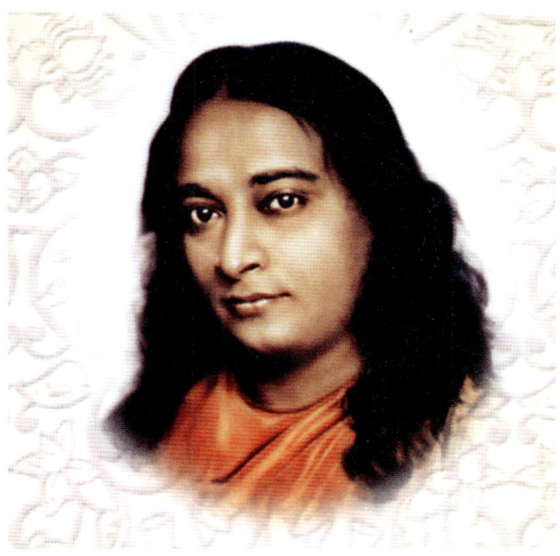

This book is dedicated with reverence to my Guru Sri Sri Paramahansa Yogananda* who has been the invisible inspiration for writing and updating this book.

To my parents and teachers who have sculpted my intellect.

To my husband, Narinder, and my children, Shruti and Rishi, who have contributed to my learning in an imperceptible way.

To my patients who have been my greatest teachers.

*Author of the book *Autobiography of a Yogi.*
Founder of Self Realization Fellowship, Mount Washington California, USA, and Yogoda Satsanga Society of India, Ranchi, Jharkhand, India.

Contributors

Adalgisa Pietropolli MD PhD
Department of Surgical Sciences
Section of Gynecology and Obstetrics
University Tor Vergata
Via Montpellier, Rome, Italy

Adam J Devall PhD
Associate Professor
Maternal Health Clinical Trials
Deputy Director
Tommy's National Centre for Miscarriage Research (Birmingham)
WHO Collaborating Centre for Global Women's Health
Department of Metabolism and Systems Science
School of Medical Sciences
College of Medicine and Health
University of Birmingham
Edgbaston, UK

Aditi Abhade MS (Obs & Gyne)
Junior Consultant
Department of Obstetrics and Gynecology
JK Women Hospital, Dombivli
Maharashtra, India

Ahmed Shelbaia MB BCh MSC MRCOG
Consultant
Department of Obstetrics and Gynecology
Luton and Dunstable University Hospital
Luton, Bedfordshire, UK

Akanshi Madan MBBS MD
Consultant
Department of Obstetrics and Gynecology
Tanvir Hospital
Hyderabad, Telangana, India

Ameet Patki MD DNB FCPS FRCOG
Medical Director
Department of IVF
Ikan Fertility Associates
Mumbai, Maharashtra, India

Anam Farooqui MBBS
Pediatrician
Biomedical Informatics Center
ICMR-National Institute for Research in Reproductive and Child Health (ICMR-NIRRCH)
Mumbai, Maharashtra, India

Arri Coomarasamy
OBE MBChB MD FRCOG FMedSci
Professor of Gynecology
Department of Medical College
University of Birmingham
Birmingham, UK

Arulmozhi Ramarajan
MD (Obs & Gyne) DGO
Consultant
Department of Obstetrics and Gynecology
Ramakrishna Medical Centre LLP
Tiruchirappalli, Tamil Nadu, India

Aruna Ashok
MBBS MS (Obs & Gyne) DNB (Obs & Gyne)
Clinical Director
A4 Hospitals and A4 Fertility Centre
Chennai, Tamal Nadu, India

Asher Bashiri MD
Full Professor
Director, Recurrent Pregnancy Loss (RPL)
Prevention Clinic and Maternity C Ward
Soroka University Medical Center
Department of Obstetrics and Gynecology
Faculty of Health Sciences
Ben-Gurion University of the Negev, Beer -Sheva, Israel
President World Congress Recurrent Pregnancy Loss (WCRPL)
President International Society Recurrent Pregnancy Loss (ISRPL)

Ashok Kumar MD PhD
Director Professor
Department of Obstetrics and Gynecology
Atal Bihari Vajpayee Institute of Medical Sciences
and Dr Ram Manohar Lohia Hospital
New Delhi, India

BS Susheela Rani
MBBS MD (Obs & Gyne) PGDMLE (Medical Law & Ethics) FICOG
Director and Consultant
Manjushree Speciality Hospital
Consultant, Sparsh Hospital
Infantry Road
President of Bangalore Society of Obstetrics & Gynaecology 2008–2009
Chairperson
BSOG PG Forum from 2000–2021
Secretary, IMS, Bangalore Chapter

Chaitanya Nagori
MD (Obs & Gyne) DGO
Director
Dr Nagori's Institute for Infertility and IVF
Ahmedabad, Gujarat, India

Chaitanya Shembekar MD FICOG
Diploma Pelviscopy FICMCH
Chairman and Managing Director
Omega Hospital
Nagpur, Maharashtra, India

Chandrashekara S
DM (Clinical Immunology and Rheumatology)
Medical Director
Department of Rheumatology and Clinical Immunology
ChanRe Rheumatology and Immunology Center and Research
Bengaluru, Karnataka, India

Chinmayee Ratha
MS (Obs & Gyne) FRCOG (UK) FICOG FIMSA
Diploma in Fetal Medicine (FMF-UK)
Director
Resolution Centre of Fetal Medicine, Hyderabad
Lead Consultant (Fetal Medicine)
KIMS Sunshine Hospitals
Hyderabad, Telangana, India

Chow-Seng Kong PhD
Postdoctoral Research Fellow
Department of Warwick Medical School
University of Warwick, UK

Deepak Modi PhD
Scientist G and Head
Molecular and Cellular Biology Lab
ICMR-National Institute for Research in Reproductive and Child Health (ICMR-NIRRCH)
Mumbai, Maharashtra, India

Durga G Rao DGO MRCOG
Infertility Specialist
Medical Director
Oasis—Centre for Reproductive Medicine
Hyderabad, Telangana, India

Duru Shah MD FICOG FCPS FICS DGO DFP
Director
Gynaecworld—The Center for Women's Health and Fertility
Consultant Gynecologist
Breach Candy Hospital and Jaslok Hospitals
Mumbai, Maharashtra, India

Emilio Piccione MD PhD
Emeritus Professor of Gynecology and Obstetrics
Department of Surgical Sciences
Tor Vergata University Medical and Surgical School of Rome
Rome, Italy

Enrico Vizza MD PhD
Professor
Department of Experimental Clinical Oncology
IRCCS Regina Elena National Cancer Institute
IRCCS Network of Neuroscience and Neurorehabilitation
Rome, Italy

Fabio Scarpellini MD PhD
Consultant
Department of Obstetrics and Gynecology
Sapienza University of Rome
Rome, Italy
CERM-Hungaria, Rome, Italy

Farhan Ali MD
Hospitalist and Internist
Internal Medicine
MultiCare Yakima Memorial Hospital
Yakima, WA-98902, USA

Gary Levy MD
Reproductive Endocrinologist and Infertility Specialist
Department of Obstetrics and Gynecology
Nevada Fertility Center
Las Vegas, NV 89118, United States

Hagit Daum MD
Department of Genetics
Hadassah Medical Organization and Faculty of Medicine
Hebrew University of Jerusalem, Israel

Harsha Bhadarka
PhD (Embryo Morphokinetics and Co-culture) Diploma in IVF and Reproductive Medicine (Kiel, Germany)
IVF Lab Director and Chief Embryologist
IVF Department
Akanksha Hospital and Research Institute
Gujarat, Ahmedabad, India

Haywood L Brown MD FACOG
Professor
Department of Obstetrics and Gynecology
University of South Florida
Tampa, Florida, USA

Henriette Svarre Nielsen MD DMSc
Chair Professor (Obstetrics and Gynecology)
Department of Medicine, University of Copenhagen
Consultant and Head of Recurrent Pregnancy Loss Unit
Department of Obstetrics and Gynecology
Copenhagen University Hospital, Amager Hvidovre Hospital
Copenhagen, Denmark

Hrishikesh D Pai
MD FRCOG (UK-HON) FCPS FICOG MSc (USA)
Founder and Medical Director
Bloom IVF Group, Lilavati Hospital IVF Center, Mumbai
Consultant Gynecologist, Lilavati Hospital IVF Center Mumbai and Fortis Hospital Bloom IVF Centre Delhi and Chandigarh
Professor
Department of Reproductive Medicine
DY Patil University
Navi Mumbai, Maharashtra, India
Past President, FOGSI (2022–2023), Trustee, FIGO Asia Oceania (2023–2025)
Chief Administrator, FOGSI Manyata Project
Postgraduate Teacher for MD and DNB Courses (1991–2018)

Isha Wadhawan MBBS MD MRCOG FAMS
Consultant
Department of Obstetrics and Gynecology
Fortis Escorts
Faridabad, Haryana, India

Israel David Gabay MD
Doctor of Medicine
Soroka University Medical Center Beer Sheva, HaDarom, Israel

J Harshini MBBS DGO DNB
Associate Consultant
Department of Obstetrics and Gynecology
Apollo Hospitals
Tiruchirappalli, Tamil Nadu, India

Jalagam Kavya Rao
MS (Obs & Gyne) FRM FIGL
Regional Medical Head and Fertility Specialist
Department of Clinical
Oasis Fertility
Hanamkonda, Telangana, India

Jayati Dureja
MBBS DNB (Obs & Gyne) Fellowship in Fetal Medicine, ICOG (Obs & Gyne) Ultrasound Certificate Course Gold Medalist, Fellowship in Clinical Genetics
Consultant
Department of Fetal Medicine
Sunrise Hospital
New Delhi, India

Jonathan Cohen MD PhD
Department of Reproductive Unit
Herzliya Medical Center, Israel
Reproductive Unit
American Hospital of Paris
Paris, France
Senior Medical Oncologist and the Director
Clinical Research Laboratory of Translational Immuno-Oncology

Judah Benjamin Smith

Jyoti Mishra MBBS MD (Obs & Gyne)
Gynecological
Endoscopic and Robotic Surgeon and Infertility Specialist
Blossom Women's Clinic
Noida, Uttar Pradesh, India

Kairavi Vyas
Microbiologist
Department of Reproductive Medicine
Akanksha Hospital and Research Institute
Anand, Gujarat, India

Kalpana P
MBBS MS (Obs & Gyne) DNB (Obs & Gyne)
Gynecologist
Department of Obstetrics and Gynecology
Women's Centre and Hospitals Pvt Ltd
Coimbatore, Tamil Nadu, India

Kamini A Rao
MBBS DGO DORCP DCH MCH FNAMS PGDMLE PhD
Chairman and Managing Director
Department of Reproductive Medicine
Dr Kamini Rao Hospitals—a unit of Medline Academics
Bengaluru, Karnataka, India

Kilian Vomstein
Department of Gynecological Endocrinology and Reproductive Medicine
Medical University of Innsbruck
Innsbruck, Austria

Kiran Kurtkoti MBBS DGO DNB
Director
Gynecologist, Infertility Specialist and Obstetrician
Department of Obstetrics
Shashwat Hospital
Pune, Maharashtra, India

Krishna Deepti Mogili
MBBS MD DNB (Obs & Gyne) MRCOG Fellowship in Reproductive Medicine
Senior Clinical Fellow
Department of Obstetrics and Gynecology
Luton and Dunstable Hospital
Luton, Bedfordshire, UK

Latha Venkatram
MBBS FRCOG (UK) MRCP (I)
Director
WMN Healthcare Services (P) Ltd
Lead Consultant
Department of Obstetrics and Gynecology
Rangadore Memorial Hospital
Bengaluru, Karnataka, India
President, Bengaluru RCOG Trust

Lindsey Ann Choi DO
Gynecologic Surgery and Obstetrics
Blanchfield Army Community Hospital
Fort Campbell, Kentucky

Liu Shuling
MBBS (Spore) RCOG MRCOG MMed (Obs & Gyne) (Spore)
Senior Consultant
Department of Reproductive Medicine
KK Women's and Children's Hospital
Singapore

Mala Arora
FRCOG (UK) FICOG DA (UK) D Obst (Ireland)
Director, Noble IVF Center
Faridabad, Haryana
Senior Consultant
Fortis La femme, New Delhi, India
Founder Director, Indian Recurrent Pregnancy Loss Foundation (IRPLF)
Vice Chairperson, International Society of Recurrent Pregnancy Loss (ISRPL)
Editor-in-Chief, International Journal of Recurrent Pregnancy Loss (IJRPL)
Past Chairperson, Indian College of Obstetricians and Gynaecologists (ICOG)
Past Vice President, Federation of Obstetric and Gynaecological Societies of India (FOGSI)

Manju Puri MD FRCOG (Hon Causa) FICOG
Director Professor
Department of Obstetrics and Gynecology
Lady Hardinge Medical College
New Delhi, India

Marco Sbracia MD
Department of Obstetrics and Gynecology
University La Sapienza
Rome, Italy
CERM-Hungaria, Rome, Italy

Martina Betti
Alleanza Controil Cancro
Rome, Italy

Mathangi T DNB (Obs & Gyne)
Consultant
Department of Obstetrics and Gynecology
Seethapathy Clinic and Hospital
Chennai, Tamil Nadu, India

Matteo Pallocca
IRCCS Regina Elena National Cancer Institute
Rome, Italy

Matthew George Apostolou
MBChB (UP) Cum Laude, PGD Acute Medicine (USW) Cum Laude
Registrar
Department of Obstetrics and Gynecology
Health Education East of England Deanery (HEEoE)
Highgate, London, UK

Mayumi Sugiura-Ogasawara
MD PhD
Professor
Department of Obstetrics and Gynecology
Graduate School of Medical Sciences and Medical School, Nagoya City University
Mizuho-ku, Nagoya, Aichi, Japan

Meenu Handa MS DNB FRM FICOG
Clinical Director
Department of Reproductive Medicine (IVF)
Cloudnine Hospital
Gurugram, Haryana, India
Secretary, Haryana ISAR

Meeta Singh MBBS MD
Consultant, Head (Obstetrics and Gynecology), Co-Director
Department of Obstetrics and Gynecology
Tanvir Hospital
Hyderabad, Telangana, India

Mirudhubashini Govindarajan
MBBS FRCS (C) FICOG
Clinical Director
Department of Obstetrics and Gynecology
Women's Centre and Hospitals Pvt Ltd
Coimbatore, Tamil Nadu, India

Mohan Raut MD DGO FCRI
Partner
Department of Clinical Reproductive Immunology
Dr Raut's Centre for Reproductive Immunology
Mumbai, Maharashtra, India

Molina Patel
MD (Obs & Gyne) Dip RM (Kiel's University, Germany)
Consultant
Akanksha Hospital and Research Institute
Anand, Gujarat, India

Moty Pansky MD
Head
Department of Gynecology
Assuta Ashdod University Hospital
Ashdod, Israel

Mrinmayi Dharmadhikari
MBBS MS MRCOG (UK) DNB (Obs & Gyne)
Consultant Obstetrician and Gynecologist
Fertility Specialist
Ashvini Maternity and Nursing Home, Panvel
Dharmadhikari Hospital
Pune, Maharashtra, India

Mugdha Raut MBBS MD (Midwifery & Gynecology) DGO
Gynecologist
Dr Raut's Maternity and Surgical Nursing Home
Mumbai, Maharashtra, India

Naama Steiner MD
Senior physician (Unit for Fertility and in-vitro Fertilization)
Department of Obstetrics and Gynecology
Soroka Medical Center
Be'er Sheva, Israel

Namrata Singh MBBS DNB
DNB Resident
Department of Obstetrics and Gynecology
Fortis Escorts
Faridabad, Haryana, India

Narinder Pal MD FRCP (UK) FRCP (Ire)
Internal Medicine
Medical Director and Consultant Physician
Department of Medicine
Noble Hospital
Faridabad, Haryana, India

Nave Kahana B Med Sc in the Joyce & Irving Gildman Medical School, MD Candidate
Faculty of Health Sciences
Ben-Gurion University of the Negev
Be'er-Sheva, Israel

Nayana Patel MD (Obs & Gyne)
Medical Director
Department of Obstetrics and Gynecology
Akanksha Hospital and Research Institute
Anand, Gujarat, India

Neelanjana Mukhopadhaya
MBBS DGO MMed FICOG FRCOG
Consultant in Gynecology
Department of Obstetrics and Gynecology
Bedfordshire Hospitals, UK
Honorary Senior Lecturer
University College Hospital, London
Member, EBCOG Standing Committee on Examinations
Past Chair, Part 1 MRCOG at the Royal College of Obstetricians and Gynaecologists

Neil J Sebire
Professor of Pathology
Department of Pediatric and Developmental Pathology
Great Ormond Street Hospital and ICH (UCL)
Trophoblastic Disease Unit
Imperial College Hospital
London, UK

Niket H Patel MD
Director
Akanksha Hospital and Research Institute Infertility Specialist and Laparoscopic Surgeon
Department of Reproductive Medicine and IVF Akanksha Hospital and Research Institute
Anand, Gujarat, India

Nikita Trehan
MBBS DNB MNAMS Fellowship in Laparoscopic Surgery
Gynecologist and Laparoscopic Surgeon
Head, Gyne Laparoscopic Surgery
Sunrise Hospital
New Delhi, India

Ole Bjarne Christiansen MD
Clinical Professor, Ledende overlæge
Aalborg University Hospital
Department of Clinical Medicine
The Faculty of Medicine
Department of Gynecology and Obstetrics
Aalborg, Denmark

Oshri Barel MD MHA FRANZCOG
Head
Department of Gynecology
Assuta Ashdod University Hospital
Ashdod, Israel

Padma Rekha Jirge
MRCOG (UK) FICOG MBA (Healthcare Management) PG DMLE (Diploma in Medical Law and Ethics)
Scientific Director
Department of Reproductive Medicine
Shreyas Multispecialty Hospital and Research Institute
and Sushrut Assisted Conception Clinic
Kolhapur, Maharashtra, India

Panayiotis Tanos MD
Department of Obstetrics and Gynecology (Ambre Balestra, Panayiotis Tanos and Stavros Karampelas)
Centre Hospitalier Universitaire Brugmann
Brussels, Belgium

Paresh Ghoghari
MD (Obs & Gyne) Dip RM (Kiel's University, Germany)
Consultant
Department of Reproductive Medicine and Reproductive Immunology
IVF Akanksha Hospital and Research Institute
Anand, Gujarat, India

Partha Sarathi Das MS MSc
Deputy Medical Director, Consultant REI
Department of Assisted Reproductive, Embryology and Genetics
Orchid Reproductive and Andrology Services
Dubai, UAE

Paul Brighton PhD
Postdoctoral Research Fellow
Department of Warwick Medical School
University of Warwick, UK

Piyush Chudasama MSc (Biochemistry)
Researcher
Sat Kaival Hospital
Akanksha Hospital and Research Institute
Anand, Gujarat, India

Pragati Oswal
MSc (Yogic Sciences) MA (Eng Lit) Current Acupressure (PGD) Masters in Reiki
Complementary and Alternative Medicine Practitioner and Researcher
Bengaluru, Karnataka, India

Priya Ranganath
MBBS MS (Obs & Gyne) DNMB-SS Medical Genetics
Consultant
Department of Clinical Genetics
The Apollo Centre of Genomic Medicine
Bengaluru, Karnataka, India

Raj Raghupathy PhD FRCPath
Professor of Immunology and Consultant Immunologist
Department of Microbiology
College of Medicine
Kuwait University
Jabriya, Kuwait

Ritu Jain
MS (Obs & Gyne) Diploma Endoscopy, Fellowship Infertility
Director
Department of Obstetrics and Gynecology
Vardhman Medicare Centre
Gurugram, Haryana, India

Rohan Krishnakumar
MS (Obs & Gyne) DNB DFP
Consultant
Department of Obstetrics and Gynecology
JK Women Hospital, Dombivli
Maharashtra, India

Rosemary A Fisher PhD FRCPath
Principal Research Fellow
Honorary Consultant Geneticist
Trophoblastic Disease Screening and Treatment Centre
Imperial College London
London, UK

S Krishnakumar MD DGO FICOG
Gynecologist
Infertility Specialist and Obstetrician
Department of Obstetrics and Gynecology
Fortis Hospital
Thane, Maharashtra, India

Saadhvi Balaji MBBS DNB (Obs & Gyne)
Fellow, Reproductive Medicine
Department of Obstetrics and Gynecology
Women's Centre and Hospitals Pvt Ltd
Coimbatore, Tamil Nadu, India

Sai Deepashri S
MBBS DGO DNB (Obs & Gyne)
Senior Resident
Department of Obstetrics and Gynecology
Sri Ramachandra Institute of Higher Education and Research
Chennai, Tamil Nadu, India

Sanjivni Khanna MD (Obs & Gyne) FICOG
Senior Director Emeritus
Department of Obstetrics and Gynecology
Fortis Hospital
New Delhi, India

Sayani Maitra MBBS MRCOG
Clinical Fellow
Department of Obstetrics and Gynecology
University Hospitals Dorset NHS Foundation Trust, UK

Seema Sharma DGO MD FRCOG FICOG
Director (Obstetrics and Gynecology)
Cloudnine Hospital
New Delhi, India
Founder Director, IRPL Foundation

Selvaraj Ravi Lakshmy MBBS
Director
Department of Fetal Medicine
Sri Lakshmi Clinic and Scan Center
Krishnagiri, Tamil Nadu, India

Sher Ali
MSc (Gold Medalist) PhD FNA FASc FNASc FSASc JCBNF MIABS
Dean, Research & Development (Senior Administrator)
Distinguished Professor
VC Office, Era University, Lucknow
Av-Humboldt Fellow, Bonn, Germany
Fulbright Fellow, USA Alumni: USA, UK, Germany and Australia
Adjunct Professor
Manipal Academy of Higher Education (MAHE) Manipal
Mangaluru, Karnataka, India
Former Dean Academics, Dean R & D
Integral University
Lucknow, Uttar Pradesh, India
Formerly Distinguished Professor
Department of Life Sciences
Sharda University
Greater Noida, Uttar Pradesh, India
Former Director
Center for Interdisciplinary Research in Basic Sciences
Jamia Millia Islamia
New Delhi, India
Formerly Senior Staff Scientist and Head
Molecular Genetics Division National Institute of Immunology
New Delhi, India

Shinobu Goto MD PhD
Professor
Department of Obstetrics and Gynecology
Graduate School of Medical Sciences and Medical School, Nagoya City University
Mizuho-ku, Nagoya, Aichi, Japan

Shira Salama
BSc in Biology and Engineering
Research Assistant
The Multidisciplinary Center for Male and Female Fertility
Tel Aviv, Israel

Shlomi Barak MD FRANZCOG
Head
Department of Reproductive Services
Assuta Ashdod University Hospital
Raanana, Israel

Shobhna Mohandas
MD DGO FICOG Dip.Endoscopy Germany
Consultant Gynecologist and Laparoscopic Surgeon
Sun Medical Centre
Thrisur, Kerala, India

Shrutika O Makde
MS (OBGY) DNB (OBGY)
Assistant Professor
Department of Obstetrics & Gynecology and Reproductive Medicine
Lokmanya Tilak Municipal Medical College and Government Hospital
Mumbai, Maharashtra, India

Sonal Panchal
MBBS MD (Radiodiagnosis) PhD
Consultant Sonography Specialist
Dr Nagori's Institute for Infertility and IVF
Ahmedabad, Gujarat, India

Sonia Malik DGO MD FICOG FIAMS
Chief Clinical Mentor
Department of Fertility and IVF
NOVA IVF and Fertility
New Delhi, India

Sreeba Balakrishanan MBBS
Resident
Department of Obstetrics and Gynecology
Atal Bihari Vajpayee
Institute of Medical Sciences
and Dr Ram Manohar Lohia Hospital
New Delhi, India

Srimathy Raman MD FRCOG CCT (UK)
Consultant
Department of Obstetrics and Gynecology
Rangadore Memorial Hospital
Bengaluru, Karnataka, India

Srividya Seshadri
MBBS MD FRCOG MSc FCRI (Fellow, Clinical Reproductive Immunology, American Society for Reproductive Immunology)
Consultant Gynecologist
Department of Reproductive Medicine and Surgery
Aria Fertility
UCL, London

Stacy Colaco PhD
Scientist (DHR Young Scientist Fellowship)
Molecular and Cellular Biology Lab
ICMR-National Institute for Research in Reproductive and Child Health
Mumbai, Maharashtra, India

Sundari N
MBBS DNB (Obs & Gyne) PGDMLE
Retd Professor and Consultant
Department of Obstetrics and Gynecology
Ramaiah Medical College, Ramaiah Memorial Hospital
Bengaluru, Karnataka, India

Sunil Jaiman
MBBS MD (Path) Dip RCPath (UK)
Assistant Professor
Pathology Discipline Director and Human Disease Foundation-I Course Director
Department of Pathology
Wayne State University School of Medicine
Detroit, Michigan, USA

T Ramanidevi
MD DGO FICS FICOG PhD
Director
Department of Obstetrics and Gynecology
Ramakrishna Medical Centre LLP
Tiruchirappalli, Tamil Nadu, India

Talya Kresch-Jaffe MD
Medical School for International Health
Faculty of Health Sciences
Ben-Gurion University of the Negev
Be'er Sheva, Israel

Tamao Kitaori
MD PhD
Professor
Department of Obstetrics and Gynecology
Graduate School of Medical Sciences and Medical School, Nagoya City University
Mizuho-ku, Nagoya, Aichi, Japan

Tanja Schlaikjær Hartwig
MD PhD PDF
Post-doctoral Researcher
Department of Gynecology and Obstetrics
Hvidovre Hospital
Copenhagen, Denmark

Tanvir Singh
MBBS Masters in Surgery—Obs & Gyne ISGE Bachelor of MIGS
Consultant
Tanvir Hospital
Hyderabad, Telangana, India

Uma Ram
DGO DNB MRCOG FRCOG
Director and Lead (Obs & Gyne)
Department of Obstetrics and Gynecology
Seethapathy Clinic and Hospital
Chennai, Tamil Nadu, India

Usha Ahluwalia
MD FRCOG LLM (Med Neg)
Retried Consultant
Bingley, West Yorkshire, England

Vageesh Ayyar D
MD DM DNB MANAMS
Professor Gr1
Department of Endocrinology
St John's Medical College and Hospital
Bengaluru, Karnataka, India

Valentina Bruno
MD PhD
Adjunct Professor
Department of Experimental Clinical Oncology
IRCCS "Regina Elena" National Cancer Institute
Rome, Italy
Adjunct Professor
Saint Camillus International University of Health and Medical Sciences
Rome, Italy

Vasilios Tanos
MD PhD
Consultant Gynecologist and Head of the Reproductive Medicine & Surgery & IVF Unit
Department of Obstetrics and Gynecology
St George's Medical School at the University of Nicosia and Aretaeio Hospital in Nicosia, Cyprus

Vyshnavi A Rao
MBBS MS (Obs & Gyne) FRM
Medical Director
Department of Reproductive Medicine
Dr Kamini Rao Hospitals
Bengaluru, Karnataka, India

Wael Saab FRCOG MD BSc
Clinical Director
Department of Reproductive Medicine
The Centre for reproductive and Genetic Health
London, UK

Wiam Saab
CRGH
Gilbert and Rose-Marie Chagoury Health Sciences Center
The Lebanese American University
Beirut, Lebanon

Yona Grossman
Honors Bachelor of Arts and Science (B Arts Sc Hons) MD Candidate
Medical School for International Health
Faculty of Health Sciences
Ben-Gurion University of the Negev
Be'er-Sheva, Israel

Yoshihara Hiroyuki MD PhD
Professor
Department of Obstetrics and Gynecology
Graduate School of Medical Sciences and Medical School, Nagoya City University
Mizuho-ku, Nagoya, Aichi, Japan

Yosuke Matsumoto MD PhD
Professor
Department of Obstetrics and Gynecology
Graduate School of Medical Sciences and Medical School, Nagoya City University
Mizuho-ku, Nagoya, Aichi, Japan

Yuval Cherlow IDF
The Tzohar Rabbinical Organization
Lod, Israel

Preface to the Fourth Edition

The field of recurrent pregnancy loss (RPL), as it stands today, is riddled with controversies. From its very definition, two versus three miscarriages, and again consecutive versus nonconsecutive losses, there is no consensus among guidelines. The workup required in every couple of RPL and the extended battery of tests that may help to unravel the diagnosis are not yet standardized. Despite guidelines on RPL published by the European Society for Human Reproduction, the American Society of Reproductive Medicine, the Royal College of Obstetricians and Gynaecologists, and many other national bodies, the reader remains confused due to the discrepancy in their recommendations.

Being of a multifactorial etiology, the domain of RPL is shared by obstetricians, specialists in assisted reproduction, endoscopists, endocrinologists, and rheumatologists. It is not surprising then that treatment consensus guidelines will need to incorporate evidence-based recommendations from different subspecialist societies, i.e. rheumatology, genetics, endocrinology, and gynecological endoscopy.

A large group of women may not identify the cause of recurrent miscarriages. The frustration of both the affected couple and the treating obstetricians leads to rampant use of empirical therapies in unexplained recurrent miscarriages. The aim of the editors is to provide data to minimize this large group of unexplained recurrent miscarriages in the coming decade.

Research in this field is also limited by the fact that the number of patients affected by RPL is small and when broken up according to different etiological factors, each center deals with a small number of patients. Hence, to collect data from multicentric studies, the research protocols need to follow standard definitions and diagnostic criteria. This has been lacking so far, hence the paucity of robust data by way of meta-analysis and systematic reviews.

The mental well-being of RPL couples has not received due attention, and it is now evident that unresolved stress may be a driver for poor obstetric outcomes. There are no guidelines on quantifying maternal stress and uniform strategies of resolving it.

We sincerely hope that this compilation will serve as a useful guide to practitioners, researchers, and postgraduate students and encourage the evolution of evidence-based treatment recommendations that can be applied globally.

The editors have made every endeavor to clarify confusions, present evidence-based recommendations, and include rarer causes of RPL, e.g., recurrent molar pregnancies and recurrent ectopic pregnancies. The section on "Case Summaries" resonates with the dilemma faced by clinicians. In short, this book reflects our lifelong commitment to improving outcomes for women facing RPL.

Mala Arora
Asher Bashiri
Neelanajana Mukhopadhaya

Preface to the First Edition (2003)

Recurrent pregnancy loss has been a gynecologist's dilemma. The causes are poorly understood and the treatment is mostly empirical. However, current research is slowly unfolding the mysteries of recurrent pregnancy loss and we are now able to categorize it and treat it appropriately in certain circumstances.

The data presented was collected over a period of six and half years and over this period the management protocol was changed according to the latest research. The cases illustrated were managed personally.

Two fields that are showing rapid advancement and knowledge are the genetic and immunological causes of recurrent pregnancy loss. It is hoped that this would take a major chunk of the as yet idiopathic causes of RPL.

It is hoped that this book will need updated editions frequently to keep the readers abreast with current research.

Mala Arora

Acknowledgments

I would like to thank my husband Dr Narinder Pal, for his immense support and personal contribution to proof read the book.

I wish to thank Pragati Singh, Development Editor at Jaypee Brothers Medical Publishers, and the entire team for their efforts to release this publication on time.

My eternal gratitude goes to the vast Cosmic Consciousness (Kutastha Chaitanya) which is the highest state of intellectual development and emotional maturity. It has been my guiding light and source of inspiration.

Mala Arora

I extend my heartfelt gratitude to the countless patients and families whose courage and resilience in the face of recurrent pregnancy loss have inspired this work. My deepest thanks go to the dedicated contributors, colleagues, and mentors whose expertise has enriched this book.

I extend my thanks to my friends, family, and specifically to my lovely children, whose unwavering support and encouragement have been my foundation.

This book is a tribute to the pursuit of hope, understanding, and compassionate care for all who walk this challenging journey.

Asher Bashiri

My gratitude to the **3Ps**
To the **P**ower that guides me
To the **P**eople who inspire and support me
For my **P**erseverance that drives me

Neelanjana Mukhopadhaya

Contents

SECTION 4: Anatomical Factors

SECTION 5: Imaging

SECTION 6: Maternal Systemic Causes

SECTION 7: Life Style Factors

SECTION 8: Miscellaneous

SECTION 9: Treatment

APPENDICES

SECTION 1

Introduction

CHAPTER

1 History, Overview, and Terminology

Mala Arora

ABSTRACT

Recurrent pregnancy loss (RPL) is mentioned in many ancient texts. However, the published literature on this subject is not more than a century old. The terminology has evolved from habitual abortions to recurrent spontaneous miscarriage (RSM). While RSM is restricted to first trimester losses, RPL is a more comprehensive term encompassing early and late miscarriages till the period of viability. The terminology used for early pregnancy events needs to be clarified and standardized in order to perform meta-analysis in this field that form the basis of generating robust evidence for guidelines.

Keywords: Recurrent spontaneous miscarriage, History of RPL, Recurrent pregnancy loss, Terminology in RPL, Interpregnancy interval.

INTRODUCTION

Percy Malpas from Liverpool, UK coined the term "habitual aborter" and published a paper in 1938 for women with three or more consecutive abortions.[1] The term is no longer used because of its negative connotations. The Royal College of Obstetricians and Gynecologists (RCOG) UK recommend to use the term *miscarriage* for a spontaneous loss of pregnancy and *abortion* for induced termination of pregnancy[2] **(Table 1)**. Miscarriage is defined as the unplanned loss of a pregnancy <24 weeks gestation or loss of a fetus weighing <500 g if the gestational age is uncertain.[2] The traditional definition of three consecutive miscarriages was proposed by Malpas and seconded by NJ Eastman[3] (Professor at Johns Hopkins Maryland USA and editor of Obstetrics and Gynecological Survey) who in 1946 worked on a community based statistical model and proposed that the group of women with two losses had a significantly better pregnancy outcome than the group with three or more pregnancy losses. Further studies by Stirrat confirmed this observation.[4] Barry Schwarz[5] in 1984 analyzed and published that the Malpas-Eastman model of recurrent aborters was flawed. Their conclusions were not based on clinical observations but on a mathematical model that had the following presumptions which were flawed:

- Women had the same miscarriage rate that did not depend on age and parity.
- Women with miscarriages could be distinctly divided into two groups—random aborters and habitual aborters.
- If habitual aborters aborted once they would surely abort a second time. He failed to recognize fetal genetic causes of miscarriage that may not be recurrent.

These factors projected a very grim prognosis for women with three miscarriages whereas recent publications confirm that at least 80% of women with recurrent pregnancy loss (RPL) will carry home a baby.

By far the most common event in a woman's obstetric career is a sporadic miscarriage, which occurs in 20–30% of women, and in <5% after the documentation of fetal cardiac activity. An estimated 23 million miscarriages occur globally every year.[6] Sporadic miscarriages do not

TABLE 1: Breakup of total number of patients visiting authors' infertility clinic according to the number of miscarriages.[8]

0	810
1	224
2	80
3	39
4	16
5	5
7	2
13	1
Total	*1,177*

TABLE 2: Outcome in patients with 0, 1, 2, 3, and 4 miscarriages.[8]

No. of abortions	Total no. of patients	No. of pregnant patients (%)	UPT + but lost to follow-up	SVD/LSCS/preterm (%)	Miscarriages (%)
0	810	197 (24.32)	81	59/116 (50.86)	57/116 (49.13)
1	224	55 (24.55)	22	17/33 (51.5)	16/33 (48.48)
2	80	25 (31.25)	8	8/17 (47.0)	4/17 (23.52)
3	39	11 (28.2)	4	3/7 (42.85)	4/7 (57.14)
4	16	5 (31.25)	0	2/5 (40.0)	3/5 (60.0)

(LSCS: lower segment cesarean section; SVD: spontaneous vaginal delivery; UPT: urine pregnancy test)

compromise future obstetric outcomes. Hence, women with a single spontaneous pregnancy loss should not be investigated,[7] as the chances of a live birth subsequently are comparable to no previous loss **(Table 2)**.

Personal data from the authors Infertility clinic is presented below. This data draws attention to the fact that a number of patients with RPL seek-assisted conception after one, two or three miscarriages **(Table 1)**.

Authors' personal observations[8] and many other observational studies[9] confirm that pregnancy outcome is no different in women with more than two and more than three miscarriages **(Table 2)**. This data showed that there is no statistically significant difference in the numbers that got pregnant, in the group with two miscarriages (25/80 = 31.2%) and the group with three miscarriages (11/39 = 28.2%). The take home baby rates were 47% in the group with two miscarriages and 42.8% in the group with three miscarriages, which is also not statistically different. With higher number of miscarriages, as the numbers get smaller it is difficult to make meaningful conclusions.

The American College of Obstetrics and Gynecology (ACOG)[10] modified the definition to two or more pregnancy losses confirmed by ultrasound or histopathology of the products of conception. The European Society for Human Reproduction and Embryology (ESHRE) special interest group for early pregnancy defined recurrent miscarriage as two or more pregnancy losses.[11] Some others consider RPL to be defined as two or more consecutive miscarriages OR three spontaneous miscarriages which may not be consecutive. Royal College of Obstetrics and Gynecology (RCOG) UK continues to define RPL as three or more consecutive pregnancy losses.[7] The 2023 FIGO guidelines also defines RPL as three consecutive pregnancy losses.[12] The lack of consensus in the definition of RPL greatly hampers research and generation of evidence from systematic reviews and meta-analysis.

TABLE 3: Summary of definitions of recurrent miscarriage used in clinical trials.

Reference	Definition of recurrent pregnancy loss
Cowchock, 1992	≥2 fetal losses
Silver, 1993	• ≥1 unexpected fetal death >12 weeks gestation OR • ≥2 unexplained first trimester losses
Kutteh, 1996	≥3 consecutive pregnancy losses
Laskin, 1997	≥2 consecutive fetal losses at <32 weeks
Rai, 1997	≥3 consecutive miscarriages
Pattison, 2000	≥3 miscarriages
Farquharson, 2002	>2 fetal losses
Triolo, 2003	≥3 consecutive fetal losses <10 weeks gestation
Clark, 2010	≥2 consecutive fetal losses at <24 weeks gestation

Source: From Bhattacharya S. Recurrent miscarriage[9] should the definition be revised? In: Arora M, Bhattacharya S, Kumari V (Eds). World Clinics Obstetrics and Gynecology: Recurrent Miscarriage. 2011. p. 136.

The ACOG and ESHRE definition of two pregnancy losses is clinically more relevant as most clinicians would start investigations for RPL after two consecutive losses. However, this would increase the prevalence of RPL to 5% as compared to previous 1% with three or more losses. It would also favorably skew the effect of treatment modalities. Hence, it was opined that for research and publication purposes, we retain the definition of three or more losses. However, this heterogeneity in definition hinders scientific research and gives birth to varying clinical practices globally.

Table 3 outlines the heterogeneity of definition in published studies.

The current definition does not include women with ectopic, molar pregnancies and pregnancy of uncertain

TABLE 4: Old and new nomenclature.[13]

Previous term	*Recommended term*
Spontaneous abortion	Spontaneous miscarriage
Threatened abortion	Threatened miscarriage
Inevitable abortion	Inevitable miscarriage
Incomplete abortion	Incomplete miscarriage
Complete abortion	Complete miscarriage
Missed abortion	Missed miscarriage
Blighted ovum	Early fetal demise
Septic abortion	Miscarriage with sepsis
Recurrent abortion	Recurrent miscarriage

location which has similar emotional consequences for the couple. Each of these conditions is known to be associated with a poor obstetric outcome and can be recurrent. Hence, the proposal is that we should include "ultrasound, histopathological *and* biochemical evidence of a pregnancy." We may have to set a minimum level of beta human chorionic gonadotropin (β-hCG) positivity so as to exclude drug-induced positive β-hCG levels in assisted reproductive technique (ART) pregnancies.

We also need to have clarity on defining early pregnancy events in a uniform manner, to facilitate meta-analysis and systematic reviews.

Table 4 outlines the new terminology which should be universally followed.[11]

Recurrent spontaneous miscarriage (RSM) is referred to as pregnancy loss of <12 weeks or first trimester loss. This comprises >80% of recurrent miscarriages. RPL encompasses both first and second trimester miscarriages. Poor/bad obstetric history is a broad term that includes miscarriages/ectopic pregnancy/molar pregnancy/stillbirths/preterm birth/neonatal deaths. It encompasses all patients with an unfavorable pregnancy outcome. It is not a robust term clinically, as it deals with varied etiological factors and management options but it effectively alerts the obstetrician to the psychological needs of the such a patient.

Recurrent implantation failure and preclinical pregnancy loss/very early pregnancy loss (VEPL) are markers of poor implantation and share an overlapping etiological spectrum with RPL. However, the current definition does not take this into consideration. Preclinical losses with documented β-hCG rise and fall are a clear indication of a failed implantation and form an overlapping etiology of both recurrent implantation failure (RIF)

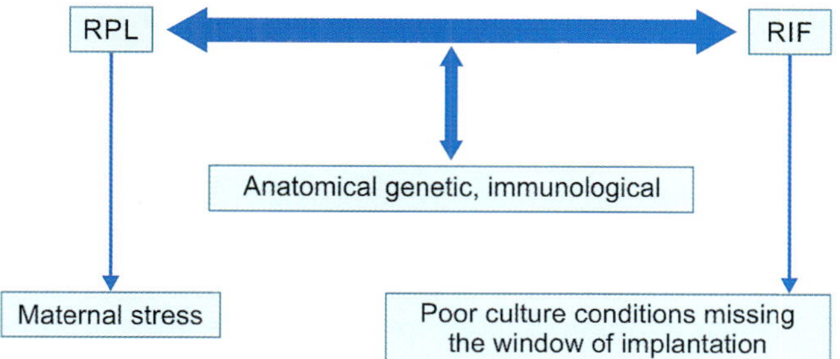

Fig. 1: Relationship of recurrent pregnancy loss (RPL) and recurrent implantation failure. (RIF: recurrent implantation failure)

and RPL. It may result from genetically abnormal embryos or a non-receptive endometrium.

It may be rational to include, the time to take home a baby from the time of first pregnancy event in the definition rather than the number of pregnancy losses alone.

Recurrent implantation failure is defined as no implantation after replacement of 4 grade-A embryos/blastocyst, in fresh and frozen embryo transfer cycles. A standard definition is still lacking. This is an entity distinct from RPL, although they both have overlapping causes as discussed above. They may be described as two ends of the same spectrum **(Fig. 1)**. Recurrent implantation failure is only relevant in the setting of assisted conception cycles, whereas RPL is usually seen in spontaneous conceptions. However, women with RIF will need to be evaluated for most causes of RPL in addition to laboratory factors as well as the synchronization of transfer with the window of implantation which is not relevant to RPL.

Recurrent pregnancy loss comprises of both early and late pregnancy losses. The spectrum encompasses:

- *Preclinical pregnancy loss:* This entity is diagnosed by performing serum β-hCG assays in the late luteal phase prior to the onset of the next menstrual cycle.
- Clinical pregnancy loss is defined as pregnancy loss following an ultrasound evidence of a gestational sac. Clinical pregnancy loss is divided into:
    - Pre-embryonic, when no fetal pole is identified (<5 weeks)
    - Embryonic, when a fetal pole is identified (5–10 weeks)
    - Fetal, >10 weeks' gestation
- First trimester loss is loss of a pregnancy <12 weeks. >80% of miscarriages occur in the first 12 weeks. This may also be addressed as recurrent miscarriages (RM) or recurrent spontaneous miscarriage (RSM).

- Mid-trimester loss occurs between 12 and 28 weeks of pregnancy. The common causes are anatomical defects and antiphospholipid syndrome. These women will benefit with a hysteroscopic evaluation
- Late fetal loss/intrauterine fetal death (IUFD)/stillbirth occurs between 28 weeks to term or of a fetus weighing >1,000 g if gestation is unknown. The most common cause is preterm labor, preterm premature rupture of membranes, preeclampsia (PE), or congenital malformations. Unexplained stillbirth (20% of all stillbirths) is even more traumatic than unexplained RPL and merits detailed investigations to ascertain a cause. Inherited thrombophilia screening becomes relevant in women with mid-trimester and late pregnancy losses.

Recurrent pregnancy loss has also been classified as:[14]

- Primary recurrent miscarriages are two or more losses with no pregnancy progressing beyond 20 weeks.
- Secondary recurrent miscarriages are two or more losses after a pregnancy that has progressed beyond 20 weeks which might have resulted in a live or stillbirth.

This division is not so important as the etiological factors and prognosis is the same in the two groups.[14] Perhaps the incidence of acquired anatomical defects such as uterine adhesions and cervical insufficiency may be higher in the secondary RPL group; hence evaluation of the uterine cavity should always be done in this group.

Table 5 defines terminology related to pregnancy loss as proposed by ESHRE—special interest group for early pregnancy.[11]

Conventionally women with RPL conceived spontaneously. However, we now have a new subgroup of women that present with infertility and RPL. They can only conceive with ART procedures. In our personal data from an infertility clinic 10% (118/1, 181) of women seeking ART are patients with two or more miscarriages. Experiencing loss of an ART pregnancy is emotionally more traumatic and these couples often have a lower threshold for investigations and treatment.

However, whether we need to investigate them after one loss or two, will depend on the time to pregnancy and the maternal age.

The link between maternal age and pregnancy loss is now well documented.[15] Maternal age of 35 and above is associated with a higher incidence of pregnancy loss; the incidence increases progressively with increasing maternal age due to the increasing incidence of aneuploidy.

TABLE 5: The European Society for Human Reproduction and Embryology (ESHRE) nomenclature of early pregnancy events.

Term	*Definition*
Biochemical pregnancy loss	Spontaneous pregnancy loss confirmed by decreasing β-hCG levels but not located on ultrasound scan
Empty sac or anembryonic pregnancy loss	Intrauterine sac with absent fetal pole/yolk sac on ultrasound
Yolk sac miscarriage	Intrauterine gestational sac and yolk sac but no fetal pole on ultrasound
Embryonic miscarriage	Intrauterine gestational sac with yolk sac and fetal pole but no cardiac activity
Fetal miscarriage	Pregnancy loss >10 weeks size with a fetal pole of CRL >33 mm on ultrasound
Ectopic pregnancy	Pregnancy visualized outside the endometrial cavity
Early pregnancy loss	Pregnancy loss <10 weeks gestational age (<8 developmental weeks)
Late pregnancy loss	>12 weeks gestation
Pregnancy of uncertain location (PUL)	• No identifiable pregnancy on transvaginal scan with a β-hCG level of 1,500 IU/L • No identifiable sac on transabdominal scan with β-hCG of 6,000 IU/L

(β-hCG: β-human chorionic gonadotropin; CRL: crown-rum length)

There is a need to constantly revise the definition, investigation, and treatment guidelines, for patients with RPL in the changing social and medical scenario, due to the following:

- Today women start their reproductive careers late and will not have the time and patience to wait for multiple losses.
- Subgroups of women that miscarry due to anatomical factors or antiphospholipid antibodies have well-defined treatment modalities that can reduce the rate of subsequent miscarriages. Hence to deny them this treatment till they have multiple pregnancy losses seems unethical.

Many women seeking pregnancy through ART may demand to have all investigations including evaluation of the uterine cavity after one miscarriage or a biochemical pregnancy.

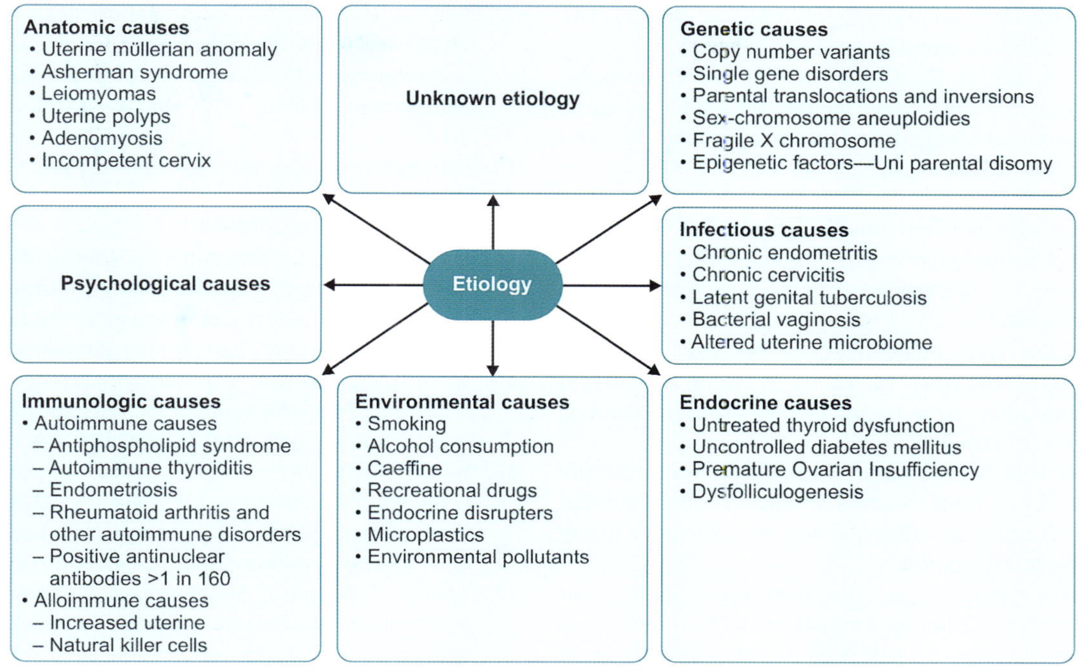

Fig. 2: Causes of recurrent pregnancy loss.

It may also be proposed that in women >37 years, one miscarriage should prompt genetic screening and replacement of a euploid embryo. Similarly, in women with RIF, abnormal gamete morphology, poor quality embryos and advanced maternal/paternal age should have sperm DNA fragmentation index (DFI) and preferably preimplantation genetic testing for aneuploidy (PGT-A) of the trophectodermal cells and replacement of only euploid embryos, prior to complete cessation of gametogenesis.

INTERPREGNANCY INTERVAL

Women with a pregnancy loss will often ask "when is it best to try again?" Although the World Health Organisation[16] has recommended 6 months interpregnancy interval between pregnancies, there are studies to suggest that a shorter interpregnancy interval in women with RPL may have better outcomes.[17,18] Having one normal period post a miscarriage is sufficient for a couple desperate to achieve their dreams of parenthood.

CONCLUSION

Definition and terminology of RPL has been revised over the past few years. However, it still needs further modifications which need to be deliberated upon.

RPL has a multifactorial etiology, hence detailed investigations are required. Genetic testing for products of conception is important and complete genomic hybridization micro array should be performed. In select cases, next generation sequencing may be required to diagnose single nucleotide polymorphism.

The author leaves you to ponder about the known causes of RPL **(Fig. 2)** and the optimistic thought that the large group unexplained miscarriages is shrinking fast due to advanced genetic testing offered to the products of conception and parental screening. Discussions in the coming chapters will promote further research to eliminate this group and discover new treatment strategies.

REFERENCES

1. Malpas P. A study of abortion sequence. J Obstet Gynecol Br Emp. 1938;45:932.
2. National institute of Child health and human development. (2012). What is pregnancy loss/miscarriage? [online] Available from:www.ncbi.nlm.nih.gov/pubmedhealth/PMH0002458. [Last accessed December, 2024].
3. Eastman NJ. Habitual abortion. In: Meigs JV, Sturgis S (Eds). Progress in Gynaecology, Volume 1. New York: Grune and Stratton; 1946.
4. Stirrat GM. Recurrent miscarriage I: Definition and epidemiology. Lancet. 1990;336:673-5.

5. Schwarz BE. Habitual Abortion Infertility. In: Aiman J (Ed). Infertility and Management. Springer; 1984.
6. Quenby S, Gallos ID, Dhillon-Smith RK, Podesek M, Stephenson MD. Miscarriage matters: the epidemiological, physical, psychological and economic costs of early pregnancy loss. Lancet. 2021;397(10285):1658-67.
7. RCOG.org. (2018). The investigation and treatment of couples with recurrent miscarriages Royal College of Obstetricians and Gynecologists green top guideline No 17. [online] Available from www.rcog.org.uk. [Last accessed December, 2024].
8. Arora M. Overview and definition in "Recurrent Pregnancy Loss" 2007. In: Arora M, Konje JC (Eds). Recurrent pregnancy Loss. New Delhi: Jaypee Brothers Medical Publishers (P) Ltd; 2007.
9. Bhattacharya S. Recurrent miscarriage: should the definition be revised? In: Arora M, Bhattacharya S, Kumari V (Eds). World Clinics Obstetrics and Gynecology Recurrent Miscarriage; 2011. p. 136.
10. Practice Committee of the American Society for Reproductive Medicine. Evaluation and treatment of Recurrent Pregnancy Loss: A committee opinion. Fertil Steril. 2012;98:1103-11.
11. ESHRE Guideline Group on RPL; Bender Atik R, Christiansen OB, et al. ESHRE guideline: recurrent pregnancy loss: an update in 2022 by the ESHRE guideline group on RPL 2022. Hum Reprod Open. 2023;2023(1):hoad002.
12. Shehata H, Elfituri A, Doumouchtsis SK, Zini ME, Ali A. FIGO Good Practice Recommendations on the use of progesterone in the management of recurrent first trimester miscarriage. Mar Int J of Gynecol Obstet. 2023;161(S1): 3-16.
13. Farquharson RG, Jauniaux E, Exalto N. Updated and revised nomenclature for description of early pregnancy events. Hum Reprod. 2005;20:3008-11.
14. Shapira E, Ratzon R, Shoham-Vardi I, Serjienko R, Mazor M, Bashiri A. Primary versus Secondary Recurrent Pregnancy loss-epidemiological characteristics, etiology and next pregnancy outcome. J Perinat Med. 2012;40:389-96.
15. Nybo Anderson AM, Wohlfahrt J, Christens P, Olsen J, Melbye M. Maternal age and fetal loss: population based register linkage study. BMJ. 2000;320:1708-12.
16. World Health Organization. (2005). Report of a WHO technical consultation on birth spacing. [online] Available from: www.who. int/making pregnancy safer/documents/ birth spacing. [Last accessed December, 2018].
17. Bentolia Y, Ratzon R, Shoham-Vardi I, Serjienko R, Mazor M, Bashiri A. Effect of interpregnancy interval on outcomes of pregnancy after recurrent pregnancy loss. J Matern Fetal Neonatal Med. 2013;26(14):1459-64.
18. Love ER, Bhattacharya S, Smith NC, Bhattacharya S. Effect of interpregnancy interval on outcomes of pregnancy after miscarriage: Retrospective analysis of hospital episode statistics in Scotland. BMJ. 2010;341:c3967.

SECTION 2

Genetic Causes

CHAPTER

2

Genetic Evaluation of Products of Conception

Chinmayee Ratha

ABSTRACT

Recurrent pregnancy loss (RPL), defined as the failure of two or more clinically recognized pregnancies before 20 weeks of gestation, remains a daunting clinical challenge even to the present day. The incidence of RPL continues to be quoted as 1–2% of all couples in the reproductive age-group, but almost 50–60% of cases of RPL remain idiopathic in etiology despite all kinds of tests. It is suspected that a significant proportion of the yet "unexplained" group may be reclassified if better genetic testing was offered. Chromosomal abnormalities contribute to a significant proportion of RPL, and the test of choice on the products of conception (POC) to detect these chromosomal abnormalities is cytogenetic microarray (CMA). Presently, the 24-chromosome comprehensive microarray is recommended, which can be done by next-generation sequencing (NGS) on various platforms. Each genetic test and technology has its own strengths and limitations. Future prospects in genetic testing of POC would be to detect either "lethal gene mutations" in the embryo itself, which could explain the failed pregnancy or the use of cell-free fetal deoxyribonucleic acid (DNA)/noninvasive prenatal testing (NIPT) to replace POC DNA studies, especially in the era of medical management of early miscarriage.

Keywords: Miscarriage, Recurrent miscarriage, Recurrent pregnancy loss, Products of conception, Genetic analysis, POC microarray.

INTRODUCTION

Commonly accepted etiologies for RPL include uterine anatomic anomalies, uncontrolled diabetes mellitus, untreated hypothyroidism, parental chromosomal abnormalities, and antiphospholipid antibody syndrome (APS), thrombophilia, genetic abnormalities or infections, but the contribution of tests in proving these etiological factors remains elusive. While the care of the woman who has suffered from the loss is directed toward her physical recovery and providing psychological support to the aggrieved couple, there remains the larger issue of providing answers for the etiology of RPL.

If the cause of pregnancy loss is ascertained, then this information is of pivotal importance for couples and may be critical for the management of their future pregnancies. Uterine anomalies when present can be detected by advanced imaging methods, and the tests for endocrine and immunological causes are well established. However, although "chromosomal and genetic" factors are definitely known to contribute to RPL, the most rational test or tests in this regard are still not defined. It is suspected that a significant proportion of the yet "unexplained" group may be reclassified if better genetic testing was offered. In a recent study on products of conception (POC) samples in cases of RPL, a comparison of definitive etiological results was done when the standard American Society for Reproductive Medicine (ASRM) protocol was followed vis-à-vis a protocol that additionally included a 24-chromsome microarray on the POC.[3] It was found that by putting together the results from the RPL evaluation and the results of genetic testing of POC provide a probable explanation for the loss in over 90% of women in their study. This study was based on retrospective data of 65,333 miscarriages and prospective evaluation of 378 women and it highlights the resurgence of interest in genetic evaluation of POC with the advent of newer genetic modalities.

There is established evidence that chromosomal abnormalities in the developing embryo are the most common cause of all pregnancy losses accounting for 70% of sporadic early pregnancy miscarriages and about 40% of RPLs. In this context, it seems rational that checking the POC in cases of RPL for chromosomal abnormalities will yield information that can explain the etiology of the condition.[4] In the era of evidence-based medicine and when the healthcare system is driven by "guidelines" for clinical practice, there is a lot of confusion regarding investigations on the POC in cases of RPL because different academic bodies have different recommendations, particularly in POC testing.

STATUS OF CURRENT GUIDELINES ABOUT PRODUCTS OF CONCEPTION GENETIC TESTING

The Royal College of Obstetricians and Gynaecologists (RCOG) green top guideline in 2023 has suggested that cytogenetic analysis should be offered on pregnancy tissue of the third and subsequent miscarriage(s) and in any second-trimester miscarriage, and this has been graded as a "grade D" recommendation.[5] This again leaves the ball in the court of the clinician because in systems where the cost-benefit analysis of a test is important, it is difficult to justify tests with low level of evidentiary support. The European Society of Human Reproduction and Embryology (ESHRE) guideline of 2017[6] mentions a conditional recommendation that "Genetic analysis of pregnancy tissue is not routinely recommended but it could be performed for explanatory purposes." There is, however, a strong recommendation that if POC evaluation is done then an array-based comparative genomic hybridization (array-CGH) is the choice of investigation as it reduces the effect of maternal cell contamination (MCC). This particular recommendation has not been changed despite an update to the ESHRE guideline published in 2022[6] for few other recommendations. The ASRM guideline on RPL[7] did not recommend routine POC genetic analysis, but restricted it only to cases in the context of therapy for RPL. It is rational to expect that many times couples opt for the investigation of the POC desperate to find an answer to the etiology of their usually "unexplained" RPL, and in such cases, appropriate testing would be imperative. Clinician's must hence be aware of what tests to offer for genetic analysis of the POC.

EXPECTED CHROMOSOMAL ABNORMALITIES IN PRODUCTS OF CONCEPTION AND SUGGESTED TESTS

It is a well-known fact that embryonic chromosomal abnormalities may be encountered in 29–60% of cases with RPL,[4] most of which are aneuploidies or abnormalities in the number of chromosomes while a few are structural abnormalities such as deletions/duplications or translocations. The common aneuploidies are trisomy, haploidy, or polyploidy. These can be detected by karyotyping, cytogenetic microarray (CMA), or in some cases by fluorescence in situ hybridization (FISH)/quantitative fluorescence polymerase chain reaction (QfPCR). Genetic risk factors for aneuploidy in the embryo include meiotic errors, mitotic errors, and abnormal parental karyotype. Maternal age has a direct correlation with the risk of embryonic aneuploidy and the risk increases from around 35% in women below 35 years to 55–85% in those above 40–45 years. Trisomies are usually the result of nondisjunction at the time of meiosis and commonly involve chromosomes 13, 16, 18, 21, and 22. Polyploidy, such as triploidy or tetraploidy, is usually caused by double spermatozoa or eggs that do not separate during maternal meiosis and are directly fertilized while tetraploidy may result from mitotic nonseparation of the fertilized ovum.

Chromosomes are carriers of genes and major structural aberrations or rearrangements also can cause lethal imbalance in the genetic material. The structural rearrangements may have arisen de novo during the process of gametogenesis or fertilization or may be inherited from parents who carry such aberrations. Usually, it is seen that couples carry balanced translocations but due to reorganization of genetic material during gametogenesis, the embryo may carry unbalanced translocations, which are mostly lethal or may cause major fetal anomalies. Even the embryos with balanced translocations may be miscarried.[8]

The test of choice on the POC to detect these chromosomal abnormalities is CMA.[9] While a karyotype also can show the major structural aberrations, it is often difficult to culture cells from the POC after a miscarriage and there are often "culture failures." The CMA is a DNA-based test, which can be performed after DNA extraction from even the nonviable tissue in POC and hence very useful in this context. The CMA can reveal microdeletions, microduplications, and unbalanced translocations but is of limited value for inversions and balanced translocations, which can be seen by karyotyping.

Reciprocal balanced translocation (RBT) is formed by a process where two chromosomes break at the same time and the broken fragments are exchanged to form two derived chromosomes, generally without increasing or decreasing genetic material, which is why the individual usually has no phenotypic alterations.

Chromosomal deletions and duplications are also known as copy number variants (CNV) and depending upon their sizes they may be classified as large CNV (≥10 Mb) and submicroscopic CNV (these are variants found in heterochromatin regions of chromosomes, including small variations in the structure, coloration intensity, and bandwidth). The large deletions and duplications can be picked up on karyotyping while CMA helps detect microscopic changes. CMA may be of limited value in some karyotypic abnormalities including balanced rearrangements, inversions, 69,XXX triploidy and low-level mosaicism.

GENETIC ABNORMALITIES IN PRODUCTS OF CONCEPTION AND SUGGESTED TESTS

Recent interest in elucidating genetic variants (including many previously recognized genes) relevant to unexplained pregnancy loss in families has led to a better understanding of implementation of POC genetic analysis. It must be clearly understood that all genetic testing modalities are not equal, and each has its own advantages and limitations.

As explained earlier, chromosomal issues are rather common causes of RPL and hence chromosomal testing is the first-line investigation in the POC of RPL. Karyotyping and FISH require viable cells, which are unlikely in the POC after miscarriage, and hence, these techniques are unsuitable due to cell-culture failure as well as an inability to detect MCC. Chromosomal microarray is a DNA-based test and can be performed on DNA extracted from POC samples. The currently suitable microarray on POC is the 24-chromosmal microarray, which can be done by different genetic platforms [i.e., CGH or single-nucleotide polymorphism (SNP) microarrays, and NGS]. SNP microarray has an advantage over array-CGH in detecting triploidy (molar pregnancies), present in 3% of all miscarriages.[10] Next-generation sequencing (NGS) can diagnose mosaic losses, with trisomy 21 and monosomy XO being the most common true mosaic fetuses after 15 weeks' gestation. NGS analysis of maternal cell-free fetal DNA (cfDNA) is presently used for noninvasive prenatal testing (NIPT) for screening for fetal aneuploidies. It has recently been proposed that cfDNA could be used as a replacement for POC genetic analysis in RPL. The use of cfDNA technology offers the advantage of not having to collect a POC sample and of much more practical sampling as in some cases women miscarry before a sample can be obtained, and it could be particularly useful if the miscarriages are managed medically.[11]

Comprehensive genetic analysis with NGS-based studies such as whole-genome sequencing (WGS) of DNA from large numbers of families (including parental and fetal DNA from affected and unaffected pregnancies) may help identify lethal genes contributing to sporadic and RPL.[9] The modes of inheritance of these genes are either compound heterozygous, de novo, autosomal-dominant or X-linked recessive. Although not a first-line investigation, NGS-based genetic tests can be particularly useful in cases of RPLs with euploid fetuses.

CLINICAL UTILITY OF PRODUCTS OF CONCEPTION GENETIC TESTING

The chromosomal abnormalities in the POC indicate the need for testing the parents for inversion or balanced translocations. In cases where chromosomal abnormalities are identified, genetic counseling can be offered to discuss the implications and potential recurrence risks in future pregnancies. In cases of recurrent POC aneuploidy, when all possible causes have already been addressed, in vitro fertilization (IVF) with preimplantation genetic testing (PGT) of embryos for aneuploidy remains an option with no evidence of potential benefit but may be an alternative to expectant management. It is important for individuals considering this option to have a thorough discussion with their healthcare provider about the potential risks and benefits. Additionally, individuals should also consider consulting with a genetic counselor to fully understand their reproductive options and the potential outcomes. Ultimately, the decision to pursue IVF with preimplantation genetic testing for aneuploidy (PGT-A) should be made carefully and with full understanding of the possible outcomes.[9] It is important to weigh the potential benefits against the potential risks and to carefully consider other options before proceeding with this treatment. **Flowchart 1** summarizes the genetic tests commonly used for POC.

Overall, elucidating genes associated with pregnancy loss has the potential to significantly impact the field of reproductive health by improving risk stratification, enhancing our understanding of normal and abnormal pregnancy, and identifying new avenues for therapeutic intervention.

CONCLUSION

If a pregnancy loss occurs, it is crucial to collect the POC for genetic testing. This can include obtaining the tissue from a dilation and curettage (D&C) procedure or from a spontaneous miscarriage. The POC after a pregnancy loss remains a very "vital" tissue, which can provide answers to the possible etiology. A stepwise, case-based rational approach to genetic testing is one of the most informative

Flowchart 1: Common genetic tests used for POC in RPL.

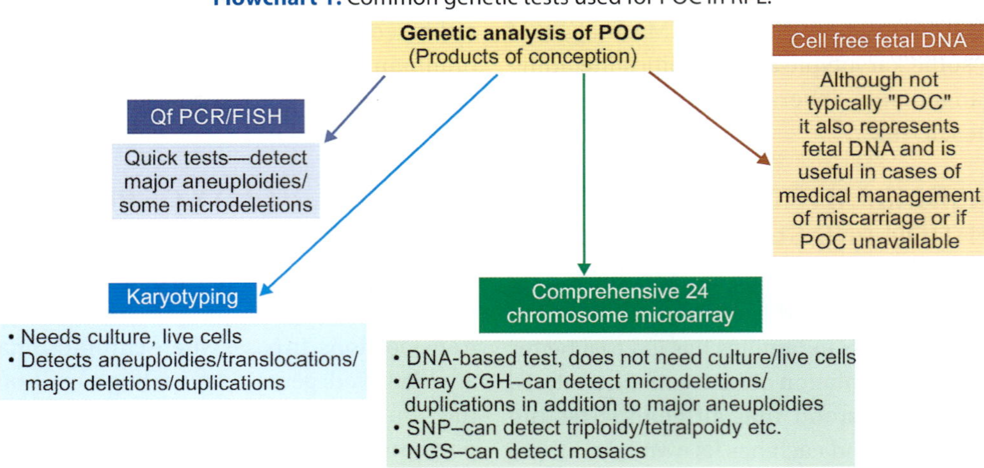

(array-CGH: array-based comparative genomic hybridization; cfDNA: cell-free fetal deoxyribonucleic acid; FISH: fluorescence in situ hybridization; NGS: next-generation sequencing; POC: products of conception; QfPCR: quantitative fluorescence polymerase chain reaction; RPL: recurrent pregnancy loss; SNP: single-nucleotide polymorphism)

and clinically relevant tests in cases of RPL. The POC can be analyzed using techniques such as QfPCR/FISH, karyotyping, chromosomal microarray analysis (CMA), and NGS to identify any chromosomal abnormalities, which cannot be detected by standard methods. There is emerging interest in the role of cfDNA to provide some answers about fetal DNA studies in case the POC sample cannot be collected. It is important for couples with RPL to work closely with their healthcare provider to determine the underlying cause of their losses. This may involve a series of tests, including genetic testing, hormone evaluations, and imaging studies. Upon identification of the causes of RPL, appropriate treatment options can be discussed.

Emotional support is crucial during this time, as the experience of RPL can be extremely difficult and stressful.[5,6] Counseling and support groups may be helpful in coping with the emotional impact of RPL.

It is also important for couples to have realistic expectations for future pregnancies. While the risk of another miscarriage may be higher for couples with RPL, many go on to have successful pregnancies with the appropriate treatment and support. To summarize, understanding the reasons behind RPL can provide a sense of closure and help couples suffering from RPL move forward with their family building goals.[12] It is important to remember that miscarriage is not typically the result of something the couple did or did not do, and that seeking help and support is a proactive step toward achieving a healthy pregnancy.

REFERENCES

1. El Hachem H, Crepaux V, May-Panloup P, Descamps P, Legendre G, Bout PE. Recurrent pregnancy loss: current perspectives. Int J Womens Health. 2017;9:331-45.
2. Li Q, Chen S, Dong X, Fu S, Zhang T, Zheng W, et al. The progress of research on genetic factors of recurrent pregnancy loss. Genet Res (Camb). 2023;2023:9164374.
3. Kutteh WH, Papas RS, Maisenbacher MK, Dahdouh EM. Role of genetic analysis of products of conception and PGT in managing early pregnancy loss. Reprod Biomed Online. 2024;49(1):103738.
4. Rosenfeld JA, Tucker ME, Escobar LF, Neill NJ, Torchia BS, McDaniel LD, et al. Diagnostic utility of microarray testing in pregnancy loss. Ultrasound Obstet Gynecol. 2015;46(4):478-86.
5. Regan L, Rai R, Saravelos S, Li TC, Royal College of Obstetricians and Gynaecologists. Recurrent miscarriage green-top guideline no. 17. BJOG. 2023;130(12):e9-39.
6. ESHRE Guideline Group on RPL, Atik RB, Christiansen OB, Elson J, Kolte AM, Lewis S, et al. ESHRE guideline: recurrent pregnancy loss: an update in 2022. Hum Reprod Open. 2023;2023(1):hoad002.
7. Practice Committee of the American Society for Reproductive Medicine. Evaluation and treatment of recurrent pregnancy loss: a committee opinion. Fertil Steril. 2012;98(5):1103-11.

8. Stephenson MD, Sierra S. Reproductive outcomes in recurrent pregnancy loss associated with a parental carrier of a structural chromosome rearrangement. Hum Reprod. 2006;21(4):1076-82.
9. Stanley KE, Giordano J, Thorsten V, Buchovecky C, Thomas A, Ganapathi M, et al. Causal genetic variants in stillbirth. N Engl J Med. 2020;383(12):1107-16.
10. Maisenbacher MK, Merrion K, Kutteh WH. Single-nucleotide polymorphism microarray detects molar pregnancies in 3% of miscarriages. Fertil Steril. 2019;112(4):700-6.
11. Yaron Y, Pauta M, Badenas C, Soler A, Borobio V, Illanes C, et al. Maternal plasma genome-wide cell-free DNA can detect fetal aneuploidy in early and recurrent pregnancy loss and can be used to direct further workup. Hum Reprod. 2020;35(5):1222-9.
12. Giouleka S, Tsakiridis I, Arsenaki E, Kalogiannidis I, Mamopoulos A, Papanikolaou E, et al. Investigation and management of recurrent pregnancy loss: a comprehensive review of guidelines. Obstet Gynecol Surv. 2023;78(5):287-301.

CHAPTER 3

Monogenic Factors

Hagit Daum

ABSTRACT

Genetic disorders causing Recurrent Pregnancy Loss (RPL) result from chromosomal copy number variants, deletions, duplications, single gene disorders, and single nucleotide polymorphism. Recently chromosomal polymorphism is also implicated. Single gene disorders e.g., point mutations in genes involved in implantation and early embryonic development can result in miscarriage. Miscarriages due to autosomal recessive genes in both partners can only be identified in highly inbred populations like the Ashkenazi Jews e.g., Smith-Lemli-Opitz syndrome. These genetic variants can only be diagnosed on the NGS platform while the parents may need exome sequencing. Both diagnosis and genetic counseling of these disorders is complex. Genetic tests are evolving and higher resolution genetic testing will soon be the norm. With the experience gained we shall be able to interpret next generation sequencing (NGS) results with greater accuracy. NGS may become the recommended test for genetic analysis of the fetus in cases of unexplained RPL.

Keywords: Single nucleotide polymorphism, Single gene disorders, Recurrent pregnancy loss.

INTRODUCTION

This chapter discusses the importance of single nucleotide variants in recurrent pregnancy loss (RPL).

Before examining the contribution of next generation sequencing (NGS) in RPL investigation, inspection of the available tests and their resolution is required **(Fig. 1)**.

Chromosomal G-banding is the lowest resolution genetic test used in the context of RPL. Applying this test, the aligned chromosomes ("karyotype") can be viewed and structural rearrangements such as reciprocal and Robertsonian translocations, inversion and also large deletions and insertions can be detected. The test resolution is 5–10 mega base-pairs. Balanced chromosomal rearrangements such as reciprocal translocation are the classical etiology investigated as the first step in the genetic exploration of RPL, even though it is not very prevalent among these couples, being up to 2–5% dependent on

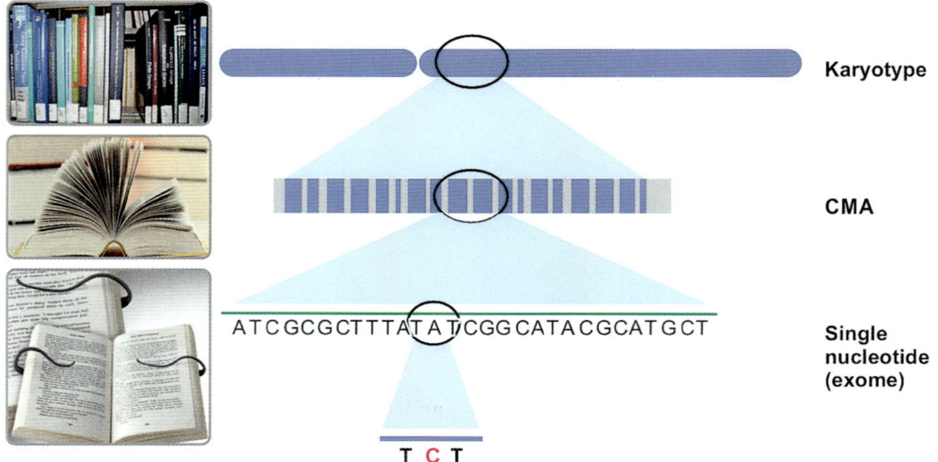

Fig. 1: The various genetic tests' resolution. If we compare every chromosome to a book, then chromosomal aberrations can be compared to a missing book or many sections of it. CMA (chromosomal microarray analysis) can detect a missing chapter and exome sequencing can detect single-letter changes.

inclusion criteria.[1-4] Since aneuploidy is the most common obstetrical complication explaining single and recurrent pregnancy loss (present in about 60% of recognized clinical pregnancies which result in a miscarriage),[4] the significance of performing chromosomal analysis on products of conception (POC) is low.

Chromosomal microarray analysis (CMA) is the next step used in the genetic investigation of RPL. The test resolution is of dozens of thousands of base-pairs, and it cannot detect balanced rearrangements. Therefore, it is used to detect copy number variations (CNV). For instance, after confirming normal parental karyotype, CMA performed on POC can detect some CNVs that might indicate a parental balanced translocation involving fragments smaller than a G-banding resolution. An algorithm for the evaluation and treatment of RPL suggests that the performance of CMA on POC at the time of the second or subsequent pregnancy loss is the first-tier genetic test.[5] Thus, normal CMA will lead to further non-genetic RPL investigation according to the ASRM (American Society for Reproductive Medicine) recommendations, while aneuploidy in POC-CMA indicates that no further investigation is needed. However, an unbalanced translocation in the POC-CMA (as represented by deletion and duplication in different loci) will dictate parental G-banding chromosomal analysis in order to diagnose the carrier of the balanced translocation.

The era of NGS provides the feasibility of sequencing all the exons or the whole genome multiple times simultaneously. This modality has the resolution of a single nucleotide variation (SNV) and can detect a "point mutation", while exome sequencing (ES) deals only with the coding regions of the genome and whole genome sequencing (WGS) deals with the whole genome. Classically, ES and WGS are used in the diagnostic process of patients with neurodevelopmental disorder[6] and/or congenital malformation/s and in recent years also for fetuses with abnormal sonographic findings.[7,8] The use of ES and WGS in the field of RPL is still restricted mostly to the research context although it seems that these platforms can be beneficial at least in some instances of RPL and/or specific populations. In this chapter we will outline the yield and lessons learned on using NGS for RPL investigation.

THE SPECTRUM OF MONOGENIC POTENTIAL IN RECURRENT PREGNANCY LOSS

Theoretically, pathogenic variants in genes that are crucial for early embryonal development lead to an "early fatal disease"—a first trimester miscarriage. In addition, a single gene defect that can cause a severe disease in humans may be embryonic-lethal in its severest form.

Fetal Monogenic Etiology

Smith-Lemli-Opitz Syndrome: The Classic Test Case

Smith-Lemli-Opitz syndrome (SLOS, OMIM #270400), is an autosomal recessive disorder characterized by the variable expression of phenotypes including multiple congenital malformations, dysmorphic features, metabolic errors, and intellectual disability. The disease is associated with biallelic variants in the *DHCR7* gene resulting in the deficiency of 7-dehydrocholesterol reductase enzyme and an impaired cholesterol metabolism. The severe extreme phenotype is associated with biallelic null variants, one being the founder null variant *DHCR7*:c.964-1G>C occurring frequently in Western Europe and, by extension, in North America. The carrier frequency of this founder variant is approximately one in 100 in the Caucasian population of North America and one in 30 in Central European populations. Based on these carrier frequencies the expected incidence of the syndrome in these populations was calculated to be between one in 1,590 and one in 17,000, respectively. However, around the world the observed prevalence and incidence are much lower. This discrepancy can be explained only in part by low ascertainment of the syndrome. It is assumed that the main cause is a high number of miscarriages before the 16 weeks of pregnancy when the incidence is in a similar range as observed at birth. Among Ashkenazi Jews (AJ) one of the populations with a high carrier frequency of the mutation, a study of couples who are carriers of c.964-1G>C reported that the actual risk for an affected child to be born is significantly <25%, probably as a result of spontaneous miscarriages of HMZ embryos.[9] In the Israeli cohort, out of 33 pregnancies of carrier couples, 14 were first or early second trimester miscarriages (42.4% observed vs. 25% expected), and 19 (57.6% observed vs. 75% expected) were of children not affected with SLOS. None of the offspring had SLOS **(Fig. 2)**. A specific family described among the couples that share the *DHCR7*:c.964-1G>C variant[9] had seven sequential unexplained first/second trimester spontaneous miscarriages, including two pregnancies with the aid of a surrogate mother. The seventh POC was tested by ES and it was found that the fetus was homozygous for the *DHCR7* variant. The eighth pregnancy was successful, and amniocentesis proved that

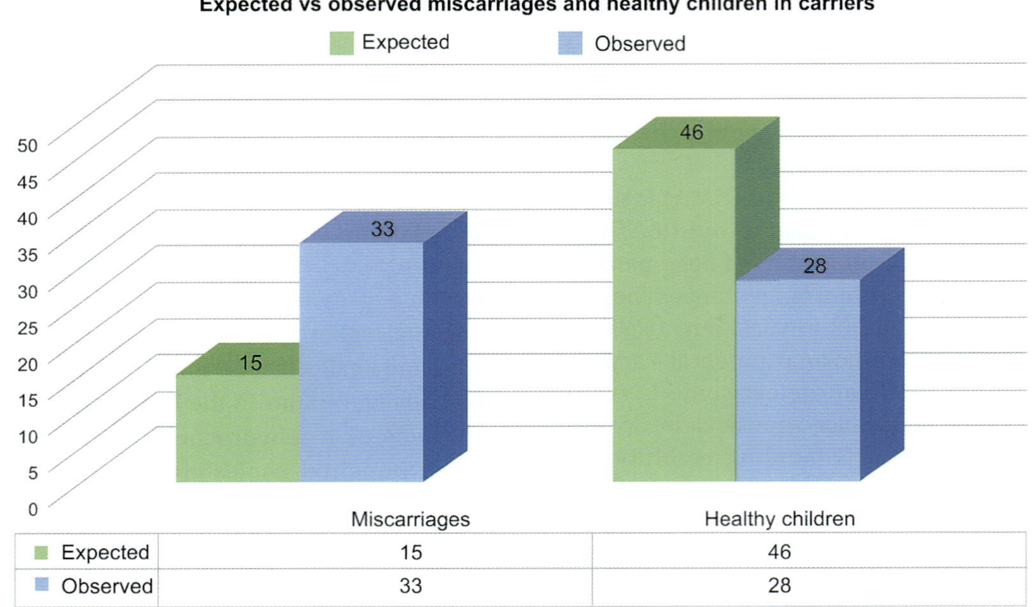

	Miscarriages	Healthy children
Expected	15	46
Observed	33	28

Fig. 2: A high ratio of observed versus expected miscarriage rate (more than doubled) in couples that share carrier state of the variant DHCR7:c.964-1G>C. It is still unexplained why the miscarriage rate exceeds 25%.
Source: Daum H, Meiner V, Michaelson-Cohen R, Sukenik-Halevy R, Zalcberg ML, Bar-Ziv A, et al. Smith-Lemli-Opitz syndrome: what is the actual risk for couples carriers of the DHCR7:c.964-1G>C variant? Eur J Hum Genet. 2020;28:938-42.

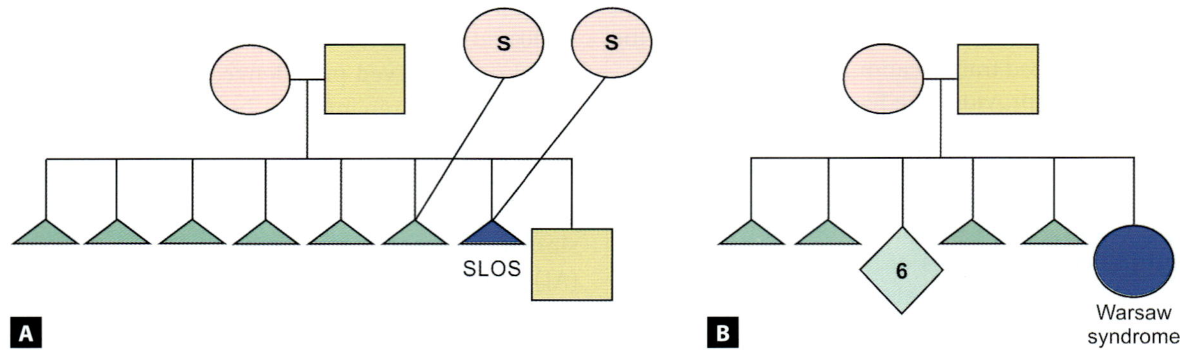

Figs. 3A and B: (A) After seven sequential first/second trimester spontaneous miscarriages, including two pregnancies with the aid of a surrogate mother, ES revealed Smith–Lemli–Opitz syndrome (SLOS) in the 7th POC. The 8th pregnancy was of a healthy fetus (diagnosed by amniocentesis). Parents are carriers of the variant DHCR7:c.964-1G>C; (B) An Ashkenazi Jewish couple had six healthy children and four unexplained miscarriages. Warsaw syndrome was diagnosed in their 7th child, shedding light on their obstetrical history. Parents are carriers of the variant DDX11:c.1763-1G>C.

the fetus was healthy regarding SLOS **(Fig. 3A)**. The rest of the fetuses were not tested but it is feasible that at least some of them were also homozygous for this variant.

Other Examples of "Early Fatal Disease"

There are a few case reports and studies describing the utility of ES in RPL investigation by the detection if biallelic/homozygous pathogenic variant/s are present in POC, most of which are of autosomal recessive mode of inheritance and are known as severe/lethal disease causatives.

Qiao et al.[10] illustrated the outcome of ES performance in three families with RPL. In one family the abortuses were compound heterozygous for variants in *DYNC2H1* (OMIM # 603297) and in another family for variants in *ALOX15* (OMIM # 152392), each variant being inherited from one of the parents. Biallelic pathogenic variants in the *DYNC2H1* gene have been frequently found in patients with asphyxiating thoracic dystrophy or short rib-polydactyly syndrome (OMIM #613091),[11] which can be prenatally lethal.[12] More than 80 damaging variants of *DYNC2H1* have been reported, mostly associated with this syndrome. Pathogenic variants in both alleles of DYNC2H1 (mouse orthologue of *DYNC2H1*) resulted in mid-gestation lethality and abnormal dorsoventral patterning of the forebrain.[13]

ALOX15 gene encodes human 12/15-lipoxygenases (12/15-LOXs), an oxidizing enzyme capable of producing reactive lipid hydroperoxides. *ALOX15* and its products are involved in many pathological conditions, such as inflammation, carcinogenesis and cardiovascular disease.[14] Association of 12/15-LOX with endoplasmic reticulum stress response was reported, which is of interest due to association of endoplasmic reticulum in stress response with early pregnancy loss.[15]

The overexpression of ALOX15 in transgenic mice showed reduced fertility with an increased miscarriage rate.[16] This gene also plays a role in spermatogenesis and ovulation and its up-regulation is associated with preeclampsia.[17]

Qiao et al.,[10] summarize that based on the information in literature, the SNVs in *ALOX15* or *DYNC2H1* could be contributory to pregnancy loss. However, functional analysis in cells from miscarriages would be needed as solid proof of this possibility (e.g., cilia function for *DYNC2H1* or biochemical assays for *ALOX15*). Unfortunately, in the case of miscarriage such studies are challenging, as they require viable cultured cells.

Srivastava et al.[18] tested 61 couples with a history of ≥2 miscarriages and 31 products of conceptions. Parents were tested by karyotype and POCs by CMA and ES. In samples of 20 couples in which POC DNA was absent or inadequate or with maternal cell contamination, couple ES was performed. Among these 20 couples, five were found to be carriers for autosomal recessive conditions: *PCNT* (primordial dwarfism type II, OMIM #210720), *MTHFR* (homocystinuria due to methylene tetrahydrofolate reductase deficiency, OMIM #236250), *ALMS1* (Alstrom syndrome, OMIM#203800), *PKD1L1* (visceral heterotaxy 8, OMIM #617205), *NEB* (arthrogryposis multiplex congenita 6, OMIM #619334), and the same couple were also carriers of variants in *INPPL1* (opsismodysplasia, OMIM #258480). It is hard to establish the prognosis of compound heterozygous offspring since not all reported variants are classified as pathogenic.

A different plausible mechanism that connects RPL with SNV suggests that some SNVs might be associated with increased risk of structural chromosomal anomalies and hence with RPL. The genes sequenced by ES by Cheng et al.[19] are involved in double-strand DNA repair and their malfunction might end in structural chromosomal anomalies. Schmid et al.[20] suggested that mosaic-variegated aneuploidy, caused by SNVs in genes such as *BUB1B* (AKA BUBR1) may be one etiology of RPL. The mechanism is related to defects of the spindle assembly checkpoint of the embryonal cells, thus characterized by random mixture of different chromosomes aneuploidy.

Maternal Monogenic Etiology

Berkay et al.[21] demonstrated the contribution of maternal ES to partially unravel the mystery of RPL (and repeated implantation failure). If we consider that early pregnancy orchestrates the immune system, embryological development, cell cycle-associated processes, developmental, implantation, placentation, coagulation, metabolism, reproductive pathways, and ovarian functions, all of which should support the developing embryo, pathogenic variants in any of involved genes can potentially end in a miscarriage **(Fig. 4)**.

Xiang et al.[22] strengthen this direction by identifying pathogenic SNVs in the *FOXA2* and *KHDC3L* genes that are involved in maternal receptivity and blastocyst implantation, angiogenesis, immune response and inflammation, cell growth and proliferation, which are functionally important processes for implantation and early pregnancy viability and development.

Maddirevula et al. (32172300) tried to decipher the monogenic basis of maternal infertility and RPL. For example, they describe a female with a history of four biochemical pregnancies that were found to be homozygous for a truncating variant in the *TLE6* gene, already linked to preimplantation embryonic lethality. Another finding was a homozygous truncating variant in *NLRP7* gene which was linked to recurrent hydatidiform mole. This woman had recurrent molar pregnancies.

A very interesting case report[23] describes two sisters, daughters of a consanguineous couple, both having repeated pregnancy loss following the diagnosis of recurrent fetal triploidy of maternal origin. ES analysis found that both sisters were homozygous for a deleterious missense variant of the cyclin B3 gene (*CCNB3*) affecting a residue conserved in mammals. Cyclin B3 malfunction is associated with the failure of oocyte second meiosis and

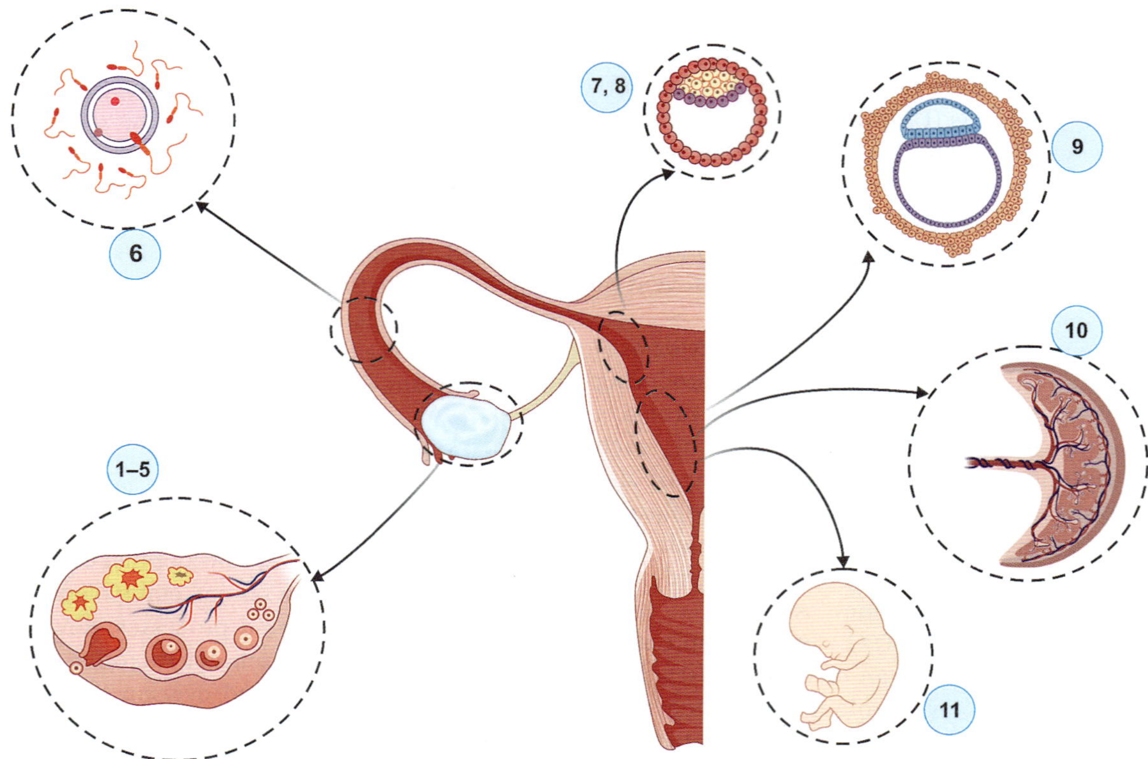

1. Oogenesis, 2. Oocyte Maturation, 3. Meiosis, 4. Metabolism, 5. Cell cycle, 6. Fertilization, 7. Implantation, 8. Immunity 9. Coagulation/Placental development, 10. Embryological development, 11. Fetal lethal variants

Fig. 4: Recurrent pregnancy loss (RPL) may be caused by point mutation in any of the crucial processes of the very early embryonic life depicted in the figure. They include gamete maturation and ovulation, fertilization, implantation etc.
Source: Berkay EG, Şoroğlu CV, Kalaycı T, Uyguner ZO, Akçapınar GB, Başaran S. A new enrichment approach for candidate gene detection in unexplained recurrent pregnancy loss and implantation failure. Mol Genet Genomics. 2023;298:253-72.

recurrent fetal triploidy, suggesting a rationale for *CCNB3* testing in RPL.

Another maternal origin of RPL was a variant in *CAPS* gene, inherited in three sisters as an HMZ variant from their consanguineous parents.[24] All three sisters experienced RPL.

Paternal Monogenic Etiology

Defective spermatogenesis can theoretically also form non-viable pregnancies if meiosis cannot be normally completed. This can also be a result of a monogenic effect in the male, thus recurring.

RECURRENT PREGNANCY LOSS IN HIGHLY INBRED POPULATIONS

A few reports and series describe unique families, in which couple shared the same deleterious variant, leading to the miscarriage of all assumed HMZ embryos. This applies mostly to highly inbred population such as in Saudi Arabia. Exome sequencing or WGS unraveled the genetic background[25-27] and provided the essence of genetic counseling and the estimated recurrence risk of 25% in every following pregnancy. One of the genes described in consanguineous families is *ASIC5*, an ion-channel, the function of which is not completely understood but it is expressed in the very various early embryonic tissues. Another gene described in the setup of RPL following clinical presentation of severe early hydrops fetalis is *CHRNA1*. Some other genes were noted in these studies as a cause of embryonic-lethal disease in an autosomal recessive manner.

While the potential of diagnoses of monogenic disorders is promising for the moment, even in highly consanguineous populations enriched for recessive disorders, a monogenic disorder is rarely found to be the etiology of RPL. In addition, a complicating frequent scenario is the identification of a variant of uncertain significance or a candidate pathogenic SNV in a gene as yet unknown to cause a disease in humans. If a variant, for example, is in a gene participating in the process of mitosis, implantation, early embryonic development etc., but is not known to be correlated with a specific disease or human phenotype, it will be difficult to offer consultation to the couple regarding the meaning of the finding, without further research.

SPECIAL POPULATIONS WHO MIGHT BENEFIT FROM NEXT GENERATION SEQUENCING INVESTIGATION FOR RECURRENT PREGNANCY LOSS

If we consider the inherited potential of a fatal disease in the offspring, then we are discussing mostly autosomal recessive (and possibly also X-linked recessive) traits. Thus, it seems reasonable that the high-risk population for RPL with an inherited monogenic background are highly inbred couples but also couples with shared ancestry.

A few examples may be found in the literature.

BRCA1 and *BRCA2*

Hereditary breast and ovarian cancer susceptibility due to *BRCA1/2* carrier state is very prevalent among AJ - up to 2.5%[28] and thus it is recently implemented in heathy AJ women screening tests in Israel.[29]

BRCA1

BRCA1 prevalent deleterious variants in AJ are c.68_69delAG (185delAG) and c.5266dupC (5382insC) with a carrier frequency of 0.75% and 0.45% respectively. Humans with validated biallelic germline mutations in *BRCA1* have not been identified, suggesting that at least one functional allele of *BRCA1* is required for human embryogenesis and development. Hence, it seems feasible that a couple will share a carrier state of *BRCA1* pathogenic variant and experience RPL of unknown etiology of all biallelic *BRCA1* embryos.

BRCA2

Fanconi anemia, complementation group D1 is also named *BRCA2*. In Genomic aggregation database (gnomAD) the variant *BRCA2*:c.5946del (c.6174 delT mutation) has a carrier frequency of 1.16%. Fanconi anemia is characterized by physical abnormalities, bone marrow failure, increased risk for malignancy, and gonadal dysgenesis. Physical abnormalities, present in approximately 75% of affected individuals, include one or more of the following—short stature, abnormal skin pigmentation, skeletal malformations of the upper and/or lower limbs, microcephaly and ophthalmic, and genitourinary tract anomalies. Progressive bone marrow failure with pancytopenia typically presents in the first decade, often initially with thrombocytopenia or leukopenia. Relevant malignancies are acute myeloid leukemia and solid tumors—particularly of the head and neck, skin, and genitourinary tract.

Very few patients have been reported as HMZ with this *BRCA2* variant and in a study of 111 Fanconi anemia patients diagnosed in Israel only one child was diagnosed as HMZ for *BRCA2*: c.5946 del.[30] Again, if the "severest end" is an early miscarriage, a "less severe scenario" regarding survival is the delivery of an offspring having a severe monogenic disease such as Fanconi anemia.

Warsaw Breakage Syndrome

Warsaw syndrome (OMIM #613398) is also a multisystemic severe disease characterized by the clinical triad of severe congenital microcephaly, growth restriction, and sensorineural hearing loss due to cochlear hypoplasia. Intellectual disability is also common. Once again, there is a discrepancy between the high rate of AJ carriers (the variant *DDX11*:c.1763-1G>C) and sick offspring. The disease seems to be rare among AJ since only two affected homozygotes have been reported in the literature. One of them was a female born to non-consanguineous parents of AJ descent. The affected child was the third of seven children. Family history was significant for four first trimester miscarriages of unknown etiology[31] **(Fig. 3B)**. Once again, the monogenic inherited undiagnosed disease could be the etiology of RPL. The implication of genetic investigation of RPL in this family is the possibility of preventing the severe disease in offspring that survive.

Congenital Amegakaryocytic Thrombocytopenia

This is a rare, autosomal recessive disease, characterized by a severely low number of megakaryocytes, the primordial form of platelets in the bone marrow. In gnomAD, the variant *MPL*: c.79+2T>A has a carrier frequency of 1.61% among AJ and a random sample of 2018 individuals of AJ descent revealed a carrier frequency of approximately

1.33%. The disease seems to be rare among AJ with only a few affected. Jalas et al. described a full-term male child of non-consanguineous AJ parents who was the fourth viable child born to a mother who had had five previous miscarriages.[32]

WHO IS THE PROBAND THAT SHOULD BE TESTED?

Evica Rajcan-Separovic reviewed reports of ES or WGS for genetic investigation following two or more miscarriages.[33] There are various familial setups for the performance of NGS in the process of RPL investigation. The ideal setup includes the parents and one or more POC. This setup actually includes validation and segregation within the family. Other setups may be more minimalistic but may be inconclusive or require validation and segregation by Sanger sequencing **(Fig. 5)**. It depicts the various familial setups for NGS investigation. One important conclusion of this section is the importance of the preservation of good quality DNA samples from POC. They may be invaluable when trying to decipher the familial painful riddle of RPL. While parental NGS can be directive, it can never be as diagnostic as the POC test. A healthy child/children of a couple experiencing RPL can promote the segregation studies since he/they should not have two abnormal alleles such as in the POC.

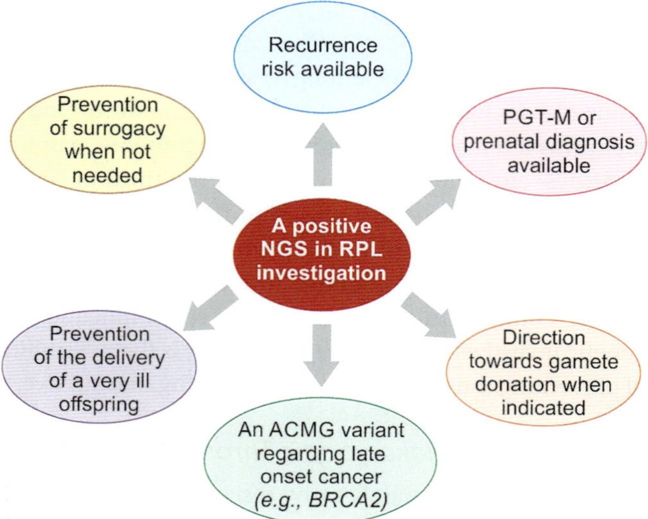

Fig. 5: The actionable aspects of next generation sequencing (NGS) diagnosis in recurrent pregnancy loss (RPL).
(ACMG: American College of Medical Genetics and Genomics; NGS: next generation sequencing; PGT-M: preimplantation genetic testing for a monogenic disease)

ACTIONABLE ASPECTS OF THE MONOGENIC DIAGNOSIS INVESTIGATION

There are several purposes for investigating RPL by NGS, especially in specific populations as mentioned above and whenever there is no etiology after the completing the investigation (uterine, endocrinological etc.).

The diagnosis of a monogenic "embryonic lethal" disease in a family can lead to a few actionable steps **(Fig. 6)**:

- The diagnosis of 25% recurrence risk of a severe disease can direct the couple to the mode of IVF with PGT-M in order to eliminate this risk in future pregnancies. The possibility of diagnosing a single gene variant as responsible for RPL, is the first step in eliminating it. The case report of Rabin et al. describes a single family with a history of RPL but also a sick child.[31]
- Ovum meiotic errors leading to the incomplete oocyte maturation may lead to RPL.[23] Hence, for example, when both sisters were HMZ for a gene variant altering their meiosis, the only way to help them was by using ovum donation. Only after molecular diagnosis was provided, this mode of action became possible.
- Fanconi anemia due to *BRCA2* biallelic pathogenic variant, is a severe disease that might be "embryonic lethal". However, the carrier state is an established cause for susceptibility for breast and ovarian cancer. This might be of utmost importance for the couple as actionable information since cautious follow-up according to written protocols may save lives. The same is true regarding the *BRCA1* carrier state.
- As mentioned above, in the minority of cases, when RPL represents the "severest end" of a monogenic disease, a sick offspring may be born with the same illness. Identification of the disease-causing variant/s can direct the couple to the process of PGT-M. However, if the pregnancy is ongoing throughout the second trimester, prenatal diagnosis should be considered in order to rule-out this monogenic disease.
- Alternative modes of pregnancy, such as surrogacy, in order to eliminate RPL, are irrelevant in situations of monogenic disease being the background of RPL. Since surrogacy is a very complicated and expensive procedure, it is worthwhile knowing when it is not required.

CONCLUSION

Genetic causes of RPL can include single gene defects, especially in highly inbred populations like the Ashkenazi Jews. In these cases NGS gives a better diagnostic yield.

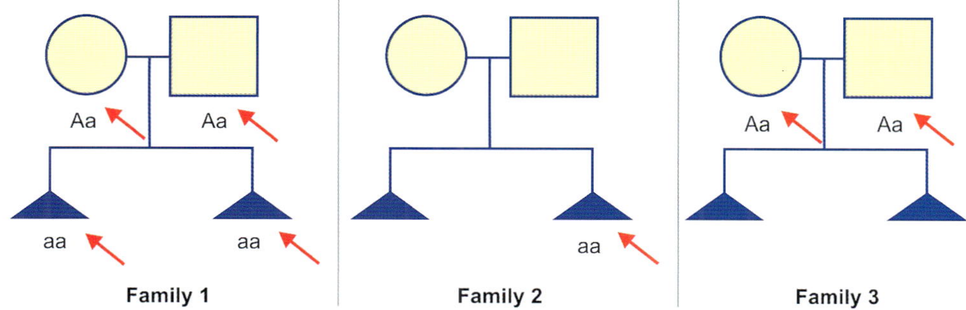

Fig. 6: Different familial setups of genetic investigation of recurrent pregnancy loss (RPL) by next generation sequencing (NGS) such as exome sequencing.

- Family 1—represents the ideal setup where there is a DNA sample of products of conceptions (POC, more than one) and the test is also performed for parents. All candidate variants are segregated within the same test.
- Family 2—represents the "economic" mode where only POC are tested. If the results are inconclusive, parents can also be tested by NGS. If the results are conclusive, then Sanger sequencing can be performed for validation.
- Family 3—represents a case where there is no POC DNA for testing. Parents can be tested by searching the monogenic etiology for RPL (i.e., if they share a carrier state for the same severe disease). If there is a POC sample, the presumed diagnosis can be validated by Sanger sequencing. If an X-linked mode of inheritance or maternal etiology for RPL is suspected, a parental test will confirm that.

Much can be learnt from analyzing the DNA of POC and segregating the results within the family. If a monogenic diagnosis is achieved, the benefit is invaluable since the mode of action for the next pregnancy is clarified. PGT-M can be applied to prevent an autosomal recessive disease in the offspring, especially if it is manifested by early lethality, but also to prevent a severe disease in the offspring.

In rare cases, the parents who are diagnosed as carriers of the lethal monogenic recessive disease (such as *BRCA* carriers), should have a specific medical follow-up.

REFERENCES

1. Priya PK, Mishra VV, Roy P, Patel H. A Study on Balanced Chromosomal Translocations in Couples with Recurrent Pregnancy Loss. J Hum Reprod Sci. 2018;11:337-42.
2. Maithripala S, Durland U, Havelock J, Kashyap S, Hitkari J, Tan J, et al. Prevalence and Treatment Choices for Couples with Recurrent Pregnancy Loss Due to Structural Chromosomal Anomalies. J Obstet Gynaecol Can. 2018;40:655-62.
3. Li S, Chen M, Zheng PS. Analysis of parental abnormal chromosomal karyotype and subsequent live births in Chinese couples with recurrent pregnancy loss. Sci Rep. 2021;11:20298.
4. Papas RS, Kutteh WH. Genetic Testing for Aneuploidy in Patients Who Have Had Multiple Miscarriages: A Review of Current Literature. Appl Clin Genet. 2021;14:321-9.
5. Popescu F, Jaslow CR, Kutteh WH. Recurrent pregnancy loss evaluation combined with 24-chromosome microarray of miscarriage tissue provides a probable or definite cause of pregnancy loss in over 90% of patients. Hum Reprod. 2018;33:579-87.
6. Alvarez-Mora MI, Rodríguez-Revenga L, Jodar M, Potrony M, Sanchez A, Badenas C, et al. Implementation of Exome Sequencing in Clinical Practice for Neurological Disorders. Genes (Basel). 2023;14.
7. Lord J, McMullan DJ, Eberhardt RY, Rinck G, Hamilton SJ, Quinlan-Jones E, et al. Prenatal exome sequencing analysis in fetal structural anomalies detected by ultrasonography (PAGE): a cohort study. Lancet. 2019;393:747-57.
8. Petrovski S, Aggarwal V, Giordano JL, Stosic M, Wou K, Bier L, et al. Whole-exome sequencing in the evaluation of fetal structural anomalies: a prospective cohort study. Lancet. 2019;393:758-67.
9. Daum H, Meiner V, Michaelson-Cohen R, Sukenik-Halevy R, Zalcberg ML, Bar-Ziv A, et al. Smith-Lemli-Opitz syndrome: what is the actual risk for couples carriers of the DHCR7:c.964-1G>C variant? Eur J Hum Genet. 2020;28:938-42.
10. Qiao Y, Wen J, Tang F, Martell S, Shomer N, Leung PC, et al. Whole exome sequencing in recurrent early pregnancy loss. Mol Hum Reprod. 2016;22:364-72.
11. Dagoneau N, Goulet M, Geneviève D, Sznajer Y, Martinovic J, Smithson S, et al. DYNC2H1 mutations cause asphyxiating thoracic dystrophy and short rib-polydactyly syndrome, type III. Am J Hum Genet. 2009;84:706-11.
12. Ellard S, Kivuva E, Turnpenny P, Stals K, Johnson M, Xie W, et al. An exome sequencing strategy to diagnose lethal autosomal recessive disorders. Eur J Hum Genet. 2015;23:401-4.
13. Huangfu D, Anderson KV. Cilia and Hedgehog responsiveness in the mouse. Proc Natl Acad Sci U S A. 2005;102:11325-30.

14. Ivanov I, Kuhn H, Heydeck D. Structural and functional biology of arachidonic acid 15-lipoxygenase-1 (ALOX15). Gene. 2015;573:1-32.
15. Gao HJ, Zhu YM, He WH, Liu AX, Dong MY, Jin M, et al. Endoplasmic reticulum stress induced by oxidative stress in decidual cells: a possible mechanism of early pregnancy loss. Mol Biol Rep. 2012;39:9179-86.
16. Dar P, Strassburger D, Shaish A, Levkovitz H, Halperin R, Harats D. Reduced reproduction with increased abortion rate in transgenic mice that overexpress 15-lipoxygenase. Gynecol Obstet Invest. 2001;52:18-21.
17. Yuan D, Ran Y, Liu Q, Zhang Y, Li H, Li P, et al. Enhancement of the HIF-1α/15-LO/15-HETE axis promotes hypoxia-induced endothelial proliferation in preeclamptic pregnancy. PLoS One. 2014;9:e96510.
18. Srivastava P, Bamba C, Chopra S, Rohilla M, Chaudhry C, Kaur A, et al. Identification of genetic alterations in couples and their products of conceptions from recurrent pregnancy loss in North Indian population. Front Genet. 2023;14:1155211.
19. Cheng Z, Cheng D, Li J, Guo L, Zhang W, Zhang C, et al. Polymorphisms Within DNA Double-Strand Breaks Repair-Related Genes Contribute to Structural Chromosome Abnormality in Recurrent Pregnancy Loss. Front Genet. 2021;12:787718.
20. Schmid M, Steinlein C, Tian Q, Hanlon Newell AE, Gessler M, Olson SB, et al. Mosaic variegated aneuploidy in mouse BubR1 deficient embryos and pregnancy loss in human. Chromosome Res. 2014;22:375-92.
21. Berkay EG, Şoroğlu CV, Kalaycı T, Uyguner ZO, Akçapınar GB, Başaran S. A new enrichment approach for candidate gene detection in unexplained recurrent pregnancy loss and implantation failure. Mol Genet Genomics. 2023;298:253-72.
22. Xiang H, Wang C, Pan H, Hu Q, Wang R, Xu Z, et al. Exome-Sequencing Identifies Novel Genes Associated with Recurrent Pregnancy Loss in a Chinese Cohort. Front Genet. 2021;12:746082.
23. Fatemi N, Salehi N, Pignata L, Palumbo P, Cubellis MV, Ramazanali F, et al. Biallelic variant in cyclin B3 is associated with failure of maternal meiosis II and recurrent digynic triploidy. J Med Genet. 2021;58:783-8.
24. Pan H, Xiang H, Wang J, Wei Z, Zhou Y, Liu B, et al. CAPS Mutations Are Potentially Associated with Unexplained Recurrent Pregnancy Loss. Am J Pathol. 2019;189:124-31.
25. Al Qahtani NH, Abdul Azeez S, Almandil NB, Fahad Alhur N, Alsuwat HS, Al Taifi HA, et al. Whole-Genome Sequencing Reveals Exonic Variation of ASIC5 Gene Results in Recurrent Pregnancy Loss. Front Med (Lausanne) 2021;8:699672.
26. Shamseldin HE, Tulbah M, Kurdi W, Nemer M, Alsahan N, Al Mardawi E, et al. Identification of embryonic lethal genes in humans by autozygosity mapping and exome sequencing in consanguineous families. Genome Biol. 2015;16:116.
27. Shamseldin HE, Swaid A, Alkuraya FS. Lifting the lid on unborn lethal Mendelian phenotypes through exome sequencing. Genet Med. 2013;15:307-9.
28. Roa BB, Boyd AA, Volcik K, Richards CS. Ashkenazi Jewish population frequencies for common mutations in BRCA1 and BRCA2. Nat Genet. 1996;14:185-7.
29. Gabai-Kapara E, Lahad A, Kaufman B, Friedman E, Segev S, Renbaum P, et al. Population-based screening for breast and ovarian cancer risk due to BRCA1 and BRCA2. Proc Natl Acad Sci U S A. 2014;111:14205-10.
30. Steinberg-Shemer O, Goldberg TA, Yacobovich J, Levin C, Koren A, Revel-Vilk S, et al. Characterization and genotype-phenotype correlation of patients with Fanconi anemia in a multi-ethnic population. Haematologica. 2020;105:1825-34.
31. Rabin R, Hirsch Y, Johansson MM, Ekstein J, Zeevi DA, Keena B, et al. Study of carrier frequency of Warsaw breakage syndrome in the Ashkenazi Jewish population and presentation of two cases. Am J Med Genet A. 2019;179:2144-51.
32. Jalas C, Anderson SL, Laufer T, Martimucci K, Bulanov A, Xie X, et al. A founder mutation in the MPL gene causes congenital amegakaryocytic thrombocytopenia (CAMT) in the Ashkenazi Jewish population. Blood Cells Mol Dis. 2011;47:79-83.
33. Rajcan-Separovic E. Next generation sequencing in recurrent pregnancy loss-approaches and outcomes. Eur J Med Genet. 2020;63:103644.

CHAPTER 4

Parental Genetic Testing

Priya Ranganath

ABSTRACT

Chromosomal translocations, inversions and ring chromosomes are implicated in couples with recurrent pregnancy loss (RPL). Inversions of chromosomes 9, 11 and 1 are commonly encountered. Parental karyotyping is indicated if the products of conception show translocation, if there is an affected child in the family and if no products of conception (POC) are available for testing as in recurrent early pregnancy losses. Other parental genetic factors are skewed X chromosome inactivation, high sperm deoxyribonucleic acid (DNA) fragmentation in male partner and monogenic disorders of genes involved in implantation. In select cases of carriers of monogenic disorders, whole exome sequencing of the couple may be required.

Keywords: Parental genetic testing, Karyotyping, Skewed X chromosome inactivation, Deletions, Duplication, Inversion, Ring chromosome, Monogenic disorders, Whole exome sequencing (WES).

INTRODUCTION

About 10–15% of all clinical pregnancies and about 30% of all pregnancies in total end in early pregnancy loss.[1] This contributes significantly to the reproductive health in a women. Based on the available evidence, up to 5% of women experience recurrent pregnancy losses. Genetic factors may contribute approximately 50% of causes of recurrent pregnancy losses.[2] The other factors include environmental factors, metabolic, hormonal factors, sperm quality, maternal and paternal age, uterine abnormalities, thrombophilia, immune, and infectious disorders. Despite the number of proposed etiologies, recurrent pregnancy loss (RPL) remains unexplained in ~45–50% of patients.[2]

THE GENETIC CONTRIBUTION IN ETIOLOGY OF RECURRENT PREGNANCY LOSS

Recurrent pregnancy loss is etiologically heterogeneous and multiple factors are suggested to contribute to the pathogenesis. The common genetic disorders include embryonic chromosomal abnormality and balanced reciprocal or Robertsonian translocation in parents.[3] Parental translocation is set to contribute approximately 5% of cases for RPL. Other genetic causes include abnormal DNA methylation, DNA fragmentation in sperms, skewed X-inactivation, chromosomal heteromorphisms, and monogenic causes.[4] The monogenic causes mainly include those factors which predispose to thrombophilia. However, apart from embryonic chromosomal abnormality and balanced translocation in couple, none of the other factors have been established as the stand-alone risk factor for RPL.

- *Fetal aneuploidies:* They are the primary cause of sporadic and recurrent pregnancy losses. Fetal aneuploidies are random errors in germ cell development. These are typically meiotic nondisjunction events in the germ cells of couples with normal parental karyotypes. Nondisjunction is the failure of homologous chromosomes to separate properly during cell division **(Fig. 1)**. Monosomy x, Trisomy 16 and 22, triploidy, and tetraploidy contribute to the most common cause for embryonic chromosomal abnormality.
- *Structural chromosomal abnormalities in couples:* Chromosomal translocations, inversions, insertions, and ring chromosomes in the couple can contribute to RPL **(Figs. 2A to F)**. Couples with RPL are 10 times more likely to have structural chromosomal abnormality.
    - Amongst the structural chromosomal rearrangements in the couple, reciprocal translocations are the most common cause. Reciprocal translocation involves exchange of chromosomal segments between two chromosomes. If this exchange occurs between acrocentric chromosomes (with short p arm) then it is called a Robertsonian translocation. During meiosis, these chromosomes (quadrivalents)

Normal
Abnormal
Abnormal
M1
M1
M1
M2
M2
M2

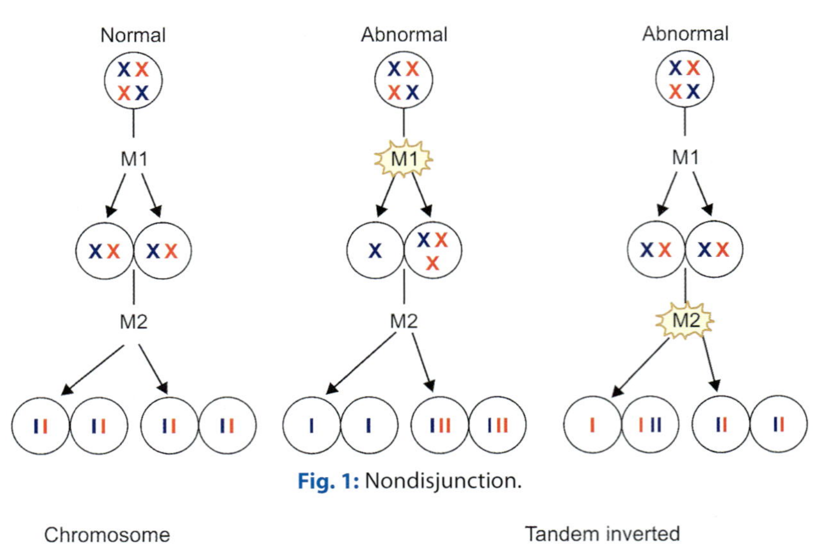

Fig. 1: Nondisjunction.

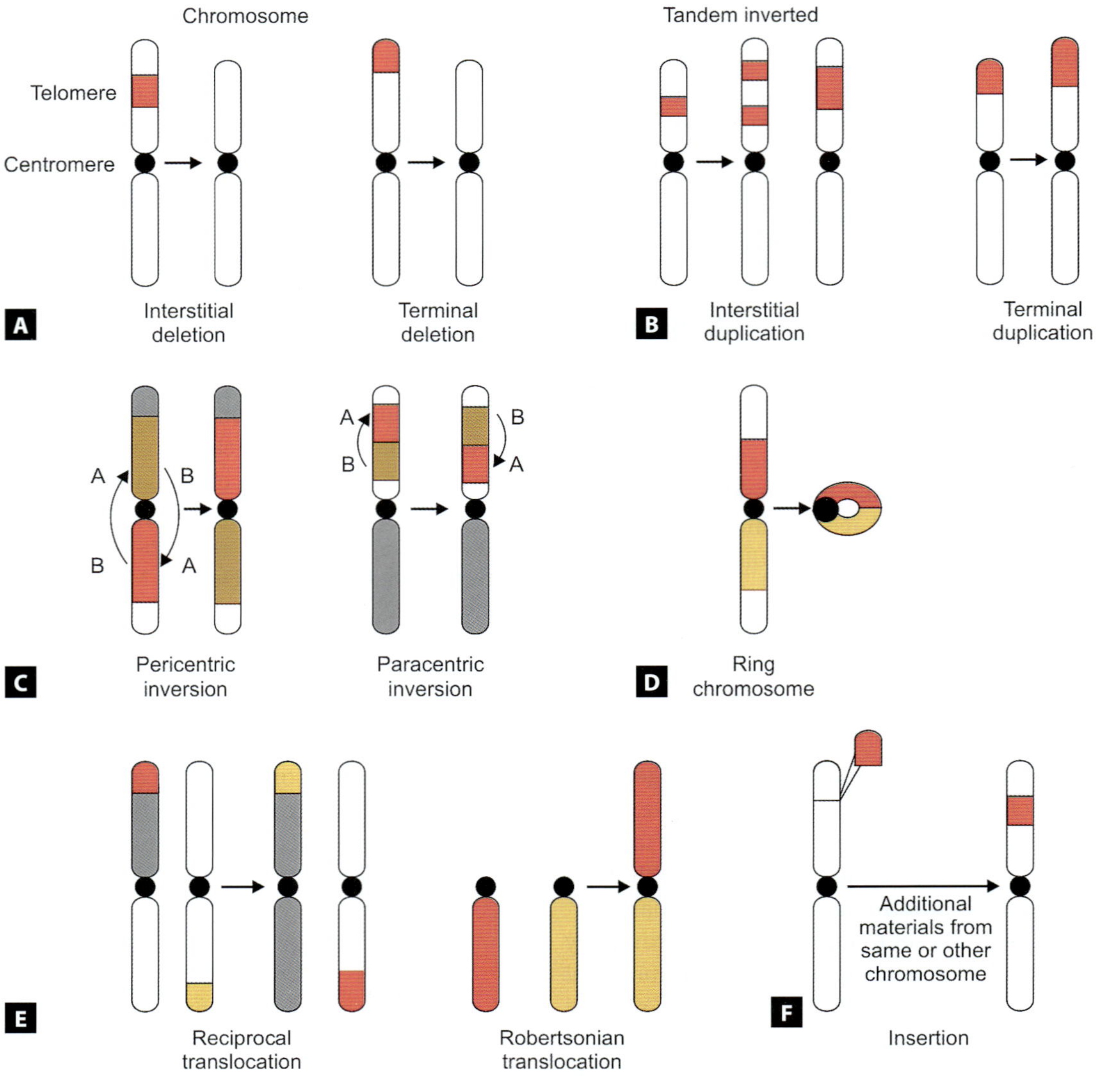

Chromosome
Telomere
Centromere
A
Interstitial deletion
Terminal deletion
Tandem inverted
B
Interstitial duplication
Terminal duplication
A
B
B
A
A
B
B
A
C
Pericentric inversion
Paracentric inversion
D
Ring chromosome
E
Reciprocal translocation
Robertsonian translocation
Additional materials from same or other chromosome
F
Insertion

Figs. 2A to F: Structural chromosomal abnormalities.

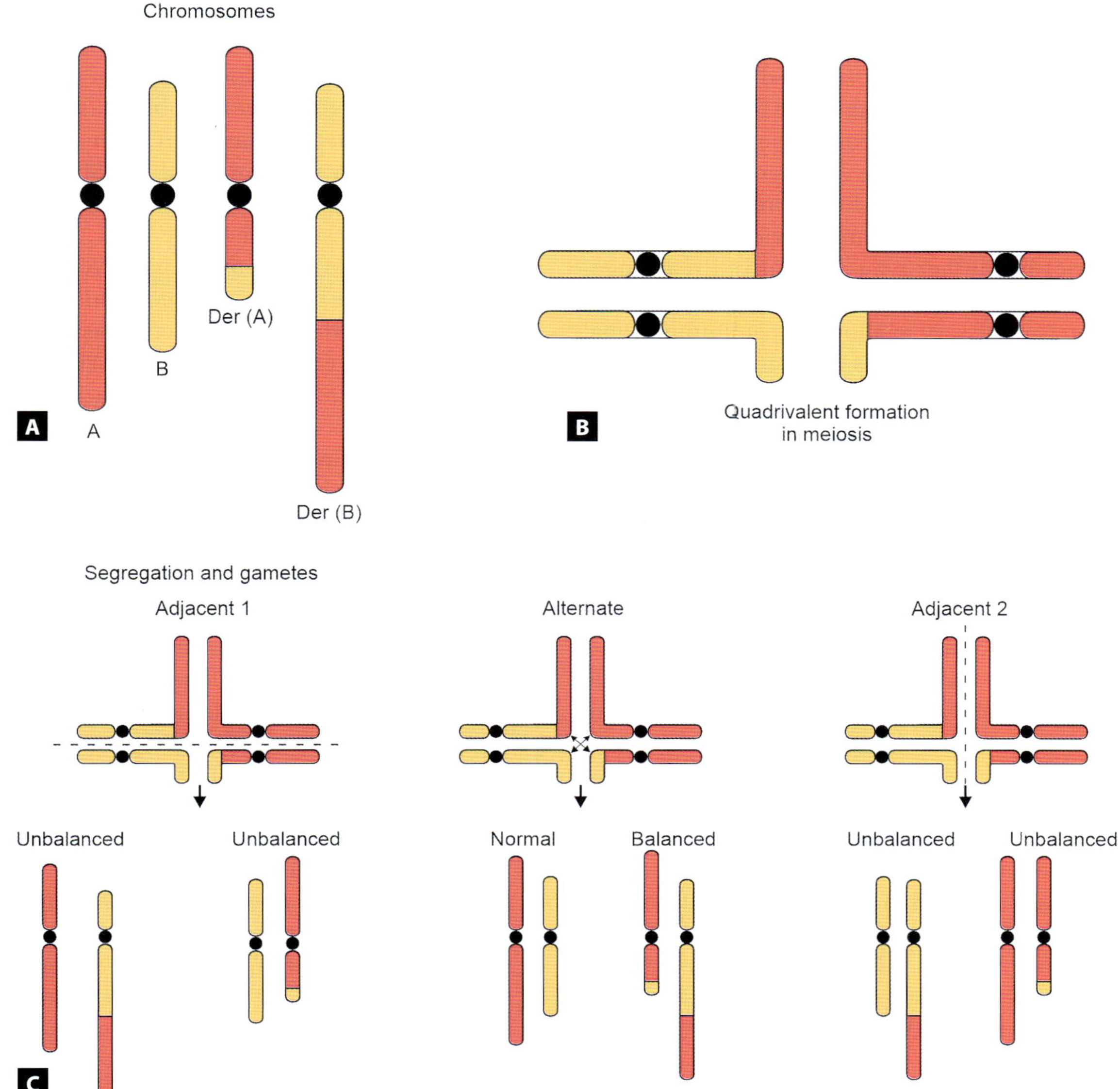

Figs. 3A to C: Segregation in balanced translocation carriers.

fail to align with their respective homologous chromosome resulting in an unbalanced derivative chromosome post segregation. This unbalanced chromosome essentially could result in gain and loss of segments of chromosomes which may involve critical genes for survival **(Figs. 3A to C)**.

Couples with balanced reciprocal translocations face a 50% chance of RPL and a 20% risk of having children with unbalanced chromosomal rearrangements.[4] The severity of imbalances influences outcomes, with larger imbalances more likely to lead to miscarriages and smaller ones increasing the risk of offspring with an unbalanced karyotype.

Genetic counseling is crucial before the next pregnancy, allowing exploration of options and informed decision-making. Prenatal diagnosis through procedures such as amniocentesis or chorionic villus sampling can detect genetic abnormalities. Couples may consider preimplantation genetic diagnosis (PGD) for specific translocations, involving the transfer of unaffected embryos. In cases where embryonic aneuploidy is certain, such as Robertsonian translocations involving homologous chromosomes, the use of donor gametes is an option. Extended family implications should be discussed, and assistance provided in informing relatives about the genetic situation. The comprehensive approach ensures that couples are well-informed, enabling appropriate planning for future pregnancies.

- An inversion chromosome (pericentric or paracentric) is another type of balanced rearrangement that can lead to unbalanced gametes because a loop is necessary to allow proper chromosomal alignment during meiosis, and recombination can occur within this loop. The unbalanced gamete from a paracentric inversion will not be viable because it will be acentric or dicentric; in contrast, the unbalanced gamete from a pericentric inversion can be viable, with resulting duplication or loss of chromosomal segments **(Fig. 4)**. Pericentric inversion in chromosomes 9, 11, and 1 are very common in normal population with prevalence of 1.0% in the population and 2.28% in RPL patients and therefore considered polymorphism. Multiple studies establish that these polymorphisms are unlikely to contribute to RPL.[5]
- It was previously thought that chromosomal heterochromatin associated polymorphisms such as 9 qh + are not associated with RPL. However, recent data is conflicting.[3,6] More case-control studies are essential to validate the significance of individual heterochromatin polymorphisms.
- Small deletions and duplications (<400 kb) are empirically not found to be associated with RPL unlike the larger CNVs.[3]

- *Monogenic causes:*
    - Many studies have evaluated the polymorphisms in genes associated with angiogenesis (VEGF, NOS) in the etiology of RPL. However, they have been unsuccessful in establishing a causal relationship.[7] Polymorphisms associated with thrombogenesis related genes such as methylenetetrahydrofolate reductase (MTHFR) C677T, Factor V (FV) G1691A, Factor II (FII) G20210A, plasminogen activator, inhibitor-1 (PAI-1) have also been implicated in RPL. Studies have been unable to establish a conclusive relationship.[8] Therefore, testing for these polymorphisms in couple with RPL is currently not recommended. Other thrombophilia related genes have also been evaluated. currently ESHRE guidelines suggest not to screen for hereditary thrombophilia except in women with additional risk factors for thrombophilia.[9] Certain human leukocyte antigen (HLA)-related polymorphisms have also been associated with RPL. HLA determination in women with RPL is not currently recommended by ESHRE in clinical practice. Cytokine polymorphism testing in RPL is not yet well established.[9]
    - Next-generation sequencing (NGS) has been widely used in research and clinical settings to investigate the genetic factors associated with RPL. Whole exome sequencing (WES) and whole genome sequencing (WGS) is a powerful tool that enables the simultaneous analysis of the protein-coding regions of the genome. Multiple WES studies have identified several novel genetic causes for euploid miscarriages. Genes essential for development, cell division, cilia function and fetal movement (KIF14, CEP55, *es*STIL, FOXP3, GLE, RYR1, DYNC2H1, ALOX15, *and* POMT1) have been evaluated as candidate genes.[10] Large scale studies and functional analysis are required to conclusively establish their significance in RPL. Further, interpretation of the identified variants and their clinical significance can be challenging, requiring further research. Currently NGS based WES or WGS is not routinely recommended in evaluation of RPL.
- *Others: Sperm DNA fragmentation, skewed x-inactivation, DNA methylation*
    - DNA fragmentation studies were considered as sperm cell can still carry a high degree of DNA damage while retaining the ability to fertilize an oocyte. Conception by sperm with a high level of DNA damage can potentially result in poor implantation or, ultimately, pregnancy loss. A newly updated RPL guideline from the European Society of Human Reproduction and Embryology (ESHRE) recommends considering DNA fragmentation analysis for diagnostic purposes rather than explanatory purpose in evaluating RPL.[9] However, management options are limited to lifestyle modification and antioxidant supplementation at present.
    - Skewed X chromosome inactivation (SXCI) and androgen receptor (AR) CAG polymorphisms have been subjects of interest in the context of RPL. The result of studies evaluating the same are conflicting which could be attributed to various factors,

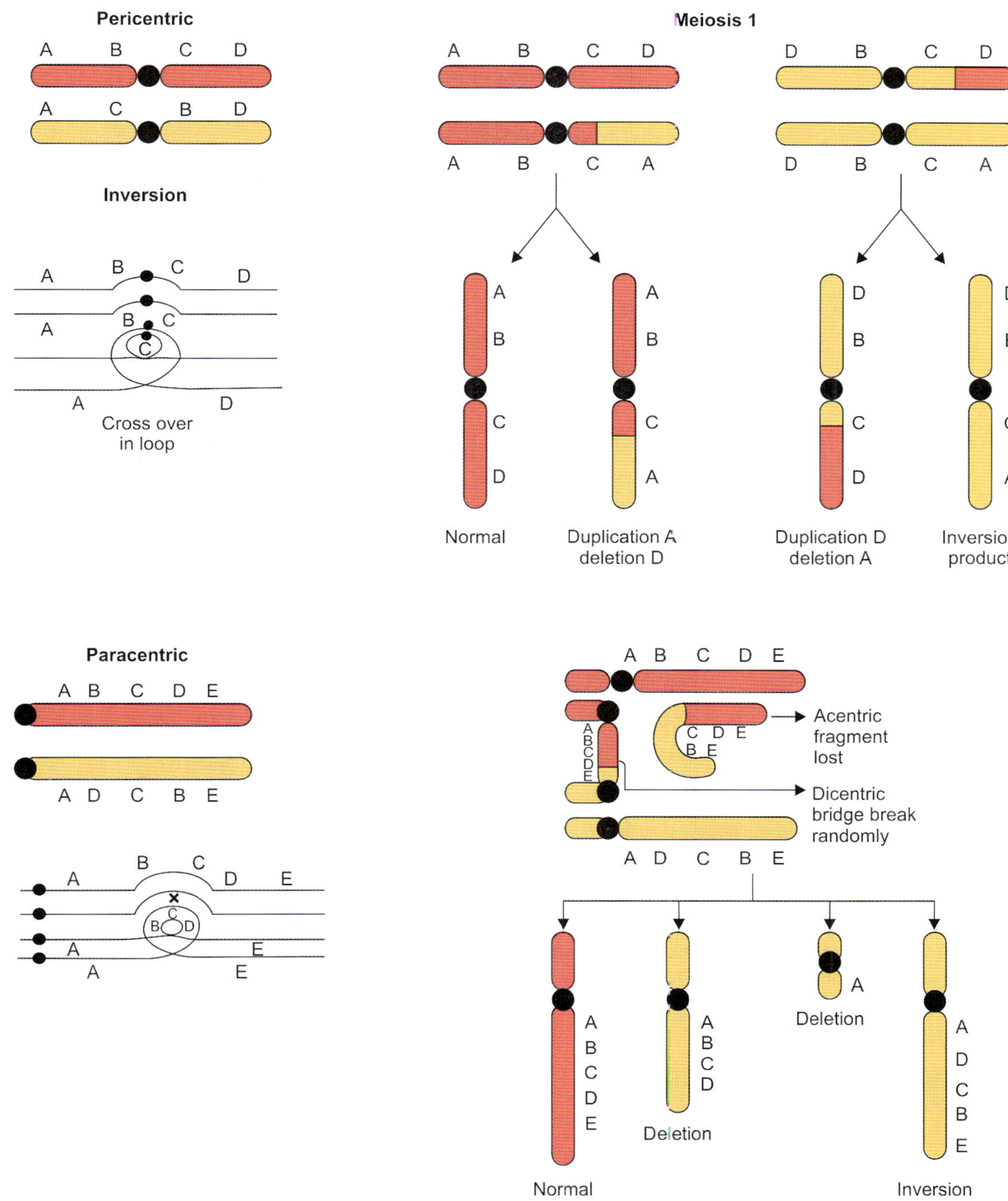

Fig. 4: Segregation in pericentric and paracentric inversions.

including differences in study design, sample sizes, population characteristics, and methodologies used to assess XCI or AR CAG polymorphisms and underlying mechanisms linking SXCI and AR CAG polymorphisms to RPL are not fully understood.[11] While there is evidence suggesting a potential link between skewed X chromosome inactivation and androgen receptor CAG polymorphisms with recurrent pregnancy loss, the conflicting results highlight the need for additional research to unravel the complexities of these associations and their underlying mechanisms.

Flowchart 1: Diagnostic algorithm for evaluation of genetic factors in recurrent pregnancy loss (RPL).

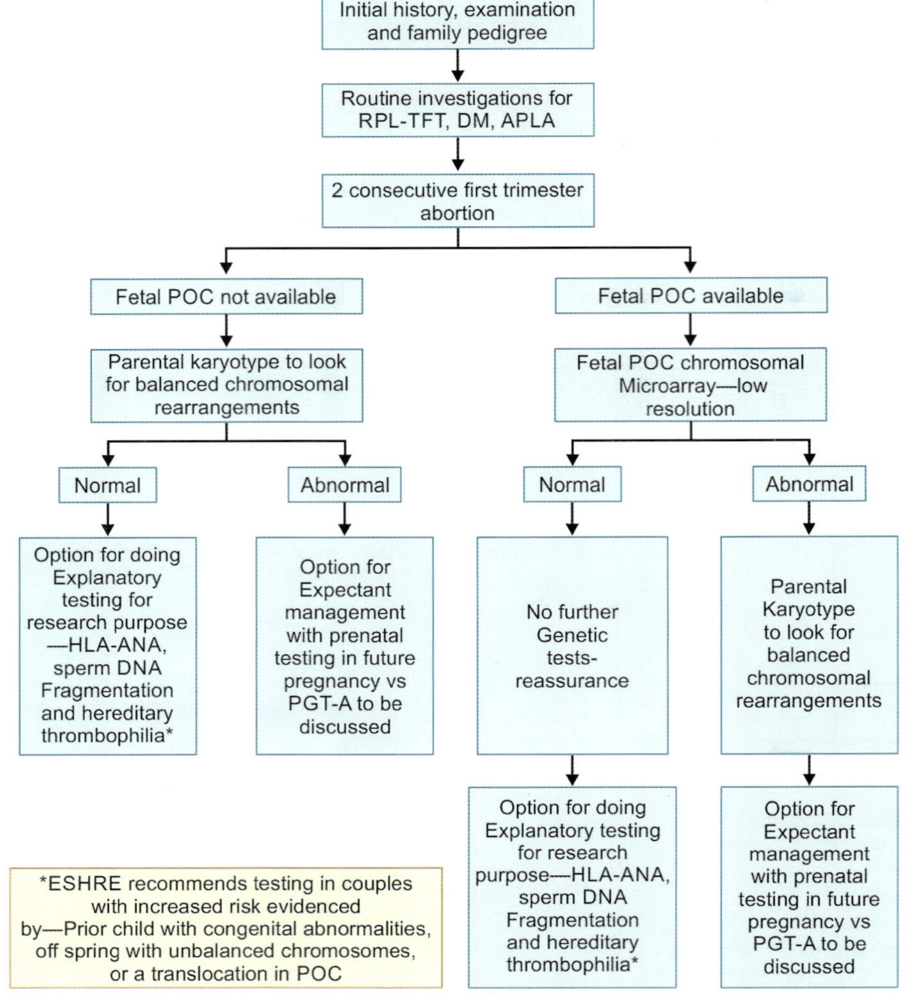

(ANA: antineutrophilic antibody; APLA: antiphospholipid antibodies; DM: diabetes mellitus; HLA: human leucocytic antigen; PGT-A: preimplantation genetic testing-aneuploidy; POC: products of conception; RPL: recurrent pregnancy loss; TFT: thyroid function test)

DIAGNOSTIC ALGORITHM FOR GENETIC EVALUATION IN RECURRENT PREGNANCY LOSS

Establishing a diagnostic algorithm for the management of RPL is essential for guiding healthcare professionals in a systematic approach to identify underlying causes and tailor effective interventions. Based on the above a diagnostic algorithm is incorporated to guide the genetic management of RPL **(Flowchart 1)**.

CONCLUSION

In conclusion, genetic evaluation plays a pivotal role in unraveling the complexities of RPL. The comprehensive assessment of genetic factors, including chromosomal abnormalities, structural rearrangements, and inherited mutations, provides valuable insights into the underlying causes of repeated pregnancy losses. By identifying these genetic abnormalities, healthcare professionals can tailor personalized treatment plans, offer informed reproductive counseling, and potentially enhance the chances of a successful pregnancy. Furthermore, ongoing advancements in genetic testing technologies continue to refine our understanding of RPL, paving the way for more targeted interventions and improved outcomes for couples facing the challenges of recurrent pregnancy loss. As research and technology progress, genetic evaluation stands as a crucial component in the multidisciplinary approach to managing and addressing the complexities of RPL, ultimately fostering hope for couples seeking to build their families.

REFERENCES

1. Ford HB, Schust DJ. Recurrent pregnancy loss: etiology, diagnosis, and therapy. Rev Obstet Gynecol. 2009;2(2):76-83.
2. Turesheva A, Aimagambetova G, Ukybassova T, Marat A, Kanabekova P, Kaldygulova L, et al. Recurrent Pregnancy Loss Etiology, Risk Factors, Diagnosis, and Management. Fresh Look into a Full Box. J Clin Med. 2023;12(12):4074.
3. Priya PK, Mishra VV, Roy P, Patel H. A Study on Balanced Chromosomal Translocations in Couples with Recurrent Pregnancy Loss. J Hum Reprod Sci. 2018;11(4):337-42.
4. Hyde KJ, Schust DJ. Genetic considerations in recurrent pregnancy loss. Cold Spring Harb Perspect Med. 2015;5(3):a023119.
5. Li Q, Chen S, Dong X, Fu S, Zhang T, Zheng W, et al. The Progress of Research on Genetic Factors of Recurrent Pregnancy Loss. Genet Res (Camb). 2023;2023:9164374.
6. Alibakhshi R, Nejati P, Hamani S, Mir-Ahadi N, Jalilian N. Cytogenetic Analysis of 570 Couples with Recurrent Pregnancy Loss: Reporting 11 Years of Experience. J Hum Reprod Sci. 2020;13(3):216-20.
7. Mrozikiewicz AE, Kurzawińska G, Ożarowski M, Walczak M, Ożegowska K, Jędrzejczak P. Polymorphic Variants of Genes Encoding Angiogenesis-Related Factors in Infertile Women with Recurrent Implantation Failure. Int J Mol Sci. 2023;24(5):4267.
8. Bigdeli R, Younesi MR, Panahnejad E, Asgary V, Heidarzadeh S, Mazaheri H, et al. Association between thrombophilia gene polymorphisms and recurrent pregnancy loss risk in the Iranian population. Systems Biol Reprod Med. 2018;64(4):274-82.
9. ESHRE Guideline Group on RPL; Bender Atik R, Christiansen OB, Elson J, Kolte AM, Lewis S, et al. ESHRE guideline: recurrent pregnancy loss: an update in 2022. Hum Reprod Open. 2023;2023(1):hoad002.
10. Wang X, Shi W, Zhao S, Gong D, Li S, Hu C, et al. Whole exome sequencing in unexplained recurrent miscarriage families identified novel pathogenic genetic causes of euploid miscarriage. Hum Reprod. 2023;38(5):1003-18.
11. Sui Y, Fu J, Zhang S, Li L, Sun X. Investigation of the role of X chromosome inactivation and androgen receptor CAG repeat polymorphisms in patients with recurrent pregnancy loss: a prospective case-control study. BMC Pregnancy Childbirth. 2022;22(1):805.

CHAPTER 5

Epigenetic Factors

Mayumi Sugiura-Ogasawara, Yosuke Matsumoto, Yoshihara Hiroyuki, Shinobu Goto, Tamao Kitaori

ABSTRACT

Genetic causes of recurrent pregnancy loss (RPL) are well known, whereas subtle genetic abnormalities have also been identified in euploid embryos of such cases. These abnormalities are imprinting defects like uniparental disomy of certain chromosomes and change in DNA methylation patterns in women with recurrent miscarriage (RM) as compared to controls. This alerts us to the fact that epigenetic factors may be playing a role in RPL when the karyotype of the miscarried embryo is euploid.

Keywords: Recurrent pregnancy loss, Recurrent miscarriage, Uniparental disomy, DNA methylation, Imprinting defects.

INTRODUCTION

Recurrent pregnancy loss (RPL) is defined as two or more pregnancy losses (death of the fetus) at any gestational age.[1-3] Recurrent miscarriage (RM) is defined as three or more consecutive clinical miscarriages occurring before 20 weeks post menstruation (before 22 weeks in Japan).[1] The Lancet series reported estimated frequencies of RM and RPL of 0.7 and 2.6%, respectively.[1] However, these frequencies depend on the age of the women, and in the Japanese population, this was found to be 1.1 and 5.0%, respectively.[4]

We describe in this chapter novel findings of epigenetic causes of miscarriage in euploid embryos. However, its association with RPL is still under researched. Meanwhile the reader needs to be reminded about the routine work-up recommended by guidelines. A Lancet review and ESHRE RPL guidelines recommend testing for antiphospholipid syndrome (APS), uterine anomalies and parental and embryonic abnormal karyotypes in clinical practice **(Table 1)**.[2,5] The Lancet review recommends evidence-based tests that provide results with prognostic value or with which treatment based on the results improves outcomes. Investigations of RM include testing for lupus anticoagulant, anticardiolipin antibodies, thyroid function, and performing a transvaginal pelvic ultrasound scan. Chromosome analysis of pregnancy tissue could also have explanatory value and selected couples can benefit from parental karyotyping. Newer genetic causes are being unfolded by research in this population. Single gene defects, single nucleotide polymorphism (SNP), uniparental disomy (UPD), chromosomal imprinting and now epigenetic factors may also play a role in recurrent

TABLE 1: Assessment of recurrent pregnancy loss.

Causes	*Recommended tests*	*Treatment*	*Controversy*
Antiphospholipid antibodies	• Lupus anticoagulant • Anticardiolipin antibodies	Aspirin and heparin	• Non-criteria obstetric APS • Refractory APS 20–30% • Occasional APLs
Congenital uterine abnormality	Ultrasonography	Surgery	• No evidence of improvement of the live birth rate
Parental genetic testing	Chromosome analysis	Genetic counseling PGT-SR	• No evidence of improvement of the live birth rate
Karyotyping of pregnancy tissue	Chromosome analysis	Genetic counseling PGT-A	• No evidence of improvement of the live birth rate
Hypothyroidism	TSH, TPO	Levothyroxine	• Subclinical hypothyroidism

miscarriage wherein the POC would be reported to have a normal genetic analysis by CGH microarray.

Antiphospholipid syndrome, uterine anomalies, and abnormal chromosomes in either partner are established causes of RPL.[6-8] In our study, only about 30% of cases had an identifiable cause and in the remaining 69%, the causes were unexplained **(Fig. 1A)**.[7] It is well-known that the cause remains unexplained in over a half of the cases.[1] An abnormal embryonic karyotype was found in 41.1% of 482 patients for whom both conventional causes and karyotypes of aborted conceptus could be examined **(Fig. 1B)**.[9] Therefore, the prevalence of truly unexplained cases with a normal embryonic karyotype was only 24.5%. The distribution of causes depends on such characteristics as the women's age or the number of previous miscarriages and these comprise the strongest risk factors.[5] Embryonic aneuploidy is the most common cause of RPL **(Fig. 1B)**. The rate of women with a normal embryonic karyotype was significantly higher in patients with RPL compared to patients with sporadic miscarriage.[10] In our previous study, the miscarriage rate increased and the normal embryonic karyotype rate decreased according to the number of previous miscarriages. The live birth rate of patients with a previous abnormal embryonic karyotype was significantly higher than that of patients with a previous normal embryonic karyotype. The embryonic karyotype can be a good predictor of subsequent success.

FOCUS ON RECURRENT EUPLOID MISCARRIAGE

Single nucleotide variants (SNVs), copy number variants (CNVs), epigenetics, and mitochondrial deoxyribonucleic acid (DNA) aberrations were reported to be associated with euploid miscarriage.[11,12] Regarding maternal SNPs, susceptibility genes implicated to date include those involved in the immune response, coagulation, metabolism, and angiogenesis.[11] Factor V Leiden and prothrombin mutations have been most frequently examined. Recently, Laisk et al. carried out a European ancestry genome-wide meta-analysis of RPL with each case defined as having a history of three or more consecutive miscarriages (n_{case} = 750), and they reported three significant genome-wide loci.[13] No clear association was ascertained between RPL and variants reported as significant in the systematic review.

As for genetic embryonic factors, putatively causative variants were found in a range of genes, including *CHRNA1* (cholinergic receptor nicotinic alpha polypeptide 1), *DYNC2H1* (dynein cytoplasmic 2 heavy chain 1), and *RYR1* (ryanodine receptor 1) by whole-exome sequencing or CNV studies.[12]

WHAT IS EPIGENETICS?

Epigenetics is defined as the study of heritable and stable changes in gene expression that occur through alterations

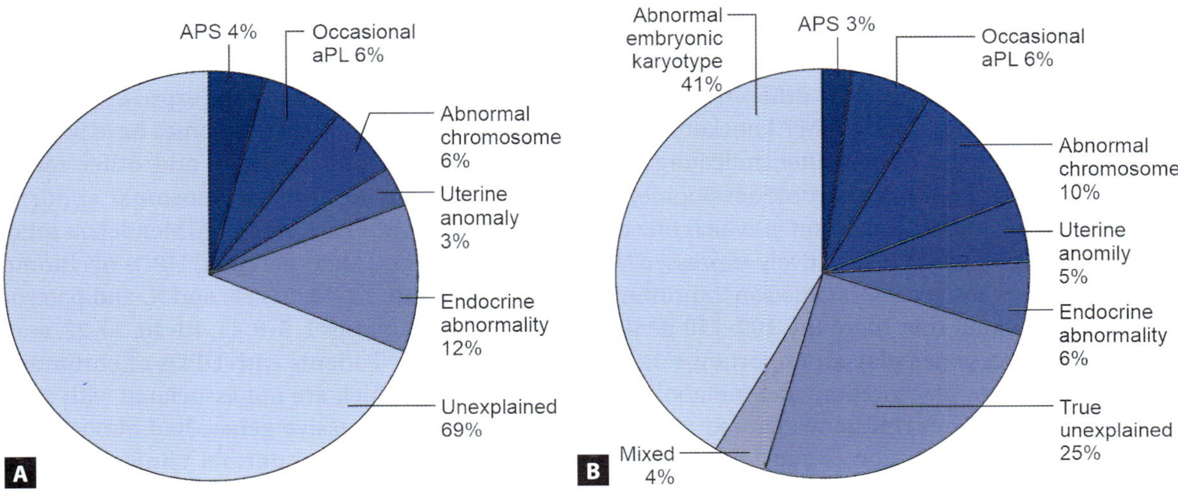

Figs. 1A and B: Comparison of the distribution of causes in 482 patients with RM, including those with an abnormal embryonic karyotype, and the 1,676 subjects of our previous study. (A) The 1,676 patients of our previous study; (B) The 482 patients with RM, including those with an abnormal embryonic karyotype.

Sources: 1. Sugiura-Ogasawara et al., Fertil Steril. 2010.[7]
2. Sugiura-Ogasawara et al., Hum Reprod. 2012.[9]

in the chromosome rather than in the DNA sequence.[14] Despite not directly altering the DNA sequence, epigenetic mechanisms can regulate gene expression through chemical modifications of DNA bases and changes to the chromosomal superstructure in which the DNA is packaged. Epigenetic features include:

- Deoxyribonucleic acid methylation
- Histone changes
- Imprinting
- Non-coding RNA sequences

Deoxyribonucleic acid methylation is a covalent modification of the nucleotide cytosine, which is heritable during cell division and is generally associated with gene silencing when methylation occurs in CpG islands of promoter sequences in which a cytosine precedes a guanosine in the 5′ to 3′ sequence.[15] DNA methylation is the best understood epigenetic modification and the clearest example of epigenetic information. This information can be copied by the enzyme DNA methyltransferase 1 (DNMT) which recognizes hemi-methylated CpG sites on newly replicated DNA and methylates the daughter-strand cytosine at the complementary CpG. Furthermore, the information can be erased, either passively during cell division or by means of an enzymatic process involving ten-eleven translocation (TET) methyl-cytosine dioxygenases, followed by glycosylation and replacement with an unmethylated cytosine.

After fertilization, cellular DNA undergoes extensive demethylation, and the level of DNA methylation is at its lowest.[16] Subsequently, the DNA undergoes cytokine-specific DNA methylation, and each cell expresses a characteristic gene that causes it to differentiate into various other cells to form tissues. DNMT knockout mice do not survive birth or die shortly thereafter, indicating that DNMT plays an important role in embryonic development.

Genome imprinting is a phenomenon in which one of the paternal or maternal genes is selectively expressed. A gene expressed from only one allele is called an imprinting gene, and it is speculated that there are 100–150 genes of this type. Imprinting genes play an important role in ontogeny, differentiation, placentation, and metabolism. Abnormal expression of imprint genes causes various diseases. Imprint gene expression is controlled within the imprinting control region (ICR), which can have a different states of DNA methylation depending on whether the father or the mother is the origin. In the IGF2/H19 (11p15.5) region, ICR1 is not methylated in the maternal allele, so the enhancer does not act, IGF2 is suppressed, and H19 is expressed. In the paternal allele, ICR1 is methylated, so IGF2 is expressed and H19 is suppressed. Epigenetic dysregulation of this region causes Beckwith-Wiedemann syndrome and Silver-Russell syndrome.[17,18]

Uniparental disomy is when the embryo expresses both chromosomes from a single parent. The classic example is hydatidiform mole where there are two sets of paternal genomes while the maternal genome is dropped. There are two types of UPD:

- *Isodisomy*—where both chromosomes from a single parent are identical copies. Its origins are often traced to a monosomic fetus that is rescued by duplication of the single parental chromosome.
- *Heterodisomy*—the two chromosomes from a single parent are non-identical. This is believed to occur in a trisomic embryo which is rescued by say the parental chromosome is dropped.

A known example is Prader-Willi and Angelman syndrome where chromosome 15 is affected.

Similarly, recessive genes may find expression in the embryo in a heterozygous couple due to uniparental disomy and be a cause of miscarriage.

Non-coding RNA sequences: These sequences may be responsible for gene expression and repressor genes thereby altering gene expression and vital protein synthesis.

EMBRYONIC EPIGENETIC FACTORS IN RECURRENT PREGNANCY LOSS

Embryonic epigenetic factors have been a focus in examining the causes of unexplained RPL. Uniparental disomies (UPDs) cause abnormal expression of imprinting genes. UPDs of various chromosomes have been detected by DNA polymorphic analysis and other methods in human individuals with chromosomal abnormalities, imprinting disturbances, and non-Mendelian inheritance of recessive genes. Maternal (mat) UPDs of chromosomes 1, 2, 4, 6, 7, 9, 10, 13–16, 21, 22, and X, and paternal (pat) UPDs of chromosomes 1, 5–8, 11, 13–16, 20–22, and X have been reported.[19] Patients with UPDs of chromosomes 1, 13, 21, and 22, which are not associated with anomalous transmission of recessive genes, had almost no clinical features. In contrast, abnormal clinical features were distinctly seen in patients with both paternal and maternal UPDs of chromosomes 14 and 15, patients with paternal UPDs of 6 and 11, and patients with mat UPDs of 2, 7, and 16. In particular, serious clinical features have been described in some cases of maternal UPD 2, paternal

UPD 14 and maternal UPD 16. Furthermore, no UPDs of chromosomes 3, 12, and 17–19 have been found in any case to date. These findings suggest that some UPD cases may also exhibit serious abnormalities before birth, including during the periods of embryogenesis and early fetal development.

We found the involvement of maternal UPD 16 and paternal UPD 14 in euploid RM.[20,21] The polymorphic patterns of microsatellites on each chromosome were analyzed in 25 of 52 POC with a euploid karyotype **(Fig. 2A)**.[20] The patterns of the microsatellites of chromosome 16 both appeared to be of maternal origin. The results also showed that the region from the distal end of the short arm to near the middle point of the long arm of chromosome 16 (pter to D16S3107) were heterozygous, and those of the remaining region of the long arm (D16S3018 to qter) were homozygous. That is, this fetus had maternal isodisomy and heterodisomy of chromosome 16, originating from a maternal, meiosis I non-disjunction of dyad 16 that accompanied a crossover at near the middle point of the long arm.

The polymorphic patterns of microsatellites on each chromosome were analyzed in 81 of 164 POC with a euploid karyotype.[21] In one of the two cases, the polymorphic patterns of chromosome 14 both appeared to be of paternal origin **(Fig. 2B)**. The patterns of the distal end of the long arm were homozygous, and those of the remaining region were heterozygous. That is, this fetus had paternal UPD 14, originating from a meiosis I nondisjunction. In the other case, the polymorphic patterns of the distal one third of the long arm of chromosome 7 were uniparental (maternal) in origin whereas those of the remaining region of this chromosome were biparental **(Fig. 2C)**. These findings thus suggested that this chromosome might have originated from a chromatid exchange between the long arms of paternal and maternal chromosome 7 at the first mitotic division. These findings suggest the possibility that some UPDs may cause euploid miscarriage. *However, the frequency of UPDs is speculated to be low in patients with RPL.*

Most complete hydatidiform moles are embryos with two paternal-derived genomes. These cystic malformations do not have a fetal component and are characterized by hydropic villous stroma and hyperplasia of chorionic villi. A *KHDC3L* mutation in components of the subcortical maternal complex of the oocyte was found in a patient with recurrent hydatidiform moles and there was found to be a genome-wide DNA methylation loss in oocytes and persistent imprinting defects after fertilization.[22]

Deoxyribonucleic acid methylation in gene regulatory regions, such as in enhancers and promoters, is closely associated with gene expression, including that of lineage-specific genes.[23,24] Dynamic epigenetic reprogramming ensures the correct development of an embryo during early embryogenesis.[25,26] Recent studies documented altered DNA methylation in certain sets of genes, such as imprinting loci, in the chorionic villi of RM, or sporadic miscarriage after *in vitro* fertilization.[27-29] In addition, a genome-wide DNA methylation analysis in decidua revealed that hypomethylation of CAMP Responsive Element Binding Protein 5 (*CREB5*) appeared to be a risk factor for RPL by causing dysfunction of trophoblast cells.[30] These studies indicate that aberrant epigenetic regulation of maternal decidua and fetal villi tissue is involved in early embryogenesis. However, information on aberrant DNA methylation in association with RM is still limited. In addition, decidua and villi have different DNA methylation profiles.[31]

We investigated genome-wide DNA methylation profiles in both chorionic villi and decidual tissues from POC of patients with euploid RM compared with the same tissues from control women who underwent artificial abortions (AAs) in the same gestational week (n = 5 each) group.[32] We found that 13,426 and 5,816 CpG sites were differentially methylated in chorionic villi and decidua, respectively. DNA methylation profiles of chorionic villi, but not decidua, in RM patients were clearly distinct from those of the AA controls **(Figs. 3A and B)**. Among the differentially methylated genes, the enhancer region of *SPATS2L* was significantly more methylated in RM patients (n = 19) than in AA controls (n = 19; mean methylation level, 52.0% vs. 28.9%, $p < 0.001$), resulting in reduced expression of SPATS2L protein in the patients. Functionally, depletion of *SPATS2L* in extra-villous trophoblast cells reduced their invasion and migration abilities. There was a clear positive correlation between DNA methylation levels in *SPATS2L* and gestational weeks in both RM and AA groups (R^2 = 0.217 and R^2 = 0.485 in RM and AA, respectively) **(Fig. 3C)**. Our data indicate that in particular, the chorionic villi of RM patients exhibit distinct DNA methylation profiles compared with normal pregnancies and that this changed DNA methylation status may impede the progression of embryo development via the altered expression of such genes as *SPATS2L* in the villi. However, all patients had live births even though the mean number of previous miscarriages was 4.7 (range 3–7, not shown). Patients with methylation abnormalities in the villi might

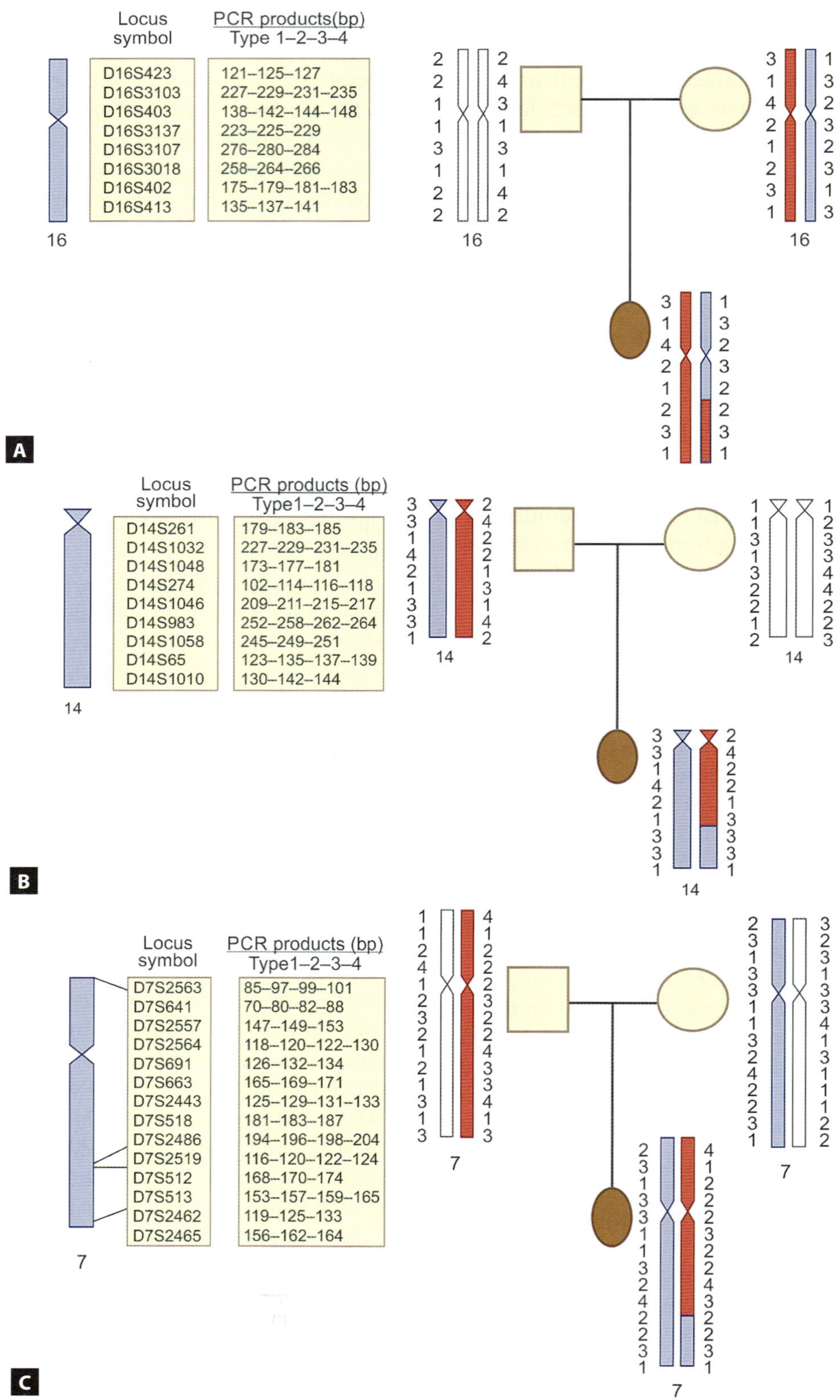

Figs. 2A to C: Uniparental disomy.

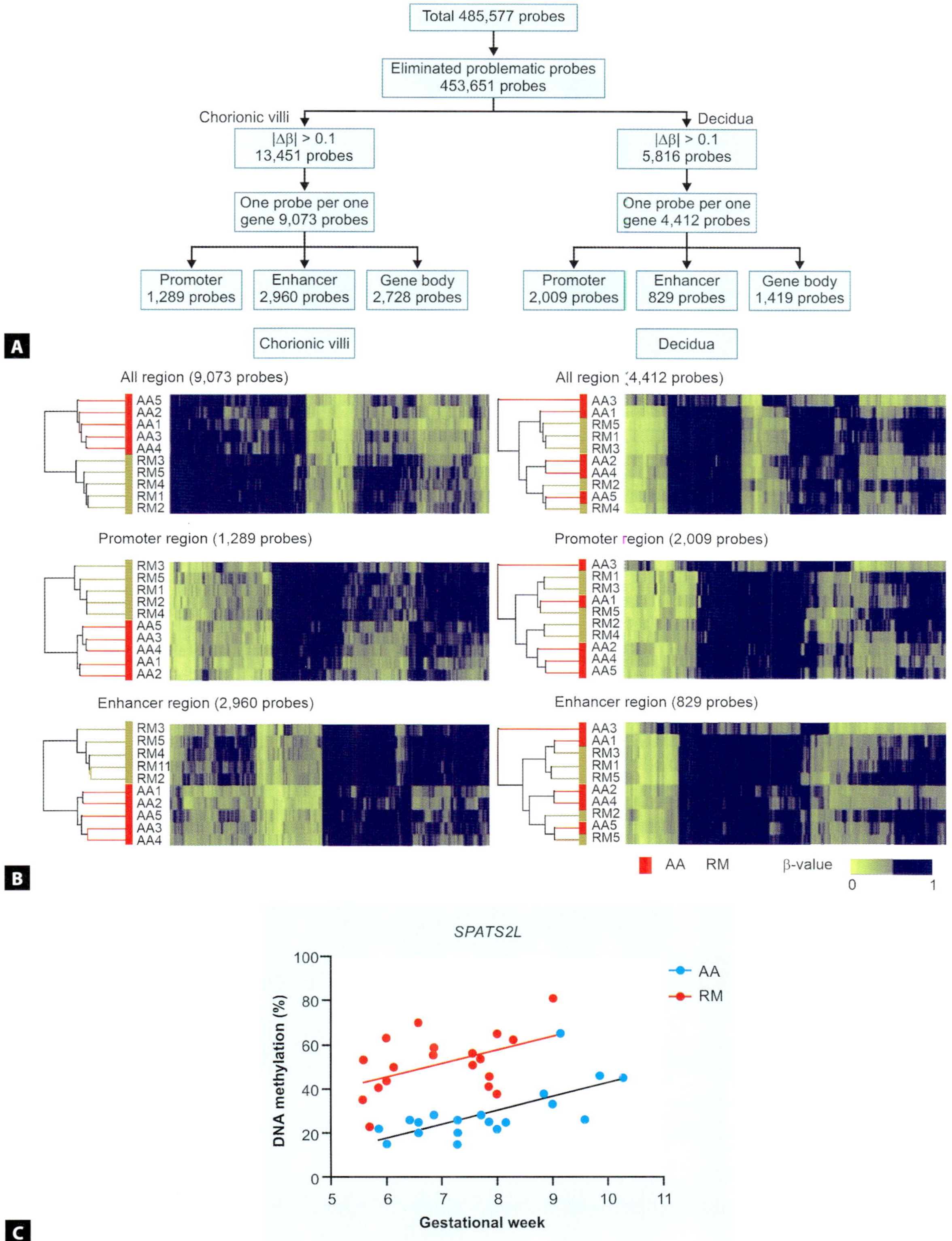

Figs. 3A to C: DNA methylation profile of chorionic villi of control AA and RM. (AA:artificial abortion; DNA: deoxyribonucleic acid; RM: recurrent miscarriage)

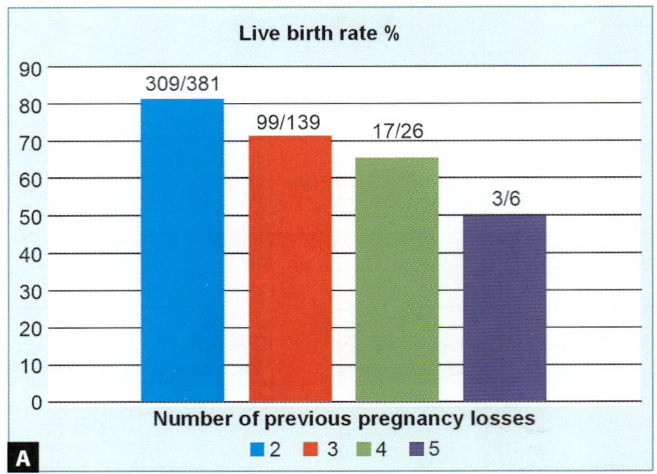

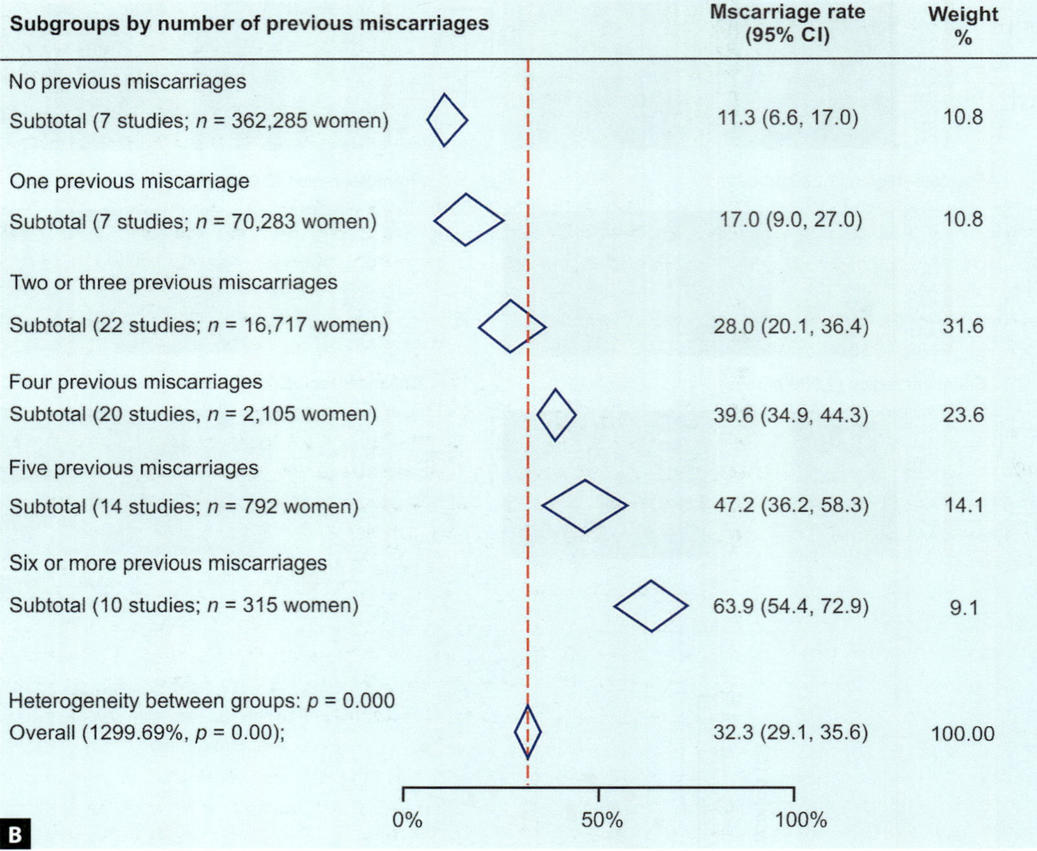

Figs. 4A and B: Live birth rate according to the number of previous pregnancy losses.
Sources: 1. Katano et al., Fertil Steril. 2013.[33]
2. Coomarasamy et al., 2021.[5]

have a favorable prognosis, as might patients with embryo aneuploidy.[10]

The rates of subsequent live birth rates in patients with an unexplained cause, including patients with an abnormal embryonic karyotype, who had previously had two, three, four, and five miscarriages were about 80%, 70%, 60%, and 50% with no medication, respectively **(Figs. 4A and B)**.[33,34] For such patients, the cumulative live birth rate was 85%, which should provide some encouragement for individuals undergoing genetic counseling.[7]

CONCLUSION

Genetic aberrations identified in miscarried euploid embryos can be single gene defects, uniparental disomy or improper DNA methylation. These epigenetic factors may be responsible for unexplained RPL. Although, these factors are currently studied in research setting only, it will open up a new avenue of investigation in unexplained RPL.

DISCLOSURE

None of the authors have any conflicts of interest to report.

REFERENCES

1. Quenby S, Gallos ID, Dhillon-Smith RK, Podesek M, Stephenson MD, Fisher J, et al. Miscarriage matters: the epidemiological, physical, psychological, and economic costs of early pregnancy loss. Lancet. 2021;397(10285):1658-67.
2. ESHRE Guideline Group on RPL; Bender Atik R, Christiansen OB, Elson J, Kolte AM, Lewis S, et al. ESHRE guideline: recurrent pregnancy loss: an update in 2022. Hum Reprod Open. 2023;2023(1):hoad002.
3. Practice Committee of the American Society for Reproductive Medicine. Definitions of infertility and recurrent pregnancy loss: a committee opinion. Fertil Steril. 2013;99:63.
4. Sugiura-Ogasawara M, Ebara T, Yamada Y, Shoji N, Matsuki T, Kano H, et al. Adverse pregnancy and perinatal outcome in patients with recurrent pregnancy loss: Multiple imputation analyses with propensity score adjustment applied to a large-scale birth cohort of the Japan Environment and Children's Study. Am J Reprod Immunol. 2019;81(1):e13072.
5. Coomarasamy A, Dhillon-Smith RK, Papadopoulou A, Al-Memar M, Brewin J, Abrahams VM, et al. Recurrent miscarriage: evidence to accelerate action. Lancet. 2021;397(10285):1675-82.
6. Farquharson RG, Pearson JF, John L. Lupus anticoagulant and pregnancy management. Lancet. 1984;28:228-9.
7. Sugiura-Ogasawara M, Ozaki Y, Kitaori T, Kumagai K, Suzuki S. Midline uterine defect size correlated with miscarriage of euploid embryos in recurrent cases. Fertil Steril. 2010;93:1983-8.
8. Sugiura-Ogasawara M, Ozaki Y, Sato T, Suzumori N, Suzumori K. Poor prognosis of recurrent aborters with either maternal or paternal reciprocal translocation. Fertil Steril. 2004;81:367-73.
9. Sugiura-Ogasawara M, Ozaki Y, Katano K, Suzumori N, Kitaori T, Mizutani E. Abnormal embryonic karyotype is the most frequent cause of recurrent miscarriage. Hum Reprod. 2012;27:2297-2303.
10. Ogasawara M, Aoki K, Okada S, Suzumori K. Embryonic karyotype of abortuses in relation to the number of previous miscarriages. Fertil Steril. 2000;73:300-4.
11. Kaur M, Kaur R, Chhabra K, Khetarpal P. Maternal candidate gene variants, epigenetic factors, and susceptibility to idiopathic recurrent pregnancy loss: A systematic review. Int J Gynaecol Obstet. 2023;162(3):829-41.
12. Colley E, Hamilton S, Smith P, Morgan NV, Coomarasamy A, Allen S. Potential genetic causes of miscarriage in euploid pregnancies: a systematic review. Hum Reprod Update. 2019;25(4):452-72.
13. Laisk T, Soares ALG, Ferreira T, Painter JN, Censin JC, Laber S, et al. The genetic architecture of sporadic and multiple consecutive miscarriage. Nat Commun. 2020;11:5980.
14. Berger SL, Kouzarides T, Shiekhattar R, Shilatifard A. An operational definition of epigenetics. Genes Dev. 2009;23(7):781-3.
15. Feinberg AP. The Key Role of Epigenetics in Human Disease Prevention and Mitigation. N Engl J Med. 2018;378(14):1323-34.
16. Shinjo K, Kondo Y. Epigenetics. J Japan Med Assoc. 2023;152:50-55.
17. Brown KW, Villar AJ, Bickmore W, Clayton-Smith J, Catchpoole D, Maher ER, et al. Imprinting mutation in the Beckwith-Wiedemann syndrome leads to biallelic IGF2 expression through an H19-independent pathway. Hum Mol Genet. 1996;5(12):2027-32.
18. Gicquel C, Rossignol S, Cabrol S, Houang M, Steunou V, Barbu V, et al. Epimutation of the telomeric imprinting center region on chromosome 11p15 in Silver-Russell syndrome. Nat Genet. 2005;37(9):1003-7.
19. Engel E. Uniparental disomies in unselected populations. Am J Hum Genet. 1998;63:962-6.
20. Kondo Y, Tsukishiro S, Tanemura M, Sugiura-Ogasawara M, Suzumori K, Sonta SI. Maternal uniparental disomy of chromosome 16 in a case of spontaneous abortion. J Hum Genet. 2004;49(4):177-81.
21. Tsukishiro S, Li QY, Tanemura M, Sugiura-Ogasawara M, Suzumori K, Sonta SI. Paternal uniparental disomy of chromosome 14 and unique exchange of chromosome 7 in cases of spontaneous abortion. J Hum Genet. 2005;4:112-7.
22. Demond H, Anvar Z, Jahromi BN, Sparago A, Verma A, Davari M, et al. A KHDC3L mutation resulting in recurrent hydatidiform mole causes genome-wide DNA methylation loss in oocytes and persistent imprinting defects post-fertilisation. Genome Med. 2019;11(1):84.

23. Kim K, Doi A, Wen B, Ng K, Zhao R, Cahan P, et al. Epigenetic memory in induced pluripotent stem cells. Nature. 2010;467:285-90.
24. Roadmap Epigenomics Concorsium. Integrative analysis of 111 reference human epigenomes. Nature. 2015;518:317-30.
25. Guo H, Zhu P, Yan L, Li R, Hu B, Lian Y, et al. The DNA methylation landscape of human early embryos. Nature. 2014;511:606-10.
26. Smith ZD, Chan MM, Humm KC, Karnik R, Mekhoubad S, Regev A, et al. DNA methylation dynamics of the human preimplantation embryo. Nature. 2014;511:611-5.
27. Hanna CW, McFadden DE, Robinson WP. DNA methylation profiling of placental villi from karyotypically normal miscarriage and recurrent miscarriage. Am J Pathol. 2013;182:2276-84.
28. Zheng HY, Tang Y, Niu J, Li P, Ye DS, Chen X, et al. Aberrant DNA methylation of imprinted loci in human spontaneous abortions after assisted reproduction techniques and natural conception. Hum Reprod. 2013;28:265-73.
29. Liu Y, Tang Y, Ye D, Ma W, Feng S, Li X, et al. Impact of Abnormal DNA Methylation of Imprinted Loci on Human Spontaneous Abortion. Reprod Sci. 2018;25:131-9.
30. Yu M, Du G, Xu Q, Huang Z, Huang X, Qin Y, et al. Integrated analysis of DNA methylome and transcriptome identified CREB5 as a novel risk gene contributing to recurrent pregnancy loss. E Bio Med. 2018;35:334-44.
31. Robinson WP, Price EM. The human placental methylome. Cold Spring Harb Perspect Med. 2015;5:a023044.
32. Matsumoto Y, Shinjo K, Mase S, Fukuyo M, Aoki K, Ozawa F, et al. Characteristic DNA methylation profiles of chorionic villi in recurrent miscarriage. Sci Rep. 2022;12(1):11673.
33. Katano K, Suzuki S, Ozaki Y, Suzumori N, Kitaori T, Sugiura-Ogasawara M. Peripheral natural killer cell activity as a predictor of recurrent pregnancy loss: a large cohort study. Fertil Steril. 2013;100(6):1629-34.
34. Devall AJ, Coomarasamy A. Sporadic pregnancy loss and recurrent miscarriage. Best Pract Res Clin Obstet Gynaecol. 2020;69:30-9.

CHAPTER

6

Cell-free Fetal DNA Testing

Tanja Schlaikjær Hartwig, Henriette Svarre Nielsen

ABSTRACT

Fetal genetic testing by cell-free fetal DNA (cffDNA) in maternal blood may be beneficial in patients with recurrent pregnancy loss (RPL). It may be possible to detect adequate fraction of fetal DNA from pregnancy week 7 onwards. There is good correlation between cffDNA test and products of conception in diagnosing aneuploidies. However fetal DNA is rapidly cleared from maternal blood within hours after miscarriage and consequently the window for testing is limited. cffDNA testing will offer noninvasive genetic testing in each pregnancy and help make a diagnosis of euploid versus aneuploid loss in couples. This chapter delves into the role of cffDNA testing in pregnancy loss, exploring its clinical significance, methodological and economical aspects, and future potential and challenges.

Keywords: Cell-free fetal DNA testing, Aneuploidy, NIPT, RPL.

INTRODUCTION

During pregnancy, both intact placental trophoblasts and cell-free fetal DNA (cffDNA) from apoptotic trophoblasts are transferred to the maternal bloodstream via the fetal-maternal interface. This pivotal discovery, described by Lo et al. in 1997,[1] has enabled noninvasive prenatal testing (NIPT) of fetal chromosomal abnormalities in ongoing pregnancies, utilizing maternal blood samples as a less invasive alternative to procedures such as chorionic villus sampling (CVS) and amniocentesis. Today, NIPT is an implemented part of prenatal screening program, and >10 million tests are performed worldwide every year.[2]

Previous cytogenetic studies using G-band karyotyping and chromosomal microarray analyzing for the investigation of fetal genetics in pregnancy loss found that 50–60% of pregnancy losses can be explained by fetal aneuploidy.[3,4] However, international guidelines do not recommend routine fetal genetic evaluation in cases of pregnancy loss.[5] A reason for this reluctancy might be the challenges of tissue-based methods as these require collection of good-quality tissue and a high risk of contamination with maternal DNA giving a high risk of inconclusive or false results reflecting the maternal karyotype. The current clinical practice of no action might also be a consequence of conventional views on pregnancy loss, founded on the high incidence of fetal aneuploidy that is considered de novo giving a decreased risk of further pregnancy loss. Consequently, literature and research on pregnancy loss typically lacks information on chromosomal status of the miscarried fetus, and in clinical practice couples are not informed about the genetic status of their loss.

Moreover, present practices do not acknowledge the link between euploid pregnancy loss and an elevated risk of subsequent losses along with potential long-term maternal health implications such as diabetes and cardiovascular disease.[6,7] Neither the promising progress in the fields of genetic and molecular diagnostics counting both whole-genome sequencing and cffDNA-based testing.

When following the current clinical recommendations on recurrent pregnancy loss (RPL) work-up, approximately 50% of RPL cases are unexplained, often leading to nonproven treatments and psychologically distress for patients.[8,9] By adding chromosomal microarray after the second loss, the number of unexplained losses was found to decline to 10% reflecting that aneuploidy is still the major reason for pregnancy loss in RPL patients[10] even though the prevalence of euploid losses increase by the number of previous losses.[11] But as the availability of pregnancy tissue is inconsistent and has decreased due to a rising practice toward medical management of miscarriage replacing surgical evacuation,[12] cffDNA-based testing might be a promising alternative.

METHODOLOGICAL ASPECTS OF cffDNA-BASED TESTING

Contrary to cytogenetic test methods such as karyotyping, chromosomal microarray, and whole-genome sequencing, cffDNA-based testing is not dependent on the collection of tissue during the miscarriage, evacuation or by CVS/amniocentesis. CffDNA-based testing is performed on 10–20 mL maternal blood drawn from a simple vein puncture. After centrifugation and DNA extraction, cfDNA fragments—both fetal and maternal—are amplified by PCR and prepared for massively parallel sequencing by adding flanking adaptors (library preparation). The DNA library is loaded to a flow cell and amplified by bridge amplification by which clusters of identical sequences are generated. The clusters are then sequenced—one base at a time—by fluorescence imaging. By image analysis, the images are transformed into FASTQ files, which is text-based lists of sequences—also referred to as reads. The reads are mapped to a human reference genome and analyzed by counting. The number of unique reads from each chromosome is aligned to a diploid reference group and the difference is expressed as a Z-score. An over- or underrepresentation of reads from a given chromosome results in a high absolute Z-score which may indicate aneuploidy. The Z-score will be increased in case of trisomy and decreased in case of monosomy. As only about ~10% of circulating cfDNA is of fetal origin and fragments from the smallest chromosome 21 represent around 1.5% of the sequenced fragments, millions of reads are needed to detect fetal trisomy 21. The number of mapped reads (sequencing depth) is associated with test reliability. **Figures 1A and B** illustrates a simplification of the workflow and bioinformatic approach of cffDNA-based testing.

Cell-free fetal DNA rapidly clears from the maternal blood after delivery[13] but in in case of pregnancy loss with pregnancy tissue still being in situ fetal DNA is still shredded to the maternal bloodstream allowing for cffDNA-based testing. Two proof-of-concept studies were published in 2020 investigating the presence of cffDNA in maternal blood after fetal demise and the potential of cffDNA-based testing.[14,15] Both studies included small cohorts of 109 and 57 women, respectively, and reported sensitivities between 57 and 82% at a 90% specificity when compared with cytogenetic results from pregnancy tissue, but both studies underscored a need for a larger cohort to support the results.

The Copenhagen Pregnancy Loss (COPL) study recently did a larger validation of cffDNA-based testing for fetal genetic evaluation in pregnancy losses occurring as early as in gestational week 5.[16] The cffDNA-based test results were validated against direct sequencing of pregnancy tissue in 333 cases of pregnancy loss and the result of cffDNA-based testing was reported for a total of 1,000 cases with a gestational age ranging from 5^{+0} to 21^{+2} weeks with a mean of 10^{+1} weeks.

Among the 1,000 cffDNA analyses, 11% (n = 112) were inconclusive due to low fetal fraction or inadequate sequencing quality. In cases with conclusive results (n = 888), 50% (n = 446) were euploid, 46% (n = 405) were aneuploid, and 4% (n = 37) revealed multiple aneuploidies **(Fig. 2)**. The most frequently identified abnormal karyotypes in the larger cffDNA sample population were trisomy 16 (n = 91), monosomy X (n = 86), and trisomy 22 (n = 41), but the panel of detected trisomies was wide.

Besides from the well-powered validation of cffDNA-based testing in pregnancy loss, Hartwig et al. report another important result, being that almost a third of women were not able to collect useful pregnancy tissue for cytogenetic testing. Likewise, Siegel et al. report a 65% success rate in chromosomal microarray analysis after home collection of pregnancy tissue.[12] These findings illustrate the difficulties of pregnancy tissue collection in early pregnancy loss and the relevance of introducing a tissue-independent alternative.

Fetal Fraction

A primary factor determining the reliability of a cffDNA test is the fraction of fetal DNA (FF) in maternal blood. If the FF is low, the cffDNA test will be inconclusive as it will reflect the maternal karyotype (no call). FF can be determined by different approaches such as (1) differential methylation, (2) single nucleotide polymorphisms (SNPs), (3) Y-chromosome counts (qPCR or sequencing based, only for male fetuses), (4) autosomal regional read (e.g., as implemented in SeqFF), (5) differences in length between cffDNA and maternal cfDNA, or (6) genome-wide nucleosome profiles. Y-based methods are found to be most accurate (but limited to males), but SeqFF is performing best in a mixed population.[17]

As FF is a ratio between circulating maternal and fetal cfDNA, it is influenced by several factors. Maternal weight has been found to be inversely associated with FF,

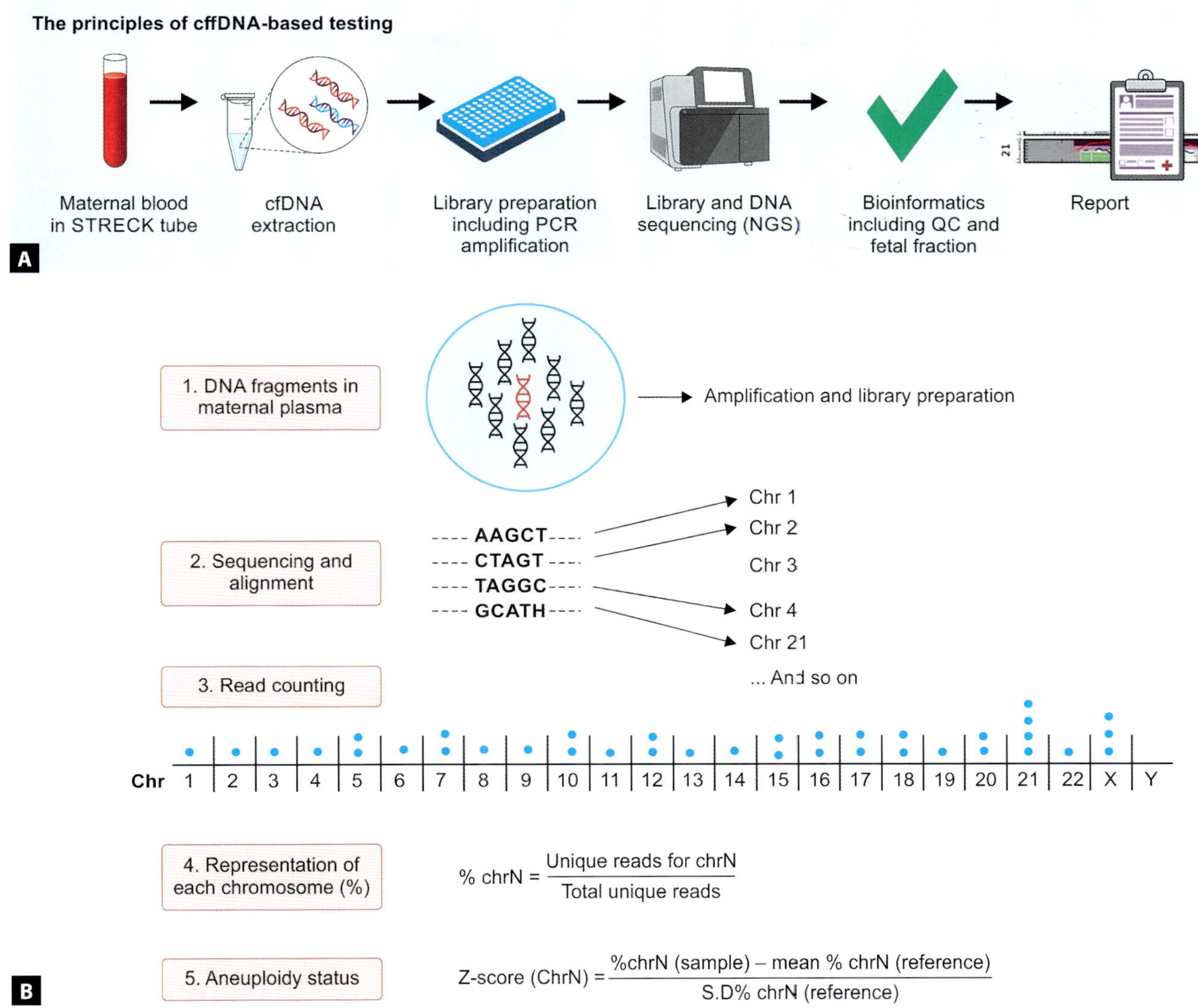

Figs. 1A and B: Illustrations of the workflow and bioinformatic principles of cffDNA-based testing. After purification of cell-free DNA fragments, they are sequenced by MPS and aligned to a human reference genome. The reads from each chromosome are counted and the differences compared to a reference group are expressed as Z-scores. An over-representation of reads from a specific chromosome indicates trisomy.
(cffDNA: cell-free fetal DNA; PCR: polymerase chain reaction; MPS: massively parallel sequencing)

probably explained by a larger proportion of maternal cfDNA due to a higher turnover of adipocytes as well as dilution of circulating cfDNA due to a larger total blood volume.[18-20] FF also depends on gestational age, to which it is positively associated. The increase of FF over the time has been found to be 0.1–0.5% per week until week 20.[19,21,22] Other potential factors impacting FF are autoimmune diseases,[23] medications (metformin and heparin),[24,25] fetal karyotype,[26,27] ethnicity,[28] parity,[28] maternal age,[28,29] smoking,[30,31] and fetal sex.[32]

Due to lower FF in the early first trimester, NIPT in ongoing pregnancies is not performed before gestational week 10/11.[33] As most pregnancy losses occur before this point, the FF might be a challenge when using cffDNA-based testing in cases pregnancy loss. On the other hand, it seems plausible that an increased fraction of trophoblasts and cffDNA is present when a pregnancy demise and the maternal immune system starts the rejection.

In the COPL cohort, the mean FF was found to be significantly lower in the cohort of pregnancy losses (mean

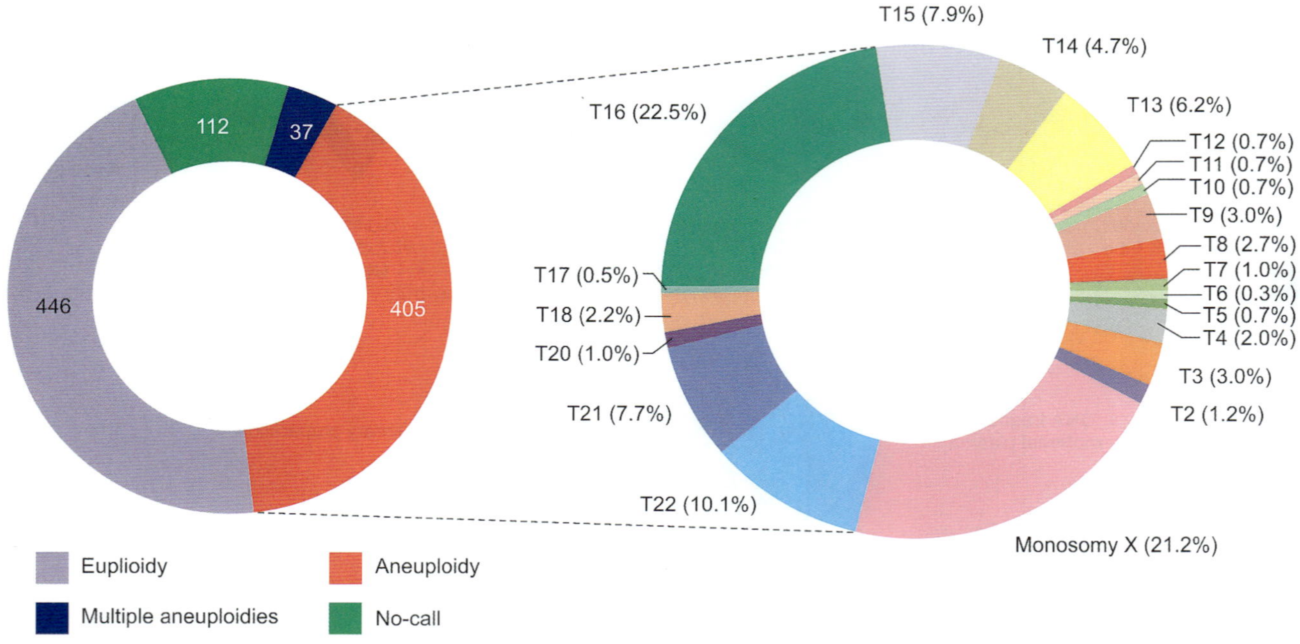

Fig. 2: Distribution of 1,000 cell-free fetal DNA-based tests results performed in Copenhagen Pregnancy Loss study.[16]

gestational age 10^{+1}) compared with a control cohort of ongoing pregnancies (mean gestational age 13^{+0}) (0.051 vs. 0–0.63 Wilcoxon $p < 0.0001$; **Figure 3A**), but when matching by gestation age, the difference between demised and living pregnancies was nonsignificant (gestational age 11 weeks plus 0 days to 11 weeks plus 6 days, Wilcoxon test $p = 0.36$; gestational age 12 weeks plus 0 days to 12 weeks plus 6 days, Wilcoxon test $p = 0.63$; gestational age 13 weeks plus 0 days to 13 weeks plus 6 days, Wilcoxon test $p = 0.56$; **Figure 3B**).

The rate of inconclusive results (no-calls) was stable at approximately 10% from gestational age 7 weeks and 0 days, whereas the no-call rate was approximately 50% in 16 pregnancy losses at earlier gestational ages.

ECONOMIC ASPECT

Despite the rapidly evolving genetic field, the cost of genome-wide cffDNA testing in ongoing pregnancies is still expensive ranging from 350 to 550£ per test. Compared to current available tissue-based methods, cffDNA-based testing is though cheaper but maintains acceptable test properties.

Considering the cost of RPL work-up suggested in international guidelines, Yaron et al. found it cost beneficial to use cffDNA-based testing to guide further work-up in RPL cases without losing diagnostic yield.[34] The economic benefits of implementing systematic cffDNA-based testing in pregnancy loss is probably not limited to the direct savings on cffDNA-based testing versus chromosomal microarray/karyotyping and further RPL work-up and treatment in cases where random aneuploidy is observed. Downstream effects, such as patient satisfaction, psychological coping, and earlier prevention of further losses are also likely to have a positive effect on the overall health economics.

CHALLENGES AND FUTURE DIRECTIONS

The rationale of fetal genetic testing in cases of pregnancy loss differs significantly from its application in ongoing pregnancies, where screening is implemented to detect rare yet serious fetal diseases. When applied to cases of pregnancy loss, the clinical purpose is to identify euploid cases to pick out those women with a potential underlying condition causing the loss. Compared to the current passive clinical practice, cffDNA therefore has the potential to accelerate and personalize the investigation of losses, but also to improve etiological research by focusing on euploid losses.

One main challenge of cffDNA-based testing in pregnancy loss is the limited window for blood sampling, as the fetal DNA rapidly clears from the maternal bloodstream after the product of conception passes.

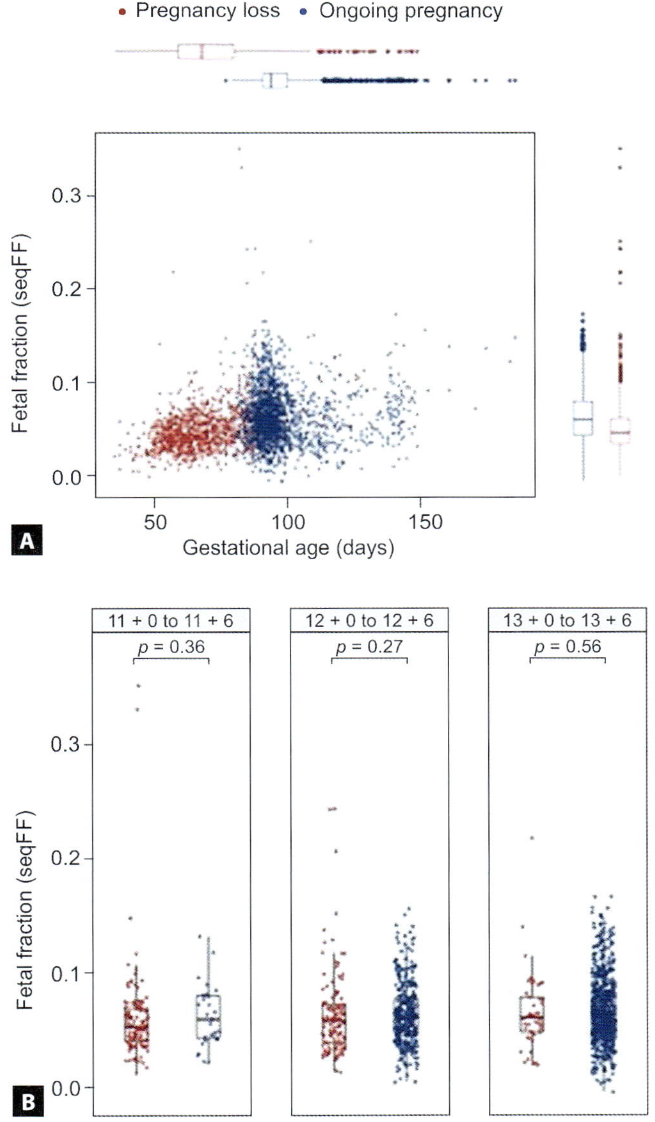

Figs. 3A and B: Fetal fraction of cell-free DNA (estimated by SeqFF) by gestational age based on last menstrual period from pregnancy losses (red) and ongoing pregnancies (blue: A) and in groups of pregnancy loss and ongoing pregnancies matched by gestational week (B).[16]

As a part of the COPL study, Hartwig et al. presented subanalysis of the fraction of cffDNA after a miscarriage and found a significant decrease within the first 24 hours after miscarriage/evacuation. When dividing the late collected samples by time after the pregnancy tissue passed, they found a significantly lower FF in samples drawn 12–24 hours after evacuation of the pregnancy tissue than in the samples drawn <6 hours after ($p = 0.008$)

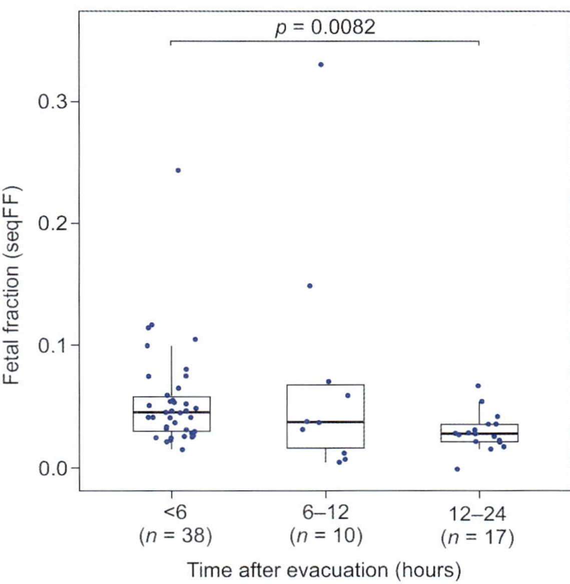

Fig. 4: Fetal fraction of cell-free DNA (estimated by SeqFF) in samples drawn <6 hours, 6–12 hours, and 12–24 hours after evacuation of pregnancy tissue in Copenhagen Pregnancy Loss study.[16]

and the no-call rate increasing from 13% in the group from which pregnancy tissue was drawn <6 hours after evacuation to 40% in the 6–12 hours group and 35% in the 12–24 hours group **(Fig. 4)**.[16] These results confirm the rapid elimination of fetal DNA in maternal blood and that cffDNA-based testing implies acute blood sampling, either during the miscarriage or immediately after. Therefore, the method is easiest applied in missed abortions.

Both cffDNA-based testing and direct sequencing of pregnancy tissue in their current forms are limited to identifying trisomies, monosomies, and sex chromosome abnormalities. These anomalies account for around 50% of sporadic first trimester pregnancy losses, while an additional approximately 10% are likely attributed to polyploidy, uniparental disomy, and copy-number variants (CNVs).[3,4,35] Consequently, approximately 10% of genetically caused losses are not detectable by cffDNA-based testing in its current form. Moreover, as described in ongoing viable pregnancies, discrepancies between cffDNA-based testing and the true fetal genetic status can arise due placental mosaicism, maternal mosaicism or CNV, vanished twin, or maternal malignancy.[36] Future advancements are expected to include increased resolution,[37] imputing and bioinformatic improvements to overcome these challenges.[38,39]

CONCLUSION

A novel, accurate, applicable, and expandable approach to genetic testing in pregnancy loss would be a key step toward improved clinical management of couples going through pregnancy loss, but also an essential step in the understanding of the underlying pathophysiology of pregnancy loss and the association with a higher risk of later disease. cffDNA-based testing in cases of pregnancy loss is a promising high-throughput approach with the potential to identify women who have experienced euploid pregnancy losses after just one or two occurrences, eliminating the necessity to collect pregnancy tissue. This method stands as an appealing alternative to the current passive approach of not conducting any investigation.

Moreover, systematic ploidy testing of pregnancy loss enables a focused approach in the search of nongenetic causes of pregnancy loss, medical managements, and the link between pregnancy loss and later-life diseases.

REFERENCES

1. Lo YM, Corbetta N, Chamberlain PF, Rai V, Sargent IL, Redman CW, et al. Presence of fetal DNA in maternal plasma and serum. Lancet. 1997;350(9076):485-7.
2. Samura O. Update on noninvasive prenatal testing: A review based on current worldwide research. J Obstet Gynaecol Res. 2020;46(8):1246-54.
3. Hardy K, Hardy PJ, Jacobs PA, Lewallen K, Hassold TJ. Temporal changes in chromosome abnormalities in human spontaneous abortions: Results of 40 years of analysis. Am J Med Genet A. 2016;170:2671-80.
4. Finley J, Hay S, Oldzej J, Meredith MM, Dzidic N, Slim R, et al. The genomic basis of sporadic and recurrent pregnancy loss: a comprehensive in-depth analysis of 24,900 miscarriages. Reprod Biomed Online. 2022;45(1):125-34.
5. ESHRE Guideline Group on RPL; Bender Atik R, Christiansen OB, Elson J, Kolte AM, Lewis S, et al. ESHRE guideline: recurrent pregnancy loss. Hum Reprod Open. 2018;2018(2):hoy004.
6. Westergaard D, Nielsen AP, Mortensen LH, Nielsen HS, Brunak S. Phenome-Wide Analysis of Short- and Long-Run Disease Incidence Following Recurrent Pregnancy Loss Using Data From a 39-Year Period. J Am Heart Assoc. 2020;9:e015069.
7. Bortoletto P, Lucas ES, Melo P, Gallos ID, Devall AJ, Bourne T, et al. Miscarriage syndrome: Linking early pregnancy loss to obstetric and age-related disorders. eBioMedicine. 2022; 81:104134.
8. Dimitriadis E, Menkhorst E, Saito S, Kutteh WH, Brosens JJ. Recurrent pregnancy loss. Nat Rev Dis Prim. 2020;6(1):98.
9. Shahine L, Lathi R. Recurrent pregnancy loss: evaluation and treatment. Obstet Gynecol Clin North Am. 2015;42:117-34.
10. Papas RS, Kutteh WH. Genetic Testing for Aneuploidy in Patients Who Have Had Multiple Miscarriages: A Review of Current Literature. Appl Clin Genet. 2021;14:321-9.
11. Ogasawara M, Aoki K, Okada S, Suzumori K. Embryonic karyotype of abortuses in relation to the number of previous miscarriages. Fertil Steril. 2000;73:300-4.
12. Siegel M, Amato P, Lee D, Wu D, Krieg S. Home collection of products of conception: Can chromosomal analysis be obtained? J Gynecol Obstet Hum Reprod. 2021;50:101810.
13. Lo YM, Zhang J, Leung TN, Lau TK, Chang AM, Hjelm NM. Rapid clearance of fetal DNA from maternal plasma. Am J Hum Genet. 1999;64:218-24.
14. Yaron Y, Pauta M, Badenas C, Soler A, Borobio V, Illanes C, et al. Maternal plasma genome-wide cell-free DNA can detect fetal aneuploidy in early and recurrent pregnancy loss and can be used to direct further workup. Hum Reprod. 2020;35(5):1222-9.
15. Colley E, Devall AJ, Williams H, Hamilton S, Smith P, Morgan NV, et al. Cell-Free DNA in the Investigation of Miscarriage. J Clin Med. 2020;9(11):3428.
16. Schlaikjær Hartwig T, Ambye L, Gruhn JR, Petersen JF, Wrønding T, Amato L, et al. Cell-free fetal DNA for genetic evaluation in Copenhagen Pregnancy Loss Study (COPL): a prospective cohort study. Lancet. 2023;401(10378):762-71.
17. van Beek DM, Straver R, Weiss MM, Boon EMJ, Huijsdens-van Amsterdam K, Oudejans CBM, et al. Comparing methods for fetal fraction determination and quality control of NIPT samples. Prenat Diagn. 2017;37(8):769-73.
18. Haghiac M, Vora NL, Basu S, Johnson KL, Presley L, Bianchi DW, et al. Increased death of adipose cells, a path to release cell-free DNA into systemic circulation of obese women. Obesity (Silver Spring). 2012;20(11):2213-9. Erratum in: Obesity (Silver Spring). 2012;20(11):2321.
19. Wang E, Batey A, Struble C, Musci T, Song K, Oliphant A. Gestational age and maternal weight effects on fetal cell-free DNA in maternal plasma. Prenat Diagn. 2013;33:662-6.
20. Juul LA, Hartwig TS, Ambye L, Sørensen S, Jørgensen FS. Noninvasive prenatal testing and maternal obesity: A review. Acta Obstet Gynecol Scand. 2020;99:744-50.
21. Hartwig TS, Ambye L, Werge L, Weiergang MK, Nørgaard P, Sørensen S, et al. Non-Invasive Prenatal Testing (NIPT) in pregnancies with trisomy 21, 18 and 13 performed in a public setting - factors of importance for correct interpretation of results. Eur J Obstet Gynecol Reprod Biol. 2018;226:35-9.
22. Kinnings SL, Geis JA, Almasri E, Wang H, Guan X, McCullough RM, et al. Factors affecting levels of circulating cell-free fetal DNA in maternal plasma and their implications for noninvasive prenatal testing. Prenat Diagn. 2015;35(8):816-22.
23. Dabi Y, Guterman S, Jani JC, Letourneau A, Demain A, Kleinfinger P, et al. Autoimmune disorders but not heparin are associated with cell-free fetal DNA test failure. J Transl Med. 2018;16(1):335.

24. Kuhlmann-Capek M, Chiossi G, Singh P, Monsivais L, Lozovyy V, Gallagher L, et al. Effects of medication intake in early pregnancy on the fetal fraction of cell-free DNA testing. Prenat Diagn. 2019;39(5):361-8.
25. Ma GC, Wu WJ, Lee MH, Lin YS, Chen M. Low-molecular-weight heparin associated with reduced fetal fraction and subsequent false-negative cell-free DNA test result for trisomy 21. Ultrasound Obstet Gynecol. 2018;51(2):276-7.
26. Rava RP, Srinivasan A, Sehnert AJ, Bianchi DW. Circulating fetal cell-free DNA fractions differ in autosomal aneuploidies and monosomy X. Clin Chem. 2014;60:243-50.
27. Zhou Y, Zhu Z, Gao Y, Yuan Y, Guo Y, Zhou L, et al. Effects of Maternal and Fetal Characteristics on Cell-Free Fetal DNA Fraction in Maternal Plasma. Reprod Sci. 2015;22(11):1429-35.
28. Galeva S, Gil MM, Konstantinidou L, Akolekar R, Nicolaides KH. First-trimester screening for trisomies by cfDNA testing of maternal blood in singleton and twin pregnancies: factors affecting test failure. Ultrasound Obstet Gynecol. 2019;53(6):804-9.
29. Revello R, Sarno L, Ispas A, Akolekar R, Nicolaides KH. Screening for trisomies by cell-free DNA testing of maternal blood: consequences of a failed result. Ultrasound Obstet Gynecol. 2016;47:698-704.
30. Ashoor G, Syngelaki A, Poon LCY, Rezende JC, Nicolaides KH. Fetal fraction in maternal plasma cell-free DNA at 11-13 weeks' gestation: Relation to maternal and fetal characteristics. Ultrasound Obstet Gynecol. 2013;41:26-32.
31. Poon LCY, Musci T, Song K, Syngelaki A, Nicolaides KH. Maternal plasma cell-free fetal and maternal DNA at 11-13 weeks' gestation: relation to fetal and maternal characteristics and pregnancy outcomes. Fetal Diagn Ther. 2013;33:215-23.
32. Palomaki GE, Kloza EM, Lambert-Messerlian GM, van den Boom D, Ehrich M, Deciu C, et al. Circulating cell free DNA testing: are some test failures informative? Prenat Diagn. 2015;35(3):289-93.
33. Miltoft CB, Rode L, Bundgaard JR, Johansen P, Tabor A. Cell-Free Fetal DNA in the Early and Late First Trimester. Fetal Diagn Ther. 2020;47:228-36.
34. Peng S, Bhatt S, Borrell A, Yaron Y. Economic impact of using maternal plasma cell-free DNA testing to guide further workup in recurrent pregnancy loss. Prenat Diagn. 2021;41:1215-21.
35. Soler A, Morales C, Mademont-Soler I, Margarit E, Borrell A, Borobio V, et al. Overview of Chromosome Abnormalities in First Trimester Miscarriages: A Series of 1,011 Consecutive Chorionic Villi Sample Karyotypes. Cytogenet Genome Res. 2017;152(2):81-9.
36. Hartwig TS, Ambye L, Sørensen S, Jørgensen FS. Discordant non-invasive prenatal testing (NIPT)—a systematic review. Prenat Diagn. 2017;37:527-39.
37. van der Meij KRM, Sistermans EA, Macville MVE, Stevens SJC, Bax CJ, Bekker MN, et al. TRIDENT-2: National Implementation of Genome-wide Non-invasive Prenatal Testing as a First-Tier Screening Test in the Netherlands. Am J Hum Genet. 2019;105(6):1091-101.
38. Curnow KJ, Wilkins-Haug L, Ryan A, Kırkızlar E, Stosic M, Hall MP, et al. Detection of triploid, molar, and vanishing twin pregnancies by a single-nucleotide polymorphism-based noninvasive prenatal test. Am J Obstet Gynecol. 2015;212(1):79.e1-9.
39. Qiao L, Zhang B, Wu X, Zhang C, Xue Y, Tang H, et al. A fetal fraction enrichment method reduces false negatives and increases test success rate of fetal chromosome aneuploidy detection in early pregnancy loss. J Transl Med. 2022;20(1):345.

CHAPTER 7

Male Factors

Shlomi Barak, Shira Salama

ABSTRACT

Sperm deoxyribonucleic acid (DNA) fragmentation has been linked to poor embryo quality and recurrent pregnancy loss (RPL). Increased DNA fragmentation is associated with life style factors like smoking, alcoholism, lack of exercise, improper diet, and disruptive sleep patterns. It is also associated with varicocele. Three types of DNA fragmentation mechanisms are improper protamination, incomplete apoptosis and oxidative stress. The assays used to measure DNA fragmentation are the TUNEL assay, sperm chromatin structure assay, sperm chromatin dispersion, and comet assay. The treatment is by correcting life style factors and administering a combination of antioxidants over a period of at least three months.

Keywords: Sperm DNA fragmentation, SDF, TUNEL, SCSA, SCD, Comet, Varicocele, Male life style factors, Antioxidants.

INTRODUCTION

Historically, research into recurrent pregnancy loss (RPL) has focused predominantly on investigating the female partner to identify potential causes. The etiology of RPL is considered multifactorial and includes genetic, endocrine, anatomical, environmental, and immunological factors. Nonetheless, despite in-depth investigations into the causes and risk factors of RPL, over half of these cases remain unexplained.[1]

Recently, there has been growing interest in the male contribution to RPL. Specifically, several meta-analyses published over the past few years have identified a clear association between high levels of sperm deoxyribonucleic acid (DNA) fragmentation (SDF) and RPL, which highlighted the potential significance of male factors in discussions about RPL.[2-4]

Advances in molecular genetics have led to a deeper understanding of the potential influence of DNA integrity on fertilization, embryo development, implantation, and pregnancy outcomes.[5]

Subsequently, this led to the creation of various SDF assays. The most commonly used are the TdT (terminal deoxynucleotidyl transferase)-mediated dUDP nick-end labeling (TUNEL) assay, the comet assay, the sperm chromatin structure assay (SCSA), and the sperm chromatin dispersion (SCD) assay.[5] Although each test is designed to detect different types of DNA damage, there is general agreement that measuring SDF offers a more precise indication of male fertility. This is mainly due to its lower biological variability compared with traditional semen analysis.[6,7]

INTEGRITY OF SPERM DEOXYRIBONUCLEIC ACID AND RECURRENT PREGNANCY LOSS

The integrity of sperm DNA may have a major impact on its fertilizing potential. The impact of SDF on reproductive success depends on the balance between the extent of DNA damage and the oocyte's DNA repair capacity. Damage to sperm DNA that exceeds the oocyte's repair capacity may influence the potential for embryo development.

Current evidence indicates a strong relationship between RPL and SDF.

Several early studies suggested that females with male partners who had high levels of SDF were at a greater risk of experiencing a miscarriage.[8-11] Although Robinson et al. and Zhao et al. collected data from couples who underwent in vitro fertilization (IVF) or intracytoplasmic sperm injection (ICSI), Zidi-Jrah et al. and Carlini et al. looked at couples who faced RPL after conceiving naturally.

A systematic review and meta-analysis of 13 prospective studies by McQueen et al. showed that male partners of women with a history of RPL had a significantly higher rate of SDF compared with the partners of fertile control women.[2]

Tan et al. summarized the evidence from 14 RPL studies and found that SDF levels were higher in the affected couples compared with fertile controls.[4]

The exact mechanism involved in RPL in couples with SDF is not clear; however, a commonly proposed mechanism involves elevated seminal oxidative stress. Jayasena et al. demonstrated a fourfold increase in levels of seminal reactive oxygen species (ROS) in the male partners of couples affected by RPL compared with the control arm.[12] Venkatesh et al. suggested that genetic/epigenetic changes in the zygote and developing embryo, consequent to increased SDF that was induced oxidatively, could cause RPL.[13]

Although the oocyte can repair some sperm DNA damage after fertilization, high levels of damage beyond the oocyte's repair capacity led to poor embryo development, implantation failure, and miscarriage.[14]

Animal studies have shown that the zygote responds to sperm DNA damage through a nonapoptotic mechanism that acts by slowing paternal DNA replication and ultimately leads to an arrest in embryonic development and a miscarriage.[15] Damage to sperm DNA can lead to the fragmentation and random distribution of paternal chromosome segments in developing embryos, which results in chaotic mosaicism. These mosaic aneuploidies, uniparental disomies, and de novo structural variation induced by damage to sperm DNA compromised fertility and led to congenital disorders when embryos escaped developmental arrest.[16]

Damage to sperm DNA in the ejaculate can result from three distinct mechanisms:

1. Improper chromatin condensation or "protamination" (i.e., faulty replacement of histones by protamines) during the last stage of spermatogenesis.
2. Incomplete apoptosis.
3. Oxidative stress that results from imbalances in ROS and antioxidant capacity.[17]

DNA damage manifests as structural changes that include base alterations, single-strand breaks (SSBs), and double-strand breaks (DSBs).

The type of DNA damage, whether it is single- or double-stranded, might influence the outcome of fertilization. DSBs had a greater impact compared with SSBs and were linked to RPL, failure of implantation, and spontaneous miscarriage following IVF or ICSI.[18] SSBs were more often associated with infertility and longer time-to-pregnancy in natural conception.[19]

Double-strand breaks are severe DNA lesions that can arise from exogenous sources, such as chemotherapeutic drugs or endogenous sources (e.g., ROS, mechanical stress, and replication aberrations). DSBs can trigger apoptosis because their repair mechanisms are more challenging than other types of DNA damage, and they cannot utilize a sister strand as a template for repair.

NATURAL REPAIR MECHANISMS FOR SPERM DEOXYRIBONUCLEIC ACID

The compact structure of mammalian sperm DNA is a result of specialized and unique chromatin packaging, which is essential for maintaining the integrity and organization of DNA from the time of spermiogenesis to fertilization. This compaction process involves the partial replacement of histones with protamines, which are proteins that are rich in arginine and cysteine; their incorporation into sperm chromatin makes the DNA highly compact and largely protected from external damage.[20,21]

Lower levels of protamines were associated with higher levels of DNA fragmentation. Furthermore, insufficient protamine remodeling, which refers to the process by which protamines are incorporated into sperm chromatin, was linked with infertility.[22]

Multiple studies have identified a positive correlation between ROS levels and DNA fragmentation.[23] Although maintaining a baseline level of physiological ROS appeared to be essential for oocyte-sperm fusion (capacitation), elevated ROS levels led to higher rates of SDF.

SPERM DEOXYRIBONUCLEIC ACID FRAGMENTATION TESTING

As mentioned, various methods have been developed to evaluate SDF. Commonly employed methods for clinical use are the TUNEL assay, the SCSA, the SCD assay, and the comet assay, which encompasses neutral, alkaline, and two-tailed (2-T) variations **(Table 1)**. Each SDF detection assay has its unique advantages and limitations. The choice of assay depends on the specific clinical scenario, available resources, and the need for detailed analysis of the integrity of sperm DNA.[24] Some assays offer high throughput and automation, and other assays provide detailed information on the type and extent of DNA damage.

In a comprehensive analysis of these assays, the alkaline comet assay was the most predictive of male infertility, followed by the TUNEL assay, the SCD assay, and the SCSA.[25]

TABLE 1: Types of assays that detect fragmentation of sperm DNA.

Assay	*Method principle*	*Detected damage*	*Advantages*	*Disadvantages*
TUNEL	• The TUNEL assay identifies DNA fragmentation by labeling the free 3′-OH termini with modified nucleotides in a template-independent manner • Fluorescein isothiocyanate is combined with dUTPs, and the resulting fluorescent signal is quantified using either flow cytometry or fluorescence microscopy. Sperm that exhibit DNA breaks emit fluorescence, and the findings are expressed as a percentage of fluorescent sperm **(Figs. 1A and B)**	SSBs and DSBs	• Providing high specificity • Considered as a more direct measure of DNA breaks compared with other assays • Can be performed on fresh or frozen samples	• The need for fluorescence microscopy or flow cytometry • May have variability in sensitivity and specificity based on the protocol used • Time-consuming
SCSA	SCSA assay measures the susceptibility of sperm DNA to denaturation in an acidic environment, followed by staining with fluorescent dye and cytometry measurement **(Figs. 2A to D)**	DSB	• Widely studied and considered simple and precise method • Can be performed on fresh or frozen-thawed samples • Highly automated and provides rapid results for a large number of samples	• Requires expensive equipment and specialized technical expertise • Indirect assay
SCD (Halo)	• SCD assesses the ability of sperm DNA to disperse chromatin loops after acid denaturation treatment • Identifies sperm with fragmented DNA that fail to produce characteristic halos postdenaturation **(Figs. 3A and B)**	SSBs and DSBs	• Simple, available, and affordable kit • Provides a visual representation of DNA fragmentation under microscopy • Can be used on low-concentrated samples	• It may require subjective interpretation of results, which can lead to variability between operators • Indirect assay • Time-consuming
Alkaline, neutral, and 2T comet	• Comet test assesses DNA damage by measuring the migration of DNA fragments from individual cells through an agarose gel under an electric field • Alkaline and neutral refer to the conditions of the test, but these require different protocols • The resulting image resembles a comet, with the tail that indicates DNA fragmentation **(Figs. 4A and B)** • The 2T comet is a modification that allows for the simultaneous detection of SSBs and DSBs **(Fig. 4B)**	SSBs and DSBs	• Can differentiate between different types of DNA damage based on methodology • Direct assay • High sensitivity and specificity	• Requires meticulous sample preparation and analysis, which lead to potential variability • Time-consuming • Requires fresh samples • Expensive

(DNA: deoxyribonucleic acid; DSB: double-strand break; SCD: sperm chromatin dispersion; SCSA: sperm chromatin structure assay; SSB: single-strand break; TUNEL: terminal deoxynucleotidyl transferase-mediated dUDP nick-end labeling)

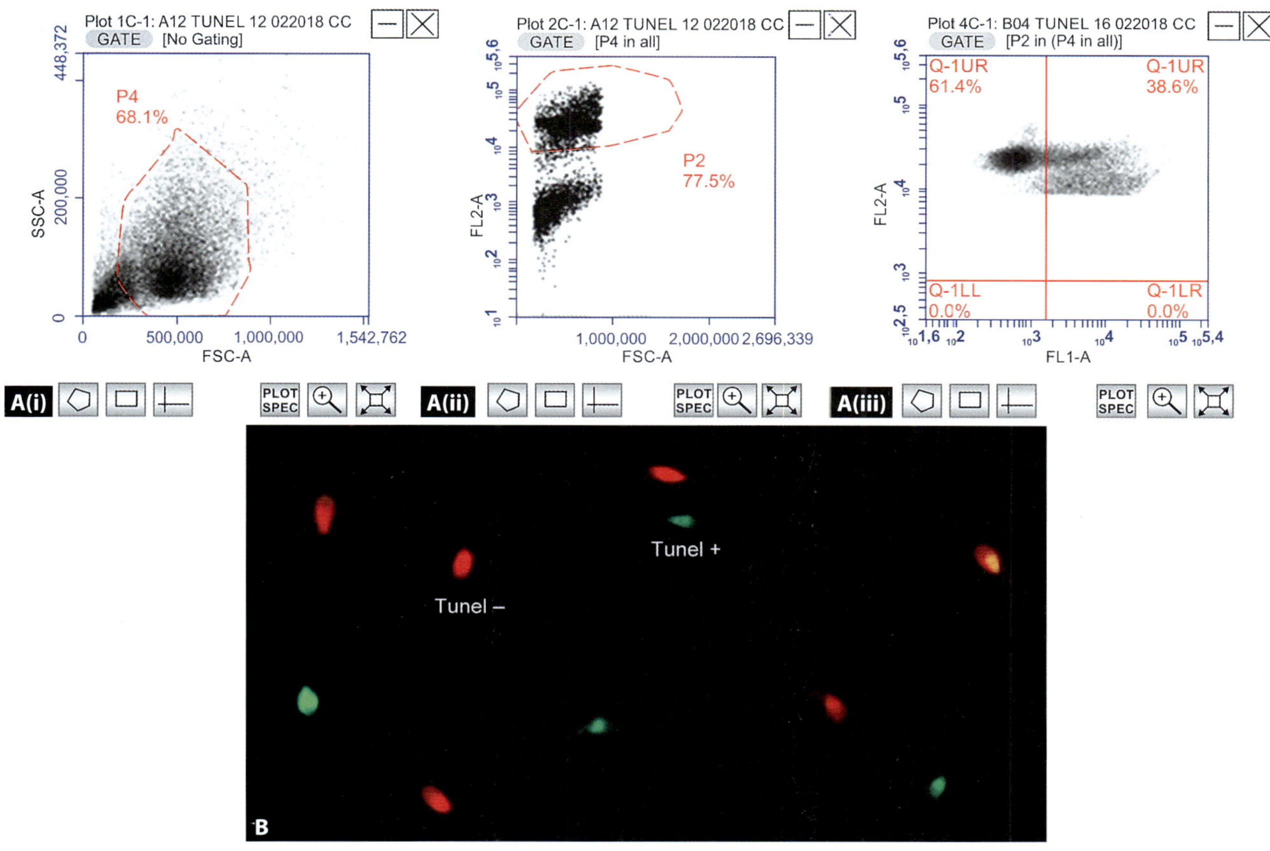

Figs. 1A(i-iii) and B: TUNEL assay. (A) TUNEL assay results using flow cytometer. (i) FSC versus side scatter (SSC-A): Gate is drawn, and small debris and larger nonsperm cells are excluded. Spermatozoa stained with PI with a flame-shaped gate are gated in the FSC versus SSC plot. (ii) FSC versus fluorescence in the red or PI channel-area (FL2-A): Gating strategy for PI-positive cells. (iii) Fluorescence in the green or FITC-area (FL1-A) versus FL2-A: Plot of a positive sample. (B) TUNEL assay resu ts in fluorescence microscopy. Digoxigenin-dUTP is incorporated into DNA breaks using a terminal transferase; antidigoxigenin-FITC is used to label the sites where digoxigenin-dUTP is present (green color). TUNEL+ represents spermatozoa presenting DNA damage. Slides were counterstained with PI (red color). TUNEL– represents spermatozoa free of DNA breaks.[26] (DNA: deoxyribonucleic acid; FITC: fluorescein isothiocyanate; FL: fluorescence; FSC: forward scatter; PI: propidium iodide; SSC: side scatter)

MANAGING HIGH SPERM DEOXYRIBONUCLEIC ACID FRAGMENTATION LEVELS—SUGGESTED STRATEGIES

The following strategies have been suggested as potential methods to reduce SDF.

Lifestyle Changes

High levels of SDF were associated with various lifestyle factors that may impact overall health negatively. These include metabolic conditions, such as diabetes mellitus, obesity, and tobacco smoking.[27]

Thus, embracing a healthy lifestyle, which includes a balanced diet, regular exercise, and refraining from smoking, may help to reduce high levels of SDF.[28]

Specifically, engaging in high-intensity exercises, following a diet rich in vegetables, fish, seafood, and whole grains (e.g., the Mediterranean diet), and reducing alcohol intake may have favorable effects on SDF. Cigarette smoking was strongly associated with high SDF,[29,30] which may be attributed to high ROS.[28,29]

Varicocele Repair

Varicocele is characterized by reflux in the spermatic vein that leads to increased scrotal temperature, which in

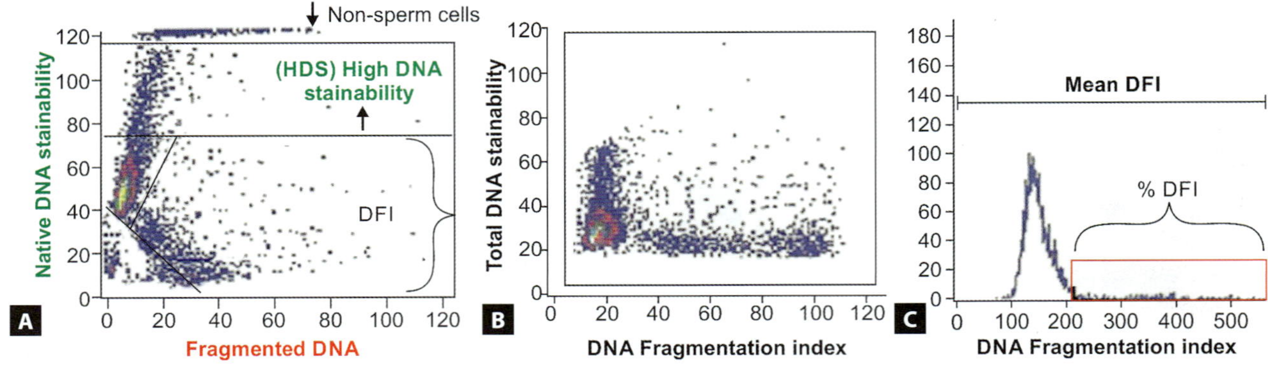

File	% DFI	% HDS	Mean DFI	Std dev DFI
1	17.66	8.40	222.4	182.2
2	18.00	8.80	224.7	186.9
Mean	17.8	8.6	223.6	184.6
Std dev	0.2	0.3	1.6	3.4

D

Figs. 2A to D: Sperm chromatin structure assay (SCSA). Test data (SCSA Diagnostics, Brookings, United States). **Left panel (A):** Raw data from a flow cytometer showing each of 5,000 spermatozoa as a single dot on a scattergram. *Y*-axis = green fluorescence with 1,024 gradations (channels) of DNA stainability (intact double-stranded DNA). *X*-axis = red fluorescence with 1,024 gradations of red fluorescence (single-strand DNA). Axes shown are 1,024/10. Line at *Y* = 75 marks the upper boundary of DNA staining of normal sperm chromatin; above that line are spermatozoa (dots) with partially uncondensed chromatin allowing more DNA stainability. Bottom left corner shows gating out of seminal debris. **Middle panel (B):** Raw data from the left panel are converted by SCSAsoft software (or equivalent) to red/red + green fluorescence. This transforms the angled sperm display in the left panel to a vertical pattern that is often critical for accurately delineating the percentage of spermatozoa with fragmented DNA. *Y*-axis = total DNA stainability versus *X*-axis = red/red + green fluorescence (DFI). **Right panel (C):** Frequency histogram of data from the middle panel showing computer gating into %DFI and Mean DFI. **Bottom box (D):** SCSAsoft software calculations of the mean of two independent measures of mean and standard deviation (std dev) of median DFI, %DFI, and %HDS (high DNA stainability).[26] (DFI: DNA fragmentation index; DNA: deoxyribonucleic acid)

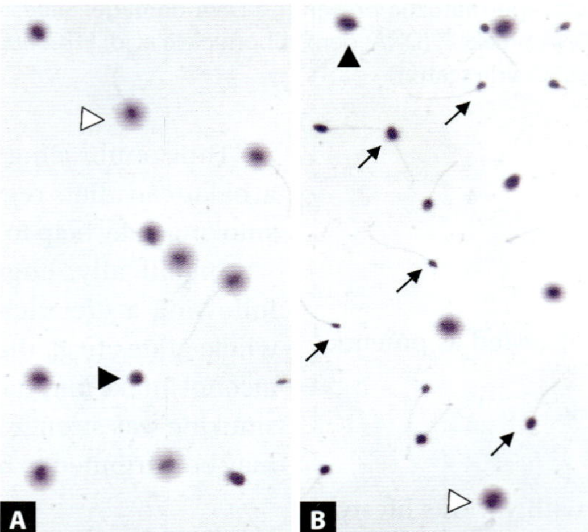

Figs. 3A and B: Sperm chromatin dispersion (SCD) test under bright-field microscopy (Halosperm, Halotech DNA, SL, Madrid, Spain). (A) Sperm sample of an individual presenting with normal level of SDF. (B) Sperm sample of a patient with varicocele presenting with elevated SDF. Open arrowheads indicate spermatozoa with halos of dispersed chromatin representing a normal DNA molecule with no fragmented DNA. Black arrowheads indicate spermatozoa with small or absent halos of dispersed chromatin, representing spermatozoa with fragmented DNA. Arrows in (B) indicate spermatozoa with fragmented-degraded DNA.[26] (DNA: deoxyribonucleic acid; SDF: sperm DNA fragmentation)

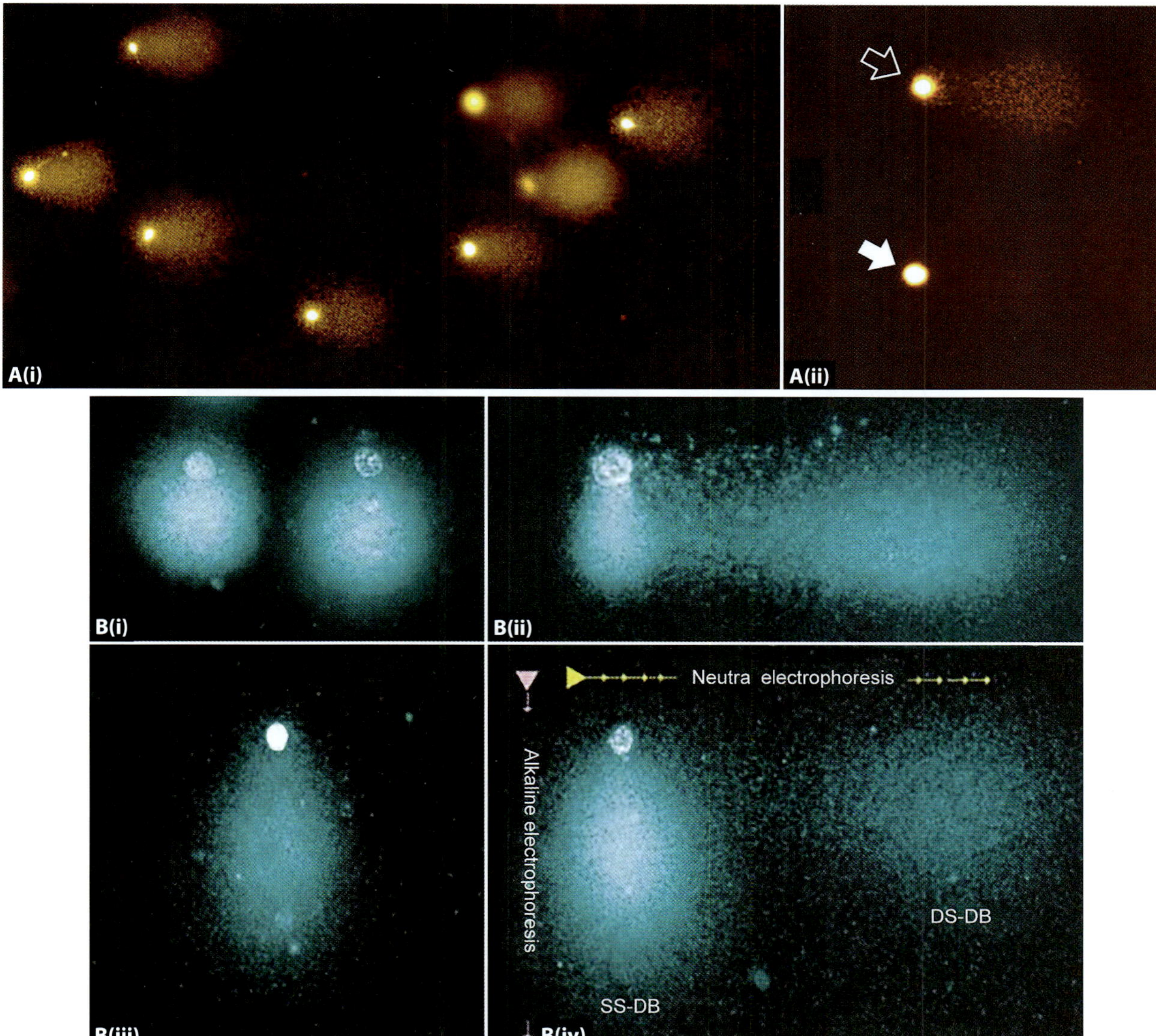

Figs. 4A(i-ii) and B(i-iv): (A) Alkaline comet assay under fluorescence microscopy. (i) Sperm sample of a patient exhibiting elevated sperm DNA fragmentation (SDF). Several comets are shown, which represent spermatozoa with DNA fragmentation. The longer and brighter the "comet" tail, the more fragmentation is present. (ii) Spermatozoon with DNA fragmentation (open arrow), and another one with a hardly visible "comet" tail (white arrow), representing a cell with minimal DNA fragmentation. As the comet test measures the amount of damage in each cell, it is rare to find a perfect spermatozoon with 0% damage, even from fertile donors. (B) Two-dimensional (two-tail) comet assay for simultaneous mapping of SS-DB (*Y*-axis) and DS-DB (*X*-axis) in spermatozoa. (i) Normal spermatozoa showing DNA displacement in the *Y*-axis due to the structural presence of alkaline-labile sites. (ii) Presence of DS-DB in the *X*-axis after electrophoresis under neutral conditions. (iii) Presence of SS-DB along the Y-axis after alkaline electrophoresis. (iv) Presence of both SS-DB and DS-DB affecting a single spermatozoon. Arrows indicate the perpendicular sense of each electrophoresis.[26] (DNA: deoxyribonucleic acid; DS-DB: double-strand DNA damage; SS-DB: single-strand DNA damage)

turn might compromise spermatogenesis. Moreover, the testicular microenvironment experiences reduced oxygen levels due to inefficient venous return, which results in heat stress and oxidative stress that affect fertility adversely and contribute to SDF.[31]

Varicocele repair significantly reduced SDF levels in patients with clinical varicocele, as reported in a recent meta-analysis.[32] Further studies are needed to establish the efficacy of varicocele repair in RPL patients with otherwise normal semen parameters and high SDF.

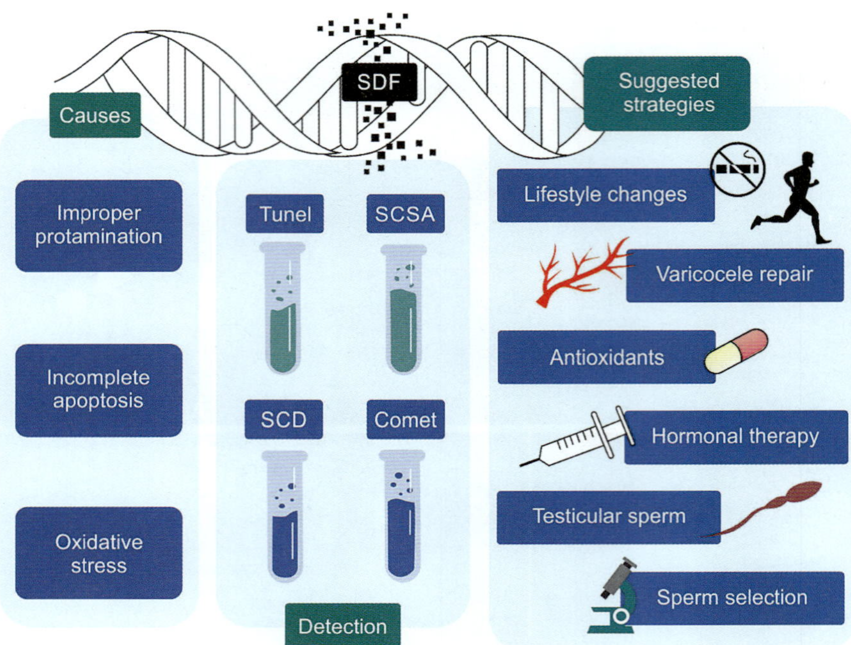

Fig. 5: A pictorial summary of this chapter includes the causes of SDF, its main detection methods, and suggested strategies for managing high SDF levels that are linked to RPL. (RPL: recurrent pregnancy loss; SCD: sperm chromatin dispersion; SCSA: sperm chromatin structure assay; SDF: sperm deoxyribonucleic acid fragmentation; TUNEL: terminal deoxynucleotidyl transferase-mediated dUDP nick-end labeling)

Antioxidants

The role of antioxidants in the management of high SDF has been explored with conflicting results.[33]

The optimal dosing, regimen length, and timing for antioxidant therapy are yet to be established.

Although the recent Cochrane Review showed that antioxidant supplementation may increase clinical pregnancy rates [odds ratio (OR) = 1.89] and live birth rates (OR = 1.43), the analysis concluded that the overall certainty of evidence was very low from the small number of randomized controlled trials (RCTs).[34]

Hormonal Therapy

Some evidence suggests that letrozole, which is a peripheral aromatase inhibitor, or direct administration of follicle-stimulating hormone (FSH), can significantly reduce SDF and contribute to a successful intrauterine pregnancy.[35,36]

Some data suggest that sequential treatment with human chorionic gonadotropin (hCG) and FSH could be effective as well.[37]

The Use of Testicular Sperm

Testicular sperm has lower levels of oxidative damage.[38]

Several studies demonstrated higher pregnancy rates and an increase in live births using testicular sperm in patients with high SDF.[39] Yet, robust RCTs are still lacking for the RPL population.

Sperm Selection and High Sperm Deoxyribonucleic Acid Fragmentation

Various methods for sperm selection have been explored to improve infertility rates in patients with high SDF who are undergoing assisted reproductive techniques. RCTs that compared common sperm selection techniques, such as density gradient centrifugation (DGC), physiologic intracytoplasmic sperm injection (PICSI), and magnetic-activated cell sorting (MACS), revealed that combining PICSI and MACS with DGC led to significantly higher implantation and pregnancy rates compared with using DGC alone.[40] Briefly, PICSI involves placing sperm on hyaluronan microdots to mimic high DNA-integrity binding, which leads to the selection of high-integrity sperm, whereas traditional ICSI relies only on morphology and motility for sperm selection. MACS separates apoptosed sperm cells by recognizing externalized phosphatidylserine residues.

Although not much is known about how effective these methods are in patients who experience RPL, healthcare professionals can discuss selection techniques with patients and acknowledge that robust studies that demonstrate the benefit of these techniques in RPL are currently lacking.

CONCLUSION

Testing for SDF in couples with RPL may help identify cases where damaged sperm chromatin plays a role in the condition. This knowledge can be valuable during patient counseling, and it can later assist in directing clinical management strategies that aim to identify and to treat the underlying causes of SDF **(Fig. 5)**.

The latest American Society for Reproductive Medicine (ASRM) guidelines now recommend evaluating SDF in addition to karyotype analysis for couples who experience RPL.[41] Similarly, the 2022 European Society of Human Reproduction and Embryology (ESHRE) guideline for RPL also acknowledges the importance of assessing SDF in such couples for diagnostic purposes, but not solely for explanatory purposes, based on emerging evidence from recent analyses.[42]

REFERENCES

1. Turesheva A, Aimagambetova G, Ukybassova T, Marat A, Kanabekova P, Kaldygulova L, et al. Recurrent pregnancy loss etiology, risk factors, diagnosis, and management. Fresh look into a full box. J Clin Med. 2023;12:4074.
2. McQueen DB, Zhang J, Robins JC. Sperm DNA fragmentation and recurrent pregnancy loss: a systematic review and meta-analysis. Fertil Steril. 2019;112(1):54-60.e3.
3. Li J, Luo L, Diao J, Li Y, Zhang S, Chen L, et al. Male sperm quality and risk of recurrent spontaneous abortion in Chinese couples: a systematic review and meta-analysis. Medicine (Baltimore). 2021;100:e24828.
4. Tan J, Taskin O, Albert A, Bedaiwy MA. Association between sperm DNA fragmentation and idiopathic recurrent pregnancy loss: a systematic review and meta-analysis. Reprod Biomed Online. 2019;38:951-60.
5. Agarwal A, Majzoub A, Esteves SC, Ko E, Ramasamy R, Zini A. Clinical utility of sperm DNA fragmentation testing: practice recommendations based on clinical scenarios. Transl Androl Urol. 2016;5(6):935-50.
6. Oleszczuk K, Giwercman A, Bungum M. Intra-individual variation of the sperm chromatin structure assay DNA fragmentation index in men from infertile couples. Hum Reprod. 2011;26(12):3244-8.
7. Erenpreiss J, Bungum M, Spano M, Elzanaty S, Orbidans J, Giwercman A. Intra-individual variation in sperm chromatin structure assay parameters in men from infertile couples: clinical implications. Hum Reprod. 2006;21(8):2061-4.
8. Robinson L, Gallos ID, Conner SJ, Rajkhowa M, Miller D, Lewis S, et al. The effect of sperm DNA fragmentation on miscarriage rates: a systematic review and meta-analysis. Hum Reprod. 2012;27;2908-17.
9. Zhao J, Zhang Q, Wang Y, Li Y. Whether sperm deoxyribonucleic acid fragmentation has an effect on pregnancy and miscarriage after in vitro fertilization/intracytoplasmic sperm injection: a systematic review and meta-analysis. Fertil Steril. 2014;102(4):998-1005.
10. Zidi-Jrah I, Hajlaoui A, Mougou-Zerelli S, Kammoun M, Meniaoui I, Sallem A, et al. Relationship between sperm aneuploidy, sperm DNA integrity, chromatin packaging, traditional semen parameters, and recurrent pregnancy loss. Fertil Steril. 2016;105(1):58-64.
11. Carlini T, Paoli D, Pelloni M, Faja F, Dal Lago A, Lombardo F, et al. Sperm DNA fragmentation in Italian couples with recurrent pregnancy loss. Reprod Biomed Online. 2017;34(1):58-65.
12. Jayasena CN, Radia UK, Figueiredo M, Revill LF, Dimakopoulou A, Osagie M, et al. Reduced testicular steroidogenesis and increased semen oxidative stress in male partners as novel markers of recurrent miscarriage. Clin Chem. 2019;65(1):161-9.
13. Venkatesh S, Thilagavathi J, Kumar K, Deka D, Talwar P, Dada R. Cytogenetic, Y chromosome microdeletion, sperm chromatin and oxidative stress analysis in male partners of couples experiencing recurrent spontaneous abortions. Arch Gynecol Obstet. 2011;284(6):1577-84.
14. Ahmadi A, Ng SC. Fertilizing ability of DNA-damaged spermatozoa. J Exp Zool. 1999;284(6):696-704.
15. Gawecka JE, Marh J, Ortega M, Yamauchi Y, Ward MA, Ward WS. Mouse zygotes respond to severe sperm DNA damage by delaying paternal DNA replication and embryonic development. PLoS One. 2013;8(2):e56385.
16. Middelkamp S, Van Tol HTA, Spierings DCJ, Boymans S, Guryev V, Roelen BAJ, et al. Sperm DNA damage causes genomic instability in early embryonic development. Sci Adv. 2020;6(16):eaaz7602.
17. García-Rodríguez A, Gosálvez J, Agarwal A, Roy R, Johnston S. DNA damage and repair in human reproductive cells. Int J Mol Sci. 2019;20:31.
18. Ribas-Maynou J, Benet J. Single and double strand sperm DNA damage: different reproductive effects on male fertility. Genes (Basel). 2019;10(2):105.
19. De Iuliis GN, Thomson LK, Mitchell LA, Finnie JM, Koppers AJ, Hedges A, et al. DNA damage in human spermatozoa is highly correlated with the efficiency of

chromatin remodeling and the formation of 8-hydroxy-2′-deoxyguanosine, a marker of oxidative stress. Biol Reprod. 2009;81(3):517-24.
20. Balhorn R. The protamine family of sperm nuclear proteins. Genome Biol. 2007;8:227.
21. Ward WS, Coffey DS. DNA packaging and organization in mammalian spermatozoa: comparison with somatic cells. Biol Reprod. 1991;44(4):569-74.
22. Gawecka JE, Ribas-Maynou J, Benet J, Ward WS. A model for the control of DNA integrity by the sperm nuclear matrix. Asian J Androl. 2015;17(4):610-5.
23. Bui AD, Sharma R, Henkel R, Agarwal A. Reactive oxygen species impact on sperm DNA and its role in male infertility. Andrologia. 2018;50(8):e13012.
24. Javed A, Talkad MS, Ramaiah MK. Corrigendum to "Evaluation of sperm DNA fragmentation using multiple methods: a comparison of their predictive power for male infertility". Clin Exp Reprod Med. 2019;46:211.
25. Ribas-Maynou J, García-Peiró A, Fernández-Encinas A, Abad C, Amengual MJ, Prada E, et al. Comprehensive analysis of sperm DNA fragmentation by five different assays: TUNEL assay, SCSA, SCD test and alkaline and neutral Comet assay. Andrology. 2013;1(5):715-22.
26. Esteves SC, Zini A, Coward RM, Evenson DP, Gosálvez J, Lewis SEM, et al. Sperm DNA fragmentation testing: summary evidence and clinical practice recommendations. Andrologia. 2021;53(2):e13874.
27. Szabó A, Váncsa S, Hegyi P, Váradi A, Forintos A, Filipov T, et al. Lifestyle-, environmental-, and additional health factors associated with an increased sperm DNA fragmentation: a systematic review and meta-analysis. Reprod Biol Endocrinol. 2023;21(1):5.
28. Humaidan P, Haahr T, Povlsen BB, Kofod L, Laursen RJ, Alsbjerg B, et al. The combined effect of lifestyle intervention and antioxidant therapy on sperm DNA fragmentation and seminal oxidative stress in IVF patients: a pilot study. Int Braz J Urol. 2022;48(1):131-56.
29. Anifandis G, Bounartzi T, Messini CI, Dafopoulos K, Sotiriou S, Messinis IE. The impact of cigarette smoking and alcohol consumption on sperm parameters and sperm DNA fragmentation (SDF) measured by Halosperm®. Arch Gynecol Obstet. 2014;290(4):777-82.
30. Amor H, Hammadeh ME, Mohd I, Jankowski PM. Impact of heavy alcohol consumption and cigarette smoking on sperm DNA integrity. Andrologia. 2022;54(7):e14434.
31. Schoor RA, Elhanbly SM, Niederberger CS. The pathophysiology of varicocele-associated male infertility. Curr Urol Rep. 2001;2(6):432-6.
32. Lira Neto FT, Roque M, Esteves SC. Effect of varicocelectomy on sperm deoxyribonucleic acid fragmentation rates in infertile men with clinical varicocele: a systematic review and meta-analysis. Fertil Steril. 2021;116(3):696-712.
33. Esteves SC, Santi D, Simoni M. An update on clinical and surgical interventions to reduce sperm DNA fragmentation in infertile men. Andrology. 2020;8:53-81.
34. de Ligny W, Smits RM, Mackenzie-Proctor R, Jordan V, Fleischer K, de Bruin JP, et al. Antioxidants for male subfertility. Cochrane Database of Syst Rev. 2022;5:CD007411.
35. Kooshesh L, Bahmanpour S, Zeighami S, Nasr-Esfahani MH. Effect of letrozole on sperm parameters, chromatin status and ROS level in idiopathic oligo/astheno/teratozoospermia. Reprod Biol Endocrinol. 2020;18(1):47.
36. Lispi M, Drakopoulos P, Spaggiari G, Caprio F, Colacurci N, Simoni M, et al. Testosterone serum levels are related to sperm DNA fragmentation index reduction after FSH administration in males with idiopathic infertility. Biomedicines. 2022;10(10):2599.
37. La Vignera S, Condorelli RA, Duca Y, Mongioi LM, Cannarella R, Giacone F, et al. FSH therapy for idiopathic male infertility: four schemes are better than one. Aging Male. 2021;23(5):750-5.
38. Ambar RF, Agarwal A, Majzoub A, Vij S, Tadros NN, Cho CL, et al. The use of testicular sperm for intracytoplasmic sperm injection in patients with high sperm DNA damage: a systematic review. World J Mens Health. 2021;39(3):391-8.
39. Tharakan T, Bettocchi C, Carvalho J, Corona G, Jones TH, Kadioglu A, et al. European Association of Urology Guidelines Panel on male sexual and reproductive health: a clinical consultation guide on the indications for performing sperm DNA fragmentation testing in men with infertility and testicular sperm extraction in nonazoospermic men. Eur Urol Focus. 2022;8(1):339-50.
40. Hozyen M, Hasanen E, Elqusi K, ElTanbouly S, Gamal S, Hussin AG, et al. Reproductive outcomes of different sperm selection techniques for ICSI patients with abnormal sperm DNA fragmentation: a randomized controlled trial. Reprod Sci. 2022;29(1);220-8.
41. Schlegel PN, Sigman M, Collura B, De Jonge CJ, Eisenberg ML, Lamb DJ, et al. Diagnosis and treatment of infertility in men: AUA/ASRM guideline part I. Fertil Steril. 2021;115(1):36-43.
42. Atik RB, Christiansen OB, Elson J, Kolte AM, Lewis S, Middeldorp S, et al. ESHRE guideline: recurrent pregnancy loss: an update in 2022. Hum Reprod Open. 2023;2023(1):hoad002.

CHAPTER 8

Y Chromosome Microdeletions

Stacy Colaco, Deepak Modi

ABSTRACT

Y chromosome microdeletions of the azoospermia factor (AZF) locus are definitely implicated in azoospermia, other microdeletions may play a role in recurrent pregnancy loss (RPL). The association of Y microdeletion and RPL is not confidently established yet. However, some studies show that microdeletions of AZF region or DYZ1 may be implicated in male partners of RPL patients.

Keywords: Y chromsome microdeletion, Recurrent miscarriage, Recurrent pregnancy loss.

INTRODUCTION

Recurrent pregnancy loss (RPL) is a heterogeneous multifactorial disorder defined as two or more clinical pregnancy losses, including embryonic and fetal loss, before gestational weeks 20–24.[1] According to estimates, 23 million cases of RPL are reported annually worldwide,[2] and in India, the prevalence of recurrent miscarriage is around 7.4%.[3] Despite thorough investigations, the cause remains elusive in 50% of cases, and the mechanism of RPL still remains poorly understood.

Although most studies associate RPL with fetal chromosomal abnormalities, female hormonal disorders or reproductive tract irregularities, in recent years, growing evidence supports the role of male factors in inducing RPL. While genomic integrity of the sperm is critical for the initiation and continuation of a successful pregnancy, other male genetic factors such as anomalies in sperm chromosome structure and number, sperm deoxyribonucleic acid (DNA) fragmentation, genetic polymorphisms, and epigenetic modifications have also been linked to RPL.[4]

ROLE OF Y CHROMOSOME IN RECURRENT PREGNANCY LOSS

The role of the Y chromosome in RPL is not yet comprehensively characterized. The human Y chromosome is bordered by two pseudoautosomal regions (PARs), PAR1 and PAR2, each located at its extremities. It is mainly composed of a short p arm bearing genes such as *SRY*, the master sex-determining gene, *ZFY*, *AMELY*, *TBL1Y*, *PCDH11Y*, and the *TSPY* repeats, and a long q arm that contains the azoospermia factor (AZF) locus and a large chunk of dense heterochromatin.[5] This heterochromatic region is composed of two highly repetitive DYZ sequence families, the DYZ1 family composed of 5,000 copies and the DYZ2 family composed of 2,000 copies. The heterochromatic region is variable in length in the normal population and was long thought to be genetically inert. However, it is now known that the DYZ1 repeat undergoes decondensation at the start of week 32 of embryonic development and is expressed onward from week 36 of embryonic development.[6] The exact role of the DYZ1 repeat in embryonic development is not yet known, but a significant increase or decrease in length of the DYZ1 repeats is associated with recurrent spontaneous miscarriage and early embryo growth arrest.[7]

WHAT ARE THE Y CHROMOSOME MICRODELETIONS?

Another common type of Y chromosome anomaly is the Y chromosome microdeletion. These submicroscopic deletions of the AZF loci occur on the long arm of the Y chromosome and are unique to infertile men. Globally, 7.5% of infertile men harbor a Y chromosome microdeletion,[5] and in India, they occur in approximately 8.5% of infertile men. The AZF locus of the Y chromosome is composed of three main regions termed AZFa, AZFb, and AZFc. These regions are rich in genes involved in spermatogenesis, and deletions in these regions lead to azoospermia or oligozoospermia. The AZFc microdeletion is the most commonly identified microdeletion globally as well as in India.[8] Another type of microdeletion called the AZFc subdeletion (gr/gr, b1/b3, and b2/b3) is also associated with infertility, with sporadic reports describing their occurrence in fertile men as well. This, however, depends on the population studied, and in the Indian milieu, the gr/gr subdeletion is found at higher frequency in infertile males who also have reduced sperm count and decreased sperm motility.[9,10] Hence, testing for gr/gr deletion in addition to testing for the Y chromosome microdeletions is imperative.[11] Presently, the European Academy of Andrology (EAA), American Society of Reproductive Medicine (ASRM), and Indian Council of Medical Research recommend testing for Y chromosome microdeletions in all men with nonobstructive azoospermia and oligozoospermia. Y chromosome microdeletions cannot be identified by standard karyotyping methods. Even today, the gold standard for diagnosing Y chromosome microdeletions remains the sequence tagged site polymerase chain reaction (STS-PCR) technique, which utilizes the multiplex polymerase chain reaction. It must be borne in mind, however, that different laboratories use different numbers and STS markers to test Y chromosome microdeletions in India;[12] hence, it remains at the discretion of the clinician to insist on testing using the appropriate markers for the population.

ANALYSIS OF STUDIES EVALUATING THE EFFECT OF Y CHROMOSOME MICRODELETIONS ON RECURRENT PREGNANCY LOSS

The complete deletion of AZFa locus is phenotypically associated with Sertoli cell-only syndrome, and complete deletion of the AZFb locus is associated with maturation arrest. However, men with AZFc microdeletion may have normozoospermia, oligozoospermia, or azoospermia. Analysis of studies describing assisted reproductive technology (ART) outcomes in couples where the male partner has an AZFc microdeletion shows that sperm retrieved from males harboring AZF deletions produce viable embryos and result in successful pregnancies.[13,14] However, other studies also report that embryos derived from sperm of men with AZFc have a high percentage of aneuploidies,[15] have lower blastocyst cleavage rate,[16] and many times are of poor quality.[17,18] Meta-analysis studies that compared ART outcomes in couples where the male partner has Y chromosome microdeletions versus men with nonobstructive azoospermia in the absence of Y chromosome microdeletion observe lower fertilization rates, clinical pregnancy rates, and live birth rates in men with Y chromosome microdeletions (unpublished results from our lab[19]).

These results are not surprising because several genes in the AZF loci are transcribed and translated in the germ cells and are also expressed in the sperm.[5] Additionally, single-cell RNA sequencing studies of human embryos also demonstrate expression of several AZF loci genes in the developing human embryo from as early as the four-cell stage up to the morula stage, with expression also seen in cells of the trophectoderm, epiblast, and placenta during later stages of embryonic development.[20,21] AZF loci genes are also expressed when embryonic stem cells differentiate into neural stem cells[22] and embryoid bodies.[23] Genes from all three AZF loci are expressed during mesoderm development (*DDX3Y*, *KDM5D*, *PRY*, and *DAZ*); those from the AZFa and AZFb loci are expressed during endoderm development (*USP9Y* and *EIF1AY*) and ectoderm development (*UTY*, *RBMY1*, and *HSFY*) in the gastrulating embryo.

Data has now emerged demonstrating that the genes of the AZF loci of the Y chromosome are also expressed in somatic tissues such as stomach, brain, heart, lungs, and spleen. The protein products of these genes are predicted to have several housekeeping functions, including those in regulation of gene transcription, translation, and regulation.[24,25] This implies that the AZF genes may have roles beyond the regulation of spermatogenesis. Indeed, clinical analysis of males harboring AZF deletions or AZF gene copy number variations (CNVs) and large-scale expression data from human cancers has demonstrated an association of the AZF genes not only with early embryonic development but also with neuropsychiatric disorders, cognitive functions, and predisposition to cancers.

Despite this knowledge, the effect of Y chromosome microdeletions in RPL still remains inconclusive. Fifteen studies till date have explored the effect of Y chromosome microdeletions on RPL, and the majority of the studies have concluded a lack of association,[26-35] while only four studies have identified an association.[36-39] A cumulative analysis of these 15 studies shows that a Y chromosome microdeletion was identified in 33 of 1,865 (1.7%) men who had RPL and in none of the 860 fertile males who had at least one live birth and no history of miscarriages. However, among the studies that have identified a positive correlation, the accuracy of the findings is questionable due to several reasons such as screening using non-European Academy of Andrology/European Molecular Genetics Quality Network (EAA/EMQN) laboratory recommended STS markers,[36-38] not reporting sperm counts of fertile and infertile men,[36,39] poor patient selection criteria and small sample size, and nonexclusion of males where the female partner has immunological, cytogenetic, or endocrine comorbidities.[36-39] Furthermore, none of the studies mentioned whether they investigated male partners of couples with RPL who had natural conception or conception via ART. The results of two independent reviews confirm that there is no significant correlation between Y chromosome microdeletions and RPL and do not recommend routine evaluation of Y chromosome microdeletions for idiopathic RPL.[35,40]

CONCLUSION

With the complete sequence of the human Y chromosome now available,[41,42] the role of the Y chromosome in human health and disease will be explored yet more comprehensively. However, in the current scenario, there is a lack of a clear-cut cause–effect relationship of Y chromosome microdeletions and RPL. Testing for Y chromosome microdeletions is not mandatory in clinical practice as yet. In the meantime, couples affected by RPL where the male partner shows the presence of Y chromosome microdeletion must be appropriately genetically counseled regarding the vertical transmission of the Y chromosome microdeletions to all male offspring. The couple and the clinician must make an informed choice of having biological parenthood at the risk of perpetuating infertility in the family.

KEY POINTS

- Genetic defects as a cause of male infertility are on the rise; hence, genetic testing is an important component in the clinical work-up for infertile males.
- Increasing studies report the effect of male factors such as anomalies in sperm chromosome structure and number, sperm DNA fragmentation, genetic polymorphisms, and epigenetic modifications in RPL.
- Association of Y chromosome microdeletions with RPL is not yet confidently established.
- Analysis of existing studies shows that only 1.7% of men in couples experiencing RPL carry a Y chromosome microdeletion.
- In cases where a Y chromosome microdeletion is suspected, screening should be performed using population-specific STS markers.
- In couples with RPL and Y chromosome microdeletion, appropriate counseling should be offered regarding vertical transmission of Y chromosome microdeletions from an infertile father to son and the perpetuation of infertility and the associated health risks in all future generations.

ACKNOWLEDGMENTS

Stacy Colaco is thankful to ICMR for the postdoctoral fellowship, and Deepak Modi's lab is supported by grants from ICMR. The manuscript bears the *NIRRH ID: OTH/1645/10-2023*.

REFERENCES

1. Dimitriadis E, Menkhorst E, Saito S, Kutteh WH, Brosens JJ. Recurrent pregnancy loss. Nat Rev Dis Primers. 2020;6:98.
2. Quenby S, Gallos ID, Dhillon-Smith RK, Podesek M, Stephenson MD, Fisher J, et al. Miscarriage matters: the epidemiological, physical, psychological, and economic costs of early pregnancy loss. Lancet. 2021;397:1658-67.
3. Standard Treatment Guidelines (2017). Management of recurrent spontaneous abortion. [online] Available from http://clinicalestablishments.gov.in/WriteReadData/3361.pdf [Last accessed December, 2024].
4. Yu W, Bao S. Association of male factors with recurrent pregnancy loss. J Reprod Immunol. 2022;154:103758.
5. Colaco S, Modi D. Genetics of the human Y chromosome and its association with male infertility. Reprod Biol Endocrinol. 2018;16:14.
6. Jehan Z, Vallinayagam S, Tiwari S, Pradhan S, Singh L, Suresh A, et al. Novel noncoding RNA from human Y distal heterochromatic block (Yq12) generates testis-specific chimeric CDC2L2. Genome Res. 2007;17:433-40.
7. Yan J, Fan L, Zhao Y, You L, Wang L, Zhao H, et al. DYZ1 copy number variation, Y chromosome polymorphism and early recurrent spontaneous abortion/early embryo growth arrest. Eur J Obstet Gynecol Reprod Biol. 2011;159:371-4.
8. Colaco S, Lakdawala A, Modi D. Role of Y chromosome microdeletions in the clinical evaluation of infertile males. MGM J Med Sci. 2017;4:79-88.
9. Sen S, Ambulkar P, Hinduja I, Zaveri K, Gokral J, Pal A, et al. Susceptibility of gr/gr rearrangements to azoospermia or oligozoospermia is dependent on DAZ and CDY1 gene copy deletions. J Assist Reprod Genet. 2015;32:1333-41.
10. Bansal SK, Jaiswal D, Gupta N, Singh K, Dada R, Sankhwar SN, et al. Gr/gr deletions on Y-chromosome correlate with male infertility: an original study, meta-analyses, and trial sequential analyses. Sci Rep. 2016;6:19798.

11. Krausz C, Navarro-Costa P, Wilke M, Tüttelmann F. EAA/EMQN best practice guidelines for molecular diagnosis of Y-chromosomal microdeletions: state of the art 2023. Andrology. 2024;12(3):487-504.
12. Sen S, Pasi AR, Dada R, Shamsi MB, Modi D. Y chromosome microdeletions in infertile men: prevalence, phenotypes and screening markers for the Indian population. J Assist Reprod Genet. 2013;30:413-22.
13. Page DC, Silber S, Brown LG. Men with infertility caused by AZFc deletion can produce sons by intracytoplasmic sperm injection, but are likely to transmit the deletion and infertility. Hum Reprod. 1999;14:1722-6.
14. Choi JM, Chung P, Veeck L, Mielnik A, Palermo GD, Schlegel PN. AZF microdeletions of the Y chromosome and in vitro fertilization outcome. Fertil Steril. 2004;81:337-41.
15. Mateu E, Rodrigo L, Martínez MC, Peinado V, Milán M, Gil-Salom M, et al. Aneuploidies in embryos and spermatozoa from patients with Y chromosome microdeletions. Fertil Steril. 2010;94:2874-7.
16. Zhang L, Mao JM, Li M, Lian Y, Lin SL, Chen LX, et al. Poor intracytoplasmic sperm injection outcome in infertile males with azoospermia factor c microdeletions. Fertil Steril. 2021;116:96-104.
17. van Golde RJ, Wetzels AM, de Graaf R, Tuerlings JH, Braat DD, Kremer JA. Decreased fertilization rate and embryo quality after ICSI in oligozoospermic men with microdeletions in the azoospermia factor c region of the Y chromosome. Hum Reprod. 2001;16:289-92.
18. Abur U, Gunes S, Ascı R, Altundag E, Akar OS, Ayas B, et al. Chromosomal and Y-chromosome microdeletion analysis in 1,300 infertile males and the fertility outcome of patients with AZFc microdeletions. Andrologia. 2019;51:e13402.
19. Li X, Li X, Sun Y, Han J, Ma H, Sun Y. Effect of Y chromosome microdeletions on the pregnancy outcome of assisted reproduction technology: a meta-analysis. Reprod Sci. 2021;28:2413-21.
20. Petropoulos S, Edsgärd D, Reinius B, Deng Q, Panula SP, Codeluppi S, et al. Single-cell RNA-seq reveals lineage and X chromosome dynamics in human preimplantation embryos. Cell. 2016;165:1012-26.
21. Yan L, Yang M, Guo H, Yang L, Wu J, Li R, et al. Single-cell RNA-seq profiling of human preimplantation embryos and embryonic stem cells. Nat Struct Mol Biol. 2013;20:1131-9.
22. Khani F, Nafian S, Mollamohammadi S, Nemati S, Shokoohian B, Hassani SN, et al. Y chromosome genes may play roles in the development of neural rosettes from human embryonic stem cells. Stem Cell Rev Rep. 2022;18:3008-20.
23. Dehkordi S, Khani F, Hassani SN, Baharvand H, Soleimanpour-Lichaei HR, Salekdeh GH. The contribution of Y chromosome genes to spontaneous differentiation of human embryonic stem cells into embryoid bodies in vitro. Cell J. 2021;23:40-50.
24. Colaco S, Modi D. Consequences of Y chromosome microdeletions beyond male infertility. J Assist Reprod Genet. 2019;36:1329-37.
25. Godfrey AK, Naqvi S, Chmátal L, Chick JM, Mitchell RN, Gygi SP, et al. Quantitative analysis of Y-chromosome gene expression across 36 human tissues. Genome Res. 2020;30:860-73.
26. Wettasinghe TK, Jayasekara RW, Dissanayake VH. Y chromosome microdeletions are not associated with spontaneous recurrent pregnancy loss in a Sinhalese population in Sri Lanka. Hum Reprod. 2010;25:3152-6.
27. Bellver J, Meseguer M, Muriel L, García-Herrero S, Barreto MA, Garda AL, et al. Y chromosome microdeletions, sperm DNA fragmentation and sperm oxidative stress as causes of recurrent spontaneous abortion of unknown etiology. Hum Reprod. 2010;25:1713-21.
28. Venkatesh S, Thilagavathi J, Kumar K, Deka D, Talwar P, Dada R. Cytogenetic, Y chromosome microdeletion, sperm chromatin and oxidative stress analysis in male partners of couples experiencing recurrent spontaneous abortions. Arch Gynecol Obstet. 2011;284:1577-84.
29. Ghorbian S, Saliminejad K, Sadeghi MR, Javadi GR, Kamali K, Amirjannati N, et al. The association between Y chromosome microdeletion and recurrent pregnancy loss. Iran Red Crescent Med J. 2012;14:358-62.
30. Pina-Aguilar RE, Martínez-Garza SG, Kohls G, Vargas-Maciel MA, Vazquez de Lara LG, Gonzalez-Ortega C, et al. Y chromosome microdeletions in Mexican males of couples with idiopathic recurrent pregnancy loss. J Obstet Gynaecol Res. 2012;38:912-7.
31. Dai R, Pan Y, Fu Y, Liu Q, Han W, Liu R. Role of male genetic factors in recurrent pregnancy loss in Northeast China. Eur J Obstet Gynecol Reprod Biol. 2018;224:6-11.
32. Kaare M, Painter JN, Ulander VM, Kaaja R, Aittomaki K. Sex chromosome characteristics and recurrent miscarriage. Fertil Steril. 2008;90:2328-33.
33. Koç G, Ulucan K, Kirac D, Ergeç D, Tarcan T, Güney AI. Molecular and cytogenetic evaluation of Y chromosome in spontaneous abortion cases. J Cell Mol Biol. 2010;7(2):45-52.
34. Lu HY, Cui YX, Xia XY, Shi YC, Yang B, Shao Y, et al. AZF microdeletions are not related with recurrent spontaneous abortion. Zhonghua Nan Ke Xue. 2008;14:1099-102.
35. Pereza N, Črnjar K, Buretić-Tomljanović A, Volk M, Kapović M, Peterlin B, et al. Y chromosome azoospermia factor region microdeletions are not associated with idiopathic recurrent spontaneous abortion in a Slovenian population: association study and literature review. Fertil Steril. 2013;99:1663-7.
36. Dewan S, Puscheck EE, Coulam CB, Wilcox AJ, Jeyendran RS. Y chromosome microdeletions and recurrent pregnancy loss. Fertil Steril. 2006;85:441-5.

37. Karaer A, Karaer K, Ozaksit G, Ceylaner S, Percin EF. Y chromosome azoospermia factor region microdeletions and recurrent pregnancy loss. Am J Obstet Gynecol. 2008;199:662.e1-5.
38. Soleimanian S, Kalantar SM, Sheikhha MH, Zaimy MA, Rasti A, Fazli H. Association between Y-chromosome AZFc region micro-deletions with recurrent miscarriage. Iran J Reprod Med. 2013;11:431-4.
39. Agarwal S, Agarwal A, Khanna A, Singh K. Microdeletion of Y chromosome as a cause of recurrent pregnancy loss. J Hum Reprod Sci. 2015;8:159-64. Erratum in: J Hum Reprod Sci. 2016;9:131.
40. Golin AP, Yuen W, Flannigan R. The effects of Y chromosome microdeletions on in vitro fertilization outcomes, health abnormalities in offspring and recurrent pregnancy loss. Transl Androl Urol. 2021;10:1457-66.
41. Rhie A, Nurk S, Cechova M, Hoyt SJ, Taylor DJ, Altemose N, et al. The complete sequence of a human Y chromosome. Nature. 2023;621:344-54.
42. Hallast P, Ebert P, Loftus M, Yilmaz F, Audano PA, Logsdon GA, et al. Assembly of 43 human Y chromosomes reveals extensive complexity and variation. Nature. 2023;621:355-64.

CHAPTER 9

Male Microbiome, Genetic, and Epigenetic Factors

Anam Farooqui, Farhan Ali, Sher Ali

ABSTRACT

Despite the scientific advancement in the area of reproductive biology, we still do not know the number of genes involved and their sequential expression, silencing, and overall regulation. The fine-tuned levels of hormones ensure the timely progress of fetal development along with the health of the mother and her emotional well-being, which tends to guarantee the normal birth of a baby. Unexplained recurrent pregnancy loss (RPL) warrants research on causative factors and the search for possible remedial measures. This review is aimed to collect, collate, and summarize all the possible known factors responsible. We have also included the other still uncharacterized factors that seem to be crucial for the sustenance of pregnancy and for eventual successful parturition. These seemingly innocuous factors include genetics, microbiomes, microplastics, environmental pollution, professional hazards, stress, nutritional deficiency, rampant food adulteration, and use of tobacco and alcohol. Notably, microplastics, which cannot be digested and may take 10–10,000 years to degrade naturally depending on their chemical composition, have been detected in nearly every part of human and animal bodies, including the brain. It is envisaged that this review will be useful for researchers, doctors, nurses, healthcare professionals, and genetic counselors. Finally, we also believe that this would enhance our overall awareness about the pregnancy and its nuances, culminating in a healthy, happy, and successful family life.

Keywords: Loss of pregnancy, Microbiomes, Hormonal imbalance, Y chromosome, Y-linked mutations, Microplastics, Exposome.

INTRODUCTION

Human reproduction is known to be highly inefficient, because nearly 70% of human conceptions do not survive to live birth.[1-4] Studies have shown that fetal aneuploidy or associated genetic factors and nongenetic factors may contribute.

Exhaustive research employing all the tools and techniques of "omics" (genomics, proteomics, metabolomics, and transcriptomics), careful assessment of hormonal profile, and detailed chromosomal analysis may provide a diagnosis. Similarly, search of genes, their organization, expression, regulation, and copy number variation together with the mutational loads from an individual pregnancy are envisaged to help uncover the likely causative factors in, as yet, unexplained pregnancy losses. We have several genes that undergo epigenetic modification, thereby silencing their expression. How many such genes are epigenetically modified resulting in loss of pregnancy is not known. The present chapter examines available information, genes suspected to be involved in sustenance of pregnancy, mutational load of the presumptive genes, hormonal fluctuation and their causes, together with the nutritional and emotional status of the pregnant females. In addition, attempts have been made to see the involvement of environmental pollution, microplastics, lifestyle, food and nutrition, and overall status of the Y chromosome.

Crucially, several questions remain to be addressed comprehensively:

- Is recurrent loss of pregnancy related to aberrant Y chromosome in males?
- Is microbiome involved in the sustenance of pregnancy?
- Is pregnancy affected by the presence of microplastics?

We have attempted to address these questions and wish to emphasize that the role of genetics in pregnancy loss extends beyond embryonic aneuploidy.

PREGNANCY AND THE HUMAN Y CHROMOSOME

The Y chromosome carries genes that determine male sex characteristics. It plays a crucial role in the development of male reproductive organs and secondary sexual characteristics during puberty. The Y chromosome is relatively small compared to the X chromosome and contains close to about 100 plus genes. One of the most well-known genes on the Y chromosome is the *SRY* gene (sex-determining region Y), which triggers the development of male characteristics during embryonic development.[5] In addition to its role in determining sex, the Y chromosome also contains genes involved in other biological functions, such as fertility and immune response.[6] However, because the Y chromosome is passed exclusively from fathers to sons without recombination with the X chromosome (except for small pseudoautosomal regions at the ends), it has a unique evolutionary history compared to other chromosomes. This has led to some interesting patterns of genetic variation and evolution in human populations. Microbiomes are present both in males and females, doing all these jobs, ensuring not only good health but also proper functions of the organs. Thus, microbiomes cannot be dissociated from pregnancy.

Recurrent pregnancy loss (RPL) may affect both male and female fetuses. However, a female fetus will not have Y chromosome in normal condition unless it is a case of Turner syndrome.[7] Startlingly, we never found a Turner case without Y chromosome in some cells. Thus, all the earlier literature prior to the discovery of polymerase chain reaction (PCR) reported XO condition for Turner cases. This is because fewer cells having an aberrant Y chromosome were not captured under the microscope. As the situation stands now, the number of Y chromosomes in a Turner case can be estimated using quantitative real-time PCR. Similarly, the entire important Y-linked loci can be ascertained by PCR. Thus, not only we can detect Y chromosome but also its aberrant status. This analysis is useful for establishing a correlation with RPL and Y-linked makers. In one RPL of a male fetus, we detected aberrant chromosomes and massive deletion of the DYZ1 region **(Fig. 1)**.

Based on our observation, we suggest sufficient copies of DYZ1 arrays are important for the sustenance of a male fetus. We have no desire to conclude that aberrant DYZ1 arrays are responsible for pregnancy loss, but this could be one of the potential candidates responsible for the loss of pregnancy, at least in some male fetuses. If this hypothesis is true, this can be substantiated by studying the father's genotype employing both FISH and PCR approaches. We are aware that fewer samples would not allow drawing an unequivocal conclusion regarding the involvement of the DYZ1 arrays in the loss of pregnancy. Nonetheless, available data provide suggestive evidence that DYZ1 is the most likely candidate gene required in its intact form for sustenance of pregnancy. This scenario warrants analysis of DYZ1 arrays in all miscarried male or female fetuses of RPL along with normal males. The analysis of DYZ1 region in a large number of normal males would establish its vulnerability with respect to its sporadic sequence deletion/aberration. The DYZ1 region of the human Y chromosome was first reported in 1976 by Cooke[8] when he observed a male-specific band of about 3.4 kb in human genomic DNA digestion with HaeIII enzyme. Normal female DNA did not show such a male-specific band. Subsequently, a Japanese scientist cloned and sequenced the DYZ1 region.[9] Further, he demonstrated that DYZ1 region has close to about 4,000–4,500 copies of its arrays in a normal male, and each array has about 3,465 base pairs. In our studies on the DYZ1 region of the Y chromosome from across the samples representing different categories of males, such as those exposed to natural background radiation or males having sex chromosome-related genetic anomalies or genetically infertile ones, showed

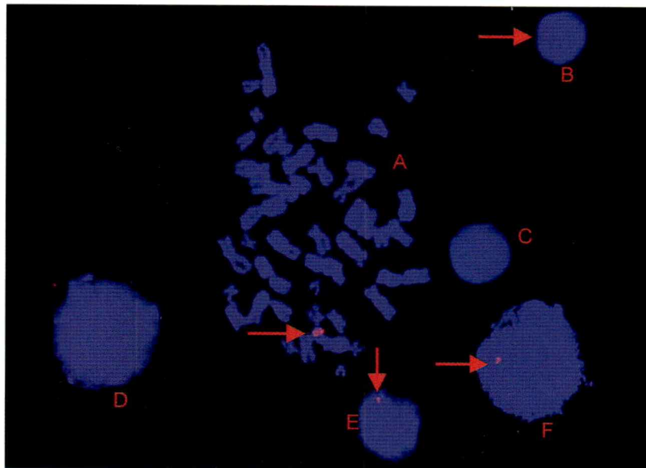

Fig. 1: A case of RPL of a male fetus showing presence of aberrant DYZ1 regions among Y chromosomes both in interphase nuclei and metaphase ones employing FISH. Note panel (A) representing metaphase chromosome showing aneuploidy and near-normal signal of the DYZ1 region on the Y chromosome [see arrow in panel (A)]. Panel (B) has minute DYZ1 signal, whereas (C) and (D) are devoid of DYZ1 signal. However, panels (E) and (F) both interphase nuclei show reduced DYZ1 signals. This establishes the heterogeneity of the DYZ1 region because of DNA sequence deletion of the human Y chromosome. Thus, all the aborted fetuses, whether male or female (Turner cases), always showed heterogeneity of the DYZ1 regions as evident from our FISH data. (DNA: deoxyribonucleic acid; FISH: fluorescence in situ hybridization; RPL: recurrent pregnancy loss)

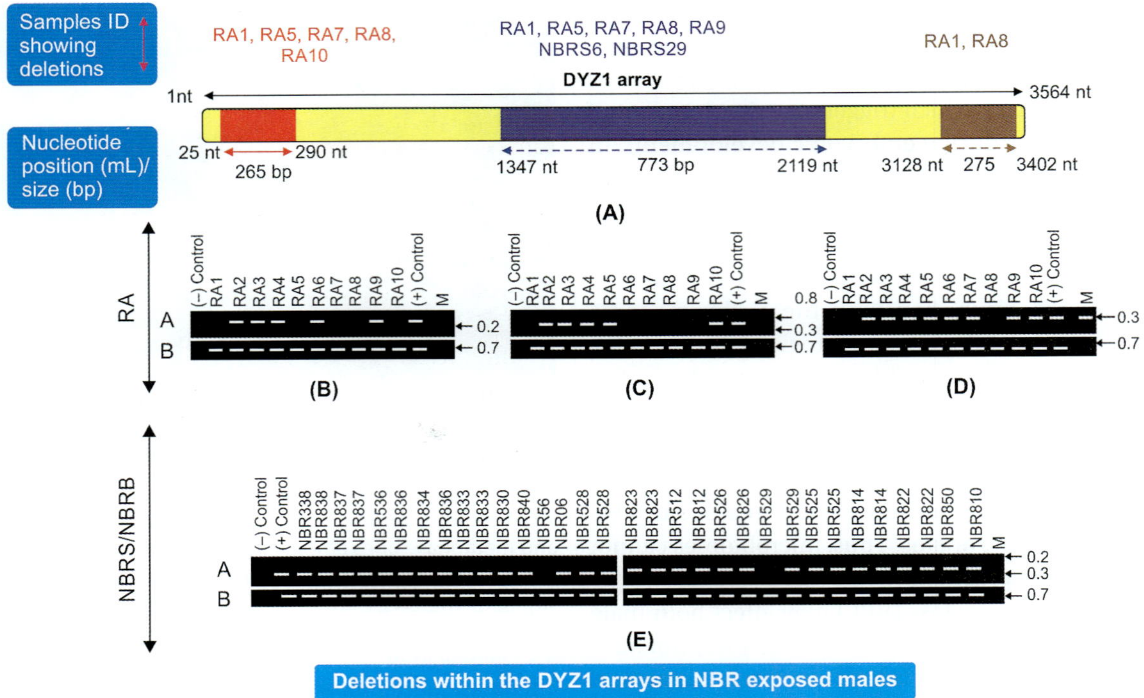

Figs. 2A to E: (A) Diagrammatic illustration of the DYZ1 array showing internal sequence deletion from the different categories of male DNA samples and microdeletion in some males. RA denotes repeated abortion, whereas NBRS denotes natural background radiation-exposed male samples. Note 265 base pair deletion (red), 773 base pair deletion (blue), and 275 base pair deletion (dark brown) in an array of DYZ1. (B to E) Shows microdeletion in some samples using PCR amplifications (top). For control, beta actin primers were used (B). (DNA: deoxyribonucleic acid; PCR: polymerase chain reaction)

heterogeneity with respect to copy number of the DYZ1 region **(Figs. 2A to E)** and frequent deletions within the copies of the arrays.

MICROBIOME AND SUSTENANCE OF PREGNANCY

The human body hosts diverse microbial communities, particularly in the gut, which are vital for maintaining overall health. These microbiomes are indispensable in regulating digestion, immunity, and even neural development. Recent research has increasingly highlighted the importance of microbiomes in pregnancy, suggesting that they play a crucial role in implantation of the embryo and fetal development.

Gut Microbiome

The human gut microbiome (GM), comprising over 500–1,500 different species of bacteria, archaea, fungi, and viruses, undergoes significant changes during pregnancy.[10] These microbiomes are not only involved in the digestion and absorption of nutrients but also play an essential role in modulating the host's immune system and metabolism. During pregnancy, the composition and diversity of GMs change, particularly in the second and third trimesters, reflecting the body's adaptation to support fetal growth and development.

Changes in the maternal GM are associated with various pregnancy complications, such as miscarriages, gestational diabetes, obesity, preeclampsia, digestive disorders, and autoimmune diseases.[11] For instance, gestational diabetes has been linked to specific changes in the GM that affect glucose metabolism.[12] Similarly, miscarriages and preeclampsia have been associated with alterations in GM composition, which may influence inflammatory pathways and immune responses.[13]

Uterine Microbiome

A balanced uterine microbiome is crucial for successful embryo implantation and placental development.[14] The uterine microbiome may also help modulate immune tolerance to the fetus, preventing immune rejection and ensuring a supportive environment for fetal growth.[15] However, dysbiosis in the uterine microbiome can lead to inflammation and disrupted implantation, increasing the risk of miscarriage. Additionally, the presence of pathogenic bacteria in the uterus can trigger inflammatory responses that may lead to miscarriage and preterm labor. These findings emphasize the importance of a healthy uterine microbiome.

Vaginal Microbiome

The vaginal microbiome, dominated by *Lactobacillus* species, plays a critical role in maintaining a healthy pregnancy by protecting against infections and contributing to the overall reproductive health of the mother.[16] Lactobacilli produce lactic acid, maintaining an acidic environment that inhibits the growth of harmful bacteria, thereby protecting the uterus against pathogens. Bacterial vaginosis (BV) is characterized by an overgrowth of harmful bacteria and a decrease in beneficial *Lactobacillus* species, leading to inflammation and disrupting the protective barrier of the vaginal epithelium. This condition is associated with an increased risk of miscarriage, premature rupture of membranes, and preterm birth.

Oral Microbiome

The oral cavity harbors a complex microbial ecosystem, which is influenced by factors such as diet, oral hygiene, and genetics. The oral microbiome is involved in digestion, immune function, and defense against pathogens. Periodontal disease due to oral dysbiosis has been linked to pregnancy complications.

Breast Milk Microbiome

The microbiome in breast milk plays a crucial role in the early colonization of the infant's GM, significantly impacting the infant's immune system and overall health. Studies have shown that bacterial species in breast milk are among the most abundant in the infant's GM, highlighting the importance of breastfeeding in establishing a healthy microbiome in early life.[17]

Microbiome Imbalances and Pregnancy Loss

Emerging evidence suggests that imbalances in microbiomes, particularly in the uterus and vagina, may contribute to RPL.[18]

Male-specific Microbiome

While the microbiome of males shares some similarities with that of females, there are certain regions and characteristics unique to males that warrant specific attention. The male urethral microbiome is dominated by *Corynebacterium* and is low in lactobacilli. Again, the prostate, a male-specific reproductive organ, harbors its own microbial community. Research into the prostate microbiome is relatively new but suggests that alterations in the prostate microbiota may be associated with conditions such as prostatitis and prostate cancer,[19] but its role in infertility has not been studied.

Changes in the microbiome may be a polygenic condition; thus, one has to know the total number of genes in the human genome and the ones that are encoded by the microbiome. Further, its role in reproduction needs to be elicited.

In a human body, there are around 30 trillion human cells, but our microbiome is estimated to have 38 trillion microbial cells, including bacteria, viruses, and fungi.[20] The human genome has 20,000–22,000 genes expressing across the tissues. However, these genes and their products are grossly inadequate for the sustenance of our body. Therefore, about 8 million genes encoded by 38 trillion microbial cells (microbiomes) are heavily involved in the upkeep of our body and ensuring homeostasis.

Strategies to promote a healthy maternal microbiome are essential. These strategies include the following aspects:

- *Diet and nutrition:* A balanced diet rich in fiber and probiotic and prebiotic foods can support a healthy GM. Prebiotics are fermented foods and fiber-rich foods on which the probiotics thrive. Probiotics are live microorganisms that confer a health benefit to the host.
- *Avoiding indiscriminate antibiotic use:* Antibiotics can disrupt the balance of microbiomes, leading to dysbiosis. Avoiding their indiscriminate use is useful in maintaining a healthy microbiome during pregnancy.
- *Stress management:* Chronic stress can negatively impact the GM. Practices such as mindfulness, yoga, and regular physical activity can help manage stress and support a healthy microbiome.
- *Hygiene practices:* Hygiene practices such as vaginal douching may be harmful in pregnancy.
- *Probiotic interventions:* Probiotics are considered safe and can provide beneficial effects on maternal, fetal, and infant health.

Understanding the adaptations of microbiomes during pregnancy and how they can be modulated may offer novel therapeutic targets to improve maternal and fetal health and better outcomes.

PREGNANCY AND EXPOSOMES

The exposome is a comprehensive concept introduced by Dr Christopher Wild in 2005, aiming to capture the totality of environmental exposures that individuals encounter throughout their lives.[21] Unlike the genome, which represents an individual's genetic makeup, the exposome encompasses all external factors to which an individual is exposed, including chemical, biological, and physical agents, as well as lifestyle factors and psychosocial stressors. This expansive framework recognizes that environmental exposures play a significant role in shaping health outcomes, often interacting with genetic factors to influence disease risk and progression. That is the reason it is advised to live in an area that is clean, green, and free from industrial pollution. Living close to nature has far-reaching positive physical and mental health consequences. Children born in such surroundings are invariably, healthy, robust, fearless, and positive toward life because they get the best exposome (adapted from Farooqui and Ali[22]).

In the context of pregnancy, the exposome takes on heightened importance due to the vulnerable nature of both the developing fetus and the pregnant mother. The exposome during pregnancy encompasses a wide range of exposures, including air pollutants, heavy metals, pesticides, endocrine-disrupting chemicals, dietary factors, psychosocial stressors, and lifestyle habits such as smoking and alcohol consumption. These exposures can originate from multiple sources, including ambient air pollution, occupational settings, household products, food and water contaminants, and personal habits of the mother. Research has shown that exposure to environmental pollutants during pregnancy can have adverse effects on maternal health and fetal development (Chapter 37).[23] Heavy metals such as lead, mercury, and arsenic can cross the placenta and interfere with fetal development, leading to neurodevelopmental deficits, cognitive impairments, and birth defects.[24] Furthermore, exposure to endocrine-disrupting chemicals during pregnancy can alter hormonal balance and contribute to reproductive disorders, developmental abnormalities, and metabolic dysregulation in both mothers and offspring. Pesticides, phthalates, bisphenols, and polycyclic aromatic hydrocarbons (PAHs) are among the chemicals of concern due to their potential to interfere with hormone function and disrupt fetal development. Metabolomics, a field that systematically analyzes metabolites in biological samples, offers a powerful tool for studying the metabolic repercussions of environmental exposures during pregnancy. By profiling metabolic changes associated with chemical exposures, researchers can identify potential biomarkers of exposure and elucidate underlying mechanisms of toxicity. Integrating exposome and metabolomic data enables researchers to uncover associations between early pregnancy exposures and later metabolic perturbations, providing insights into the link between environmental exposures and adverse health outcomes of pregnancy.

IMPACT OF ENVIRONMENTAL POLLUTANTS ON PREGNANCY AND FETAL HEALTH

Exposure to various pollutants, including air pollution, water contaminants, heavy metals, pesticides, and endocrine-disrupting chemicals, has been associated with an increased risk of miscarriage and pregnancy complications. Water contaminants, such as lead, mercury, arsenic, microplastics, and industrial chemicals, can also pose risks to reproductive health. These pollutants can accumulate in the body over time and may interfere with hormonal balance, impair fertility, cause erectile dysfunctions (ED), affect eukaryotic transcriptional machinery (ETM), and increase the risk of pregnancy complications.

Despite the growing body of research in this field, discrepancies and disagreements persist among studies investigating the impact of prenatal pollution exposure. Causal mediation analysis has emerged as a valuable tool in elucidating the pathways through which air pollution affects pregnancy outcomes, including its loss.

Metabolomic markers offer insights into the molecular pathways linking arsenic exposure to adverse birth outcomes, highlighting the multifaceted nature of environmental toxicity. Epigenetic changes and nitrosative stress in the placenta further underscore the intricate interplay between environmental pollutants and fetal development, with potential implications for long-term health outcomes.[25] Exposure to air pollution during the critical developmental window of the first 1,000 days of life can have enduring effects on lung development and immune system function, predisposing children to respiratory disorders such as asthma. Particulate matter (PM) exposure, in particular, has been linked to adverse outcomes such as low birth weight and impaired lung function, highlighting the importance of addressing air pollution during pregnancy.

Nicotine exposure from maternal smoking or environmental tobacco smoke (ETS) poses significant risks to fetal health, increasing the likelihood of obstetric complications and childhood respiratory diseases. Incentive-based smoking cessation programs in pregnancy may offer promise.

Noise pollution has emerged as a pervasive health risk, with potential implications for fetal development and congenital hearing loss. Growing urbanization has exacerbated this issue, necessitating interventions to mitigate noise-related health risks.

Exposure to environmental toxins such as *endocrine-disrupting chemicals and mycotoxins* during pregnancy can have far-reaching consequences for maternal and fetal health (Chapter 37).

Below is a comprehensive overview of the effects of various air pollutants on pregnancy outcomes and potential mechanisms of harm.

Mercury Exposure and Lung Development

Mercury exposure during pregnancy poses significant risks to fetal neurodevelopment, emphasizing the importance of monitoring environmental mercury levels.

Aromatic Hydrocarbon Pollution and Placental Function

Aromatic hydrocarbon pollution can disrupt endocrine and metabolic processes in the human placenta, potentially compromising fetal development.

Particulate Matter

Particulate matter, including $PM_{2.5}$ and PM_{10}, consists of tiny particles suspended in the air, originating from sources such as vehicle exhaust and industrial emissions.[26] These particles can penetrate the placental barrier, exposing the developing fetus to harmful substances. Research suggests that exposure to PM during pregnancy is associated with increased risks of spontaneous miscarriage and stillbirth. Mechanisms of harm may include inflammation, oxidative stress, and disruption of placental function, ultimately leading to adverse pregnancy outcomes.

Nitrogen Dioxide

Nitrogen dioxide (NO_2) is primarily emitted from vehicle engines and industrial activities. Exposure to NO_2 during pregnancy may increase the risk of spontaneous miscarriage and stillbirth, *albeit* to a lesser extent than other pollutants. Mechanisms of harm may involve placental dysfunction and impaired fetal development.

Sulfur Dioxide

Sulfur dioxide (SO_2) is a byproduct of combustion processes. Studies indicate that exposure to SO_2 during pregnancy is associated with increased risks of spontaneous miscarriage and stillbirth. The mechanisms of harm may include oxidative stress, inflammation, and disruption of placental function.

Carbon Monoxide

Carbon monoxide (CO), produced by incomplete combustion of fossil fuels, poses a risk of spontaneous miscarriage. Exposure during the third trimester has been associated with increased risks of stillbirth. Mechanisms of harm may involve impaired oxygen delivery to the fetus, leading to hypoxia along with placental dysfunction, oxidative stress, and inflammation.

Ozone

Exposure to elevated levels of ozone (O_3) during pregnancy may increase the risk of spontaneous miscarriage and stillbirth, although further research is needed to clarify this relationship. Mechanisms of harm may involve oxidative stress, inflammation, and disruption of placental function, similar to other air pollutants.

Cooking Smoke

Exposure to cooking smoke, particularly from solid fuels such as wood and coal, as in a barbecue, is a significant indoor air pollutant. Studies have shown that exposure to cooking smoke is associated with higher risks of spontaneous miscarriage and stillbirth.[27]

MICROPLASTICS AND LOSS OF PREGNANCY

Plastic pollution has become an urgent global issue, with projections indicating a significant escalation in plastic leakage into the environment and water bodies. The COVID-19 pandemic further exacerbated this problem, leading to a surge in single-use plastics, particularly in healthcare settings where personal protective equipment became essential.

The term "plastic" is derived from the Greek word πλαστικός (plastikos), meaning "capable of being shaped or molded." Most contemporary plastics are primarily derived from fossil fuel-based chemicals such as natural gas or petroleum. In 2019, global plastic production reached 460 million tons, and it is expected to surge to 1.2 billion tons by 2060.

The major components of plastics include:

- Polypropylene (PP)
- Polyethylene (PE)
- Polyethylene terephthalate (PET)
- Polystyrene (PS)
- Polyvinyl chloride (PVC)
- Polyvinyl chloride acetate (PVCA)

Additionally, copolymers, which are made up of two or more monomer species, are more complex components and take ages to degrade on their own.

In 2004, Richard Thompson OBE FRS, a Professor of Marine Biology and Director of the Marine Institute at the University, first described the long-term accumulation of plastics and coined the term "microplastics" in his landmark paper, "Lost at Sea: Where Is All the Plastic?"[28] The history of plastic usage includes the invention of the first plastic-handled toothbrush in 1927 and the creation of modern manual toothbrushes with the invention of nylon by the DuPont Company in 1938. With a global population of approximately 7.53 billion, and assuming the weight of a single toothbrush is 20 g, an estimated 29.4 billion toothbrushes are produced each year, resulting in 600 million kilograms of plastic toothbrush waste annually. A potential remedy for this waste issue is the use of wood as the handle, and a natural toothbrush made from the *Salvadora persica* tree. Miswak not only has antibacterial properties that help control dental plaque but also serves as an effective and natural alternative to plastic toothbrushes.

The aviation industry has also used plastics at a large scale. An Airbus A380, for instance, has approximately 4 million parts produced by 1,500 companies across 30 countries. Plastics have played a crucial role in the rapid development of aeronautical engineering, leading to innovations such as Boeing's 787 Dreamliner, often referred to as the "plastic airplane" due to its extensive use of plastic components. At any given time, around 16,000 planes are in the sky. The annual global production of plastics has doubled since the start of the 21st century, reaching nearly 400 million metric tons in 2021. Despite an average lifespan of 10 years for plastic products, they can take up to 1,000 years to decompose based on their chemical composition and polymer nature.

Microplastics, defined as plastic particles between 1 and 1,000 μm[29] or 1 and 5,000 μm, and nanoplastics, which range from 1 to 1,000 nm, have become ubiquitous in the environment.[30] An estimated 358 trillion microplastic particles float on the surface of the world's oceans, with countless more in deeper waters. Microplastics are often mistaken for food by marine life, posing significant ecological risks. They have been detected in human samples, indicating exposure through ingestion, inhalation, and skin contact **(Fig. 3)**. Research has shown that microplastics can cause oxidative stress, DNA damage, organ dysfunction, metabolic disorders, immune responses, neurotoxicity, and reproductive and developmental toxicity in humans. Epidemiological studies suggest a link between microplastic exposure and various chronic diseases.

Carcinogens and endocrine-disrupting chemicals found in plastics have been linked to various health issues, ranging from infertility and miscarriage to obesity, diabetes, and cancer. Microplastics and nanoplastics, resulting from the degradation of larger plastic objects, have become pervasive pollutants in the environment. These particles have been detected in various human

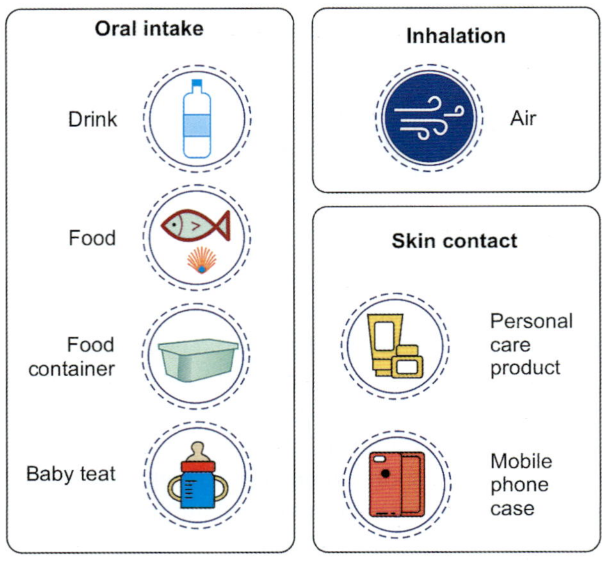

Fig. 3: Pathways of human exposure to microplastics.

tissues, indicating their ability to infiltrate the human body. Recent findings, including the presence of microplastics in human placenta and meconium, raise significant concerns about their potential impact on reproductive health. Maternal exposure to certain types of microplastics has been associated with adverse outcomes such as fetal growth restriction and altered placental metabolism.[31] A recent study addressed the research gap concerning the effects of PE, one of the most widely produced plastics, on pregnancy outcomes. The study investigated the impact of maternal exposure to PE micro- and nanoplastics on fetal growth and placental function using a mouse model. While fetal growth remained unaffected, the study revealed a significant effect on placental function, suggesting potential adverse pregnancy outcomes.

Recent studies have detected microplastic particles in human placental tissues, raising concerns about their potential impact on fetal development. Maternal exposure to microplastics, especially those containing endocrine-disrupting chemicals found in personal care products, may affect fetal growth and placental function, contributing to pregnancy loss. Studies have shown that microplastics can accumulate in fetal organs, leading to oxidative stress, metabolic disruptions, and alterations in immune responses. Animal studies have demonstrated that ingestion of microplastics leads to inflammation in the intestine, affecting immune responses and increasing oxidative stress levels, which can impact fetal development and contribute to pregnancy loss. Studies have shown that maternal exposure to PE microplastics alters immune-related factors and gut microbiota composition, potentially increasing the risk of adverse pregnancy outcomes.

Gene dysregulation: While specific genes have been implicated in certain cases of pregnancy loss, such as genes involved in blood clotting disorders (e.g., factor V Leiden mutation) or immune system dysregulation [e.g., human leukocyte antigen (*HLA*) genes], there is no single set of genes that can account for all cases of pregnancy loss. Moreover, many cases of pregnancy loss may involve complex interactions between multiple genetic and environmental factors. The *HLA* genes, which play a crucial role in the immune system's function, have been of particular interest in pregnancy loss research. Variations in *HLA* genes have been associated with an increased risk of pregnancy complications, including recurrent miscarriage and preeclampsia. These genes encode proteins involved in immune responses, including the recognition and rejection of foreign tissues, such as those of the fetus during pregnancy.

Literature currently suggests that genetics has only 10% role to play, whereas the environment plays 90% role in health and disease.

- Environmental pollutants such as microplastics can interact with genetic predispositions, increasing the risk of adverse pregnancy outcomes.
- Environment may alter genotype owing to sporadic mutations.

Protecting maternal and fetal health from the pervasive threat of microplastics requires interdisciplinary efforts, robust research, and effective public health interventions. Integrating genetic and microbiome research with studies on environmental exposures such as microplastic exposure is essential. Some microbes thrive in the presence of microplastics, while others are negatively impacted. Acetylcholinesterase (AChE), an enzyme influenced by sex hormones and certain drugs, plays a critical role in breaking down the neurotransmitter acetylcholine at neuromuscular junctions.[32] This, along with other health implications, is depicted in **Figure 4**.

Large-scale recycling, banning single-use plastic, and promotion of nonplastic materials for everyday items, such as paper, jute, or cotton bags, and encouraging responsible disposal and recycling practices are important.

EPIGENETICS

Epigenetics refers to changes in gene expression that do not involve alterations to the underlying DNA sequence and may play a role in pregnancy loss, although the exact mechanisms are not fully understood (Chapter 37). These changes can be influenced by various factors, including environmental exposures, lifestyle, and maternal health during pregnancy.

Alterations in the epigenetic regulation of genes involved in embryonic development, placental function, and immune response may contribute to pregnancy loss. For example, changes in DNA methylation, histone modifications and microribonucleic acid (miRNA) expression patterns have been implicated in pregnancy complications. These epigenetic alterations can affect the expression of genes critical for proper embryo implantation, placental development, and fetal growth.

Factors such as maternal age, exposure to environmental toxins, stress, nutrition, and lifestyle habits

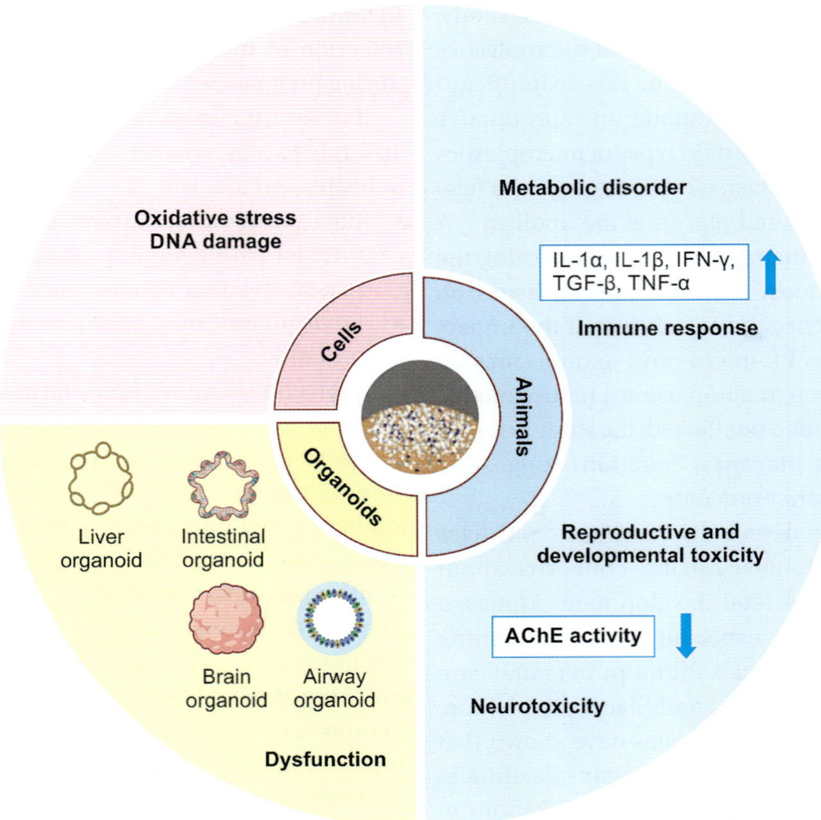

Fig. 4: Toxic effects of microplastics. (AChE: acetylcholinesterase; IFN-γ: Interferon gamma; IL: interleukin; TGF-β: transforming growth factor beta; TNF-α: tumor necrosis factor alpha)

can influence epigenetic modifications during pregnancy. Additionally, certain medical conditions, such as diabetes and obesity, have been associated with epigenetic changes that may increase the risk of pregnancy loss.

The field of epigenetics in reproductive health is still evolving. Understanding how epigenetic mechanisms contribute to pregnancy loss may lead to the development of new diagnostic tools and therapeutic interventions to improve pregnancy outcomes.

DEPRESSION, ANXIETY, AND STRESS

Chronic stress, in particular, may have a cumulative effect on reproductive health over time. Prolonged exposure to stressors can lead to dysregulation of the hypothalamic-pituitary-adrenal (HPA) axis, which plays a key role in regulating stress responses and hormone production. Dysregulation of the HPA axis can disrupt menstrual cycles, ovulation, and implantation, potentially increasing the risk of pregnancy loss.[33]

Additionally, stress can influence behaviors and lifestyle factors that may indirectly affect pregnancy outcomes. For example, individuals experiencing high levels of stress may be more likely to engage in unhealthy coping mechanisms such as smoking, excessive drinking, or poor dietary habits, which can negatively impact fertility and pregnancy.

Stress can trigger physiological responses in the body, including the release of stress hormones such as cortisol and adrenaline. These hormones can affect the function of the reproductive system by disrupting hormonal balance, altering blood flow to the uterus, and impacting immune function. It is important to note that the relationship between stress and pregnancy loss is complex and multifaceted. Not all individuals who experience stress will have pregnancy complications, and many factors contribute to pregnancy outcomes. However, managing stress through techniques such as relaxation exercises, mindfulness, therapy, and social support may be beneficial for overall well-being and reproductive health.

AUTOSOMAL GENES, ABERRANT SIGNAL TRANSDUCTION, AND PREGNANCY

Aberrant signal transduction, which refers to disruptions in the normal processes by which cells communicate and respond to signals, can indeed contribute to pregnancy loss. Signal transduction pathways play crucial roles in various aspects of reproductive physiology, including fertilization, implantation, and embryonic development. Dysregulation of these pathways can disrupt normal cellular functions and increase the risk of pregnancy complications, including miscarriage.

Several signaling pathways are essential for successful pregnancy, including those involving hormones such as progesterone, estrogen, and human chorionic gonadotropin (hCG), as well as growth factors, cytokines, and cell adhesion molecules. Abnormalities in these signaling pathways can impair embryo implantation, placental development, and fetal growth, leading to pregnancy loss. For example, abnormalities in the progesterone signaling pathway can disrupt the maintenance of the uterine lining and increase the risk of miscarriage. Similarly, dysregulation of signaling pathways involved in trophoblast invasion and placental development can lead to placental insufficiency and pregnancy loss. The maternal immune system undergoes complex changes during pregnancy to tolerate the developing fetus while still providing protection against infection. Dysregulation of immune signaling pathways can lead to immune dysfunction, inflammation, and autoimmune reactions that may contribute to pregnancy complications, including miscarriage. Various factors can contribute to aberrant signal transduction during pregnancy, including genetic factors, hormonal imbalances, environmental exposures, and underlying medical conditions such as diabetes, autoimmune disorders, or infections. Additionally, lifestyle factors such as smoking, alcohol consumption, poor nutrition, and stress can also affect signaling pathways and increase the risk of pregnancy loss.

Understanding the role of aberrant signal transduction in pregnancy loss is essential for developing new diagnostic tools and identifying potential therapeutic targets.

CONCLUSION

There is no easy and simple way to uncover and establish the genes and causative factors responsible for the loss of pregnancy. However, it is possible to screen the couple for all the known mutations that have been putatively implicated with the loss of pregnancy. The list includes the following categories:

- Y chromosome linked known loci responsible for loss of pregnancy
- Autosomal genes known to sustain pregnancy
- Gene interactomes that are involved in regulating pregnancy
- Microbiomes that are implicated in the sustenance of pregnancy
- Microplastics that are known to affect growth and development of fetus and loss of pregnancy
- Stress, pollution, depression, and unhealthy lifestyle that are known to be the cause of loss of pregnancy
- Defective spermatozoa that could be the cause of loss of pregnancy
- Contaminated food, water, overdose of medicine, wrong medicine, and abuse of substances and alcohol could be the cause of loss of pregnancy.

There could be more such reasons for pregnancy failure. Systematic work on every single aspect will require massive funding and mega infrastructural facilities. This will generate a large quantum of data that needs to be managed and interpreted. For this purpose, artificial intelligence (AI), deep learning, and machine learning tools of bioinformatics may be used. Network-based analysis will help find out the actual culprit and not the suspected ones. In this context, data mining and data annotation based on the publication are envisaged to be of great relevance.

REFERENCES

1. Hyde KJ, Schust DJ. Genetic considerations in recurrent pregnancy loss. Cold Spring Harb Perspect Med. 2015;5:a023119.
2. El Hachem H, Crepaux V, May-Panloup P, Descamps P, Legendre G, Bouet PE. Recurrent pregnancy loss: current perspectives. Int J Womens Health. 2017;9:331-45.
3. Melo P, Dhillon-Smith R, Islam MA, Devall A, Coomarasamy A. Genetic causes of sporadic and recurrent miscarriage. Fertil Steril. 2023;120:940-4.
4. Parikh FR, Athalye AS, Naik NJ, Naik DJ, Sanap RR, Madon PF. Preimplantation genetic testing: its evolution, where are we today? J Hum Reprod Sci. 2018;11:306-14.
5. Pathak D, Baksi A, Vasan SS, Dighe RR. Molecular and functional characterization of human sex-determining region on the Y chromosome variants using protamine 1 promoter. DNA Cell Biol. 2024;43:12-25.
6. Ali S. Genomics of Y chromosome. In: Arora M, Konje JC (Eds). Recurrent Pregnancy Loss. New Delhi: Jaypee Brothers Medical Publishers (P) Ltd.; 2007. p. 32.

7. Premi S, Srivastava J, Panneer G, Ali S. Startling mosaicism of the Y-chromosome and tandem duplication of the SRY and DAZ genes in patients with Turner syndrome. PLoS One. 2008;3:e3796.
8. Cooke H. Repeated sequence specific to human males. Nature. 1976;262:182-6.
9. Nakahori Y, Yamada M, Nakagome Y. Very low rate Y-chromosome mosaicism (1:5,400) detectable by a novel probe enzyme combination. Jap J Human Genet. 1989;34:203-8.
10. Parizadeh M, Arrieta MC. The global human gut microbiome: genes, lifestyles, and diet. Trends Mol Med. 2023;29:789-801.
11. Lu X, Shi Z, Jiang L, Zhang S. Maternal gut microbiota in the health of mothers and offspring: from the perspective of immunology. Front Immunol. 2024;15:1362784.
12. Kuang YS, Lu JH, Li SH, Li JH, Yuan MY, He JR, et al. Connections between the human gut microbiome and gestational diabetes mellitus. Gigascience. 2017;6:1-12.
13. Cornelius DC. Preeclampsia: from inflammation to immunoregulation. Clin Med Insights Blood Disord. 2018;11:1179545X1775232.
14. Sehring J, Beltsos A, Jeelani R. Human implantation: the complex interplay between endometrial receptivity, inflammation, and the microbiome. Placenta. 2022;117:179-86.
15. Bardos J, Fiorentino D, Longman RE, Paidas M. Immunological role of the maternal uterine microbiome in pregnancy: pregnancies pathologies and alterated microbiota. Front Immunol. 2020;10:2823.
16. Holdcroft AM, Ireland DJ, Payne MS. The vaginal microbiome in health and disease—what role do common intimate hygiene practices play? Microorganisms. 2023;11:298.
17. Notarbartolo V, Giuffrè M, Montante C, Corsello G, Carta M. Composition of human breast milk microbiota and its role in children's health. Pediatr Gastroenterol Hepatol Nutr. 2022;25:194-210.
18. Jiang I, Yong PJ, Allaire C, Bedaiwy MA. Intricate connections between the microbiota and endometriosis. Int J Mol Sci. 2021;22:5644.
19. Porter CM, Shrestha E, Peiffer LB, Sfanos KS. The microbiome in prostate inflammation and prostate cancer. Prostate Cancer Prostatic Dis. 2018;21:345-54.
20. Sender R, Fuchs S, Milo R. Revised estimates for the number of human and bacteria cells in the body. PLoS Biol. 2016;14:e1002533.
21. Niedzwiecki MM, Miller GW. The exposome paradigm in human health: lessons from the Emory exposome summer course. Environ Health Perspect. 2017;125:064502.
22. Farooqui A, Ali S. Nuances of Restlessness and Epistemology of Happiness. New Delhi: Aargon Press; 2024.
23. Gómez-Roig MD, Pascal R, Cahuana MJ, García-Algar O, Sebastiani G, Andreu-Fernández V, et al. Environmental exposure during pregnancy: influence on prenatal development and early life: a comprehensive review. Fetal Diagn Ther. 2021;48:245-57.
24. Zinia SS, Yang KH, Lee EJ, Lim MN, Kim J, Kim WJ, et al. Effects of heavy metal exposure during pregnancy on birth outcomes. Sci Rep. 2023;13:18990.
25. Saenen ND, Martens DS, Neven KY, Alfano R, Bové H, Janssen BG, et al. Air pollution-induced placental alterations: an interplay of oxidative stress, epigenetics, and the aging phenotype? Clin Epigenetics. 2019;11:124.
26. Thangavel P, Park D, Lee YC. Recent insights into particulate matter (PM2.5)-mediated toxicity in humans: an overview. Int J Environ Res Public Health. 2022;19:7511.
27. Islam S, Mohanty SK. Maternal exposure to cooking smoke and risk of low birth weight in India. Sci Total Environ. 2021;774:145717.
28. Thompson RC, Olsen Y, Mitchell RP, Davis A, Rowland SJ, John AW, et al. Lost at sea: where is all the plastic? Science. 2004;304:838.
29. Hartmann NB, Hüffer T, Thompson RC, Hassellöv M, Verschoor A, Daugaard AE, et al. Are we speaking the same language? Recommendations for a definition and categorization framework for plastic debris. Environ Sci Technol. 2019;53:1039-47.
30. Frias JPGL, Nash R. Microplastics: finding a consensus on the definition. Mar Pollut Bull. 2019;138:145-7.
31. Panneerselvam D, Murugesan A. Maternal microplastic exposure during pregnancy and risk of gestational diabetes mellitus associated with gut dysbiosis. Med Microecol. 2023;18:100091.
32. Pilz W. Acetylcholinesterase. In: Bergmeyer HU (Ed). Methods of Enzymatic Analysis. Amsterdam: Elsevier; 1965. pp. 765-70.
33. Joseph D, Whirledge S. Stress and the HPA axis: balancing homeostasis and fertility. Int J Mol Sci. 2017;18:2224.

CHAPTER

10 Preimplantation Genetic Screening

Durga G Rao, Kavya Rao Jalagam

ABSTRACT

Preimplantation genetic screening is subdivided into preimplantation genetic testing for aneuploidy (PGT-A), PGT-SR for structural defects, and PGT-M for monogenic disorders. PGT-HLA is for couples who plan a pregnancy for the cure of a lethal disease in the elder sibling. Aneuploidy is an established cause of recurrent pregnancy loss (RPL). Currently, the success rates of IVF with PGT are not better than spontaneous pregnancy. With improvement in biopsy techniques and standardization of noninvasive PGT, this equation may change.

Keywords: PGT-A, PGT-SR, PGT-M, PGT-HLA, RPL.

INTRODUCTION

Genetic abnormalities are most commonly implicated in recurrent first-trimester miscarriages. In this chapter, the role of preimplantation genetic screening in avoiding genetic causes of recurrent pregnancy loss (RPL) is described in detail.

EMBRYONIC GENETIC CAUSES OF RECURRENT PREGNANCY LOSS

Miscarriage may be due to numerical chromosomal abnormalities, which arise due to meiotic nondisjunction, i.e., when homologous chromosomes or sister chromatids fail to separate properly resulting in chromosomal disorders. (e.g., trisomy or monosomy), or aberrant fertilization (e.g., triploidy), or embryogenesis (e.g., tetraploidy).

Another reason for miscarriages is structural chromosomal abnormalities (e.g., translocations and inversions) arising from the inheritance of a derivative chromosome[1] (the chromosome resulting from a translocation).

However, an increasing number of previous miscarriages in a woman are most likely to be associated with euploid products of conception (POC),[2] implying that there could be other reasons for miscarriage, rather than embryonic, in higher-order miscarriages. According to Ogasawara et al.,[2] as the number of miscarriages increases, the embryo involved is more likely to be euploid.

In a small study, it was shown that irrespective of the number of prior miscarriages, the probability of a euploid embryo remains the same, which denotes that a higher number of miscarriages in a woman does not mean higher aneuploidy.

In some pregnancies with euploid embryo miscarriages, the embryo was diagnosed with morphological defects on embryoscopy, which explains why some euploid embryos still miscarry. Unfortunately, morphological defects leading to miscarriage cannot be picked by genetic analysis.

Women with RPL have been known to be associated with higher aneuploid embryos than normal fertile controls.[1,2] But if a woman has aneuploid embryo miscarriage diagnosed by analysis of POC, it is likely that it was sporadic, and she may have a better pregnancy outcome in her next conception and should be counseled and reassured appropriately.

Nussbaum et al.[3] observed that the karyotypic abnormalities that are more likely to result in a miscarriage are:

- Polyploid embryos
- 45,X
- Trisomy 16, 18, 21, and other trisomies
- Structural anomalies

Unbalanced rearrangements in chromosomes have a higher risk of miscarriage, but balanced rearrangement, 47,XXY, 47,XXX, and 47,XYY have a lower incidence of miscarriage.

Meiotic Differences between Sperm and Oocyte

Oocytes, which develop synaptic defects in the prophase 1 or metaphase 1, still have the ability to retain viability. Also, oocytes have a longer duration until ovulation in which genetic insults such as disturbances in the synaptonemal complex and loss of cohesion between homologs and sister chromatids can occur. Whereas, in comparison, in spermatocytes, synaptic defects cause apoptosis and cannot retain viability.

Many of these aneuploidies are derived as a function of maternal age[4] probably because spermatocytes with synaptic defects in the pachytene phase of prophase 1 or metaphase 1 undergo apoptosis, unlike the oocytes with similar defects, which retain the viability.

Structural Chromosomal Rearrangements

Mostly 2–5% of the couples who had RPL are found to have structural chromosomal abnormalities compared to 0.2% of the general population. A translocation can be reciprocal in which exchange occurs between two chromosomes with double-strand breakage and nonhomologous end joining or by recombination,[5] or it may be Robertsonian, wherein two acrocentric chromosomes (chromosomes 13, 14, 15, 21, and 22) break and recombine with the long arms fusing at the centromere to form a separate chromosome.[5] With repeated cell divisions, the short-arm rearrangement is lost **(Figs. 1A to F)**.

Patients with these translocations are phenotypically normal unless the breakpoint involves a critical gene. But the gametes from these individuals may be unbalanced resulting in miscarriage.[5] The probability of translocation increases with the increase in miscarriages.

The association between the type of parental chromosomal rearrangement and risk of subsequent miscarriage also appears dependent on the type of rearrangement, as miscarriage rates for parents with reciprocal translocations, inversions, Robertsonian translocations, and other types of chromosomal anomalies have been shown to be 54%, 49%, 34%, and 27% respectively.[1,6]

Some translocations can be missed by karyotyping as they could not be picked up because of the sub-resolution and some owing to the similar banding patterns and/or comparable sizes shared by the two segments exchanged.

Inversions result in two double-stranded breakages in a single chromosome and subsequent reversal of the intervening segment. The individual as such is phenotypically normal, but unbalanced gametes may result because a loop is necessary for chromosomal alignment during meiosis and recombination can occur in the loop.[5]

Why do Euploid Embryos Fail to Implant?

A major factor in the failed implantation of euploid embryos is poor quality blastocyst that is either a low quantity inner cell mass or trophectoderm quality.

A blastocyst at day 6 or 7, developing late from a morula, and a spontaneous blastocyst collapse were all associated with poorer reproductive outcomes, even if the embryo is euploid.

Multiple vitrification-warming cycles, which may need to be done if the decision of preimplantation genetic testing (PGT) was taken after vitrifying embryos, meaning embryos will have to be thawed, biopsied, and then vitrified again. Once results are obtained, the embryo has to undergo a re-thaw for performing the embryo transfer (ET), which could reduce implantation rates.

Why do Euploid Embryos Miscarry?

In some instances of pregnancy loss, though the POC may show euploid karyotype, there may be aberrations in the genes that may be responsible for pregnancy loss but are not currently known or cannot be assessed. These include single-nucleotide variants (SNVs) that affect individual genes and are detectable by next generation sequencing, or small sub-microscopic aberrations that affect a cluster of genes and are detectable by microarray analysis. SNVs may follow an autosomal-recessive or X-linked pattern of inheritance, and thus, have a high-recurrence risk.[7]

Copy number variants (CNVs) may unmask a recessive mutation in a relevant gene or involve dosage-sensitive genes, where loss or gain of copies affects the gene function. Many of these genes are involved in the early development of the embryo and may lead to embryonic lethality when they are functionally "knocked out," resulting in pregnancy loss.[8] Carrier screening of couples with the help of next-generation sequencing (NGS)-based exome sequencing will identify such risks.

Skewed X-chromosome inactivation has also been implicated in euploid RPL.[9,10] A normal female is a mosaic with one-half of the cells expressing paternal

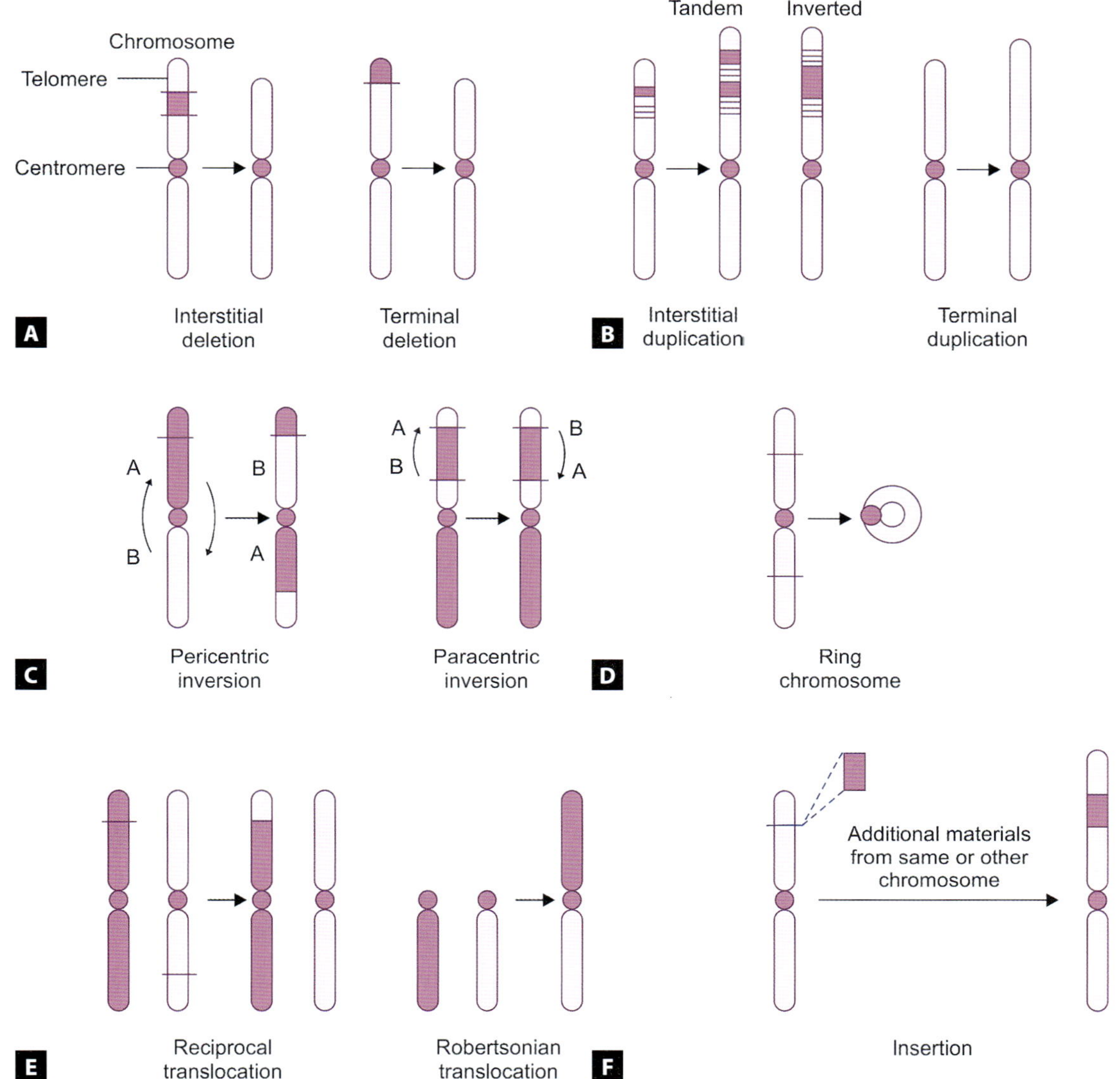

Figs. 1A to F: Types of structural chromosomal rearrangements: (A) Deletions; (B) Duplications; (C) Ring chromosomes; (D) Isochromosomes; (E) Robertsonian translocations; and (F) Reciprocal translocations.

X-chromosome and the other half-expressing maternal X-chromosome. In some cases, the inactivation is such that almost all the somatic cells inactivate only the paternal or maternal X-chromosome, resulting in skewed X-chromosome inactivation. A systematic review in 2015 says that there is no association found between X-chromosome inactivation up to 80–90% with RPL, but X-chromosome inactivation >90% is found to have an association with three or more pregnancy losses.[10,11]

In recurrent molar pregnancies, autosomal-recessive mutations in the genes encoding the cell machinery that labels the parental origin of the two sets of chromosomes are implicated. These genes include *NLRP7, C6orf221, NLRP2* and are usually euploid.[9,12-14]

In addition, there are multiple maternal genotypes associated with RPL in genes such as coagulation genes (e.g., *ANAX5, F2, F5, F13A1, MTHFR, MTRR, MTR, PAI1,* and *VEGFA*), human leukocyte antigen (HLA) polymorphisms (e.g., HLA-G, HLA-DRB1, and HLA-DQB1), immune function-related interleukin (IL) genes [e.g., *IL2, IL3, IL10, IL18, IL21, PROLR2,* and tumor necrosis factor alpha (TNF-α)], and genes affecting oxidative stress and antiapoptosis response in placental trophoblast cells (e.g., SOD2, MDM2).

INVESTIGATIONS FOR GENETIC CAUSES

The two investigations that need to be done for evaluating genetic causes of repeated miscarriages are parental karyotyping and genetic analysis of POC.

When Should Parental Karyotyping be Considered?

Parental karyotyping should be considered under following conditions:

- Previous birth of a child with congenital abnormalities
- Offspring with unbalanced chromosome abnormalities in the family
- Detection of a translocation in the pregnancy tissue

Parental karyotyping can also be done based on the genetic history in other cases.

The European Society of Human Reproduction and Embryology (ESHRE) 2022 does not recommend routine testing of the POC, but it may be considered for explanatory purposes. Routine parental karyotyping is not recommended, but may be considered after individual assessment of the risk.[15] The American Society for Reproductive Medicine (ASRM), on the other hand, recommends genetic testing of the POC and parental karyotyping in RPL patients.[2]

The Royal College of Obstetricians and Gynaecologists (RCOG) recommends cytogenetic analysis on pregnancy tissue on the third and subsequent consecutive pregnancy loss(es). If unbalanced structural chromosome abnormality is found, parental karyotyping is indicated.[6]

Testing the Products of Conception

Conventional metaphase karyotyping by G-banding or Giemsa staining may actually underestimate the proportion of abnormality in the POC due to culture failure and maternal cell contamination resulting in false negatives. Newer techniques for genetic testing such as complete genomic hybridization (CGH) and single nucleotide polymorphism (SNP) microarray are beneficial in this aspect.[1]

Approximately 55–60% of miscarriages are likely to have a chromosomal anomaly and this is detected by doing chromosomal microarray (CMA) on the POC. So, CMA of POC can be advised in women with a history of previous miscarriages to evaluate the correct incidence of unexplained RPL as some of them would have been because of chromosomally abnormal pregnancies.

The advantages of CMA are:

- Better resolution of 10–100 kb
- Can be performed on nonviable tissue such as paraffin-fixed samples
- No culture failure
- Does not require living cells
- Low chance of maternal cell contamination

But the drawback is that it cannot detect balanced translocation and low-level mosaicism. International guidelines differ in their recommendations for genetic studies in patients with RPL as shown in **Table 1**. Comparison between conventional karyotyping and complete genomic hybridization microarray (CGH MA) for POC, CGH is superior to karyotyping **(Table 2)**.

Whole Genome Sequencing and Whole Exome Sequencing

Whole genome sequencing (WGS) involves the sequencing of the entire genome and is the most extensive sequencing method. Exome can be sequenced, i.e., the protein-coding region of the genome constituting approximately 1% of the human genome and estimated to account for 85% of the mutations associated with the disease.[3,9] Usually, whole exome sequencing (WES) is

TABLE 1: International guidelines on genetic testing.

Genetics	*ESHRE*	*DGGG/OEGGG/SGGG*	*ASRM*	*RCOG*
Analysis of parents	In case of increased genetic risk	Parents to be tested	Parents to be tested	Parents to be tested only with evidence of chromosomal disorder in the aborted material
Analysis of embryo	Not recommended	Optional	Not mentioned	Recommended from the third miscarriage

(ASRM: American Society of Reproductive Medicine; DGGG: German Society for Gynecology and Obstetrics; ESHRE: European Society of Human Reproduction and Embryology; OEGGG: Austrian Society for Gynecology and Obstetrics; RCOG: Royal College of Obstetricians and Gynaecologists; SGGG: Swiss Society for Gynecology and Obstetrics)

TABLE 2: Comparison between CGH and karyotyping.

Conventional karyotyping by G-banding	***CGH microarray/SNP array***
Resolution only up to 10 MB	<10 MB
Requires cell culture, high-culture failure rate due to nonviable fetal cells, and high-bacterial contamination	No cell culture is required—so culture failure, contamination, overgrowth of maternal cells, selection against mosaic cell lines
Labor intensive and requires manual microscopic work, and highly qualified trained personnel who can pick up chromosomal rearrangements	Not labor intensive, has no user variability, less time. This is mostly automated and analysis tools are available for the detection of CNVs
Inability to detect submicroscopic deletions, duplications of clinical significance such as CNV, SNV	Microdeletions and microduplications can be detected
Possible false negative results due to maternal cell contamination	Cannot avoid, but labs can rule out maternal cell contamination by running maternal DNA alongside
	Reanalysis of tissues fixed in formalin can be done
	The parental origin of aneuploidy can be known. This is only to prove pathogenicity. For example, if the CNV identified is a variant of uncertain significance, and the parent also carries the same, it is not implicated as pathogenic
	CMA also detects loss of heterozygosity, which is an indication of the possibility of a recessive condition in the product, and further testing such as exome sequencing is required

(CGH: complete genomic hybridization; CMA: chromosomal microarray; CNV: copy number variants; DNA, deoxyribonucleic acid; SNP: single nucleotide polymorphism; SNV: single-nucleotide variants)

preferred as it is cheaper and has a smaller manageable set of data still covering comprehensively the coding regions of deoxyribonucleic acid (DNA). WGS analyzes the whole genome and can detect large structural variants, insertions and deletions, single nucleotide variants (SNV), and CNV.[9]

ROLE OF PREIMPLANTATION GENETIC TESTING FOR ANEUPLOIDY IN RECURRENT PREGNANCY LOSS

Preimplantation genetic testing for aneuploidy (PGT-A) is a technique that allows the identification of chromosomally normal embryos before their transfer into the uterus during an assisted reproductive technology (ART) cycle. By selecting euploid embryos, PGT-A aims to increase the chances of successful implantation, reduce miscarriage rates, and improve live birth rates (LBR).

Preimplantation genetic testing is one of the advanced technologies that can improve reproductive outcomes. There have been a lot of developments with PGT in terms of both clinical application and laboratory aspects for embryo biopsy and genetic screening since its first report in 1990. The updated version is 3.0 as suggested by the ESHRE special interest group. The terminologies of preimplantation genetic screening (PGS) and preimplantation genetic diagnosis (PGD)[16] have changed over the years and are currently together referred to as PGT.

Preimplantation genetic testing is divided into four subtypes as mentioned below:

1. *PGT-A (aneuploidy):* It is used to determine the number of chromosomes in an embryo.
2. *PGT-SR (structural rearrangement):* It screens for structural rearrangements such as translocations, inversions, and deletions in an embryo.
3. *PGT-M (monogenic):* It screens for monogenic disorders such as cystic fibrosis, cancer (autosomal-dominant disorders), Huntington's disease, thalassemia, sickle-cell anemia, hemophilia, Fragile X syndrome, etc.
4. *PGT-HLAs typing:* HLA-matched embryo selection via PGT can help couples who already have an affected child with malignancy, genetic disorder, or an acquired disorder. The affected child can be treated with stem-cell therapy from an HLA-matched sibling.

The change in terminology to PGT along with the usage of comprehensive chromosomal screening (CCS) methods such as NGS has been termed the PGT 3.0 version by the Preimplantation Genetic Diagnosis International Society (PGDIS).

Preimplantation genetic testing for aneuploidy has been proposed as an intervention because the best implantation rates are possible with a transfer of a single euploid embryo with the added advantage of reducing multiple pregnancies, miscarriage rates, time to pregnancy, and live birth. PGT-A is recommended in the case of women with RPL wherein the etiology is idiopathic.

Preimplantation genetic testing-SR can have a therapeutic role in women with a history of RPL where the parental karyotype indicates a structural rearrangement.

Preimplantation genetic testing-SR involves a targeted approach when known chromosomal abnormalities are present in parental genomes and plays a key role in balanced parental translocation diagnosed by karyotyping and in the presence of unbalanced translocation or inversion detected on POC genetic testing.[17,18]

Multiple pregnancies, which are associated with increased risks for both the mother and the developing fetus, can be reduced by the transfer of a euploid embryo after PGT-A.

In couples with RPL and structural chromosomal rearrangements, the 2018 systematic review states that natural conception has similar pregnancy outcomes compared with in vitro fertilization (IVF)–PGD and IVF/intracytoplasmic sperm injection (ICSI) should not be the first-line treatment in view of the cost and unproven benefits.[19]

American Society for Reproductive Medicine, 2018—A Committee Opinion on Preimplantation Genetic Testing for Aneuploidy

The amplification of various tests is shown in **Table 3**.

Future studies are warranted to determine, if any platforms are superior. PGT is done by performing a biopsy on an expanded blastocyst, developed either on day 5 or 6.

ROLE OF PREIMPLANTATION GENETIC TESTING IN RECURRENT PREGNANCY LOSS

Canadian guidelines 2021 state that, in patients with RPL, there is insufficient evidence to recommend PGT-A over expectant management to improve LBR, decrease early pregnancy loss, and decrease time to LBR.[20] These recommendations are based on a single retrospective cohort study published in 2016 by Murugappan et al.[21]

The American Society for Reproductive Medicine also states that there is no evidence suggesting an improved LBR using PGT-A in RPL patients, again due to lack of well-designed and powered studies.

The European Society of Human Reproduction and Embryology guidelines on RPL 2022 also state that the limited evidence for PGT-A in couples with RPL shows no clear benefit of treatment (very low quality evidence).[22] Genetic counseling is advised for all couples with abnormal fetal or parental karyotypes. Those with abnormal fetal or parental karyotypes should be informed about the possible treatment options.

Recently, however, UK Human Fertilisation and Embryology Authority (HFEA) data collection assessing the outcomes of PGT-A and non-PGT-A cycles between 2016 and 2018 has demonstrated the significant benefit of PGT-A compared to morphological selection.[23]

Sacchi et al. studied 2,538 couples undergoing 2,905 egg collections (control group), 308 (PGT-A), and 106 (dropout group, consenting for PGT-A but withdrawing due to poor embryological outcome). Findings reported an improved LBR per transferred embryo (40.3 vs. 11.0%) compared to the control group.[24] These findings

TABLE 3: Comparison of PGT testing.

	FISH	*aCGH*	*qPCR*	*NGS*	*SNP*
CCS	–	+	–	+	+
Minimal resolution	–	6 MB	>20 mb	3 mb	2 mb
Balanced aberrations	Limited	–	–		–
Unbalanced aberrations	+	+		+	+
Single gene defects	–	–	+	+	+/–
Mosaicism	No	4%	No	21%	
Time required		24 hours	4 hours	16 hours	72 hours
For		PGT-A/SR	PGT-M	PGT-A	PGT-SR

(aCGH: array comparative genomic hybridization; CCS: comprehensive chromosomal screening; FISH: fluorescence in-situ hybridization; NGS: next-generation sequencing; PGT-A/SR: preimplantation genetic testing for aneuploidy/structural rearrangement; PGT-M: preimplantation genetic testing for monogenic; qPCR: quantitative polymerase chain reaction)

TABLE 4: Studies published on PGT-A in RPL.

S. no.	References	Study group	CPR	OPR	LBR	BLPR	MR
1.	Kim et al.[28]	RPL PGT-A	73%	65%	62%	–	15%
		RPL	61%	55%	41%	–	32%
2.	Lei et al.[29]	RPL PGT-A	–	46%	44.9%	–	15.7%
		RPL	–	25.1%	25.1%	–	34.6%
3.	Sato et al.[30]	RPL PGT-A	66.7%	–	52.4%	12.5%	14.3%
		RPL	29.7%	–	21.6%	45%	20%
4.	Sui et al.[31]	RPL PGT-A	51.3%	49.57%	43.48%	–	1.74%
		RPL	31.41%	19.87%	18.59%	–	11.54%
5.	Bhatt et al.[32]	RPL PGT-A	–	–	47.7%	9.9%	10.8%
		RPL	–	–	33.6%	11.5%	12.6%
6.	Pantou et al.[33]	RPL PGT-A	–	–	50%	0%	18.1%
		RPL	–	–	12.5%	7.1%	75%
7.	Pavlovic et al.[34]	RPL PGT-A	58.8%	–	44.3%	–	12.4%
		RPL	45.6%	–	32%	–	12.2%

(BLPR: biological pregnancy loss rate; CPR: clinical pregnancy rate; LBR: live birth rate; MR: miscarriage rate; OPR: ongoing pregnancy rate; PGT-A: preimplantation genetic testing for aneuploidy; RPL: recurrent pregnancy loss)

support the notion that PGT-A facilitates the selection of chromosomally normal embryos, resulting in improved pregnancy outcomes.[25,26] The ability to identify and transfer euploid embryos with a higher likelihood of successful implantation and ongoing development contributes to the increased clinical pregnancy and LBRs observed in the PGT-A group.

A retrospective study was conducted by us at OASIS Fertility in 2020, including 112 idiopathic RPL patients (patients with previous two or more pregnancy losses). Eighty-two patients underwent PGT-A (study group) and 30 patients did not undergo PGT-A (control group). The study group underwent elective euploid single embryo transfer (eSET) whereas the control group underwent transfer of two blastocysts [double embryo transfer (DET)]. We found a marked reduction in the miscarriage rate with PGT-A in RPL patients (9.68 vs. 23.33%)[27] and no multiple pregnancy, showing an advantage of the intervention.

Kim et al.[28] and Lei et al.[29] showed that miscarriage rates were reduced and LBRs increased in unexplained RPL due to PGT-A. Sato et al.[30] showed that PGT improved the LBR per embryo transfer and biochemical rate. Sui et al.[31] also gave the same conclusions. **Table 4** summarizes the studies published on PGT-A in RPL. (See also Appendix 1 Case 12)

LIMITATIONS OF STUDIES OF PREIMPLANTATION GENETIC TESTING FOR ANEUPLOIDY IN RECURRENT PREGNANCY LOSS

The data from some published studies is limited by:
- Small numbers for analysis in published studies
- Retrospective nature of studies
- Different platforms of CCS in different studies
- Some studies being included conducted FISH (fluorescence in situ hybridization) for genetic evaluation
- Inclusion of studies where biopsy was done on day 3

Pitfalls of PGT-A[20,35,36] are summarized in **Table 5**.

MOSAICISM

The presence of two (or more) distinct cytogenetic populations of cells in an embryo or individual derived from a single fertilized oocyte is defined as mosaicism (Spinner and Conlin, 2014).[37] It is the result of postzygotic errors, i.e., chromosome segregation errors occurring during the first mitotic divisions. Embryos diagnosed as mosaic based on trophectoderm analysis may be fully euploid, fully aneuploid, mosaic for a euploid, and an aneuploid cell line, or mosaic for two or more different

TABLE 5: Pitfalls of PGT-A.

Error category	*Examples*
Human error	• Mislabeling • Misinterpretation of results/report • Transfer of the wrong embryo
Technical factors	• DNA contamination • DNA amplification error • CCS platform used • Biopsy technique leading to embryo wastage • No DNA detected/noninformative embryos • Poor survival post-thaw • Advanced skill and infrastructure requirement • Sensitivity for detection of chromosomal abnormality <3–10 Mb, which means any abnormality beyond this sensitivity can't be detected accurately
Intrinsic embryo factors	Mosaicism leading to discard of potentially euploid embryos
Others	• Costly intervention • Risk of having no blastocyst in women of advanced maternal age • Natural conception around the time of ET

(CCS: comprehensive chromosome screening; DNA: deoxyribonucleic acid; ET: embryo transfer)
Sources: Munné et al.[35] and Wilton et al.[36]

abnormal cell lines, if inner cell mass were to be tested. This might result in the discarding of normal embryos or the transfer of abnormal embryos resulting in negative results. This is one of the hindrances in advocating PGT on a wider scale.

RETROSPECTIVE ANALYSIS OF UNEXPLAINED RECURRENT PREGNANCY LOSS

Personal data of OASIS clinic from 2014 to 2022 is summarized in **Table 6**.

Box 1 depicts the odds ratio and confidence interval (CI) for live births in PGT versus non-PGT cohort.

Box 2 depicts the odds ratio and CI for miscarriage rates in PGT versus non-PGT cohort.

TABLE 6: Personal data from OASIS clinic.

RPL with PGT—160 patients	*Control group – RPL – No PGT – 168 patients*
Miscarriage—8/127 = 6.6%	Miscarriage—35/168 = 21%
Live birth—88/127 = 69%	Live birth—76/168 = 45%
Negative—31/127 = 24.4%	Negative—57/168 =34%
Drop-out after 1st ET = 21%	Drop-out after 1st ET = 26%
2nd ET—2 +ve	2nd ET—23+ ve
71% cumulative live birth 59% cumulative live birth	

(ET: embryo transfer; PGT: preimplantation genetic testing; RPL: recurrent pregnancy loss)

BOX 1: Live births in PGT versus non-PGT cohort.

LBR—71% ($n = 127$) versus 59% ($n = 168$)
- Odds ratio: 0.5899
- 95% CI: 0.3610–0.9637
- *Z* static: 2.108
- Significance level, $p = 0.035$

(CI: confidence interval; LBR: live birth rate)

BOX 2: Miscarriage rates in PGT versus non-PGT cohort.

PGT group: 6.7% versus non-PGT group: 29%
- Odds ratio: 0.1692
- 95% CI: 0.0684–0.4186
- *Z* statistic: 3.845
- Significance level, $p = 0.0001$

(CI: confidence interval; LBR: live birth rate; PGT preimplantation genetic testing)

Study Conclusion

Our studies show that the cumulative LBR is higher with PGT-A intervention than with no intervention. Miscarriage following PGT-A is lower than when no intervention is used but the drawback is that few may not reach the ET stage.

Study Limitations

- The cost of intervention is not analyzed.
- Time to pregnancy between the two groups is not evaluated.

CONCLUSION

Recurrent pregnancy loss is rather an emotionally and psychologically distressing situation for the couple. However, the outcomes for livebirth are reasonably good with expectant management even after a history of recurrent miscarriages. The evidence, though at present, is trending toward recommending IVF/ICSI and PGT in a subset of couples with recurrent aneuploid losses to improve live birth outcomes. But, PGT-A might only improve outcomes per embryo transfer and not per cycle started as a significant proportion of patients may not even reach the embryo transfer stage. However, with increasing evidence, it can be said that PGT-A reduces the risk of further miscarriages in these women, as opposed to just IVF/ICSI or expectant management.

It may be considered safely when a female partner has a normal ovarian reserve producing a high number of oocytes and blastocysts that may be available for biopsy. In older patients and women with diminished ovarian reserve, few oocytes are retrieved and the selection technique of PGT-A may become counterproductive. So PGT-A should be utilized in this group with proper counseling and explanations of the possibility of cycle cancellation but with the advantage of improved implantation and reduced miscarriage risk if a euploid embryo were to be transferred. PGT-A is associated with improvement in live birth and clinical pregnancy in women with RPL undergoing frozen embryo transfer (FET), with the largest difference noted in the group of women with age >42 years.[38]

In the fertile RPL patient population, there does not appear to be a clear benefit to proceeding directly with fertility treatment. Patients could be encouraged to attempt spontaneous conception for at least 6 months.[39,40]

A single attempt at PGT was compared with 6 months of attempting spontaneous conception. PGT is not effective in improving LBR or decreasing clinical miscarriage rate compared with expectant management, except in those PGT cycles that complete the transfer of a euploid embryo, where the LBR is greater.[41]

Success rates with PGT are limited by the high incidence of cycles that intend to perform PGT, but cancel PGT cycle, due to no blastocysts[42] developing, or cycles that do not reach transfer due to nonavailability of an euploid embryo, and a higher no transfer rate is seen in women over 35 years of age. Counseling RPL patients on their treatment options should include not only success rates with PGT per euploid embryo transferred, which is increased and reduced miscarriages but also LBR per initiated PGT cycle.

The role of PGT in RPL patients will be further established by a study that is currently being undertaken.[43] More well-designed randomized and adequately powered studies in the future are needed for establishing firmly the role of PGT, in unexplained RPL.

REFERENCES

1. Practice Committee of the American Society for Reproductive Medicine. Evaluation and treatment of recurrent pregnancy loss: a committee opinion. Fertil Steril. 2012;98(5):1103-11.
2. Ogasawara M, Aoki K, Okada S, Suzumori K. Embryonic karyotype of abortuses in relation to the number of previous miscarriages. Fertil Steril. 2000;73(2):300-4.
3. Nussbaum RL, McInnes RR, Willard HF. Principles of clinical cytogenetics and genome analysis. In: Cohn R, Scherer S, Hamosh A (Eds). Thompson & Thompson Genetics and Genomics in Medicine, 8th edition. Philadelphia: Elsevier; 2016. pp. 57-74.
4. Royal College of Obstetricians and Gynaecologists. (2011). The investigation and treatment of couples with recurrent first-trimester and second-trimester miscarriage. Green-top Guideline No. 17. [online] Available from https://www.rcog.org.uk/media/3cbgonl0/gtg_17.pdf. [Last accessed December, 2024].
5. Hunt PA, Hassold TJ. Sex matters in meiosis. Science. 2002;296(5576):2181-3.
6. Kaser D. The status of genetic screening in recurrent pregnancy loss. Obstet Gynecol Clin North Am. 2018;45(1):143-54.
7. Choi M, Scholl UI, Ji W, Liu T, Tikhonova IR, Zumbo P, et al. Genetic diagnosis by whole exome capture and massively parallel DNA sequencing. Proc Natl Acad Sci U S A. 2009;106(45):19096-101.
8. Wilson R, Geyer SH, Reissig L, Rose J, Szumska D, Hardman E, et al. Highly variable penetrance of abnormal phenotypes in embryonic lethal knockout mice. Wellcome Open Res. 2017;1:1.
9. Colley E, Hamilton S, Smith P, Morgan NV, Coomarasamy A, Allen S. Potential genetic causes of miscarriage in euploid pregnancies: a systematic review. Hum Reprod Update. 2019;25(4):452-72.
10. Bagislar S, Ustuner I, Cengiz B, Soylemez F, Akyerli CB, Ceylaner S, et al. Extremely skewed X-chromosome inactivation patterns in women with recurrent spontaneous abortion. Aust N Z J Obstet Gynecol. 2006;46(5):384-7.
11. Sui Y, Chen Q, Sun X. Association of skewed X chromosome inactivation and idiopathic recurrent spontaneous abortion: a systematic review and meta-analysis. Reprod Biomed Online. 2015;31(2):140-8.
12. Andreasen L, Christiansen OB, Niemann I, Bolund L, Sunde L. NLRP7 or KHDC3L genes and the etiology of molar pregnancies and recurrent miscarriage. Mol Hum Reprod. 2013;19(11):773-81.
13. Aghajanova L, Mahadevan S, Altmae S, Stavreus-Evers A, Regan L, Sebire N, et al. No evidence for mutations in NLRP7, NLRP2 or KHDC3L in women with unexplained recurrent pregnancy loss or infertility. Hum Reprod. 2015;30(1):232-38.

14. Manokhina I, Hanna CW, Stephenson MD, McFadden DE, Robinson WP. Maternal NLRP7 and C6orf221 variants are not a common risk factor for androgenetic moles, triploidy and recurrent miscarriage. Mol Hum Reprod 2013;19(8):539-44.
15. ESHRE Guideline Group on RPL, Atik RB, Christiansen OB, Elson J, Kolte AM, Lewis S, et al. ESHRE guideline: recurrent pregnancy loss: an update. Hum Reprod Open. 2023'Mar2;2023(1):hoad002.
16. Kort JD, McCoy RC, Demko Z, Lathi RB. Are blastocyst aneuploidy rates different between fertile and infertile populations? J Assist Reprod Genet. 2018;35(3):403-8.
17. Viotti M. Preimplantation genetic testing for chromosomal abnormalities: aneuploidy, mosaicism, and structural rearrangements. Genes (Basel). 2020;11(6):602.
18. ESHRE PGT Consortium Steering Committee, Carvalho F, Coonen E, Goossens V, Kokkali G, Rubio C, et al. ESHRE PGT consortium good practice recommendations for the organisation of PGT. Hum Reprod Open. 2020;2020(3):hoaa021.
19. Iews M, Tan J, Taskin O, Alfaraj S, AbdelHafez FF, Abdellah AH, et al. Does preimplantation genetic diagnosis improve reproductive outcome in couples with recurrent pregnancy loss owing to structural chromosomal rearrangement? A systematic review. Reprod Biomed Online. 2018;36(6):677-85.
20. Chan C, Ryu M, Zwingerman R. Preimplantation genetic testing for aneuploidy: A Canadian Fertility and Andrology Society Guideline. Reprod Biomed Online. 2021;42(1):105-16.
21. Murugappan G, Shahine LK, Perfetto CO, Hickok LR, Lathi RB. Intent to treat analysis of in vitro fertilization and preimplantation genetic screening versus expectant management in patients with recurrent pregnancy loss. Hum Reprod. 2016;31(8):1668-74.
22. Practice Committees of the American Society for Reproductive Medicine and the Society for Assisted Reproductive Technology. The use of preimplantation genetic testing for aneuploidy (PGT-A): a committee opinion. Fertil Steril. 2018;109(3):429-36.
23. Sanders KD, Silvestri G, Gordon T, Griffin DK. Analysis of IVF live birth outcomes with and without preimplantation genetic testing for aneuploidy (PGT-A): UK Human Fertilisation and Embryology Authority data collection 2016–2018. J Assist Reprod Genet. 2021;38(12):3277-85.
24. Sacchi L, Albani E, Cesana A, Smeraldi A, Parini V, Fabiani M, et al. Preimplantation genetic testing for aneuploidy improves clinical, gestational, and neonatal outcomes in advanced maternal age patients without compromising cumulative live-birth rate. J Assist Reprod Genet. 2019;36(12):2493-504.
25. Yang Z, Liu J, Collins GS, Salem SA, Liu X, Lyle SS, et al. Selection of single blastocysts for fresh transfer via standard morphology assessment alone and with array CGH for good prognosis IVF patients: results from a randomized pilot study. Mol Cytogenet. 2012;5(1):24.
26. Mastenbroek S, Twisk M, van der Veen F, Repping S. Preimplantation genetic screening: a systematic review and meta-analysis of RCTs. Hum Reprod Update. 2011;17(4):454-66.
27. Mantravadi K, Mathew S, Soorve S, Rao DG, Karunakaran S. Does pre-implantation genetic testing for aneuploidy optimise the reproductive outcomes in women with idiopathic recurrent pregnancy loss? Fertil Steril. 2020;114(3):e437.
28. Kim JG, Murugappan G, Lathi RB, Kort JD, Hanson BM, Tiegs AW, et al. Preimplantation genetic testing for aneuploidy (PGT-A) reduces miscarriage and improves live birth rates in recurrent pregnancy loss patients. Fertil Steril. 2019;112:e401.
29. Lei CX, Ye JF, Sui YL, Zhang YP, Sun XX. Retrospective cohort study of preimplantation genetic testing for aneuploidy with comprehensive chromosome screening versus nonpreimplantation genetic testing in normal karyotype, secondary infertility patients with recurrent pregnancy loss. Reprod Dev Med. 2019;3(4):205-12.
30. Sato T, Sugiura-Ogasawara M, Ozawa F, Yamamoto T, Kato T, Kurahashi H, et al. Preimplantation genetic testing for aneuploidy: a comparison of live birth rates in patients with recurrent pregnancy loss due to embryonic aneuploidy or recurrent implantation failure. Hum Reprod. 20191;34(12):2340-8. PMID 31811307.
31. Sui YL, Lei CX, Ye JF, Fu J, Zhang S, Li L, et al. In vitro fertilization with single-nucleotide polymorphism microarray-based preimplantation genetic testing for aneuploidy significantly improves clinical outcomes in infertile women with recurrent pregnancy loss: a randomized controlled trial. Reprod Dev Med. 2020;4(1):32-41.
32. Bhatt SJ, Marchetto NM, Roy J, Morelli SS, McGovern PG. Pregnancy outcomes following in vitro fertilization frozen embryo transfer (IVF-FET) with or without preimplantation genetic testing for aneuploidy (PGT-A) in women with recurrent pregnancy loss (RPL): a SART-CORS study. Hum Reprod. 2021;36(8):2339-44.
33. Pantou A, Mitrakos A, Kokkali G, Petroutsou K, Tounta G, Lazaros L, et al. The impact of preimplantation genetic testing for aneuploidies (PGT-A) on clinical outcomes in high risk patients. J Assist Reprod Genet. 2022;39(6):1341-9.
34. Pavlovic ZJ, Gallahan S, Papri S, Widra EA, Plosker S, Imudia AN, et al. Analysis of pregnancy outcomes in patients with idiopathic recurrent pregnancy loss who utilized preimplantation genetic testing for aneuploidy. Fertil Steril. 2023;120:e77-8.
35. Munné S, Alikani M, Ribustello L, Colls P, Martínez-Ortiz PA, McCulloh DH, et al. Euploidy rates in donor egg cycles significantly differ between fertility centers. Hum Reprod. 2017;32(4):743-9.

36. Wilton L, Thornhill A, Traeger-Synodinos J, Sermon KD, Harper JC. The causes of misdiagnosis and adverse outcomes in PGD. Hum Reprod. 2009;24(5):1221-8.
37. Bhatt SJ, Marchetto NM, Roy J, Morelli SS, McGovern PG. Pregnancy outcomes following in vitro fertilization frozen embryo transfer (IVF-FET) with or without preimplantation genetic testing for aneuploidy (PGT-A) in women with recurrent pregnancy loss (RPL): a SART-CORS study. Hum Reprod. 2021;36(8):2339-44.
38. Spinner NB, Conlin LK. Mosaicism and clinical genetics. Am J Med Genet C Semin Med Genet. 2014;166C(4):397-405. PMID: 25424979.
39. Perfetto CO, Murugappan G, Lathi RB. Time to next pregnancy in spontaneous pregnancies versus treatment cycles in fertile patients with recurrent pregnancy loss. Fertil Res Prac. 2015;1:5.
40. Liu XY, Fan Q, Wang J, Li R, Xu Y, Guo J, et al. Higher chromosomal abnormality rate in blastocysts from young patients with idiopathic recurrent pregnancy loss. Fertil Steril. 2020;113(4):853-64.
41. Murugappan G, Shahine LK, Perfetto CO, Hickok LR, Lathi RB. Intent to treat analysis of in vitro fertilization and preimplantation genetic screening versus expectant management in patients with recurrent pregnancy loss. Hum Reprod. 2016;31(8):1668-74.
42. Franssen MT, Korevaar JC, van der Veen F, Leschot NJ, Bossuyt PM, Goddijn M. Reproductive outcome after chromosome analysis in couples with two or more miscarriages: index [corrected]-control study. BMJ. 2006;332(7544):759-63.
43. Lei C, Sui Y, Ye J, Lu Y, Xi J, Sun Y, et al. Comparison of PGS2.0 versus conventional embryo morphology evaluation for patients with recurrent pregnancy loss: a study protocol for a multicentre randomised trial. BMJ Open. 2020;10(10):e036252.

CHAPTER 11

Hysteroembryoscopy

Vasilios Tanos, Panayiotis Tanos

ABSTRACT

Hysteroembryoscopy in cases of missed miscarriage provides insight into the site of implantation, the gestational sac and embryo morphology. It allows us to remove the intact embryo for anatomical studies by embryo-pathologist as well as detailed genetic analysis. The learning curve for this technique is not too steep and the information provided may offer an explanation in hitherto unexplained pregnancy loss. It is akin to an vivo autopsy of the embryo. Newer techniques of sonoembryology and 3D HD US will help to identify anomalies of internal organs as well.

Keywords: Hysteroembryoscopy, In vivo autopsy, Sonoembryology, 3D HD US.

INTRODUCTION

Dr Bjorn Westin in 1954 performed hysteroembryoscopy (HEpy) in three embryos, before termination of pregnancy during early second trimester. He used the McCarthy's 10 mm telescope. Two cases were performed under GA and one with local anesthesia. He reported active embryo extremities movements and he counted over 30 swallowing movements per minute.[1] However, the introduction of fetal sonography, the big diameter of hysteroscopes and the high risk of abortion did not permit the development of hysteron-embryoscopy those earlier years.

The recent optic and instrument technological advances offer excellent visualization with smaller diameter telescopes enabling better and more accurate diagnostic capabilities. Also enable minimal operative procedures to the fetus with less complications for the fetus and the mother. Small diameter hysteroscopes can be progressed into the cervical canal reaching the endometrial cavity and search for the implantation of the pregnancy sac, its content (embryo, umbilical cord, and yolk sac) and the surrounding decidua. Hysteroembryoscopy can be used for an in-situ autopsy of an embryo in sporadic as well as in repeated pregnancies loss. Such an autopsy of a miscarriage embryo can provide useful information regarding the morphology of the embryo ruling out anatomical defects and by collecting the embryo and sending it to cytogenetic analysis anticipating an accurate embryo karyotyping. It is well known that the karyotype after collection of products of conception by D&C is unreliable because the risk maternal tissue contamination of female embryos is up to 22%.[2]

IMAGING VERSUS HYSTEROEMBRYOSCOPY

Embryo sonography 2D/4D can verify normal structures and isolate organ anomalies. Even more impressive is the recent use of sonoembryology by three-dimensional high definition live silhouette ultrasound (3D HD US) allowing by a "see through" fashion to observe the internal organs of an embryo during first trimester.[3] Hence, new challenges in diagnosis and treatment of embryo and fetal medicine are anticipated. This new diagnostic imaging modality is still at the very early stage and more results will be needed to indicate the accuracy of this technology. We speculate that 3D HD US will be focusing mainly for the live early pregnancy evaluation and less for the miscarriage cases since early missed abortions embryo shrinking and tissue decomposition affects images clarity. The accurate information received from imaging during live affected embryos, HEpy can be probably used for repair small tissue defects and provide an access to gene therapy. The huge advances made in molecular biology and human genetics also expected to contribute to accurate antenatal diagnosis by isolating fetal DNA from the maternal circulation at the very early stage of pregnancy. A good example might be the correction of a beta thalassemia affected embryo at gestational age of 6 weeks when the hematopoietic system is still under development allowing molecular changes and probably correction to the globin chains.

Spontaneous miscarriages (SM) occur between 15 and 20% in spontaneous pregnancies, up to 35% in IVF pregnancies and 1–3% in women with repeated pregnancy loss (RPL). The causes varied and multifactorial etiology has been repeatedly reported. The genetic anomalies and predominantly the trisomies prevail among all the reasons of missed abortions.[4,5]

INDICATION FOR HYSTEROEMBRYOSCOPY

- Interest of the parturient to know the cause of her embryo death
- Women with missed abortion with chronic diseases under treatment
- Women with missed abortion, treated with teratogenic medication around fertilization and/or after 5 weeks of GA
- First trimester and early stage second trimester missed abortions
- Women with repeated pregnancy loss
- Women with missed abortion and history of coagulation problems
    - Phospholipid syndrome
    - Heparin treatment during pregnancy
    - Bleeding during the pregnancy
    - Thrombophilia
- Women with missed abortion and family history with genetic and somatic defects
- Women with missed abortion and suspected embryo anomalies reported by sonography
- Miscarriage after IUI/IVF/ovum donation
- Cervical pregnancy for diagnosis and treatment

Spontaneous miscarriages (SM): In our modern society women initiate their family planning later in life after the age of 35, hence, they cannot afford to have multiple miscarriages; neither to lose time by having several attempts of pregnancy expecting to take home a baby only by chance. In addition, like all other pathologies, doctors are expected to explain to the patients the factors leading to the health problem and treatment usually is directed by the causation of the disease. Similarly, a patient with a miscarriage is expecting to know the reason of her loss and what the doctor will do to prevent another abortion. To the best of our knowledge and experience, after 600 hysteroembryoscopies results the reason of the miscarriage can be diagnosed in 95% of the cases, hence it is justified to proceed to routine HEpy after every miscarriage. When a woman is pregnant for the first time over the age of 35 with an abortion probably HEpy becomes even more essential as an in-situ autopsy tool.

All women with a miscarriage always ask if they did something wrong to stop the embryo development. In case of medication, they would like to know if medicines affected their embryo and surrounding environment. HEpy can diagnose with a high accuracy embryo somatic anomalies, cord and yolk sac anomalies, defective implantation, endometrial cavity irregularities and bleedings.

Repeated pregnancy loss: Majority of studies have observed that women with three or more miscarriages more often have:

- Genetic abnormalities 3–5% (recurrent aneuploidy, structural chromosomal abnormalities, Mendelian, and polygenic factors)
- Uterine hereditary anatomical abnormalities and acquired uterine pathologies 15–20%
- Immunologic abnormalities 15–25% (alloimmune aspects, opposing paternal histocompatibility, anti-fetal and other antibodies), antiphospholipid antibody syndrome, hereditary thrombophilia
- Endocrine and metabolic disorders 5–8% (diabetes, hypothyroidism, polycystic ovarian syndrome, luteal phase defect, obesity, and severe nutritional deprivation) even
- Environmental factors 5–10% (smoking, alcohol, caffeine, and occupational exposures). About 40% of RPL cannot yet identify the etiology and are defined as unexplained.

Clinically we observe three major groups of patients with RPL. (1) Older nulliparous women, with or without infertility problem. The miscarriage occurs during 5–10 weeks of gestational age and most often aneuploidy (trisomy) and less frequently deletions and insertions are diagnosed. The RPL is attributed to the aged oocytes and IVF combined with an ovum donation program proved to be very efficient treatment. (2) Patients presenting high blood pressure or antiphospholipid antigen syndrome or anticardiolipin syndrome and usually treated with low molecular heparin (LMH), aspirin and cortisone. The RPL in this category occurs at progressively earlier gestational age and severe utero—placental vascular insufficiency leading to miscarriage. (3) Younger multiparous women, prone to intermittent fetal loss around the tenth weeks of gestational age. In 3% of the cases, parental unbalanced chromosomal translocation is present. However, the great majority of these patients have no firm diagnosis and are treated empirically.[6,7]

Early sporadic or repeated pregnancy losses might present other and/or more genetic causes. RPL mainly concerns pregnancies around 8 weeks' gestation and aneuploidies account for less than half of recurrent spontaneous abortions. Information about early aborted embryos remains very limited.[8] Cytogenetic analysis of abortion specimens from couples with recurrent miscarriage has shown that the percentage of chromosomally normal abortions is significantly higher in women (<36 years old) with recurrent miscarriage than in women (<36 years old) in the general population.[8,9] Detection of a chromosomally normal miscarriage conveys an increased risk for a subsequent chromosomally normal miscarriage.[10] However, the detection of a previous aneuploid abortion has not been proven to increase the chance of a subsequent aneuploid miscarriage.[11,12] Many RPL cases that have been diagnosed and treated may experience a consequent miscarriage during next pregnancy.

Cervical ectopic pregnancy: Hysteroembryoscopy provides direct visualization of the CP enabling the assessment of the implantation site and treatment modality. Hysteroscopic surgery allows prevention of bleeding by injecting vasoconstrictors and hemostasis control by direct vessel coagulation. Preservation of fertilization potential and short hospitalization facilitate fast return of menstrual period and future conception. Operative hysteroscopy can be used as a sole treatment option in early <8-week CPs safely.[13]

We have published four patients with early CP between 5 and 7 weeks were successfully managed with operative hysteroscopy. Three out of four patients had at least one risk factor for cervical ectopic pregnancy. Two patients were diagnosed on routine examinations and the other two presented with vaginal spotting and pelvic pain. Mechanical hysteroscopy was used in three patients while one case was managed by a 10-mm resectoscope. Three women discharged home on the same day and one patient 24 hours after the operation. Literature review revealed 16 publications of cervical pregnancy managed with operative hysteroscopy. 14 articles demonstrated single case reports and two papers were CP case series. Hysteroscopic surgery was successfully reported in 12 cases as a sole treatment, in seven cases after failure of methotrexate treatment and in eight cases as a combined treatment with uterine artery embolization. Our case series demonstrated that operative hysteroscopy can be used as a sole treatment in early, less than 8-week CPs with safety. Literature review demonstrated that most of the early first trimester CP cases were treated by hysteroscopy and the rest after failure of methotrexate treatment or in combination with uterine artery embolization.[13]

TECHNIQUE OF HYSTEROEMBRYOSCOPY

Patient Preparation

- Preoperative trans-vaginal ultrasound checks for—endometrial thickness, absence of the embryo heart-beat, implantation site, umbilical cord, embryo early anomalies, yolk sac (allantois) and amniotic fluid density especially to rule out bleeding **(Figs. 1A to D)**.
- Arrange and confirm availability of the genetic laboratory before HEpy
- Be sure that you have the correct collection container
- Confirm the way of transportation

Patient position and anesthesia: The patients are placed in a lithotomy position. There is no need and is strictly prohibited to use the Trendelenburg position as in hysteroscopy. All patients can have the option to undergo the embryoscopy procedure with or without sedation or general anesthesia. According to patients demand the majority of them do not want neither, need sedation or general anesthesia for embryoscopy. However, when the telescope of 5 mm with a working channel is inserted to extract the embryo, the patients can undergo general anesthesia. The rest of the patients may receive general anesthesia from the beginning of the procedure. The vast majority 98% of the cases manage to undergo a successful HEpy procedure after good visualization without any complications, reaching complete diagnosis of the cause of the miscarriage.

Instruments: Embryoscopy can usually be performed using a 5 mm, double way, rigid hysteroscope of 30° angle and a 5Fr working channel. The hysteroscope is introduced transcervical and progressed under vision within the uterine cavity. Using an automated fluid distention pump, warm normal saline is used to distend the uterine cavity. The intrauterine pressure is set at 70 mm Hg and can be increased to 100 mm Hg until optimal visualization of the endometrial structures.

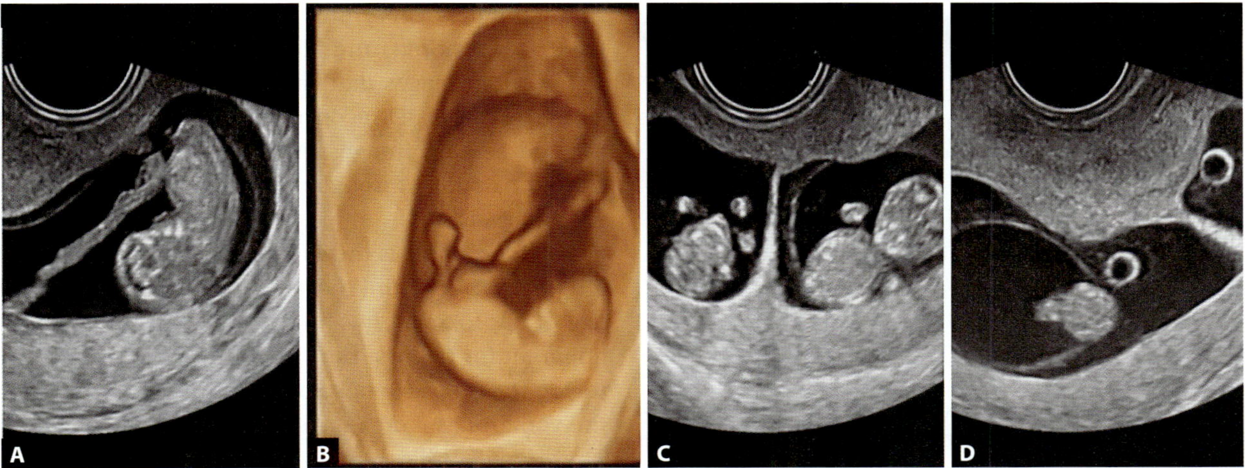

Figs. 1A to D: Detailed preoperative transvaginal scan A–D, left to right. (A) Fetus and umbilical cord; (B) position of placenta; (C) fetal heart beat and anatomy check; (D) yolk sac or allantois.

The decidua, the pregnancy sac location and characteristics are carefully visualized, and observations are noted immediately. The whole procedure is recorded in a video.

Procedure: The hysteroscope is carefully inserted into the cervical canal and progresses slowly in the endometrial cavity following fluid distention. The cervical canal is soft and progression of a 5-mm diameter telescope is smooth and atraumatic. Once the endometrial cavity dilatation is established, observation of the decidua, cornua, ostia, and pregnancy sac are performed. Frequently cornua are covered by thickened decidua so cannot be seen. Meticulous inspection of the decidua for possible defects, clottings, identification of the implantation location, and pregnancy sac external characteristics are noted.

The next step is to identify a thin area of the chorion. Using the tip of 5Fr scissors a small point hit at the area of interest opens a small hole, enabling the introduction of the telescope within the pregnancy sac. Most often embryos could be observed through the amniotic membrane (extraceolomic embryoscopy) while in the bigger gestational age the telescope could be introduced intramniotically. The amniotic surface, the external embryo characteristics including head, face, spine, chest abdominal wall, upper and lower limbs, umbilical cord, and the yolk sac could be easily observed and thoroughly examined.

Using the scissors, the small embryo mass can be detached from its uterus attachment by excising the umbilical cord form the placental site point of attachment. Using a 5Fr grasper and holding the umbilical cord the embryo can be evacuated from the endometrial cavity together with the hysteroscope under continuous vision, transferred directly in a sterile container with normal saline or culture medium and send to the laboratory for karyotyping. The patient can then be given general anesthesia cervical dilatation followed and suction curettage clears the endometrial cavity.[14,15] The summary and steps of the HEpy procedure is presented in **Box 1**.

Video-documentation of embryoscopies helps investigators to cooperate with an experienced anatomist—embryopathologist for the final diagnosis of embryo phenotype. By principle the embryo developmental stage can be assessed by Carnegie embryo development staging and compared with the reported gestational age derived from the last menstrual period and weekly trans-vaginal sonography CRL measurements. The embryoscopic findings can be classified into normal development embryos according to their gestational age and abnormal according to morphological defects.

CARNEGIE EMBRYO STAGING SYSTEM FOR EVALUATION OF THE EMBRYO MORPHOLOGY

Carnegie stages are a system used by embryologists to describe the apparent maturity of embryos. An embryo is assigned a Carnegie stage (numbered from 1 to 23) based on its external features. This staging system is not dependent on the chronological age nor the size of the embryo. There are 837 sections through the embryo.

BOX 1: Hysteroembryoscopy procedure by steps.

Targets of the HEpy inspection:
- Evaluate embryo development according to morphology (Carnegie staging system is used)
- Evaluation of the pregnancy sac and its contents characteristics
- Correlation of the embryo morphology (external characteristics) in situ and its genetic analysis (karyotype)

Embryoscopy findings following a structured and meticulous examination:
- Using the 5Fr scissors the pregnancy sac and chorion can be open
- Allows the telescope to enter and visualize the embryo through the amniotic membrane
- Most of the cases the final diagnosis about the embryo, umbilical cord, and yolk sac condition are managed transamniotically
- Embryo close-up examination
- In cases that the embryo should further need to be manipulated in order to be able to establish the final diagnosis the amniotic membrane is incised and the hysteroscope approaches the area of interest

Operative manipulations for better embryo visualization and evacuation:
- Using the hysteroscope's inward flow valve, by opening and closing it, works as fluid jet to push and turn the embryo to its best viewing position. Similarly, a 5Fr grasper can be used to turn the embryo however, touching the embryo can also cause damage to the tissues since it is very fragile and in many cases, manipulations can cause a complete destruction of its integrity. Hence less you touch the embryo more is the chance to evacuate it in its complete structure
- Using 5Fr scissors the umbilical cord is incised close to the endometrium site, grasped, and pulled outwards by a hysteroscopic grasper

Embryo evacuation tips and tricks:
- Most difficult part of HEpy is embryo evacuation
- Small and/or macerated embryos are collected and engaged within the grasper space and pull it through the 5Fr working channel
- The bigger embryos (1–2 cm) pulled by the umbilical cord or from the head and evacuated (using 5 mm or 8 mm diameter scopes, enabling the passage of the embryo through the cervical lumen)
- The evacuation is completed under vision until the embryo is placed in the NS or culture medium and send to cytogenetic laboratory
- Occasionally the whole hysteroscope is removed together with the grasping forceps and the embryo since its bigger diameter prevents the cervical canal to collapse and destroy the tissue or disable the evacuation process

Approximately every fifth or sixth section was digitally captured, restored, and labeled. The database contains 147 section images that can be viewed at four magnifications. Several 3D reconstructions were produced from aligned section images. Animations of the 3D reconstructions and flythroughs of the aligned section images are also available.

Good example is the Stage 18 embryos have a greatest length of 13–17 mm and an estimated postfertilization age of approximately 44 days. Many structures become apparent for the first time during this stage. In the head region the tip of the nose becomes discernable as well as the vomeronasal organ, eyelids, and nasolacrimal ducts. The auricular hillocks begin to form parts of the definitive external ear. The mammary glands appear in the surface ectoderm on the side of the thorax. Metacarpals are evident as rays of precartilage condensations, or cartilage, in the hand plate and intermetacarpal notches are present at the periphery of the plate. Similarly, metatarsals appear as rays of precartilage condensations or cartilage in the foot plate with intermetatarsal notches at the periphery of the foot plate. The phallus and genital tubercle (glans penis and glans clitoris) are evident for the first time. Many individual muscles and cartilages that were earlier blastema can be identified.[16,17]

SYNOPSIS OF EXPERIENCE AND RESULTS OF HYSTEROEMBRYOSCOPY OF SPONTANEOUS MISCARRIAGE AND REPEATED PREGNANCY LOSS

Chromosomal abnormalities diagnosed in 70% of SM and 72% of RPL cases while morphological defects observed in 79% and 80.4%, respectively **(Table 1)**. The most frequent reason for genetic abnormalities were Trisomies 62% in SM and 58.3% in RPL. Among miscarriage after artificial reproductive treatments Trisomies encountered 71.3% as reported by Qin et al. 2013 **(Table 2)**. Non-embryological cause of loss found 13% in SM and 10% RPL including decidua hematoma, umbilical cord, and implantation defects **(Table 3)**. Comparing embryo karyotypes among spontaneous miscarriages between three different clinical studies of HEpy the incidence of abnormal chromosomal aberration was 70–77% and for normal phenotype and karyotype was between 7 and 13 % **(Table 4)**.

In 10.6% of the spontaneous missed abortions and 5.9% of the RPL cases HEpy failed to diagnose a clear cause

TABLE 1: Correlation of the embryo external characteristics (phenotype) and embryo genetic analysis (karyotype) after HEpy examination.

Embryo status	*Spontaneous miscarriages (94) (%)*	*RPL (51) (%)*
Normal morphology and karyotype	13	15.7
Normal morphology and abnormal karyotype	7	4
Abnormal morphology and normal karyotype	17	13.7
Abnormal morphology and abnormal karyotype	62	66.7

Source: Tanos et al. 2019.[13]

TABLE 2: Embryo genetic analysis in spontaneous miscarriages and repeated pregnancy loss as compared to ART.

Embryo karyotype	*Spontaneous miscarriages (94) (%)*	*RPL (51) (%)*	*3278 ART abortion cases Qin et al. (2013) (%)*
Normal	30	29	51.1
Abnormal	70	72	48.9
Trisomies	62	58.3	71.3
Turner syndrome	21	19.4	Not reported
Tetrasomies	10	15.4	0.9
Monosomy	4	2.8	7.3
Mosaic	3	4	2.4

of the miscarriage indicating other unknown etiological factors such as myometrial, anatomical, and dysfunctional abnormalities.[14,15]

CONTEMPORARY PRACTICE ON REPEATED PREGNANCY LOSS AND HYPERCOAGULABILITY STATE

Immunological factors seem to be more complex than previously appreciated. Coagulopathies including thrombophilia are diagnosed in less cases than before, due to improved technologies and disease understanding **(Figs. 2A and B)**. RPL-specialized clinics approach patients in a systematic way (usage of standardized investigation protocols). However, many RPL cases are still treated arbitrarily using aspirin/steroids and/or LMH, although this treatment is not supported by the literature for all RPL patients. HEpy results contribute to management decision and especially on individual cases. Our series 18% were receiving LMH postulating that their past cause of RPL was hypercoagulability state. HEpy revealed that most embryos had chromosomal abnormalities ensuring patients that the problem of their loss was not the followed treatment. Future directions opt to investigate biomolecular markers (risk factors for RPL due to multifactorial etiology, SNPs, copy number of variations, gene/protein expression, epigenetic whole-genome analysis).[4]

TABLE 3: Non-embryonal factors contributing to miscarriage—umbilical cord and decidua characteristics.

Defect/abnormality	*Spontaneous miscarriages (94)*	*RPL (51)*
Umbilical cord defect	5	3
Decidua hematoma/ implantation defect	7	2
Disputed reason	4	1
Unknown reason	6	2
Overall	22 (23.4%)	8 (15.7%)

TABLE 4: Comparison of embryo karyotypes between spontaneous miscarriages.

Embryo karyotype	*Philipp T et al. Hum Rep. (2003)*	*Robberecht C et al. J Pren Dg. (2012)*	*Tanos V et al. (2016)*
	203 cases missed abortions %	51 cases missed abortions %	94 cases missed abortions %
Abnormal karyotype	75	77	70
Normal pheno- and karyotype	7	12	13

CONCLUSION

Embryoscopy seems to be a valuable method for accurate diagnosis of the cause during first trimester SM and RPL and can be especially useful for future treatment purposes **(Figs. 3 and 4)**. The diagnosis about the cause of the miscarriage alleviates women pain about their loss, relieve their stress from future uncertainty, encourage, and accelerate effort for another pregnancy. Standardization of RPL patients' clinical characteristics criteria and treatment protocols are imperative to perform clinical studies with reliable results.

Hysteroembryoscopy might have an added value in the armamentarium of modern RPL specialized clinics. The

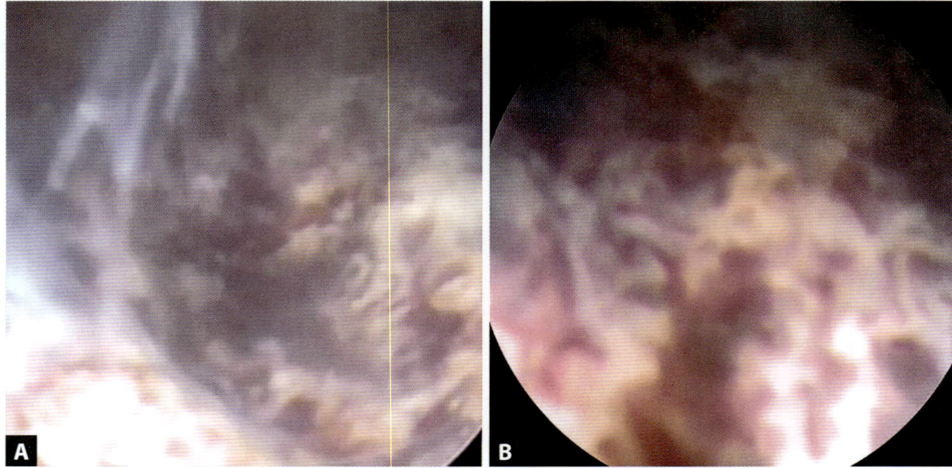

Figs. 2A and B: Decidua fresh blood coagulum next to old clot.

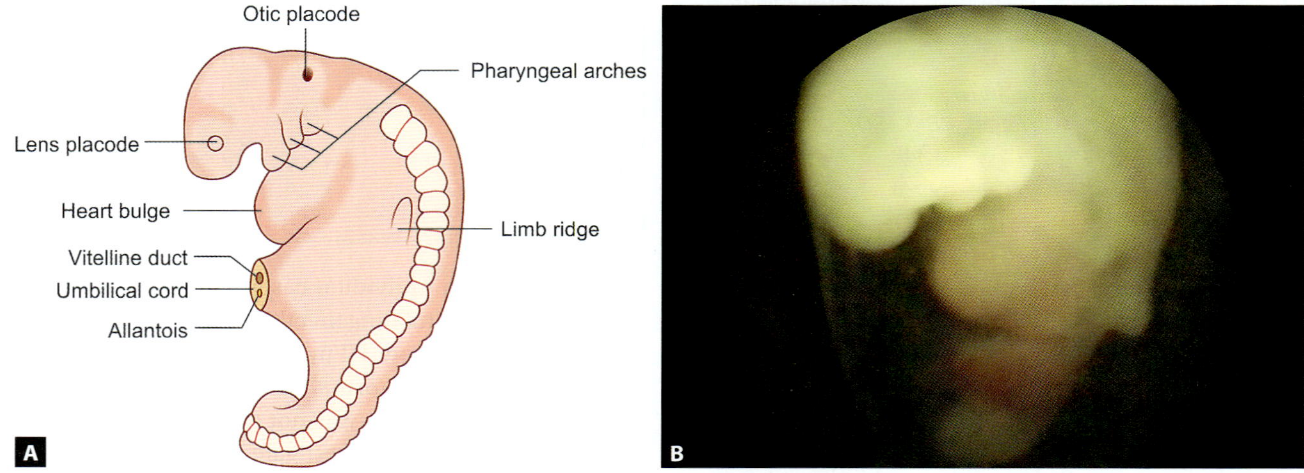

Figs. 3A and B: 28 days embryo.

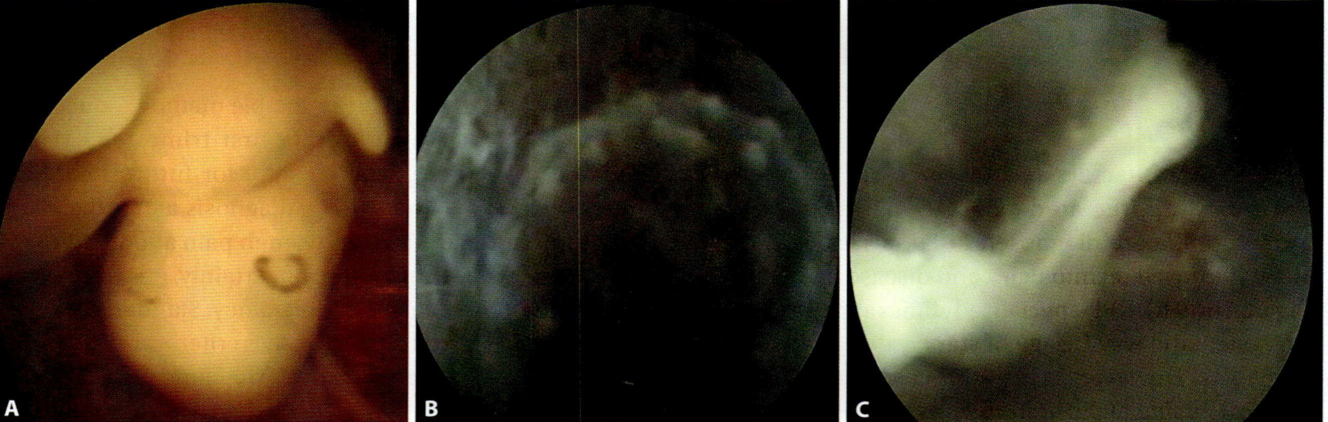

Figs. 4A to C: Embryo morphological and karyotype abnormalities. (A) Embryo left eye maldevelopment and defective upper limbs; (B) malformed allantois from an embryo with abnormal karyotype; (C) sticky embryo.

combination of 4D sonography, in situ embryo autopsy together with embryo genetic analysis can probably enlighten our knowledge about the cause of SM and RPL.

REFERENCES

1. Westin B. Hysteroscopy In early pregnancy. Lancet. 1954;2:872.
2. Canhao P, Falcao F, Ferro JM. Thrombolytics for cerebral sinus thrombosis: a systematic review. Cerebrovasc Dis. 2003;15:159-66.
3. Pooh RK. Recent Advances in 3D Ultrasound, Silhouette Ultrasound, and Sonoangiogram in Fetal Neurology. Donald School J Ultrasound Obstet Gynecol. 2016;10(2):193-200.
4. Hardy K, Hardy PJ. 1st trimester miscarriage: four decades of study. Transl Pediatr. 2015;4(2):189-200.
5. Rull K, Nagimaja L, Laan M. Genetics of recurrent miscarriage: challenges, current knowledge, future directions. Front Genet. 2012;3:34.
6. Crotti L, Tester DJ, White WM, Bartos DC, Insolia R, Besana A, et al. Long QT syndrome—associated mutations in intrauterine fetal death. JAMA. 2013;309(14):1473-82.
7. Stephenson MD, Sierra S. Reproductive outcomes in recurrent pregnancy loss associated with a parental carrier of a structural chromosome rearrangement. Hum Reprod. 2006;21(4):1076-82.
8. Robberecht C, Pexsters A, Jan D, Fryns JP, D'Hooghe T, Vermeesch JR. Cytogenetic and morphological analysis of early products of conception following hystero-embryoscopy from couples with recurrent pregnancy loss. Prenat Diagn. 2012;32:933-42.
9. Carp HJA, Toder V, Orgad S, Aviram A, Danieli M, Mashiach S, Barkai G. Karyotype of the abortus in recurrent miscarriage. Fertil Steril. 2001;75:678-82.
10. Stephenson MD, Awartani KA, Robinson WP. Cytogenetic analysis of miscarriages from couples with recurrent miscarriage: a case-control study. Hum Reprod. 2002;17:446-51.
11. Warburton D, Neugut RH, Lustenberger A, Nicholas A, Kline J. No association between spermicide use and trisomy at prenatal diagnosis. New Engl J Med. 1987;317(8):478-82.
12. Frias AE Jr, Luikenaar RA, Sullivan AE, Lee RM, Porter TF, Branch DW, Silver RM. Poor obstetric outcome in subsequent pregnancies in women with prior fetal death. Obstet Gynecol. 2004;104(3):521-6.
13. Tanos V, El-Akhras S. Kayia Hysteroscopic Management of Cervical Pregnancy: Case Series and Review of the Literature Journal. J Gynecol Obstetr Human Reprod. 2019;48(4):247-53.
14. In: Tanos V. Role of Embryoscopy Fetal Karyotyping and Placental Biopsy. In: Arora M, Mukhopadhaya N (Eds). Recurrent Pregnancy Loss; 3rd edition. Jaypee Brothers Medical Publishers; 2018. pp. 289-95.
15. Tinelli A, Alonso PL, Haimovich S. Hysteroscopy. In: Tanos V (Ed). Hystero-embryoscopy. Springer Intern Publishing AG; 2017.
16. Laitman JT, Smith HF. The Anatomical Record digests new findings on the twists and turns and surprises of the gastrointestinal system in a new Special Issue. Anatom Immune Gastrointest Syst. 2023;306(5):937-40.
17. DiCaglio S. Staging Embryos: Pregnancy, Temporality and the History of the Carnegie Stages of Embryo Development. Body Society; 2017.

SECTION

3 Endometrial Factors

CHAPTER 12

Chronic Endometritis

Mirudhubashini Govindarajan, Kalpana P, Saadhvi Balaji

ABSTRACT

Chronic endometritis is associated with the unexplained RPL. It may be asymptomatic or cause mild symptoms. A wide variety of pathogens are implicated, mostly gram-negative bacteria and cocci. However, the commensals of the vagina like *Gardnerella* and *Mycoplasma hominis* are also implicated. Diagnosis is by imaging (ultrasound, sonohysterogram), hysteroscopy, and finally by endometrial biopsy and demonstration of plasma cells by special CD138 immunostaining. Microbial cultures are not of help but RT-PCR may be helpful in identifying the organisms. Treatment is with directed antibiotics and probiotics. Intrauterine antibiotic infusions have been tried in resistant cases. Other unproven modalities are platelet rich plasma infusion and low intensity laser destruction.

Keywords: Chronic endometritis, Plasma cells. CD138, Antibiotics, Probiotics, Prebiotics, Hysteroscopy, Intrauterine antibiotic infusion.

INTRODUCTION

Endometrium is a dynamic tissue that undergoes proliferation, differentiation, and sloughing repeatedly during a woman's reproductive life. In the past, it was assumed that the endometrium did not harbor any micro-organisms. This concept of "sterile endometrium" has now been refuted. Like all other mucocutaneous surfaces of the human body, the uterus has also been found to harbor a rich flora of aerobic and anaerobic bacteria.

Uterine microbiota however differs from that of vaginal microflora. It is a colony consisting of bacteria, yeast, and viruses, of which anaerobes are the most dominant. This colony more closely resembles the oral microbiota. This fact explains the association between periodontal diseases and reproductive problems. Alteration or overgrowth of these commensals has the potential to cause disease.[1,2]

ENDOMETRITIS—THE PROBLEM

Endometritis is a term that refers to infection and inflammation of the endometrium and can be either acute or chronic.

Acute Endometritis

Acute endometritis (AE) is the familiar entity that occurs due to ascending bacterial infection from the vagina or cervix. It is characterized by endometrial microabscesses and infiltration of neutrophils in superficial epithelium and glandular lumen. Antibiotic treatment with cefexime, metronidazole, and azithromycin is the effective treatment. However, AE is not usually associated with long-term fertility issues unless it is associated with tubal or pelvic inflammation.

Chronic Endometritis

Chronic endometritis (CE) on the other hand refers to a continuous, prolonged mild inflammation of the endometrium with infiltration of plasma cells in endometrial stroma due to microbial colonization. It is most often clinically silent and hence rarely suspected or diagnosed.

PREVALENCE

Reported prevalence of CE varies widely from 0.2% to 46%. Differences in diagnostic criteria may be responsible for this large variation in reported prevalence. Women diagnosed with CE are likely to have a 60% increased risk of infertility. Around 45% of infertile couple with recurrent implantation failure (RIF)/recurrent pregnancy loss (RPL) have been diagnosed to have CE in some studies.[3-6]

ETIOLOGY

The most common microbes involved in CE are *Streptococcus* species, *Escherichia coli*, *Enterococcus faecalis*, *Staphylococcus* species, *Mycoplasma*/*Ureaplasma* species (*Mycoplasma genitalium*, *Mycoplasma hominis*, and *Ureaplasma urealyticum*), *Proteus* species, *Klebsiella pneumoniae*, *Pseudomonas aeruginosa*, *Gardnerella vaginalis*, Corynebacterium, and yeasts (*Saccharomyces cerevisiae*) and candida species. In South Asian countries, *Mycobacterium tuberculosis* is an important pathogen, which causes chronic granulomatous endometritis with multiple caseating granulomas and lymphocytic infiltration. *Chlamydia trachomatis* and *Neisseria gonorrhoeae* are more likely to be associated with AE.[7-9]

CLINICAL FEATURES

In CE, around 25% of women may be totally asymptomatic, while others can present with some pelvic discomfort, spotting, leukorrhea, hypomenorrhea, secondary amenorrhea, or infertility.

CHRONIC ENDOMETRITIS—EFFECT ON FERTILITY

Successful pregnancy requires:

- Normal and functional embryo.
- Receptive endometrium.
- Embryo-endometrial interaction.

In CE, two out of the three *endometrium* and *interaction* are adversely affected.

Chronic endometritis is the outcome of altered endometrial microbiota, which in turn is secondary to dysbiosis and decreased lactobacilli in the lower genital tract. The altered micro-organisms in the cavity form a *"Biofilm"* as a strategy against host immune response. Biofilm is a syntrophic consortium or layer of micro-organisms, in which the cells stick to one another and to the mucosal surface.

CHRONIC ENDOMETRITIS—PATHOPHYSIOLOGY

Chronic endometritis starts a cascade of adverse events, which negatively affect the uterine receptivity:

- Cytokine dysregulation
- Leukocyte infiltration
- Altered uterine contractility
- Altered vascularization
- Altered decidualization
- Altered autophagy

Cytokine Dysregulation

- *Interleukin 11 (IL-11):* It helps in trophoblastic invasion and decidualization. Its expression is downregulated in CE.
- *CCL4:* A chemokine involved in attracting natural killer (NK) cells and macrophages important for implantation. CE downregulates its expression.
- *Insulin-like growth factor 1 (IGF1):* It is responsible for estrogen-mediated endometrial proliferation in proliferative phase. Activity is downregulated in CE.
- CE upregulates BCL-2 and BAX, which are responsible for increased antiapoptotic activity, leading to micropolyp formation.
- Selectin E expression is altered in CE, leading to inappropriate trophoblast invasion.
- CE enhances CXCL3 and CXCL1 expression in endometrial glandular epithelium, responsible for the recruitment of circulation of B lymphocytes into the endometrium and sustaining the inflammation.
- IL-17 activity is increased and anti-inflammatory modulators IL-10 and transforming growth factor beta 1 (TGF-β1) are decreased, resulting in impaired implantation **(Fig. 1)**.

Leukocyte Infiltration

- In normal endometrium, B cells can be found only in endometrial stroma. In CE, B cells are recruited into the functional layer. Some of these cells differentiate into plasma cells, which are pathognomonic of CE.
- Aberrant immune responses of immunoglobulin M (IgM), IgG, and IgA.
- Uterine natural killer (uNK) cells decrease during secretory phase in CE-affected endometrium.

Altered Uterine Contractility

Altered leukocytes and paracrine factors affect the junctional zone, inducing altered uterine peristalsis, especially in mid-luteal and periovulatory phases, causing retrograde contractility.

Altered Vascularization

- High vascular density with endothelial proliferation and swelling
- Hyaline thickening of vascular wall with luminal occlusion
- Small vessel thrombosis

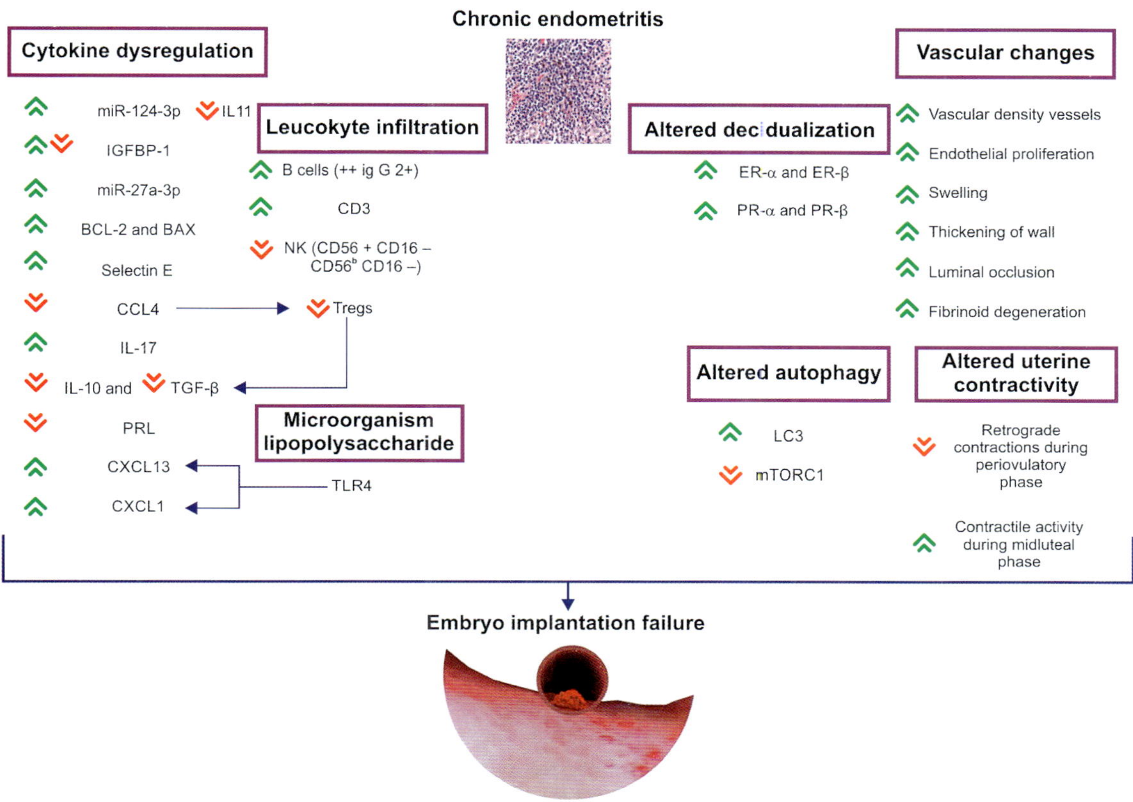

Fig. 1: Chronic endometritis pathway. (ER: estrogen receptor; IGFBP-1: insulin-like growth factor-binding protein-1; IgG: immunoglobulin G; IL: interleukin; NK: natural killer; PR: progesterone receptor; TGF: transforming growth factor)

Altered Decidualization

- There is an increase in Ki-67 (kiel antigen), which is a marker of cell proliferation, and also the expressions of estrogen receptor (ER)-α and ER-β and progesterone receptor (PR)-α and PR-β are higher in CE.
- These altered sex steroid function and endometrial proliferation lead to *"out of phase"* morphology of the endometrium **(Fig. 2)**.[10]

Numerous studies have evaluated the relationship of CE with adverse reproductive outcomes, such as implantation failure, RPLs, miscarriages, preterm births, and preterm prelabor rupture of membranes (PTPROM). The prevalence of CE may be as high as 60% in women with RIF/RPL.[11-14]

In summary, the various factors that play a role in negative outcomes are:

- Decreased endometrial receptivity due to direct microbe effect and decreased αvβ3 integrin
- Altered immune response due to abnormal microenvironment
- Decreased response to oral steroids
- Increased endometrial stromal sclerosis and decrease fibrous tissue remodeling
- Altered uterine contractility in mid-luteal and periovulatory phases along with decreased retrograde fallopian tube contractility
- Altered vascularization—increased vascular density and endothelial proliferation. Hyaline wall thickening occurs causing luminal occlusion. Micropolyps may represent developing vasculopathy. Increased vascular density can increase the oxygen tension, which can lead to more reactive oxygen species (ROS) production and resultant altered endometrial receptivity.
- Increase in autophagy leading to proinflammatory response.

DIAGNOSTIC MODALITIES

Symptomatology does not help in diagnosis of CE, as a quarter of the affected patients lack specific symptoms. Various modalities available for diagnosis of CE are:

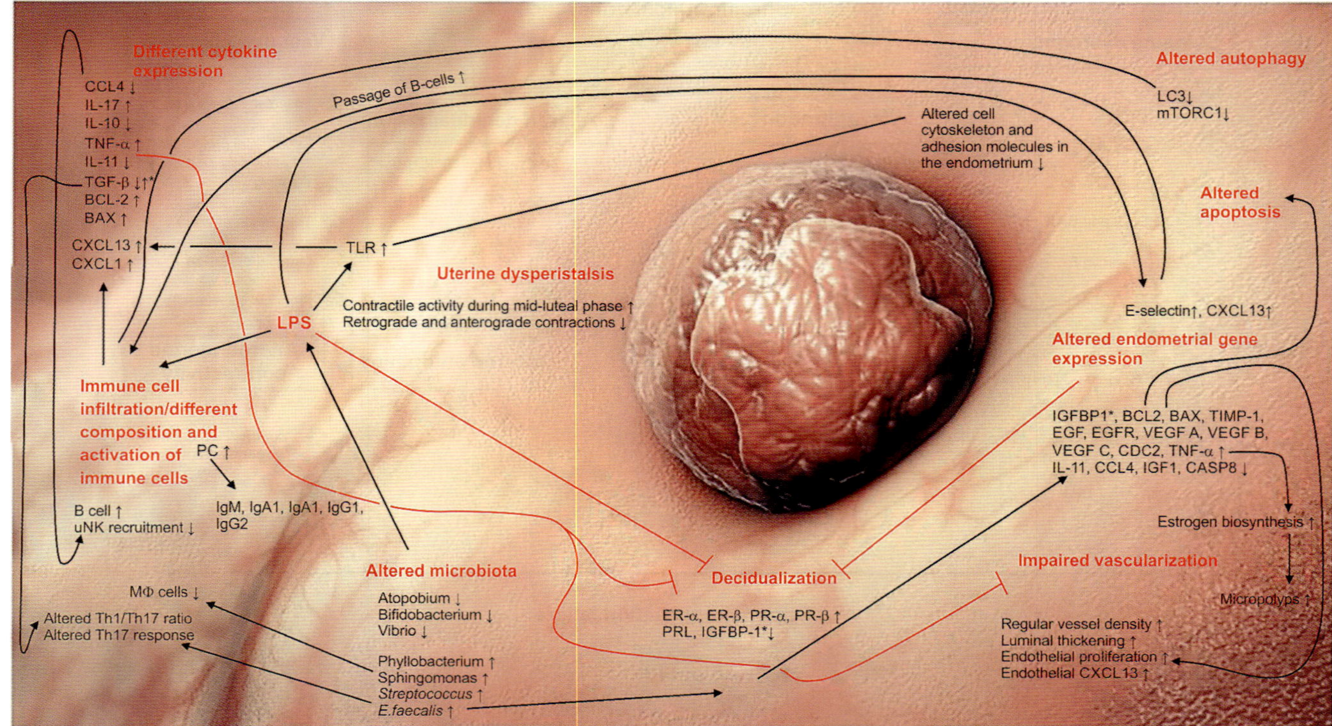

Fig. 2: Pathophysiology of CE. (CE: chronic endometritis; ER: estrogen receptor; IGFBP-1: insulin-like growth factor-binding protein-1; IgM: immunoglobulin M; IL: interleukin; LPS: lipopolysaccharides; PC: plasma cell; PR: progesterone receptor; PRL: prolactin; TGF: transforming growth factor; TLR: toll-like receptor; uNK: uterine natural killer)

Source: Murtinger M, Wirleitner B, Spitzer D, Bralo H, Miglar S, Schuff M. Diagnosing chronic endometritis: when simplification fails to clarify. Hum Reprod Open. 2022;2022(3):hoac023.

Imaging

Ultrasonography

The features of endometritis are not specific and include a tender and enlarged uterus identified with the transvaginal probe in association with:

- Thickened and heterogenous endometrium
- Intracavitary/cul de sac fluid
- Increased vascularity on Doppler ultrasound
- Loss of well-defined interface between the endometrium and myometrium.[15]

Hysterosalpingography

Hysterosalpingography (HSG) is contraindicated in cases of acute infections and, if done, may show irregular endometrial cavity and intravasation of contrast in vascular and lymphatic systems. In CE, HSG may not reveal any specific findings. Filling defect and low cavity volume may be seen occasionally.

Sonohysterogram

Sonohysterogram can reveal thin and irregular endometrium, hyperechoic spots due to calcification and fibrosis. Linear echogenic bridges and loculated fluid-filled cavity may be seen. On 3D ultrasound, micropolyps can be visualized as multiple isoechoic, round structures diffusely located inside endometrial cavity.[16]

Magnetic Resonance Imaging

- *T2:* The uterus may be enlarged with overall high signal intensity.
- *T1 C+ (Gd):* It can show intense enhancement of the uterus.[15]

Diagnostic Hysteroscopy

Hysteroscopy: It is an essential basic test for ruling out CE in patients with RIF and RPL. CE on hysteroscopy is characterized by:[16]

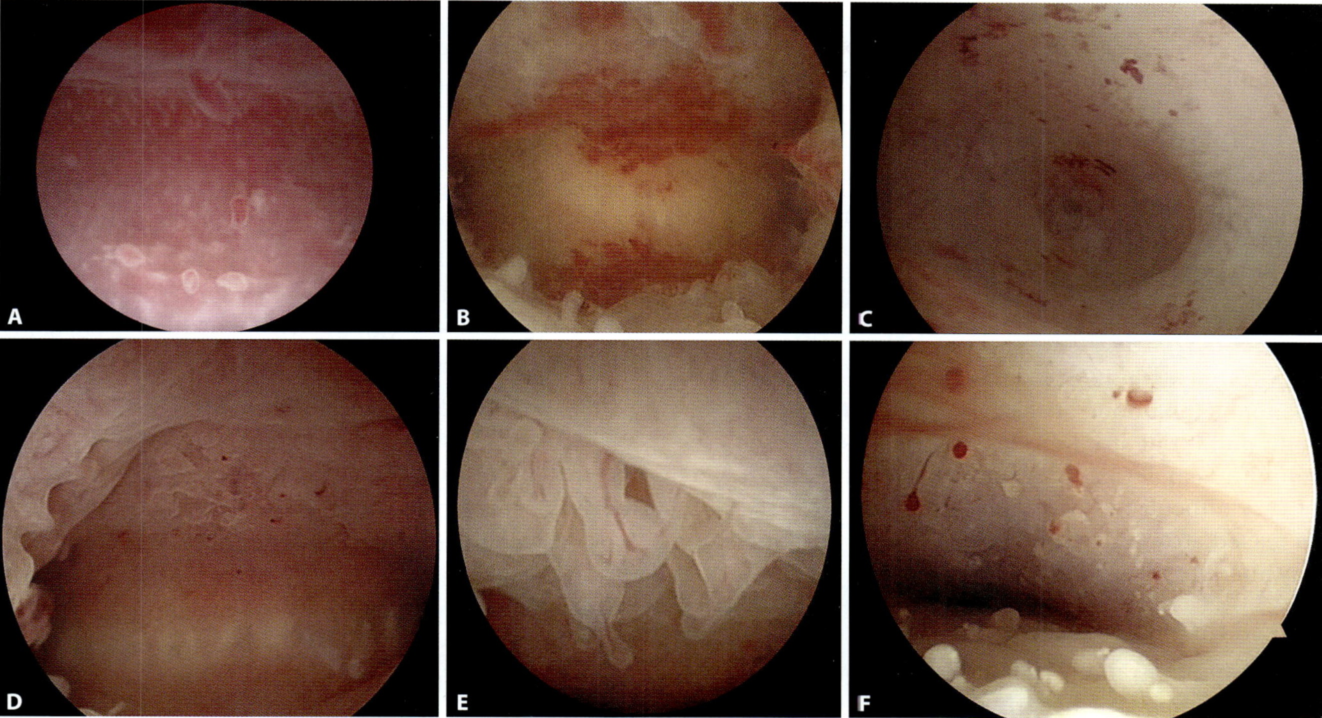

Figs. 3A to F: Chronic endometritis in hysteroscopy.

- *Strawberry appearance:* Large areas of hyperemic endometrium with white central points **(Fig. 3A)**
- *Focal hyperemia:* Small areas of hyperemic endometrium **(Fig. 3B)**
- *Hemorrhagic spots:* Focal red areas with sharp and irregular borders possibly in continuity with capillary **(Fig. 3C)**.
- *Focal or diffuse micropolyps:* <1 mm in size with a distinct connective vascular axis distributed on focal area or on all endometrial surfaces **(Figs. 3D and E)**
- Thick and pale appearance of the endometrium in the follicular phase owing to stromal oedema (a normal finding in the secretory phase) **(Fig. 3F)**.

Endometrial Biopsy and Histopathology

Chronic endometritis is characterized by the presence of endometrial stromal plasma cell (ESPC). These cells have a high nucleus to cytoplasm ratio, basophilic cytoplasm, and a peculiar heterochromatin rearrangement of nucleus known as *clock face chromatin/spoke wheel pattern.*

Morphological features of plasmacytes can be similar to stromal fibroblasts and mononuclear leukocytes in the endometrium. This may create difficulty in diagnosis.

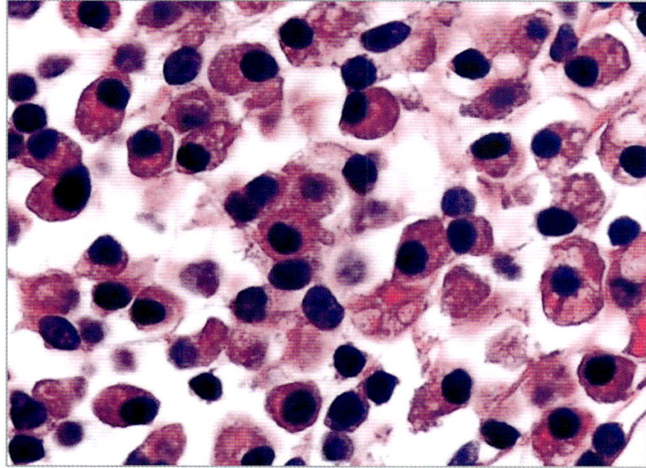

Fig. 4: Plasma cells in stroma by hematoxylin and eosin (H&E) staining.

Plasma cells can be identified by hematoxylin and eosin (H&E) stain or by CD138 immunohistochemistry (IHC) testing **(Fig. 4)**.

The biopsy should be taken during the proliferative phase of cycle by 3 mm Novak's curette, as the prevalence of CE is more during that phase. In secretory phase, 15% of the samples taken show plasma cells only in the basal layers of stroma, resulting in a missed diagnosis. Full-thickness biopsy is preferred over superficial and should preferably be done under hysteroscopic guidance.

Other Inflammatory Findings in the Endometrium

Besides the presence of plasma cells, other inflammatory findings may be the presence of neutrophils, macrophages and lymphocytes **(Table 1)**.

Hematoxylin and Eosin (H&E) Staining

Glandular-stromal dis-synchrony and endometrial eosinophil infiltration are also seen in CE **(Fig. 5)**.

Endometrial stromal plasma cell closely resembles mononuclear leukocytes and fibroblasts, and it may be very difficult to differentiate them on H&E staining. Increased stromal cell infiltration in the endometrium may interfere with ESPC identification.[17]

CD138 Immunostaining

CD138 immunostaining is also known as syndecan-1. It is a transmembrane-type heparin-sulfate proteoglycan and is most specific for diagnosis of CE. CD138 immunostaining is superior to conventional tissue staining using H&E with less interobserver (96% vs. 68%) and intraobserver variability.

TABLE 1: Inflammatory findings in the endometrium.

Histopathological finding	*Cause*
Glandular lumen neutrophils	Frank bacterial infection necessitating antibiotics
Glandular lumen macrophages	Indicative of pelvic endometriosis
Mixture of lymphocytes and macrophages	Immunological response to autoantigen
Classic tubercular lesion	Due to *Mycobacterium tuberculosis* infection

The number of plasma cells needed to make a diagnosis of CE is not well defined. The presence of one or more CD138+ ESPC in one microscopic high-power field or >5 CD138 + ESPC in at least one out of three sections can be used as a diagnostic criterion for CE. Sensitivity of diagnosing CE varies with the type of method used, being 13% with H&E stain and 56% with IHC staining.

More recent studies have shown that even one plasma cell in 10 HPF is significant. Even with one plasma cell, decreased clinical pregnancy rate, live birth rate, and increased miscarriage rate have been demonstrated. Dana et al. compared the prevalence of CE in women with RPL and controls and found that plasma cells were rarely found in biopsy from healthy controls but both plasma cells and endometrial stromal changes were present only in the RPL group. Based on these findings, they proposed that CE should be defined *as the presence of one or more plasma cells per 10 HPFs detected by either H&E or CD138 staining in the setting of endometrial stromal changes* so as to maximize sensitivity and specificity and limit false positives.[18]

Drawback

Sometimes endometrial epithelial cells constitutively express CD138 on their plasma membrane, leading to false positive diagnosis of CE.

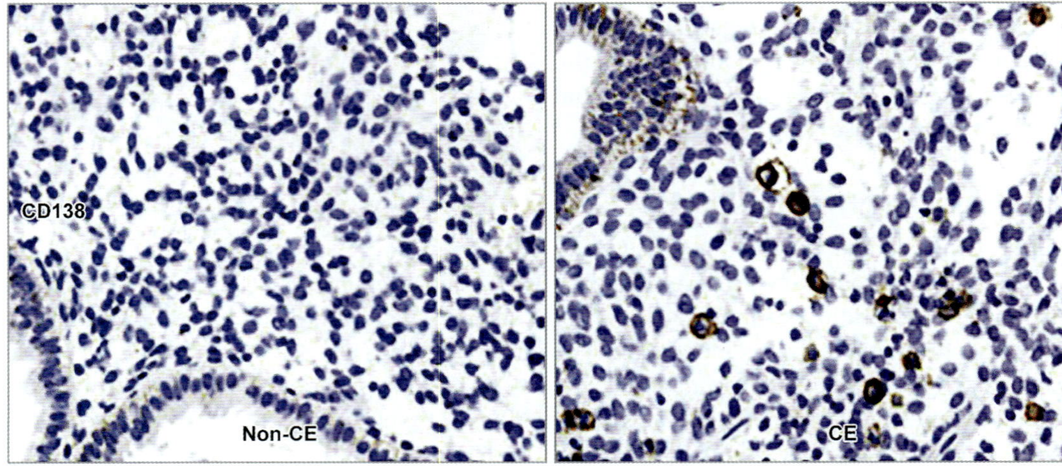

Fig. 5: Plasma cells by IHC–CD138 staining. (CE: chronic endometritis; IHC: immunohistochemistry)

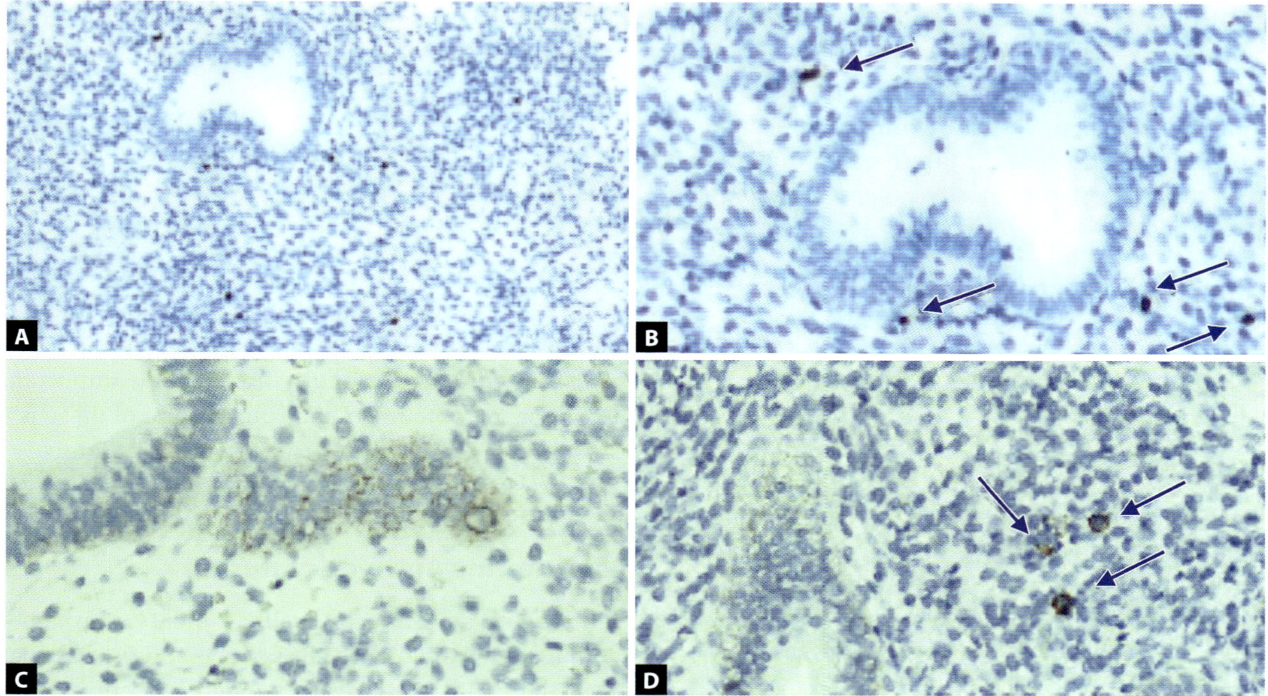

Figs. 6A to D: (A and B) MUM-1 and (C and D) CD138 stains demonstrate the presence of plasma cells within the endometrial stroma (blue arrows).

Multiple Myeloma Oncogene 1 Immunostaining

Multiple myeloma oncogene 1 (MUM-1) IHC has been evaluated in the diagnosis of CE. MUM-1 is a protein, normally expressed in plasma cells, and activates B and T cells. Cicinelli et al. in their study compared MUM-1 and CD138 and found that sensitivity and specificity of MUM-1 are 93.48 and 85% when compared to CD138, whose sensitivity and specificity are 89 and 80%. Also, MUM-1 allowed the identification of higher number of plasma cells/HPF than CD138 **(Figs. 6A to D)**.[19]

According to recent studies, MUM-1 shows a minor background staining compared to CD138 and a higher interobserver agreement. Therefore, the concomitant use of both IHC-CD138 and IHC MUM-1 may potentially compensate for the shortcomings of each method in the histopathologic diagnosis of CE.

Microbiology—Regular Microbial Culture, Molecular Microbiology

Regular microbial cultures are not useful.

Both culture and reverse transcription polymerase chain reaction (RT PCR) cannot identify organisms in up to 50% of cases.

The main limitations related to endometrial culture include:

- Risk of contamination from vaginal bacteria
- Limited culture ability of selected micro-organisms
- Delays in culturing bacteria
- Long turnaround time

Real-time Polymerase Chain Reaction or Next-generation Sequencing 16S Ribosome Sequencing

In this technique, microbes are detected using a comprehensive panel of primers. It can detect organisms even when tissue histopathology is negative.

This technology is feasible, faster, accurate, and more informative than regular culture.

EMMA (Endometrial Microbiome Metagenomic Analysis) and ALICE (Analysis of Infectious Chronic Endometritis)

These tests are based on next-generation sequencing (NGS). However, recent randomized control trials (RCTs) have not shown any benefits for the above tests in the diagnosis of CE.[20]

Inflammatory Markers

Various noninvasive inflammatory markers, cytokines, metalloproteinases, and micro-RNAs, such as miR27a-3p and miR124-3p, can assess the endometrial inflammatory milieu. They are however in the research domain, and there is still a lack of evidence to support or recommend their routine use in clinical diagnosis.

COMPARATIVE DIAGNOSTIC EFFICACY

The comparative diagnostic accuracy of each modality is mentioned in **Table 2**.

EVALUATION AND TREATMENT OF CHRONIC ENDOMETRITIS

Flowchart 1 summarizes the evaluation and treatment of chronic endometritis.

Cicinelli et al.[22] describe the treatment based on the microbiological profile and recommended the treatment mentioned in **Table 3**.

TABLE 2: Diagnostic modality and accuracy.

Diagnostic modality	***Diagnostic accuracy***
Histopathology	60.8%
Hysteroscopy	67.8%
Culture	66.15%
Molecular tests	76.92%

MICROBIOLOGICAL PROFILE-BASED TREATMENT OF CHRONIC ENDOMETRITIS

Microbiota Regulator

Pro- and Prebiotic Administration/Microbiota Transplants

Lactobacilli-dominant environment has a better implantation rate than non-lactobacilli-dominated one. Several strategies for modifying endometrial microbial composition such as pro- and prebiotic administration and microbiota transplants are gaining importance. However, the core microbial composition of these is not standardized, and there are no standard protocols for diagnosis of dysbiosis.[7,23]

Intrauterine Antibiotic Infusion

It involves systemic as well as local approach for administering antibiotics in CE. The main risk associated is off label antibiotic usage, which can contribute to antibiotic resistance.[24,25]

If CE is persistent, antibiotic treatment may need to be repeated even up to three times. There is no difference in the LBR between women who got cured in the first versus who got treated in third time. Around 25% patients needed a third course of antibiotic before they were completely cured.[26]

Flowchart 1: Evaluation and treatment of chronic endometritis.[21]

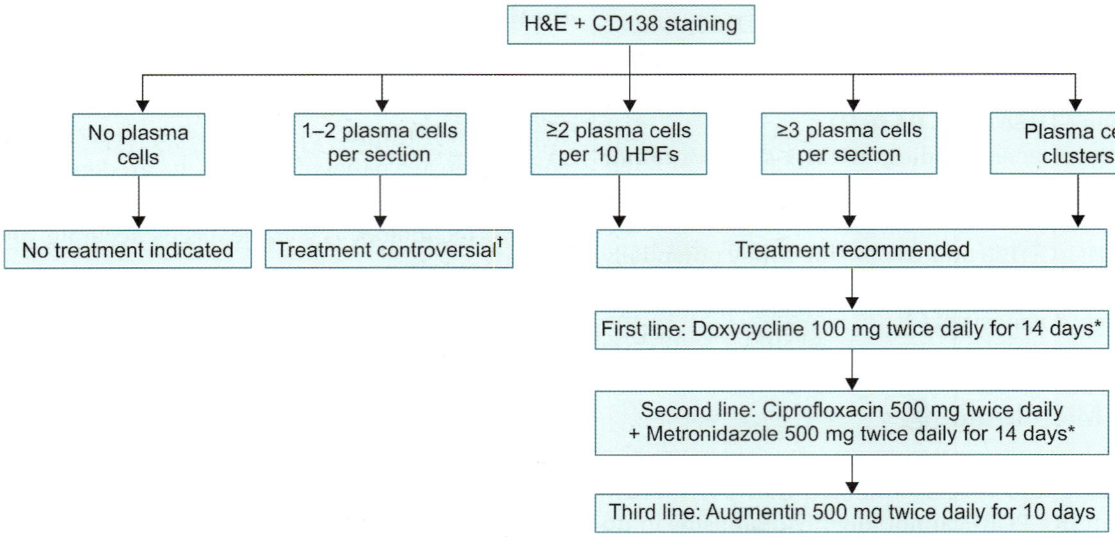

H&E + CD138 staining

- No plasma cells → No treatment indicated
- 1–2 plasma cells per section → Treatment controversial†
- ≥2 plasma cells per 10 HPFs → Treatment recommended
- ≥3 plasma cells per section → Treatment recommended
- Plasma cell clusters → Treatment recommended

Treatment recommended → First line: Doxycycline 100 mg twice daily for 14 days* → Second line: Ciprofloxacin 500 mg twice daily + Metronidazole 500 mg twice daily for 14 days* → Third line: Augmentin 500 mg twice daily for 10 days

(H&E: hematoxylin & eosin stain; CD138: cell differentiation 138; HPF: high power field)

TABLE 3: Treatment based on micro-organism.

Micro-organism	*Treatment*
Gram-negative	Ciprofloxacin 500 mg twice a day for 10 days
Gram-positive	Amoxicillin + clavulanate 1 g twice a day for 8 days
Mycoplasma/ Ureaplasma	Fosfomycin 1 g twice a day for 12 days
Resistant	Minocycline 100 mg twice a day for 12 days
Negative culture	Injection ceftriaxone 250 mg intramuscular single dose + Tablet doxycycline 100 mg BD for 14 days + Tablet metronidazole 500 mg BD for 14 days

FUTURE PROSPECTS IN CHRONIC ENDOMETRITIS

Chronic endometritis is characterized by the abnormal distribution of immune cells impeding implantation. Many recent researchers have suggested the term "impaired inflammatory state of endometrium (IISE)" as a better term. Recently, many studies have evaluated the possible role of adjuvants, which act on inflammatory processes. Some of the newer advancements in diagnosis and of CE are described here.

Narrow Band Imaging Hysteroscopy

It is a real-time endoscopic imaging technique aimed at improving the visualization of vascular network and texture of mucosal surface and hence improving tissue characterization and diagnosis. The technique improves the specificity of diagnosis and helps to take the biopsy from the appropriate areas. There is a higher concordance between hysteroscopy and histopathological findings when this technique is used compared to hysteroscopy alone.[27]

Anti-inflammatory Therapy

Nonsteroidal anti-inflammatory drugs inhibit the proinflammatory cytokines involved in CE by inhibiting the COX pathway and decreasing prostaglandin synthesis. This anti-inflammatory effect can be used as a mode of pathogenetic therapy. However, further research is still needed in this area.[28,29]

Progestogens

Various studies have shown a reduced expression of progesterone receptor in patients with CE. The action of progesterone is mediated by interaction via progesterone receptor membrane component 1 (PGRMC1), which is deficient in patients with CE. Interaction between the hormone and target organs is impaired in inflammation. Anti-inflammatory therapy may need to be administered first followed by hormonal therapy with progestogens.[30]

Intrauterine Treatment with Autologous Platelet-rich Plasma

Platelet-rich plasma acts by increasing the apoptosis of proinflammatory cells and decreasing prostaglandins, matrix metalloproteinases. The expression and synthesis of IL-1 receptor antagonist, tumor necrosis factor receptor (TNFR), IL-4, IL-10, TGF-β, and lipoxins is augmented, which decreases uterine stroma inflammation.[6]

Low Intensity Intravascular Laser Irradiation of Blood

It acts by balancing proinflammatory and anti-inflammatory cytokines. It increases the oxygen tension, decreases carbon dioxide, and hence augments metabolism and tissue regeneration.[31]

CONCLUSION

Chronic endometritis is not an uncommon problem, though the diagnosis may be missed in most cases. It is usually silent or mildly asymptomatic and lacks systemic manifestations or localizing findings on examination. CE has significant negative effect on local immune mechanism, resulting in adverse local inflammatory response that adversely impacts implantation, resulting in RIF or RPL. The diagnostic criteria for CE are not well defined hence, accurate diagnosis can be challenging. Definitive treatment has proven to be beneficial in improving the reproductive outcomes.

REFERENCES

1. Sirota I, Zarek SM, Segars JH. Potential influence of the microbiome on infertility and assisted reproductive technology. Semin Reprod Med. 2014;32:35-42.
2. González A, Vázquez-Baeza Y, Knight R. SnapShot: the human microbiome. Cell. 2014;158:690-1.
3. Boggess KA, Tita A, Jauk V, Saade G, Longo S, Clark EAS, et al.; Cesarean Section Optimal Antibiotic Prophylaxis

Trial Consortium. Risk Factors for Post cesarean Maternal Infection in a Trial of Extended-Spectrum Antibiotic Prophylaxis. Obstet Gynecol. 2017;129:481-5.

4. Chaim W, Bashiri A, Bar-David J, Shoham-Vardi I, Mazor M. Prevalence and clinical significance of postpartum endometritis and wound infection. Infect Dis Obstet Gynecol. 2000;8:77-82.
5. Singh N, Sethi A. Endometritis - Diagnosis, Treatment and its impact on fertility - A Scoping Review. JBRA Assist Reprod. 2022;26(3):538-46.
6. Cicinelli E, Matteo M, Tinelli R, Lepera A, Alfonso R, Indraccolo U, et al. Prevalence of chronic endometritis in repeated unexplained implantation failure and the IVF success rate after antibiotic therapy. Hum Reprod. 2015;30:323-30.
7. Haggerty CL, Hillier SL, Bass DC, Ness RB; PID Evaluation and Clinical Health study investigators. Bacterial vaginosis and anaerobic bacteria are associated with endometritis. Clin Infect Dis. 2004;39(7):990-5.
8. Cicinelli E, De Ziegler D, Nicoletti R, Colafiglio G, Saliani N, Resta L, et al. Chronic endometritis: correlation among hysteroscopic, histologic, and bacteriologic findings in a prospective trial with 2190 consecutive office hysteroscopies. Fertil Steril. 2008;89:677-84.
9. Cicinelli E, De Ziegler D, Nicoletti R, Tinelli R, Saliani N, Resta L, et al. Poor reliability of vaginal and endocervical cultures for evaluating microbiology of endometrial cavity in women with chronic endometritis. Gynecol Obstet Invest. 2009;68:108-15.
10. B Giovanni, Vitagliano A, Andrisanil1 A, Santarsiero CMF, Cicinelli R, N Claudia, et al. Chronic endometritis and altered embryo implantation: a unified pathophysiological theory from a literature systematic review. J Assist Reprod Genet. 2020;37:2897-911.
11. Zolghadri J, Momtahan M, Aminian K, Ghaffarpasand F, Tavana Z. The value of hysteroscopy in diagnosis of chronic endometritis in patients with unexplained recurrent spontaneous abortion. Eur J Obstet Gynecol Reprod Biol. 2011;155:217-20.
12. Oliveira FG, Abdelmassih VG, Diamond MP, Dozortsev D, Nagy ZP, Abdelmassih R. Uterine cavity findings and hysteroscopic interventions in patients undergoing in vitro fertilization-embryo transfer who repeatedly cannot conceive. Fertil Steril. 2003;80:1371-5.
13. Bouet PE, El Hachem H, Monceau E, Gariepy G, Kadoch IJ, Sylvestre C. Chronic endometritis in women with recurrent pregnancy loss and recurrent implantation failure: prevalence and role of office hysteroscopy and immunohistochemistry in diagnosis. Fertil Steril. 2016;105:106-10.
14. Kasius JC, Fatemi HM, Bourgain C, Sie-Go DM, Eijkemans RJ, Fauser BC, et al. The impact of chronic endometritis on reproductive outcome. Fertil Steril. 2011;96:1451-6.
15. Laifer-Narin SL, Kwak E, Kim H, Hecht EM, Newhouse JH. Multimodality imaging of the postpartum or post termination uterus: evaluation using ultrasound, computed tomography, and magnetic resonance imaging. Curr Probl Diagn Radiol. 2014;43:374-85.
16. Cicinelli E, Vitagliano A, Kumar A, Lasmar RB, Bettocchi S, Haimovich S; International Working Group for Standardization of Chronic Endometritis Diagnosis. Unified diagnostic criteria for chronic endometritis at fluid hysteroscopy: proposal and reliability evaluation through an international randomized-controlled observer study. Fertil Steril. 2019;112(1):162-73.
17. Kasius JC, Broekmans FJ, Sie-Go DM, Bourgain C, Eijkemans MJ, Fauser BC, et al. The reliability of the histological diagnosis of endometritis in asymptomatic IVF cases: a multicenter observer study. Hum Reprod. 2012;27:153-8.
18. McQueen DB, Maniar KP, Hutchinson A, Confino R, Bernardi L, Pavone ME. Redefining chronic Endometritis: the importance of endometrial stromal changes. Fertil Steril. 2021;116(3):855-61.
19. Cicinelli E, Haimovich S, De Ziegler D, Raz N, Ben-Tzur D, Andrisani A, et al.; International Working Group for Standardization of Chronic Endometritis Diagnosis. MUM-1 immunohistochemistry has high accuracy and reliability in the diagnosis of chronic endometritis: a multi-centre comparative study with CD138 immunostaining. J Assist Reprod Genet. 2022;39:219-26.
20. T Bamford, D Polson, P Lowe, C Easter, A Coomarasamy. P-350 Endometrial receptivity analysis (ERA) and microbiome testing for recurrent implantation failure (RIF): a matched case control study. Human Reproduction. 2022;37(1).
21. Strug MR, Hartup LA, Ryan E, Lathi RB. Unveiling the silver lining: a narrative review of clinical evaluation and management of chronic endometritis and its impact on fertility. F&S Reviews. 2024;5(2).
22. Cicinelli E, Matteo M, Tinelli R, Pinto V, Marinaccio M, Indraccolo U, et al. Chronic endometritis due to common bacteria is prevalent in women with recurrent miscarriage as confirmed by improved Chronic endometritis in repeated IVF failures from pregnancy outcome after antibiotic treatment. Reprod Sci. 2014;21:640-7.
23. Molina NM, Sola-Leyva A, Saez-Lara MJ, Plaza-Diaz J, Tubić-Pavlović A, Romero B, et al. New Opportunities for Endometrial Health by Modifying Uterine Microbial Composition: Present or Future? Biomolecules. 2020;10(4):593.
24. Pantos K, Simopoulou M, Maziotis E, Rapani A, Grigoriadis S, Tsioulou P, et al. Introducing intrauterine antibiotic infusion as a novel approach in effectively treating chronic endometritis and restoring reproductive dynamics: a randomized pilot study. Sci Rep. 2021;11(1):15581.

25. Sfakianoudis K, Simopoulou M, Nikas Y, Rapani A, Nitsos N, Pierouli K, et al. Efficient treatment of chronic endometritis through a novel approach of intrauterine antibiotic infusion: a case series. BMC Womens Health. 2018; 18:197.
26. Espinós JJ, Fabregues F, Fontes J, García-Velasco JA, Llácer J, Requena A, et al.; Spanish Infertility SWOT Group (SISG). Impact of chronic endometritis in infertility: a SWOT analysis. Reprod Biomed Online. 2021;42(5):939-51.
27. Samodelkin EI, Mercucheva NG, Kosareva PV, Nesterova LY. The role of prostaglandins and Cyclooxygenase in pathogenesis of chronic endometritis. Patol Fiziol Eksp Ter. 2017;61(2):98-100.
28. Sekulovski N, Whorton AE, Shi M, MacLean JA, Hayashi K. Endometriotic inflammatory microenvironment induced by macrophages can be targeted by niclosamide. Biology of Reproduction. 2019;100(2):398-408.
29. Bayer-Garner IB, Nickell JA, Korourian S. Routine syndecan-1 immunohistochemistry aids in the diagnosis of chronic endometritis. Arch Pathol Lab Med. 2004;128(9):1000-3.
30. Chang Y, Li J, Chen Y, Wei L, Yang X, Shi Y, et al. Autologous platelet-rich plasma promotes endometrial growth and improves pregnancy outcome during in vitro fertilization. Int J Clin Exp Med. 2015;8(1):1286-90.
31. Konoplya AA, Gavrish SA, Konoplya AI, Loktionov AL. The application of intravascular laser irradiation of blood for the correction of the immune disturbances in patients presenting with chronic endometritis. Vopr Kurortol Fizioter Lech FizKult. 2016;93(5):19-22.

CHAPTER 13

Latent Tuberculosis

Sonia Malik

ABSTRACT

Tubercular infection continues to rage as one of the leading cause of death in females. 25% of pulmonary tuberculosis patients suffer from female genital tuberculosis. Genital tuberculosis goes through various stages depending upon the immunological status of the female. It presents as active disease when the immune system is weak and remains in a latent state in the woman if the immune system is strong. Latent tuberculosis is defined as the state of TB when there are no symptoms, and the disease is picked up only on testing. Latent tuberculosis can be activated any time when the immunity is low. This can be seen in pregnancy, conditions like diabetes, if the patient has medications like steroids and infections like HIV. Recently, tuberculosis has been recognized as a disease causing miscarriages, preterm labor and even recurrent pregnancy loss. Two cases are presented, emphasizing the need to recognize latent tuberculosis as a cause of recurrent pregnancy loss.

Keywords: Latent tuberculosis, Immunology, Pregnancy, Recurrent pregnancy loss.

INTRODUCTION

One-third of the world's population harbors the *Mycobacterium* tubercle bacillus according to World Health Organization (WHO) statistics.[1] It kills two million people each year and around eight million new cases of tuberculosis (TB) are detected each year. The resurgence of TB the world over is probably due to frequent travel across countries, the breakdown of health services, the spread of the human immunodeficiency virus human immunodeficiency virus (HIV)/immunodeficiency syndrome (AIDS), and the emergence of multidrug-resistance bacteria. Extrapulmonary TB is now recognized as a major health hazard and genital TB forms an underdiagnosed part of it. Genital TB affects women of all age groups but in the reproductive age group, it can cause infertility in a fair number of cases. The actual incidence of genital TB is not known because of its subtle presentation. It is estimated that 5% of females presenting themselves in infertility clinics worldwide have genital TB and the majority (80–90%) of women are in the age group of 20–40 years but older women are also known to harbor it.[2]

Female genital TB is almost always secondary to TB elsewhere in the patient's body. 8–15% of women suffering from pulmonary TB may have genital TB.[3] The future course of the disease depends upon the virulence of the organism and the immune response mounted by the host.

In the case of a low-virulence organism and a good immune response, the disease is contained and lies latent for many years. If the organism is highly virulent or the host is immunocompromised, the disease spreads. The spread may be hematogenous, lymphatic, or a direct extension from a contiguous focus.[4] Hematogenous spread is generally from the lungs while lymphatic spread is known to occur from a primary abdominal lesion in the intestine or kidneys. Some references to a direct spread by venereal transmission are also found in the literature.[5] Tubes are the likely source of initial infection in the majority of the cases and both tubes are involved in 85–100% of cases.[2,5,6] The uterus is said to be involved in 50–70% of cases predominantly affecting the endometrium and occasionally the myometrium.[2,5] Indian studies have quoted an endometrial involvement of up to 99.5% of cases of genital TB.[7] Ovaries may be involved in 20–30% of cases.[5]

Active TB arises only in 10% of the infected individuals[8] and generally, a clinically asymptomatic latent persistent infection develops.[9] These latently infected individuals harbor dormant yet viable bacilli that are capable of reactivating themselves to cause disease. In the presence of normal host defense or antimycobacterial drugs, the bacilli are converted to metabolically inactive nonacid-fast granular forms. These represent cell wall deficient variants which may remain dormant but may also revert back to the parent acid-fast bacilli when immunocompromised, thus causing the disease to persist despite chemotherapy.[10]

LATENT TUBERCULOSIS

It has long been known that intracellular organisms like viruses can evade the host by transforming themselves into inert forms that can survive within the cells under minimally conducive survival conditions. The concept of TB continuing to remain in the body as a latent infection was first understood when it was realized that TB is rampant in patients with HIV. The disease was found to surface when the immunity of the person was found to be low. Further experiments on guinea pigs where similar conditions were created confirmed that the inert forms of the organism lying within the subcutaneous fat of the animal replicated into active forms under favorable conditions.[11]

Hence, TB can be present in broadly in two forms: (1) Active and (2) latent. With a better understanding of the pathogenesis and progression in the study of this disease, it has been found that TB evolves as a disease after passing through various stages from lying latent to a fully active virulent disease. Chan & Flynn et al.[12] elaborated upon the etiopathology of the various stages of the infection, how it evades the host immune system and survives in the body, and in situations where the host response breaks down, the organism starts getting activated thus progressing from a dormant stage to an active form. So, it was a continuum rather than a sudden change. Many studies have elaborated upon conditions associated with latent TB—one noteworthy being the activation of the disease when antitumor necrosis factor alpha (anti-TNFα) drugs were given to patients of arthritis or uveitis.[13]

This reiterated the concept that it was the immune system of the host that kept a check on the disease. However, none of the studies mention pregnancy or related physiological states that may allow one to understand the presentation of this form of extrapulmonary disease in women.

PREGNANCY HORMONES, IMMUNE SYSTEM, AND TUBERCULOSIS

Medhawar[14] based his hypothesis and later findings of the immune system and immunomodulation on the state of pregnancy and likened it to allograft acceptance or rejection. This formed the basis of present-day transplant medicine. Taking a cue from the same, we hypothesized[10] that it was the heightened immune system of the infected mother (in this case with TB) that was controlling the infection and also at the same time not accepting the foreign proteins of the sperm or embryo as its own leading to infertility. New research is now pointing toward the same and in fact, has demonstrated the specific cytokines that get upregulated and downregulated depending upon the hormonal status of the patient in pregnancy. If the hormonal milieu is normal, the pregnancy continues uninterrupted but if it is disturbed, it not only affects the cytokine cascade and immune system but also the microbiome within the uterus. *Mycobacterium tuberculosis (M. tb)* is a known microbe that is known to reside in the reproductive tract and cause irreparable damage if not detected early. Hence, these new insights into the immune system and how it orchestrates pregnancy are worth considering.

During pregnancy, the maternal immune system undergoes transient modification in order to promote tolerance to fetal antigens **(Table 1)**.[15] Apart from a Th1/Th2 shift, to maintain maternal-fetal tolerance, pregnancy is also accompanied by changes in the Th17/Treg cell balance, resulting in a reduction of Th17 and expansion of Treg responses. Reduced proportions of Treg cells and an increase in the Th17/Treg ratio have been observed in women with a history of recurrent spontaneous abortion.[16] Thus, the balance between Th17 and Treg cells is crucial for a successful pregnancy outcome. Hence, Tregs play an important role in regulating the maternal immune system to tolerate the fetus, which expresses paternal antigens. Studies have demonstrated high numbers of Tregs in decidua and the periphery, in mice and humans, during pregnancy.[17,18] Pregnancy-related complications such as miscarriage and preeclampsia have also been associated with reduced expression of Tregs in the placental decidua.[19,20] Further supporting that Treg cells are central for the maintenance of pregnancy. Expansion of Tregs in decidua and periphery during pregnancy suppresses maternal Th1/Th17 activity.[21] The mechanism behind the suppressive effect of Tregs is not completely understood. It has been proposed that the Treg responses are mediated in a cell-contact-dependent manner through the recognition of costimulatory molecules that suppress the activity of effector T cells.[22] Fetomaternal tolerance is generated after the Treg cells recognize fetal antigens by maternal antigen-presenting cells (APCs) and tolerance is established in an antigen-specific manner.[22] Another Treg suppressive mechanism is by production of regulatory and anti-inflammatory cytokines, such as transforming growth factor-beta (TGF-β) and interleukin-10 (IL-10). Pregnancy enhances the expression of these cytokines which can stimulate the expansion and suppressive

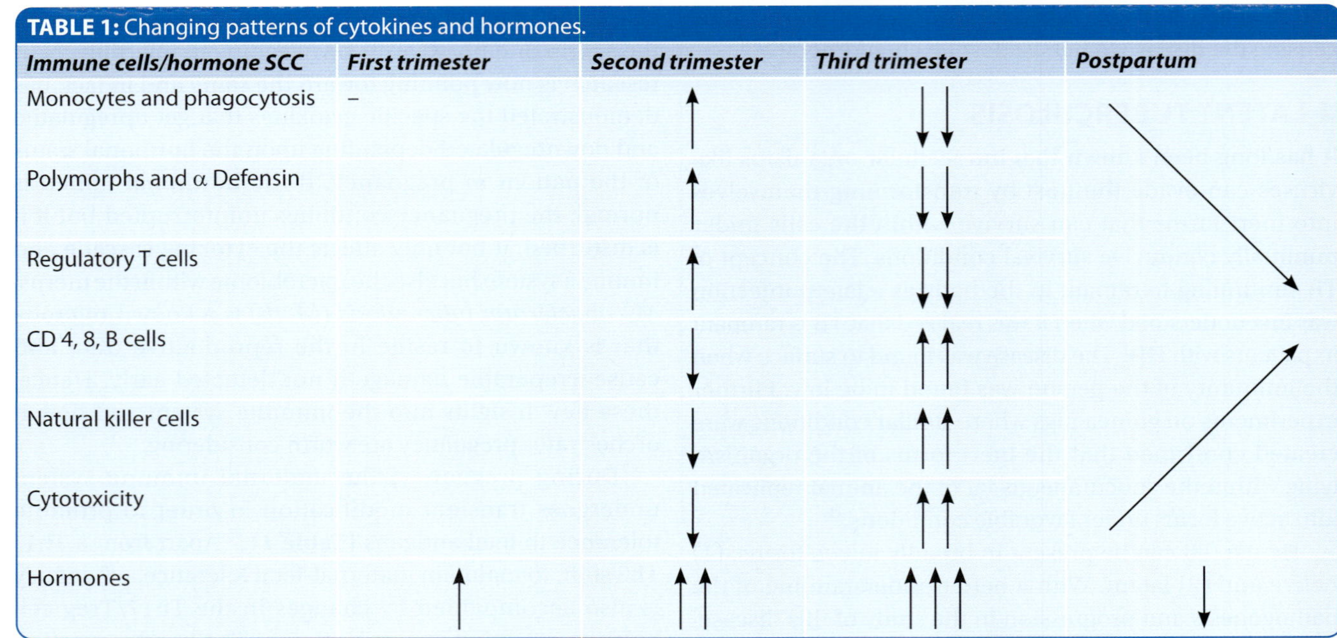

TABLE 1: Changing patterns of cytokines and hormones.

Immune cells/hormone SCC	*First trimester*	*Second trimester*	*Third trimester*	*Postpartum*
Monocytes and phagocytosis	–	↑	↓↓	↘
Polymorphs and α Defensin		↑	↓↓	↘
Regulatory T cells		↑	↓↓	↘
CD 4, 8, B cells		↓	↑↑	↗
Natural killer cells		↓	↑↑	↗
Cytotoxicity		↓	↑↑	↗
Hormones	↑	↑↑	↑↑↑	↓

activity of Tregs and prevent immunological rejection of the fetus. TGF-β is an important factor in establishing early embryo development, trophoblastic differentiation, and proliferation in human fetuses.

In addition, trophoblasts, which develop in the placenta, induce fetomaternal tolerance by expressing an inhibitory enzyme called indoleamine 2,3-dioxygenase (IDO). IDO suppresses the secretion and activity of maternal immune cells[23] Furthermore, trophoblasts induce immune suppression through the secretion of regulatory cytokines, such as TGF-β and IL-10.[24]

EFFECT OF PREGNANCY

Stewart made his observations on TB in pregnancy[25,26] that are true to this day: (1) Both pregnancy and TB can have adverse effects on each other and are linked with poor outcomes, (2) outcomes are variable and extremely difficult to predict early in pregnancy, and management decisions should be made on a case-by-case basis, and (3) for all populations, there should be special provision made for pregnant women with TB. Worldwide, an estimated 900 million women have a latent *Mycobacterium tuberculosis* infection (LTBI), and pregnant women with LTBI are more likely to progress developing active tuberculous disease than men.[27]

It has been observed by obstetricians that pregnancy is associated with a more active and rapid onset of TB and also more rapid progression of TB disease compared with the non-pregnant state. Moreover, the postpartum period may be associated with an increased risk of TB reactivation. LTBI was estimated to be present in up to nearly one-half of foreign-born pregnant women tested in the USA[28] and recently Sustained Attention to Response Task (SART) has advised that the latent disease should be looked for in infertile patients of foreign origin who present to the infertility clinics of the US. Immunological changes associated with pregnancy favor the reactivation of mycobacterial infection. In the late stages of pregnancy, a whole range of modifications in both cellular and humoral immunity have been observed.[29,30]

Increased levels and activity of phagocytes and plasmacytoid dendritic cells have been reported with respect to cellular immunity, and simultaneously a down-regulated natural killer (NK) cell cytotoxicity by progesterone-induced blocking factor and interleukin (IL)-10, and also a decrease in interferon-gamma (IFN-γ) production, indicate a generally suppressed innate cellular response.[31,32]

Th1 cytokines (IFN-γ and IL-12) are down-regulated thus also changing the adaptive response, however, reports on Th2 responses are conflicting. Humoral immunity shows increased levels of complement proteins and acute phase reactants and also increased T-cell-dependent immunoglobulin production· Such changes favor the activation of viral as well as other opportunist infections like TB **(Table 1)**. This also explains why pregnant women who are HIV-positive and have LTBI are more likely to progress to active TB disease.[33]

ACTIVATION OF LATENT FEMALE GENITAL TUBERCULOSIS TO DISEASE (FIG. 1)

Females with LMTB and their labile immune system are therefore at an increased risk of progression to full-blown active TB yet, a large number may not develop TB, either because of an efficient immune system or because they are no longer infected with live bacteria.

There is also increasing evidence that the familial genetics of the host also influence its disease manifestations, fulminant spread, and outcomes.[34] An attempt to make an infertile patient pregnant may also activate the latent infection.[35,36]

Reactivation can also be initiated during surgical manipulation and has been observed postlaparoscopy, hysteroscopy, hysterosalpingography,[37,38] and pelvic surgery.[39] High steroid levels and increased vascularity during ovarian stimulation are thought to be the triggering factors in the infertile population going through in vitro fertilization (IVF). Empirical use of steroids and immunotherapies is common in infertile patients with recurrent implantation failure and recurrent pregnancy loss, and these also increase the risk for reactivation.[40] The risk factors for reactivation are presented in **Box 1**.

Immunocompromise always remains the most important cause of reactivation of dormant bacterium as seen in HIV-positive individuals.[41] Recently there have been papers attributing recurrent pregnancy loss (RPL) and recurrent implantation failure (RIF) to female genital tuberculosis (FGTB). A systematic review of 624 cases described cases of RIF found to be positive for TB showed a lower pregnancy rate and RIF after embryo transfer.[42]

In another retrospective analysis of RPL, patients were found to have a lower pregnancy rate and higher miscarriage rate in patients affected by FGTB. Live birth was higher (75%) in the group that did not have tubercular involvement of the genital tract.[43]

The author's personal case series reported a success rate of 41.6% and an abortion rate of only 8.4% after the detection of FGTB and treatment with antitubercular treatment (ATT) in patients with unexplained pregnancy losses.[44]

Tuberculosis is known as the Great Masquerade. In this context, we cite two cases that explain how latent FGTB escapes diagnosis and leads to multiple pregnancy loss.

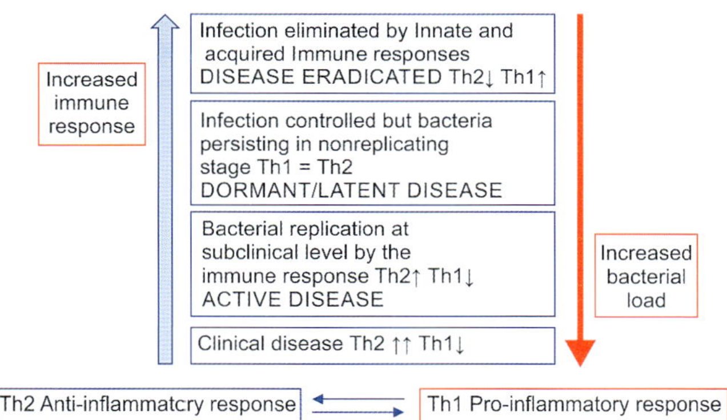

Fig. 1: Phases of tuberculosis.

BOX 1: Risk factors for reactivation of latent to active disease.

Risk factors for reactivation

- *Host factors:*
  - Host resistance an inflammation
  - Compromised immunity due to noncommunicable disease, such as diabetes type 2 and pregnancy
  - Characteristics of immune activation and inflammation
  - Genetics
  - HIV coinfection
  - Therapy using TNF-alpha
- *Pathogen factors:*
  - Pathogen species and load
  - Degree of pathogen replication
  - Type of pathology
  - Spread of lesions

CASES

Case 1

A 34-year-old CA; with a 31-year-old husband has been married for 4 years and has been trying for pregnancy for 2.5 years.

Menstrual history: Period lasts for 3 days/28–30 days/regular/mild pain. Last menstrual period 19/02/24

The patient has been receiving supportive therapy in the form of progesterone, Human chorionic gonadotropin (hCG), aspirin, intralipid, and low molecular weight heparin.

Past history: Not significant medical or surgical history

Family history: Father—alcoholic pancreatitis—followed by type 3 diabetes mellitus (DM)

Husband history: Not significant, no addiction.

Infertility treatment done so far: Ovulation induction done with clomiphene citrate—not conceived in that cycle.

TABLE 2: Obstetric history case 1.

Spontaneous/IVF conception	***Beta-hCG***	***USG Findings***	***Miscarriage***
Spontaneous conception	300	No gestational sac	Spontaneous
Spontaneous conception	Positive	6 weeks gestational sac with faint cardiac activity initially and later absent cardiac activity	MTP
Spontaneous conception	Positive	• 8 weeks-subchorionic hemorrhage • Cardiac activity 145 beats/min • 10 weeks—no cardiac activity	10 weeks bleeding P/V MTP microarray normal
Spontaneous conception	500	No gestational sac	Spontaneous
Spontaneous conception	100	No gestational sac	Spontaneous
Spontaneous conception	200	No gestational sac	Spontaneous
• IVF conception • PGTA-Euploid	1,054	• Gestational sac seen • No fetal pole	Spontaneous

(IVF: in vitro fertilization; MTP: medical termination of pregnancy; PGTA: preimplantation genetic testing for aneuploidy; P/V: per vaginum)

Diagnosis of 34-year-old POA7 with recurrent pregnancy loss was made.

All investigations were normal except that they all showed growth retardation in the pregnancies that were supported and grew a little bit.

TABLE 3: Investigations case 1.

Investigation	***Results***
MRI	Slightly concave uterine fundal contour, with increased intercornual distance s/o partial bicornuate, bilateral ovaries normal
MLPA for SMA, CAH, DMD	• Husband-carrier of likely pathogenic variant in *NPHP4* gene • Wife-carrier of likely pathogenic variant in *MYO7A* gene • Noncarriers of SMA
• CD3 • CD19 • $CD16^{+}56$	• 78.9% • 11.8% • 8.82%
Karyotype	• *Wife:* 46,XX • *Husband:* 46,XY
HLA typing	Normal
• FBS • PPBS	• 86 • 101
• Anti-TPO antibodies • TSH	• 87.05 • 1.5
Factor V Leiden mutation	Not detected
Lupus anticoagulant	Absent
Factor viii activity	Normal
Anticardiolipin antibodies	Negative
Anti-beta-2 glycoprotein-	Negative
Prolactin	19.13
AMH	1.01
Blood grouping and typing	Both partners-A positive

(AMH: anti-Müllerian hormone; CAH: congenital adrenal hyperplasia; DMD: Duchenne muscular dystrophy; FBS: fasting blood sugar; HLA: human lymphocyte antigen; MLPA: multiplex ligation-dependent probe amplification; MRI: magnetic resonance imaging; PPBS: postprandial blood sugar; SMA: smooth muscle antibody; TPO: thyroid peroxidase; TSH: thyroid stimulating hormone)

Case 2

A 32-year-old lady married to a 34-year-old man for the past 3 years. Started trying soon after they got married.

Mensuration cycle normal 4/28 days, past history normal, no surgical or medical history. Family history: Grandmother had pulmonary TB.

TABLE 4: Obstetric history of case 2.

Spontaneous/IVF conception	*Beta-hCG*	*USG Findings*	*Miscarriage*
Spontaneous	Positive	Missed miscarriage corresponding to 7 weeks	MTP
Spontaneous	Positive	At 10 weeks, USG findings corresponding to 7.4 weeks with absent cardiac activity	MTP
Spontaneous	Positive	• NT scan normal • USG 2 days prior to the abortion for a slightly shortened cervix of 1.8 cm and ascites in the abdomen	Spontaneous second-trimester miscarriage at 16 weeks

(hCG: human chorionic gonadotropin; MTP: medical termination of pregnancy; NT: nuchal translucency; USG: ultrasonography)

TABLE 5: Obstetric history of case 2.

Investigation	*Results*
Karyotype	• *Wife:* 46,XX • *Husband:* 46,XY
HLA typing	Normal
• FBS • PPBS	• 80 mg/dL • 94 mg/dL
• Anti-TPO antibodies • TSH	• Negative • 2.5
Factor V Leiden mutation	Not detected
Lupus anticoagulant	Absent
Factor viii activity	Normal
Anticardiolipin antibodies	Negative
Anti-beta-2 glycoprotein-	Negative
Prolactin	20.2
AMH	2.23
Blood grouping and typing	Both partners-B positive

In both these cases, an endometrial biopsy revealed a positive polymerase chain reaction (PCR) and tuberculosis nucleic acid amplification testing (TB NAAT). On giving appropriate treatment, both patients conceived and carried on till full term they delivered at term giving birth to female babies.

These cases highlight the importance of testing for genital TB in recurrent pregnancy loss. The infection had gone unnoticed because it was latent TB.

The definition of latent TB comprises of incubating actively replicating bacteria in the absence of clinical symptoms. Similarly, active TB is characterized by diverse presentations, ranging from small granulomas, and caseous lesions containing variable numbers of bacteria, to liquefied cavities with a massive load of replicating organisms to miliary disease. The question then arises whether every patient should positive for the disease be treated or if it is only the active disease that requires treatment. What then is the marker that can differentiate between the two states: active or latent?

TABLE 6: STW for the management of female genital tuberculosis.

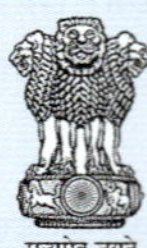

Department of Health Research
Ministry of Health and Family Welfare, Government of India

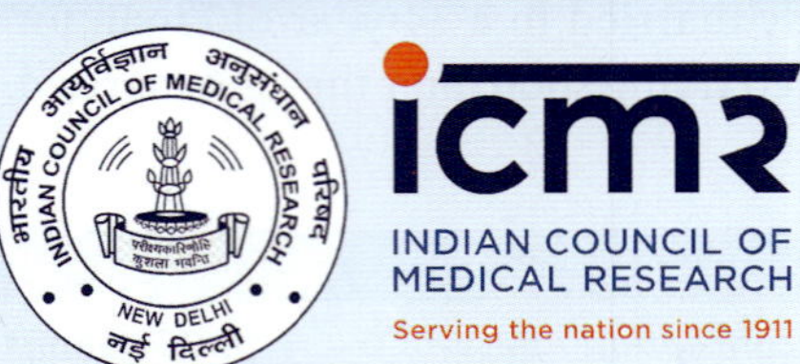

Standard Treatment Workflow (STW) for the Management of Female Genital Tuberculosis ICD-10-A18.17

	Suspect	
WHEN TO SUSPECT?	Consider the following symptoms in history: • H/O infertility (primary or secondary) • Chronic lower abdominal or pelvic pain • Amenorrhea or other menstrual disturbances • Abnormal vaginal discharge • Constitutional symptoms of TB (low grade fever, weight loss, etc.) • Other symptoms related to extragenital TB (abdominal, CNS, bone and lymph nodes etc.) In addition, standard investigations for TB to be carried out	*Clinical examination*: • General physical examination • Pelvic Examination (cervical growth, uterine size and mobility, adnexal tenderness, and mass) *Abdominal and pelvic USG (TVS)*: • Uterus, adnexa and pelvis to be evaluated preferably by transvaginal scan • Endometrial cavity and vascularity to be looked carefully with color Doppler *Specific investigations*: • Endometrial sampling or biopsy with Pipelle device or Karman cannula (4 mm) for microbiological and histopathological examination • *Endoscopy*: – Hysteroscopy and laparoscopy to evaluate the uterus, adnexa, and other pelvic organs along with the lower abdomen – Laparoscopic biopsy from peritoneum or abdominal/pelvic lesions • MTB diagnosis from biopsy specimen (endometrium and other tissues) by: – Smear microscopy (AFB smear) and culture – Gene Xpert or other NAAT – HPE of biopsy specimen

(H/O: history of; HPE: histopathology examination; MTB: Mycobacterium tuberculosis; NAAT: nucleic acid amplification test; TB: tuberculosis; TVS: transvaginal ultrasound scan; USG: ultrasonography)

TESTS FOR LATENT TUBERCULOSIS INFECTION

So, LTBI may be defined as a state of persistent immune response to *M. tb* antigens detected by biomarkers that may:

- Either be an indicator of a normal biological process
- Pathological process
- Pharmacological response to therapeutic intervention.

In infectious diseases, biomarkers can either be host or pathogen-derived, and in TB infection these markers can be used for diagnostic and prognostic tools, monitoring of anti-TB treatment success and evaluation of vaccine response by the tuberculin skin test (TST) or by interferon-alpha release assay (IGRA) without evidence of clinically manifest TB.[9]

Although there is advancement in the understanding of FGTB, it is still a challenge to diagnose genital TB despite a battery of tests being present. Female genital TB is a paucibacillary disease hence it is very difficult to find the bacteria within the tract. An acid-fast bacillus (AFB) culture or presence of bacteria in the tissue or fluid is even today considered the gold standard. A positive PCR or a NAAT like Gene Xpert is also now considered a standard test for extrapulmonary TB recommended in the Index

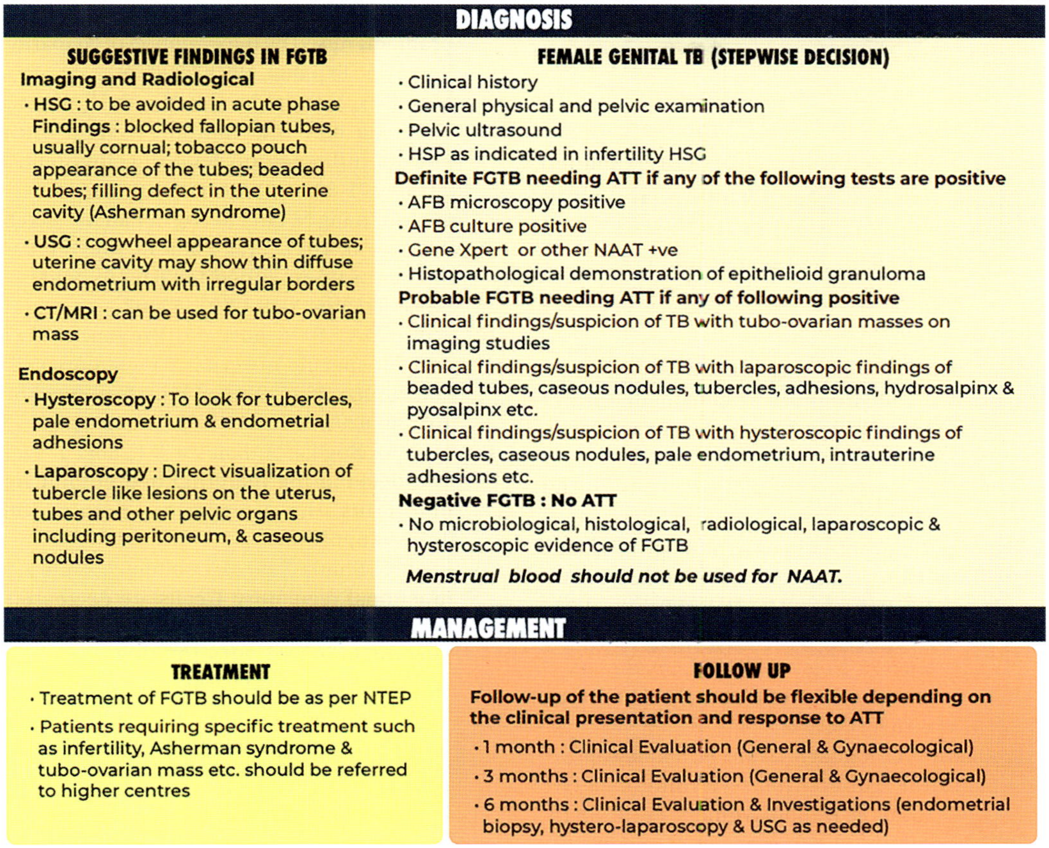

Fig. 2: Standard treatment workflow for genital tuberculosis. (AFB: Acid–fast bacilli, ATT: antituberculosis therapy; CNS: central nervous system; CT: computed tomography; FGTB: female genital tuberculosis; FNAC: fine-needle aspiration cytology; HSE: histopathology examination; HSG: hysterosalpingography; MRI: magnetic resonance imaging; MTB: Mycobacterium tuberculosis; NAAT: nucleic acid amplification test; NTEP: National Tuberculosis Elimination Programme; PCR: polymerase chain reaction; TB: tuberculosis; TVS: transvaginal scan; USG: ultrasonography)

TB guidelines issued by the Indian Ministry of Health and Family Welfare in 2016.[45]

Indirect evidence such as ultrasound, magnetic resonance imaging (MRI), laparoscopy, and hysteroscopy, are used as diagnostic modalities for making a diagnosis. The pickup rate of most tests is poor ranging from 5 to 7% and many cases of early disease are missed.[45] An algorithmic approach using multiple tests, signs, and symptoms has been advocated[40,46] by workers.

This, however, still does not solve the problem of detecting the stage of the disease.

A promising more specific test is an updated version of the QFT-GIT that contains peptides that are intended to specifically induce a $CD8^+$ T-cell response in addition to the $CD4^+$ T-cell response. The rationale is that *M. tb*-specific $CD8^+$ T-cells are more frequently detected in people with active TB disease compared to LTBI, they are associated with a recent exposure to TB, and they decline when patients receive anti-TB treatment. The first data on the performance of QuantiFERON TB Plus in a multicenter European study was reported recently.[47] Yet another promising test is the TSPOT. TB which is also based on the IFN-γ levels. This test has been effectively used to detect LTBI in infertile patients undergoing IVF in order to rule out latent infection.[48]

Other biomarkers in addition to this have also been reported and seen as the future in the diagnosis of FGTB.

A recent guideline issued in 2022 by ICMR and the Ministry of Health and Family Welfare, defines a standard treatment workflow (STW) for the management of FGTB wherein the disease is defined according to the signs and symptoms and a positive definitive test like AFB culture is positive **(Tables 6 and Fig. 2)**.[49,50]

CONCLUSION

Genital TB in its latent form can play havoc with the reproductive tract. This can range from infertility to ectopic pregnancy to RIF to RPL. LGTB must always be kept in mind when confronted with a case of unexplained RPL. A battery of tests needs to be performed including an endometrial biopsy for AFB culture, PCR, TB NAAT, and histopathology. Treatment with ATT gives good results.

REFERENCES

1. World Health Organization. WHO Fact sheet No. 104. (2002). [Online] Available from ww.whoint/mediacentre/factsheet/who104/eu/index.html [Last accessed December, 2024].
2. Schaefer G "Female genital tuberculosis. Clin Obstet Gynecol. 1976;19(1):223-39.
3. Arora VK, Gupta R. Relevance of DOTS strategy in female genital tuberculosis. Obst Gynae Today. 2002;7(4):179-83.
4. Miller JW, Gilmour HM, Robertson HH. Vulval Tuberculosis. Tubercle. 1979;60(3):173-6.
5. Nogales-Ortiz F, Tarancón I, Nogales FF Jr. The pathology of female genital tuberculosis. A 31-year study of 1436 cases. Obstet Gynaecol. 1979;53(4):422-8.
6. Parikh F R, Nadkarni S G, Kamat SA, Naik N, Soonawala SB, Parikh RM. Genital Tuberculosis—a major pelvic factor causing infertility in Indian Women. Fertil Steril. 1997;67(3):497-500
7. Agarwal J, Gupta JK. Female Genital Tuberculosis—a retrospective clinico-pathologic study 501 cases. Indian J Pathol Microbiol. 1994;37(2):232.
8. Stead WW. Pathogenesis of a first episode of chronic pulmonary tuberculosis in man: recrudescence of residuals of the primary infection or exogenous reinfection? Am Rev Resp Dis. 1967;95(5):729-74.
9. Stead WW, Kerby GR, Schlueter DP, Jordahl CW. The clinical spectrum of primary tuberculosis in adults. Confusion with reinfection in the pathogenesis of chronic tuberculosis. Ann Intern Med. 1968;68(4):731-45.
10. Chandrasekhar S, Ratnam S. Studies on cell-wall deficient non-acid fast variants of Mycobacterium tuberculosis. Tuber Lung Dis. 1992;73(5):273-9.
11. Malik S. Genital tuberculosis and implantation in assisted reproduction. Rev Gynaecol Pract. 2003;3(3):160-4.
12. Wira CR, Fahey JV. A new strategy to understand how HIV infects women: identification of a window of vulnerability during the menstrual cycle. AIDS (London, England). 2008;22(15):1909.
13. Chan J, Flynn J. The immunological aspects of latency in tuberculosis. Clinical immunology. 2004;110(1):2-12.
14. Stenger S. Immunological control of tuberculosis: role of tumour necrosis factor and more. Ann Rheum Dis. 2005;64(Suppl 4):iv24-8.
15. Medawar PB. Some immunological and endocrinological problems raised by the evolution of viviparity in vertebrates. Symp Soc Exp Biol. 1953;7:320-38.
16. Morelli S, Mandal M, Goldsmith LT, Kashani BN, Ponzio NM. The maternal immune system during pregnancy and its influence on fetal development. Res Rep Biol. 2015;6:171-89.
17. Qian J, Zhang N, Lin J, Wang C, Pan X, Chen L, et al. Distinct pattern of Th17/Treg cells in pregnant women with a history of unexplained recurrent spontaneous abortion. Biosci Trends. 2018;12(2):157–67.
18. Kahn DA, Baltimore D. Pregnancy induces a fetal antigen-specific maternal T regulatory cell response that contributes to tolerance. Proc Natl Acad Sci U S A. 2010; 107(20):9299-304.
19. Mori M, Bogdan A, Balassa T, Csabai T, Szekeres-Bartho J. The decidua-the maternal bed embracing the embryo-maintains the pregnancy. Semin Immunopathol. 2016;38(6):635-49.
20. Inada K, Shima T, Ito M, Ushijima A, Saito S. Helios-positive functional regulatory T cells are decreased in decidua of miscarriage cases with normal fetal chromosomal content. J Reprod Immunol. 2015;107:10-9.
21. Sasaki Y, Sakai M, Miyazaki S, Higuma S, Shiozaki A, Saito S. Decidual and peripheral blood $CD4^{+}CD25^{+}$ regulatory T cells in early pregnancy subjects and spontaneous abortion cases. Mol Hum Reprod. 2004;10(5):347-53.
22. Saito S, Nakashima A, Shima T, Ito M. Th1/Th2/Th17 and Regulatory T-Cell Paradigm in Pregnancy. Am J Reprod Immunol. 2010;63(6):601-10.
23. Tsuda S, Nakashima A, Shima T, Saito S. New paradigm in the role of regulatory T cells during pregnancy. Front Immunol. 2019;10:573.
24. Chang RQ, Li DJ, Li MQ. The role of indoleamine-2,3-dioxygenase in normal and pathological pregnancies. Am J Reprod Immunol. 2017;79(4):e12786.
25. Guzeloglu-Kayisli O, Kayisli UA, Taylor HS. The role of growth factors and cytokines during Implantation: endocrine and paracrine interactions. Semin Reprod Med. 2009;27(1):62-79.
26. Stewart DA. Pregnancy and Tuberculosis: Part 2.-The Treatment of Tuberculosis Complicated by Pregnancy. Can Med Assoc J. 1922;12(2):103-6.
27. Stewart DA. Pregnancy and tuberculosis: Part I-The effects of pregnancy on tuberculosis. Can Med Assoc J. 1922;12(1):1-3.
28. Malhamé I, Cormier M, Sugarman J, Schwartzman K. Latent Tuberculosis in Pregnancy: A Systematic Review Isabelle Malhamé, Maxime Cormier, Jordan Sugarman, Kevin Schwartzman. PLoS One. 2016; 11(5): e01548259.
29. ASRM Press release. (2017). SART is the primary organization of professionals dedicated to the practice of assisted reproductive technologies (ART) in the United States. [Online] Available from www.sart.org [Last accessed December, 2024].

30. Zenner D, Kruijshaar ME, Andrews N, Abubakar I. Risk of tuberculosis in pregnancy: a national, primary care-based cohort and self-controlled case series study. Am J Respir Crit Care Med. 2012;185(7):779-84.
31. Gupta A, Nayak U, Ram M, Bhosale R, Patil S, Basavraj A, et al., Byramjee Jeejeebhoy Medical College-Johns Hopkins University Study Group. Postpartum tuberculosis incidence and mortality among HIV-infected women and their infants in Pune, India, 2002-2005. Clin Infect Dis. 2007;45(2):2419-9.
32. Kraus TA, Engel SM, Sperling RS, Kellerman L, Lo Y, Wallenstein S, et al. Characterizing the pregnancy immune phenotype: results of the viral immunity and pregnancy (VIP) study. J Clin Immunol. 2012;32(2):300-11.
33. Singh N, Perfect JR. Immune reconstitution syndrome and exacerbation of infections after pregnancy. Clin Infect Dis. 2007;45(9):1192-9.
34. Pazos M, Sperling RS, Moran TM, Kraus TA. The influence of pregnancy on systemic immunity. Immunol Res. 2012;54(1-3):254-61.
35. Shanmugalakshmi S, Pitchappan RM. Genetic basis of tuberculosis susceptibility in India. Indian J Pediatr. 2002;69(Suppl 1):S25-8.
36. Huang HJ, Xiang DR, Sheng JF. Exacerbation of latent genital tuberculosis during in vitro fertilisation and pregnancy. Int J Tuberc Lung Dis. 2009;13(7):921.
37. Annamraju H, Ganapathy R, Webb B. Pelvic tuberculosis reactivated by in vitro fertilization egg collection? Fertil Steril. 2008;90(5):2003.e1-3.
38. Singh N, Sharma A, Dadhwal V, Gupta N, Mittal S. Postoperative flare-up of genital tuberculosis: a clinical reality. [Int J Tuberc Lung Dis. 2008;12(8):981-3.
39. Forseyl J, Caul E, Paul I, Hull M. Chlamydia trachomatis, tubal disease and the incidence of symptomatic and asymptomatic infection following hysterosalpingography. Hum Reprod. 1990;5(4):444-7.
40. Jha AA, Ballal R, Aditya G. Reactivation of tuberculosis following major abdominal surgery. J Health All Sci NU. 2016;6(4):87-8.
41. Mahajan N, Naidu P, Kaur SD. Insight into the diagnosis and management of subclinical genital tuberculosis in women with infertility. J Hum Reprod Sci. 2016;9(3):135-44.
42. Sullivan ZA, Wong EB, Ndung'u T, Kasprowicz VO, Bishai WR. Latent and Active Tuberculosis Infection Increase Immune Activation in Individuals Co-Infected with HIV. EBioMedicine. 2015;2(4):334-40.
43. Xinzhuan Jia, Lan Wei, Na Zhang, Bolin Zheng, Mengya Li, Hongxia Wang, et al. A retrospective analysis of the effect of latent tuberculosis infection on clinical pregnancy outcomes of in vitro fertilization-fresh embryo transferred in infertile women Open Med (Wars). 2023;18(1): 20230870.
44. Bagchi B, Chatterjee S, Chowdhury RG. Role of latent female genital tuberculosis in recurrent early pregnancy loss: A retrospective analysis. Int J Reprod Biomed. 2019;17(12):929-34.
45. Sharma SK, Ryan H, Sachdeva KS, Singh AD, Mohan A, Sarin R, et al. Index-TB Guidelines: Guidelines on extrapulmonary tuberculosis for India. Indian J Med Res. 2017;145(4):448-63.
46. Thangappah R, Paramasivan C, Narayanan S. Evaluating PCR, culture & histopathology in the diagnosis of female genital tuberculosis. Indian J Med Res. 2011;134(1):40-6.
47. Jindal U. An algorithmic approach to female genital tuberculosis causing infertility. Int J Tuberc Lung Dis. 2006;10(9):1045-50.
48. Petruccioli E, Scriba TJ, Petrone L, Hatherill M, Cirillo DM, Joosten SA, et al. Correlates of tuberculosis risk: predictive biomarkers for progression to active tuberculosis. Eur Resp J. 2016;48(6):1751-63.
49. Jia X, Wei L, Zhang N, Zheng B, Li M, Wang H, et al. A retrospective analysis of the effect of latent tuberculosis infection on clinical pregnancy outcomes of in vitro fertilization-fresh embryo transferred in infertile women. Open Med (Wars). 2023;18(1):20230870.
50. Indian Council of Medical Research, Department of Health Research, Ministry of Health and Family Welfare, Government of India. (2022). Standard Treatment Workflows of India, 2022, Special Edition on Paediatric and Extrapulmonary Tuberculosis. https://www.icmr.gov.in/icmrobject/uploads/STWs/1725964681_paediatric_tuberculosis_all.pdf [Last accessed December, 2024].

CHAPTER 14

Cytokines: Success or Failure of Pregnancy

Raj Raghupathy

ABSTRACT

Cytokines are small protein molecules that are secreted to control the growth and activity of other immune cells. They are classified into proinflammatory (TNF-α, IFN-γ, and IL-2 also called Th1) and anti-inflammatory (IL-4, IL-5, IL-6, and IL-10 also called Th2) cytokines.

During pregnancy the cytokine shift from proinflammatory to anti-inflammatory is vital for successful implantation. Failure of this shift in cytokine secretion in the decidua may lead to unexplained RPL. Progesterone may be responsible for the dominance of Th2 response in pregnancy. Besides this, increased number of natural killer cells and presence of Th17 cells which secrete IL-17, is also associated with an inflammatory response and RPL

Keywords: Cytokines, Th1, Th2, Interleukins, TNF alpha, Interferon gamma, Natural killer cells.

INTRODUCTION

From conception until delivery, pregnancy is fraught with numerous potential complications ranging from spontaneous miscarriage and preeclampsia to intrauterine growth restriction, intrauterine fetal death, and preterm delivery. The incidence of early pregnancy loss postimplantation can be as high as 31%.[1] The most common cause of pregnancy loss is sporadic spontaneous miscarriage,[2] defined as a clinically detectable loss of the fetus occurring before 20 weeks of gestation. About one out of every five pregnant women undergoes one or more spontaneous miscarriages.[3] Recurrent spontaneous miscarriage (RSM), or the occurrence of three or more spontaneous miscarriages, is a "sentinel risk marker" for several pregnancy complications, such as preterm birth, intrauterine fetal growth restriction, placental abruption, and stillbirth in future pregnancies.[3] RSM has been attributed to "known" etiologies such as anatomic abnormalities, chromosomal aberrations, infections, and endometrial dysfunction;[2,4] however, the etiology of as much as 60% of RSM remains "unknown" or "unexplained."[1-5] This has spurred extensive and intensive research directed at unraveling potential immunologic causes of spontaneous miscarriage.

Several humoral immune etiologic factors have been proposed for RSM over the years; these include antibodies to phospholipids, spermatozoa, and trophoblasts, and a deficiency of blocking antibodies.[1,2] Of these, only antiphospholipid antibodies have been confirmed as etiologic agents but are estimated to be responsible for only about 3% of the cases.[6] This led to research on *cellular* immunity (as opposed to *humoral* immunity) mediated by cellular effectors and/or cytokines secreted by them, and these have been shown to have significant deleterious effects on the conceptus.

Elucidating the roles, in pregnancy, of maternal T lymphocytes, macrophages, natural killer (NK) cells, as well as cytokines produced by them, has been aided significantly by our understanding of immune responses. The delineation of the subsets of T helper (Th) cells provides a framework for understanding how the immune system handles responses to different types of pathogens and antigenic stimuli.

Th1/Th2/Treg/Th17 REACTIVITY AND CYTOKINES

One of the most significant advances in immunology has been the delineation of the subsets of CD4$^+$ Th cells, of which Th1, Th2, T regulatory (Treg), and Th17 are the major ones; these Th cell subsets have different patterns of cytokine production and different roles in immune responses. Each subset mediates immune responses that are effective at handling certain types of pathogens but can be ineffective or even pathological if made in response to other types of pathogens.[7]

Th1 cells secrete the pro-inflammatory cytokines interferon (IFN)-γ, tumor necrosis factor (TNF)-α, and interleukin (IL)-2; these Th1-type cytokines activate macrophages and cell-mediated immune responses that are involved in defense against intracellular pathogens and in cytotoxic and delayed-type hypersensitivity reactions. In general, Th1 cytokines mediate strong cellular immunity and inflammatory reactions and are implicated in graft rejection, autoimmunity, and cytotoxicity.[8] On the contrary, Th2 lymphocytes produce the anti-inflammatory cytokines IL-4, IL-5, IL-10, and IL-13; these are cytokines that generally stimulate strong antibody responses and thus contribute to immune defense against extracellular infections.[8] Th1 and Th2 lymphocytes tend to inhibit each other; thus, individuals with strong Th1 responses tend to have poor Th2 reactivity and vice versa. Which type of reactivity, Th1 or Th2, is activated first may influence the subsequent outcome; if a particular T cell subset is activated first or preferentially in a response, it can suppress the development of the other subset. The overall effect is that certain responses are dominated by either humoral (Th2) or cell-mediated (Th1) immunity.

While Th1 and Th2 represent two polarized subsets that play important roles in immune responses, Treg and Th17 are two other important T cell subsets. Treg cells, as the name suggests, are cells that regulate the functions of several other cells; they suppress immune responses such as the proliferation of other T cells and thus play critical roles in maintaining homeostasis and in preventing autoimmune reactions. The immunoregulatory capability of Treg cells is attributed to the immunosuppressive cytokines IL-10 and transforming growth factor beta (TGF-β).[9] Th17 cells are pro-inflammatory and defined by their production of the inflammatory cytokine IL-17. These cells are developmentally different from Th1 and Th2 cells and play robust immunopathogenic roles in autoimmune and inflammatory disorders.[10]

MATERNAL IMMUNE STATUS DURING NORMAL PREGNANCY

Humoral immune responses are enhanced during pregnancy, while cell-mediated immunity such as delayed-type hypersensitivity, NK activity, responses to intracellular infections, and the severity of cell-mediated autoimmune disorders and inflammatory reactions are downregulated.[11] Clinical evidence indicates that pregnant women undergo immunological changes consistent with a weakening of Th1 responses and a strengthening of Th2 responses. Higher levels of IL-10, an anti-inflammatory Th2 cytokine, are produced by placental cells from pregnant women compared with nonpregnant women.[12] On the other hand, significantly reduced expression of IL-2 and IFN-γ messenger ribonucleic acid (mRNA) has been demonstrated during normal human pregnancy with Th1/Th2 ratios revealing a shift to a pronounced Th2 status.[13] Increased numbers of IL-4-producing T cells were demonstrated in normal pregnant women compared to nonpregnant women. In contrast, IFN-γ and IL-2-producing T cells were significantly reduced in pregnancy, suggestive of toward dominance of Th2 reactivity in pregnancy.[14] These studies on human pregnancy, along with extensive studies on animal models, led to the conclusion that successful pregnancy is correlated with, and even depends on, preferential stimulation of Th2 cytokine-producing T cells.[10-14]

Relevance of Cytokines to Pregnancy Loss

Cellular immunity mediated by effector cells and cytokines released by them has significant deleterious effects on the conceptus. The pro-inflammatory Th1-type cytokines TNF-α, IFN-γ, and IL-2 figure prominently among cytokines that contribute adversely to the survival of the conceptus. The administration of pregnant mice with IL-2 or IFN-γ or TNF-α results in abortions, while antibodies to TNF-α reduce abortion rates in mice that are prone to natural, immunologically mediated resorptions. The cytokines IFN-γ and TNF-α have been shown to hinder the growth of human trophoblasts in vitro;[15] they have also been shown to cause the apoptotic death of human primary villous trophoblast cells.[16] Soon an intriguing nexus between inflammatory Th1 cytokines and pregnancy failure was noticed[17] as researchers observed interesting connections between successful pregnancy and Th2 immunity. Wegmann et al.[11] were the first to make the insightful proposal that the conceptus protects itself by secreting Th2 cytokines, which downregulate harmful Th1 cytokines.

CYTOKINE PROFILES IN RECURRENT SPONTANEOUS MISCARRIAGE

Numerous studies have shown convincingly that the cytokine profile in women with RSM are different from those in women with healthy pregnancies. Hill's laboratory reported higher levels of pro-inflammatory Th1 cytokines secreted by peripheral blood lymphocytes from women with unexplained recurrent miscarriage when stimulated with a trophoblast antigen preparation secrete compared to lymphocytes from healthy pregnant controls.[18,19] Supernatants of such stimulated lymphocytes had embryotoxic activity; 66% of women with RSM had embryotoxic activity while none of the healthy controls did, and this embryotoxicity was shown to be due to the cytotoxic, inflammatory cytokine IFN-γ.[18,19] These researchers concluded that Th1 immunity to trophoblast antigens is associated with unexplained recurrent miscarriage and may play a role in reproductive failure, while Th2 immunity is the normal, healthy maternal immune response to trophoblast, contributing to healthy, successful pregnancy.[18]

Studies in our laboratory have shown higher levels of anti-inflammatory Th2 cytokines IL-4, IL-5, IL-6, and IL-10 produced by peripheral lymphocytes from healthy pregnant women compared to women with unexplained RSM. On the other hand, higher levels of the pro-inflammatory Th1 cytokines TNF-α, IFN-γ, and IL-2 are produced by women with RSM than by healthy pregnant women.[20,21] This was substantiated by our studies on maternal immune reactivity to placental antigens stimulated either by coculturing maternal lymphocytes with autologous placental cells or by exposing maternal lymphocytes to a trophoblast antigen preparation.[22] This dominance of inflammatory cytokines in RSM as opposed to a stronger Th2-bias in healthy pregnancy was supported by our observation that the ratios of inflammatory (Th1) cytokines to anti-inflammatory (Th2) cytokines were higher in women undergoing unexplained RSM group compared to women undergoing a normal pregnancy.[20-22]

An important question arises: Has a cause-and-effect relationship been demonstrated between cytokines and pregnancy loss? Studies on animals have shown that the injection of Th1 cytokines results in abortions,[23] but what we have in humans at present is a strong *association* between maternal cytokine profiles and pregnancy outcomes. One study came close to showing a cause-and-effect relationship; decreased production of the anti-inflammatory cytokines IL-4 and IL-10 and increased production of the inflammatory cytokines IFN-γ and IL-2 were observed in women with RSM 1–2 weeks *before* any upcoming pathology could be detected.[24]

What Is the Evidence for Local Production of Th2 Cytokines in Healthy Pregnancy?

The studies described above show persuasively that maternal cytokine profiles in the peripheral blood are skewed toward a pro-inflammatory bias in women with RSM. Is there evidence for a similar bias in the *local* environment, that is, at the maternal–fetal interface? Indeed, the situation in the maternal periphery is mirrored by reactivity at the maternal–fetal interface; endometrial expression of pro-inflammatory cytokines was shown to be upregulated, and anti-inflammatory cytokines downregulated in women with idiopathic recurrent miscarriage compared to controls.[25,26] Lower levels of Th2 cytokine-producing T cell clones were measured in the decidua of women with unexplained RSM than from women with normal pregnancy.[27] Th2 cytokines have been detected in postpartum human placental tissue,[28] amniotic fluid,[29] endometrium and decidua of early pregnancy,[30] and in supernatants from cultures of endometrial cells, decidual stroma,[31] cytotrophoblast,[28] and amnion epithelial cells.[31] Levels of IL-6 and IL-10 were substantially higher in endometrial biopsy tissues during pregnancy than in the nonpregnant state. Peri-implantation endometrial tissues were found to have predominantly Th2 cytokines, while Th1 cytokines were absent.[32] Similarly, IL-10 production by endometrial stromal cells was shown to be about a 100-fold higher during gestation than in the absence of pregnancy.[28]

How does Th2 reactivity become dominant in the decidua during normal gestation? Trophoblast cells produce IL-4 and IL-10, which induce Th2 cells,[27,33] and these cytokines activate more Th2 cells. Saito et al.[34,35] suggest that the high levels of IL-10 in the decidua of healthy pregnancies could help induce strong Th2-type responses. Indeed, levels of IL-10 are significantly higher in healthy pregnancy compared to unexplained RSM.[36] Furthermore, progesterone may well have an influential role in this process,[37] an aspect that is discussed in greater detail later in this chapter. Dealtry et al.[38] reported the expression of IL-13 by human trophoblast cells and suggest that the expression of Th2 cytokines at the fetomaternal interface implies changes in cytokine balance during the establishment and maintenance of pregnancy. IL-13, an anti-inflammatory Th2 cytokine, is proposed to limit local inflammatory reactions at the site of implantation and within the placenta during pregnancy.[38]

So, Is There a Th1 Bias in Unexplained Recurrent Spontaneous Miscarriage?

Vince and Johnson[39] posed the provocative question: "Is there a Th2 bias in human pregnancy?" to which Guilbert[40] answered rather nimbly that "there is a bias against Th1 cytokine expression and function in pregnancy"; a bias against Th1 reactivity can be tantamount to a bias in favor of Th2 reactivity given their antagonistic natures. A bias away from Th1 cytokines downregulates the more harmful (i.e., pro-inflammatory) form and cross-upregulates a pregnancy-conducive (i.e., anti-inflammatory) type of maternal immune reactivity.[40] The absolute levels of cytokines *per se* are not as important as the *relative* levels of Th1 and Th2 cytokines, their receptors and antagonists; when relative levels of Th1 and Th2 cytokines are calculated, evidence emerges for a pro-Th2 bias in cytokine balance in healthy pregnancy and a pro-Th1 bias in unexplained RSM.[41]

The notion that Th1 is "bad" for pregnancy and that Th2 is "good," based on several lines of evidence indicating a Th1 to Th2 shift, is perhaps a little too simplistic. Bates et al.[42] argue that cytokines do not act in isolation but are an integral part of a complex regulatory network in which modulatory interactions maintain homeostasis between the conceptus and the maternal immune system. If this delicate balance is adversely affected, immunoregulatory mechanisms may be insufficient to restore homeostasis and may lead to pregnancy failure.[42] Zourbas et al.[43] reported the expression of the cytokines IL-11, IL-12, IL-13, and IL-15 at the murine fetomaternal interface. While IL-13 is a Th2 cytokine and IL-12 is an inflammatory cytokine with Th1-cytokine-like properties, IL-11 has Th2-like anti-inflammatory properties, and IL-15 is not a Th2 cytokine. Thus, they question whether cytokine profiles in pregnancy and RSM really fit the Th1 or Th2 paradigm; they suggest that pregnancy may be better viewed in the context of anti-inflammatory (IL-4, IL-10, IL-11, and IL-13) and pro-inflammatory (IFN-γ, TNF-α, IL-2, IL-12, and IL-15) cytokines, rather than Th1–Th2 cytokines. As the pattern of expression of these cytokines is rather complex, it is difficult to reconcile with a pure and simple Th1 or Th2 paradigm. Chaouat et al. state that even though the Th1–Th2 paradigm has been useful in the analysis of the fetomaternal relationship, it is an oversimplification.[44] They suggest that the maternal–fetal relationship consists of a series of intricate mutual cytokine interactions governing selective immune regulation and that it would be inappropriate to classify a cytokine as exclusively "good" or "bad," but that cytokine expression occurs in sequential windows, with precise timing and tuning.

Laird et al.[45] emphasize that despite the apparent controversies in this area, there is clear evidence for an alteration in the ratio of Th1 and Th2 cytokines produced by peripheral blood mononuclear cells (PBMCs) and decidual T cells; they suggest that variations in the data could be due to the compartment of cells studied (peripheral blood vs. endometrium vs. decidua) and the timing of sampling. Thus, substantial literature exists to suggest an increased pro-inflammatory cytokine bias in recurrent miscarriage.[17,19-27,32,34,35,45] Most reports support the contention that women with recurrent miscarriage produce elevated levels of pro-inflammatory or Th1 cytokines, while women with healthy pregnancy have decreased Th1 cytokines and increased anti-inflammatory Th2 cytokines; there is thus an increased pro-inflammatory cytokine bias in unexplained recurrent miscarriage.[46]

How might Th1 immunity be induced in pregnant women? The predominance of certain cytokines at the time of differentiation of T cells drives naïve T cells toward Th1 or Th2 dominated populations. IFN-γ and IL-12 promote Th1 differentiation, whereas IL-4 is the dominant factor in determining Th2 polarization.[8] IL-12 could well play a key Th1-inducing role in pregnancy loss; IL-12 is produced in response to infections, thus IL-12 produced during infectious diseases, even subclinical infections, may bring about a shift toward strong Th1 reactivity. IFN-γ produced in viral infections and in response to stimulus by IL-12 is a strong promoter of Th1 development. In the infection scenario, the conceptus has been described as an "innocent bystander" as the mother and her fetus try to contend with infections using an appropriately robust pro-inflammatory or Th1 immune reaction, which may end up being detrimental to the fetus.[47] Indeed, we have shown that women with a history of RSM have substantially higher levels of IL-12 compared to healthy pregnant women.[21] Furthermore, reduced immunosuppression at the maternal–fetal interface has been suggested to induce a Th1 shift. Levels of TGF-β2, an immunosuppressive cytokine, are decreased in the decidual tissue of women with recurrent miscarriage compared to decidual tissue from healthy pregnant women.[48,49] TGF-β2 is proposed to suppress antifetal immune reactivity, and thus any decrease in levels of this cytokine may lead to an increase in Th1 reactivity. Considering that TGF-β is produced by Treg cells, it is not surprising that animal and human experiments have shown decreased numbers and/or function of Treg cells. The transfer of Treg cells from normal pregnant mice has been reported to help prevent miscarriage in mice. At the maternal–fetal interface, Treg cells are proposed to help sustain an environment that is conducive to the success of pregnancy by the secretion of immunosuppressive cytokines such as IL-10 and TGF-β.[49] Treg cells could thus play important roles by averting the development of strong Th1 reactivity.

How Could Th1 and Th17 Immunity Affect Pregnancy?

The trophoblast is resistant to killing by cytotoxic T lymphocytes, conventional NK cells, and conventional macrophages. At the same time, elevated activity of NK cells in the blood and in the uterus has been shown to be associated with miscarriage and also to be predictive of RSM.[50] NK cells, like activated Th1 cells, are known to release cytokines deleterious to the trophoblast.[51] Hill and Choi[52] describe Th1-mediated mechanisms as "immunodystrophism"; they suggest that cells in the decidua could respond to trophoblast invasion with a Th1-dominated response, which is detrimental to early placental differentiation and growth and embryonic development. Decidual NK cells produce high levels of IFN-γ,[51] which activate decidual macrophages that then secrete toxic levels of nitric oxide. Decidual macrophages activated by Th1 cytokines also appear to be important players; their levels are elevated in spontaneous miscarriage, and they may mediate trophoblast apoptosis.[52,53]

The detrimental actions of Th1 cytokines in pregnancy would thus be to damage the conceptus directly and to also indirectly damage the placenta by activating cellular effectors such as NK cells and macrophages; the protective role of Th2 cytokines would be to counteract Th1 cytokines and to suppress the Th1-NK-macrophage system. Th1 cytokines, such as TNF-α and IFN-γ have been shown to directly damage the conceptus by apoptosis of trophoblast cells,[54,55] by inhibiting the secretion of the placental growth-stimulating cytokine granulocyte-macrophage colony-stimulating factor (GM-CSF) from the uterine epithelium and by activating coagulation mechanisms that may lead to vasculitis affecting blood supply to the implanted embryo, a process termed as "cytokine-triggered vascular autoamputation."[56] Anti-inflammatory cytokines such as IL-4 and IL-10 and immunosuppressive cytokines such as TGF-β2 may well have critical roles in this equation by inhibiting the fgl2 response to Th1 cytokines. Furthermore, IL-12, a Th1-inducing cytokine, increases IFN-γ levels, T cell cytotoxicity, and NK cell activation, and IL-12 could mediate abortion by activating NK cells and/or T cell cytotoxicity.[57]

While Th1 cytokines have numerous inflammatory and/or cytotoxic effects, they are not "bad guys" all the time. Depending on the stage of gestation in which they are produced and their relative levels vis-à-vis other cytokines, they may actually be saviors and not assassins. Low levels of IFN-γ are not only not deleterious to pregnancy but appear to be essential for the implantation of the embryo as well as for the viability of decidual cells.[58] Likewise, TNF has been reported to play key roles in early pregnancy events.[50] Cytokines are pluripotent mediators, and their functions are influenced by their concentrations as well as the levels of their receptors and antagonists, because of which their actions may seem inconsistent. It is suggested that cytokines should be considered within a "physiological context"; *when* and *where* these cytokines are produced and their relative levels are very important factors that need to be considered.

Recent studies implicate Th17 cells in recurrent miscarriage, via the secretion of IL-17, which activates strong inflammatory reactions.[59] Treatment of pregnant mice results in fetal loss, which suggests that this inflammatory cytokine is harmful to pregnancy.[60] In humans, levels of Th17 are elevated in the peripheral blood and decidua of RSM patients.[61] Moreover, the frequency of unexplained RSM has been shown to be associated with an increase in serum IL-17 levels[62] and elevated Th17/Treg ratios both in blood and at the fetal–maternal interface.[63] Our laboratory has demonstrated significantly increased production of IL-17 by peripheral blood lymphocytes from women with unexplained RSM compared to healthy pregnant women.[64] Thus, it would be fair to say that the older Th1/Th2 paradigm[11,17] has now evolved into the Th1/Th2/Th17/Treg paradigm,[35] in which Th2 and Treg cells help sustain maternal tolerance to fetoplacental antigens, while Th1 and Th17 cells can mediate spontaneous miscarriage.[46]

Is there a relationship between cytokines in the peripheral blood and cytokines in the local vicinity of the fetus? If pregnancy affects alterations both in the uterus and in the periphery, then it is entirely plausible that maternal Th2 cells in the periphery may boost Th2 immunity in the uterus. Likewise, if maternal immune reactivity becomes Th1-dominant in the periphery, for example, as a result of an infection or due to genetic causes or hormonal changes, it is likely that this Th1 reactivity could result in a shift in the uterine environment toward Th1-type reactivity. T cells in the periphery and T cells at the maternal–fetal interface have been suggested to interact and communicate with each other in determining the type and extent of the immune response, resulting in alterations in the Th1:Th2 ratio in the uterus.[65]

How Is Th2-bias Sustained in Normal Pregnancy?

The initiation of a shift toward Th2 bias and the subsequent maintenance of it is mediated by cytokines and hormones. IL-10 appears to be the most critical cytokine for initiating and maintaining a Th2 bias; this anti-inflammatory, immunosuppressive cytokine interferes with antigen presentation, downregulates cytokine production by Th1 cells, and directly or indirectly inhibits NK responses.[66]

Cytotrophoblast and syncytiotrophoblast cells have been shown to preferentially secrete IL-10.[67] Chaouat et al.[68] refer to the placenta as a "strong Th2 cytokine shield" based on their demonstration of high levels of IL-10 in trophoblast cells; they also showed that the injection of abortion-prone mice with IL-10 results in a reversal in high rates of abortion.[69] Thus, IL-10 produced by trophoblast cells and Treg cells, uterine NK cells, and monocytes are proposed to help maintain immunologic tolerance of the fetus.[70] IL-10 also attenuates fetal growth restriction and fetal death induced by lipopolysaccharide, suggesting that IL-10 produced in the placenta helps to counteract detrimental pro-inflammatory cytokines. Piccinni and Romagnani[71] opine that T cell cytokines play critical roles in the regulation of both fetal survival and rejection, influenced by hormones. The role of hormones in promoting the differentiation of Th cells or in favoring the shifting of already differentiated Th cells from one cytokine profile to another has also been suggested.[71,72] Progesterone at concentrations comparable to those at the maternofetal interface favors the development of human T cells producing Th2-type cytokines.[72] Thus, the high levels of progesterone present at the maternofetal interface during gestation may contribute, at least partially, to the development of a robust Th2-type profile, which nurtures successful pregnancy. Choi et al. showed that progesterone inhibits the production of Th1 cytokines by peripheral blood cells stimulated with trophoblast antigens.[73]

In addition to its direct effect on cytokine production, progesterone has been shown to mediate immunomodulation via the induction of production of an immunomodulatory protein, progesterone-induced blocking factor (PIBF). Szekeres-Bartho and colleagues demonstrated that lymphocytes from pregnant women produce PIBF when exposed to progesterone. This factor inhibits various cell-mediated immune reactions.[74-76] PIBF induces Th2-biased cytokine production in lymphocytes from women with unexplained RSM,[77] and thus brings about a shift Th1→Th2 cytokine bias. The percentage of PIBF-positive lymphocytes is significantly reduced in women prone to pregnancy loss, preterm labor (PTL), and threatened miscarriage. PIBF-treated spleen cells from nonpregnant female mice produce significantly more IL-4 and IL-10 than those in the absence of PIBF,[78] and PIBF prevents fetal resorptions in a murine model of pregnancy loss.[79] Thus, activation and maturation of maternal T cells in pregnancy occur in an environment that is gradually progesterone-enriched as gestation progresses. This would result in T cell activation and differentiation in the presence of lower concentrations of IL-2 and IFN-γ and higher concentrations of IL-4 and IL-10, an environment that favors the development of Th2.[71] Piccinni and Romagnani suggest that high levels of progesterone at the maternal–fetal interface at the start of pregnancy orient maternal immune reactivity toward Th2 dominance;[71] these Th2 cytokines would then downregulate the potentially antagonistic Th1 response, thus preventing fetal rejection.

Can We Redirect Cytokine Responses Toward a Pregnancy-conducive Profile?

The demonstration of a possible association between RSM and maternal Th1 cytokine bias led to the consideration of the therapeutic possibility of redirecting or modulating the cytokine balance in such a manner as to downregulate pro-inflammatory cytokines such as IFN-γ and TNF-α, thereby creating a setting that is more conducive to the success of pregnancy. One approach would be to use a hormone such as progesterone. This pregnancy-related hormone has long been known to be indispensable for the establishment of the endometrium, and thus indispensable to pregnancy; but it is now being recognized as also contributing immunologically to the success of pregnancy by interacting with the maternal immune system. More than 45 years ago, Siiteri et al.[80]

described progesterone as "nature's immunosuppressant" based on their studies that revealed immunosuppressive properties of progesterone. Indeed, progesterone has been shown to suppress the activation and proliferation of lymphocytes[81] and to prolong the survival of allografts when administered locally.[82] Studies have demonstrated that progesterone favors the development of human T cells producing Th2 cytokines,[72] and it also blocks the production of Th1 cytokines by lymphocytes responding to in vitro stimulation with a trophoblast antigen extract.[73]

The association between pro-inflammatory cytokines and recurrent miscarriage on the one hand[17,19-25,32,45,47,65,82] and the fascinating immunological capabilities of progesterone on the other[72,73,80-83] led us to ask a provocative question: Can progestogens be used to downregulate Th1 pro-inflammatory cytokine reactivity with the objective of preventing or treating recurrent miscarriage? We have investigated the immunomodulatory capabilities of progesterone and dydrogesterone (6-dehydro-9β and 10α-progesterone) (Duphaston), an orally administered progestogen, which is similar to endogenous progesterone in terms of molecular structure and pharmacologic effects but is substantially more potent than natural progesterone, with a high affinity for the progesterone receptor.[84]

We have shown that PBMC from women with a history of unexplained RSM, when cultured in the presence of dydrogesterone or progesterone, produce significantly lower levels of the Th1 pro-inflammatory cytokines IFN-γ and TNF-α. On the other hand, levels of IL-4 and IL-6, both Th2 cytokines, are significantly elevated in the presence of dydrogesterone or progesterone.[85] Th1:Th2 cytokine ratios in cultures containing dydrogesterone are markedly reduced, indicating a decrease in Th1 cytokine bias. We have recently reported that dydrogesterone also suppresses the production of the powerful inflammatory cytokine IL-17; given the association of high levels of IL-17 with unexplained RSM, the ability of dydrogesterone to inhibit the production of IL-17 is significant.[64] We also showed that the progesterone receptor antagonist RU486 reverses the effects of dydrogesterone and progesterone, demonstrating that the effect of dydrogesterone and progesterone mediated via the progesterone receptor.[85] Once administered to subjects, dydrogesterone is converted into its major metabolite 20α-dihydrodydrogesterone (20α-DHD); thus, in circulation, dydrogesterone is present as DHD. We showed that this metabolite suppresses the production of the pro-inflammatory cytokines IFN-γ, TNF-α, and upregulates the production of the anti-inflammatory cytokine IL-4, showing that this metabolite retains the immunomodulatory effects of the parent molecule dydrogesterone.[86]

As mentioned above, progestogens bring about their cytokine-modulating effects in two ways: One is the direct Th1-inhibiting effect on lymphocytes, and the second is the indirect route via PIBF, discovered by Szekeres-Bartho et al.[87] PIBF induces a Th2-dominant cytokine response by facilitating the production of IL-4 and IL-10, thus altering the Th1:Th2 balance in favor of pregnancy. Studies on humans[88] and animals[89,90] suggest that progestogens could contribute to the success of pregnancy through the actions of PIBF. Animal studies indicate important roles for PIBF in the sustenance of pregnancy; fetal wastage induced by the transfer of NK cells is corrected by the administration of PIBF.[91]

There is therefore ample justification to support supplementation with progestogens in the therapeutic management of unexplained RSM, based on their direct and indirect effects on cytokine profiles.[71-92]

A Cochrane review showed that progesterone supplementation reduces the rate of miscarriage without any adverse effects.[93] A systematic review of progesterone supplementation in RSM showed a significant beneficial effect.[91] Choi et al.[73] had suggested that potentially immunosuppressive doses of progesterone may benefit individuals in whom the etiology of RSM is related to maternal Th1 cytokine predominance. Several studies have explored the benefits of supplementation with oral progesterone in treating miscarriage.[93-95] However, progesterone administered orally is poorly absorbed, is subjected to first-pass mechanism, has a short biologic half-life,[96] loses much of its bioactivity,[97] and is cleared rapidly.[98] On the contrary, the orally active progestogen, dydrogesterone, is superior from this perspective, as it does not suffer from these drawbacks; as mentioned above, dydrogesterone retains immunomodulatory activity even after it is converted to its major metabolite upon oral administration.[86] Moreover, the antiandrogenic properties of dydrogesterone helps to avoid the masculinization of female fetuses.[99,100]

Dydrogesterone supplementation has been shown to be beneficial in recurrent miscarriage. A randomized, placebo-controlled double-blind study by Kumar et al. demonstrated a significant decrease in the number of miscarriages and an increase in the mean gestational age at delivery after supplementation with dydrogesterone.[101] A systematic review of randomized trials on dydrogesterone by Carp showed a rate of miscarriage of 10.5% miscarriage after dydrogesterone treatment and a miscarriage rate of 23.5% in control women; he concluded that there is a significant reduction of 29% in the odds for miscarriage with dydrogesterone when compared to standard care.[102] A systematic review and meta-analysis of 10 randomized controlled trials revealed a lower risk of recurrent miscarriage as well as a higher rate of live births in women who received progestogen supplementation when compared to those who did not.[103] Thus, dydrogesterone is an immune-modulator that shifts the balance from a Th1 or pro-inflammatory cytokine bias toward a Th2 or anti-inflammatory bias, a milieu that is favorable to the success of pregnancy. Dydrogesterone can therefore be considered for effective, safe, and orally administered immunomodulatory therapy in unexplained RSM.

CONCLUSION

Future research will no doubt be directed at the complete characterization of cytokine networks at the maternal–fetal interface, and elucidating factors that stimulate undesirable Th1 reactivity and those that sustain favorable Th2 immunity. It would be of immense benefit to develop new preventive and therapeutic options for shifting the maternal immune response toward a pattern that is conducive to successful pregnancy. Research described in this chapter indicates that dydrogesterone has immunomodulatory capabilities. It induces a cytokine shift from pro-inflammatory cytokine dominance toward an anti-inflammatory bias; this cytokine profile is favorable to successful pregnancy. Thus, progestogens could be considered for effective and orally administered therapy for immunologically mediated recurrent miscarriage. The assessment of "personal cytokine profiles" in women with recurrent miscarriage may point to an immunologic etiology. Such women could benefit from immunomodulation of cytokine profiles by supplementation with progestogens, based on the personal cytokine profile of each patient.

REFERENCES

1. Schummers L, Oveisi N, Ohtsuka MS, Hutcheon JA, Ahrens KA, Liauw J, et al. Early pregnancy loss incidence in high-income settings: a protocol for a systematic review and meta-analysis. Syst Rev. 2021;10(1):274.
2. Larsen EC, Christiansen OB, Kolte AM, Macklon N. New insights into mechanisms behind miscarriage. BMC Med. 2013;11:154.
3. Quenby S, Gallos ID, Dhillon-Smith RK, Podesek M, Stephenson MD, Fisher J, et al. Miscarriage matters: the epidemiological, physical, psychological, and economic costs of early pregnancy loss. Lancet. 2021;397(10285):1658-67.
4. Dimitriadis E, Menkhorst E, Saito S, Kutteh WH, Brosens JJ. Recurrent pregnancy loss. Nat Rev Dis Primers. 2020;6(1):98.
5. Ford HB, Schust DJ. Recurrent pregnancy loss: etiology, diagnosis and therapy. Rev Obstet Gynecol. 2009;2(2):76-83.
6. Schreiber K, Radin M, Sciascia S. Current insights in obstetric antiphospholipid syndrome. Curr Opin Obstet Gynecol. 2017;29(6):397-403.
7. Zielinski CE. T helper cell subsets: diversification of the field. Eur J Immunol. 2023;53(12):e2250218.
8. Ruterbusch M, Pruner KB, Shehata L, Pepper M. In vivo CD4+ T cell differentiation and function: revisiting the Th1/Th2 paradigm. Annu Rev Immunol. 2020;38:705-25.
9. Sakaguchi S, Mikami N, Wing JB, Tanaka A, Ichiyama K, Ohkura N. Regulatory T cells and human disease. Annu Rev Immunol. 2020;38:541-66.
10. Stockinger B, Omenetti S. The dichotomous nature of T helper 17 cells. Nat Rev Immunol. 2017;17(9):535-44.
11. Wegmann TG, Lin H, Guilbert L, Mosmann TR. Bidirectional cytokine interactions in the maternal-fetal relationship: is successful pregnancy a Th2 phenomenon? Immunol Today. 1993;14(7):353-6.
12. Hanna N, Hanna I, Hleb M, Wagner E, Dougherty J, Balkundi D et al. Gestational age-dependent expression of IL-10 and its receptor in human placental tissues and isolated cytotrophoblasts. J Immunol. 2000;164(11):5721-8.
13. Kruse N, Greif M, Moriabadi NF, Marx L, Toyka KV, Rieckmann P. Variations in cytokine mRNA expression during normal human pregnancy. Clin Exp Immunol. 2000;119(2) 317-22.
14. Reinhard G, Noll A, Schlebusch H, Mallmann P, Ruecker AV. Shifts in the TH1/TH2 balance during human pregnancy correlate with apoptotic changes. Biochem Biophys Res Commun. 1998;245(3):933-8.
15. Haimovici F, Hill JA, Anderson DJ. The effects of soluble products of activated lymphocytes and macrophages on blastocyst implantation events in vitro. Biol Reprod. 1991;44(1):69-76.
16. Pijnenborg R, Luyten C, Vercruysse L, Keith Jr JC, Van Assche FA. Cytotoxic effects of tumour necrosis factor (TNF)-alpha and interferon-gamma on cultured human trophoblast are modulated by fibronectin. Mol Hum Reprod. 2000;6(7):635-41.
17. Raghupathy R. Th1-type immunity is incompatible with successful pregnancy. Immunol Today. 1997;18(10):478-82.
18. Hill JA, Anderson DJ, Polgar K. T helper 1-type cellular immunity to trophoblast in women with recurrent spontaneous abortions. J Am Med Assoc. 1995;273(24):1933-58.

19. Lee J, Choi BC, Cho C, Hill JA, Baek KH, Kim JW. Trophoblast apoptosis is increased in women with evidence of TH1 immunity. Fertil Steril. 2005;83(4):1047-9.
20. Makhseed M, Raghupathy R, Azizieh F, Al-Azemi MM, Hassan NA, Bandar A. Mitogen-induced cytokine responses of maternal peripheral blood lymphocytes indicate a differential Th-type bias in normal pregnancy and pregnancy failure. Am J Reprod Immunol. 1999;42(5):273-81.
21. Raghupathy R, Makhseed M, Azizieh F, Omu A, Gupta M, Farhat R. Cytokine production by maternal lymphocytes during normal human pregnancy and in unexplained recurrent spontaneous abortion. Hum Reprod. 2000;15(3):713-8.
22. Raghupathy R, Makhseed M, Azizieh F, Hassan N, Al-Azemi M, Al-Shamali E. Maternal Th1- and Th2-type reactivity to placental antigens in normal human pregnancy and unexplained recurrent spontaneous abortions. Cell Immunol. 1999;196(2):122-30.
23. Chaouat G, Menu E, Clark DA, Dy M, Minkowski M, Wegmann TG. Control of fetal survival in CBA x DBA/2 mice by lymphokine therapy. J Reprod Fertil. 1990;89(2):447-57.
24. Marzi M, Vigano A, Trabattoni D, Villa ML, Salvaggio A, Clerici E, et al. Characterization of type 1 and type 2 cytokine production profile in physiologic and pathologic human pregnancy. Clin Exp Immunol. 1996;106(1):127-33.
25. Banerjee P, Ghosh S, Dutta M, Subramani E, Khalpada J, Roychoudhury S, et al. Identification of key contributory factors responsible for vascular dysfunction in idiopathic recurrent spontaneous miscarriage. PLoS One. 2013;8(11):e80940.
26. Ticconi C, Pietropolli A, Di Simone N, Piccione E, Fazleabas A. Endometrial immune dysfunction in recurrent pregnancy loss. Int J Mol Sci. 2019;20(21):5332.
27. Logiodice F, Lombardelli L, Kullolli O, Haller H, Maggi E, Rukavina D, et al. Decidual interleukin-22-producing CD4+ T cells (Th17/Th0/IL-22+ and Th17/Th2/IL-22+, Th2/IL-22+, Th0/IL-22+), which also produce IL-4, are involved in the success of pregnancy. Int J Mol Sci. 2019;20(2):428.
28. Roth I, Corry DB, Locksley RM, Abrams JS, Litton MJ, Fisher SJ. Human placental cytotrophoblasts produce the immunosuppressive cytokine interleukin 10. J Exp Med. 1996;184(2):539-48.
29. Greig PC, Herbert WN, Robinette BL, Teot LA. Amniotic fluid interleukin-10 concentrations increase through pregnancy and are elevated in patients with preterm labor associated with intrauterine infection. Am J Obstet Gynecol. 1995;173(4):1223-7.
30. Sharma S, Godbole G, Modi D. Decidual control of trophoblast invasion. Am J Reprod Immunol. 2016;75(3):341-50.
31. Jones CA, Williams KA, Finlay-Jones JJ, Hart PH. Interleukin-4 production by human amnion epithelial cells and regulation of its activity by glycosaminoglycan binding. Biol Reprod. 1995;52(4):839-47.
32. Lim KJ, Odukoya OA, Ajjan RA, Li TC, Weetman AP, Cooke ID. The role of T-helper cytokines in human reproduction. Fertil Steril. 2000;73(1):136-42.
33. Piccinni MP, Beloni L, Livi C, Maggi E, Scarselli G, Romagnani S. Defective production of both leukemia inhibitory factor and type 2 T-helper cytokines by decidual T cells in unexplained recurrent abortions. Nat Med. 1998;4(9):1020-4.
34. Saito S. Cytokine network at the feto-maternal interface. J Reprod Immunol. 2000;47(2):87-103.
35. Saito S, Nakashima A, Shima T, Ito M. Th1/Th2/Th17 and regulatory T-cell paradigm in pregnancy. Am J Reprod Immunol. 2010;63(6):601-10.
36. Azizieh FY, Raghupathy R. IL-10 and pregnancy complications. Clin Exp Obstet Gynecol. 2017;44(2):252-8.
37. Piccinni MP, Lombardelli L, Logiodice F, Kullolli O, Romagnani S, Le Bouteiller P. T helper cell mediated-tolerance towards fetal allograft in successful pregnancy. Clin Mol Allergy. 2015;13(1):9.
38. Dealtry GB, O'Farrell MK, Fernandez N. The Th2 cytokine environment of the placenta. Int Arch Allergy Immunol. 2000;123(2):107-19.
39. Vince GS, Johnson PM. Is there a Th2 bias in human pregnancy? J Reprod Immunol. 1996;32(2):101-4.
40. Guilbert LJ. There is a bias against type 1 (inflammatory) cytokine expression and function in pregnancy. J Reprod Immunol. 1996;32(2):105-10.
41. Azizieh F, Dingle K, Raghupathy R, Johnson K, VanderPlas J, Ansari A. Multivariate analysis of cytokine profiles in pregnancy complications. Am J Reprod Immunol. 2018;79(3):e12818.
42. Bates MD, Quenby S, Takakuwa K, Johnson PM, Vince GS. Aberrant cytokine production by peripheral blood mononuclear cells in recurrent pregnancy loss? Hum Reprod. 2002;17(9):2439-44.
43. Zourbas S, Dubanchet S, Martal J, Chaouat G. Localization of pro-inflammatory (IL-12, IL-15) and anti-inflammatory (IL-11, IL-13) cytokines at the foetomaternal interface during murine pregnancy. Clin Exp Immunol. 2001;126(3):519-28.
44. Chaouat G, Ledée-Bataille N, Dubanchet S, Zourbas S, Sandra O, Martal J. Th1/Th2 paradigm in pregnancy: paradigm lost? Cytokines in pregnancy/early abortion: reexamining the TH1/TH2 paradigm. Int Arch Allergy Immunol. 2004;134(2):93-119.
45. Laird SM, Tuckerman EM, Li TC. Cytokine expression in the endometrium of women with implantation failure and recurrent miscarriage. Reprod Biomed Online. 2006;13(1):13-23.
46. Piccinni MP, Raghupathy R, Saito S, Szekeres-Bartho J. Cytokines, hormones and cellular regulatory mechanisms favoring successful reproduction. Front Immunol. 2021;12:717808.
47. Clark DA, Blois S, Kandil J, Handjiski B, Manuel J, Arck PC. Reduced uterine indoleamine 2,3-dioxygenase versus increased Th1/Th2 cytokine ratios as a basis for occult

and clinical pregnancy failure in mice and humans. Am J Reprod Immunol. 2005;54(4):203-16.

48. Lea RG, Underwood J, Flanders KC, Hirte H, Banwatt D, Finotto S, et al. A subset of patients with recurrent spontaneous abortion is deficient in transforming growth factor beta-2-producing "suppressor cells" in uterine tissue near the placental attachment site. Am J Reprod Immunol. 1995;34(1):52-64.
49. Alijotas-Reig J, Llurba E, Gris JM. Potentiating maternal immune tolerance in pregnancy: a new challenging role for regulatory T cells. Placenta. 2014;35(4):241-8.
50. Guerrero B, Hassouneh F, Delgado E, Casado JG, Tarazona R. Natural killer cells in recurrent miscarriage: an overview. J Reprod Immunol. 2020;142:103209.
51. Erlebacher A. Immunology of the maternal-fetal interface. Ann Rev Immunol. 2013;31:387-411.
52. Hill JA, Choi BC. Immunodystrophism. Evidence for a novel alloimmune hypothesis for recurrent pregnancy loss involving Th1-type immunity to trophoblast. Sem Reprod Med. 2000;18(4):401-5.
53. Zhao QY, Li QH, Fu YY, Ren CE, Jiang AF, Meng YH. Decidual macrophages in recurrent spontaneous abortion. Front Immunol. 2022;13:994888.
54. Yui J, Garcia-Lloret M, Wegmann TG, Guilbert LJ. Cytotoxicity of tumour necrosis factor-alpha (TNF-α) and gamma-interferon (IFN-γ) against primary human placental trophoblasts. Placenta. 1994;15(8):819-28.
55. Zhang L, Zhao M, Jiao F, Xu X, Liu X, Jiang Y, et al. Interferon gamma is involved in apoptosis of trophoblast cells at the maternal-fetal interface following Toxoplasma gondii infection. Int J Infect Dis. 2015;30:10-6.
56. Knackstedt MK, Zenclussen AC, Hertwig K, Hagen E, Dudenhausen JW, Clark DA, et al. Th1 cytokines and the prothrombinase fgl2 in stress-triggered and inflammatory abortion. Am J Reprod Immunol. 2003;49(4):210-20.
57. Hayakawa S, Nagai N, Kanaeda T, Karasaki-Suzuki M, Ishii M, Chishima F, et al. Interleukin-12 augments cytolytic activity of peripheral and decidual lymphocytes against choriocarcinoma cell lines and primary culture human placental trophoblasts. Am J Reprod Immunol. 1999;41(5):320-9.
58. Micallef A, Grech N, Farrugia F, Schembri-Wismayer P, Calleja-Agius J. The role of interferons in early pregnancy. Gynecol Endocrinol. 2014;30(1):1-6.
59. Mills KHG. IL-17 and IL-17-producing cells in protection versus pathology. Nat Rev Immunol. 2023;23(1):38-54.
60. Xu WM, Xiao ZN, Wang XB, Huang Y. IL-17 induces fetal loss in a CBA/J×BALB/c mouse model, and an anti-IL-17 antibody prevents fetal loss in a CBA/J×DBA/2 mouse model. Am J Reprod Immunol. 2016;75:51-8.
61. Wang WJ, Hao CF, Yi-Lin, Yin GJ, Bao SH, Qiu LH, et al. Increased prevalence of T helper 17 (Th17) cells in peripheral blood and decidua in unexplained recurrent spontaneous abortion patients. J Reprod Immunol. 2010;84:164-70.
62. Fu B, Tian Z, Wei H. Th17 cells in human recurrent pregnancy loss and pre-eclampsia. Cell Mol Immunol. 2014;11(6):56470.
63. Qian J, Zhang N, Lin J, Wang C, Pan X, Chen L, et al. Distinct pattern of Th17/Treg cells in pregnant women with a history of unexplained recurrent spontaneous abortion. Biosci Trends. 2018;12:157-67.
64. AbdulHussain G, Azizieh F, Makhseed M, Raghupathy R. Effects of progesterone, dydrogesterone and estrogen on the production of Th1/Th2/Th17 cytokines by lymphocytes from women with recurrent spontaneous miscarriage. J Reprod Immunol. 2020;140:103132.
65. Arck PC, Rose M, Hertwig K, Hagen E, Hildebrandt M, Klapp BF. Stress and immune mediators in miscarriage. Hum Reprod. 2001;16:1505-11.
66. Saraiva M, Vieira P, O'Garra A. Biology and therapeutic potential of interleukin-10. J Exp Med. 2020;217(1):e20190418.
67. Naruse K, Innes BA, Bulmer JN, Robson SC, Searle RF, Lash GE. Secretion of cytokines by villous cytotrophoblast and extravillous trophoblast in the first trimester of human pregnancy. J Reprod Immunol. 2010;86(2):148-50.
68. Chaouat G, Cayol V, Mairovitz V, Dubanchet S. Localisation of the Th2 cytokines IL-3, IL-4, IL-10 at the murine feto maternal interface during pregnancy. In: Gupta SK (Ed). Reproductive Immunology. New Delhi: Narosa Publishing House; 1999. p. 61.
69. Chaouat G, Assal Meliani A, Martal J, Raghupathy R, Elliott JF, Mosmann T, et al. IL-10 prevents naturally occurring fetal loss in the CBA x DBA/2 mating combination, and local defect in IL-10 production in this abortion-prone combination is corrected by in vivo injection of IFN-tau. J Immunol. 1995;154(9):4261-8.
70. Thaxton JE, Sharma S. Interleukin-10: a multi-faceted agent of pregnancy. Am J Reprod Immunol. 2010;63:482-91.
71. Piccinni MP, Romagnani S. Regulation of foetal allograft survival by hormone-controlled Th1- and Th2-type cytokines. Immunol Res. 1996;15(2):141-50.
72. Piccinni MP, Giudizi MG, Biagiotti R, Beloni L, Giannarini L, Sampognaro S, et al. Progesterone favors the development of human T helper cells producing Th2-type cytokines and promotes both IL-4 production and membrane CD30 expression in established Th1 cell clones. J Immunol. 1995;155(1):128-33.
73. Choi BC, Polgar K, Xiao L, Hill JA. Progesterone inhibits in-vitro embryotoxic Th1 cytokine production to trophoblast in women with recurrent pregnancy loss. Hum Reprod. 2000;15(Suppl. 1):46-59.
74. Check JH, Arwitz M, Gross J, Szekeres-Bartho J, Wu CH. Evidence that the expression of progesterone-induced blocking factor by maternal T-lymphocytes is positively correlated with conception. Am J Reprod Immunol. 1997;38(1):6-8.
75. Laskarin G, Tokmadzić VS, Strbo N, Bogović T, Szekeres-Bartho J, Randić L, et al. Progesterone induced blocking

factor (PIBF) mediates progesterone induced suppression of decidual lymphocyte cytotoxicity. Am J Reprod Immunol. 2002;48(4):201-9.
76. Polgár B, Nagy E, Mikó É, Varga P, Szekeres-Barthó J. Urinary progesterone-induced blocking factor concentration is related to pregnancy outcome. Bio Reprod. 2004;71(5):1699-705.
77. Raghupathy R, Al-Mutawa E, Al-Azemi M, Makhseed M, Azizieh F, Szekeres-Bartho J. Progesterone-induced blocking factor (PIBF) modulates cytokine production by lymphocytes from women with recurrent miscarriage or preterm delivery. J Reprod Immunol. 2009;80(1-2):91-9.
78. Szekeres-Bartho J, Wegmann TG. A progesterone-dependent immunomodulatory protein alters the Th1/Th2 balance. J Reprod Immunol. 1996;31:81-95.
79. Szekeres-Bartho J, Chaouat G. Lymphocyte-derived, progesterone-induced blocking factor corrects resorption in a murine abortion system. Am J Reprod Immunol. 1990;23(1):26-8.
80. Siiteri PK, Febres F, Clemens LE, Chang RJ, Gondos B, Stites D. Progesterone and maintenance of pregnancy: is progesterone nature's immunosuppressant? Ann N Y Acad Sci. 1977;286:384-97.
81. Stites DP, Bugbee S, Siiteri PK. Differential actions of progesterone and cortisol on lymphocyte and monocyte interaction during lymphocyte activation—relevance to immunosuppression in pregnancy. J Reprod Immunol. 1983;5(4):215-28.
82. Kwak-Kim J, Bao S, Lee SK, Kim JW, Gilman-Sachs A. Immunological modes of pregnancy loss: inflammation, immune effectors, and stress. Am J Reprod Immunol. 2014;72(2):129-40.
83. Piccinni MP. T cells in normal pregnancy and recurrent pregnancy loss. Reprod Biomed Online. 2006;13(6):840-4.
84. Schindler A. Dydrogesterone: a unique progestogen. Maturitas. 2009;65(Suppl. 1):S1.
85. Raghupathy R, Al Mutawa E, Makhseed M, Azizieh F, Szekeres-Bartho J. Modulation of cytokine production by dydrogesterone in lymphocytes from women with recurrent miscarriage. BJOG. 2005;112(8):1096-101.
86. Raghupathy R, Al-Azemi M. Modulation of cytokine production by the dydrogesterone metabolite dihydrodydrogesterone. Am J Reprod Immunol. 2015;74(5):419-26.
87. Szekeres-Bartho J. The role of progesterone in feto-maternal immunological cross talk. Med Princ Pract. 2018;27(4):301-7.
88. Kalinka J, Szekeres-Bartho J. The impact of dydrogesterone supplementation on hormonal profile and progesterone-induced blocking factor concentrations in women with threatened abortion. Am J Reprod Immunol. 2005;53(4):166-71.
89. Szekeres-Bartho J, Polgar B, Kozma N, Miko E, Par G, Szereday L, et al. Progesterone-dependent immunomodulation. Chem Immunol Allergy. 2005;89:118-25.
90. Szekeres-Bartho J, Polgar, B. PIBF: the double edged sword. Pregnancy and tumor. Am J Reprod Immunol. 2010;64(2):77-86.
91. Szekeres-Bartho J, Balasch T. Progestagen therapy for recurrent miscarriage. Hum Reprod Update. 2008;14(1):27-35.
92. Szekeres-Bartho J, Kilar F, Falkay G, Csernus V, Török A, Pacsa AS. The mechanism of the inhibitory effect of progesterone on lymphocyte cytotoxicity: I. Progesterone-treated lymphocytes release a substance inhibiting cytotoxicity and prostaglandin synthesis. Am J Reprod Immunol Microbiol. 1985;9(1):15-8.
93. Haas DM, Ramsey PS. Progestogen for preventing miscarriage. Cochrane Database Syst Rev. 2013;(10):CD003511.
94. Wahabi HA, Abed Althagafi NF, Elawad M, Al Zeidan RA. Progestogen for treating threatened miscarriage. Cochrane Database Syst Rev. 2011;12:CD005943.
95. Ismail AM, Abbas AM, Ali MK, Amin AF. Peri-conceptional progesterone treatment in women with unexplained recurrent miscarriage: a randomized double-blind placebo-controlled trial. J Matern Fetal Neonatal Med. 2018;31:388-94.
96. Stanczyk FZ. Pharmacokinetics of progesterone administered by the oral and parenteral routes. J Reprod Med. 1999;44(2 Suppl.):141-7.
97. Simon JA, Robinson DE, Andrews MC. The absorption of oral micronised progesterone: the effect of food, dose proportionality and comparison with intramuscular progesterone. Fertil Steril. 1993;60(1):26-33.
98. Maxson WS, Hargrove JT. Bioavailability of oral micronized progesterone. Fertil Steril. 1985;44(5):622-6.
99. Schindler AE. Progestational effects of dydrogesterone in vitro, in vivo and on the human endometrium. Maturitas. 2009;65(Suppl. 1):S3-11.
100. Mirza FG, Patki A, Pexman-Fieth C. Dydrogesterone use in early pregnancy. Gynecol Endocrinol. 2016;32:97-106.
101. Kumar A, Begum N, Prasad S, Aggarwal S, Sharma S. Oral dydrogesterone treatment during early pregnancy to prevent recurrent pregnancy loss and its role in modulation of cytokine production: a double-blind, randomized, parallel, placebo-controlled trial. Fertil Steril. 2014;102(5):1357-63.
102. Carp H. A systematic review of dydrogesterone for the treatment of recurrent miscarriage. Gynecol Endocrinol. 2015;31(6):422-30.
103. Saccone G, Schoen C, Franasiak JM, Scott Jr RT, Berghella V. Supplementation with progestogens in the first trimester of pregnancy to prevent miscarriage in women with unexplained recurrent miscarriage: a systematic review and meta-analysis of randomized, controlled trials. Fertil Steril. 2017;107:430-8.e3.

CHAPTER

15

Uterine Natural Killer Cells

Chow-Seng Kong, Paul Brighton

ABSTRACT

Uterine natural killer cells are component of the innate immune system. They peak at the time of implantation and during the first trimester. They play a key role in secreting cytokines, interleukins, chemokines, and growth factors. They also play a role in angiogenesis and vascular remodeling.

The link between increased number of uterine natural killer cells and miscarriage has been established in some studies. The mechanism of miscarriage is poorly understood in these patients. Further studies need to clarify the exact role played by uterine natural killer cells in recurrent miscarriages.

Keywords: Uterine natural killer cells, Decidual natural killer cells, Endometrial natural killer cells, Recurrent miscarriage, Implantation.

INTRODUCTION

Natural killer (NK) cells are integral players of the innate immune system, serving as key defenders against various pathological conditions without the need for prior sensitization. Targets include both virally infected cells and those transformed by malignancy or stress.[1] In addition to their presence in the peripheral blood, NK cells also localize in diverse nonlymphoid tissues such as the liver, lungs, intestine, and reproductive tissues, including the endometrium and decidua of pregnancy.[2-4] Unlike their circulating counterparts, these NK cells are profoundly influenced by the specific microenvironment of the host tissue, leading to the development of unique phenotypes and functions. Thus, these NK cells are referred to as tissue-resident NK cells.[5,6] The intricate relationship between NK cells and the tissue environment highlights the versatile roles they play beyond their traditional function in immune defense. In this chapter, we highlight our current understanding of tissue-resident NK cells in reproductive tissue and explore their significance in implantation and pregnancy. Understanding their physiological and pathological roles is crucial, as this could provide mechanistic insights underlying the immune-mediated causes of reproductive failure, and potentially offer avenues for clinical interventions.

UTERINE NATURAL KILLER CELLS

In the endometrium and decidua of pregnancy, a wide range of both innate and adaptive immune cells coexist. This cellular landscape includes B cells, dendritic cells, monocytes, macrophages, T cells, neutrophils, and most notably, a predominant population of NK cells.[3,7] These tissue-resident NK cells exhibit distinct features and functions within this unique microenvironment, and thus are denoted as uterine natural killer (uNK) cells, endometrial NK cells, or decidual NK cells.[6,8]

Unique Molecular Features of Uterine Natural Killer Cells

One characteristic that separates uNK cells from their circulating counterparts is the expression of CD56 and CD16. Unlike the $CD56^{dim}CD16^{+}$ peripheral blood NK cells, uNK cells are characterized by a high density of CD56 and an absence of CD16 on their cell surface ($CD56^{bright}CD16^{-}$).[9] Additionally, uNK cells express specific tissue-residency markers, such as CD9, CD49a, and CD69, which are notably absent in peripheral blood NK cells.[3,10]

Temporal Expression of Uterine Natural Killer Cells

Uterine NK cells are particularly intriguing due to dynamic changes within the endometrium. This not only varies

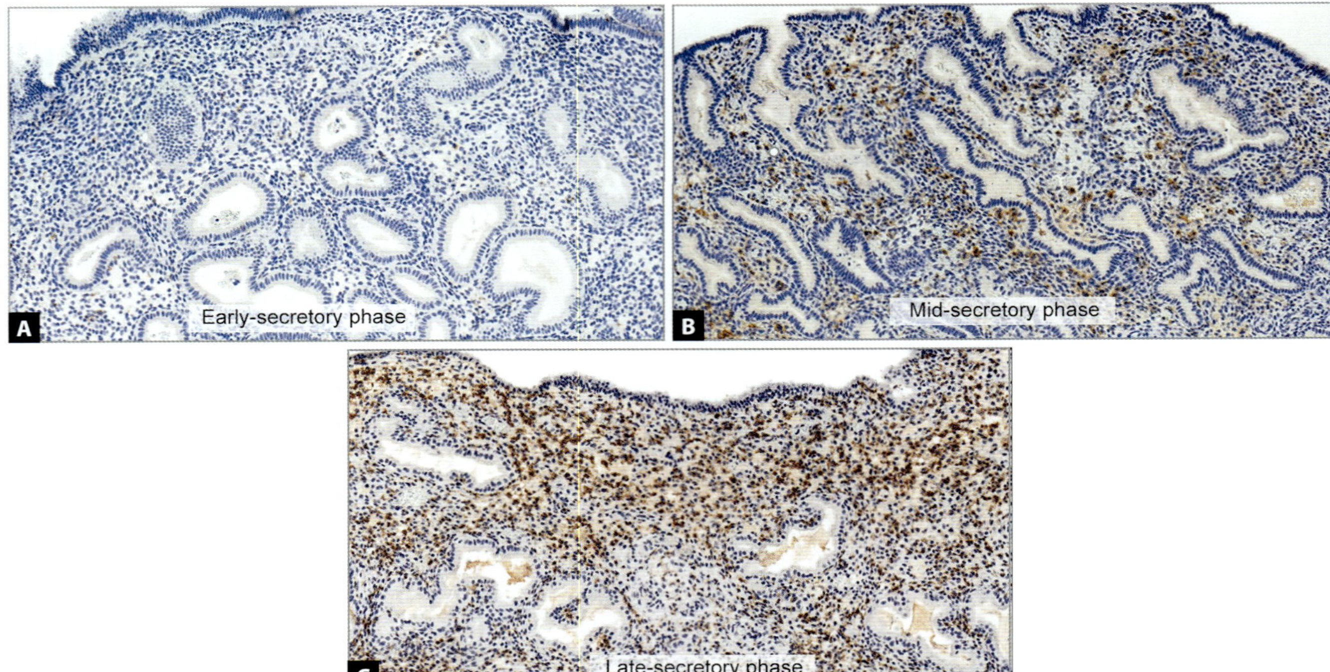

Figs. 1A to C: uNK cell staining in human endometrium. Representative images depicting the accumulation of uNK cells throughout the secretory phase of the cycle. (uNK: uterine natural killer)

between women but also fluctuates dramatically from one cycle to the next. The most notable change, however, is the phasic accumulation observed throughout the secretory phase of the menstrual cycle.[2] During the proliferative phase, uNK cell numbers remain relatively low.[2] However, around 3–5 days postovulation, and in conjunction with the process of decidualization during the mid-secretory phase, the number of uNK cells expands significantly to constitute approximately 30–40% of endometrial stromal cells (EnSC)[2] **(Figs. 1A to C)**. If embryo implantation occurs, uNK cells continue to expand in situ, peaking during the first trimester, where astonishingly, they account for 70% of total leukocytes. As pregnancy progresses, a portion of uNK cells (~50% of total leukocytes) persists into the later stages of gestation, where a concomitant and proportional increase in the number of T cells is observed.[8,11-13] Although uNK cells become less abundant in the decidua toward term, studying this decline becomes challenging due to a lack of available pregnancy tissues beyond elective termination. In nonconception cycles where pregnancy does not occur, the uNK cell levels rapidly decrease as they are sloughed off with the menstruating tissue, decreasing to basal levels at the start of new cycle.[11]

The timely regulation of uNK cells highlights their essential role in temporal-dependent processes across the menstrual cycle and pregnancy. They emerge as essential immunomodulators, contributing significantly to the complex and finely tuned mechanisms that underpin successful reproduction.[2,7]

FUNCTIONS OF UTERINE NATURAL KILLER CELLS IN PREGNANCY ESTABLISHMENT

The dynamic expression of uNK cells has captured considerable interest among researchers and clinicians who endeavor to understand their physiological and pathological roles in embryo implantation and early placental formation. Indeed, several pertinent roles have emerged, including trophoblast invasion, angiogenesis, vascular remodeling, and immune tolerance.[4,14-16]

Uterine natural killer cells have emerged as prolific producers of various cytokines, including interleukins, chemokines, and growth factors. Indeed, cytokine secretions such as interleukin-8 (IL-8), C-X-C motif chemokine ligand 10 (CXCL10), transforming growth factor beta (TGF-β), interferon gamma (IFN-γ), and vascular endothelial growth factor (VEGF) directly interact with receptors expressed within primary trophoblasts to regulate their migration and invasion.[14,15] The crosstalk between uNK cells and trophoblasts balances the tissue microenvironment of pro- and antiinvasive cytokines. Thus, both the extent and depth of invasion can be regulated depending on the stage and the specific context of the pregnancy.

In addition, uNK cells have important roles in angiogenesis and vascular remodeling, promoting vascular growth and transformation in the endometrium during and after implantation.[17] Vascularization of the endometrium is essential to increase blood supply, nurturing and maintaining fetal growth. Adaptations involve enlargement of spiral arteries from initially small and narrow vessels to those that are wider and low-resistant. uNK cells coordinate the initial phases of vascular remodeling by abundantly secreting angiogenic factors, including matrix metalloproteinases and angiopoietin, which degrade the extracellular matrix and disrupt vascular endothelial cells, respectively.[18,19] Subsequently, endovascular trophoblasts invade the decidual arteries and displace endothelial cells lining the arterial wall. It is no surprise, therefore, that uNK cells are seen to accumulate around spiral arteries on histochemical analysis.[20]

IMMUNE TOLERANCE

Natural killer cells express a diverse array of surface receptors, including those known to both inhibit and activate NK activity. This diverse repertoire guarantees that NK cells mount a precise and balanced response upon interaction with ligands expressed by neighboring cells. For example, in virally infected or malignant cells, the pathological ligands tip the balance toward activating signals, overpowering inhibitory cues to cause rapid lysis of target cells without the need for antibodies.

One distinctive characteristic of human pregnancy is deep hemochorial placentation, where the entire embryo is embedded in the decidua and extravillous trophoblasts (EVT) invade beyond the inner third of myometrium. Owing to the presence of a semi-allogeneic embryo, immune tolerance becomes indispensable for a successful pregnancy. In other words, the maternal immune system must effectively recognize and tolerate trophoblast cells during implantation.[21,22] Unfortunately, there exists a misconception, most likely due to the natural role of circulating NK cells, that uNK cells can attack the embryos, leading to pregnancy loss. This has however been refuted and is widely considered to be inaccurate because maternal tissues employ several strategies to suppress the effector function of uNK cells. In humans, EVT express classical major histocompatibility complex (MHC) class I molecules, such as human leukocyte antigen-C (HLA-C), as well as nonclassical MHC molecules such as HLA-E and HLA-G.[21,23,24] HLA-E interacts with the inhibitory receptor CD94-NKG2A, while HLA-G interacts with inhibitory receptors such as leukocyte immunoglobulin-like receptor B1 (LILRB1) and killer immunoglobulin-like receptors (KIR), including KIR2DL4.[12] All these engagements suppress uNK cells, ensuring the semi-allogeneic fetus will not be attacked. Of note, HLA-A and -B are absent in EVT, offering additional protection to trophoblast cells by minimizing their visibility and shielding them from attack by maternal cytotoxic T cells.[3,12]

Table 1 summarizes the immune tolerance mechanisms employed by uNK cells at the maternal–fetal interface.

Cytotoxicity of Uterine Natural Killer Cells

In contrast to peripheral blood NK cells, uNK cells have long been considered to possess poor cytotoxicity. This perception was based on weak cytolysis against K562 cells, a standard cell line derived from chronic myelogenous leukemia and widely used in cancer biology.[31,32] In addition, the observation that uNK cells naturally downregulate their cytotoxicity in acceptance of a genetically distinct fetus may also have contributed to this perception. However, recent evidence challenges this notion, revealing that uNK cells possess specific cytotoxic capabilities, particularly within the peri-implantation endometrium and during infection.[2,33,34]

During decidualization in the mid-secretory endometrium, a distinct subpopulation of acute senescent decidual cells emerges. These cells play a crucial role in triggering an acute inflammatory response, preparing the endometrium for embryo implantation.[2,7] However, persistent expression of cellular senescence can transform senescent cells from an acute to a chronic phenotype. Chronic senescence can overwhelm the endometrium with inflammatory factors and matrix metalloproteinases, leading to tissue breakdown and subsequent menstruation.[35,36] In the context of a conception cycle, preventing the emergence of chronic senescence is therefore vital. uNK cells play an active role in this objective by triggering granule exocytosis

TABLE 1: The immune tolerance mechanisms employed by uNK cells at the maternal–fetal interface.

Immune tolerance mechanism	*Description*
Immature immunological synapse	Functional assessment in vitro reveals that uNK cells lack the ability to form an immunological synapse. This deficiency prevents the polarization of the microtubule-organizing center and cytolytic granules toward the target cells[25]
Tim-3–Galectin-9 interaction	Tim-3 receptor is expressed by both uNK cells and T cells. Upon engagement with inhibitory ligand Galectin-9 on trophoblast cell, the uNK cytotoxicity was greatly impaired[26]
uNK cells–T cells crosstalk	uNK cells secrete interferon-γ and dampen the inflammatory response triggered by T helper 17 cells[27]
Engagement between CD39 and CD73	CD39, an enzyme that functions to hydrolyze extracellular nucleotide, can inhibit the uNK cell cytotoxicity through interaction with CD73 expressed by trophoblast cells. The engagement can convert the adenosine triphosphate (ATP) molecule into immunosuppressive adenosine[12]
Production of TGF-β	Immunosuppressive factor produced TGF-β, produced by trophoblast cells, has been shown to transform the peripheral blood NK cells into uNK cell-like phenotype and subsequently reduce the cytotoxicity[28,29]
Presence of Treg cells	Increased levels of Treg cells were observed in decidua in later pregnancy; depletion of Treg cells in patients experiencing recurrent miscarriages[30]

(TGF-β: transforming growth factor beta; Treg: regulatory T; uNK: uterine natural killer)

and eliminating senescent decidual cells, effectively transforming the pro-inflammatory cycling endometrium into an anti-inflammatory decidua of pregnancy. Failures here can lead to persistent chronic senescent activity, promoting the breakdown of the maternal-fetal interface and miscarriage.[2,35] Additionally, uNK cells serve as biosensors in assessing embryo quality at implantation. A recent study demonstrated that the secretome from low-fitness embryos that failed to implant inhibited the cytotoxicity of uNK cells, whereas the secretome from high-fitness embryos that resulted in live births has no impact on uNK cell activity.[33] In response to infections, uNK cells also function as defenders, ensuring maternal and fetal well-being. For example, uNK cells can form nanotubules connecting them with *Listeria monocytogenes* (Lm)-infected trophoblasts, through which antibacterial granulysin is transferred, eliminating Lm without harming the trophoblasts.[34]

These diverse cytotoxic functions, encompassing senescent clearance-mediated tissue transformation, embryo biosensing, and anti-infection, challenge previous assumptions about uNK cell cytotoxicity. They emphasize their context and time-dependent roles in maintaining tissue homeostasis, shedding new light on their complex contributions to successful pregnancy.

UTERINE NATURAL KILLER CELL HETEROGENEITY

The diverse functions of uNK cells underscore their intricate and essential role in reproduction. Yet, a fundamental question arises as to how uNK cells efficiently perform numerous tasks within strict time constraints. Perhaps the question could be answered by the recent advancements in single-cell ribonucleic acid (scRNA) sequencing, a molecular technique widely used to analyze transcriptomic profiles in individual cells from complex biological samples.[3] These experiments, combined also with immunohistochemical and flow cytometry analysis, have demonstrated that not all uNK cells are identical. In fact, these cells can be delineated into three distinct subpopulations: uNK1, uNK2, and uNK3, with different molecular features, profiles, and functions.[3,10] Notably, uNK1 cells are relatively larger in size compared to uNK2 and uNK3 cells, and express unique biomarkers, including KIR, LILRB1, and CD39. This unique receptors/antigen repertoire reflects the subpopulation's role in immune tolerance.[3,21] This is further supported by spatial localization, in which uNK1 cells reside near the EVT. In contrast, uNK2 cells, mid-sized between uNK1 and uNK3 cells, are characterized by increased expression of Annexin A1 and integrin beta chain-2 (ITGB2). In contrast, uNK3 cells express unique markers such as C-X-C chemokine receptor (CXCR)-4 and CCL5, and produce IFN-γ, a factor known to be involved in vascular remodeling in murine model.[3,12,14]

A recent study has revealed that this heterogeneity represents the differentiation status of uNK cell subpopulations. Functional assessment in vitro shows

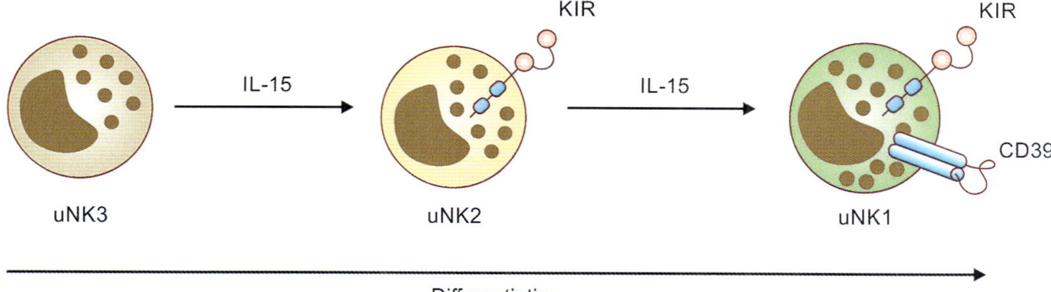

Fig. 2: uNK cell differentiation. Differentiation trajectory of uNK cell subpopulations in response to IL-15. (IL-15: interleukin-15; KIR: killer immunoglobulin-like receptors; uNK: uterine natural killer)

how uNK cells undergo cellular proliferation in response to interleukin-15 (IL-15). Continuous treatment of IL-15 can lead to the emergence of uNK2 cells that express KIR on the cell surface (KIR+CD39$^-$), which subsequently differentiate to upregulate CD39 on the cell surface, indicating transition to uNK1 cells (KIR+CD39$^+$).[10] The linear differentiation trajectory of uNK cell subpopulations is shown in **Figure 2**.

In fact, the trajectory of differentiation from the in vitro model can be extended in vivo, where the temporal regulation of these uNK cell subpopulations is shown across the menstrual cycle and throughout pregnancy. In the cycling endometrium, uNK3 cells constitute the major subpopulation, accounting for about 40–60% of total uNK cells. However, their prevalence diminishes as the cycle progresses toward the late-secretory phase. In the event of conception, uNK1 cells predominate in the decidua during the first trimester of pregnancy, constituting approximately 55% of total uNK cells. Although the abundance of uNK cells in the decidua basalis decreases as gestation unfolds, uNK3 cells resurge as the prominent subpopulation, comprising approximately 70% of total uNK cells in the third trimester of pregnancy.[11] This fluctuation reflects the need for different uNK cell subpopulations across different stages of the reproductive process. Functional studies have revealed that subpopulations exhibit the ability to degranulate and secrete cytokines. Indeed, from transcriptomic analysis, uNK3 cells appear to have proinflammatory characteristics, while uNK1 cells demonstrate immunomodulatory properties, coupled with an enhanced angiogenic capacity.[10]

Combined, these findings reflect the need for distinct uNK cell subpopulations in executing temporally sensitive functions at different stages of the reproductive process.

UTERINE NATURAL KILLER CELL LEVELS AND REPRODUCTIVE FAILURES

Immune dysregulation has been posited as a potential cause of miscarriage, although the precise mechanisms underlying this theory remain inadequately understood.[2,9,37,38] Ample evidence has dispelled the concept that the uNK cells are capable of "killing" trophoblasts,[9,39] but another concept has emerged, suggesting that uNK cells might contribute to miscarriage by overloading the endometrium with angiogenic factors, leading to excessive vascularization and oxidative stress.[40] In support of this, some studies demonstrate that increased levels of uNK cells can contribute to an excessive inflammatory response in the cycling endometrium.[37,41] Of note, the hypothesis emerged based on the observation from recurrent miscarriage (RM) patients, where increased levels of uNK cells have been noted.

Numerous research groups have diligently investigated the link between uNK cell levels and reproductive failures over the past few decades. However, the findings have not always aligned Differences in results stem from the use of diverse biomarkers, variations in quantification techniques (such as immunohistochemistry vs flow cytometry), and differing methods of measurement (such as number of uNK cells/mm^2 vs number of cells/μL). Additionally, the absence of a standardized reference range to normalize the temporal expression to each day of the menstrual cycle adds to the complexity of interpreting results.[2] Indeed, it is crucial to highlight that numerous studies comparing uNK cell levels between patients with RM and fertile subjects often focus on the specific timeframe known as the "implantation window." This approach aims to control for timing-related issues. However, even minor discrepancies in this narrow timeframe can distort data significantly.

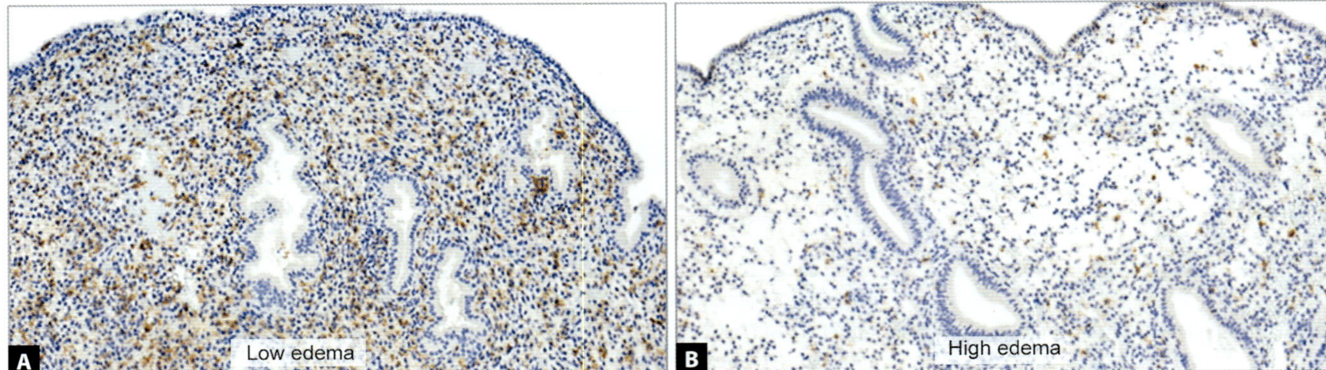

Figs. 3A and B: Reduced uNK cells in endometrial tissue edema. Images are representative of the relative levels of uNK cells in human endometrium in the presence of tissue edema. (uNK: uterine natural killer)

To overcome this issue, a daily uNK cell reference range was established from nearly 2,000 patients.[2] This approach revealed depletion of uNK cell levels in RM patients, contradicting prior findings without adequate normalization. Further, it is important to acknowledge that the quantification of uNK cells can be influenced by the presence of edema frequently observed in the mid-secretory endometrium[9] **(Figs. 3A and B)**. Consequently, depending on unvalidated diagnostic methods, uNK cell quantitation can frequently result in the mismanagement of patients and underscores the necessity for validated and standardized approaches for quantification. Implementing such rigorous methods is essential to guarantee precise assessments and to make appropriate medical decisions for individuals navigating reproductive challenges.[9,42]

IMMUNOTHERAPY

Immunotherapy has often been considered as part of the treatment options in trying to improve pregnancy outcomes. The treatment options include intravenous use of immunoglobulin, intralipid, intrauterine infusion of granulocyte colony-stimulating factor, subcutaneous administration of tumor necrosis factor alpha (TNF-α) inhibitors, leukemia inhibitory factor, and oral administration of glucocorticoids.[43-45] Despite these options, accurately diagnosing patients suffering from immune-mediated pregnancy failures remains challenging due to the absence of standardized criteria. Consequently, the true efficacy of these immunotherapies remains ambiguous. Importantly, given the heterogeneity across uNK cells, how these therapies affect uNK cell function is hard to predict.

CONCLUSION

Decidual uterine NK cell population plays a complex yet significant role in reproductive health. The population of uNK rises during implantation and in the first trimester of pregnancy thereby signifying a supportive role in placentation. However, various subtypes of uNK cells (uNK1, uNK2, uNK3) play different roles during implantation and fetal development.

REFERENCES

1. Moretta A, Bottino C, Mingari MC, Biassoni R, Moretta L. What is a natural killer cell? Nat Immunol. 2002;3(1):6-8.
2. Brighton PJ, Maruyama Y, Fishwick K, Vrljicak P, Tewary S, Fujihara R, et al. Clearance of senescent decidual cells by uterine natural killer cells in cycling human endometrium. Elife. 2017;6:e31274.
3. Vento-Tormo R, Efremova M, Botting RA, Turco MY, Vento-Tormo M, Meyer KB, et al. Single-cell reconstruction of the early maternal-fetal interface in humans. Nature. 2018;563(7731):347-53.
4. Santoni A, Carlino C, Gismondi A. Uterine NK cell development, migration and function. Reprod Biomed Online. 2008;16(2):202-10.
5. Sharkey AM, Xiong S, Kennedy PR, Gardner L, Farrell LE, Chazara O, et al. Tissue-specific education of decidual NK cells. J Immunol. 2015;195(7):3026-32.
6. Moffett-King A. Natural killer cells and pregnancy. Nat Rev Immunol. 2002;2(9):656-63.
7. Lucas ES, Vrljicak P, Muter J, Diniz-da-Costa MM, Brighton PJ, Kong CS, et al. Recurrent pregnancy loss is associated with a pro-senescent decidual response during the peri-implantation window. Commun Biol. 2020;3(1):37.
8. Trundley A, Moffett A. Human uterine leukocytes and pregnancy. Tissue Antigens. 2004;63(1):1-12.

9. Moffett A, Shreeve N. First do no harm: uterine natural killer (NK) cells in assisted reproduction. Hum Reprod. 2015;30(7):1519-25.
10. Strunz B, Bister J, Jonsson H, Filipovic I, Crona-Guterstam Y, Kvedaraite E, et al. Continuous human uterine NK cell differentiation in response to endometrial regeneration and pregnancy. Sci Immunol. 2021;6(56):eabb7800.
11. Whettlock EM, Woon EV, Cuff AO, Browne B, Johnson MR, Male V. Dynamic changes in uterine NK cell subset frequency and function over the menstrual cycle and pregnancy. Front Immunol. 2022;13:880438.
12. Moffett A, Shreeve N. Local immune recognition of trophoblast in early human pregnancy: controversies and questions. Nat Rev Immunol. 2022;23:222-35.
13. Williams PJ, Searle RF, Robson SC, Innes BA, Bulmer JN. Decidual leucocyte populations in early to late gestation normal human pregnancy. J Reprod Immunol. 2009;82(1):24-31.
14. Ashkar AA, Di Santo JP, Croy BA. Interferon gamma contributes to initiation of uterine vascular modification, decidual integrity, and uterine natural killer cell maturation during normal murine pregnancy. J Exp Med. 2000;192(2):259-70.
15. Lash GE, Schiessl B, Kirkley M, Innes BA, Cooper A, Searle RF, et al. Expression of angiogenic growth factors by uterine natural killer cells during early pregnancy. J Leukoc Biol. 2006;80(3):572-80.
16. Colucci F. The role of KIR and HLA interactions in pregnancy complications. Immunogenetics. 2017;69(8-9):557-65.
17. El-Azzamy H, Dambaeva SV, Katukurundage D, Salazar Garcia MD, Skariah A, Hussein Y, et al. Dysregulated uterine natural killer cells and vascular remodeling in women with recurrent pregnancy losses. Am J Reprod Immunol. 2018;80(4):e13024.
18. Das SK, Yano S, Wang J, Edwards DR, Nagase H, Dey SK. Expression of matrix metalloproteinases and tissue inhibitors of metalloproteinases in the mouse uterus during the peri-implantation period. Dev Genet. 1997;21(1):44-54.
19. Naruse K, Lash GE, Innes BA, Otun HA, Searle RF, Robson SC, et al. Localization of matrix metalloproteinase (MMP)-2, MMP-9 and tissue inhibitors for MMPs (TIMPs) in uterine natural killer cells in early human pregnancy. Hum Reprod. 2009;24(3):553-61.
20. Greenbaum S, Averbukh I, Soon E, Rizzuto G, Baranski A, Greenwald NF, et al. A spatially resolved timeline of the human maternal–fetal interface. Nature. 2023;619(7970):595-605.
21. Apps R, Gardner L, Sharkey AM, Holmes N, Moffett A. A homodimeric complex of HLA-G on normal trophoblast cells modulates antigen-presenting cells via LILRB1. Eur J Immunol. 2007;37(7):1924-37.
22. Vacca P, Cantoni C, Vitale M, Prato C, Canegallo F, Fenoglio D, et al. Crosstalk between decidual NK and CD14+ myelomonocytic cells results in induction of Tregs and immunosuppression. Proc Natl Acad Sci U S A. 2010;107(26):11918-23.
23. Kovats S, Main EK, Librach C, Stubblebine M, Fisher SJ, DeMars R. A class I antigen, HLA-G, expressed in human trophoblasts. Science. 1990;248(4952):220-3.
24. Shreeve N, Depierreux D, Hawkes D, Traherne JA, Sovio U, Huhn O, et al. The CD94/NKG2A inhibitory receptor educates uterine NK cells to optimize pregnancy outcomes in humans and mice. Immunity. 2021;54(6):1231-44.e4.
25. Kopcow HD, Allan DS, Chen X, Rybalov B, Andzelm MM, Ge B, et al. Human decidual NK cells form immature activating synapses and are not cytotoxic. Proc Natl Acad Sci U S A. 2005;102(43):15563-8.
26. Sun J, Yang M, Ban Y, Gao W, Song B, Wang Y, et al. Tim-3 is upregulated in NK cells during early pregnancy and inhibits NK cytotoxicity toward trophoblast in galectin-9 dependent pathway. PLoS One. 2016;11(1):e0147186.
27. Fu B, Li X, Sun R, Tong X, Ling B, Tian Z, et al. Natural killer cells promote immune tolerance by regulating inflammatory TH17 cells at the human maternal-fetal interface. Proc Natl Acad Sci U S A. 2013;110(3):E231-40.
28. Cerdeira AS, Rajakumar A, Royle CM, Lo A, Husain Z, Thadhani RI, et al. Conversion of peripheral blood NK cells to a decidual NK-like phenotype by a cocktail of defined factors. J Immunol. 2013;190(8):3939-48.
29. Keskin DB, Allan DS, Rybalov B, Andzelm MM, Stern JN, Kopcow HD, et al. TGFbeta promotes conversion of CD16+ peripheral blood NK cells into CD16-NK cells with similarities to decidual NK cells. Proc Natl Acad Sci U S A. 2007;104(9):3378-83.
30. Keller CC, Eikmans M, van der Hoorn MP, Lashley LEELO. Recurrent miscarriages and the association with regulatory T cells; A systematic review. J Reprod Immunol. 2020;139:103105.
31. King A, Birkby C, Loke YW. Early human decidual cells exhibit NK activity against the K562 cell line but not against first trimester trophoblast. Cell Immunol. 1989;118(2):337-44.
32. Rouas-Freiss N, Goncalves RM, Menier C, Dausset J, Carosella ED. Direct evidence to support the role of HLA-G in protecting the fetus from maternal uterine natural killer cytolysis. Proc Natl Acad Sci U S A. 1997;94(21):11520-5.
33. Kong CS, Ordonez AA, Turner S, Tremaine T, Muter J, Lucas ES, et al. Embryo biosensing by uterine natural killer cells determines endometrial fate decisions at implantation. FASEB J. 2021;35(4):e21336.
34. Crespo AC, Mulik S, Dotiwala F, Ansara JA, Sen Santara S, Ingersoll K, et al. Decidual NK cells transfer granulysin to selectively kill bacteria in trophoblasts. Cell. 2020;182(5):1125-39.e18.
35. Muter J, Kong CS, Brosens JJ. The role of decidual subpopulations in implantation, menstruation and miscarriage. Front Reprod Health. 2021;3:804921.

36. Di Micco R, Krizhanovsky V, Baker D, d'Adda di Fagagna F. Cellular senescence in ageing: from mechanisms to therapeutic opportunities. Nat Rev Mol Cell Biol. 2021;22(2):75-95.
37. Giuliani E, Parkin KL, Lessey BA, Young SL, Fazleabas AT. Characterization of uterine NK cells in women with infertility or recurrent pregnancy loss and associated endometriosis. Am J Reprod Immunol. 2014;72(3):262-9.
38. Fukui A, Funamizu A, Fukuhara R, Shibahara H. Expression of natural cytotoxicity receptors and cytokine production on endometrial natural killer cells in women with recurrent pregnancy loss or implantation failure, and the expression of natural cytotoxicity receptors on peripheral blood natural killer cells in pregnant women with a history of recurrent pregnancy loss. J Obstet Gynaecol Res. 2017;43(11): 1678-86.
39. Apps R, Murphy SP, Fernando R, Gardner L, Ahad T, Moffett A. Human leucocyte antigen (HLA) expression of primary trophoblast cells and placental cell lines, determined using single antigen beads to characterize allotype specificities of anti-HLA antibodies. Immunology. 2009;127(1): 26-39.
40. Quenby S, Nik H, Innes B, Lash G, Turner M, Drury J, et al. Uterine natural killer cells and angiogenesis in recurrent reproductive failure. Hum Reprod. 2009;24(1):45-54.
41. Wang F, Qualls AE, Marques-Fernandez L, Colucci F. Biology and pathology of the uterine microenvironment and its natural killer cells. Cell Mol Immunol. 2021;18(9):2101-13.
42. Bagkou Dimakou D, Tamblyn J, Justin C, Coomarasamy A, Richter A. Diagnosis and management of idiopathic recurrent pregnancy loss (RPL): current immune testing and immunomodulatory treatment practice in the United Kingdom. J Reprod Immunol. 2022;153:103662.
43. Quenby S, Kalumbi C, Bates M, Farquharson R, Vince G. Prednisolone reduces preconceptual endometrial natural killer cells in women with recurrent miscarriage. Fertil Steril. 2005;84(4):980-4.
44. Wong LF, Porter TF, Scott JR. Immunotherapy for recurrent miscarriage. Cochrane Database Syst Rev. 2014;2014(10):CD000112.
45. Achilli C, Duran-Retamal M, Saab W, Serhal P, Seshadri S. The role of immunotherapy in in vitro fertilization and recurrent pregnancy loss: a systematic review and meta-analysis. Fertil Steril. 2018;110(6):1089-100.

CHAPTER

16

Endometrial Microbiome

Kilian Vomstein

ABSTRACT

Endometrial microbiome is of very low biomass and is best studied by culture independent methods like quantitative polymerase chain reaction (qPCR), 16S rRNA sequencing and shotgun metagenomic sequencing. Alterations of the endometrial microbiome has been demonstrated in patients with recurrent pregnancy loss (RPL) when compared with controls. Endometrial dysbiosis will affect the immune environment, thereby hampering the implantation process. Therapeutic interventions include prebiotics and probiotics. Of all the strains of probiotic Lactobacilli, *Lactobacillus crispatus* is most abundant in the healthy endometrium. In resistant cases microbiome transplant has also been effective.

Keywords: Endometrial microbiome, Dysbiosis, *Lactobacillus iners*, Probiotics, Prebiotics, *Lactobacillus crispatus*.

INTRODUCTION

Even after a thorough examination into different risk factors, a significant number of cases of recurrent pregnancy loss (RPL) still lack a clear explanation. This uncertainty poses a hurdle for both medical practitioners and academics. The human microbiome, encompassing trillions of microorganisms living on and within our bodies, has been recognized as a significant influencer of numerous health aspects.[1] It consists of bacteria, viruses, fungi, archaea, and other microbial entities that form complex ecosystems in different body sites. The microbiome has been extensively studied in the gut, skin, and oral cavity, demonstrating its profound impact on metabolic processes, immune regulation, and disease pathogenesis.[1] Lately, the focus has shifted toward the possible role of the microbiome in aspects of reproductive health, encompassing fertility, outcomes of pregnancy, and disorders related to gynecology.[2]

The vaginal microbiome has a significant part in reproductive health. Its structure and steadiness have an impact on vaginal pH, immune system reactions, and vulnerability to infections. Disruption in the balance of the vaginal microbiome has been associated with unfavorable reproductive results,[3-5] including pregnancy loss.[6,7]

The term "endometrial microbiome" refers to microorganisms present within the endometrium or the uterine cavity. Historically, it was hypothesized to be a sterile environment, yet recent progress in molecular sequencing techniques has disclosed a complex microbial ecosystem existing within the uterine cavity. The bacterial abundance in the uterus is projected to be 100 to 10,000-fold less compared to the vagina. Therefore, the uterine (endometrial) microbiome is recognized as an area characterized by a low microbial biomass.[8] Dysbiosis in the endometrial microbiome has been associated with impaired IVF outcomes and (recurrent) pregnancy loss.[9-11] However, the role of the endometrial microbiome has been questioned lately, due to the contradicting results of studies, which may have caused differences in sequencing- and sampling techniques. Therefore, this chapter aims to shed light on these differences and show, how and why an endometrial microbiome might exist and influence reproductive outcomes in RPL.

MICROBIOME

Methods to Study the Microbiome

Analyzing the microbiome requires sophisticated methodologies that can characterize the complex microbial communities and their functional activities.

Culture-dependent Methods

Culture-dependent methodologies, necessitating the growth of microorganisms on diverse culture media for targeted species identification, have been historically used but present certain restrictions. They are insufficient in encapsulating the total biodiversity of the microbiome due to the inherent difficulties associated with culturing microorganisms. While these techniques permit the isolation and characterization of specific species from distinct sites, they exhibit a bias toward the culturable constituents of the microbiome, potentially resulting in an under-representation of the authentic microbial diversity.

Culture-independent Methods

Culture-independent methodologies leverage sophisticated molecular techniques for the direct examination of the genetic content of microorganisms, bypassing the necessity for cultivation. These techniques provide a broader and unbiased evaluation of the composition and functionality of the microbial community.

Quantitative polymerase chain reaction (qPCR): qPCR is a common technique in microbiome studies for its speed, sensitivity, and specificity. It amplifies and quantifies targeted deoxyribonucleic acid (DNA) sequences using specific primers and fluorescent probes, which allows for accurate quantification of the target organism in a sample. It is especially useful for detecting changes in microbial abundance related to various conditions. The method can detect and quantify low-abundance organisms and is faster and more cost-effective than many sequencing approaches. It has been used to assess the abundance of key species in the female reproductive tract. However, its targeted approach may limit the ability to capture the full diversity and complexity of the microbiome.

16S rRNA gene sequencing: The method of 16S rRNA gene sequencing is extensively used for microbial community profiling, targeting the highly preserved areas of the bacterial 16S *rRNA* gene. Distinct characteristics are exhibited in the sequencing analysis of different regions of the 16S *rRNA* gene, such as V2, V3, and V4. For instance, an evaluation of the vaginal microbiome, comparing V1-2 and V3-4 hyper-variable regions, demonstrated the V3-4 region identified more taxa with greater diversity than the V1-2 region, which failed to detect certain significant species of the female lower genital tract.[12] These regions are amplified through polymerase chain reaction (PCR) and sequenced using high-throughput platforms, and the sequences obtained are categorized into operational taxonomic units (OTUs) or species-level taxa. This method yields information regarding the relative abundance and diversity of bacterial taxa in the sample. Although 16S *rRNA* gene sequencing allows for a comprehensive overview of microbial community composition, it offers limited resolution at the species level. Nonetheless, it is the most frequently employed method in contemporary microbiome research.[13]

Shotgun metagenomic sequencing: The shotgun approach involves randomly fragmenting and subsequently sequencing all DNA from a specific environmental sample, thereby providing an impartial perspective of the community's genomic content.[14] The resulting sequences, or "reads," are assembled into longer sequences (contigs) and, ultimately, into complete or near-complete genomes. This approach offers insights into both the taxonomic structure and the metabolic capabilities of the community.[15]

A key strength of shotgun metagenomics lies in its capability to apprehend the broad functional diversity encoded within microbial genomes. It surpasses mere taxonomic profiling by uncovering the metabolic pathways and functional genes existent in the community. Hence, this approach can shed light on possible ecological roles and interactions among community constituents, thereby enriching our comprehension of microbiome dynamics and resilience.[16] In addition, shotgun metagenomics can identify all forms of microorganisms, which encompasses bacteria, archaea, viruses, and eukaryotic microbes, in contrast to 16S *rRNA* gene sequencing which is confined to bacteria and archaea. Furthermore, it can accomplish superior resolution down to the strain level, a substantial progression given the functional variation that is present at this level.[17]

Despite its advantages, shotgun metagenomic sequencing also presents unique challenges. The enormous volume of data generated can be computationally intensive to analyze and necessitates advanced bioinformatics skills.[18] Additionally, it necessitates comprehensive and well-curated reference databases for taxonomic designation and functional annotation. However, numerous microbial species, particularly from nonmodel or inadequately studied environments, remain uncharacterized, resulting in a multitude of sequences being unassignable.[19] A further challenge is the issue of DNA contamination, which can originate from the host in host-associated microbiomes or from the environment and reagents used in the DNA extraction and sequencing process.[20] Therefore, a properly designed experimental layout and stringent data-cleaning procedures are essential to counteract these problems. Despite these obstacles, the progression of sequencing technologies and bioinformatics tools persistently enhances the accessibility and utility of shotgun metagenomics. Given its unparalleled capacity to capture the intricacy of microbial communities, shotgun metagenomic sequencing will unquestionably remain a principal instrument in microbiome research.

In conclusion, these methodologies offer diverse strategies for an all-encompassing study of the female microbiome. Each technique carries its own strengths and limitations, and the selection of a method is reliant on the research objectives, sample types, and available resources. The use of multiple methods can yield a more comprehensive picture of the female microbiome and its potential associations with RPL, thus facilitating a deeper understanding of microbial dysbiosis and its impact on reproductive health.

ENDOMETRIAL MICROBIOME

Traditionally, the endometrium was believed to be a sterile environment; however, recent advancements in molecular techniques have revealed the presence of a complex and dynamic microbial ecosystem in this niche. Endometriosis, chronic endometritis, dysfunctional endometrial bleeding, endometrial malignancy or hyperplasia, and poor assisted reproductive technology (ART) results have all been linked to an altered endometrial microbiome composition.[8,21]

By using qPCR, Mitchell et al. identified bacteria in 95% of endometrial samples from asymptomatic women undergoing hysterectomies, thereby describing the upper vaginal tract microbiome[22] with the most prevalent species being *Lactobacillus iners*, *Prevotella* spp., and *Lactobacillus crispatus*. Notably, the microbiome of the upper vaginal canal differed from that of the lower genital tract both numerically and qualitatively, although the qPCR results only focused on a small subset of these bacteria. Using 16s rRNA sequencing, Moreno and colleagues investigated the uterine and vaginal microbiome in 13 fertile women.[10] This paper illustrated and somehow manifested, that *Lactobacillus* spp. was the dominant species in the endometrial fluid of fertile, healthy women. Other prevalent species detected in the uterine microbiomes of healthy reproductive-age women included *Gardnerella*, *Bifidobacterium*, *Streptococcus*, and *Prevotella*. Further, it was shown in a cohort of 35 infertile women that an endometrium not dominated by *Lactobacillus* (<90% *Lactobacillus* spp.) during the receptive phase correlated significantly with decreased chances of implantation, ongoing pregnancy, and live births.[10] Nonetheless, it should be noted that despite the identification of taxa in the endometrium, which was absent in the vaginal samples and vice versa, statistical analysis revealed no significant distinction between the endometrial and vaginal microbiome. These findings were corroborated by a subsequent international multi-center study conducted by the same group, which analyzed endometrial fluid and biopsies in 342 patients.[9] Moreover, studies that obtained endometrial biopsies through hysterectomy[23] or laparoscopy[24] (and thereby reducing the contamination risk from the vagina and cervix) concluded that *Lactobacillus* does not dominate the uterine cavity and instead bacteria such as *Pseudomonas*, *Acinetobacter*, *Vagococcus*, and *Sphingobium* contribute most to the endometrial microbiome. Still, indications for hysterectomy or laparoscopy included the presence of uterine fibroids, dysfunctional bleeding, endometrial hyperplasia, etc. and the patients were significantly older than in the studies including infertile couples. Additionally, the patients in these studies were notably older compared to those involved in studies focusing on infertile couples. These underlying conditions introduce significant heterogeneity, making direct comparisons between these studies nearly impossible. This emphasizes the unique complexities involved in analyzing the endometrial microbiome in comparison to other body sites.[25] One of the primary challenges encountered in studying the endometrial microbiome is the limited microbial biomass present. The bacterial load in the endometrium is typically lower compared to other body sites such as the vagina, gut, or skin. This scarcity of microbial material poses difficulties in obtaining an adequate amount of microbial DNA for comprehensive analysis. To accurately detect and characterize the endometrial microbiome, sensitive, and optimized techniques and controls are required.

An additional concern in endometrial sampling is the risk of contamination. The endometrium is located within the uterus, which is not directly exposed to the external environment. Consequently, precautions must be taken during sample collection to minimize contamination from the more accessible vaginal or cervical microbiota. This highlights the importance of employing appropriate controls in endometrial microbiome studies. Negative controls should be included to account for any background contamination that may occur during sample processing. Positive controls are also essential to verify the efficiency and sensitivity of the sequencing and analysis methods employed. Taken together, by implementing meticulous sampling procedures and employing well-designed control measures, researchers can better differentiate the true endometrial microbiota from potential contaminants, ensuring the reliability and accuracy of endometrial microbiome studies.[25]

CURRENT STUDIES ON THE MICROBIOME AND RECURRENT PREGNANCY LOSS

A growing body of evidence suggests that shifts in the microbiome, particularly within the vaginal and endometrial environments, may be implicated in RPL. A total of five studies have especially investigating the endometrial microbiome in RPL **(Table 1)**.

In a longitudinal setup, with a sampling of endometrial flushing in three different cycle phases, an analysis of 20 RPL, 20 RIF, and 10 healthy controls showed a higher diversity during the luteal phase in RIF and RPL patients.[11] In this study, RPL patients showed a higher abundance of *Proteobacteria* and *Dialister* in the endometrium. When analyzing endometrial fluid and endometrial biopsies, another study could show a higher prevalence of *Anaerobacillus*, *Erysipelothrix,* and *Hydrogenophilus* spp., while no differences were seen in endometrial tissue.[26] Diverging results were reported by Masucci, when analyzing endometrial biopsies. They identified a higher bacterial diversity in controls than in RPL patients; however, when looking at different taxa, no differences were found.[27] In contrast, Peuranpää et al. found a decreased prevalence of *Lactobacillus* spp. in endometrial samples from RPL patients,[28] supporting the results of Moreno with a lower chance of reproductive success when *Lactobacillus* are decreased in the endometrium.[9,10] A Chinese study followed their patients for up to 14 months after an endometrial biopsy.[29] The authors could show that patients with an increase in *Ureplasma* spp. had a higher risk of preterm delivery and pregnancy loss, than the patients that did not show more *Ureaplasma*. Interestingly, Peuranpää also found a strong correlation between endometrial and vaginal microbial composition, questioning the need of performing an endometrial biopsy for microbiome analysis.[28]

MICROBIOME-IMMUNE LINK

Embryo implantation is a complex process that involves several critical steps for the establishment of a pregnancy. It begins with apposition, where the blastocyst attaches to the uterine epithelium, followed by adhesion, where firm attachment is achieved through specific molecular interactions. Invasion then occurs as trophoblast cells penetrate the endometrial tissue, migrating into the uterine stromal layer. Decidualization, a transformation of the endometrial stromal cells into specialized decidual cells, supports the growing embryo. Angiogenesis, the formation of new blood vessels, is essential for establishing a sufficient blood supply to the developing embryo. Immunomodulation is another crucial aspect, ensuring immune tolerance by the maternal system to prevent rejection of the embryo. Finally, placenta formation occurs, as trophoblast cells differentiate and create the placental structure. The placenta serves as the interface between the maternal and fetal circulatory systems, facilitating nutrient exchange and waste removal. These intricate steps collectively contribute to the successful attachment, invasion, establishment of maternal blood supply, and placenta formation necessary for a healthy pregnancy.[30,31] This requires an orchestration of angiogenesis,[30] decidualization[32] and an adaptive immune response adaptability.[31]

Investigating the intricate immunological mechanisms behind successful pregnancy is necessary to comprehend the function of the immune system in the link between the reproductive tract microbiota and RPL. The need for the maternal immune system to accept the semiallogeneic fetus, which shares just half of the mother's genetic material, while still being able to mount effective responses against possible infections, is one of the primary challenges during pregnancy. The fragile equilibrium is influenced by the reproductive tract's microbiota, which is crucial in controlling maternal immune responses.[33]

At the fetomaternal interface in a healthy state, the interaction between bacteria and immune cells involves three potential mechanisms that contribute to maintaining a healthy balance: Firstly, innate immune cells and epithelial cells produce antimicrobial peptides, which help protect the local tissue lining from potential infections. This serves as a barrier defense mechanism. Secondly, antigen-presenting cells interact with bacteria and initiate an immune response. This response involves activating immune cells, such as uterine natural killer (NK) cells and indirectly influencing T-cells. The activation of uterine NK (uNK) cells and the development of T-cell subsets, characterized by a high number of regulatory Tregs, a low number of Th-17, and a shift from Th1 to Th2 cytokine-producing cells, are the result of this microbiome-host

TABLE 1: Studies on the endometrial microbiome and RPL.

Study		Population	Specimen	Method	Results
Peuranpää 2022	2022	47 RPL (≥3 losses, 23 parous, 23 nulliparous) 39 control (male factor infertility, six parous, six nulliparous)	• Vaginal swab • Endometrial biopsy	16s rRNA V3–V4 (Illumina MiSeq)	*L. crispatus* less abundant in endometrial samples of RPL, *G. vaginalis* more abundant in vaginal and endometrial samples of RPL. Vaginal and endometrial microbial compositions correlated strongly
Shi 2022	2022	• 67 RPL (≥2 losses) • Follow-up for >14 months	• *Vagina:* Nugent score • Endometrial biopsy	16s rRNA V4 (Illumina MiSeq)	Increase in *Ureaplasma* species in the endometrium showed a higher risk of preterm delivery and miscarriage
Vomstein 2022	2022	• 20 RPL (≥3 losses) • 20 RIF • 10 control (healthy, never pregnant)	Endometrial fluid	16s rRNA V3–V4 (Illumina MiSeq)	In the control group, a significant decrease of species richness and evenness was shown around ovulation which remained at this lower level during the luteal phase. This loss of diversity during the menstrual cycle was not apparent in RIF and RM patients. A higher similarity was seen in taxonomic distribution between RM and RIF patients compared to the control group. In the luteal phase, RPL with higher abundance of *Proteobacteria* and *Dialister* and a lower abundance of *Gardnerella*.
Liu 2022	2022	• 25 RPL (≥2 losses) • 25 control (male factor infertility)	• Vaginal swab • Cervical fluid • Endometrial fluid • Endometrial biopsy	16s rRNA V3-V4 (Illumina NovaSeq)	• No difference in alpha diversity between RPL and control in vaginal, cervical, or endometrial samples. • *Vagina:* No sign of the difference in specific taxa between RPL and control • *Cervix:* Bacteroidetes and *Crenarchaeota* sign. Higher abundance in RPL. Higher abundance of *Atopobium*, *Staphylococcus* spp., and *Cutibacterium* in RPL. • *Endometrial tissue:* No significant difference between RPL and control. • *Endometrial fluid: Anaerobacillus*, *Erysipelothrix*, and *Hydrogenophilus* spp. sign. Lower abundance in RPL. The bacillus sign is higher in RPL
Masucci 2023	2023	40 RPL (≥2 losses; 20 HLA-DQ2/DQ8 positive, 20 HLA-DQ2/DQ8 negative) Seven control (healthy, HLA-DQ2/DQ8 negative, previous live birth)	• Vaginal swab • Endometrial biopsy	16s rRNA V3-V4 (Illumina MiSeq)	• *Endometrium:* Higher diversity in control than in RPL. No significant differences concerning different taxa. • *Vagina:* No difference in diversity between RPL and control • *L. iners* more prevalent in RPL women—in endometrial and vaginal samples.

(HLA: human leukocyte antigen; RPL: recurrent pregnancy loss; rRNA: ribosomal ribonucleic acid)

interaction,[31] which supports processes like implantation, angiogenesis (blood vessel formation), and remodeling of spiral arteries. Thirdly, bacterial metabolites stimulate a local immune response, contributing to the mechanisms mentioned earlier. However, in cases of dysbiosis, where the balance of bacteria is disrupted, these mechanisms can be disturbed. A disruption of the local barrier and epithelium occurs, making it vulnerable to damage. This damage triggers a signaling cascade that leads to a switch in the immune response, characterized by a shift toward a Th1 cytokine response. This altered immune response can impact angiogenesis, spiral artery remodeling, and the function of uterine NK cells ultimately leading to incorrect implantation and placentation **(Fig. 1)**.[31]

In general, bacterial infections have the ability to trigger an immunological reaction against the pathogen,

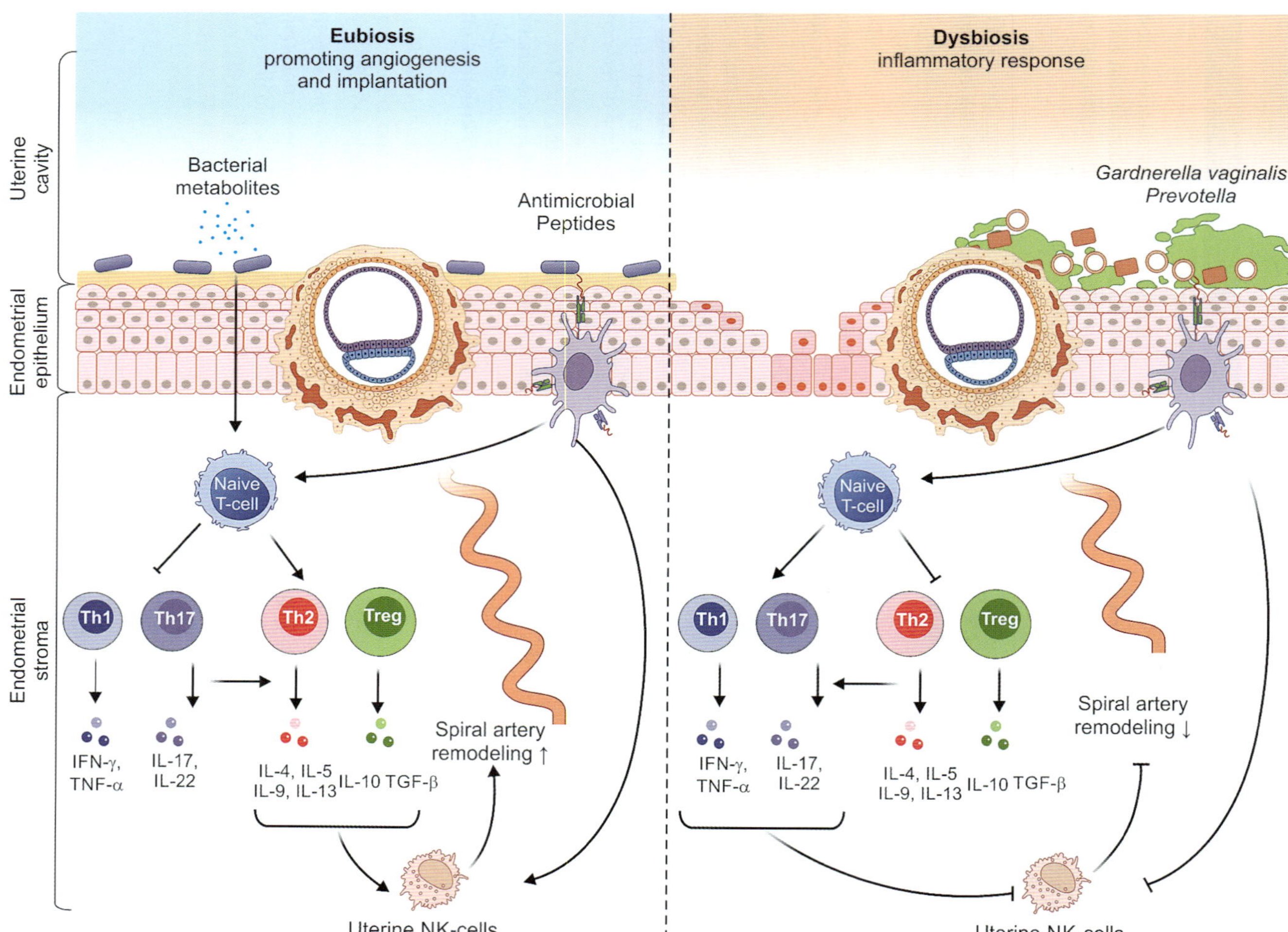

Fig. 1: Proposed mechanism of the interaction between the endometrial microbiome and its influence on the implantation and the immune system.

Note:

Left, eubiosis: There are three potential mechanisms of the interaction between bacteria driving eubiosis and the local immune cells at the fetomaternal interface: (1) Innate immune cells and epithelial cells produce antimicrobial peptides protecting the local epithelium, (2) antigen-presenting cells interact with the bacteria and trigger a response of the immune cells—directly inducing uterine NK-cells and indirectly by interacting with T-cells, leading toward a Th-2 shift that supports implantation, angiogenesis, and spiral artery remodeling, and (3) bacterial metabolites induce a local immune response, leading to the aforementioned mechanisms.

Right, dysbiosis: In dysbiosis, these mechanisms are disturbed: (1) The local barrier and epithelium are destroyed. (2) thereby, a signal cascade is being induced, leading to a switch to Th1-cytokine response, altered angiogenesis, and spiral artery remodeling by impacting uterine NK-cell function.

Source: Figure created with BioRender.com, adapted from.[31]

which can result in excessive inflammation and damage the fetal-placental unit's cellular components.[33-35] Certain bacteria, such as *Lactobacillus* species, which predominate in a healthy vaginal microbiota, have been shown to support an anti-inflammatory environment conducive to pregnancy.[36] Using vaginal epithelial cell culture, it could even be shown, that *L. crispatus*, and not *L. jensenii* were able to reduce the secretion of IL-6 and IL-8.[36] On the other hand, a change toward a pro-inflammatory state has been linked to an increased relative abundance of *Gardnerella* and *Ureaplasma* species in the vagina, as found in (recurrent) pregnancy loss.[6] This proinflammatory response is characterized by an increased production of proinflammatory cytokines including TNF-α, IL-17, IL-1, and IL-6 as well as a decrease in Tregs. Grewal et al. found that the proinflammatory cytokines IL-1, IL-6, and TNF- α were increased in women with a depleted vaginal microbiome and a pregnancy loss when comparing the cervicovaginal secretions of these women to those of women who delivered at term.[6] This is in line with findings in women undergoing a cervical cerclage, where a *Lactobacillus*-depleted microbiome was also linked with inflammation.[37] An aberrant immune profile was observed in women experiencing RPL who were screened for *Gardnerella vaginalis*. The prevalence of *Gardnerella vaginalis* and gram-negative anaerobes was significantly higher in RPL patients with elevated peripheral natural killer (pNK) cell levels compared to patients with normal pNK cell levels.[38]

Recent research suggests that the gut microbiota also has a role in influencing the immune system of the host. Commensal bacteria, which are bacteria that coexist with the host without causing harm, are crucial for the development and proper functioning of the host's immune response. They can influence both the innate and adaptive branches of the immune system.[39] Certain elements of the gut microbiota, for example, can influence T cell development into regulatory T cells or effector T cells, which can have far-reaching effects on immunological responses throughout the body.[40] However, future research will need to show that these alterations have an influence on reproductive outcomes.

These results highlight the possibility that the (reproductive tract) microbiome might influence immune responses during pregnancy as well as the potential contribution of microbial dysbiosis to RPL through its effects on immunological balance. Additional investigation into the microbiome-immune interface in relation to RPL may provide important information for the creation of microbiota-based treatment approaches to rebalance the immune system and enhance the success of pregnancies.

MICROBIOME-BASED INTERVENTIONS IN RECURRENT PREGNANCY LOSS: CURRENT CHALLENGES AND FUTURE DIRECTIONS

Diagnostics

It is progressively becoming clearer how microbiota might be used to diagnose RPL. There may be microbial indicators for RPL based on differences in the vaginal and endometrial microbiome between women with RPL and those who had uncomplicated pregnancies. As a result, microbial profiling shows potential as a new diagnostic method for RPL, providing information on an individual's susceptibility to miscarriage. These methods can be helpful in locating variations from the typical microbiota that can be related to RPL. While taking into consideration potential confounders such as the ploidy status of a pregnancy loss, the period of the menstrual cycle, sexual activity,[41] and usage of contraceptives or other medications,[42] further research is required to uncover distinct microbiological signatures of RPL.

Innovative Approaches for Modulating the Microbiome in the Context of Reproductive Health

Bacterial vaginosis has been treated with antibiotics and antimicrobials. However, antibiotics should only be used with caution because of their broad scope, risk of resistance, and potential adverse effects on beneficial microorganisms. Probiotics and prebiotics may provide a safer and more focused strategy in this situation. The microbiota may be modified with probiotics, which are live beneficial bacteria, and prebiotics, which encourage the growth of beneficial bacteria. Some probiotics may have a role in avoiding RPL, according to early research suggesting they might increase pregnancy rates in women using assisted reproductive technology.[43] Notably, in a recent case study of our group, a vaginal microbiota transplant in a woman with RPL resulted in dysbiosis resolution, symptom improvement, and confirmed donor-strain *L. crispatus* engraftment without antibiotic pretreatment.[44] Moreover, after the transplant, the mother gave birth to a healthy baby at term. However, in order to verify these results and determine the most efficient strains and doses, additional thorough clinical trials are required.

CONCLUSION

The study of the microbiome's function in RPL is a quickly developing area that has several potential research directions. It will be necessary to do studies that clarify the processes by which the microbiome interacts with the immune system and affects pregnancy outcomes. Additionally, long-term studies monitoring changes in the microbiome in connection to RPL and during various phases of pregnancy are required. Here, a precise definition of RPL and clearly defined control cohorts are essential.

Personalized microbial treatment research may also lead to new therapeutic opportunities. As our knowledge of the microbiome expands, we might be able to create (personalized) probiotic therapies that will encourage a microbiota that is favorable for a healthy pregnancy. This may fundamentally alter how RPL caused by microbial dysbiosis is managed.

REFERENCES

1. Human Microbiome Project C. Structure, function and diversity of the healthy human microbiome. Nature. 2012;486(7402):207-14.
2. Koedooder R, Mackens S, Budding A, Fares D, Blockeel C, Laven J, et al. Identification and evaluation of the microbiome in the female and male reproductive tracts. Human Reprod Update. 2019;25(3):298-325.
3. Skafte-Holm A, Humaidan P, Bernabeu A, Lledo B, Jensen JS, Haahr T. The Association between Vaginal Dysbiosis and Reproductive Outcomes in Sub-Fertile Women Undergoing IVF-Treatment: A Systematic PRISMA Review and Meta-Analysis. Pathogens (Basel, Switzerland). 2021;10(3):295.
4. Haahr T, Zacho J, Brauner M, Shathmigha K, Skov Jensen J, Humaidan P. Reproductive outcome of patients undergoing in vitro fertilisation treatment and diagnosed with bacterial vaginosis or abnormal vaginal microbiota: a systematic PRISMA review and meta-analysis. BJOG. 2019;126(2):200-7.
5. Haahr T, Jensen JS, Thomsen L, Duus L, Rygaard K, Humaidan P. Abnormal vaginal microbiota may be associated with poor reproductive outcomes: a prospective study in IVF patients. Hum Reprod. 2016;31(4):795-803.
6. Grewal K, Lee YS, Smith A, Brosens JJ, Bourne T, Al-Memar M, et al. Chromosomally normal miscarriage is associated with vaginal dysbiosis and local inflammation. BMC Med. 2022;20(1):38.
7. Al-Memar M, Bobdiwala S, Fourie H, Mannino R, Lee YS, Smith A, et al. The association between vaginal bacterial composition and miscarriage: a nested case-control study. BJOG. 2020;127(2):264-74.
8. Baker JM, Chase DM, Herbst-Kralovetz MM. Uterine Microbiota: Residents, Tourists, or Invaders? Front Immunol. 2018;9:208.
9. Moreno I, Garcia-Grau I, Perez-Villaroya D, Gonzalez-Monfort M, Bahceci M, Barrionuevo MJ, et al. Endometrial microbiota composition is associated with reproductive outcome in infertile patients. Microbiome. 2022;10(1):1.
10. Moreno I, Codoner FM, Vilella F, Valbuena D, Martinez-Blanch JF, Jimenez-Almazan J, et al. Evidence that the endometrial microbiota has an effect on implantation success or failure. Am J Obstet Gynecol. 2016;215(6):684-703.
11. Vomstein K, Reider S, Bottcher B, Watschinger C, Kyvelidou C, Tilg H, et al. Uterine microbiota plasticity during the menstrual cycle: Differences between healthy controls and patients with recurrent miscarriage or implantation failure. J Reprod Immunol. 2022;151:103634.
12. Graspeuntner S, Loeper N, Kunzel S, Baines JF, Rupp J. Selection of validated hypervariable regions is crucial in 16S-based microbiota studies of the female genital tract. Sci Rep. 2018;8(1):9678.
13. Knight R, Vrbanac A, Taylor BC, Aksenov A, Callewaert C, Debelius J, et al. Best practices for analysing microbiomes. Nat Rev Microbiol. 2018;16(7):410-22.
14. Sharpton TJ. An introduction to the analysis of shotgun metagenomic data. Front Plant Sci. 2014;5:209.
15. Quince C, Walker AW, Simpson JT, Loman NJ, Segata N. Shotgun metagenomics, from sampling to analysis. Nat Biotechnol. 2017;35(9):833-44.
16. Gilbert JA, Dupont CL. Microbial metagenomics: beyond the genome. Ann Rev Mar Sci. 2011;3:347-71.
17. Truong DT, Franzosa EA, Tickle TL, Scholz M, Weingart G, Pasolli E, et al. MetaPhlAn2 for enhanced metagenomic taxonomic profiling. Nat Methods. 2015;12(10):902-3.
18. Wooley JC, Godzik A, Friedberg I. A primer on metagenomics. PLoS Comput Biol. 2010;6(2):e1000667.
19. Almeida A, Mitchell AL, Boland M, Forster SC, Gloor GB, Tarkowska A, et al. A new genomic blueprint of the human gut microbiota. Nature. 2019;568(7753):499-504.
20. Salter SJ, Cox MJ, Turek EM, Calus ST, Cookson WO, Moffatt MF, et al. Reagent and laboratory contamination can critically impact sequence-based microbiome analyses. BMC Biol. 2014;12:87.
21. Molina NM, Sola-Leyva A, Saez-Lara MJ, Plaza-Diaz J, Tubic-Pavlovic A, Romero B, et al. New Opportunities for Endometrial Health by Modifying Uterine Microbial Composition: Present or Future? Biomolecules. 2020;10(4):593.
22. Mitchell CM, Haick A, Nkwopara E, Garcia R, Rendi M, Agnew K, et al. Colonization of the upper genital tract by vaginal bacterial species in nonpregnant women. Am J Obstet Gynecol. 2015;212(5):611.e1-9.
23. Winters AD, Romero R, Gervasi MT, Gomez-Lopez N, Tran MR, Garcia-Flores V, et al. Does the endometrial cavity have a molecular microbial signature? Sci Rep. 2019;9(1):9905.

24. Chen C, Song X, Wei W, Zhong H, Dai J, Lan Z, et al. The microbiota continuum along the female reproductive tract and its relation to uterine-related diseases. Nat Commun. 2017;8(1):875.
25. Molina NM, Sola-Leyva A, Haahr T, Aghajanova L, Laudanski P, Castilla JA, et al. Analysing endometrial microbiome: methodological considerations and recommendations for good practice. Hum Reprod. 2021;36(4):859-79.
26. Liu FT, Yang S, Yang Z, Zhou P, Peng T, Yin J, et al. An Altered Microbiota in the Lower and Upper Female Reproductive Tract of Women with Recurrent Spontaneous Abortion. Microbiol Spectr. 2022;10(3):e0046222.
27. Masucci L, D'Ippolito S, De Maio F, Quaranta G, Mazzarella R, Bianco DM, et al. Celiac Disease Predisposition and Genital Tract Microbiota in Women Affected by Recurrent Pregnancy Loss. Nutrients. 2023;15(1):221.
28. Peuranpää P, Holster T, Saqib S, Kalliala I, Tiitinen A, Salonen A, et al. Female reproductive tract microbiota and recurrent pregnancy loss: a nested case-control study. Reprod Biomed Online. 2022;45(5):1021-31.
29. Shi Y, Yamada H, Sasagawa Y, Tanimura K, Deguchi M. Uterine endometrium microbiota and pregnancy outcome in women with recurrent pregnancy loss. J Reprod Immunol. 2022;152:103653.
30. Chen X, Liu S, Tan Q, Shoenfeld Y, Zeng Y. Microbiome, autoimmunity, allergy, and helminth infection: The importance of the pregnancy period. Am J Reprod Immunol. 2017;78(2):e12654.
31. Al-Nasiry S, Ambrosino E, Schlaepfer M, Morre SA, Wieten L, Voncken JW, et al. The Interplay Between Reproductive Tract Microbiota and Immunological System in Human Reproduction. Front Immunol. 2020;11:378.
32. Mori M, Bogdan A, Balassa T, Csabai T, Szekeres-Bartho J. The decidua-the maternal bed embracing the embryo-maintains the pregnancy. Seminars in immunopathology. 2016;38(6):635-49.
33. Mor G, Aldo P, Alvero AB. The unique immunological and microbial aspects of pregnancy. Nat Rev Immunol. 2017;17(8):469-82.
34. Romero R, Espinoza J, Goncalves LF, Kusanovic JP, Friel L, Hassan S. The role of inflammation and infection in preterm birth. Semin Reprod Med. 2007;25(1):21-39.
35. Straszewski-Chavez SL, Abrahams VM, Mor G. The role of apoptosis in the regulation of trophoblast survival and differentiation during pregnancy. Endocrine reviews. 2005;26(7):877-97.
36. Spurbeck RR, Arvidson CG. Lactobacilli at the front line of defense against vaginally acquired infections. Future Microbiol. 2011;6(5):567-82.
37. Kindinger LM, MacIntyre DA, Lee YS, Marchesi JR, Smith A, McDonald JA, et al. Relationship between vaginal microbial dysbiosis, inflammation, and pregnancy outcomes in cervical cerclage. Sci Transl Med. 2016;8(350):350ra102.
38. Kuon RJ, Togawa R, Vomstein K, Weber M, Goeggl T, Strowitzki T, et al. Higher prevalence of colonization with Gardnerella vaginalis and gram-negative anaerobes in patients with recurrent miscarriage and elevated peripheral natural killer cells. J Reprod Immunol. 2017;120:15-9.
39. Belkaid Y, Hand TW. Role of the microbiota in immunity and inflammation. Cell. 2014;157(1):121-41.
40. Ivanov, II, Atarashi K, Manel N, Brodie EL, Shima T, Karaoz U, et al. Induction of intestinal Th17 cells by segmented filamentous bacteria. Cell. 2009;139(3):485-98.
41. Gajer P, Brotman RM, Bai G, Sakamoto J, Schutte UM, Zhong X, et al. Temporal dynamics of the human vaginal microbiota. Sci Transl Med. 2012;4(132):132ra52.
42. Krog MC, Hugerth LW, Fransson E, Bashir Z, Andersen A, Edfeldt G, et al. The healthy female microbiome across body sites: effect of hormonal contraceptives and the menstrual cycle. Hum Reprod. 2022;37(7):1525-43.
43. Lopez-Moreno A, Aguilera M. Vaginal Probiotics for Reproductive Health and Related Dysbiosis: Systematic Review and Meta-Analysis. J Clin Med. 2021;10(7):1461.
44. Wrønding T, Vomstein K, Bosma EF, Mortensen B, Westh H, Heintz JE, et al. Antibiotic-free vaginal microbiota transplant with donor engraftment, dysbiosis resolution and live birth after recurrent pregnancy loss: a proof of concept case study. EClinicalMedicine. 2023;61:102070.

SECTION

4 Anatomical Factors

CHAPTER 17

Endometriosis

T Ramanidevi, J Harshini, Arulmozhi Ramarajan

ABSTRACT

Endometriosis is a common inflammatory disorder affecting women of reproductive age group. It is commonly associated with infertility but may also be associated with recurrent pregnancy loss (RPL), post-treatment of infertility. Its clinical presentation is varied, but even in its mildest forms, it can cause immune dysregulation in pregnancy and compromise implantation rates. Diagnosis of mild peritoneal disease poses a dilemma and may require laparoscopy which is not only diagnostic but also therapeutic. Medical suppression therapy with depot GnRH agonist will also improve pregnancy outcomes.

Keywords: Endometriosis, RPL, Laparoscopy.

INTRODUCTION

Endometriosis is a chronic inflammatory disease, which is estrogen-dependent and progesterone-resistant, affecting the women of reproductive age-group, where there is presence of endometrial-like tissue (stroma and gland) outside the uterine cavity. Two main problems caused by endometriosis are infertility and pelvic pain.

In approximately 25–40% of women with infertility, the probable cause could be endometriosis. Similarly, endometriosis leads to subfertility in 40% of the women, and they often need assisted reproductive technology (ART) to conceive. Currently, the pregnancy rates after ART are at par with male and tubal factors of infertility. Let us see in this chapter how recurrent miscarriages occur in endometriosis and how to overcome them.

ENDOMETRIOSIS AND RECURRENT MISCARRIAGE

There are conflicting results in varying studies regarding recurrent miscarriages in endometriotic patients. Boje et al. published a nationwide cohort study among 295,630 controls and 29,563 individuals with endometriosis in which they studied how recurrent pregnancy loss (RPL) occurs in endometriosis patients.[1] This study reported that early RPL was associated with endometriosis. Women who conceived spontaneously with endometriosis had higher incidence of recurrent miscarriage.[2] There is also increased incidence of ectopic pregnancy, preterm labor, intrauterine growth retardation (IUGR), and placental complications among those who conceived with endometriosis.[2]

Recurrent Pregnancy Loss in Endometriosis

Endometriosis and associated chronic endometritis can lead to RPL. Adenomyosis is associated with endometriosis in varying proportions ranging from 5 to 80%.[3] Associated adenomyosis can be an important cause for RPL. A 2002 meta-analysis of ART success rates in endometriosis patients showed a lower clinical pregnancy rate, when compared to tubal and male factors, because of varying reasons including lowered number of oocytes retrieved, lowered fertilization and implantation rates, and increased miscarriages.[4]

Recent studies showed controversial results,[5] and miscarriage rates and implantation rates, post ART for endometriosis, are found to be equal with other factors, with euploid embryo transfer (ET).[6,7] Natural pregnancies occurring in endometriosis patients are associated with higher rate of pregnancy loss rather than pregnancy through ART, which may be because the gametes are exposed to abnormal peritoneal factors with increased reactive oxygen species for a longer period during spontaneous conception.

Early Pregnancy Loss: What does the Evidence Show?

Endometriosis causes endometriotic proliferation, immunomodulation, angio-neurogenesis, progesterone resistance, and hyperestrogenic state that will impair embryo-endometrial dialogues and also lead to early miscarriages.[8] Progesterone resistance is the hallmark for endometriosis. There are multiple mechanisms causing RPL in endometriosis.

- *Oocyte and embryo quality:*
  - Altered oocyte quality and embryo quality
  - Embryo aneuploidy (more so in natural conception than ART conception in endometriosis patients)
- *Endometrial factors:*
  - Altered window of implantation (WOI)
  - Impaired decidualization of endometrium due to progesterone resistance
- *Toxic pelvic factors:*
  - Ectopic endometriotic lesions leading to increased pro-inflammatory cytokines in endometrium
- *Defective placentation*

Oocyte and Embryo Quality

Oocyte quality is altered due to aberrant follicular environment, which can cause maturational defects.[9] Alteration in the meiotic bundle can increase the rate of aneuploidy.[10,11] In patients with endometriosis having spontaneous conception, abnormal oocyte quality and ovarian function can be a reason for RPL. However, a study by Juneau et al.[6,12] showed equal euploidy rates in endometriosis and nonendometriosis patients undergoing ART.

Endometrial Effects—Altered Window of Implantation and Poor Decidualization

According to Wilcox et al.,[13] there is increased pregnancy loss when women implant outside the WOI. In endometriosis, there is:

- Delayed WOI
- Retarded progesterone-induced histologic decidual transformation
- Stunted pinopode formation
- Disrupted balance among glycodelin, integrins, mucin I, and leukemia-inhibiting factor[14] leading to RPL

These endometrial alterations are linked to inflammation-mediated histological changes.[15,16] Progesterone resistance is a known mechanism in endometriosis, which was discovered by using deoxyribonucleic acid (DNA) microarray analysis.[17] There is increase in estradiol (E2) receptor dominance even during the secretory phase.[18]

Inflammation in the endometrium is the basis for impaired implantation. Hyperestrogenic milieu persists in the secretory phase due to deficiency of 17-hydroxylase (OH) dehydrogenase enzyme, which converts estradiol to estrone, and this leads to progesterone resistance.[19] This also causes suboptimal WOI. Lessey et al.[20] have studied increased expression of *BCL6* gene, which causes altered endometrial receptivity. There is overexpression of aromatase enzyme in endometriosis patients, which is also a predictor of implantation failure in fresh ET cycles. The hyperestrogenic status is a potential inhibitor of α-5 β-3 integrin, which is needed for embryo implantation.[21,22] Estradiol-induced cyclooxygenase stimulates prostaglandin E2, providing a pro-inflammatory status.[23] Hypoxia-induced factor is overexpressed in endometrium and it is linked with inflammatory cytokines.[24] Freitag et al.[25] could not find any association with increased natural killer (NK) cells in endometriosis patients. They concluded that chronic endometritis was the cause of recurrent miscarriages in endometriosis. Recurrent implantation failure is more common in fresh ET cycles compared to frozen embryo transfer (FET) cycles.[26] FET cycles have results that are comparable to tubal and male factors.[6] Downregulation with gonadotropin-releasing hormone (GnRH) analogues modulates immune mechanism, suppresses estrogen, and promotes implantation.

CHRONIC ENDOMETRITIS

Chronic endometritis is defined as the inflammation of the endometrium, which is often asymptomatic and can occasionally present with abnormal uterine bleeding (AUB), pelvic discomfort, and leukorrhea.[27] Altered endometrial microbiota is a cause for chronic endometritis as well as endometriosis. 16s ribonucleic acid (RNA) analysis will be helpful in the diagnosis of chronic endometritis. Hysteroscopy showing hyperemia, polyps, and micropolyps are evidence of chronic endometritis.[28,29] Plasma cells within the endometrial stroma can be picked up by immunohistochemistry (IHC) CD138, which is gaining popularity.[30,31] Chronic endometritis leads to reduced endometrial receptivity and therefore causes infertility, implantation failure, and RPL. The outcome improves after treating with appropriate antibiotics such as doxycycline for 2–3 weeks.

Chronic endometritis causes both cellular and biochemical alterations leading to RPL. Endometrial inflammation alters endometrial receptivity during WOI between day 20 and 24.[32] In cases of chronic endometritis, quality, organization, and distribution of leukocytes in the endometrium are altered. B-lymphocytes increase in number both in the functional layer of endometrium and basal layer.[33] Significant variation of CD68, macrophages, CD8, T cells, and regulatory T (Treg) cells is seen. Contrasting results are seen in uterine NK cells that regulate trophoblastic invasion and vascular remodeling. Similar to chronic inflammatory diseases such as rheumatoid arthritis and irritable bowel syndrome (IBS), interleukin (IL) and tumor necrosis factor alpha (TNF-α) are highly expressed in chronic endometritis. TNF-α increases the local estrogen biosynthesis, which is the leading cause of chronic endometritis. There is abnormal microenvironment for recruitment of circulating B cells in the endometrial stromal compartment. The endometrial B cells differentiate into stromal endometrial plasmacytes, which increase the levels of multiple immunoglobulins with predominance of immunoglobulin G2 (IgG2).[34] This will lead to negative impact on implantation. Genes involved in promoting receptivity and decidualization are downregulated in chronic endometritis. Expression of microRNA (Mi) 643 is decreased. TNF-α receptor-associated factor 6 (TRAF6) protein level enhances the expression of nuclear factor kappa light chain enhancer of activated B cells (NF-kB), which is pro-inflammatory and negatively impacts implantation. Enhancing the expression of Mi R643, which attenuates lipopolysaccharide (LPS)-induced inflammatory response by targeting TRAF6, can be a novel method for treating chronic endometritis.[35] Uterine contractility in patients with chronic endometritis shows altered pattern around periovulatory and mid-luteal phase. These findings are similar to endometriosis. Despite above derangements, if an embryo implants, the possibility of miscarriage is high in endometriosis due to the altered biochemical milieu.

IMMUNOMODULATION

Maternal immunomodulation is a key step in the successful implantation. There is a shift from type 2 T helper (Th2) to Th1 pro-inflammatory status. In RPL, there is dysregulation of T-cell function with the imbalance in Th1/Th17 versus Th2/Treg cells, where the Th1/T17 has pro-inflammatory status and Th2/Treg cells are anti-inflammatory. The adaptive immune response fails in endometriosis. Immunological aberration in endometriosis explains immunosurveillance evasion, implantation, proliferation, and angiogenesis of ectopic endometrial tissue. Decreased T-cell activity, NK cell cytotoxins, polyclonal activation of cells, increased antibody production, increased activation of macrophages, and changes in inflammatory mediation have been described. This will also increase the loss of euploid embryos.

Activated macrophages can secrete proinflammatory cytokines such as IL 1B, IL6, IL8 and TNF-α into the peritoneum, which triggers venous thromboembolism during pregnancy. A Scottish cohort study comparing proven endometriosis (5,375 patients) versus nonendometriosis patients (8,710) shows that endometriosis predisposes to increased pregnancy loss.[35,36]

Autoimmune disease is common between endometriosis and RPL. There is a strong correlation between autoimmune diseases such as rheumatoid arthritis, Hashimoto's thyroiditis, IBS, and endometriosis.

RECURRENT PREGNANCY LOSS AND PHENOTYPES OF ENDOMETRIOSIS

Study by FitzSimmons et al. showed slightly increased spontaneous miscarriage rates among endometriosis patients,[37] irrespective of the varying phenotypes. Among the phenotypes, endometrioma has the least miscarriage rate when compared to deep infiltrating endometriosis (DIE) and superficial endometriosis. Patients who underwent in vitro fertilization (IVF) for endometriosis had higher incidence of previous spontaneous miscarriages. Barbosa et al. studied 18 studies where 2,324 patients were included and found small-to-moderate increase in the risk of miscarriage among women with endometriosis [relative risk (RR) 1.31, 95% confidence interval (CI) 1.07–1.59].[38,39]

Management of Recurrent Pregnancy Loss

Endometriosis is generally managed medically or surgically or both. Endometriosis-associated pelvic pain is suppressed by hormonal management, which is contra-reproductive. Infertility has to be managed through surgery if there is associated pain. If the patient is not having pain, fertility can be restored through ART procedures such as ovulation induction (OI) and/or intrauterine insemination (IUI), or IVF. Women with RPL should undergo surgical optimization of the pelvis and remove toxic peritoneal factors, prior to ART cycles, to prevent miscarriage. A systematic review of various treatment regimens was published in 2020.[40]

Recurrent pregnancy loss patients can also benefit by immunological treatment such as intravenous immunoglobulins (IVIG) if it is started before ART. Optimization of autoimmune disorders should be done prior to infertility treatment (See Appendix 1 Case 5).

It is proposed to screen all patients with RPL for endometriosis, especially superficial peritoneal endometriosis or DIE. It may be possible to prevent RPL by reverting the inflammatory changes in endometriosis both medically and surgically. Additionally, hyperestrogenism can be addressed by GnRH agonist, which modulates uterine NK cells, suppresses pro-inflammation, and promotes anti-inflammation. In patients where associated adenomyosis is present, GnRH analogues combined with aromatase inhibitors might help in reducing the junctional zone (JZ) thickness and uterine volume and this can promote better implantation. Thus, miscarriage rates can be decreased by reducing toxic factors by surgical resection, treating chronic endometritis and adenomyosis, controlling autoimmune diseases, pituitary downregulation, and adequate luteal support.

Segmented Assisted Reproductive Technology Cycle

Sallam et al. in 2006 showed GnRH downregulation followed by ART improved the outcome by fourfold.[41] But this protocol may require higher doses of gonadotrophins for ovarian stimulation. Improvement in vitrification techniques and good embryo survival rates has led to segmented IVF cycles. This is especially beneficial in patients with endometriosis and RPL. In a controlled study, it was observed that the number of oocytes retrieved in the presence of endometrioma was not different from a control population.42 In this protocol, controlled ovarian stimulation and oocyte retrieval are done followed by prolonged downregulation with GnRH agonist and FET, which improves pregnancy outcome. Several studies have confirmed better success rates of segmented cycles, in women with endometriosis. This allows the ART clinic to harvest better number of oocytes after ovarian hyperstimulation, then proceed to complete surgical excision of endometriotic lesions. Sequential embryo transfer can be done post surgical optimization of pelvis.

CONCLUSION

The following salient points summarize the pathophysiology and treatment modalities to improve pregnancy outcome and reduce the incidence of RPL.

- Altered oocyte/embryo quality is noted in endometriosis patients.
- Pelvic toxicity should be corrected surgically prior to embryo transfer, thereby reducing RPL.
- Chronic endometritis associated with endometriosis should be treated with antibiotics.
- Segmented ART cycles are ideal to achieve good pregnancy rates and reduce RPL.
- In segmented cycles, ART results are at par with the male and tubal factors.
- Adequate luteal support is mandatory in view of progesterone resistance.
- Surgical excision is indicated prior to embryo transfer to reduce the toxic factors in the pelvis; also among patients with associated pain, if not controlled medically.

REFERENCES

1. Boje AD, Egerup P, Westergaard D, Bertelsen MMF, Nyegaard M, Hartwell D, et al. Endometriosis is associated with pregnancy loss: a nationwide historical cohort study. Fertil Steril. 2023;119(5):826-35.
2. Breintoft K, Pinnerup R, Henriksen TB, Rytter D, Uldbjerg N, Forman A, et al. Endometriosis and risk of adverse pregnancy outcome: a systematic review and meta-analysis. J Clin Med. 2021;10(4):667.
3. Pirtea P, Cicinelli E, De Nola R, de Ziegler D, Ayoubi JM. Endometrial causes of recurrent pregnancy losses: endometriosis, adenomyosis, and chronic endometritis. Fertil Steril. 2021;115(3):546-60.
4. Barnhart K, Dunsmoor-Su R, Coutifaris C. Effect of endometriosis on in vitro fertilization. Fertil Steril. 2002;77(6):1148-55.
5. Pirtea P, de Ziegler D, Ayoubi JM. Children born from frozen embryo transfers: is there a difference? Fertil Steril. 2020;114(3):502-3.
6. Juneau C, Kraus E, Werner M, Franasiak J, Morin S, Patounakis G, et al. Patients with endometriosis have aneuploidy rates equivalent to their age-matched peers in the in vitro fertilization population. Fertil Steril. 2017;108(2):284-8.
7. Bishop LA, Gunn J, Jahandideh S, Devine K, Decherney AH, Hill MJ. Endometriosis does not impact live-birth rates in frozen embryo transfers of euploid blastocysts. Fertil Steril. 2021;115(2):416-22.
8. de Ziegler D, Pirtea P, Carbonnel M, Poulain M, Cicinelli E, Bulletti C, et al. Assisted reproduction in endometriosis. Best Pract Res Clin Endocrinol Metab. 2019;33(1):47-59.
9. Pellicer A, Oliveira N, Ruiz A, Remohí J, Simón C. Exploring the mechanism(s) of endometriosis-related infertility: an analysis of embryo development and implantation in

assisted reproduction. Hum Reprod. 1995;10(Suppl. 2): 91-7.

10. Mandelbaum J, Anastasiou O, Lévy R, Guérin JF, de Larouzière V, Antoine JM. Effects of cryopreservation on the meiotic spindle of human oocytes. Eur J Obst Gynecol Reprod Biol. 2004;113(Suppl. 1):S17-23.
11. De Santis L, Cino I, Rabellotti E, Calzi F, Persico P, Borini A, et al. Polar body morphology and spindle imaging as predictors of oocyte quality. Reprod Biomed Online. 2005;11(1):36-42.
12. Zhao R, Wang J, Zhang X, Chen Y. MiR-643 inhibits lipopolysaccharide-induced endometritis progression by targeting TRAF6. Cell Biol Int. 2020;44(4):1059-67.
13. Wilcox AJ, Baird DD, Weinberg CR. Time of implantation of the conceptus and loss of pregnancy. N Engl J Med. 1999;340(23):1796-9.
14. Creus M, Balasch J, Ordi J, Fábregues F, Casamitjana R, Quinto L, et al. Integrin expression in normal and out-of-phase endometria. Hum Reprod. 1998;13(12):3460-8.
15. Li X, Large MJ, Creighton CJ, Lanz RB, Jeong JW, Young SL, et al. COUP-TFII regulates human endometrial stromal genes involved in inflammation. Mol Endocrinol. 2013;27(12):2041-54.
16. Savaris RF, Groll JM, Young SL, DeMayo FJ, Jeong JW, Hamilton AE, et al. Progesterone resistance in PCOS endometrium: a microarray analysis in clomiphene citrate-treated and artificial menstrual cycles. J Clin Endocrinol Metab. 2011;96(6):1737-46.
17. Gregory CW, Wilson EM, Apparao KBC, Lininger RA, Meyer WR, Kowalik A, et al. Steroid receptor coactivator expression throughout the menstrual cycle in normal and abnormal endometrium. J Clin Endocrinol Metab. 2002;87(6): 2960-6.
18. Bulun SE, Zeitoun KM, Takayama K, Sasano H. Estrogen biosynthesis in endometriosis: molecular basis and clinical relevance. J Mol Endocrinol. 2000;25(1):35-42.
19. Lessey BA, Castelbaum AJ, Buck CA, Lei Y, Yowell CW, Sun J. Further characterization of endometrial integrins during the menstrual cycle and in pregnancy. Fertil Steril. 1994;62(3):497-506.
20. Lessey BA, Castelbaum AJ, Sawin SW, Buck CA, Schinnar R, Bilker W, et al. Aberrant integrin expression in the endometrium of women with endometriosis. J Clin Endocrinol Metab. 1994;79(2):643-9.
21. Somkuti SG, Yuan L, Fritz MA, Lessey BA. Epidermal growth factor and sex steroids dynamically regulate a marker of endometrial receptivity in Ishikawa cells. J Clin Endocrinol Metab. 1997;82(7):2192-7.
22. Wu MH, Lu CW, Chuang PC, Tsai SJ. Prostaglandin E2: the master of endometriosis? Exp Biol Med (Maywood). 2010;235(6):668-77.
23. Kim BG, Yoo JY, Kim TH, Shin JH, Langenheim JF, Ferguson SD, et al. Aberrant activation of signal transducer and activator of transcription-3 (STAT3) signaling in endometriosis. Hum Reprod. 2015;30(5):1069-78.
24. McQueen DB, Perfetto CO, Hazard FK, Lathi RB. Pregnancy outcomes in women with chronic endometritis and recurrent pregnancy loss. Fertil Steril. 2015;104(4):927-31.
25. Freitag N, Pour SJ, Fehm TN, Toth B, Markert UR, Weber M, et al. Are uterine natural killer and plasma cells in infertility patients associated with endometriosis, repeated implantation failure, or recurrent pregnancy loss? Arch Gynecol Obstet. 2020;302(6):1487-94.
26. Bourdon M, Santulli P, Maignien C, Gayet V, Pocate-Cheriet K, Marcellin L, et al. The deferred embryo transfer strategy improves cumulative pregnancy rates in endometriosis-related infertility: a retrospective matched cohort study. PLoS One. 2018;13(4):e0194800.
27. Greenwood SM, Moran JJ. Chronic endometritis: morphologic and clinical observations. Obstet Gynecol. 1981;58(2):176-84.
28. Moreno I, Cicinelli E, Garcia-Grau I, Gonzalez-Monfort M, Bau D, Vilella F, et al. The diagnosis of chronic endometritis in infertile asymptomatic women: a comparative study of histology, microbial cultures, hysteroscopy, and molecular microbiology. Am J Obstet Gynecol. 2018;218(6): 602.e1-16.
29. Moreno I, Codoñer FM, Vilella F, Valbuena D, Martinez-Blanch JF, Jimenez-Almazán J, et al. Evidence that the endometrial microbiota has an effect on implantation success or failure. Am J Obstet Gynecol. 2016;215(6): 684-703.
30. Resta L, Palumbo M, Rossi R, Piscitelli D, Fiore MG, Cicinelli E. Histology of micro polyps in chronic endometritis. Histopathology. 2012;60(4):670-4.
31. Liu Y, Chen X, Huang J, Wang CC, Yu MY, Laird S, et al. Comparison of the prevalence of chronic endometritis as determined by means of different diagnostic methods in women with and without reproductive failure. Fertil Steril. 2018;109(5):832-9.
32. Chen X, Liu Y, Zhao Y, Cheung WC, Zhang T, Qi R, et al. Association between chronic endometritis and uterine natural killer cell density in women with recurrent miscarriage: clinical implications. J Obst Gynaecol Res. 2020;46(6):858-63.
33. Kitaya K. Prevalence of chronic endometritis in recurrent miscarriages. Fertil Steril. 2011;95(3):1156-8.
34. Kitaya K, Tada Y, Hayashi T, Taguchi S, Funabiki M, Nakamura Y. Comprehensive endometrial immunoglobulin subclass analysis in infertile women suffering from repeated implantation failure with or without chronic endometritis. Am J Reprod Immunol. 2014;72(4):386-91.
35. Saraswat L, Ayansina DT, Cooper KG, Bhattacharya S, Miligkos D, Horne AW, et al. Pregnancy outcomes in women with endometriosis: a national record linkage study. BJOG. 2017;124(3):444-52.

36. Devi TR, Devi CA. Fertility and pregnancy following surgical management of endometriosis. Bangladesh J Fertil Steril. 2021;1(1):04-17.
37. FitzSimmons J, Stahl R, Gocial B, Shapiro SS. Spontaneous abortion and endometriosis. Fertil Steril. 1987Apr;47(4):696-8.
38. Barbosa MA, Teixeira DM, Navarro PA, Ferriani RA, Nastri CO, Martins WP. Impact of endometriosis and its staging on assisted reproduction outcome: systematic review and meta-analysis. Ultrasound Obstet Gynecol. 2014;44(3):261-78.
39. Devi TR, Basheer M, Deepika A, Sangavi D. Couple's battle to achieve parenthood. Int Res J Pharm Med Sci. 2022;5(2):62-4.
40. Hodgson RM, Lee HL, Wang R, Mol BW, Johnson N. Interventions for endometriosis-related infertility: a systematic review and network meta-analysis. Fertil Steril. 2020;113(2):374-82.e2.
41. Sallam HN, Garcia-Velasco JA, Dias S, Arici A. Long-term pituitary down-regulation before in vitro fertilization (IVF) for women with endometriosis. Cochrane Database Syst Rev. 2006;2006(1):CD004635.
42. Ozgur K, Bulut H, Berkkanoglu M, Coetzee K. Reproductive outcomes of segmented in vitro fertilization in patients diagnosed with endometriomas. J Minim Invasive Gynecol. 2018;25(1):105-10.

CHAPTER 18

Adenomyosis

Sanjivni Khanna, Sai Deepashri S

ABSTRACT

Adenomyosis is a disease of the junctional zone of the uterus, presenting as diffuse or focal lesions in the uterus. It may rarely present as juvenile cystic or adult cystic adenomyosis. It is associated with poor implantation rates and RPL. For focal disease treatment can be surgical. Medical management is advocated with aromatase inhibitors, both GnRH agonist and GnRH antagonist like elagolix.

Keywords: Adenomyosis focal diffuse, Juvenile cystic, Adult cystic adenomyosis, GnRH agonist, GnRH antagonist, Aromatase inhibitors, Elagolix.

INTRODUCTION

Adenomyosis, a condition that affects the very organ which would nest a pregnancy safely, is likely to reduce fertility, leading to miscarriages, and other adverse pregnancy outcomes. Poor outcomes may occur despite the rescue and salvaging processes meted out by the body's recourse to fight adversity. Therapeutic intervention could assist in achieving the best possible results.

ADENOMYOSIS AND ITS ASSOCIATION WITH INFERTILITY, IMPLANTATION FAILURE, AND MISCARRIAGE

Often considered an enigma, adenomyosis is characterized by benign invasion of the myometrium by ectopic endometrium.[1,2] It is essentially a disease of the endomyometrial junction and should be comprehended as a "two-component" disease consisting of:

1. Ectopic endometrial glands and stroma in the muscle wall of the uterus
2. Secondary hyperplastic and hypertrophic changes in the myometrium[3]

Both epithelial and stromal components of the heterotopic endometrium are present in the invading tissue, and the invasion occurs at least 2.5 mm below the endomyometrial interface.[4] The areas of the ectopic endometrium may be present widely throughout the myometrium, or restricted to a focal location in the form of an adenomyoma.[5] The posterior uterine wall is more frequently involved than the anterior, while other areas such as the cornua or the cervical orifice are infrequently affected by adenomyosis.[5-7]

Factors indicating the severity of the disease include the magnitude of symptoms, the number of adenomyotic foci, and the depth of invasion into the myometrium the most invading focus lies.[2] Levgur et al. proposed a grading system, describing the depth of adenomyotic lesions:

- Deep >80% in depth within the myometrium
- *Intermediate:* 40–80% deep
- *Superficial:* <40% deep

Many symptoms are related to the depth of invasion of ectopic endometrium within the myometrium.

Junctional zone (JZ) is an area of importance for the function of the uterus, and also in relation to pathologic conditions, notably, adenomyosis.[8] This compartment within the uterus is located at the endomyometrial interface, also known as the "archi-myometrium" or the inner myometrium, as revealed by magnetic resonance imaging (MRI) >2 decades ago.[9] Disturbances in the structure or function of the JZ before conception can lead to fertility-related issues and obstetrical complications, as pointed out by observational studies.[10] Thickening of the JZ has been associated with dysperistalsis.[11]

Adenomyosis has varied presentations:

- Abnormal uterine bleeding
- Dysmenorrhea
- Chronic pelvic pain
- Dyspareunia
- Uterine enlargement **(Fig. 1)**[12,13]

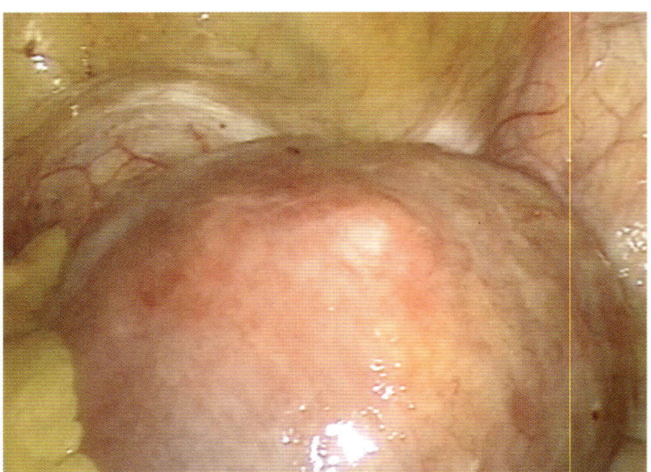

Fig. 1: Laparoscopic view of a large globular adenomyotic uterus with small leiomyoma.

Adenomyosis typically manifests more frequently after the age of 30 years. Consequently, it is increasingly encountered in women who are planning pregnancies later in life.

The condition is often discovered during the assessment for infertility.[14] A strong link exists between adenomyosis and infertility according to many investigational studies.[1,15-18] The mechanisms underlying infertility in adenomyosis are not well understood.[19] Adenomyosis has been reported to be present, on the basis of three-dimensional (3D) transvaginal ultrasonography (TVUS), in 38% of women with recurrent pregnancy loss (RPL), and 35% of women with recurrent implantation failure (RIF).[20] A higher prevalence of adenomyosis has been linked with miscarriage in other studies as well.[21,22]

The exact manner in which adenomyosis influences the outcomes of assisted reproductive technology (ART) remains unclear.[20] Some reports suggest a negative impact,[23-26] while others have not documented such an association, indicating that adenomyosis may not significantly affect the outcomes of in vitro fertilization (IVF) and embryo transfer (ET).[1,27,28] Additionally, adenomyosis may exert less adverse effects on IVF/intracytoplasmic sperm injection (ICSI) cycles in women with endometriosis, treated with long-term pituitary downregulation before the procedure.[29] However, there may be a significant negative effect of adenomyosis on the likelihood of conception and live birth.[25,30]

Link between Adenomyosis, Endometriosis, and Myomas

It is interesting to note that there is a strong association between adenomyosis and endometriosis. The former condition was observed to be present in conjunction with endometriosis in 27% women and according to other studies, the two conditions may coexist in 54–90% of cases, especially in infertile women.[1,31,32] Adenomyosis may be found in coexistence with endometriosis in 70% infertile women.[32] Co-occurrence of adenomyosis with endometriosis has been seen in one-third women with surgically treated endometriosis.[33-35] The depth of invasion of adenomyosis is linked to the extent of endometriosis when the two conditions coexist.[34]

Adenomyosis could be present simultaneously with endometriosis in younger women, which may indicate a common pathogenesis.[36-40] Adenomyosis may be compounded by leiomyomas as well.[41-44] In a retrospective study, Güzel and colleagues evaluated 129 women operated for treatment resistant "menometrorrhagia." Histopathology revealed that both conditions coexisted in patients with greater mean ages, early age at menarche and gravidity, and that these patients had significantly lower preoperative hemoglobin.[44]

PREVALENCE AND TYPES

Adenomyosis may occur at any age from adolescence to later reproductive years.[45,46] The prevalence has been observed to vary from 1 to 70%.[2,46] This wide range is probably accounted for by a lack of standard criteria for diagnosis, both on imaging assessments, and histopathological analyses.[47,48]

Cystic adenomyosis, similar to other manifestations of the disease, usually occurs in women who are over the age of 30 years and are multiparous.[49] However, even young girls may be affected by this form, and when it presents in women younger than 30 years, it is >1 cm in size, lies independent of the endometrial lining, and (often) causes severe dysmenorrhea, it is named as *juvenile cystic adenomyosis (JCA)*. The age cutoff is used to differentiate it from *adult cystic adenomyosis*.[50-52]

PREDISPOSING FACTORS

The predisposing factors are enumerated in **Table 1**.

TABLE 1: Factors which predispose to the development of adenomyosis.[5,8,41,47,53-56]

Factor	Estrogen excess[5,8,41,47]	Trauma during uterine surgery[8,47,53]	Treatment with tamoxifen[54-56]
Clinical situations	Early menarche (≤10 years)	Pregnancy termination	Selective binding to estrogen receptors—stimulatory to normal and ectopic endometrial tissue
	Short cycles (≤24 days)	Dilatation and curettage	
	Higher parity (higher estrogen levels/ trophoblast invasion into myometrium during implantation)	Previous cesarean delivery	
	Oral contraceptives ± elevated body mass index (BMI)	Other uterine surgery	

PATHOGENESIS

The precise mechanism underlying the pathogenesis of adenomyosis remains elusive. Several theories have been proposed:

- Direct invasion of the endometrium into the myometrium[5,57-60]
- Misplaced embryologic pluripotent Müllerian remnants[5,57,61-63]
- Invagination of the basalis endometrium along the lymphatic system of the myometrium[5,57]
- Displacement of bone marrow stem cells.[5,64,65]

Various mechanisms disrupt fertility in adenomyosis,[65] including:

- Abnormal uterotubal transport and disruption of endometrial function and receptivity.
- An enlarged uterus and anatomical distortions can hinder sperm migration, embryo transfer, and implantation potential.
- Myometrial hyperactivity, irregular muscle contractions, and distorted calcium circulation affect uterine contractility and sperm progression.
- Distortions of the uterine cavity may impair uterotubal transport.
- Adenomyosis-associated changes worsen endometrial receptivity, affecting the implantation window.
- Molecular level abnormalities include reduced expression of implantation-associated molecules like HOXA10 and LIF.
- Downregulation of (orphan nuclear receptor) NR4A receptor and (fork head box protein) FOXO1A leads to incorrect decidualization.
- Abnormal expression of integrins and osteopontin (OPN) may be responsible for IVF failure.
- Chronic inflammation in adenomyosis alters cytokine expression and cellular immunity in the endometrium.
- Increased levels of pro- and antioxidative cytokines such as Cu, Zn-super oxide dismutase (SOD) and manganese SOD (Mn-SOD) contribute to inflammation.
- Abnormal high levels of nitric oxide negatively impact sperm transport, implantation, and decidualization.

CLINICAL SYMPTOMATOLOGY

Careful attention to the following symptoms will raise a suspicion for adenomyosis:

- *Abnormal uterine bleeding:*[57,66-68] Seen in 40–60%
- *Dysmenorrhea:*[57,67,68] present in 15–30%
- *Dyspareunia:* Affects 7–10%[68]
- *Chronic pelvic pain* in 76.9%[69-72]
- *Diffuse uterine enlargement*[73]
- *Irregular contour of uterus*[5,15,60]
- *Uterus tender to palpation*[72]
- *Infertility:*[68] Approximately in 12%
- *Coexisting leiomyomas:*[41-44] These may be found in 50% cases.
- *Endometriosis:*[74] In 25%
- *Endometrial polyps* may coexist in 7% women.[5,15,60,74]

CLASSIFICATION OF ADENOMYOSIS

This is based on the extent of myometrial invasion seen on histology.[75]

- *Diffuse adenomyosis:* Endometrial glands and stroma scattered throughout the myometrium[60]
- *Focal adenomyosis:* A localized area embedded within the myometrium.[60,76] This type can be further categorized as:
  - *Adenomyoma:* A lesion which infiltrates a restricted area of the myometrium.[76,77]
  - *Cystic adenomyosis:* A single adenomyotic cyst present in the myometrium.[78] In women younger than 30 years it is called JCA.

- *Polypoid adenomyomas:* These are polypoidal masses[75] which may be typical or atypical polypoid adenomyomas.[76,79]
- *Rarer forms:*
  - Adenomyoma of the endocervix
  - Retroperitoneal adenomyomas.[46,80]

DIAGNOSIS

The diagnosis rests upon imaging studies with TVUS, 3D-TVUS, and MRI. 3D-TVUS and MRI display the endomyometrial junction, clearly. The JZ, which is the innermost part of myometrium near the endometrium, shows up as a thin hypoechoic zone on TVUS and a low signal band abutting the endometrium on an MRI.[3]

Imaging Methods (Table 2)

- Transvaginal ultrasonography:
  - *Two-dimensional transvaginal ultrasonography:* The two-dimensional (2D) features which suggest adenomyosis include:[9,81-86]
    - Globally enlarged uterus **(Fig. 1)**[2,82,87,88]
    - Asymmetrical enlargement of the uterus[87] **(Fig. 2)**
    - Heterogeneous echotexture of the myometrium[5] **(Fig. 2)**
    - Linear striations in the myometrium **(Fig. 2A)**[87]
    - Poorly defined endomyometrial junction or pseudowidening of the endometrium may be evident **(Fig. 2B)**.[89]
    - A diffuse spread of small vessels within the myometrium may also be observed on power Doppler ultrasound **(Fig. 2C)**.[91] These vessels do not follow the course of the arcuate and uterine arteries.[87]
    - An adenomyoma may be seen as a focal circumscribed nodular collection of ectopic endometrium, commonly identified on the posterior uterine wall.[89]
    - Myometrial cysts **(Fig. 2A)** may be observed in 50% of patients. They are dilated glands or foci of hemorrhage in the heterotopic endometrium.[89]

TABLE 2: Diagnosis of adenomyosis: Imaging methods.[5,8,41,47,53-56,88-92]

Modality	*2D-TVUS*	*3D-TVUS*	*MRI*
Characteristic features	Globular/globally enlarged uterus[2,82]	Accurate assessment of the JZ	Large, regular, and asymmetric uterus[81]
	Enlarged uterine fundus (approximately 12 cm uterine length)[87,88]	Coronal view: Hypoechoic area surrounding endometrium[9]	Abnormal myometrial signal intensity
	Asymmetrical enlargement[87]	Better visualization of JZ (vs. 2D-TVUS)[9]	JZ thickening[67,89]
	Heterogeneous echotexture of the myometrium[5]		High signal intensity myometrial foci on T1-weighted images[67,89]
	Linear striations in the myometrium[87,90]		Bright foci within areas of low-signal intensity within myometrium (T2 weighted)[89]
	Poorly defined endomyometrial junction, pseudowidening[89]		Linear striations radiating from endometrium to myometrium, pseudowidening
	Diffuse spread of small vessels within the myometrium[91]		Lack of contour, mass effect, ill-defined margins between normal and abnormal myometrium, and elliptical shape of low-signal intensity in myometrium[89]
	Adenomyoma		
	Myometrial cysts[89]		
	Appearance of "question mark sign"[92]		

(2D: two dimensional; 3D: three dimensional; TVUS: transvaginal ultrasonography; JZ: junctional zone; MRI: magnetic resonance imaging)

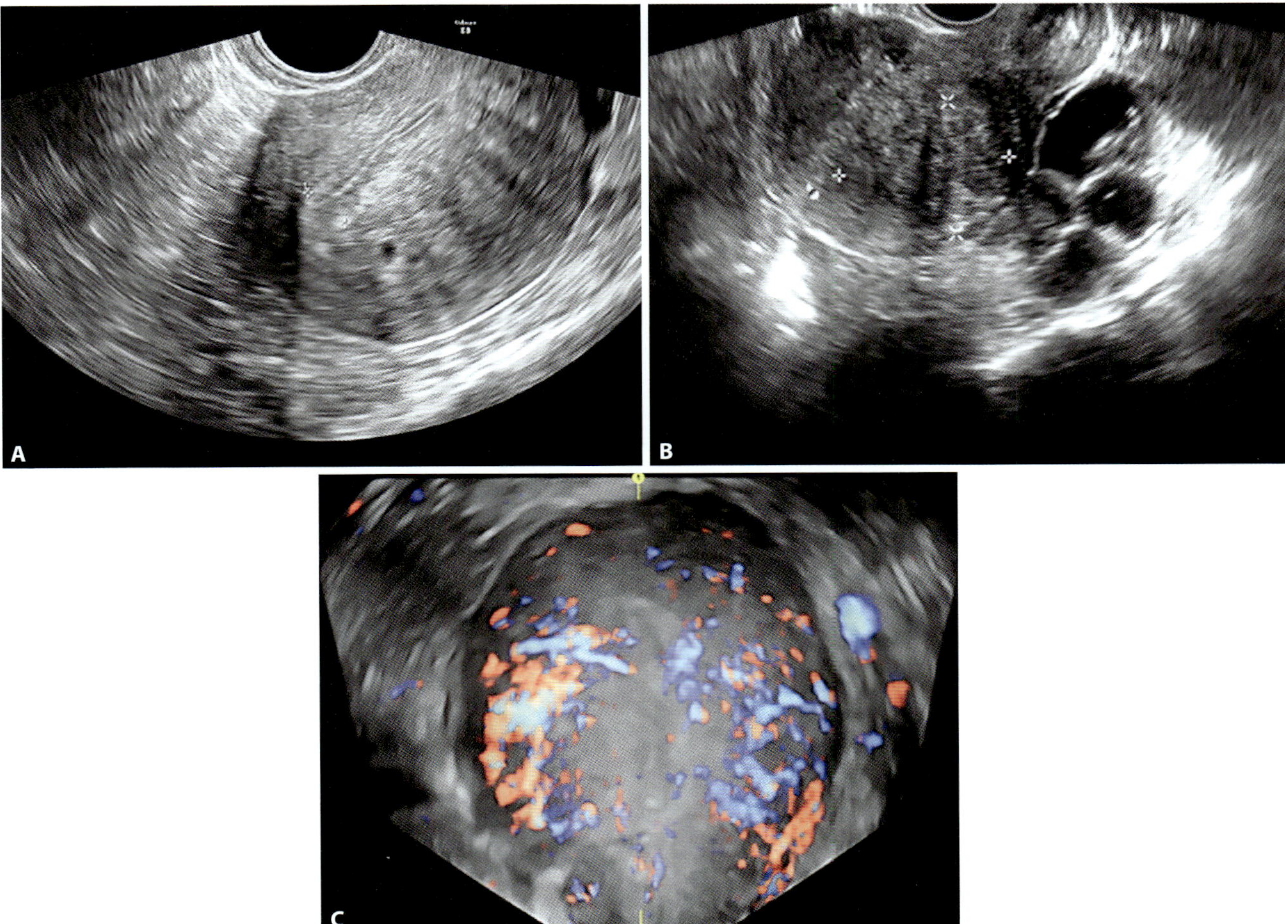

Figs. 2A to C: Diagnosis of adenomyosis—transvaginal ultrasonography (TVUS). (A) Adenomyotic changes of posterior wall with focal posterior wall thickening, myometrial cysts, and loss of endomyometrial interface with pseudowidening of the cavity (*Courtesy:* Dr Rajeev Choudhary); (B) TVUS showing thickened posterior myometrium with areas of altered echo pattern and an ill-defined hypoechoic lesion suggestive of an adenomyoma (*Courtesy:* Dr Puneet Jain, Dr Pankaj Kumar, and Dr Vineet Sethia); and (C) Coronal reformat of the uterus showing diffusely increased vascularity on power Doppler (*Courtesy:* Dr Rajeev Choudhary).

- A "question mark" sign of the uterus may be manifested due to the uterine corpus becoming flexed backward, with the cervix directed to the front.[92]

- *Three-dimensional transvaginal ultrasonography:* Assessment of JZ is performed on a 3D-TVUS coronal view. The JZ appears as a hypoechoic area surrounding the endometrium. All planes of the JZ can be seen clearly with volume contrast imaging (VCI) with 2–4 mm slices.[9]

A 3D-TVUS offers slightly better visualization of the JZ compared with 2D-TVUS,[9,93] especially early adenomyosis.[2,91]

Mavrelos D et al. noted the following ultrasonic features **(Table 3)**. An "adenomyosis score" **(Table 3)** was calculated and women were placed in categories. Each of the seven ultrasonic features of adenomyosis was given the value 0 when absent or 1 when present, thereby allotting a minimum score of 0 and maximum of 7. In women with a score of 4 or more, the chance of pregnancy is halved.[94]

- *Magnetic resonance imaging:* The observations on MRI include **(Figs. 3A to C)**:
  - A large, regular, or asymmetric uterus[82]
  - Abnormal myometrial signal intensity
  - Junctional zone thickening[66,89]
  - High-signal intensity myometrial foci on T1-weighted images[67,89]

TABLE 3: Ultrasonic features in adenomyosis.[94]

1	Asymmetrical myometrial thickening
2	Parallel shadowing
3	Linear striations
4	Myometrial cysts
5	Hyperechoic islands
6	Adenomyomas
7	Irregular endomyometrial junction
A score of 0 is given when absent or 1, when present	

- Bright foci within areas of low-signal intensity[89]
- Linear striations represent penetration of the basal endometrium into the myometrium
- Pseudowidening of the endometrium
- Lack of contour, mass effect, ill-defined margins between normal and abnormal myometrium, and elliptical shaped low-signal intensity in the myometrium.[89]

Diagnostic Accuracy of Imaging Modalities

A meta-analysis on the precision of ultrasound in the diagnosis of adenomyosis revealed a sensitivity of 82.5% and specificity of 84.6%, with a positive likelihood ratio

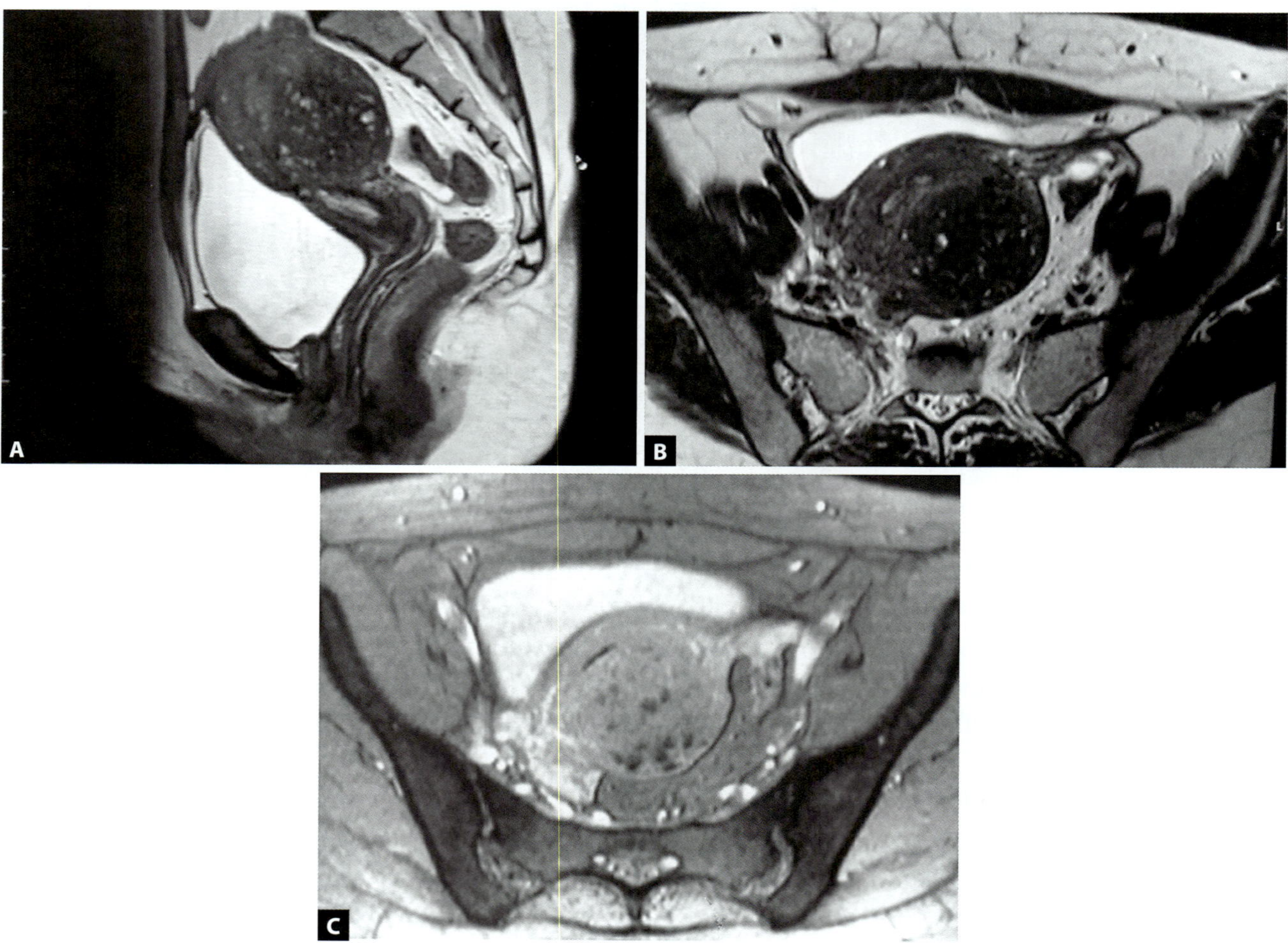

Figs. 3A to C: Diagnosis of adenomyosis—MRI. (A) T2-weighted sagittal MRI image showing heterogeneous signal intensity with multiple T2 hyperintense foci suggestive of adenomyoma (*Courtesy:* Dr Puneet Jain, Dr Pankaj Kumar, and Dr Vineet Sethia); (B) T2-weighted axial MRI image showing an adenomyoma with typical, poorly defined margins. The endometrium is pushed anteriorly (*Courtesy:* Dr Puneet Jain, Dr Pankaj Kumar, and Dr Vineet Sethia); and (C) MEDIC sequence axial MRI image showing multiple punctate foci of blooming (hemorrhage) in an adenomyoma (*Courtesy:* Dr Puneet Jain, Dr Pankaj Kumar, and Dr Vineet Sethia).

of 4.7 and negative likelihood ratio of 0.26, comparable to MRI.[95] Leiomyomas can affect adversely the ability of ultrasound to diagnose adenomyosis, which can be as low as 33%.[96] TVUS is as accurate as MRI, but in presence of leiomyomas the sensitivity of TVUS was lower, and thus, MRI would be preferable.[82]

Ascher et al. and Dueholm et al. had observed that MRI proves superior to TVUS for diagnosis of adenomyosis.[96,97] Another study and a systematic review have also shown MRI to be very accurate in the diagnosis of adenomyosis.[98,99]

THE JUNCTIONAL ZONE (TABLE 4)

The JZ may show focal or diffuse thickening and represent smooth muscle hyperplasia.[100] The thickness of a normal JZ has been noted to be approximately 4 mm and varies during the cycle by 0.9 mm.[101] Patients with adenomyosis have a mean JZ thickness of 15 mm versus 7 mm in nonadenomyotic uterus.[100]

Adenomyosis is diagnosed when the JZ thickness was 12 mm or greater and ruled out if maximal junction zone thickness of 8 mm or less.[100] Other studies take 10 mm (JZmax) as a cutoff.[32] It has been suggested by Gordts that >8 mm and <12 mm can be taken as hyperplasia, or stage 0 of adenomyosis.[102,103] It would be appropriate to look for JZ changes in women with RPL and RIF.[3]

TABLE 4: Junctional zone changes in adenomyosis.[99-102]

Conditions	*JZ thickness*
Normal	• 4 mm (±0.9 mm during cycles[101]) • Maximum thickness of junctional zone (JZmax) ≤ 8 mm
Hyperplasia (stage 0 adenomyosis)	8–12 mm[102,103]
Adenomyosis	JZmax ≥ 12 mm[100]

(JZ: junctional zone)

HISTOLOGY (FIGS. 4A TO D)

Hysteroscopy

It has been suggested by some authors that hysteroscopic assessment may be a useful investigation.[104] The procedure

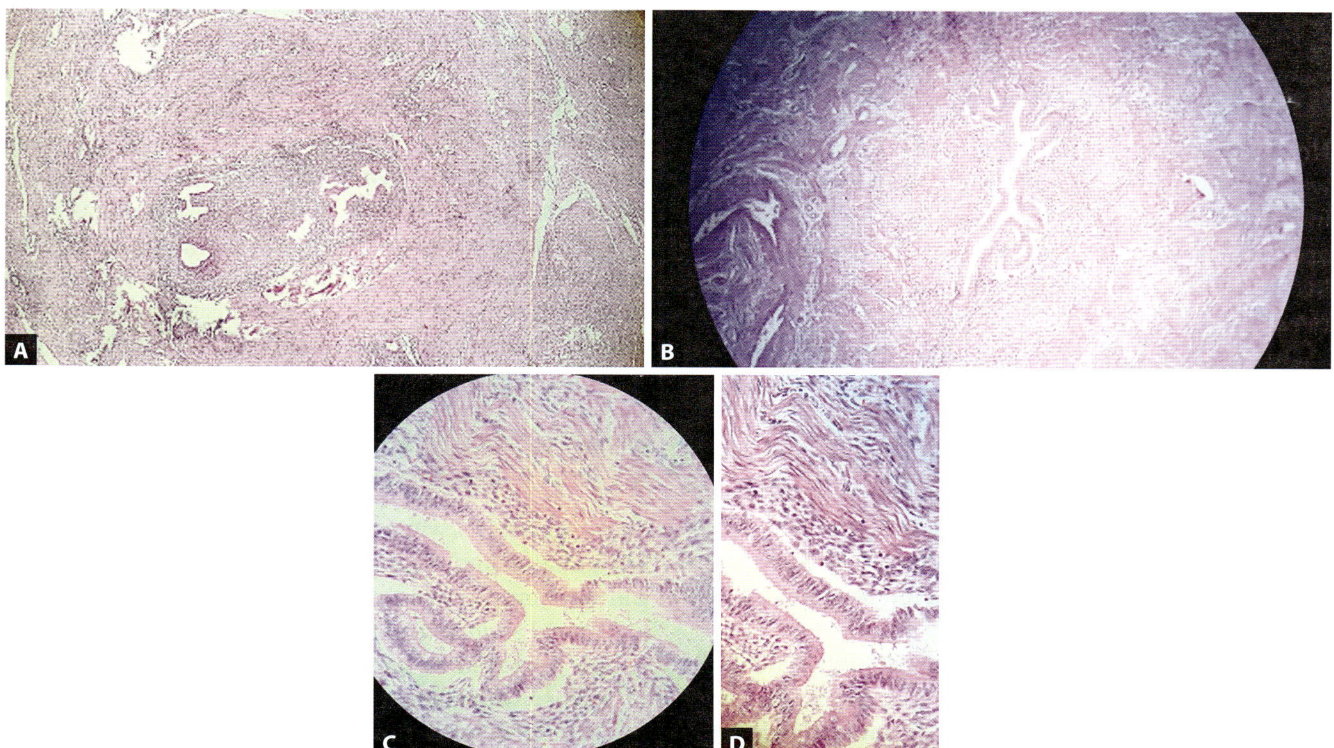

Figs. 4A to D: Histolopathological features of adenomyosis. (A and B) 5X H&E images showing well-circumscribed adenomyoma with smooth muscle fibers, islands of endometrial glands, and stroma (*Courtesy:* Dr Karn Bhardwaj); (C) A 40X H&E images of adenomyoma (*Courtesy:* Dr Karn Bhardwaj); and (D) zoomed 40X H&E images of adenomyoma (*Courtesy:* Dr Karn Bhardwaj). (H&E: hematoxylin and eosin).

allows visualization of the uterine cavity, enables assessment for other prevailing abnormalities, and permits obtaining endometrial or myometrial biopsies under direct vision.[105]

Hysteroscopic findings in adenomyosis include:[105]

- An irregular endometrium
- Endometrial defects
- Cystic/hemorrhagic lesions
- Altered vascularization

Diagnosis of adenomyosis can be missed if it lies deeper than the biopsy sites or is located at areas that are not biopsied.[5]

Laparoscopic Biopsy

Myometrial needle biopsies can be obtained at laparoscopy for the diagnosis of adenomyosis.[2,106] The sensitivity of a single myometrial biopsy was between 8 and 18.7%.[107] Sensitivity increased with the number of biopsies and the depth of adenomyosis. They reported a sensitivity of two random biopsies to be between 2.3 and 56%.[108]

ADENOMYOSIS: RECURRENT PREGNANCY LOSS AND RECURRENT IMPLANTATION FAILURE

No studies have examined natural conception in women with adenomyosis. With ART, there is decreased implantation and increased early miscariages.[3] There are decreased clinical, viable, ongoing pregnancy, and live-birth rates and significantly increased miscarriage rates.[21,25,30,109]

In women undergoing oocyte donation, higher miscarriage rates and lower term pregnancy rates are observed.[1]

A significantly greater prevalence of adenomyosis was observed in women with two previous miscarriages.[20] It is also possible that adenomyosis may have been caused by uterine interventions, which can damage the endomyometrial interface and facilitate endometrium migration into the myometrium.[110]

In their study, Campo et al. concluded that there was lower uterine receptivity and lower implantation rates in adenomyosis.[110] The results of IVF have brought forth conflicting conclusions in women with adenomyosis.[40] Few studies, reporting the outcome of IVF/ICSI in women treated before 2007, concluded that adenomyosis, as diagnosed with ultrasound, did not affect the results of the procedure.[28,29] However, it was observed that when long-term pituitary downregulation protocols are used for IVF/ICSI, the presence of adenomyosis and the implantation rates improved.

TABLE 5: Correlation of JZ thickness with pregnancy rates after IVF.[24]

Thickness	*Pregnancy rate*
JZ thickness <7 mm	63%
JZmax thickness <10 mm	63%
JZ thickness >7 mm	26%
JZmax thickness >10 mm	14%

(IVF: in vitro fertilization; JZmax: maximum thickness of junctional zone)

Shukla et al. showed that surrogates exhibited significantly higher clinical pregnancy and live birth rates compared to the adenomyotic infertile patients. Adenomyosis decreases implantation potential, leading to poorer pregnancy rates.[111,112]

An observation of a higher prevalence of adenomyosis was found among women with RIF, suggesting poorer endometrial receptivity.[20] Poorer pregnancy rates after ART in women with adenomyosis have been noted in many studies,[24-26,30] whereas others did not find this association.[1,27-29] This disparity may be because of limited sample sizes and varying ART procedures.[20] **Table 5** correlates the pregnancy rates with JZ thickness.

Diffuse adenomyosis has a worse prognosis compared to focal adenomyosis.[21] Adenomyosis was associated with an increased risk of 2nd trimester miscarriage, preterm delivery, preeclampsia, and placental malposition, thereby leading to poor perinatal outcomes **(Table 6)**.[113,114]

MECHANISMS RESPOSIBLE FOR LOWERING FERTILITY RATES

The mechanisms, which may lead to a negative impact on implantation and continuation of pregnancies in women with adenomyosis, could include the following:

- *Altered endometrial receptivity markers:* Few markers are observed to be altered in the endometrium of women with adenomyosis.[40,111,115]
- *Structural and functional defects in the eutopic endometrium and the myometrial junctional zone:* These have been shown to exist in adenomyosis.[87] Nerve fibers are lost at the endometrial-myometrial interface, which may account for some of the defects.[11,116]

TABLE 6: Evidence table: Pregnancy outcomes following IVF in adenomyosis.

Authors (year)	*Study design*	*No. of cases, controls*	*Diagnosis*	*Inference with respect to pregnancy outcome*
Salim et al. (2012)[30]	Prospective	275 (19 Adeno, 256 Co) underwent IVF/ICSI	TVUS	• Pregnancy rate in Adeno (22.2%) versus Co (47.2%) • Miscarriage rate in Adeno (50.0%) versus Co (2.8%)
Thalluri et al. (2012)[25]	Retrospective	213 (38 Adeno, 175 Co) underwent IVF	TVUS	• Pregnancy rate in Ca (23.6%) versus Co (44.6%) • Viable pregnancy in Adeno group
Martínez-Conejero et al. (2011)[1]	Retrospective, matched cohort	152 Adeno, 147 Co, IVF with donor oocytes	TVUS and MRI	• Term pregnancy rate in Adeno (26.8%) versus Co (37.1%) • Miscarriage rate in Adeno (13.1%) versus Co (7.2%)
Costello et al. (2011)[28]	Retrospective	201 (37 Adeno, 164 Co) underwent IVF/ICSI	TVUS	• No difference in live-birth rates (29.7 vs. 26.1%) • No differences in ovarian response, embryological parameters, or clinical outcomes
Youm et al. (2011)[26]	Retrospective	413 IVF-ET; divided on myometrial thickness into groups A (<2 cm), B (2–2.49 cm), and C (≥2.49 cm)	TVUS	Adeno (35.8%) in group B: Implantation (12.4 vs. 27.2%), pregnancy (34.5 vs. 63.5%), and birth rates (17.2 vs. 53.8%); and abortion rates (50 vs. 12.1%) compared those without these myometrial thickening of >2.50 cm and sonographic findings of adenomyosis are associated with adverse outcomes of IVF-ET.
Maubon et al. (2010)[24]	Prospective	152 IVF	MRI	JZ thickness > 7 mm, JZmax > 10 mm had 95.8% implantation failure versus others (37.5%).
Mijatovic et al. (2010)[29]	Retrospective	74 infertile women (27% Adeno) IVF/ICSI with prior GnRHa	Surgical	No adverse effects of Adeno on IVF outcomes in infertile women with proven endometriosis pretreated with long-term GnRHa.

(Adeno: adenomyosis; Ca: cases; Co: controls; ET: embryo transfer; GnRHa: gonadotropin-releasing hormone analog; ICSI: intracytoplasmic sperm injection; IVF: in vitro fertilization; JZmax: maximum thickness of junctional zone; MRI: magnetic resonance imaging; TVUS: transvaginal ultrasonography)

- *Disturbed uterine peristalsis:* This alteration may cause reduced embryo implantation. However, controversy surrounds this probability.[87,117] Adenomyosis may lead to abnormal contractility, or the latter could contribute to the pathogenesis of adenomyosis.[118]
- *Abnormal concentrations of free radicals:* Nitric oxide, superoxide, and other free radicals have been observed to be present in excess, which may alter implantation and increase the risk of early miscarriage.[86,111]
- *Altered endometrial vascularization:* The total surface area of capillaries in the endometrium, when measured per mm^2, may be elevated by >10 times, in both the proliferative as well as the secretory phase. This fact is, incidentally, related to hypermenorrhea, as well.[111]

MANAGEMENT IN WOMEN DESIRING CONCEPTION

Assisted reproductive technology post depot gonadotropin-releasing hormone (GnRH) agonist suppression or short-term medical treatment can be offered. Surgery may be indicated in selected cases.

Medical Therapies

A recent review discusses the medical treatment of adenomyosis.[118] The following therapies will help women desiring fertility:

- *Aromatase inhibitors*—therapy with letrozole 2.5 mg daily for up to 12 weeks compared favorably with depot GnRH injection of 3.6 mg for reducing the volume of adenomyoma.[119]
- *Antiplatelet therapy:* In mice experiments a trial of antiplatelet therapy with ozagrel showed beneficial results of reduction in adenomyosis.[120]
- Gonadotropin-releasing hormone analogs (GnRHa) are also likely to bring about a beneficial effect by reducing adenomyosis.[3,117]
- Combinations of gonadotropin-releasing hormone (GnRH) analogs (such as elagolix with estradiol and

norethindrone, and relugolix with estradiol and norethindrone)[121-124] have been approved for individuals with uterine fibroids and those with both fibroids and adenomyosis. Nonetheless, the effectiveness of these treatments has not been specifically investigated in cases of isolated adenomyosis. Elagolix was found to be less effective than depot GnRH agonist in adenomyosis.

Gonadotropin-releasing Hormone Analog Treatment

Medication with GnRHa with add-back estrogen therapy has resulted in many pregnancies following the treatment.[122] GnRH agonist treatment has been observed to have a positive effect on the markers of endometrial implantation.[123] They induce antiproliferative effect on tissues, cause apoptosis in lesions, and decrease inflammatory reaction and angiogenesis.[123]

Women undergoing frozen ET following long-term GnRH agonist therapy showed significantly higher rates of clinical and ongoing pregnancies as compared to those who were not treated with GnRHa.[125,126] It may be prudent to harvest oocytes and freeze embryos prior to downregulation to improve clinical pregnancy rates.

Uterus-preserving Surgical Treatment

Indications for Surgery

Indications for conservative surgical treatment include:

- Focal adenomyoma[127]
- Failures of IVF treatment, especially in women ≤39 years of age.[128]

Progress in surgical techniques of minimal access surgery has improved outcomes in adenomyosis.[129] The adenomyotic tissue is known to bury deep into the myometrium, often making complete excision of the lesion difficult.[130] An attempt at removing this tissue is invariably accompanied by removal of the adjacent normal myometrium and may prove destructive for the uterine wall, possibly leaving behind weak areas.[75] Moreover, recurrence of adenomyosis may be quick to follow.[131]

Uterus-sparing Techniques

Various surgical procedures can be performed.[132] Laparoscopic route is preferred over laparotomy. The procedures could include:[75]

- Complete excision of the adenomyotic lesion:
  - *Adenomyomectomy:* Performed in cases of localized adenomyosis.[133] The procedure can also be carried out in some cases of diffuse adenomyosis with a careful reconstruction of the uterine wall, thereby maintaining the integrity of the latter.[133]
  - Cystectomy may be carried out in cystic focal adenomyosis.[51,134,135]

  Following adenomyomectomy, the defect may be closed in layers, as performed conventionally.[77,132,136,137] Modifications in the reconstruction of uterine wall by U-shaped suturing,[137] overlapping flaps,[138] or the triple flap method may be utilized.[133]
- *Cytoreductive procedure/partial adenomyomectomy:* This method is utilized in diffuse adenomyosis. The procedure aims to preserve a critical amount of healthy myometrium.[131,139,140]

  In order to carry out cytoreductive surgery or partial adenomyomectomy, various techniques may be employed, including:
- The classic technique, such as the transverse H incision technique,[138] wedge resection of the uterine wall,[140] or an asymmetric dissection of the uterus.[131] Standard closure techniques are typically followed.

  The majority of documented cases involving the removal of diffuse adenomyosis have been through open surgery, which likely addresses specific challenges encountered during these operations. To overcome these difficulties, Dr. Hisao Osada, a reproductive surgeon from Japan, introduced a laparoscopic-assisted open surgical technique in 2011. This technique emphasizes thorough removal of the adenomyotic tissue, employs preventive measures for control of blood loss, and reconstructs the uterine wall using a triple-flap method. Relative to other surgical methods for treating diffuse adenomyosis, the Osada technique[133,141] has demonstrated superior results in terms of pregnancy outcomes.
- A laparoscopic-assisted vaginal method for excision has been described.[75]
- Robotic adenomyomectomy has also been performed, including for cases of juvenile cystic adenomyosis (JCA).[142,143]

Preoperative assessment by imaging is mandated to map the location and the size/extent of the lesion.[75]

- *Nonexcisional techniques:* Laparoscopic electrocoagulation of adenomyomata and uterine artery occlusion.[140,144,145] The effect on fertility and the outcome of a scarred uterus are yet to be reported.[146,147] These treatment options cannot, as yet, be recommended routinely for women desiring fertility.

- *Operative hysteroscopy:* Utilizing a resectoscope to selectively resect adenomyotic lesions via hysteroscopy has been performed. However, it is not a first-line treatment option for women with adenomyosis. It may be a viable recourse only in selected cases in which the adenomyotic lesion is focal and subendometrial.[148,149]

Natural conception has proved successful following conservative surgery. Clinical pregnancies resulted in 30% women, attempting conception after surgery, either by natural or assisted conception according to a study by Saremi et al.[132] Osada et al. have also reported natural conception following adenomyomectomy.[133]

MEDICAL OR SURGICAL TREATMENT OF ADENOMYOSIS

Both medical and surgical management plans exist for cases with poor fertility and/or pregnancy losses.[2] Recourse to surgery is exceptional and not the routine in infertile patients. There is a propensity of weakening the myometrial wall with the excision of the adenomyosis which leads to a higher risk of uterine rupture during subsequent pregnancy.[20] Pre-IVF treatment with the use of GnRHa is less invasive and may prove safer and more reasonable in many cases of adenomyosis who wish to conceive.[21]

CONTROL OF SYMPTOMS FOLLOWING SURGERY

The outcome of patients following surgery is summarized in **Table 7**.

FERTILITY AFTER SURGICAL TREATMENT

Conservative surgical techniques for adenomyosis may result in alterations to the uterine anatomy, pelvic adhesions, intrauterine adhesions, and reduced uterine capacity.[75] These outcomes may hinder postoperative pregnancy rates.[130]

Despite these challenges, a crude delivery rate exceeding 70% has been reported following cytoreductive surgery.[75] This figure can be compared with approximately 50% pregnancy rates following surgical treatment of myomas, and it can be concluded that cytoreductive surgery for adenomyosis offers a reasonably good outcome with respect to subsequent fertility.[149] It should be noted that prospective controlled studies for the burden on fertility caused by adenomyosis are lacking.[150-152]

Conception rates after partial excision of adenomyosis are reported as 46.8%, while those following complete excision are 60.5%.[75] However, total clinical pregnancy rate of 31.4% was reported following uterus-sparing surgery for adenomyosis in one study.[128] Upon grouping the cases into ≤39 years and ≥40 years age groups, the clinical pregnancy rates of 41.3% and 3.7%, respectively, were observed. Clinical pregnancy rates among the ≥40 years group were significantly lower, and in majority of the pregnancies, miscarriages followed.[128]

Miscarriage rates after partial excision are reported as 26.7% and following complete excision of adenomyosis are 16.9% indicating increased fertility after surgery for adenomyosis.[75] Combined treatment with conservative surgery and GnRHa versus GnRHa treatment alone revealed that surgery is associated with an increase in pregnancy rates.[132,133]

Role of Gonadotropin-releasing Hormone Analog in Conjunction with Fertility-preserving Surgery

The role of GnRHa in women undergoing fertility preservation surgery for adenomyosis is unclear.[75] The propounded benefits of employing these agents include a reduction in the vascularity of the uterus, anemia, and operative bleeding.[75,136] An impaired ability to recognize adenomyotic areas, and differentiate them from the normal myometrium can, however, occur with these agents.[136] Also, associated is an increased likelihood of an unintentional entry into the endometrium.[136]

Assisted Reproductive Technology Postsurgery

Majority of studies permitted attempts at conception after 3 months following surgery for adenomyosis.[50,131] Following operative intervention for adenomyosis, ART increased conception rates compared with natural cycles.[134] A single ET is preferred in order to avoid the risk of uterine rupture with multiple pregnancies.[151]

Uterine Rupture

The risk of uterine rupture during pregnancy and labor exists following conservative surgery for adenomyosis, as the uterus may have diminished tensile strength.[151-153] Safer operative procedures and ensuring adequate healing of the uterine wound after surgical intervention have been

TABLE 7: Evidence table: Outcomes after surgery for adenomyosis.

Authors (year)	*Study design*	*Surgical intervention*	*Number of cases*	*Dysmenorrhea*	*Menorrhagia*	*Pregnancy rate*	*Miscarriage*
Saremi et al. (2012)[132]	Prospective	Adenomyomectomy	103 severe adeno	In 40%	In 65%	21/70 (30%)	4/21 (19%)
Osada et al. (2011)[133]	Prospective	Adenomyomectomy (triple flap method)	104 adeno	Preoperative VAS 10–1.67 (2 years postoperative)	Preoperative VAS 10–2.87 (2 years postoperative)	16/26 (61.5%)	2/26 (12.5%)
Al Jama (2011)[148]	Retrospective	GnRHa versus GnRHa + Sx	40; (A) GnRHa-22 (B) GnRHa + Sx-18	(B) In 15/18 (83.3%)	(B) In 15/18 (83.3%)	3/22 (13.6%) in (A) 8/18 (44.4%) in (B)	1/2 (50%) in (A) 2/8 (25%) in (B)
Sun et al. (2011)[140]	Retrospective	Modified adenomyomectomy, wedge resection	24	In 91.2% (complete resection), in 88.9% (incomplete resection)	In 40% (complete resection), in 50% (incomplete resection)	3/8 (37.5%)	5/8 (62.5%)
Nishida et al. (2010)[130]	Retrospective	Cons Sx	44	9.4–0.8	Improvement	2/2; one normal, one ectopic	
Wang et al. (2009)[131]	Retrospective	Cons Sx ± GnRHa (A), GnRHa only (B)	65; 28(A), 37(B)	(A) > (B)		3-year pregnancy, delivery rates in (A) versus (B) (46.4 vs. 10.8% and 32.1 vs. 8.1%)	4/13 (14.3%) in (A)
Takeuchi et al. (2006)[137]	Prospective	Laparoscopic adenomyomectomy and hysteroplasty	14 adeno	VAS 2.5		2/8 (25%)	
Fujishita et al. (2004)[138]	Retrospective	Old classical reduction versus transverse H incision	Old (5) versus new H incision (6)	Old (18%) new H incision (55%)		2/4 (50%)	

(Adeno: adenomyosis; Cons Sx: conservative surgery; GnRHa: gonadotropin-releasing hormone analog; Sx: surgery; VAS: visual analog scale)

proposed.[130] It was observed that peripartum hysterectomy may be required in some cases.[153]

CONCLUSION

Adenomyosis may play a significant causative role in RPL and RIF. Maintaining a high index of suspicion for the disease possesses deep significance. History of implantation failure and/or miscarriages often dictate an active approach by medical and/or surgical options. The benefits of treatment choices need to be confirmed by comparative studies in this group of women. Both medical and surgical treatment modalities ask for time prior to attempting pregnancy. Hence, oocyte freezing prior to treating adenomyosis is advisable. Without the application of either or both treatment forms, pregnancy outcomes are often poor.

ACKNOWLEDGMENT

The author wishes to acknowledge the efforts of Dr Vishesh Khanna in compilation, editing, and preparation of the manuscript. Crucial inputs from Dr Jyoti Chakraverty, Dr Puneet Jain, Dr Pankaj Kumar, Dr Vineet Sethia, Dr Karn Bhardwaj, Dr Rajeev Choudhary, Dr Mamta Mittal, Dr Sonal Sharma, Dr Priyanka Suhag, and Dr Sai Deepashri have also helped in the completion of this article.

REFERENCES

1. Martínez-Conejero JA, Morgan M, Montesinos M, Fortuño S, Meseguer M, Simón C, et al. Adenomyosis does not affect implantation, but is associated with miscarriage in patients undergoing oocyte donation. Fertil Steril. 2011;96(4):943-50.
2. Struble J, Reid S, Bedaiwy MA. Adenomyosis: a clinical review of a challenging gynecologic condition. J Minim Invasive Gynecol. 2016;23(2):164-85.
3. Dueholm M. Uterine adenomyosis and infertility, review of reproductive outcome after in vitro fertilization and surgery. Acta Obstet Gynecol Scand. 2017;96(6):715-26.
4. Wang PH, Su WH, Sheu BC, Liu WM. Adenomyosis and its variance: adenomyoma and female fertility. Taiwan J Obstet Gynecol. 2009;48(3):232-8.
5. Garcia L, Isaacson K. Adenomyosis: review of the literature. J Minim Invasive Gynecol. 2011;18(4):428-37.
6. Benson RC, Sneeden VD. Adenomyosis: a reappraisal of symptomatology. Am J Obstet Gynecol. 1958;76(5):1044-57.
7. Emge LA. The elusive adenomyosis of the uterus. Its historical past and its present state of recognition. Am J Obstet Gynecol. 1962;83:1541-63.
8. Levgur M, Abadi MA, Tucker A. Adenomyosis: symptoms, histology, and pregnancy terminations. Obstet Gynecol. 2000;95(5):688-91.
9. Exacoustos C, Manganaro L, Zupi E. Imaging for the evaluation of endometriosis and adenomyosis. Best Pract Res Clin Obstet Gynaecol. 2014;28(5):655-81.
10. Brosens I, Derwig I, Brosens J, Fusi L, Benagiano G, Pijnenborg R. The enigmatic uterine junctional zone: the missing link between reproductive disorders and major obstetrical disorders? Hum Reprod. 2010;25(3):569-74.
11. Kissler S, Hamscho N, Zangos S, Wiegratz I, Schlichter S, Menzel C, et al. Uterotubal transport disorder in adenomyosis and endometriosis—a cause for infertility. BJOG. 2006;113(8):902-8.
12. Tamai K, Togashi K, Ito T, Morisawa N, Fujiwara T, Koyama T. et al. MR imaging findings of adenomyosis: correlation with histopathologic features and diagnostic pitfalls. Radiographics. 2005;25(1):21-40.
13. Nadella SP, Oshodi C, Castellanos ME. Incidence of adenomyosis in chronic pelvic pain patients undergoing hysterectomy. J Minim Invasive Gynecol. 2017;24(7):S68.
14. Matalliotakis IM, Katsikis IK, Panidis DK. Adenomyosis: what is the impact on fertility? Curr Opin Obstet Gynecol. 2005;17(3):261-4.
15. Azziz R. Adenomyosis: current perspectives. Obstet Gynecol Clin North Am. 1989;16(1):221-35.
16. Leyendecker G, Kunz G. Endometriosis and adenomyosis. Zentralbl Gynakol. 2005;127:288-94.
17. Leyendecker G, Kunz G, Kissler S, Wildt L. Adenomyosis and reproduction. Best Pract Res Clin Obstet Gynaecol. 2006;20(4):523-46.
18. Ben Hamouda S, Ouerdiane N, Ben Zina H, Masmoudi A, Ennine I, Bouguerra B, et al. Adenomyosis at hysterectomy. Tunis Med. 2007;85:559-62.
19. Tomassetti C, Meuleman C, Timmerman D, D'Hooghe T. Adenomyosis and subfertility: evidence of association and causation. Semin Reprod Med. 2013;31(2):101-8.
20. Puente JM, Fabris A, Patel J, Patel A, Cerrillo M, Requena A, et al. Adenomyosis in infertile women: prevalence and the role of 3D ultrasound as a marker of severity of the disease. Reprod Biol Endocrinol. 2016;14(1):60.
21. Younes G, Tulandi T. Effects of adenomyosis on in vitro fertilization treatment outcomes: a meta-analysis. Fertil Steril. 2017;108(3):483-90.e3.
22. Sharma S, Bathwal S, Agarwal N, Chattopadhyay R, Saha I, Chakravarty B. Does presence of adenomyosis effect reproductive outcome—a retrospective analysis of 607 patients having endometriosis, endometriosis with adenomyosis and only adenomyosis who underwent IVF/ICSI. Fertil Steril. 2015;104(3 Suppl):e160.
23. Ballester M, d'Argent EM, Morcel K, Belaisch-Allart J, Nisolle M, Daraï E. Cumulative pregnancy rate after ICSI-IVF in patients with colorectal endometriosis: results of a multicentre study. Hum Reprod. 2012;27(4):1043-9.
24. Maubon A, Faury A, Kapella M, Pouquet M, Piver P. Uterine junctional zone at magnetic resonance imaging: a predictor of in vitro fertilization implantation failure. J Obstet Gynaecol Res. 2010;36(3):611-8.

25. Thalluri V, Tremellen KP. Ultrasound diagnosed adenomyosis has a negative impact on successful implantation following GnRH antagonist IVF treatment. Hum Reprod. 2012;27(12):3487-92.
26. Youm HS, Choi YS, Han HD. In vitro fertilization and embryo transfer outcomes in relation to myometrial thickness. J Assist Reprod Genet. 2011;28(11):1135-40.
27. Benaglia L, Cardellicchio L, Leonardi M, Faulisi S, Vercellini P, Paffoni A, et al. Asymptomatic adenomyosis and embryo implantation in IVF cycles. Reprod Biomed Online. 2014;29(5):606-11.
28. Costello MF, Lindsay K, McNally G. The effect of adenomyosis on in vitro fertilisation and intra-cytoplasmic sperm injection treatment outcome. Eur J Obstet Gynecol Reprod Biol. 2011;158(2):229-34.
29. Mijatovic V, Florijn E, Halim N, Schats R, Hompes P. Adenomyosis has no adverse effects on IVF/ICSI outcomes in women with endometriosis treated with long-term pituitary down-regulation before IVF/ICSI. Eur J Obstet Gynecol Reprod Biol. 2010;151(1):62-5.
30. Salim R, Riris S, Saab W, Abramov B, Khadum I, Serhal P. Adenomyosis reduces pregnancy rates in infertile women undergoing IVF. Reprod Biomed Online. 2012;25(3):273-7.
31. Bazot M, Fiori O, Darai E. Adenomyosis in endometriosis—prevalence and impact on fertility. Evidence from magnetic resonance imaging. Hum Reprod. 2006;21(4):1101-2.
32. Kunz G, Beil D, Huppert P, Noe M, Kissler S, Leyendecker G. Adenomyosis in endometriosis—prevalence and impact on fertility. Evidence from magnetic resonance imaging. Hum Reprod. 2005;20(8):2309-16.
33. Bazot M, Darai E, Hourani R, Thomassin I, Cortez A, Uzan S, et al. Deep pelvic endometriosis: MR imaging for diagnosis and prediction of extension of disease. Radiology. 2004;232:379-89.
34. Larsen SB, Lundorf E, Forman A, Dueholm M. Adenomyosis and junctional zone changes in patients with endometriosis. Eur J Obstet Gynecol Reprod Biol. 2011;157(2):206-11.
35. Exacoustos C, Luciano D, Corbett B, De Felice G, Di Feliciantonio M, Luciano A, et al. The uterine junctional zone: a 3-dimensional ultrasound study of patients with endometriosis. Am J Obstet Gynecol. 2013;209(3):248.e1-7.
36. Benagiano G, Brosens I. The history of endometriosis: identifying the disease. Hum Reprod. 1991;6(7):963-8.
37. Benagiano G, Brosens I. History of adenomyosis. Best Pract Res Clin Obstet Gynaecol. 2006;20(4):449-63.
38. Benagiano G, Brosens I. Who identified endometriosis? Fertil Steril. 2011;95(1):13-6.
39. Benagiano G, Brosens I, Carrara S. Adenomyosis: new knowledge is generating new treatment strategies. Womens Health (Lond). 2009;5(3):297-311.
40. Benagiano G, Brosens I, Habiba M. Structural and molecular features of the endomyometrium in endometriosis and adenomyosis. Hum Reprod Update. 2014;20(3):386-402.
41. Templeman C, Marshall SF, Ursin G, Horn-Ross PL, Clarke CA, Allen M, et al. Adenomyosis and endometriosis in the California Teachers Study. Fertil Steril. 2008;90(2):415-24.
42. Taran FA, Weaver AL, Coddington CC, Stewart EA. Understanding adenomyosis: a case control study. Fertil Steril. 2010;94(4):1223-8.
43. Nomelini RS, Ferreira FA, Borges RC, Adad SJ, Murta EF. Frequency of endometriosis and adenomyosis in patients with leiomyomas, gynecologic premalignant, and malignant neoplasias. Clin Exp Obstet Gynecol. 2013;40(1):40-4.
44. Güzel Aİ, Akselim B, Erkılınç S, Kokanalı K, Tokmak A, Dolmuş B, et al. Risk factors for adenomyosis, leiomyoma and concurrent adenomyosis and leiomyoma. J Obstet Gynaecol Res. 2015;41(6):932-7.
45. Ryan GL, Stolpen A, Van Voorhis BJ. An unusual cause of adolescent dysmenorrhea. Obstet Gynecol. 2006;108(4):1017-22.
46. Farquhar C, Brosens I. Medical and surgical management of adenomyosis. Best Pract Res Clin Obstet Gynaecol. 2006;20(4):603-16.
17. Parazzini F, Vercellini P, Panazza S, Chatenoud L, Oldani S, Crosignani PG. Risk factors for adenomyosis. Hum Reprod. 1997;12:1275-9.
48. Vercellini P, Parazzini F, Oldani S, Panazza S, Bramante T, Crosignani PG. Adenomyosis at hysterectomy: a study on frequency distribution and patient characteristics. Hum Reprod. 1995;10(5):1160-2.
49. Takeda A, Sakai K, Mitsui T, Nakamura H. Laparoscopic management of juvenile cystic adenomyoma of the uterus: report of two cases and review of the literature. J Minim Invasive Gynecol. 2007;14(3):370-4.
50. Kriplani A, Mahey R, Agarwal N, Bhatla N, Yadav R, Singh MK. Laparoscopic management of juvenile cystic adenomyoma: four cases. J Minim Invasive Gynecol. 2011;18(3):343-8.
51. Takeuchi H, Kitade M, Kikuchi I, Takeuchi H, Kitade M, Kikuchi I, Kumakiri J, Kuroda K, Jinushi M. Diagnosis, laparoscopic management, and histopathologic findings of juvenile cystic adenomyoma: a review of nine cases. Fertil Steril. 2010;94(3):862-8.
52. Dogan E, Gode F, Saatli B, Seçil M. Juvenile cystic adenomyosis mimicking uterine malformation: a case report. Arch Gynecol Obstet. 2008;278(6):593-5.
53. Riggs JC, Lim EK, Liang D, Bullwinkel R. Cesarean section as a risk factor for the development of adenomyosis uteri. J Reprod Med. 2014;59(1-2):20-4.
54. Cohen I, Beyth Y, Tepper R, Figer A, Shapira J, Cordoba M, et al. Adenomyosis in postmenopausal breast cancer patients treated with tamoxifen: a new entity? Gynecol Oncol. 1995;58(1):86-91.
55. Cohen I, Beyth Y, Shapira J, Tepper R, Fishman A, Cordoba M, et al. High frequency of adenomyosis in postmenopausal breast cancer patients treated with tamoxifen. Gynecol Obstet Invest. 1997;44(3):200-5.

56. Green AR, Styles JA, Parrott EL, Gray D, Edwards RE, Smith AG, et al. Neonatal tamoxifen treatment of mice leads to adenomyosis but not uterine cancer. Exp Toxicol Pathol. 2005;56(4-5):255-63.
57. Ferenczy A. Pathophysiology of adenomyosis. Hum Reprod Update. 1998;4(4):312-22.
58. Ostrzenski A. Extensive iatrogenic adenomyosis after laparoscopic myomectomy. Fertil Steril. 1998;69(1):143-5.
59. Ota H, Igarashi S, Hatazawa J, Tanaka T. Is adenomyosis an immune disease? Hum Reprod Update. 1998;4(4):360-7.
60. Bergeron C, Amant F, Ferenczy A. Pathology and physiopathology of adenomyosis. Best Pract Res Clin Obstet Gynaecol. 2006;20(4):511-21.
61. Bedaiwy MA, Dahoud W, Skomorovska-Prokvolit Y, Liua JH,·Falconeb T, Mesianoa S. Expression of progesterone receptor isoforms-A and -B in adenomyosis. Fertil Steril. 2013;100(3 Suppl 1):S387.
62. Matsumoto Y, Iwasaka T, Yamasaki F, Sugimori H. Apoptosis and Ki-67 expression in adenomyotic lesions and in the corresponding eutopic endometrium. Obstet Gynecol. 1999;94(1):71-7.
63. Propst AM, Quade BJ, Gargiulo AR, Nowak RA, Stewart EA. Adenomyosis demonstrates increased expression of the basic fibroblast growth factor receptor/ligand system compared with autologous endometrium. Menopause. 2001;8(5):368-71.
64. Sasson IE, Taylor HS. Stem cells and the pathogenesis of endometriosis. Ann N Y Acad Sci. 2008;1127:106-15.
65. Szubert M, Koziróg E, Olszak O, Krygier-Kurz K, Kazmierczak J, Wilczynski J. Adenomyosis and Infertility-Review of Medical and Surgical Approaches. Int J Environ Res Public Health. 2021;18(3):1235.
66. Du H, Taylor HS. Stem cells and female reproduction. Reprod Sci. 2009;16(2):126-39.
67. Bragheto AM, Caserta N, Bahamondes L, Petta CA. Effectiveness of the levonorgestrel-releasing intrauterine system in the treatment of adenomyosis diagnosed and monitored by magnetic resonance imaging. Contraception. 2007;76(3):195-9.
68. Huang FJ, Kung FT, Chang SY, Hsu TY. Effects of short-course buserelin therapy on adenomyosis. A report of two cases. J Reprod Med. 1999;44(8):741-4.
69. McCausland AM. Hysteroscopic myometrial biopsy: its use in diagnosing adenomyosis and its clinical application. Am J Obstet Gynecol. 1992;166(6 Pt 1):1619-26.
70. Koike H, Egawa H, Ohtsuka T, Yamaguchi M, Ikenoue T, Mori N. Correlation between dysmenorrheic severity and prostaglandin production in women with endometriosis. Prostaglandins Leukot Essent Fatty Acids. 1992;46(2):133-7.
71. Parker JD, Leondires M, Sinaii N, Premkumar A, Nieman LK, Stratton P. Persistence of dysmenorrhea and nonmenstrual pain after optimal endometriosis surgery may indicate adenomyosis. Fertil Steril. 2006;86(3):711-5.
72. Shrestha A, Sedai LB. Understanding clinical features of adenomyosis: a case control study. Nepal Med Coll J. 2012;14(3):176-9.
73. Levgur M. Diagnosis of adenomyosis: a review. J Reprod Med. 2007;52(3):177-93.
74. McElin TW, Bird CC. Adenomyosis of the uterus. Obstet Gynecol Annu. 1974;3:425-41.
75. Grimbizis GF, Mikos T, Tarlatzis B. Uterus-sparing operative treatment for adenomyosis. Fertil Steril. 2014;101(2):472-87.
76. Gilks CB, Clement PB, Hart WR, Young RH. Uterine adenomyomas excluding atypical polypoid adenomyomas and adenomyomas of endocervical type: a clinicopathologic study of 30 cases of an underemphasized lesion that may cause diagnostic problems with brief consideration of adenomyomas of other female genital tract sites. Int J Gynecol Pathol. 2000;19(3):195-205.
77. Grimbizis GF, Mikos T, Zepiridis L, Theodoridis T, Miliaras D, Tarlatzis BC, et al. Laparoscopic excision of uterine adenomyomas. Fertil Steril. 2008;89(4):953-61.
78. Wang JH, Wu RJ, Xu KH, Lin J. Single large cystic adenomyoma of the uterus after cornual pregnancy and curettage. Fertil Steril. 2007;88(4):965-7.
79. Mazur MT. Atypical polypoid adenomyomas of the endometrium. Am J Surg Pathol. 1981;5:473-82.
80. Gilks CB, Young RH, Clement PB, Hart WR, Scully RE. Adenomyomas of the uterine cervix of endocervical type: a report of ten cases of a benign cervical tumor that may be confused with adenoma malignum [corrected]. Mod Pathol. 1996;9(3):220-4.
81. Dueholm M. Transvaginal ultrasound for diagnosis of adenomyosis: a review. Best Pract Res Clin Obstet Gynaecol. 2006;20(4):569-82.
82. Bazot M, Cortez A, Darai E, Rouger J, Chopier J, Antoine JM, et al. Ultrasonography compared with magnetic resonance imaging for the diagnosis of adenomyosis: correlation with histopathology. Hum Reprod. 2001;16(11):2427-33.
83. Reinhold C, Tafazoli F, Wang L. Imaging features of adenomyosis. Hum Reprod Update. 1998;4:337-49.
84. Bromley B, Shipp TD, Benacerraf B. Adenomyosis: sonographic findings and diagnostic accuracy. J Ultrasound Med. 2000;19(8):529-34.
85. Kepkep K, Tuncay YA, Göynümer G, Tutal E. Transvaginal sonography in the diagnosis of adenomyosis: which findings are most accurate? Ultrasound Gynecol Obstet. 2007;30(3):341-5.
86. Van den Bosch T, Dueholm M, Leone FP. Terms, definitions and measurements to describe sonographic features of myometrium and uterine masses: a consensus opinion from the Morphological Uterus Sonographic Assessment (MUSA) group. Ultrasound Obstet Gynecol. 2015;46(3):284-98.
87. Alabiso G, Alio L, Arena S, Barbasetti di Prun A, Bergamini V, et al. Adenomyosis: What the patient needs. J Minim Invasive Gynecol. 2016;23(4):476-88.

88. Sakhel K, Abuhamad A. Sonography of adenomyosis. J Ultrasound Med. 2012;31:805-8.
89. Reinhold C, Tafazoli F, Mehio A, Wang L, Atri M, Siegelman ES, et al. Uterine adenomyosis: endovaginal US and MR imaging features with histopathologic correlation. Radiographics. 1999;19:S147-60.
90. Shwayder J, Sakhel K. Imaging for uterine myomas and adenomyosis. J Minim Invasive Gynecol. 2014;21(3):362-76.
91. Exacoustos C, Brienza L, Di Giovanni A, Szabolcs B, Romanini ME, Zupi E, et al. Adenomyosis: three-dimensional sonographic findings of the junctional zone and correlation with histology. Ultrasound Obstet Gynecol. 2011;37(4):471-9.
92. Di Donato N, Bertoldo V, Montanari G, Zannoni L, Caprara G, Seracchioli R. Question mark form of uterus: a simple sonographic sign associated with the presence of adenomyosis. Ultrasound Obstet Gynecol. 2015;46(1):126-7.
93. Andres MP, Borrelli GM, Ribeiro J, Baracat EC, Abrão MS, Kho RM. Transvaginal ultrasound for the diagnosis of adenomyosis: systematic review and meta-analysis. J Minim Invasive Gynecol. 2017;S1553-4650(17):31113-5.
94. Mavrelos D, Holland TK, O'Donovan O, Khalil M, Ploumpidis G, Jurkovic D, et al. The impact of adenomyosis on the outcome of IVF-embryo transfer. Reprod Biomed Online. 2017;35(5):549-54.
95. Meredith SM, Sanchez-Ramos L, Kaunitz AM. Diagnostic accuracy of transvaginal sonography for the diagnosis of adenomyosis: systematic review and meta-analysis. Am J Obstet Gynecol. 2009;201(1):107.e1-6.
96. Dueholm M, Lundorf E, Hansen ES, Sørensen JS, Ledertoug S, Olesen F. Magnetic resonance imaging and transvaginal ultrasonography for the diagnosis of adenomyosis. Fertil Steril. 2001;76(3):588-94.
97. Ascher SM, Arnold LL, Patt RH, Schruefer JJ, Bagley AS, Semelka RC, et al. Adenomyosis: prospective comparison of MR imaging and transvaginal sonography. Radiology. 1994;190(3):803-6.
98. Togashi K, Ozasa H, Konishi I, Itoh H, Nishimura K, Fujisawa I, et al. Enlarged uterus: differentiation between adenomyosis and leiomyoma with MR imaging. Radiology. 1989;171(2):531-4.
99. Champaneria R, Abedin P, Daniels J, Balogun M, Khan KS. Ultrasound scan and magnetic resonance imaging for the diagnosis of adenomyosis: systematic review comparing test accuracy. Acta Obstet Gynecol Scand. 2010;89(11):1374-84.
100. Reinhold C, McCarthy S, Bret PM, Mehio A, Atri M, Zakarian R, et al. Diffuse adenomyosis: comparison of endovaginal US and MR imaging with histopathologic correlation. Radiology. 1996;199(1):151-8.
101. Hoad CL, Raine-Fenning NJ, Fulford J, Campbell BK, Johnson IR, Gowland PA. Uterine tissue development in healthy women during the normal menstrual cycle and investigations with magnetic resonance imaging. Am J Obstet Gynecol. 2005;192(2):648-54.
102. Tocci A, Greco E, Ubaldi FM. Adenomyosis and 'endometrial-subendometrial myometrium unit disruption disease' are two different entities. Reprod Biomed Online. 2008;17(2):281-91.
103. Gordts S, Brosens JJ, Fusi L, Benagiano G, Brosens I. Uterine adenomyosis: a need for uniform terminology and consensus classification. Reprod Biomed Online. 2008;17(2):244-8.
104. Gordts S, Campo R, Brosens I. Hysteroscopic diagnosis and excision of myometrial cystic adenomyosis. Gynecol Surg. 2014;11(4):273-8.
105. Molinas CR, Campo R. Office hysteroscopy and adenomyosis. Best Pract Res Clin Obstet Gynaecol. 2006;20(4):557-67.
106. Fernández C, Ricci P, Fernández E. Adenomyosis visualized during hysteroscopy. J Minim Invasive Gynecol. 2007;14(5):555-6.
107. Popp LW, Schwiedessen JP, Gaetje R. Myometrial biopsy in the diagnosis of adenomyosis uteri. Am J Obstet Gynecol. 1993;169(3):546-9.
108. Brosens JJ, Barker FG. The role of myometrial needle biopsies in the diagnosis of adenomyosis. Fertil Steril. 1995;63(6):1347-9.
109. Vercellini P, Consonni D, Dridi D, Bracco B, Frattaruolo MP, Somigliana E. Uterine adenomyosis and in vitro fertilization outcome: a systematic review and meta-analysis. Hum Reprod. 2014;29(5):964-77.
110. Leyendecker G, Bilgicyildirim A, Inacker M, Stalf T, Huppert P, Mall G, et al. Adenomyosis and endometriosis. Re-visiting their association and further insights into the mechanisms of auto-traumatisation. An MRI study. Arch Gynecol Obstet. 2015;291(4):917-32.
111. Campo S, Campo V, Benagiano G. Adenomyosis and infertility. Reprod Biomed Online. 2012;24(1):35-46.
112. Shukla A, Chattopadhyay R, Ghosh S, Haseena S, Goswami S, Chakravarty B. Evaluation of the pregnancy outcomes with surrogacy in infertile women with adenomyosis following failed intracytoplasmic sperm injection (ICSI). Fertil Steril. 2013;100(3):S389
113. Brosens I, Pijnenborg R, Benagiano G. Defective myometrial spiral artery remodelling as a cause of major obstetrical syndromes in endometriosis and adenomyosis. Placenta. 2013;34(2):100-5.
114. Hashimoto A, Iriyama T, Sayama S, Nakayama T, Komatsu A, Miyauchi A, et al. Adenomyosis and adverse perinatal outcomes: increased risk of second trimester miscarriage, preeclampsia, and placental malposition. J Matern Fetal Neonatal Med. 2018;31(3):364-9.
115. Garavaglia E, Audrey S, Annalisa I, Stefano F, Iacopo T, Laura C, et al. Adenomyosis and its impact on women fertility. Iran J Reprod Med. 2015;13(6):327-36.
116. Quinn M. Uterine innervation in adenomyosis. J Obstet Gynaecol. 2007;27(3):287-91.

117. Kunz G, Leyendecker G. Uterine peristaltic activity during the menstrual cycle: characterization, regulation, function and dysfunction. Reprod Biomed Online. 2002;4(Suppl 3):5-9.
118. Mehasseb MK, Bell SC, Pringle JH, Habiba MA. Uterine adenomyosis is associated with ultrastructural features of altered contractility in the inner myometrium. Fertil Steril. 2010;93(7):2130-6.
119. Badawy AM, Elnashar AM, Mosbah AA. Aromatase inhibitors or gonadotropin-releasing hormone agonists for the management of uterine adenomyosis: a randomized controlled trial. Acta Obstet Gynecol Scand. 2012;91(4):489-95. Erratum in: Acta Obstet Gynecol Scand. 2021.
120. Zhu B, Chen Y, Shen X, Liu X, Guo SW. Anti-platelet therapy holds promises in treating adenomyosis: experimental evidence. Reprod Biol Endocrinol. 2016;14(1):66.
121. Pontis A, D'Alterio MN, Pirarba S, de Angelis C, Tinelli R, Angioni S. Adenomyosis: a systematic review of medical treatment. Gynecol Endocrinol. 2016;32(9):696-700.
122. Khan KN, Kitajima M, Hiraki K, Fujishita A, Nakashima M, Masuzaki H. Decreased expression of human heat shock protein 70 in the endometria and pathological lesions of women with adenomyosis and uterine myoma after GnRH agonist therapy. Eur J Obstet Gynecol Reprod Biol. 2015;187:6-13.
123. Khan KN, Kitajima M, Hiraki K, Fujishita A, Nakashima M, Ishimaru T, et al. Cell proliferation effect of GnRH agonist on pathological lesions of women with endometriosis, adenomyosis and uterine myoma. Hum Reprod. 2010;25(11):2878-90.
124. Kavoussi SK, Esqueda AS, Jukes LM. Elagolix to medically treat a uterine adenomyoma: A case report. Eur J Obstet Gynecol Reprod Biol. 2020;247:266-267.
125. Niu Z, Chen Q, Sun Y, Feng Y. Long-term pituitary downregulation before frozen embryo transfer could improve pregnancy outcomes in women with adenomyosis. Gynecol Endocrinol. 2013;29(12):1026-30.
126. Younes G, Tulandi T. Conservative surgery for adenomyosis and results: a systematic review. J Minim Invasive Gynecol. 2017;S1553-4650(17):30402-8.
127. Kishi Y, Yabuta M, Taniguchi F. Who will benefit from uterus-sparing surgery in adenomyosis-associated subfertility? Fertil Steril. 2014;102(3):802-7.e1.
128. Mikos T, Downes E. Ambulatory Gynecology: what can we do? Best Pract Res Clin Obstet Gynaecol. 2005;19(5):647-61.
129. Koo YJ, Im KS, Kwon YS. Conservative surgical treatment combined with GnRH agonist in symptomatic uterine adenomyosis. Pak J Med Sci. 2011;27(2):365-70.
130. Nishida M, Takano K, Arai Y, Ozone H, Ichikawa R. Conservative surgical management for diffuse uterine adenomyosis. Fertil Steril. 2010;94(2):715-9.
131. Wang PH, Fuh JL, Chao HT, Liu WM, Cheng MH, Chao KC. Is the surgical approach beneficial to subfertile women with symptomatic extensive adenomyosis? J Obstet Gynaecol Res. 2009;35(3):495-502.
132. Saremi A, Bahrami H, Salehian P, Hakak N, Pooladi A. Treatment of adeno-myomectomy in women with severe uterine adenomyosis using a novel technique. Reprod Biomed Online. 2014;28(6):753-60.
133. Osada H, Silber S, Kakinuma T, Nagaishi M, Kato K, Kato O. Surgical procedure to conserve the uterus for future pregnancy in patients suffering from massive adenomyosis. Reprod Biomed Online. 2011;22(1):94-9.
134. Protopapas A, Millingos S, Markaki S, Loutradis D, Haidopoulos D, Sotiropoulou M, et al. Cystic uterine tumors. Gynecol Obstet Invest. 2008;65(4):275-80.
135. Hyams LL. Adenomyosis, its conservative surgical treatment (hysteroplasty) in young women. N Y State J Med. 1952;52(22):2778-84.
136. Dubuisson JB, Fauconnier A, Deffarges JV, Norgaard C, Kreiker G, Chapron C. Pregnancy outcome and deliveries following laparoscopic myomectomy. Hum Reprod. 2000;15(4):869-73.
137. Takeuchi H, Kitade M, Kikuchi I, Shimanuki H, Kumakiri J, Kitano T, et al. Laparoscopic adeno-myomectomy and hysteroplasty: a novel method. J Minim Invasive Gynecol. 2006;13(2):150-4.
138. Fujishita A, Masuzaki H, Khan KN, Kitajima M, Ishimaru T. Modified reduction surgery for adenomyosis. A preliminary report of the transverse H incision technique. Gynecol Obstet Invest. 2004;57(3):132-8.
139. Wood C. Surgical and medical treatment of adenomyosis. Hum Reprod Update. 1998;4(4):323-36.
140. Sun AJ, Luo M, Wang W, Chen R, Lang JH. Characteristics and efficacy of modified adeno-myomectomy in the treatment of uterine adenomyoma. Chin Med J (Engl). 2011;124(9):1322-6.
141. Lu C, Corbett C, Elliott JE, Evans D. Fertility-sparing surgery for diffuse adenomyosis: a narrated, stepwise approach to the Osada procedure. Fertil Steril. 2022;118(3):588-90.
142. Akar ME, Leezer KH, Yalcinkaya TM. Robot-assisted laparoscopic management of a case with juvenile cystic adenomyoma. Fertil Steril. 2010;94(3):e55-6.
143. Phillips DR, Nathanson HG, Milim SJ, Haselkorn JS. Laparoscopic bipolar coagulation for the conservative treatment of adeno-myomata. J Am Assoc Gynecol Laparosc. 1996;4(1):19-24.
144. Wood C. Adenomyosis: difficult to diagnose, and difficult to treat. Diagn Ther Endosc. 2001;7(2):89-95.
145. Kang L, Gong J, Cheng Z, Dai H, Liping H. Clinical application and midterm results of laparoscopic partial resection of symptomatic adenomyosis combined with uterine artery occlusion. J Minim Invasive Gynecol. 2009;16(2):169-73.
146. Wang CJ, Yen CF, Lee CL, Soong YK. Laparoscopic uterine artery ligation for treatment of symptomatic adenomyosis. J Am Assoc Gynecol Laparosc. 2002;9(3):293-6.

147. Di Spiezio Sardo A, Calagna G, Santangelo F, Zizolfi B, Tanos V, Perino A, et al. The role of hysteroscopy in the diagnosis and treatment of adenomyosis. Biomed Res Int. 2017;2017:2518396.
148. Al Jama FE. Management of adenomyosis in subfertile women and pregnancy outcome. Oman Med J. 2011;26(3):178-81.
149. Somigliana E, Vercellini P, Daguati R, Pasin R, De Giorgi O, Crosignani PG. Fibroids and female reproduction: a critical analysis of the evidence. Hum Reprod Update. 2007;13(5):465-76.
150. Wada S, Kudo M, Minakami H. Spontaneous uterine rupture of a twin pregnancy after a laparoscopic adenomyomectomy: a case report. J Minim Invasive Gynecol. 2006;13(2):166-8.
151. Levgur M. Therapeutic options for adenomyosis: a review. Arch Gynecol Obstet. 2007;276(1):1-15.
152. Wang CJ, Yuen LT, Chang SD, Lee CL, Soong YK. Use of laparoscopic cytoreductive surgery to treat infertile women with localized adenomyosis. Fertil Steril. 2006;86(2):462.e5-8.
153. Coghlin DG. Pregnancy with uterine adenomyoma. Can Med Assoc J. 1947;56:315-6.

CHAPTER 19

Congenital Uterine Malformations

Meeta Meeta, Tanvir Tanvir, Akanshi Madan

ABSTRACT

Congenital uterine malformations (CUMs) or congenital uterine anomalies (CUAs) are a consequence of inadequate formation, differentiation of the Müllerian ducts. There are different types and varied presentations of CUAs.[1] Recurrent pregnancy loss (RPL) is defined as two or more failed clinical pregnancies before 20 weeks gestation and the frequent causes are immunologic and anatomic abnormalities. The association of CUAs and poor reproductive outcomes is accepted, the role in infertility is not clearly established. Clinically, it is important to diagnose the type of CUA, which is individually associated with varying types of adverse outcomes. Data suggests that women with canalization defects are frequently associated with repeated early pregnancy loss, complete septate being the leading cause followed by bicornuate and unicornuate uterine anomalies. Women with unification defects seem to be associated with adverse obstetric and neonatal outcomes throughout the course of pregnancy. Currently, there are no universal standards for the classification of CUA subtypes. Septate is the major cause of RPL amongst the CUM. It is suggested to use Congenital Uterine Malformation by Experts (CUME) criteria for defining septum in clinical practice and research, which is simple and reproducible. The combination of gynecological examination and two-dimensional (2D) ultrasound (US) could be recommended as the current standard for the evaluation of asymptomatic women; 3D US could be considered the standard supplemented by other techniques in complex cases.The ASRM and French guidelines recommend septum resection in case of septate uteri associated with RPL.

Keywords: Congenital uterine malformations, Congenital uterine anomalies, RPL, Hysteroscopic correction, septum resection.

INTRODUCTION

Congenital uterine malformations (CUMs) or congenital uterine anomalies (CUAs) are the result of abnormalities in the formation, differentiation of the Müllerian ducts, of fusion, or in the resorption of the septum. There are different types and varied presentations of CUAs.[1] Recurrent pregnancy loss (RPL) is defined as two or more failed clinical pregnancies before 20 weeks gestation and may be caused by genetic, endocrinologic, anatomic, and immunologic abnormalities.[2] The most common causes of RPL include both autoimmune factors and anatomical abnormalities. Anatomic uterine anomalies causing poor reproductive outcomes include CUMs such as septate, bicornuate, didelphic, and unicornuate uteri and acquired defects of the uterus are fibroids, adenomas, adhesions, and polyps.

There is agreement on the association of CUAs and poor reproductive outcomes such as recurrent miscarriages, preterm delivery, fetal malpresentation, and fetal growth restriction. preeclampsia and stillbirth. The role of CUAs in infertility is not established. Clinically, it is important to diagnose the type of CUA, which is individually associated with varying types of adverse outcomes. Data suggests that women with canalization defects are frequently associated with repeated early pregnancy loss, complete septate being the leading cause followed by bicornuate and unicornuate uterine anomalies. Women with unification defects seem to be associated with adverse obstetric and neonatal outcomes throughout the course of pregnancy.[3]

PREVALENCE AND REPRODUCTIVE OUTCOMES

Müllerian duct anomalies (MDAs) occur in up to 7% of the general population,[1] and in almost one-third of women with a renal anomaly.[4,5] The reported population prevalence rates of CUAs have wide variation ranging from 0.06 to 38%.[6-9]

The explanation for the observed wide variation is due to a number of factors. CUAs may be asymptomatic, hence reported prevalence depends on the population studied. The population studied may be unselected or women with a history of infertility, including those undergoing in vitro fertilization (IVF) treatment and poor reproductive outcomes. Moreover, there is no universally accepted classification of mullein duct abnormalities, nor for diagnosis or management of CUAs.

2011 systematic review[10] reported the prevalence rate of CUAs to be 5.5% in an unselected population, 13.3% in those with a history of recurrent miscarriage, and 24.5% in those with miscarriage and infertility. The investigations used for diagnosis in the studies may be optimal tests that are capable of accurately identifying and classifying CUAs accurately while suboptimal tests can identify and differentiate most but not all anomalies. The most frequently reported malformation was the arcuate uterus, followed by the septate.

2021 Systematic review and meta-analysis state that women with CUAs had an over threefold increased risk of miscarriage than those with a normal uterus. Septate uterus is three times more common in women with RPL, with a twofold increase in cases of bicornuate uterus. Unicornuate and uterus diadelphous do not seem to be associated with RPL.[10]

A the study examined the impact of CUAs on reproductive outcomes after IVF and intracytoplasmic sperm injection (embryo transfer over a period of 10 years). They concluded that women with canalization defects were more likely to experience spontaneous first-trimester pregnancy loss than women with normal uteri 19.8% versus 5.3% as were women with unification defects 19.8% vs 7.6%.[11]

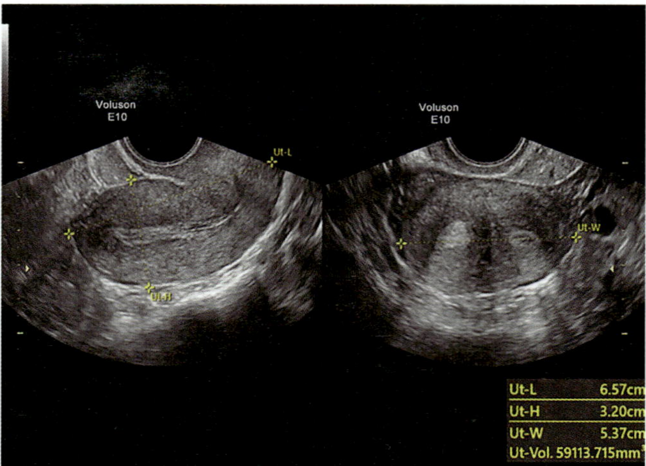

Fig. 1: Partial septate transvaginal ultrasound in sagittal and transverse plane.
Courtesy: Meeta, Tanvir Hospital.

SEPTATE UTERUS

The septate uterus is a result of incomplete or no resorption of the uterovaginal septum after the fusion of the Müllerian ducts. The presentation can be varied. Uterine septa range from small septa projecting from the uterine fundus into the uterine cavity **(Figs. 1 and 2)** to complete septa that extend to the internal cervical os, dividing the uterus in two with a single cervix. The septum may continue through the cervix partially or completely dividing a single cervix into two cervical canals **(Fig. 3)**. The cervical septum may incompletely divide the cervix, resulting in the appearance

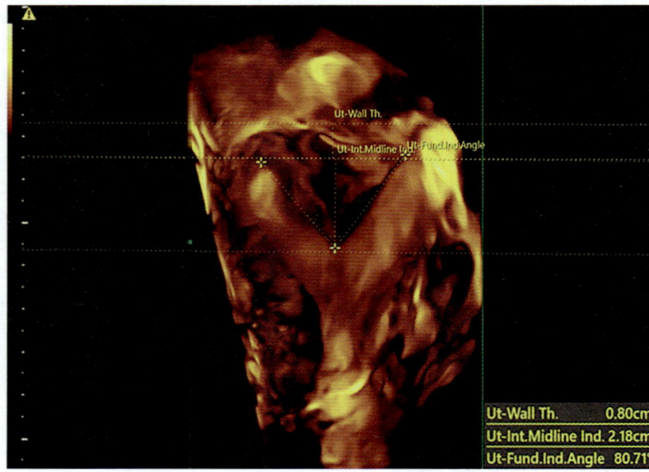

Fig. 2: Partial septate—transvaginal ultrasound (TVS) in coronal plane.
Courtesy: Meeta, Tanvir Hospital.

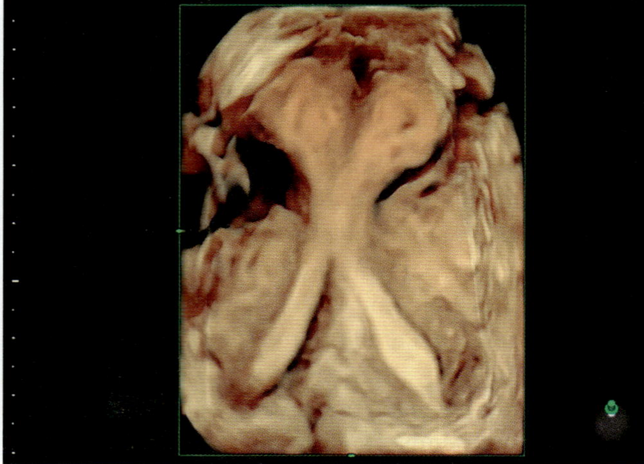

Fig. 3: Complete septum—transvaginal ultrasound in the coronal plane.
Courtesy: Meeta, Tanvir Hospital.

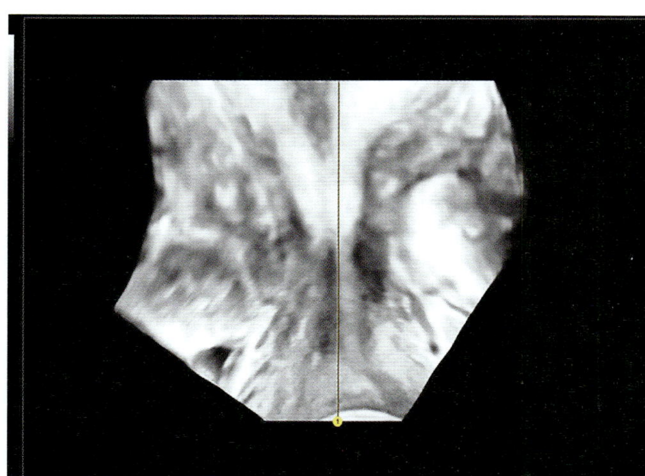

Fig. 4: Complete septum—extending up to the vagina—transvaginal ultrasound (TVS) in the coronal plane.
Courtesy: Meeta, Tanvir Hospital.

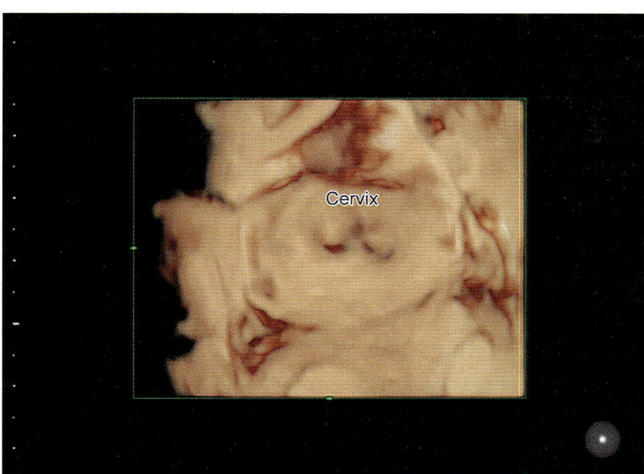

Fig. 5: Complete septum—demonstrating two cervices on transvaginal ultrasound (TVS) coronal view.
Courtesy: Meeta, Tanvir Hospital.

of a single external cervical os, despite division at the level of the upper cervix. Two cervical canals can result from two types of anomalies: a double cervix, a duplication of a normal cervix, and a septate cervix, in which a septum partially or completely divides a single cervix into two cervical canals **(Figs. 4 to 6)**. Both may exist with a septate uterus, duplication being rare. Septa may also be segmental, resulting in partial communication between the two sides. The size and shape of the septum can vary by width, length, and vascularity, although most have not been categorized systematically, and definitions are not standardized.[12,13]

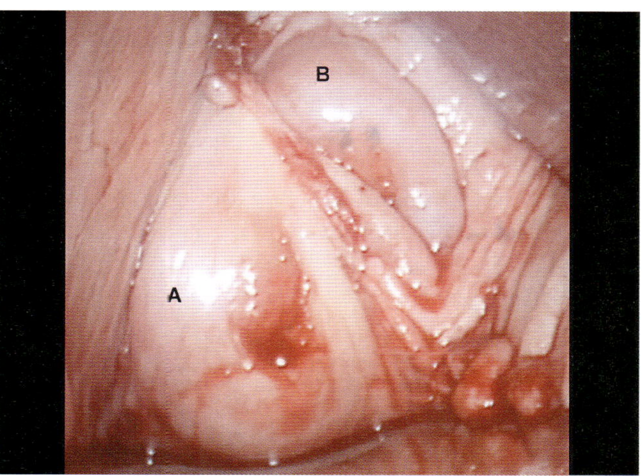

Fig. 6: Complete septum-demonstrating two cervices on clinical examination.
Courtesy: Meeta, Tanvir Hospital.

Prevalence

It is the most common congenital anomaly of the uterus, comprising approximately 55% of all anomalies.[14] A septate uterus is the most common type of congenital anomaly among patients with RPL 5.3%% and rises to 15.4% in association with infertility.[3]

Subseptate or septate uteri, have a prevalence of 2.3% in the unselected population when optimal tests are used to define their presence, and suboptimal tests gave a prevalence of 0.2% in an unselected population; a 10-fold reduction in prevalence. The prevalence of canalization defects in various high-risk populations diagnosed by suboptimal tests was consistent with those diagnosed by optimal tests. In one prospective study, the risk of miscarriage in women with septate uterus increased with each loss from approximately 11–40% after three or more pregnancy losses.[15]

Reproductive Outcome

Investigations of the impact of a septate uterus on reproductive outcomes are limited and comprised primarily of observational and descriptive studies with only RCT that have not added to the understanding[13,16] **(Table 1)**.

They indicate a wide range of prevalence in the high-risk group from 5.3 to 38%. This wide range reflects the differences in diagnostic criteria for RPL as studies have included women with two, three, or more miscarriages.

TABLE 1: Septate and subseptate uterus with reproductive and obstetric results systematic reviews with meta-analysis.

Study	Sub-analysis	Clinical pregnancy	1st trimester miscarriage	2st trimester miscarriage	Preterm birth	Fetal mal-presentation	C-section
Chan 2011 (RR*)	NA^	0.86 (0.77–0.96)	2.89 (2.02–4.14)	3.74 (1.57–8.91)	2.14 (1.48–3.11)	6.24 (4.05–9.62)	NA
Venetis 2014 (RR)	NA	0.86 (0.77–0.96) natural gestations	2.65 (1.39–5.06)	2.95 (1.51–5.77)	2.11 (1.51 to 2.94)	–	NA
Kim 2021 (OR**)	Subseptate	–	4.36 (2.64–7.21)	–	3.15 (1.34–7.4)	11.42 (3.74–34.86)	5.91 (1.59–21.95)
	Septate	0.45 (0.21-0.95)	2.55 (1.33–4.91)	4.33 (2.52– 7.43)	2.93 (2.01–4.28)	11.49 (5.24–25.17)	4.84 (2.33–10.02)
Panagio-topoulos 2022 (OR)	NA	–	–	–	4.06 (2.89–5.70)	13.76 (5.52–34.32)	5.19 (1.84–14.62)

*RR = Relative Risk; **OR = Odds Ratio; ^NA = Not Available

A systematic review of 3,805 women with CUAs reported that those with canalization defects, such as septate and partial septate uteri, appeared to have the poorest reproductive performance and an increased risk of first-trimester miscarriage with an odds ratio of 2.89 (2.02–4.14).[17] Compared with those with a partial septate uterus, women with a complete septate uterus have poorer outcomes throughout their pregnancies.[18] In one study first-trimester miscarriage occurred more often among embryos implanted on the septum than those implanted elsewhere on the uterine walls.[19]

Systematic reviews on the pathophysiology of the intrauterine septum concluded that there was no clear biological basis for the impaired reproductive outcomes in women with a septate uterus.[20,21] The septum is made of endometrium, myometrial tissue, and fibrous tissue which is vascularized and the endometrial lining contains glands and stroma corresponding to the menstrual phase of the endometrium. Differences in the histology of the endometrium make it vulnerable to pregnancy loss. The composition of the uterine septum is variable; the more vascularized muscular septum may result in higher or uncoordinated uterine contractions while the less vascularized fibrous septum may interfere with implantation. There may also be a factor of reduced uterine volume due to the septum. In a study by Fasiclla et al., showed that the septum was made of islands of muscle fibers and irregularly arranged collagen tissue similar to myomas.[22] Gene expression of the septum could account for the increased risk of reproductive waste observed after implantation in the septum.[23,24] CUAs are caused by *HOX* gene mutations, although the mechanism is most likely polygenic. The gene expression of *HOXA 10* genes, shown to be important in the early implantation of an embryo, seems to be altered in women with a septate uterus in two studies. Gross chromosomal rearrangements are unlikely to produce the CUAs associated with RPL.[25]

UNIFICATION CONGENITAL UTERINE ANOMALIES

Unification defects include bicornuate, unicornuate, and didelphic uteri. Bicornuate uteri are uncommon in the unselected population 0.3%; unicornuate uterus is significantly more common in women with a history of miscarriage 0.5%, and in women with miscarriage in association with infertility 3.1%.[3]

BICORNUATE UTERUS

This anomaly is a result of incomplete fusion of the uterine horns at the level of the fundus. The distinguishing aspect of this anomaly is the presence of two separate but communicating endometrial cavities and a single cervix **(Figs. 7A to C)**. It represents 10% of Müllerian duct anomalies. The external uterus has a sagittal cleft of variable length. The cleft extends to the internal cervical os in the complete bicornuate and to a lesser degree in the partial bicornuate uteri. The degree of incomplete Müllerian fusion appears to affect reproductive outcomes.

Bicornuate uteri may be classified into two subtypes, depending on the level of the caudal extension of fundal

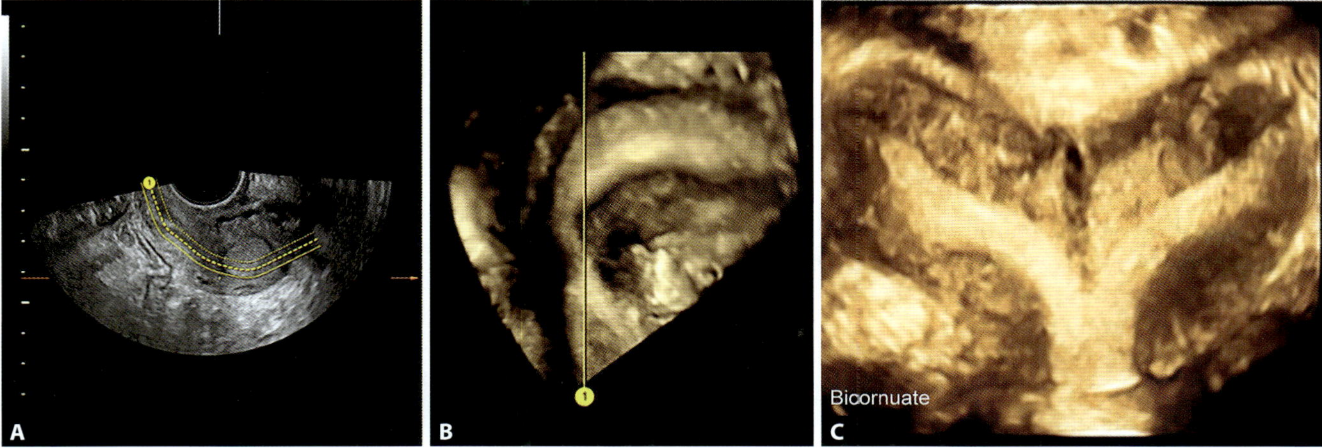

Figs. 7A to C: (A and B) Unicornuate uterus—transvaginal ultrasound (TVS) banana-shaped in the transverse and coronal plane; (C) Bicornuate uterus—transvaginal ultrasound (TVS) fundal indentation in the coronal plane.
Courtesy: Meeta, Tanvir Hospital.

indentation: bicornuate unicollis if at the level of the internal cervical os, bicornuate bicollis if at the level of the external cervical os. The horns of this uterus are not fully developed and are thus smaller than those of a didelphic uterus.

All women with CUAs had a higher rate of second-trimester miscarriage than that women with a normal uterus. Women with bicornuate uterus showed an RPL prevalence of 1.2% versus 0.3% in normal women.[10]

A systemic review showed that women with bicornuate uteri have an increased risk of both first-trimester pregnancy loss and second-trimester pregnancy loss.[26]

Women with bicornuate uterus showed a significant increase in second-trimester miscarriage while women with unicornuate or didelphys uterus did not show this association.[26]

UNICORNUATE UTERUS

Unicornuate uterus showed a prevalence of 0.5% in the high-risk group versus 0.03–0.1% in the unselected population **(Fig. 8)**.

The prevalence for didelphys uteri was 0.03–0.3% in the unselected population and a prevalence of 0.2% in women with miscarriage.[3] Women with unicornuate uterus or didelphys uterus did not show an increased prevalence of second-trimester miscarriage.[26]

ARCUATE UTERUS

The prevalence of arcuate and didelphic uteri do not differ in women with early RPL and the general population

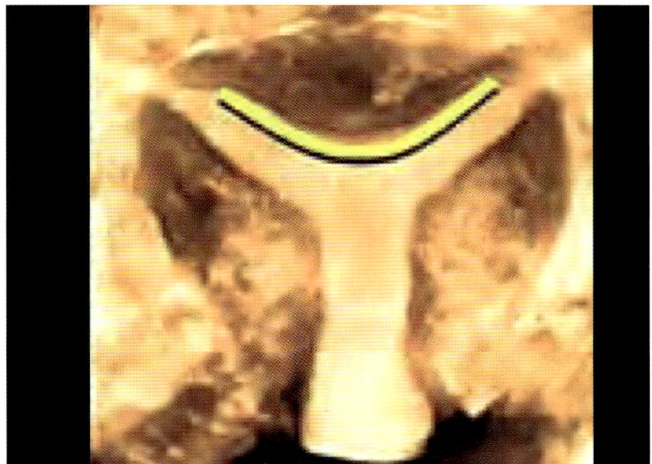

Fig. 8: Arcuate uterus—indentation depth of endometrial cavity <10 mm.

because neither uterine anomaly represents a cause for early RPL. The arcuate uterus is a simple change in the uterine cavity shape with no external dimpling. As a consequence, term delivery rates were almost 80% with a live birth rate of 82.7% and no impact on reproduction. Based on data, an arcuate uterus is considered a variant and not a CUA. Arcuate uterus is the most common in the unselected population 3.9%, and its prevalence is not increased in RPL as diagnosed by an optimal test. Suboptimal tests gave a prevalence for arcuate uteri of 2.2% in the unselected population and indicated a higher prevalence of 8.9% in women with miscarriages.[3]

A systematic review and meta-analysis in 2021 indicated that the risk of first-trimester miscarriage was not significantly different between women with an arcuate uterus and those with a normal uterus, who had a higher rate of second-trimester miscarriage than that in women with a normal uterus.[10]

T-SHAPED OR DYSMORPHIC UTERUS

The T-shaped uterus may be of primary origin or secondary to intrauterine adhesion syndrome.[27] It has been suggested that it may be related to reproductive failure, such as infertility and recurrent miscarriage.[28]

According to the Congenital Uterine Malformation by Experts (CUME) group, three sonographic criteria should be present for reliable and accurate diagnosis of a T-shaped uterus[29] **(Fig. 9)**:

- T-angle ≤40°
- Lateral indentation depth ≥7 mm
- Lateral indentation angle ≤130°

The presence of two of the above three criteria is defined as borderline. T-shaped uterus, whereas the lack or presence of only one of the above criteria is defined as a normal uterus with respect to lateral uterine morphology.

CLASSIFICATION SYSTEMS

Different classification systems have been developed to standardize terminology and diagnosis for good understanding and to improve clinical management **(Fig. 10)**. Currently, there are no universal standards for the classification of CUA subtypes. The availability of noninvasive simple tests has changed the landscape for diagnosis. The observational and retrospective data have differences in sensitivity and specificity with respect to the diagnostic tests used, which inevitably affects the classification and diagnosis of CUA subtypes. Hence, there is a need for universal classification systems and standardized tests for counseling patients and determining the management strategies of CUA patients.

Historically, the first classifications for CUAs were described by Cruveilher, Foerster, and von Rokitansky in

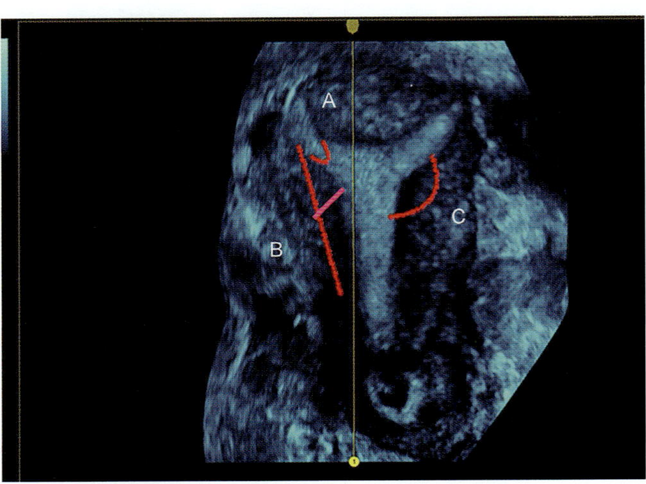

Fig. 9: Criteria for diagnosis T-shaped uterus according to CUME. A: T-angle ≤40°; B: Lateral indentation depth ≥7 mm; and C: Lateral angle ≤130°.
Courtesy: Meeta, Tanvir Hospital.

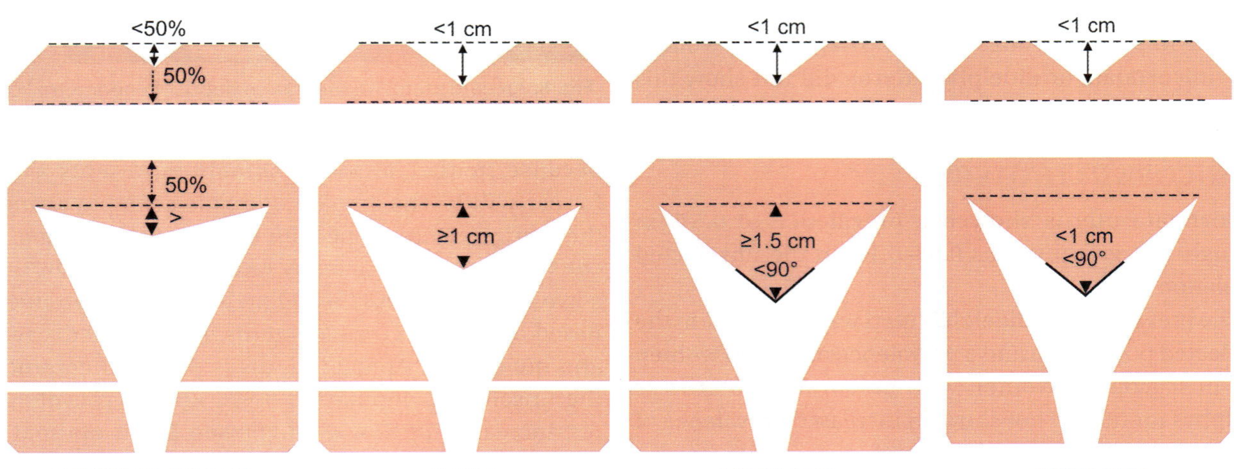

Fig. 10: Classification of the septate uterus by various organizations. *ESHRE/ESGE 2016:* Indentation (I) to wall thickness (I–WT) ratio >50%, *CUME 2018:* Septal length >10 mm, Septal angle <140° and I–WT >110%, *ASRM 2016:* Septal angle <90° and septal length >15 mm, *ASRM 2021:* Septal angle <90° and septal length >10 mm. (ESHRE: European Society of Human Reproduction and Embryology; ESGE: European Society for Gynaecological Endoscopy)

the mid-19th century.[30] American Fertility Society (AFS) Classification from 1988 has been the most recognized and utilized, and is based on Buttram and Gibbons classification described in 1979.[31,32] The advantages are that in the AFS classification, anomalies are represented as simple drawings within each group. The AFS classification has been criticized for its focus primarily on uterine anomalies, with the exclusion of those of the vagina and cervix, its lack of clear diagnostic criteria, and its inability to classify complex aberrations.

The European Society of Human Reproduction and Embryology (ESHRE)—European Society for Gynaecological Endoscopy (ESGE) developed a classification based primarily on uterine anatomy, with cervical and vaginal anomalies classified as independent supplementary subclasses to precisely identify each anomaly.[33]

Congenital Uterine Malformation by Experts (CUME) defined septate and T-shaped uterus, and are considered to be the best for clinical use.[34]

Comparing various outcomes of septum applying the ESHRE/ESGE, American Society for Reproductive Medicine (ASRM), and CUME definitions, patients received a diagnosis from the same group of observers showed a prevalence of septate uteri of 5% when the ASRM criteria were used, 12% when the CUME criteria were used, and 31% when the ESHRE/ESGE criteria were used. ASRM underestimates and ESHRE/ESGE overestimates the prevalence of septa that leads to under or overcorrection of the septum. It is suggested to use CUME criteria for defining septum in clinical practice and research, which is simple and reproducible.[35]

The ASRM Müllerian Anomalies Classification 2021 (MAC2021) classifies Müllerian anomalies into nine categories and relies on simple diagrams and descriptive terminology to identify anomalies of uterine, cervical, and vaginal origin. The ASRM MAC2021 tool is an interactive electronic format hosted on the ASRM website accessed through a laptop or personal computer and an Apple iPad. The tool is designed with three main levels, moving from general to specific, and is interactive.[36]

The classification of the AFS are class V (Va—the complete and Vb—the partial). In the ESGE and the ESHRE's new classification system of septate uteri are classified as class U2, (U2a—the partial and U2b—the complete).

DIAGNOSIS

Over a period of years, the methods to identify CUAs uterine anomalies have included: suggestive history, pelvic examination, dilation and curettage (D&C), hysterosalpingography (HSG), laparotomy or other abdominal surgeries, laparoscopy, hysteroscopy two-dimensional or three-dimensional (3D) transabdominal or transvaginal ultrasonography alone or with saline infusion sonohysterography (SHG) and magnetic resonance imagining (MRI).

Müllerian anomalies in general may be associated with renal anomalies in approximately 11–30% of individuals. However, data do not exist to suggest an association between septate uterus and renal anomalies and, as such, it is not necessary to evaluate the renal system in all patients with a uterine septum.[37]

The combination of gynecological examination and two-dimensional (2D) US could be recommended as the current standard for the evaluation of asymptomatic women; 3D US could be considered the standard for diagnosis of female genital anomalies supplemented by MRI, hysteroscopy, and laparoscopy in complex ones or in diagnostic dilemmas.[38]

ULTRASOUND

Pooled sensitivity and specificity were 83 and 99% for two-dimensional transvaginal ultrasonography, 94 and 100% for two-dimensional transvaginal sonohysterography, and 98 and 100% for 3D transvaginal ultrasound (TVS), respectively.[39]

Recommendations on Performing the Ultrasound

Three-dimensional TVS with the coronal view is considered the gold standard for the assessment of CUAs as it is less invasive and can classify the varying types of uterine anomalies correctly[40] **(Table 2)**.

- The endometrial wall and the outline of the cavity are best visualized in the midcycle or luteal phase; the endometrial thickness should be at least 5 mm **(Fig. 11)**.
- Leiomyomata, adenomyosis, and the presence of an IUD may compromise the evaluation of the endometrial contour.
- Similarly, diagnosis of CUA during pregnancy or menstrual bleeding should be avoided.
- Obtain an image of the uterus in a midsagittal plane in 2D.
- The serial sagittal plane should span from beyond the outer margin of one side of the uterus to the other including both cervix and uterine body if feasible.

TABLE 2: CUME—diagnosis of CUMs by 3D ultrasonography.

Normal	***Fundal contour***	***External contour***
Accurate	Concave fundal indentation with a central point of indentation at an obtuse angle	Uniformly convex or with indentation <10 mm
Subseptate	Presence of septum, which does not extend to the cervix, with a central point of the septum at an acute angle	Uniformly convex or with indentation <10 mm
Septate	Presence of uterine septum that completely divides the cavity from fundus to cervix	Uniformly convex or with indentation <10 mm
Bicornuate	Two well-formed uterine cornua	Fundal indentation >10 mm dividing the two cornua
Unicornuate with or without rudimentary horn	Single well-formed uterine cavity with a single interstitial portion of fallopian tube and concave fundal contour	—

(CUMs: congenital uterine malformations; CUME: congenital uterine malformation by experts)

- Transverse planes from the cervix to beyond the uterine fundal level should be taken systematically. Visualization of two endometrial cavities on a transverse plane is indicative of CUA.
- In cases of vaginal obstruction or stenosis, if the woman consents, transrectal ultrasound with a vaginal probe or transperineal could be performed to evaluate the vaginal canal and uterus.
- Transperineal 2D ultrasound may provide information on the vaginal cavity, especially in the presence of imperforate hemivagina.
- 3D gives the coronal plane of the uterus. Normal uterus with no indentation at the funds and the uterine cavity **(Fig. 11)**. Arcuate uterus is considered a normal variant with an indentation of an endometrial cavity of <10 mm **(Fig. 12)**.
- The reconstructed coronal plane of the uterus might show the cavity and the external uterine profile as well as the tubal angle and the junctional zone, if possible, along all the endometrium and cavity. This view classifies bicornuate septate or partial septate uteri correctly.

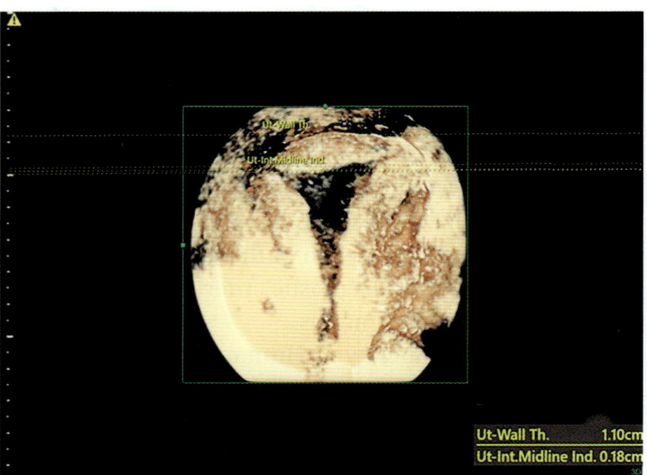

Fig. 11: Normal uterus coronal view no indentation at the fundus nor the endometrium.
Courtesy: Meeta, Tanvir Hospital.

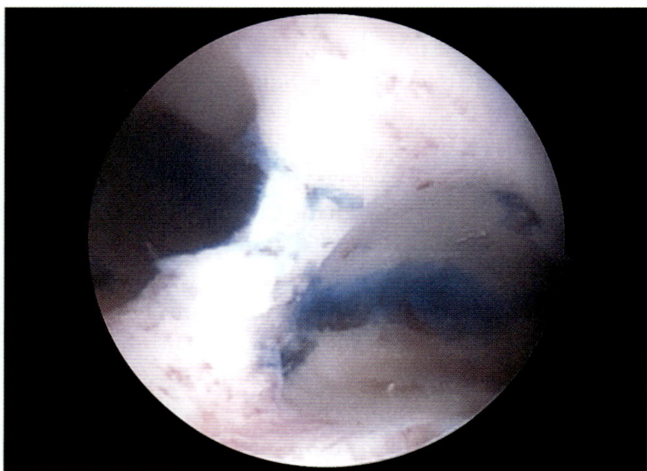

Fig. 12: Hysteroscopic view of partial septum following methylene blue test.
Courtesy: Tanvir, Tanvir Hospital.

- Uterus didelphys (complete bicorporeal), although very rare, also shows two endometrial cavities in the transverse plane of conventional 2D ultrasound, but 3D ultrasound, with a clinical demonstration of two cervices or two vaginas on speculum examinations, can confirm the diagnosis.
- A banana-shaped uterine cavity and a single interstitial portion of the fallopian tube in the coronal plane is seen using 3D ultrasound.
- Save a 3D volume for off-line analysis.
- Sonovaginocervicography aids in the maximum complicated and sophisticated evaluation of the

female genital tract in one visit. It is done after filling the vagina with gel or saline.

Three-dimensional Sonohysterography

New methods like 3D sonohysterography as well as automatic volume estimation, aid in giving newer ways of morphology evaluation, assessing variations in uterine cavity volume, symmetry, extent of deformity, and surgical anatomic outcomes.[39]

MAGNETIC RESONANCE IMAGING

Magnetic resonance imaging provides highly reliable and objective information and can be used for diagnosis in cases of complex and obstructing anomalies with the exception of assessment of the tubes.

HYSTEROSCOPY

It provides highly reliable information for the anatomical status of the vagina, cervical canal and the uterine cavity aa well as the tubal ostia. It is minimally invasive giving the additional opportunity of treating and differential diagnosis of T-shaped uterus. Electronic storage of the procedure is possible for reevaluation are advantageous.[41]

Combined Laparoscopy and Hysteroscopy

Combined laparoscopic and hysteroscopic examination is the gold standard for assessing CUAs, especially for differentiating between the bicornuate and the septate uterus. Laparoscopy also is required to complete the diagnostic workup of infertility and provides an opportunity to treat any coexisting pathology, such as endometriosis. Hysteroscopic metroplasty is performed best under laparoscopic guidance.

MANAGEMENT

The objective to treat CUMs is to increase live births at term, by restoring the normal volume and shape of the endometrial cavity and cervical canal as much as possible.

SEPTATE

Many women with a uterine septum have an uncomplicated reproductive outcome yet, there is fair evidence that CUMs contribute to RPLs. The current standard of care is hysteroscopic metroplasty or transcervical division of the uterine septum. In experienced hands, the procedure is simple, safe, and cost-effective in an outpatient setting, and reduces the rates of adverse obstetric outcomes related to the presence of the septum. However, the management of the septate uterus is under considerable debate.[42]

There is concurrence in the following situations:

- Asymptomatic women with successful reproductive outcomes are not treated, only documented.
- The main indication is in patients with RPL since observational studies have shown improved reproductive outcomes **(Table 1)**.

The debate and universally accepted solutions are not available for the following questions.

- Who should be treated?
- When should they be treated?
- Standardization in classification, diagnosis, pathology, and techniques of hysteroscopic resection.
- Evidence of reproductive outcomes after resection.

The value of uterine septum surgery to optimize fertility and fecundity was experimentally assessed in The Randomized Uterine Septum Trial (TRUST), which concluded that septum resection does not improve reproductive outcomes, which was against conclusions from previous studies. It is a multicenter study including 10 centers, with a sample size of 80, and the study lasted for a decade.[16]

Limitations of the TRUST Study

- Whether most patients had an incomplete septum or an arcuate uterus?
- All septate uteri were placed in a single group. We know there are subtypes of septa based on anatomic, histologic, or cytoarchitectural features that may impact fertility and pregnancy outcomes differently.[20]
- There was no uniformity in the criteria for diagnosis and management techniques.
- Another variable was the lack of standardization for complete resection.
- Inclusion and exclusion criteria changed twice during the study.
- Subgroup analysis on the outcomes concerning pregnancy loss, ongoing pregnancy, preterm birth, and fetal malposition was not done.
- Follow-up hysteroscopy was done only in 69% of the patients.

CURRENT CONSENSUS FOR TREATMENT OF SEPTET UTERUS

Hence, in the case of septum, the systematic reviews may be superior to the observations of the randomized clinical trial. The ASRM and French guidelines recommend septum resection in case of septate uteri associated with RPL.[43,44] However, the Royal College of Obstetricians and Gynaecologists concludes that there is insufficient evidence for justifying surgical correction of septate uteri.[45] Likewise, the ESHRE guidelines conclude that the net value of septum resection should be evaluated in further randomized controlled trials.[33] The consensus from ASRM states that hysteroscopic septum incision is associated with a reduction in subsequent miscarriage rates and improvement in live-birth rates in patients with a history of RPL (evidence level Grade C).[46]

Operative Tips

Preoperative endometrial suppression by progesterone therapy is not used routinely, but may improve visualization and operative precision

The procedure is preferably performed in the early proliferative phase of the menstrual cycle. The length of the uterine septum may vary from a small septum of 1 cm to a large septum extending from the fundus to the internal cervical os.

A variety of hysteroscopic instruments can be used for the division of a uterine septum including:

- Microscissors **(Figs. 11 to 13)**
- Bipolar electrosurgical needle
- Resectoscope with an operating loop

A systematic review and network meta-analysis suggest that hysteroscopic septoplasty with scissors is associated with higher pregnancy rates compared to the resectoscope.[47] Keeping both the tubal ostia under vision as a guiding point, a transverse incision of the uterine septum should be made just in the middle of it, equidistant from the anterior and posterior uterine walls **(Figs. 14 and 15)**.

The procedure is considered complete when both the ostia are visualized in a panoramic view with free side-to-side movement of the hysteroscope **(Fig. 16)**.

Concurrent use of intraoperative 3DUS reduces the incidence of suboptimal septal resections at hysteroscopic metroplasty.[48]

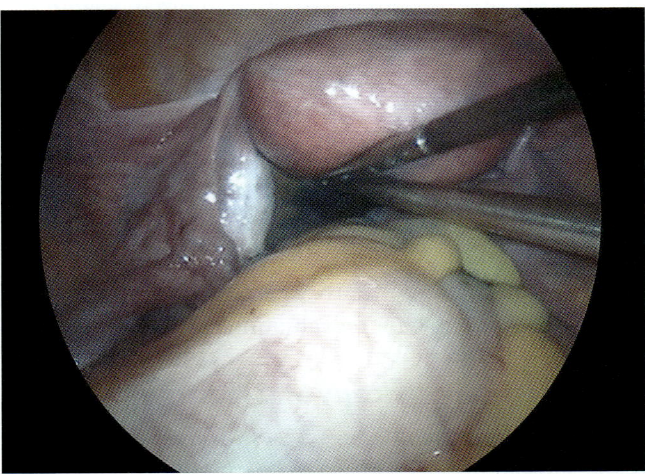

Fig. 14: Hysteroscopic view of partial septum following methylene blue test.
Courtesy: Tanvir, Tanvir Hospital.

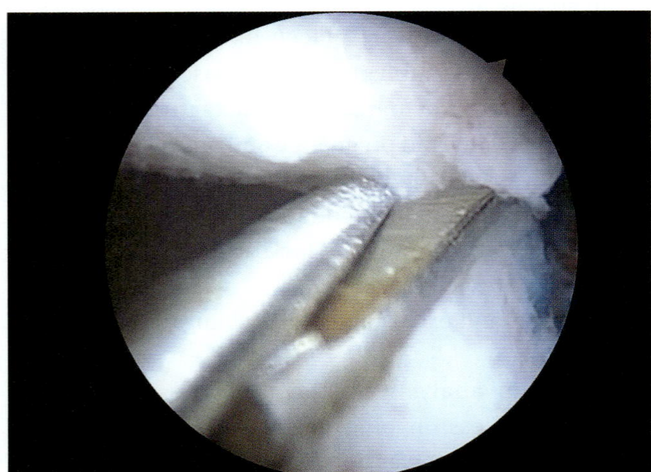

Fig. 13: Partial septum, cut with scissors.
Courtesy: Tanvir, Tanvir Hospital.

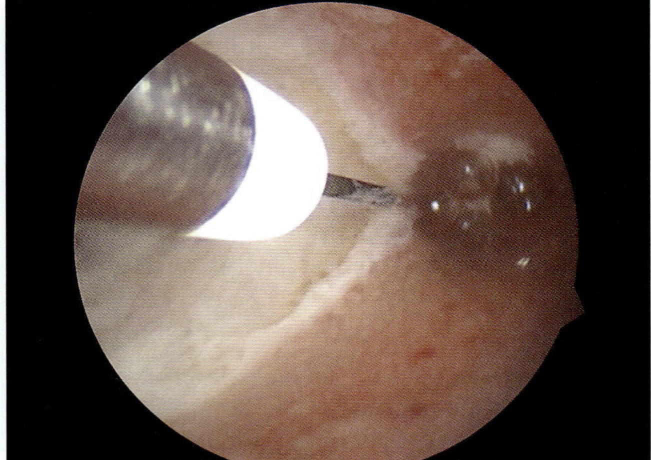

Fig. 15: Septum is excised until both ostia are visualized.
Courtesy: Tanvir, Tanvir Hospital.

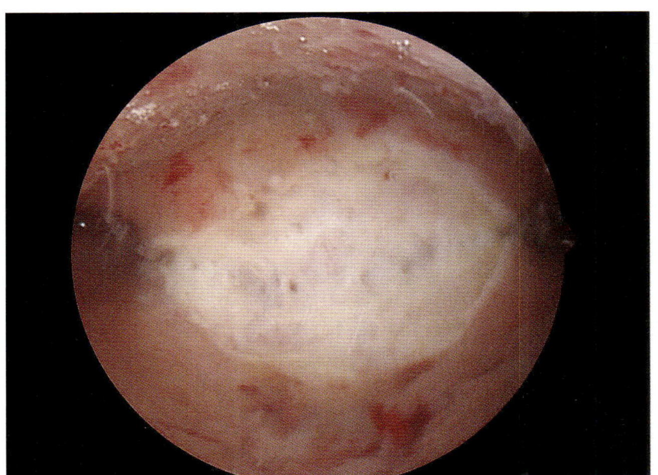

Fig. 16: Final view after septum resection.
Courtesy: Tanvir, Tanvir Hospital.

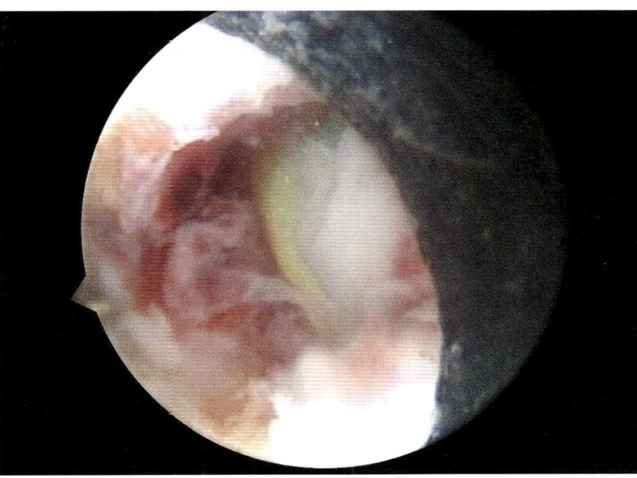

Fig. 18: Foley's catheter was placed on the right side of the septum. An incision is made with Collin's knife of a 16 Fr miniresectoscope from the left side just above the internal os in the midline until the catheter bulb is seen.
Courtesy: Tanvir, Tanvir Hospital.

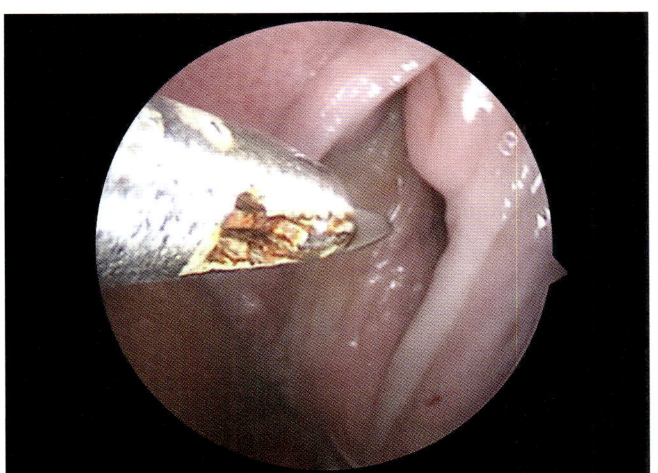

Fig. 17: Vertical vaginal septum, cut with 5 Fr hysteroscopic scissors.
Courtesy: Tanvir, Tanvir Hospital.

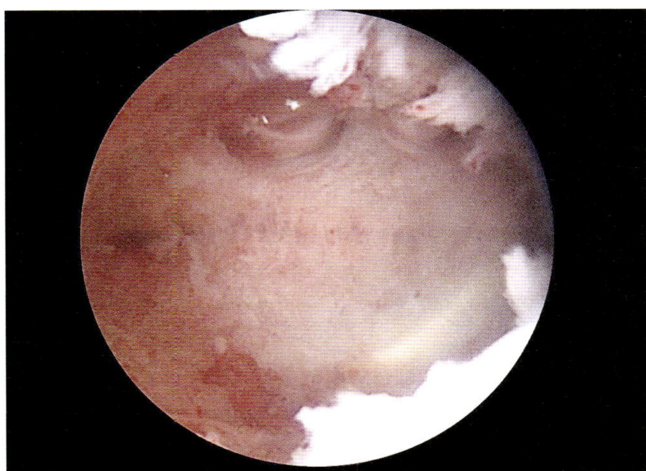

Fig. 19: Hysteroscopic view following septal selection.
Courtesy: Tanvir, Tanvir Hospital.

COMPLETE SEPTATE UTERUS

There are two schools of thought, some prefer to retain the septum below the internal os for fear of intraoperative bleeding and cervical incompetence **(Figs. 17 to 19)**. Few recommend resecting the cervical septum in all cases of complete uterine septum since it makes the procedure safer, and faster with similar obstetric outcomes.[49,50]

POSTOPERATIVE MANAGEMENT

- Prophylactic antibiotics.
- Hormonal therapy with estrogen is generally not needed, some prefer intrauterine autocross-linked hyaluronic acid gel to prevent intrauterine adhesions.
- Follow-up examination of the uterine cavity by ultrasound in all patients undergoing hysteroscopic

metroplasty after one to three months will be decisive in identifying patients deserving a second step metroplasty.[51]

Endometrial reepithelialization of the cut surface can occur centripetally by the proliferation of endometrial tissue and centrifugally from the base of the remaining glands to the margin of the incision. The available evidence suggests that the uterine cavity is healed by two months postoperatively. There is insufficient evidence to advocate a specific length of time before a woman should conceive.[51]

- *Residual septa:* The presence of a residual septum 0.5–1.0 cm in length may not influence outcomes adversely.[52]

COMPLICATIONS

Surgical and obstetrical complications of hysteroscopic metroplasty have been described as follows:[53]

- Complications associated with the distension medium
- Traumatic complications
- *Hemorrhage:* This is rare and may be seen in cases with a wide septum. The average blood loss is 20–25 mL. Bleeding may be tackled by placing an inflated foley catheter which acts as a tamponade for approximately 6 hours, cervical injection of vasopressin, or fundal injection of vasopressin through the laparoscope.
- Postoperative intrauterine adhesions
- *Obstetric complications:* Uterine rupture in subsequent pregnancy. Few cases have been reported, and dystocia leading to an increased incidence of cesarean section.

BICORNUATE AND DIDELPHIC UTERI

Traditionally, abdominal metroplasty was performed to unify or restore the shape of the uterus and remains the only surgical treatment available for women with unification defects such as bicornuate or didelphic uteri. Evidence on improving reproductive outcomes following abdominal metroplasty for unification defects in the uteri of women with past histories of repeated pregnancy loss or preterm deliveries is very limited. Only one controlled study of 21 women with bicornuate uteri, 13 of whom did not undergo surgery and eight who underwent abdominal metroplasty, records no improvement in obstetric outcomes.[54]

There is a divided opinion on treating a didelphic uterus and bicornuate uterus by performing laparoscopic metroplasty in women with RPL for whom no other cause can be identified.[55,56]

UNICORNUATE UTERUS

Metroplasty is not recommended for a unicornuate uterus, although surgical removal of an existing rudimentary horn is recommended to reduce dysmenorrhea and other menstrual complications and to avoid the risk of a corneal ectopic pregnancy.[56]

T-SHAPED UTERUS

Expectant management should be considered the most appropriate choice for women with a T-shaped uterus based on current research. A systematic review regarded the available evidence of very low quality on the diagnosis, prevalence, clinical relevance, and particularly interventions.[57]

CONCLUSION

Anatomic uterine anomalies causing poor reproductive outcomes include CUMs, such as septate, bicornuate, didelphic, and unicornuate uteri. Septate is the major cause of RPL amongst the CUM. 3D ultrasonography has emerged as the gold standard for the diagnosis of simple CUM, and MRI is used for complex cases. There is a need for a universal classification system for CUM. Presently, the CUME classification is simple, reproducible, and may not over or underdiagnose septum. Hysteroscopic metroplasty is safe, simple, and cost-effective for tackling septum in RPLs as an office procedure. The consensus from ASRM states that hysteroscopic septum incision is associated with a reduction in subsequent miscarriages and improvement in live birth rates in patients of RPL.

REFERENCES

1. Breech LL, Laufer MR. Developmental abnormalities of the female reproductive tract. Curr Opin Obstet Gynecol. 1999;11(5):441-50.
2. Jaslow CR, Carney JL, Kutteh WH. Diagnostic factors identified in 1020 women with two verses three or more recurrent pregnancy losses. Fertil Steril. 2010;93(4):1234-43. doi: 10.1016/j.fertnstert.2009.01.166. Epub 2009 Mar 31. PMID: 19338986.
3. Chan YY, Jayaprakasan K, Zamora J, Thornton JG, Raine-Fenning N, Coomarasamy A. The prevalence of congenital uterine anomalies in unselected and high-risk populations: a systematic review. Hum Reprod Update. 2011;17(6):761-71.
4. Bhagavath B, Ellie G, Griffiths KM, Winter T, Alur-Gupta S, Richardson C, et al. Uterine malformations: an update of diagnosis, management, and outcomes. Obstet Gynecol Surv. 2017;72(6):377-92.
5. O'Flynn O'Brien KL, Bhatia V, Homafar M, Gong YY, Winsten MT, Gerber J, et al. The Prevalence of Müllerian

Anomalies in Women with a Diagnosed Renal Anomaly. J Pediatr Adolesc Gynecol. 2021;34(2):154-60.
6. Simón C, Martinez L, Pardo F, Tortajada M, Pellicer A. Müllerian defects in women with normal reproductive outcome. Fertil Steril. 1991;56(6):1192-3.
7. Makino T, Hara T, Oka C, Toyoshima K, Sugi T, Iwasaki K, et al. Survey of 1120 Japanese women with a history of recurrent spontaneous abortions. Eur J Obstet Gynecol Reprod Biol. 1992;44(2):123-30.
8. Acién P. Incidence of mullerian defects in fertile and infertile women. Hum Reprod. 1997;12(7):1372-6.
9. Guimarães Filho HA, Mattar R, Pires CR, Araujo Júnior E, Moron AF, Nardozza LM. Prevalence of uterine defects in habitual abortion patients attended on at a university health service in brazil. Arch General. Obstet. 2006;274(6):345-8.
10. Kim MA, Kim HS, Kim YH. Reproductive, Obstetric and neonatal outcomes in women with congenital uterine anomalies: a systematic review and meta-analysis. J Clin Med. 2021;10(21):4797.
11. Kang J, Qiao J. Impact of congenital uterine anomalies on reproductive outcomes of IVF/ICSI-embryo transfer: a retrospective study. Eur J Med Res. 2024 Jan 11;29(1):48.
12. Sugi MD, Penna R, Jha P, Põder L, Behr SC, Courtier J, et al. Müllerian duct anomalies: role in fertility and pregnancy. Radiographics. 2021;41(6):1857-75.
13. Homer HA, Li TC, Cooke ID. The septate uterus: a review of management and reproductive outcome. Fertil Steril. 2000;73(1):1-14.
14. Troiano RN. Magnetic resonance imaging of mulerian duct anomalies of the uterus. Top Magn Reson Imaging. 2003;14(4):269-79.
15. Magnus MC, Wilcox AJ, Morken NH, Weinberg CR, Håberg SE. Role of maternal age and pregnancy history in risk of miscarriage: prospective register based study. BMJ. 2019;364:l869.
16. Rikken JFW, Kowalik CR, Emanuel MH, Bongers MY, Spinder T, Jansen FW, et al. Septum resection versus expectant management in women with a septate uterus: an international multicentre open-label randomized controlled trial. Hum Reprod. 2021;36(5):1260-7.
17. Chan YY, Jayaprakasan K, Tan A, Thornton JG, Coomarasamy A, Raine-Fenning NJ. Reproductive outcomes in women with congenital uterine anomalies: a systematic review. Ultrasound Obstet General. 2011;38(4):371-82.
18. Fox NS, Roman AS, Stern EM, Gerber RS, Saltzman DH, Rebarber A. Type of congenital uterine anomaly and adverse pregnancy outcomes. J Matern Fetal Neonatal Med. 2014;27(9):949-5.
19. Fedele L, Dorta M, Brioschi D, Giudici MN, Candiani GB. Pregnancies in septate uteri: outcome in relation to site of uterine implantation as determined by sonography. AJR Am J Roentgenol. 1989;152(4):781-4.
20. Rikken JFW, Leeuwis-Fedorovich NE, Letteboer S, Emanuel MH, Limpens J, van der Veen F, et al. The pathophysiology of the septate uterus: a systematic review. BJOG. 2019;126(10):1192-9.
21. Noventa M, Spagnol G, Marchetti, Saccardi C, Bonaldo G, Laganà AS, et al. Uterine Septum with or without Hysteroscopic Metroplasty: Impact on Fertility and Obstetrical Outcomes-A Systematic Review and Meta-Analysis of Observational Research. J Clin Med. 2022;11(12):3290.
22. Fascilla FD, Resta L, Cannone R, De Palma D, Ceci OR, Loizzi V, et al. Resectoscopic metroplasty with uterine septum excision: a histologic analysis of the uterine septum. J Minim Invasive Gynecol. 2019;27(6):1287-94.
23. Dabirashrafi H, Bahadori M, Mohammad K, Alavi M, Moghadami-Tabrizi N, Zandinejad K, et al. Septate uterus: new idea on the histologic features of the septum in this abnormal uterus. Am J Obstet Gynecol. 1995;172(1 Pt 1): 105-7.
24. Fedele L, Bianchi S, Marchini M, Franchi D, Tozzi L, Dorta M. Ultrastructural aspects of endometrium in infertile women with septate uterus. Fertil Steril. 1996;65(4):750-2.
25. Daniilidis A, Papandreou P, Grimbizis GF. Uterine septum and reproductive outcome. From diagnosis to treatment. How, why, when? Facts Views Vis Obgyn. 2022;14(1):31-6.
26. Venetis CA, Papadopoulos SP, Campo R, Gordts S, Tarlatzis BC, Grimbizis GF. Clinical implications of congenital uterine anomalies: a meta-analysis of comparative studies. Reprod Biomed Online. 2014;29(6):665-83.
27. Fernandez H, Garbin O, Castaigne V, Gervaise A, Levaillant JM. Surgical approach to and reproductive outcome after surgical correction of a T-shaped uterus. Hum Reprod. 2011;26(7):1730-4.
28. Ducellier-Azzola G, Lecointre L, Hummel M, Pontvianne M, Garbin O. Hysteroscopic enlargement metroplasty for T-shaped uterus: 24 years' experience at the Strasbourg Medico-Surgical and Obstetrical Centre (CMCO). Eur J Obstet Gynecol Reprod Biol. 2018;226:30-4.
29. Ludwin A, Coelho Neto MA, Ludwin I, Nastri CO, Costa W, Acién M, et al. Congenital Uterine Malformation by Experts (CUME): diagnostic criteria for T-shaped uterus. Ultrasound Obstet Gynecol. 2020;55(6):815-29.
30. Doerr W. [Jean Cruveilhier, Carl v. Rokitansky, Rudolf Virchow. Fundaments of pathology, thoughts on the 100th anniversary of Rokitansky's death]. Virchows Arch A Pathol Anat Histol. 1978;378(1):1-16.
31. American Fertility Society. The American Fertility Society classifications of adnexal adhesions, distal tubal occlusion, tubal occlusion secondary to tubal ligation, tubal pregnancies, müllerian anomalies and intrauterine adhesions. Fertil Steril. 1988;49(6):944-55.
32. Buttram VC Jr, Gibbons WE. Müllerian anomalies: a proposed classification. (An analysis of 144 cases). Fertil Steril. 1979:32(1):40-6.
33. Grimbizis GF, Gordts S, Di Spiezio Sardo A, Brucker S, De Angelis C, Gergolet M, et al. The ESHRE/ESGE consensus

on the classification of female genital tract congenital anomalies. Hum Reprod. 2013;28(8):2032-44.
34. Ludwin A, Martins WP, Nastri CO, Ludwin I, Coelho Neto MA, Leitão VM, et al. Congenital Uterine Malformation by Experts (CUME): better criteria for distinguishing between normal/arcuate and septate uterus? Ultrasound Obstet. Gynecol. 2018;51(1):101-9.
35. Ludwin A, Ludwin I, Coelho Neto MA, Nastri CO, Bhagavath B, Lindheim SR, et al. Septate uterus according to ESHRE/ESGE, ASRM and CUME definitions: association with infertility and miscarriage, cost and warnings for women and healthcare systems. Ultrasound Obstet Gynecol. 2019;54(6):800-14.
36. Pfeifer SM, Attaran M, Goldstein J, Lindheim SR, Petrozza JC, Rackow BW, et al. ASRM müllerian anomalies classification 2021. Fertil Steril. 2021;116(5):1238-52.
37. Jonaityte G, Kagan KO, Prodan NC, Hoopmann M. How to do a 3D uterus ultrasound? Arch Gynecol Obstet. 2023;307(6):1839-45.
38. Grimbizis GF, Di Spiezio Sardo A, Saravelos SH, Gordts S, Exacoustos C, Van Schoubroeck D, et al. The Thessaloniki ESHRE/ESGE consensus on diagnosis of female genital anomalies. Hum Reprod. 2016;31(1):2-7.
39. Alcázar JL, Carriles I, Cajas MB, Costa S, Fabra S, Cabrero M, et al. Diagnostic performance of two-dimensional ultrasound, two-dimensional sonohysterography and three-dimensional ultrasound in the diagnosis of septate uterus-a systematic review and meta-analysis. Diagnostics (Basel). 2023;13(4):807.
40. Salim R, Woelfer B, Backos M, Regan L, Jurkovic D. Reproducibility of three-dimensional ultrasound diagnosis of congenital uterine anomalies. Ultrasound Obstet Gynecol. 2003;21(6):578-82.
41. Mencaglia L, Tantini C. Hysteroscopic treatment of septate and arcuate uterus. Gynaecol Endosc. 1996;5:151-4.
42. Carrera M, Pérez Millan F, Alcázar JL, Alonso L, Caballero M, Carugno J, et al. Effect of hysteroscopic metroplasty on reproductive outcomes in women with septate uterus: systematic review and meta-analysis. J Minim Invasive Gynecol. 2022;29(4):465-75.
43. Practice Committee of the American Society for Reproductive Medicine. Evaluation and treatment of recurrent pregnancy loss: a committee opinion. Fertil Steril. 2012;98(5):1103-11.
44. Huchon C, Deffieux X, Beucher G, Capmas P, Carcopino X, Costedoat-Chalumeau N, et al. Pregnancy loss: French clinical practice guidelines. Eur J Obstet Gynecol Reprod Biol. 2016;201:18-26.
45. The Royal College of Obstetricians and Gynaecologists. (2011). The investigation and treatment of couples with recurrent first-trimester and second trimester miscarriage. Green-top Guideline. [Online] Available from https://www.rcog.org.uk/media/3cbgonl0/gtg_17.pdf [Last accessed December, 2024].
46. Practice Committee of the American Society for Reproductive Medicine. Uterine septum: a guideline. 2016;106(3):530-40.
47. Kalaitzopoulos DR, Themeli MZ, Grigoriadis G, Alterio MD, Vitale SG, Angioni S, et al. Fertility, pregnancy and perioperative outcomes after operative hysteroscopy for uterine septum: a network meta-analysis. Arch Gynecol Obstet. 2024;309(3):731-44.
48. Muzii L, Galati G, Mattei G, Romito A, Di Donato V, Palaia I, et al. Intraoperative Three-Dimensional Transvaginal Ultrasound for Hysteroscopic Metroplasty: a Controlled Study. Reprod Sci. 2023;30(11):3372-8.
49. Parsanezhad ME, Alborzi S, Zarei A, Dehbashi S, Shirazi LG, Rajaeefard A, et al. 2006. Hysteroscopic metroplasty of the complete uterine septum, duplicate cervix, and vaginal septum. Fertil Steril. 2006;85(5):1473-7.
50. Wang Z, An J, Su Y, Liu C, Lin S, Zhang J, et al. Reproductive outcome of a complete septate uterus after hysteroscopic metroplasty. J Int Med Res. 2020;48(3):300060519893836.
51. Casadio P, Magnarelli G, La Rosa, Alletto A, Arena A, Fontana E, et al. Uterine Fundus Remodeling after Hysteroscopic Metroplasty: A Prospective Pilot Study. J Clin Med. 2021;10(2):260.
52. Fedele L, Bianchi S, Marchini M, Mezzopane R, DiNola G, Tozzi L. Residual uterine septum of less than 1 cm after hysteroscopic metroplasty does not impair reproductive outcome. Hum Reprod. 1996;11(4):727-9.
53. Agostini A, De Guibert F, Salari K, Crochet P, Bretelle F, Gamerre M. Adverse obstetric outcomes at term after hysteroscopic metroplasty. J Minim Invasive Gynecol. 2009;16(4):454-7.
54. Maneschi F, Marana R, Muzii L, Mancuso S. Reproductive performance in women with bicornuate uterus. Acta Eur Fertil. 1993;24(3):117-20.
55. Alborzi S, Asadi N, Zolghadri J, Alborzi S, Alborzi M. Laparoscopic metroplasty in bicornuate and didelphic uteri. Fertil Steril. 2009;92(1):352-5.
56. Taylor E, Gomel V. The uterus and fertility. Fertil Steril. 2008;89(1):1-16.
57. Coelho Neto MA, Ludwin A, Petraglia F, Martins WP. Definition, prevalence, clinical relevance and treatment of T-shaped uterus: systematic review. Ultrasound Obstet Gynecol. 2021;57(3):366-77.

CHAPTER

20

Intrauterine Pathologies

S Krishnakumar, Shrutika O Makde, Aditi Abhade, Rohan Krishnakumar

ABSTRACT

Intrauterine pathologies are associated with recurrent pregnancy loss (RPL). The T-shaped uterus or dysmorphic uterus, submucous myomas, polyps and intrauterine adhesions lead to implantation disorders. Hysteroscopy serves as a gold standard for both diagnosis and management of these conditions. The hysteroscopic procedures, precautions, and pregnancy outcomes, post correction are outlined in this chapter

Keywords: Hysteroscopy, RPL, T-shaped uterus, Dysmorphic uterus, CUME, Submucous Myoma, Intrauterine adhesions, Endometrial polyp.

INTRODUCTION

The prevalence of anatomical uterine anomalies in women experiencing RPL varies from 15 to 42% according to different studies.[1-5] Congenital uterine anomalies, mainly septate uterus, are associated with 7–28% of RPL.[4,6,7] Acquired uterine anomalies are associated with 6–15% of RPL.[5] These include:

- Submucosal myomas
- Endometrial polyps
- Intrauterine adhesions (IUAs)

In this chapter, we shall restrict ourselves to the etiology and management of RPL due to only one of the congenital anomalies of uterus—the T-shaped uterus (U1) anomalies and the acquired uterine anomalies.

T-SHAPED UTERUS

Here, the cavity of the uterus is similar to the alphabet "T", indicating a narrow cavity and reduced volume, which may contribute to infertility and poorer reproductive outcome.[4,8] In 1977, Kaufman et al. first reported T-shaped uterus as a diethylstilbestrol (DES)—exposure-related condition. DES use is being banned for pregnant women, but T-shaped uterus still occurs with some unknown mechanism. The reported prevalence of T-shaped uterus varies from 0.2 to 10%. Today, T-shaped uterus can be seen because of the following reasons:[9]

- *Primary:* Congenital Müllerian anomaly[1-3]
- *Secondary:* IUAs (lateral walls)
- *Tuberculosis:* The primary T-shaped uterus **(Fig. 1)**

The classic T-shaped uterus has a narrow uterine cavity due to thickened lateral walls involving two-thirds of the uterine corpus and one-third of the cervix, with both tubal ostia invisible. The normal uterine cavity is shown in **Figure 2**.

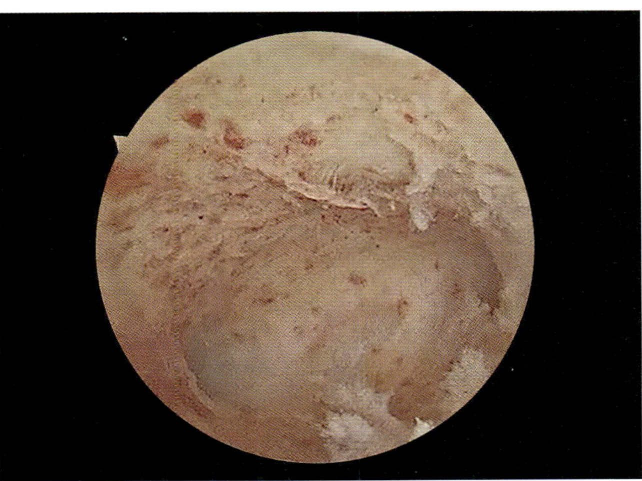

Fig. 1: Hysteroscopy finding of a classic T-shaped uterus where bilateral ostia are not visualized from the level of internal os.

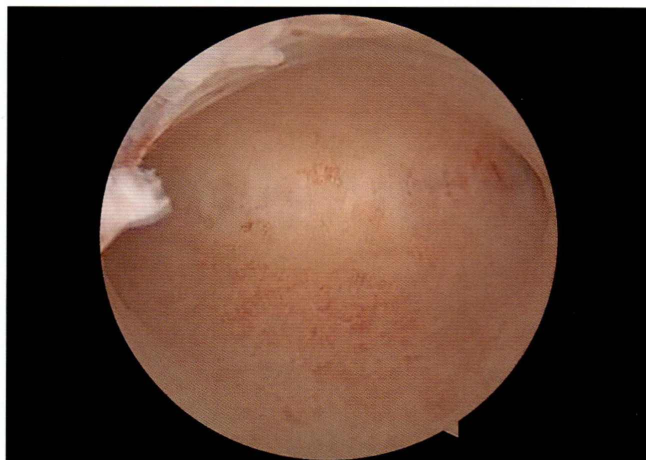

Fig. 2: Hysteroscopic findings in normal uterus where bilateral ostia can be visualized from the level of internal os.

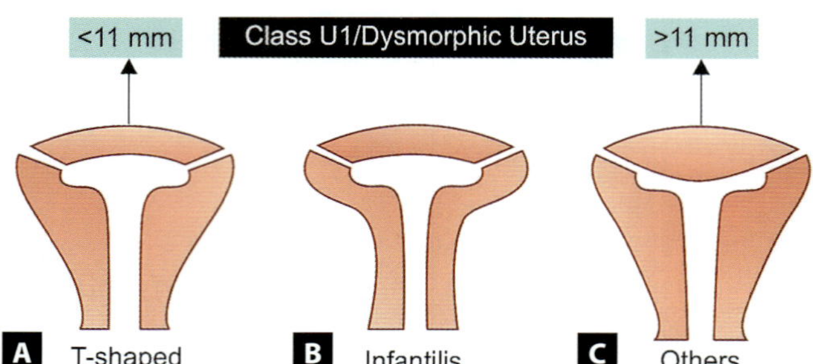

Figs. 3A to C: Illustration of dysmorphic uterus according to ESHRE and ESGE. (ESGE: European Society for Gynaecological Endoscopy; ESHRE: European Society of Human Reproduction and Embryology)

TABLE 1: Categorization of dysmorphic uterus.

T-shaped uterus (U1a)	***Uterus infantilis (U1b)***	***Others (T-shaped and subseptus U1c)***
Narrow uterine cavity due to thickened lateral walls	Narrow uterine cavity without thickened lateral walls	Include all minor deformities of the uterine cavity
Correlation corpus: Two-thirds versus cervix one-third	*Correlation corpus:* One-third versus cervix two-thirds	

A new classification of uterine malformation recently published by the European Society of Human Reproduction and Embryology (ESHRE) and the European Society for Gynaecological Endoscopy (ESGE) describes a new category defined as "dysmorphic uterus" for the T-shaped and its variants. The dysmorphic uterus is categorized as a class 1 uterine anomaly. This class incorporates three different subgroups of anomalies: (1) U1a (T-shaped uterus), (2) U1b (infantilis uterus), and (3) U1c (T-shaped uterus with partial septum)[10] **(Table 1 and Figs. 3A to C)**.

As described by Alonso et al., there are three subtypes for class U1a: (1) A classical T-shaped uterus defined as class U1a in ESHRE/ESGE classification, (2) a Y-shaped uterus **(Fig. 4B)** that has a fundal septum or subseptum and reduced interostial distance with the thickened lateral uterine walls, and (3) an I-shaped uterus **(Fig. 4A)** that defines a narrow tubular cavity.[11]

T-shaped Uterus and Reproductive Outcomes

Many studies have reported poor reproductive outcomes when this malformation is present. T-shaped uterus is associated with high rate of first-trimester miscarriage (47%) and a low rate of full-term delivery (21%). Many further studies have demonstrated that a dysmorphic uterus may account for reproductive failure when surgical correction is not undertaken.[12] Few studies have been published assessing pregnancy outcome after surgical treatment.[12,13] The various hypotheses for the poor reproductive outcomes suggested are:

- Narrowed uterine cavity
- Uncoordinated and aggravated muscular activity
- Abnormal expression of the endometrial proteins that play a role in endometrial implantation[14]

Diagnosis

The recent development of highly sensitive three-dimensional (3D) imaging and hysteroscopic surgery has enabled accurate diagnosis and treatment of uterine malformations with a minimally invasive approach, resulting in decreased morbidity.[15]

Today with advances in imaging, a 3D transvaginal (TV) ultrasonography (USG) is considered the gold standard for diagnosing congenital uterine anomalies and should be done during the luteal phase of the cycle (day 21–25). This is considered the optimal time to examine patients for uterine anomalies as the endometrium appears thick and echogenic clearly differentiating the uterine cavity from the surrounding myometrium.[14]

The Congenital Uterine Malformations by Experts (CUME) group has identified the best measurements **(Figs. 5A to C)** with good diagnostic test accuracy and fair-to-moderate interobserver reliability.[16] The cutoffs values for these measurements are:

- Lateral-indentation angle ≤130°
- Lateral-indentation depth ≥7 mm
- T-angle ≤40°

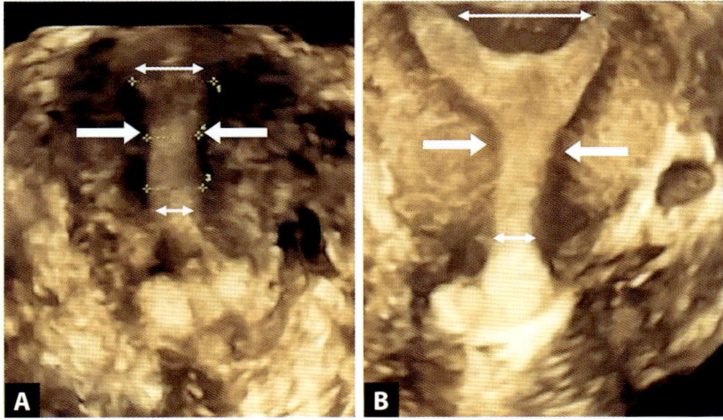

Figs. 4A and B: (A) I-shaped uterus; and (B) T-shaped uterus as described by Lui Alonso.

A T-shaped uterus is defined when all three criteria are present on a 3D uterine scan **(Figs. 6A to C)**.[16]

Using the above strict criteria, it should be much easier to study the prevalence of T-shaped uterus and assess its clinical relevance and not wrongly treat any narrow looking cavity as T- shaped uterus.

These three Congenital Uterine Malformations by Experts (CUME)[16] criteria for defining T-shaped uterus aid in determination of the prevalence, clinical implications, and management of women with this morphology and assessment of postsurgical morphologic outcome with sufficient accuracy and reliability and with a known probability of disease following negative and positive test results.

For the secondary type of T-shaped uterus, there will be history of instrumentation inside the uterine cavity, which can lead to lateral wall adhesions, only with associated scanty menstrual cycle or a past infection of tuberculosis.

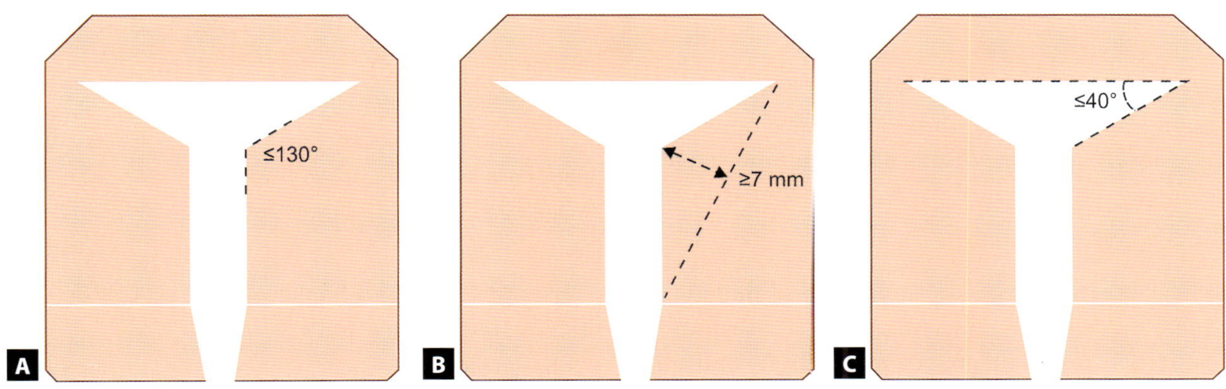

Figs. 5A to C: Congenital Uterine Malformations by Experts (CUME) criteria to define T-shaped uterus.

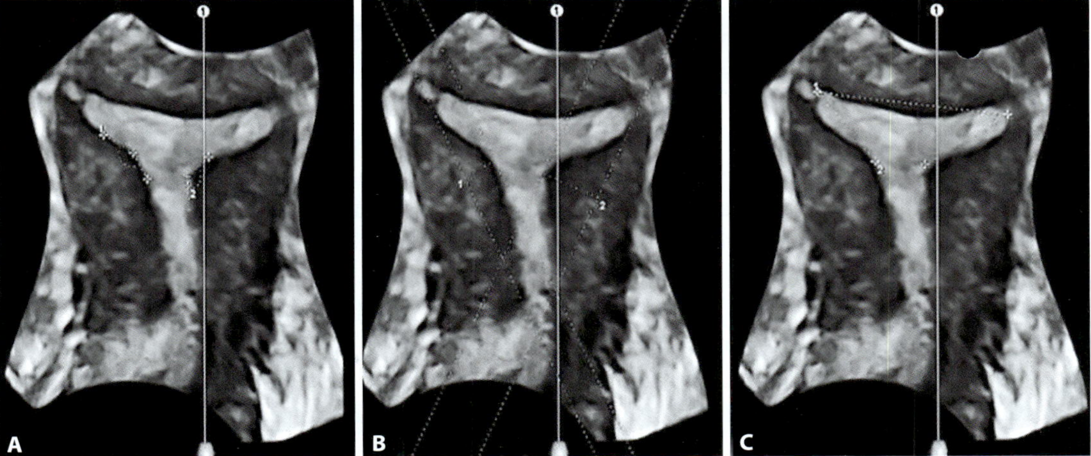

Figs. 6A to C: Measurements in three-dimensional ultrasonography (3D-USG) to define a T-shaped uterus.

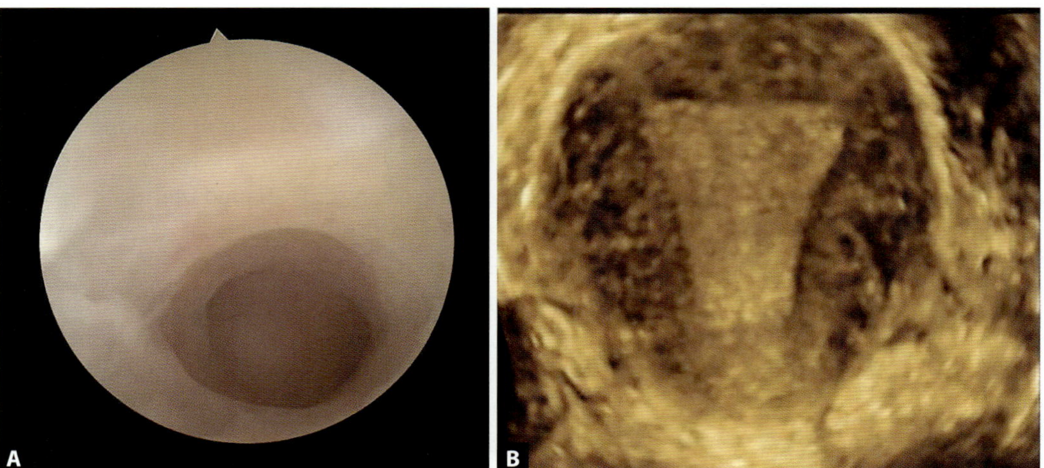

Figs. 7A and B: Secondary T-shaped uterus (hysteroscopic view) showing a narrow uterine cavity with three-dimensional ultrasonography (3D-USG) revealing normal muscle thickness.

The 3D-USG picture will reveal a normal uterine muscle thickness but a hysteroscopic view of narrow cavity as shown in **Figures 7A and B**.

Management of T-shaped Uterus

Significant improvement in the reproductive outcome of patients with dysmorphic uterus has been reported after hysteroscopic correction of dysmorphic uterus in case series.[17]

Şükür et al. retrospectively evaluated the reproductive outcome of 62 women with a T-shaped uterus undergoing lateral metroplasty with conventional 26-F resectoscope and reported a clinical pregnancy rate of 59.7% and a live birth rate of 75.6% after surgery.[18]

The recent advancement of hysteroscopic surgery has not only enabled accurate diagnosis but also treatment of uterine malformations with a minimally invasive approach, resulting in decreased morbidity and improved results.[12]

Ducellier-Azzola et al. confirmed reproductive improvement in patients with a T-shaped uterus after hysteroscopic metroplasty, with a significantly increased rate of live births (60 vs. 2.5%) and a reduced rate of early spontaneous miscarriage (22 vs. 78.3%).[19]

In a recent large multicenter study, conducted by Dr Attilio Sardo et al.,[20] a total of 214 patients with dysmorphic uterus were enrolled. The main baseline characteristics of these patients are summarized in **Table 2**.

The final reproductive outcome of the study is given in **Table 3**.

TABLE 2: Baseline characteristics of patients in the study conducted by Attilio et al.

Baseline patient characteristics (n = 214)	
Characteristic	*Value*
Age (in years), mean ± SD	36 ± 3.7
Caucasian ethnicity, n (%)	214 (100)
Body mass index (kg/m^2), mean ± SD	23.7 ± 5.4
Indications for surgery n (%)	
Primary infertility	166 (77.6)
Repeated spontaneous abortions (>2)	48 (22.4)
Subtypes of dysmorphic uteri n (%)	
T-shaped uterus	124 (57.9)
Tubular-shaped (infantilis uterus)	39 (18.3)
T-shaped with subseptum uterus	51 (23.8)

(SD: standard deviation)

Apart from improving pregnancy rate in spontaneous and assisted reproductive technology (ART), of particular interest is the improvement of term birth rate in patients with repeated miscarriage to 72.4% and a drop in miscarriage rate to 21.6%. The technique described by Attilio Sardo[20] to incise the lateral wall and subsequent increase on isthmic diameters can be well appreciated in **Figure 8**.

In modern-day hysteroscopy, the following are the techniques to do lateral metroplasty:

- 5-F scissors **(Fig. 9A)**
- 5-F electrodes, preferably bipolar

TABLE 3: Final reproductive outcomes in the study conducted by Attilio et al.

Outcome	Primary infertility number (%)	RPL number (%)	Total number (%)
Number	166	48	214
Clinical pregnancy	119/166 (71.6%)	37/48 (71%)	156/214 (72.9%)
Miscarriage rate	23/119 (19.3%)	8/37 (21.6%)	31/156 (19.9%)
Live birth rate/pregnancy	96/119 (80.6%)	29/37(78.3%)	125/156 (80.1%)
Delivery >34 weeks	91/96 (94.7%)	27/29 (93.1%)	118/125 (94.4%)

(RPL: recurrent pregnancy loss)

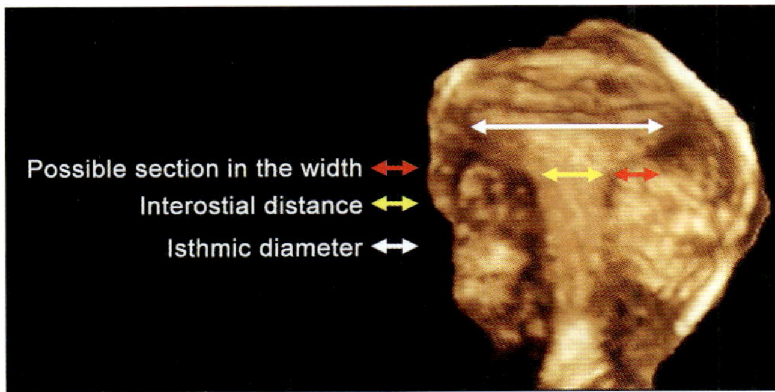

Fig. 8: Technique described by Attilio Sardo to incise the lateral wall to increase on isthmic diameters.

- Miniature resectoscope (15–16-F, bipolar): Here both Collins knife **(Fig. 9B)** or the loop could be used.

The above-mentioned techniques avoid the use of dilation of cervix, which apart from avoiding chances of perforation and false passage, decreases the chances of cervical incompetence significantly. Successful completion of the above procedures has been described in outpatient technique also **(Figs. 10A to D)**. However, there remains a lack of evidence on the impact of outpatient hysteroscopic correction of dysmorphic uterus in women reproductive failure.

FIBROIDS

The prevalence of fibroids and RPL varies from 0.5 to 1.3%, depending on the study.[4,22] Various mechanisms by which leiomyomas may adversely affect pregnancy development have been described. These include:

- Altered uterine contractility and disturbances in endometrial cytokine expression
- Abnormal vascularization and chronic endometrial inflammation
- Mechanical stretch of the endometrium and/or myometrium altering varying gene expressions.[23] *HOXA-10* levels have been reported to be reduced in the endometrium of women with submucous leiomyomas, not only in the tissue around the leiomyomas themselves but also elsewhere in the endometrial cavity.[24]

As per the International Federation of Gynecology and Obstetrics (FIGO) classification **(Table 4)**, fibroids altering the anatomy of the uterine cavity (FIGO 0–2) are susceptible of causing RPL. Submucosal fibroids (FIGO 0–2) have the strongest association with lower ongoing pregnancy rates and miscarriages, but according to certain reports, a correlation also exists between intramural fibroids and low-fertility outcomes.[25] Indeed, the size of intramural myomas can augment the risk of RPL, especially when myomas are >4 cm, a point of view that remains controversial according to certain researchers.[26] The presence of multiple fibroids is a significant predictor of miscarriage and RPL.[9] Subserosal myomas are not associated with miscarriages and/or poor fertility outcomes.[26]

Diagnosis

- *Ultrasound:* A good transvaginal ultrasound can pick most of the myomas and their relation to the endometrium. Recent introduction of 3D ultrasound has given additional benefits for proper mapping of fibroids and also for picking up congenital uterine anomalies in patients with RPL.
- *Sonohysterography:* It can also delineate submucosal myomas, and in the case of totally or partially intramural myomas (FIGO 3–5), it can indicate the proximity of intramural myomas to the endometrial cavity with high accuracy.
- *Magnetic resonance imaging (MRI):* It can be used as a second diagnostic test when ultrasound is not sufficiently informative and at times provides extra information, particularly on the number of myomas, size, and relationship with the serosal surface.

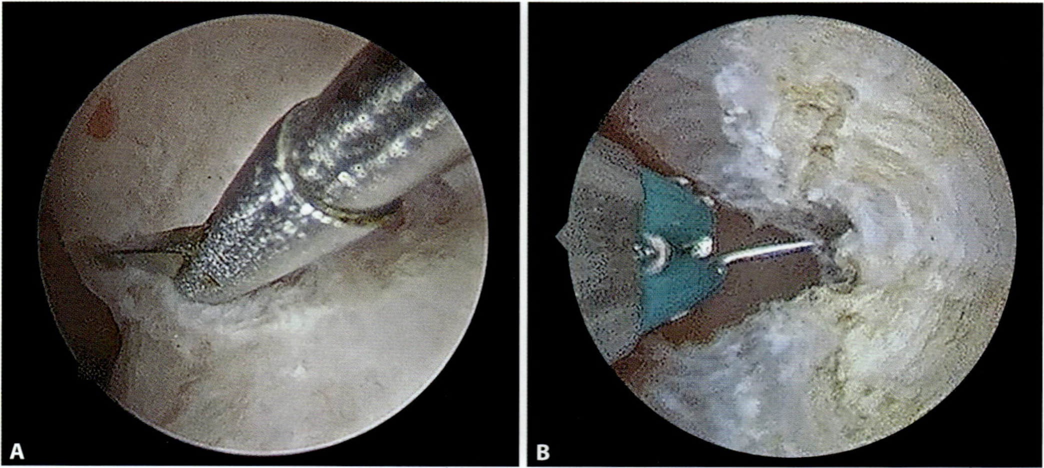

Figs. 9A and B: (A) 5-F scissors; and (B) Collins knife being used for lateral wall metroplasty.

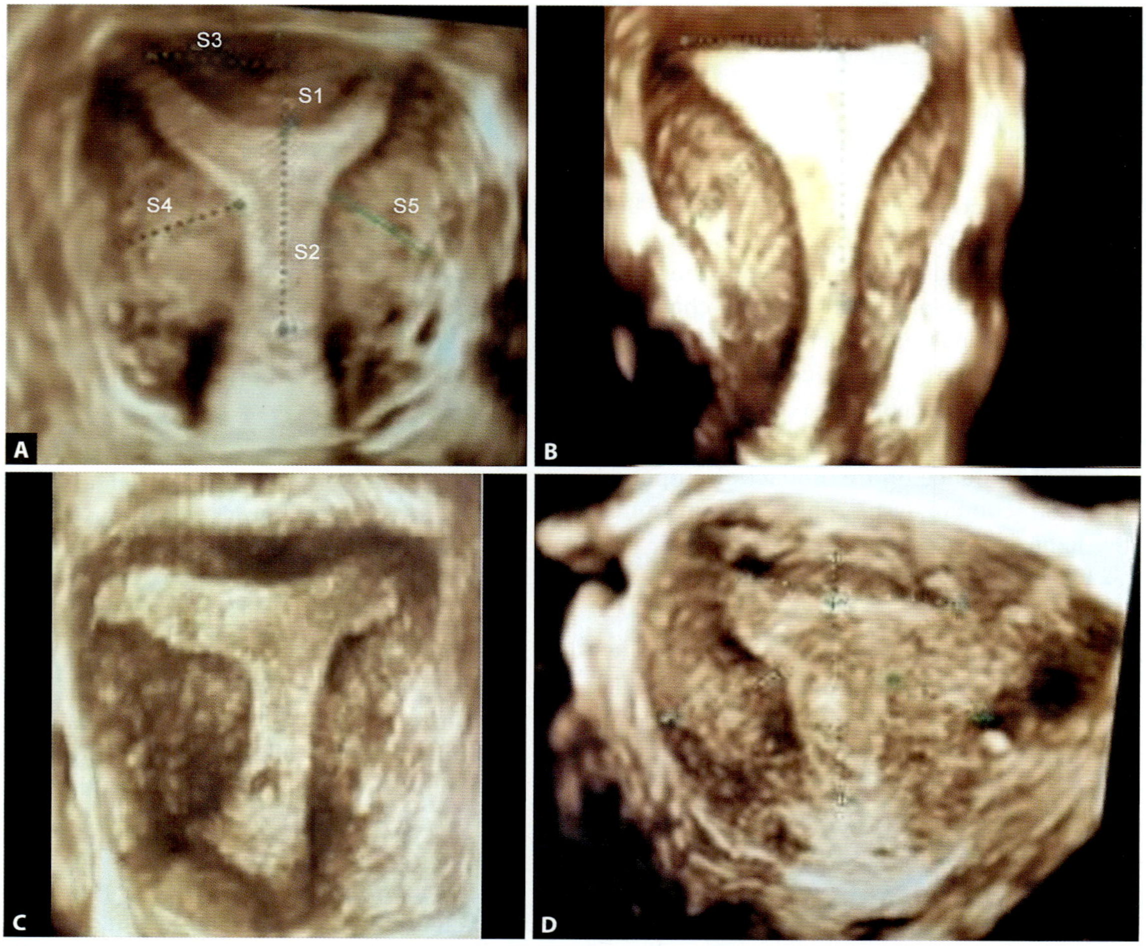

Figs. 10A to D: Preoperative and postoperative three-dimensional ultrasonography (3D-USG) image of: (A and B) Y-shaped uterus; and (C and D) T-shaped uterus.[21]

TABLE 4: FIGO classification of leiomyoma.[27]

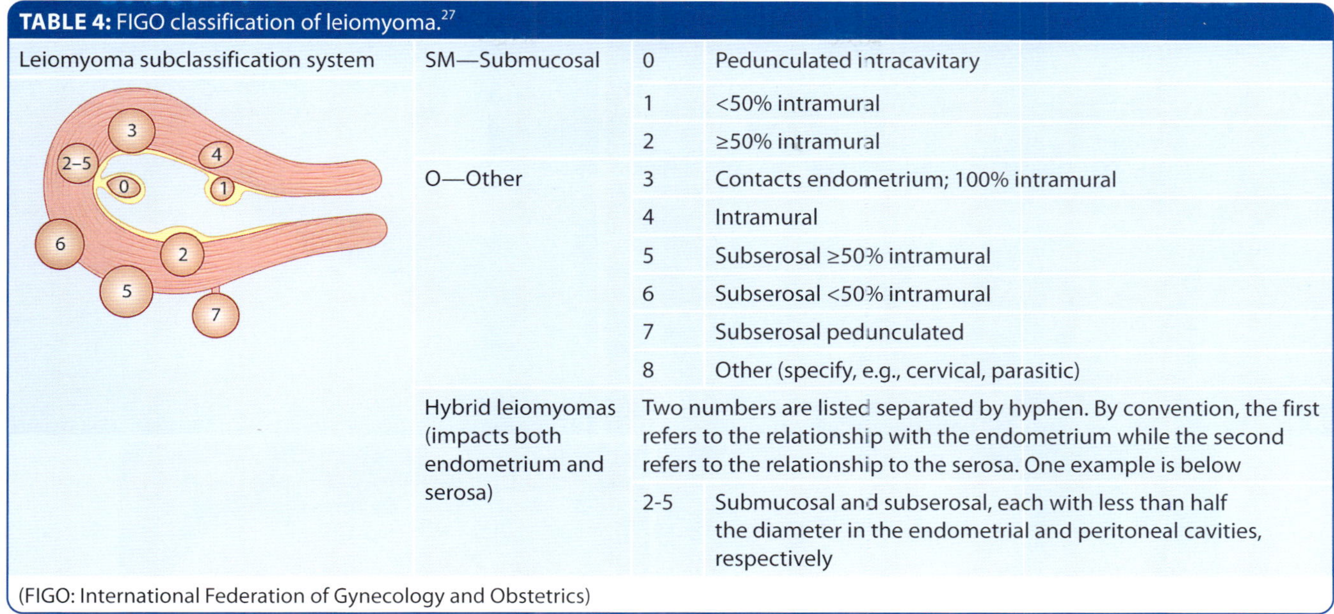

Leiomyoma subclassification system			
	SM—Submucosal	0	Pedunculated intracavitary
		1	<50% intramural
		2	≥50% intramural
	O—Other	3	Contacts endometrium; 100% intramural
		4	Intramural
		5	Subserosal ≥50% intramural
		6	Subserosal <50% intramural
		7	Subserosal pedunculated
		8	Other (specify, e.g., cervical, parasitic)
	Hybrid leiomyomas (impacts both endometrium and serosa)	Two numbers are listed separated by hyphen. By convention, the first refers to the relationship with the endometrium while the second refers to the relationship to the serosa. One example is below	
		2-5	Submucosal and subserosal, each with less than half the diameter in the endometrial and peritoneal cavities, respectively

(FIGO: International Federation of Gynecology and Obstetrics)

Management of Myomas with Recurrent Pregnancy Loss

Management of myomas has always been controversial regarding improving fertility or reproductive outcome. Myomectomy improves the chances of pregnancies in case of submucosal myomas, but the data are insufficient to support a true decrease in pregnancy losses and even less for the possible cure of RPL.[26] No clear benefit of surgery has been demonstrated for intramural myomas with no impact on the uterine cavity.

Though surgical removal of intramural fibroids is not recommended by international guidelines, one has to weigh other factors of RPL, age, and anxiety of the patient. In the presence of larger fibroids beyond 5 cm or multiple fibroids, myomectomy is offered to the patient. Today, laparoscopic myomectomy **(Figs. 11A to D)** is the preferred approach in most of the cases, taking care to do contained morcellation of the myoma tissues. A waiting period of minimum 3 months is to be followed postlaparoscopic myomectomy.

Hysteroscopy is the route commonly employed for submucosal myomas type 0–2 that are <4 cm **(Fig. 12)**. A two-stage procedure may be adopted in difficult cases. The various techniques for hysteroscopic myomectomy include:

- *Conventional slicing method:* This is routinely done with 22–26-F resectoscope. The chances of thermal damage and intravasation of fluid is more with this method. Since energy is used, the chances of IUAs are also more.
- *Hysteroscopic tissue retrieval systems (HTRS):* (Intrauterine morcellators) **(Fig. 13)**—The main advantage of this technique is that no energy is used, which may result in less damage to the endometrium and decreased incidence of adhesions. Its role is proven in type 0 and type 1 myomas but is of doubtful value in type 2 myomas. The other potential benefit is that it can be carried out in office settings.
- *Enucleation:* The enucleation technique was described by Mazzon in 1995 and Lasmar in 2001. These techniques have the same basis for enucleation, but Mazzon fragments the nodule until it reaches its intramural portion followed by mobilization using a "cold loop." Lasmar enucleates the entire fibroid followed by slicing it.

This technique involves incision of the endometrium around the submucosal myoma to reach the pseudocapsule (Lasmar) or reaching the plane by slicing the myoma close to the myometrium (Mazzon). Fibrous beams are to be sectioned after arriving at the pseudocapsule. The mobilization of the myoma progressively frees it from the myometrium without significant bleeding and thermal damage, with a low risk of intravasation, as the myometrial vessels are not cut. The mobilization of the myoma with its enucleation can be performed without energy with the use

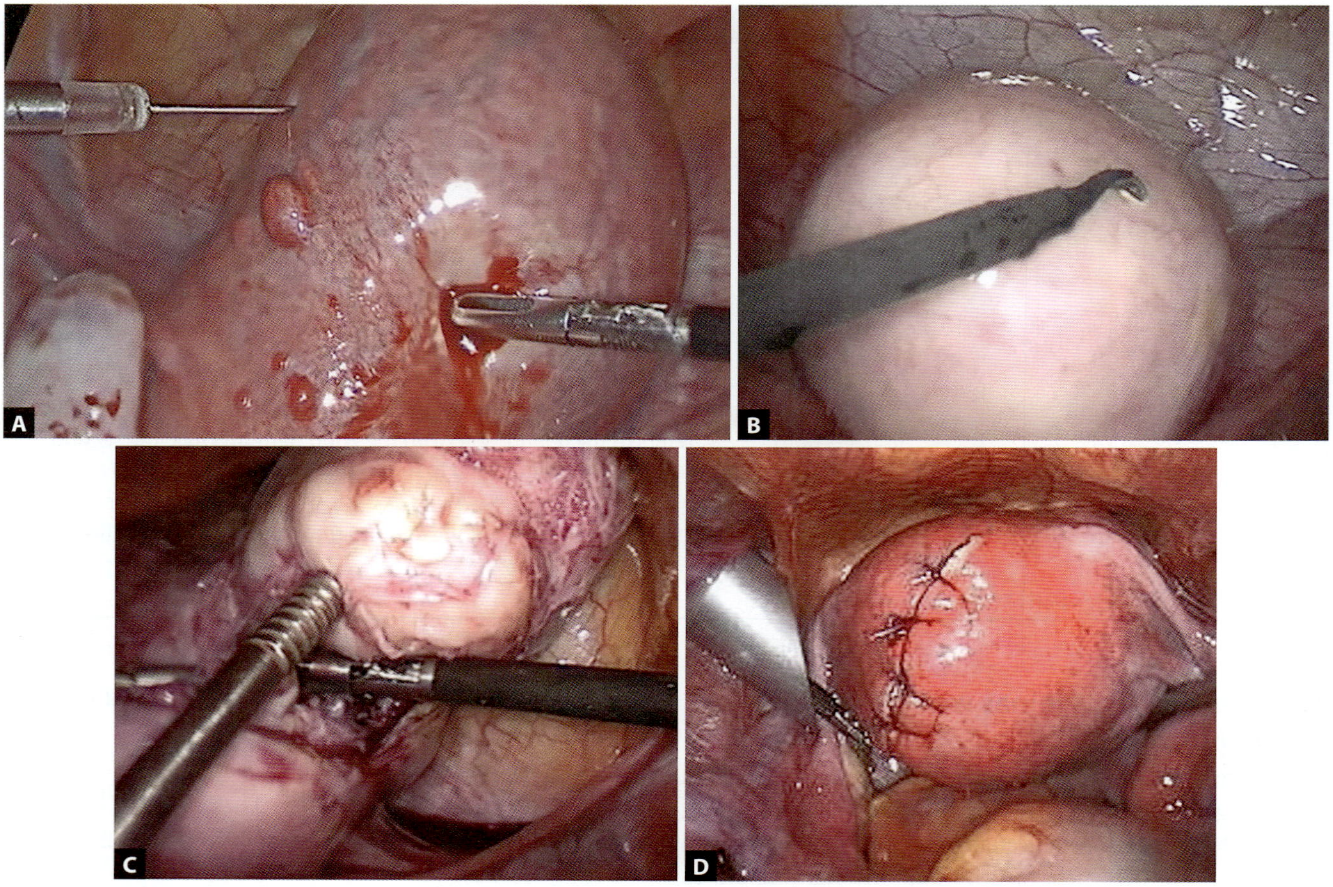

Figs. 11A to D: (A) Injection of vasopressin in pseudocapsule; (B) Incision over the myoma; (C) Enucleation of myoma along the pseudocapsule; and (D) Suturing the myoma bed.

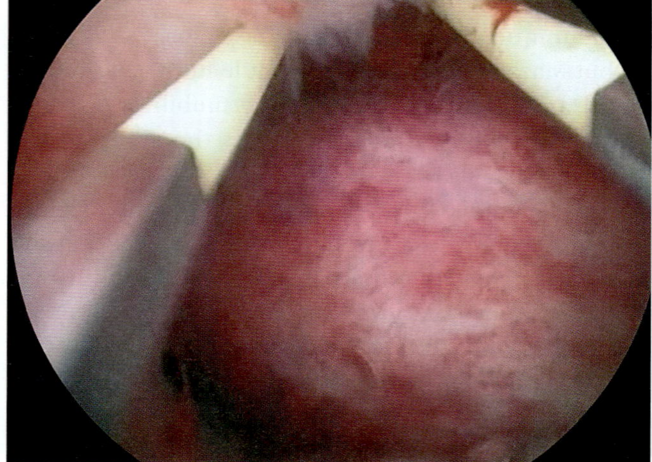

Fig. 12: Resectoscopic slicing for submucosal fibroid.

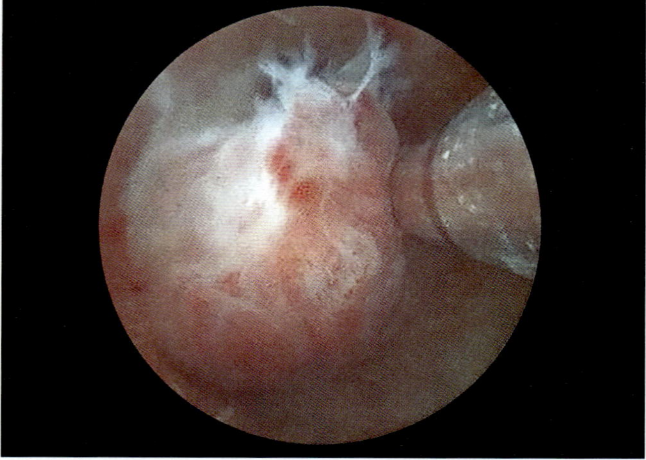

Fig. 13: Type 0 myoma and tissue retrieval system being used for myomectomy.

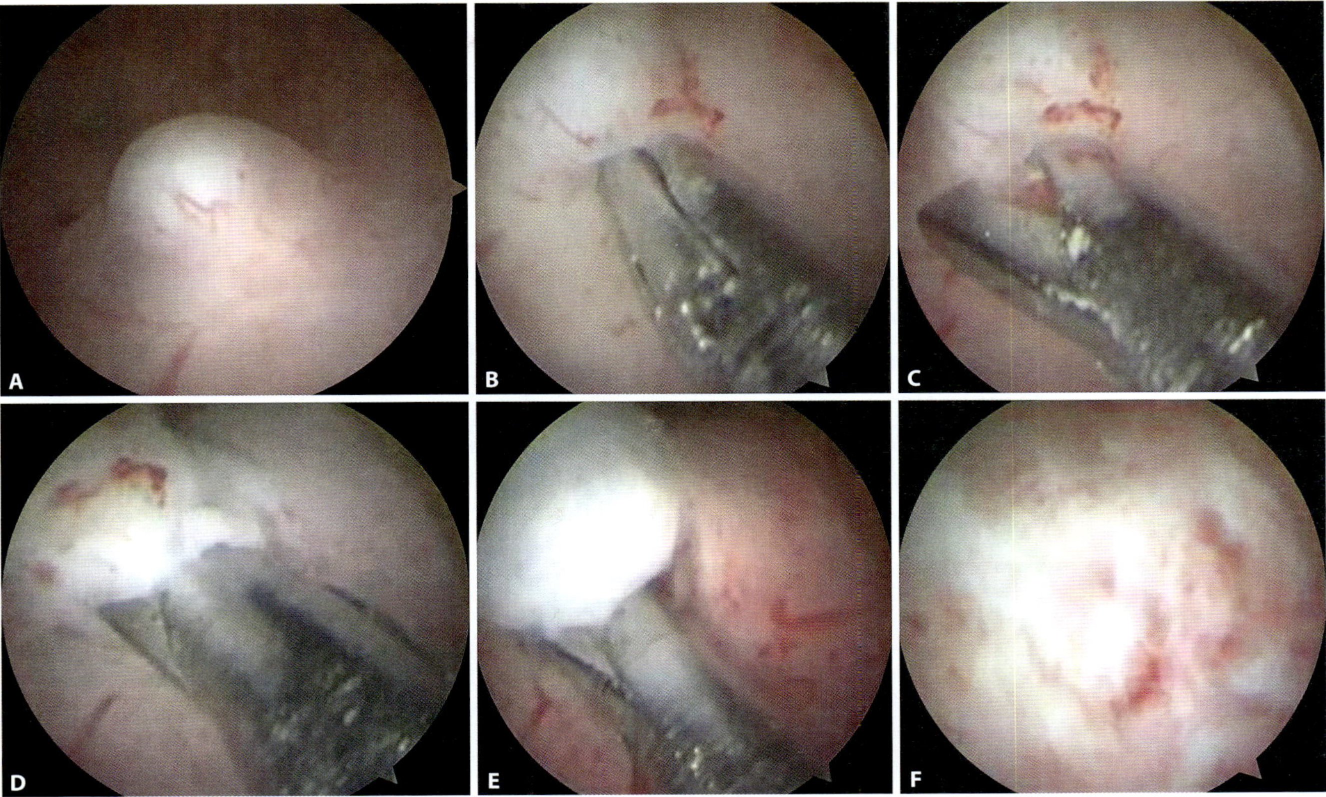

Figs. 14A to F: Stepwise hysteroscopic enucleation of the myoma.

of scissors being more appropriate in the outpatient clinic and Collins loop in hospital hysteroscopy **(Figs. 14A to F)**. As an outpatient procedure, a multicenter study has been published, which describes myoma enucleation without extraction, leaving the myoma for spontaneous expulsion that may take a few weeks.[28] As per the systematic review published by Ugo Indraccolo and Vittorio Bini, there is still no single hysteroscopic technique proven to be unequivocally superior to others for treating submucous fibroids with intramural development in one-surgical step.[29]

Apart from inherent complications during various methods of hysteroscopic myomectomy, postoperative adhesions can develop, necessitating a relook hysteroscopy before the patient is allowed to go for a pregnancy.[29]

Similar postoperative complications and cesarean rates have been observed with abdominal myomectomy and laparascopic myomectomy.[30]

ENDOMETRIAL POLYPS

The prevalence of endometrial polyps related to RPL varies from 1.6 to 6%,[4,22] but there is no clear evidence showing an association with RPLs. The morphology of endometrial polyps varies considerably, from millimeters to centimeters in the largest dimension, sessile or pedunculated in shape, and single or multiple in number. Their impact on fertility could be mainly due to:

- Mechanical interference
- Increased release of molecules such as glycodelin, inflammatory markers, and aromatase
- Decreased levels of *HOXA*-10 and 11 messenger ribonucleic acid (RNA)

Diagnosis

- Ultrasound should be able to pick up most of the polyps.
- Sonohysterography may be useful in 20–30% of cases not picked by USG.

Management

Universally accepted recommendations have not been accepted for polyp management. Endometrial polyps are commonly removed when identified as clinicians may not know when these findings negatively impact early pregnancy development. Hysteroscopy is the gold standard in removing endometrial polyps, which could be done either in operating room or as an outpatient procedure by one of the following methods:

- *5-Fr scissors or electrodes:* In case of larger polyps, the slicing of the polyps may be required to be sliced before they could be removed **(Fig. 15)**.
- *Resectoscope:* Any resectoscope varying from 15 to 26-F can be used for the resection of the polyps, but it is always preferred to use the smallest resectoscope **(Figs. 16A and B)**.

INTRAUTERINE ADHESIONS

The prevalence of IUAs in RPL varies from 1.3 to 9.6%.[31] Except for genital Koch's, IUA is totally an iatrogenic disease caused by traumatic denudation of the basalis layer of the endometrium. Dilation and curettage (D&C) was always considered the only culprit for this condition, especially done for obstetric conditions such as termination of pregnancy and postpartum bleeding.[3] Infection of the endometrium is an important cause of IUAs. The number of D&Cs is also a significant factor in increasing the severity of adhesions. In a country like India, the incidence can be much more than reported because of following factors: (1) High number of both therapeutic and illegal abortions; (2) Use of sharp curettage for performing the same; (3) Higher incidence of genital tuberculosis and puerperal infection; and (4) Lower awareness of the clinical condition till now. With the widespread use of hysteroscopy for intrauterine surgery, the number of reported cases of IUA has been increasing.[32] The reported incidence of adhesions after various intrauterine surgery is shown in **Table 5**.

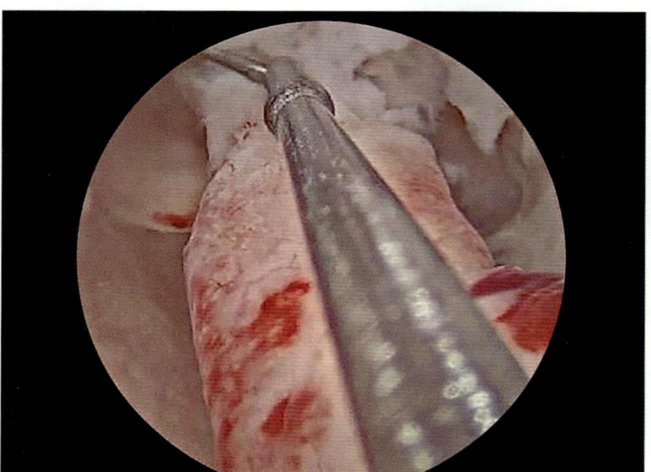

Fig. 15: Use of hysteroscopic scissors for polypectomy.

There are no studies assessing IUAs as a cause—or a consequence—of RPL. However, the presence of moderate-to-severe IUAs may greatly affect fertility and predisposes to pregnancy and obstetrical complications. IUAs may lead to pregnancy loss due to insufficient endometrial development for supporting the fetoplacental growth.[9]

Diagnosis

Apart from a strong suspicion with the classic history of hypomenorrhea, following any surgical intervention inside the uterine cavity and subfertility, the following are the routine investigations done to confirm the diagnosis:

- Hysteroscopy is the most accurate method for diagnosis of IUAs and should be the investigation of choice when available.[7] It provides a real-time view of the cavity and

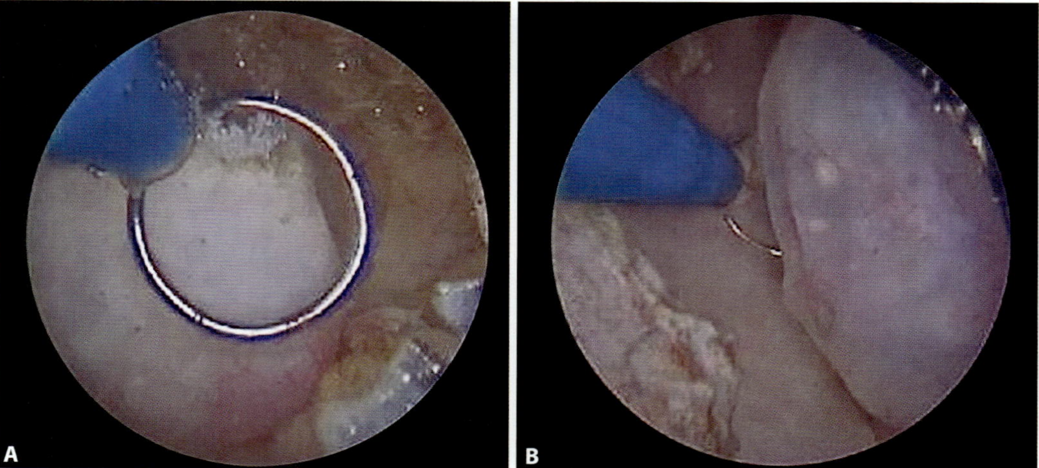

Figs. 16A and B: Mini resectoscope for polypectomy.

helps classify the location and extent of the disease.[33] It can be performed as an outpatient procedure with ability to treat at the same time **(Figs. 17A to D)**.

- If hysteroscopy is not available, hysterosalpingography (HSG)[33] and hysterosonography are reasonable alternatives.[34] On HSG-filling defects with homogenous opacity clinches the diagnosis of IUA. Transvaginal ultrasound alone may not be enough, but combined with sonohysterogram, it yields result similar to HSG.[34] Doppler sonography has shown promise for diagnosis and follow-up postadhesiolysis.[35]
- Magnetic resonance imaging is rarely used because of unproven diagnostic ability and expense involved.

TABLE 5: Reported incidence of adhesions after intrauterine surgery.

Procedure	*Reported cases of IUA*
D&C	19.1%
Uterine septal incision	6.7%
Single myoma resection	31.3%
Multiple myoma resection	45.5%
Diagnostic hysteroscopy	1.6%

(D&C: dilation and curettage; IUA: intrauterine adhesion)
Source: Khan Z, Goldberg JM. Hysteroscopic management of Asherman's syndrome. J Minim Invasive Gynecol. 2018;25(2):218-28.

Management

No guideline exists about the proper management of IUAs. Hysteroscopic surgery is now the treatment of choice for Asherman's syndrome (AS), because it can be performed under vision with minimal trauma.[36]

Today with increasing application of miniature hysteroscopes (2.9 mm, 2.7 mm, and 1.9 mm) with overall diameter of operative sheath reduced to 3.5 mm, even in very difficult cases of cervical stenosis and adhesions it is easy to negotiate and complete a good job inside the uterine cavity. Adhesiolysis is done starting inferiorly and advancing cephalically until the uterine architecture has

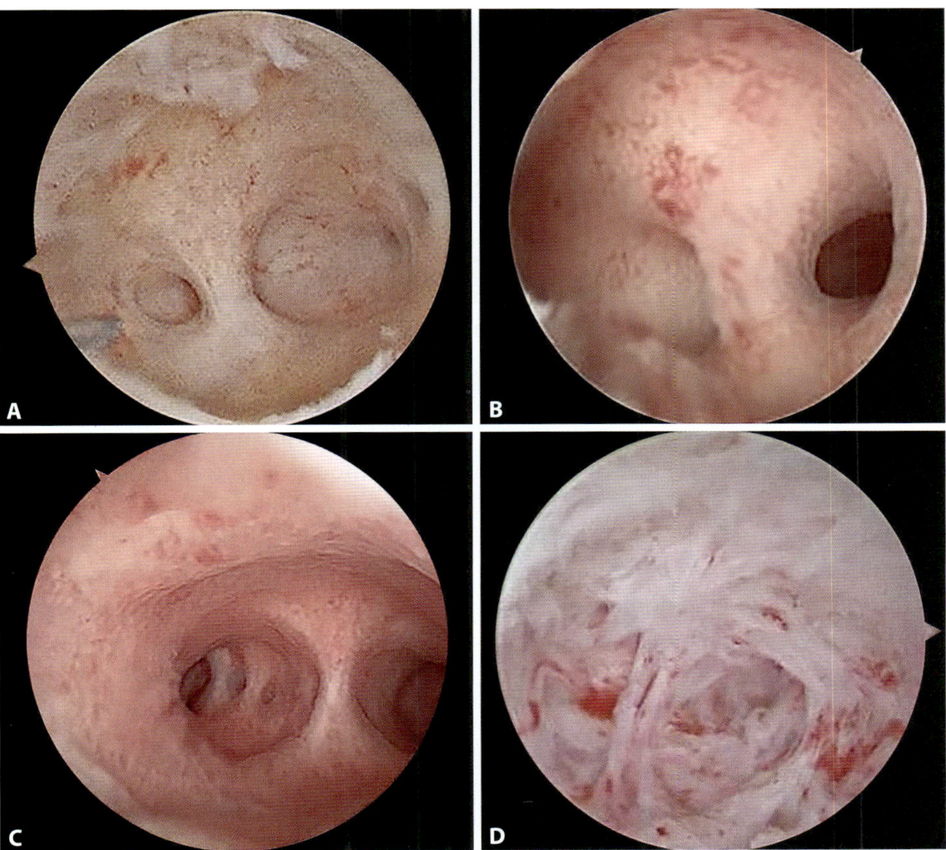

Figs. 17A to D: Hysteroscopic views of various intrauterine adhesions.

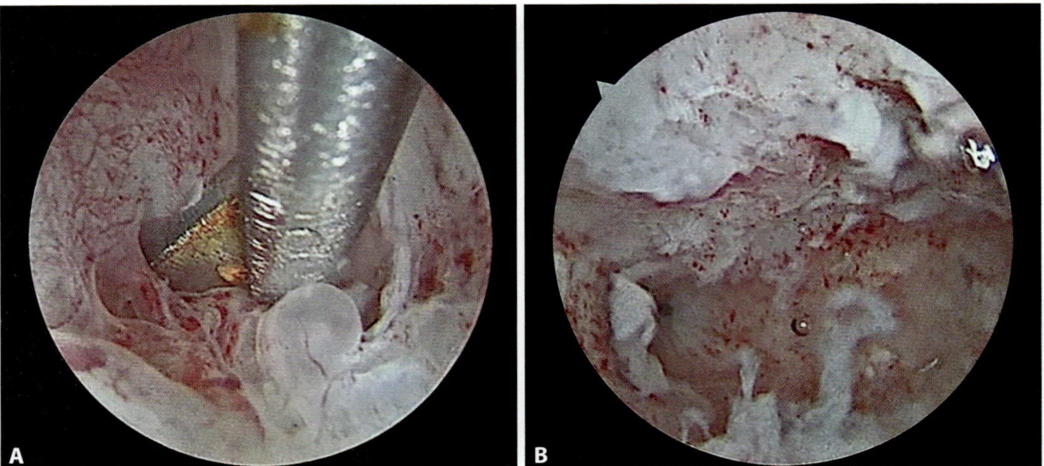

Figs. 18A and B: (A) Hysteroscopic scissors for adhesiolysis; and (B) Hysteroscopic view after adhesiolysis.

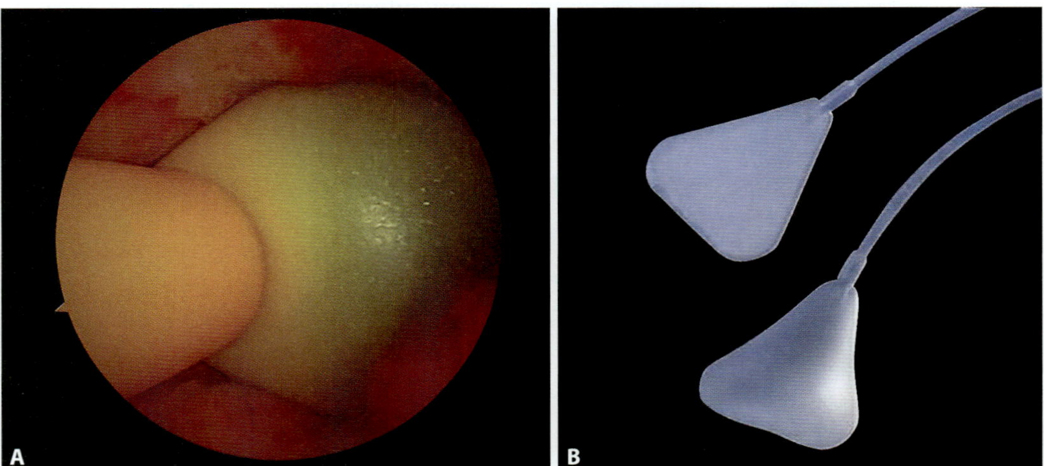

Figs. 19A and B: Physical barriers used after adhesiolysis.

been normalized. It can be performed through operative hysteroscopy by using:

- Hysteroscopic scissors (5-F and 7-F) **(Figs. 18A and B)**
- Bipolar needle

The main advantage of using scissors for adhesiolysis is that it avoids complications related to energy sources and possibly minimizes the destruction of endometrium. In a recent meta-analysis published by Yang et al. comparing cold scissors versus electrosurgery found a significant lower recurrence rate, shorter operating time, and higher menstrual flow with cold scissors over electrosurgery.[37]

Hysteroscopic diode lasers—the diode laser with a fiber of 1,470 nm—can also be used for adhesiolysis, but as mentioned avoid energy sources as far as possible and use mechanical methods such as scissors.

None of these techniques has been compared with others; consequently, there is no available evidence that one method is superior. But as with any repair surgery, results will be better in the first sitting, and any subsequent attempts, there will be a fall in the prognosis.

But it is also important to counsel all patients with severe adhesions that a second-look hysteroscopy will give better prognosis. Ultrasound, fluoroscopy, and laparoscopy are adjunctive interventions to aid adhesiolysis, but there is no data to suggest that these prevent perforation or improve surgical outcomes.

The recurrence is common and may occur in 30–66% of women treated for IUAs.[38] The postoperative strategies to prevent IUA include barriers (physical/gel) **(Figs. 19A and B)** to separate the opposing walls with or without the use of estrogen preparations and adjuvants to regenerate the endometrium faster.

Guidelines for Secondary Prevention of Intrauterine Adhesions[38]

The following American Association of Gynecologic Laparoscopists (AAGL) and ESGE practice guidelines on their use seem to be useful at this point of time:

- The use of an intrauterine device (IUD), stent, or catheter appears to reduce the rate of postoperative adhesion reformation. There are limited data regarding subsequent fertility outcomes when these barriers are used (grade A).
- The risk of infection appears to be minimal when a solid barrier is used compared with no treatment (grade A).
- There is no evidence to support or refute the use of preoperative, intraoperative, or postoperative antibiotic therapy in surgical treatment of IUAs (grade C).
- If an IUD is used postoperatively, it should be inert and have a large surface area such as a Lippes loop. IUDs that contain progestin or copper should not be used after surgical division of IUAs (grade C).
- Semisolid barriers such as hyaluronic acid and auto-cross-linked hyaluronic acid gel reduce adhesion reformation. At this time, their effect on posttreatment pregnancy rates is unknown (grade A).
- Following hysteroscopic-directed adhesiolysis, postoperative hormone treatment using estrogen, with or without progestin, may reduce recurrence of IUAs (grade B).
- The role of medications designed as adjuvants to improve vascular flow to the endometrium has not been established. Consequently, they should not be used outside rigorous research protocols (grade C).
- Stem-cell treatment may ultimately provide an effective adjuvant approach to the treatment of AS; however, evidence is very limited and this treatment should not be offered outside rigorous research protocols (grade C).

The initial severity of adhesions appears to strongly correlate with reproductive outcome, with severe adhesions having the highest rate of recurrence.[39] Precautions must also be taken to prevent such recurrences after hysteroscopic resections of IUAs.[40] These precautions include, notably, practicing second-look office hysteroscopy for identifying and easily removing newly formed IUAs approximately 4 weeks after surgery, and also strict follow-up with sonography for endometrial thickness and blood flow. The pregnancy rate of 66% and live birth rate of 61% are being reported after adhesiolysis with postoperative adjuvants including one or a combination of IUD, balloon, estrogen, and hyaluronic acid of moderate-to-severe AS. The success rate, defined as normal menstruation, was 95%.[38]

Many recent studies have suggested that after hysteroscopic adhesiolysis, women have increased risk of serious perinatal complications, such as placenta previa, placental abruption, or morbidly adherent and retained placenta.[14] Also, other complications including postpartum hemorrhage and neonatal complications, including preterm birth, intrauterine growth restriction (IUGR), and stillbirth were reported.[41-43] In a recent study published in the *Human Reproduction* by Mára et al. have reported that surgical treatment for moderate-to-severe AS is associated with a number of serious perinatal complications and increased risks of preterm delivery, though without impacts on intrauterine growth and outcomes of the neonate. The most serious complications reported in AS patients were retained placenta requiring manual or surgical removal and associated postpartum hemorrhage, which were observed in 46.7% and 31.7% patients, respectively, especially after D&C performed postpartum and after repeated hysteroscopy treatments preceding the index pregnancy.[44]

The severity of perinatal morbidity of patients after postpartum D&C suggests that conservative or noninvasive retained products of conception (RPOC) management should be considered to avoid unnecessary surgery and minimize the damage to endometrium to decrease the incidence of IUAs. If D&C is unavoidable, use of hysteroscopic techniques instead of blind curettages in order to minimize the damage to the uterus as well as to minimize the risk of repeated procedures is advocated.[44]

A novel technique as described by Shi et al. is intermittent balloon dilation therapy on 2nd and 6th weeks following adhesiolysis **(Fig. 20)** is cheap, feasible, and effective, and has been suggested in order to decrease the adhesions reformation rate with significant results.[45]

CONCLUSION

Recurrent pregnancy loss is a complication having significant impact on the couple. With the advent of newer and easier modalities of diagnosis such as 3D-USG, the easily correctable causes of RPL can be effectively

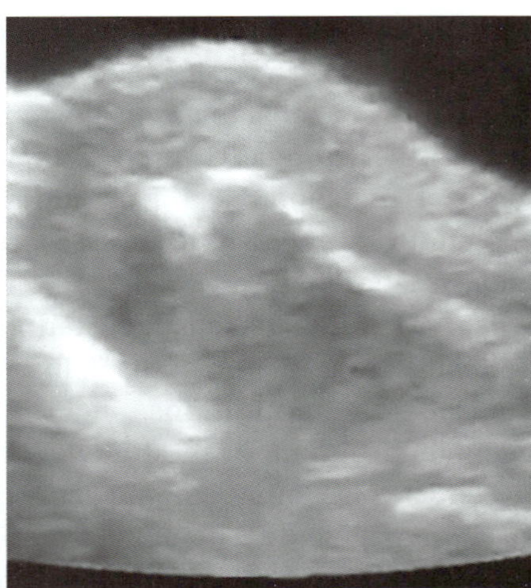

Fig. 20: Use of intermittent balloon dilation under ultrasonography (USG) guidance.

diagnosed with accuracy. Hysteroscopic approach to correction of submucosal myomas and polyps is well known, but hysteroscopic correction of T-shaped has opened new horizons in management of RPL. Early and timely hysteroscopic treatment of IUA is important for better long-term results. With easy and effective diagnostic techniques and minimally invasive procedures to treat the same, a good obstetric career can be provided to women with RPL.

REFERENCES

1. ESHRE Guideline Group on RPL, Atik RB, Christiansen OB, Elson J, Kolte AM, Lewis S, et al. ESHRE guideline: recurrent pregnancy loss. Hum Reprod Open. 2018;2018(2):hoy004.
2. Rock JA, Zacur HA. The clinical management of repeated early pregnancy. Fertil Steril. 1983;39(2):123-40.
3. van Dijk MM, Kolte AM, Limpens J, Kirk E, Quenby S, van Wely M, et al. Recurrent pregnancy loss: diagnostic workup after two or three pregnancy losses? A systematic review of the literature and meta-analysis. Hum Reprod Update. 2020;26(3):356-67.
4. Medrano-Uribe FA, Enríquez-Pérez MM, Reyes-Muñoz E. Prevalence of uterine anatomical anomalies in Mexican women with recurrent pregnancy loss (RPL). Gac Med Mex. 2016;152(6):163-6.
5. Hooker AB, Lemmers M, Thurkow AL, Heymans MW, Opmeer BC, Brölmann HAM, et al. Systematic review and meta-analysis of intrauterine adhesions after miscarriage: prevalence, risk factors and long-term reproductive outcome. Hum Reprod Update. 2014;20(2):262-78.
6. Ono S, Yonezawa M, Watanabe K, Abe T, Mine K, Kuwabara Y, et al. Retrospective cohort study of the risk factors for secondary infertility following hysteroscopic metroplasty of the uterine septum in women with recurrent pregnancy loss. Reprod Med Biol. 2018;17(1):77-81.
7. Seckin B, Sarikaya E, Oruc AS, Celen S, Cicek N. Office hysteroscopic findings in patients with two, three, and four or more, consecutive miscarriages. Eur J Contracept Reprod Health Care. 2012;17(5):393-8.
8. Practice Committee of the American Society for Reproductive Medicine. Definitions of infertility and recurrent pregnancy loss: a committee opinion. Fertil Steril. 2020;113(3):533-5.
9. Carbonnel M, Pirtea P, de Ziegler D, Ayoubi JM. Uterine factors in recurrent pregnancy losses. Fertil Steril. 2021;115(3):538-45.
10. Grimbizis GF, Gordts S, Di Spiezio Sardo A, Brucker S, De Angelis C, Gergolet M, et al. The ESHRE/ESGE consensus on the classification of female genital tract congenital anomalies. Hum Reprod. 2013;28(8):2032-44.
11. Alonso L, Haimovich S, Di Spiezio Sardo A, Carugno J. Dysmorphic uterus: do we need a T-Y-I subclassification? J Minim Invasive Gynecol. 2020;27(1):4-6.
12. Di Spiezio Sardo A, Campo R, Zizolfi B, Santangelo F, Furst RM, Di Cesare C, et al. Long-term reproductive outcomes after hysteroscopic treatment of dysmorphic uteri in women with reproductive failure: an European multicenter study. J Minim Invasive Gynecol. 2020;27(3):755-62.
13. Pacheco LA, Laganà AS, Garzon S, Garrido AP, Gornés AF, Ghezzi F. Hysteroscopic outpatient metroplasty for T-shaped uterus in women with reproductive failure: results from a large prospective cohort study. Eur J Obstet Gynecol Reprod Biol. 2019;243:173-8.
14. Zhang Y, Zhu Y, Ge B, Sui M, Zheng Z, Sun J. Reproductive outcome of hysteroscopic metroplasty for women with T-shaped uterus: a retrospective study. Reprod Health. 2022;19(1):78.
15. Di Spiezio Sardo A, Zizolfi B, Bettocchi S, Exacoustos C, Nocera C, Nazzaro G, et al. Accuracy of hysteroscopic metroplasty with the combination of presurgical 3-dimensional ultrasonography and a novel graduated intrauterine palpator: a randomized controlled trial. J Minim Invasive Gynecol. 2016;23(4):557-66.
16. Ludwin A, Coelho Neto MA, Ludwin I, Nastri CO, Costa W, Acién M, et al. Congenital uterine malformation by experts (CUME): diagnostic criteria for T-shaped uterus. Ultrasound Obstet Gynecol. 2020;55(6):815-29.
17. Uyar E, Usal D, Selam B, Cincik M, Bagis T. IVF outcomes after hysteroscopic metroplasty in patients with T-shaped uterus. Fertil Res Pract. 2019;5:15.
18. Şükür YE, Yakıştıran B, Özmen B, Sönmezer M, Berker B, Atabekoğlu C. Hysteroscopic corrections for complete septate and T-shaped uteri have similar surgical and reproductive outcome. Reprod Sci. 2018;25(12):1649-54.
19. Ducellier-Azzola G, Lecointre L, Hummel M, Pontvianne M, Garbin O. Hysteroscopic enlargement metroplasty for T-shaped uterus: 24 years' experience at the Strasbourg

medico-surgical and obstetrical centre (CMCO). Eur J Obstet Gynecol Reprod Biol. 2018;226:30-4.
20. Di Spiezio Sardo A, Campo R, Zizolfi B, Santangelo F, Meier Furst R, Di Cesare C, et al. Long-Term Reproductive Outcomes after Hysteroscopic Treatment of Dysmorphic Uteri in Women with Reproductive Failure: An European Multicenter Study. J Minim Invasive Gynecol. 2020;27(3):755-62. PMID: 31146029.
21. Dilbaz B, Mert SA, Diktas EG, Kose C, Ustun YE. The effect of hysteroscopic metroplasty on fertility in T-shaped and Y-shaped dysmorphic uterus. Eur J Contracept Reprod Health Care. 2022;27(5):384-9.
22. Galamb Á, Pethő B, Fekete D, Petrányi G, Pajor A. Uterine anomalies in women with recurrent pregnancy loss. Orv Hetil. 2015;156(27):1081-4.
23. Norian JM, Owen CM, Taboas J, Korecki C, Tuan R, Malik M, et al. Characterization of tissue biomechanics and mechanical signaling in uterine leiomyoma. Matrix Biol. 2012;31(1):57-65.
24. Rackow BW, Jorgensen E, Taylor HS. Endometrial polyps affect uterine receptivity. Fertil Steril. 2011;95(8): 2690-2.
25. Horcajadas JA, Goyri E, Higón MA, Martínez-Conejero JA, Gambadauro P, García G, et al. Endometrial receptivity and implantation are not affected by the presence of uterine intramural leiomyomas: a clinical and functional genomics analysis. J Clin Endocrinol Metab. 2008;93(9): 3490-8.
26. Pritts EA, Parker WH, Olive DL. Fibroids and infertility: an updated systematic review of the evidence. Fertil Steril. 2009;91(4):1215-23.
27. Munro MG, Critchley HOD, Fraser IS, FIGO Menstrual Disorders Working Group. The FIGO classification of causes of abnormal uterine bleeding in the reproductive years. Fertil Steril. 2011;95(7):2204-8, 2208.e1-3.
28. Tinelli A, Favilli A, Lasmar RB, Mazzon I, Gerli S, Xue X, et al. The importance of pseudocapsule preservation during hysteroscopic myomectomy. Eur J Obstet Gynecol Reprod Biol. 2019;243:179-84.
29. Indraccolo U, Bini V, Favilli A. Likelihood of accomplishing an in-patient hysteroscopic myomectomy in a one-step procedure: a systematic review and meta-analysis. Biomed Res Int. 2020;2020:4208497.
30. Tian YC, Long TF, Dai YM. Pregnancy outcomes following different surgical approaches of myomectomy. J Obstet Gynaecol Res. 2015;41(3):350-7.
31. Yu D, Wong YM, Cheong Y, Xia E, Li TC. Asherman syndrome—one century later. Fertil Steril. 2008;89(4): 759-79.
32. Khan Z, Goldberg JM. Hysteroscopic management of Asherman's syndrome. J Minim Invasive Gynecol. 2018;25(2):218-28.
33. Magos A. Hysteroscopic treatment of Asherman's syndrome. Reprod Biomed Online. 2002;4(Suppl. 3):46-51.
34. Soares SR, dos Reis MMB, Camargos AF. Diagnostic accuracy of sonohysterography, transvaginal sonography, and hysterosalpingography in patients with uterine cavity diseases. Fertil Steril. 200;73(2):406-11.
35. Yan L, Wang A, Bai R, Shang W, Zhao Y, Wang W, et al. Application of SonoVue combined with three-dimensional color power angiography in the diagnosis and prognosis evaluation of Intrauterine adhesion. Eur J Gynecol Reprod Biol. 2016;198:68-72.
36. Kodaman PH, Arici A. Intra-uterine adhesions and fertility outcome: how to optimize success? Curr Opin Obstet Gynecol. 2007;19(3):207-14.
37. Yang L, Wang L, Chen Y, Guo X, Miao C, Zhao Y, et al. Cold scissors versus electrosurgery for hysteroscopic adhesiolysis: a meta-analysis. Medicine (Baltimore). 2021;100(17):e25676.
38. AAGL practice report: practice guidelines on intrauterine adhesions developed in collaboration with the European Society of Gynaecological Endoscopy (ESGE). Gynecol Surg. 2017;14(1):6.
39. McComb PF, Wagner BL. Simplified therapy for Asherman's syndrome. Fertil Steril. 1997;68(6):1047-50.
40. Newton JR, MacKenzie WE, Emens MJ, Jordan JA. Division of uterine adhesions (Asherman's syndrome) with the Nd-YAG laser. Br J Obstet Gynaecol. 1989;96(1):102-4.
41. Deans R, Vancaillie T, Ledger W, Liu J, Abbott JA. Live birth rate and obstetric complications following the hysteroscopic management of intrauterine adhesions including Asherman syndrome. Hum Reprod. 2018;33(10):1847-53.
42. Feng Q, Gao B, Huang H, Woo JJ, Zou L, Zhao X, et al. Obstetrical outcome in the third trimester after hysteroscopic adhesiolysis. Ann Transl Med. 2020;8(4):51.
43. Baradwan S, Shafi D, Baradwan A, Bashir MS, Al-Jaroudi D. The effect of endometrial thickness on pregnancy outcome in patients with Asherman's syndrome post-hysteroscopic adhesiolysis. Int J Womens Health. 2018;10:77-82.
44. Mára M, Borčinová M, Lisá Z, Boudová B, Richtárová A, Kužel D. The perinatal outcomes of women treated for Asherman syndrome: a propensity score-matched cohort study. Hum Reprod. 2023;38(7):1297-304.
45. Shi X, Saravelos SH, Zhou Q, Huang X, Xia E, Li TC. Prevention of postoperative adhesion reformation by intermittent intrauterine balloon therapy: a randomised controlled trial. BJOG. 2019;126(10):1259-66.

CHAPTER 21

Arteriovenous Malformations

Sayani Maitra, Neelanjana Mukhopadhaya

ABSTRACT

Arteriovenous malformations are a rare complication of miscarriage, post dilatation and curettage. Although rare, they demand mention as they can lead to severe hemorrhage. Classically, these lesions were treated surgically by hysterectomy, whereas uterine artery embolization is the current preferred option in young patients, to preserve fertility. Medical management with GnRH analogs, progesterones and oral contraceptives is of limited value. Data on fertility outcomes after noninvasive therapies is limited at present.

Keywords: AV malformations, Retained placenta, Uterine artery embolization, GnRH agonists.

INTRODUCTION

Uterine arteriovenous malformations (*UAVMs*) are a rare but potential cause of recurrent pregnancy loss (RPL).[1] Only very few cases of UAVM are reported in literature, which have resulted in a live birth after conservative management. Recent research has cast a spotlight on the interconnection between UAVM and RPL, prompting a nuanced investigation into the pathophysiology, treatment modalities, and the underlying impact of UAVM on pregnancy outcomes.

Uterine arteriovenous malformations result from the formation of multiple arteriovenous fistulous communications within the uterus without an intervening capillary network.[2] This direct arteriovenous shunt formation potentially compromises the endometrial environment critical for the success of pregnancies. In the first weeks of gestation, trophoblast cells penetrate inside the decidua, reaching the myometrium and invading maternal spiral arteries. This is necessary to regulate the supply of oxygen in this period. Paradoxically, it is known that excessive vascularization produces an increased rate of flow of oxygen that could be detrimental to the embryo. Therefore, the presence of a continuous flow to the intervillous space is associated with early pregnancy loss.[3]

INCIDENCE

Recurrent miscarriage is defined as the loss of three or more consecutive pregnancies, affecting 1% of couples trying to conceive.[4,5] The prevalence of uterine anomalies in recurrent miscarriage populations ranges between 1.8% and 37.6%.[6,7] The reported incidence of arteriovenous malformation (AVM) is increasing.

PATHOGENESIS

A UAVM consists of a proliferation of vascular channels with fistula formation and an admixture of small, capillary-like channels. The size of these vessels can vary considerably.[8]

The vascular endothelial growth factors are the main growth factors involved in vasculogenesis and angiogenesis;[9,10] other factors involved are acidic and basic fibroblast growth factors (FGFs)—FGF1 and FGF2[11]—and placental growth factor.[12]

Uterine arteriovenous malformations are classified as congenital or acquired.[13]

Congenital UAVMs tend to have multiple feeding arteries, a central nidus (a tangle of vessels with histologic characteristics of both arteries and veins), and numerous large draining veins.[14] It is believed to arise from arrested vascular embryologic development, resulting in anomalous differentiation in the capillaries and abnormal communication between arteries and veins.

Acquired or traumatic UAVMs (also called arterio-venous fistulas) represent multiple small arteriovenous fistulas between the intramural arterial branches and the myometrial venous plexus. Acquired AVM is more common and usually follows uterine trauma. These AVMs are more common and are characterized by abnormal communication between uterine arteries and the myometrial venous plexus, deep within the myometrium and endometrium.[14] The incorporation of necrotic villi in the venous sinuses of scar tissue is thought to cause acquired UAVM.[15]

Acquired AVMs are associated with conditions, such as:[8,14,16]

- Multiple pregnancies
- Miscarriage
- *Previous surgery:*
  - Dilation and curettage
  - Termination of pregnancy
  - Cesarean section
- Also associated with infection, retained products of conception (RPOC),[17] gestational trophoblastic disease (GTD),[17] and gynecological malignancies.[18]

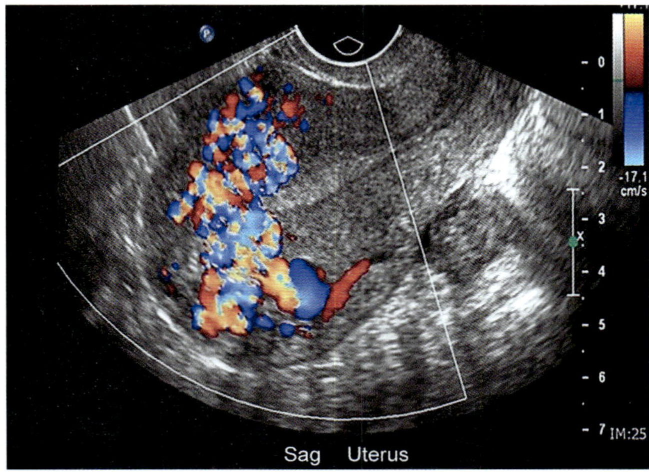

Fig. 1: Sagittal view of the uterus obtained by transvaginal ultrasound, demonstrating bidirectional Doppler flow over the hypoechoic areas of the fundus and representing blood flow in the uterine arteriovenous malformation.

DIAGNOSIS

Clinical Presentation

The clinical presentation of UAVMs varies—the classical clinical feature is intermittent, heavy vaginal bleeding, which may be life-threatening in young women.[19]

Radiographic Features

Ultrasound

Gray scale sonographic appearances can be nonspecific with a range of manifestations, including the areas of subtle myometrial inhomogeneity, tubular spaces within the myometrium, an intramural uterine, endometrial, or cervical mass-like region, or sometimes as prominent parametrial vessels. The extent of the mass effect, however, is minimal.[15,20]

Color Doppler ultrasound typically shows a low resistance [resistive index (RI) ~0.2–0.5], high-velocity flow pattern[21] **(Fig. 1)**.

Magnetic Resonance Imaging

Magnetic resonance imaging (MRI) shows multiple serpentine flow-related signal voids typically seen in the uterine wall, endometrial cavity, and parametrium on T1- and T2-weighted images. **(Figs. 2A to D)** Contrast-enhanced dynamic magnetic resonance (MR) angiography can depict complex serpentine abnormal vessels that enhance as intensely as normal vessels and show early venous return.[22]

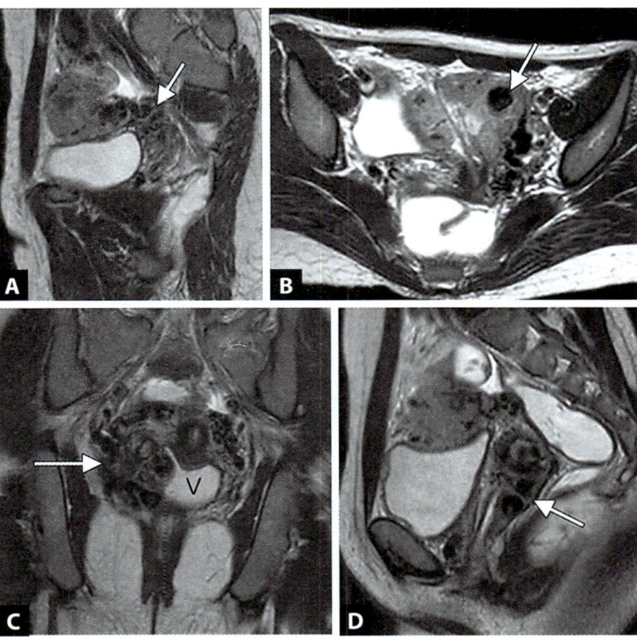

Figs. 2A to D: Pelvic MRI—sagittal (A and D), axial (B), and coronal (C) T2-weighted turbo spin-echo (TSE) sequences. The images show the uterus increased in volume, with multiple vascular-like serpiginous structures characterized by flow void (arrow on A). In the fundus/left lateral wall of the uterus, a round-shaped lesion with similar characteristics corresponding to a voluminous arteriovenous fistula (arrow on B). Also, the presence of prominent parametrial vessels is observed at right (arrows on C and D). (V: vaginal cavity distended by gel; MRI: magnetic resonance imaging)

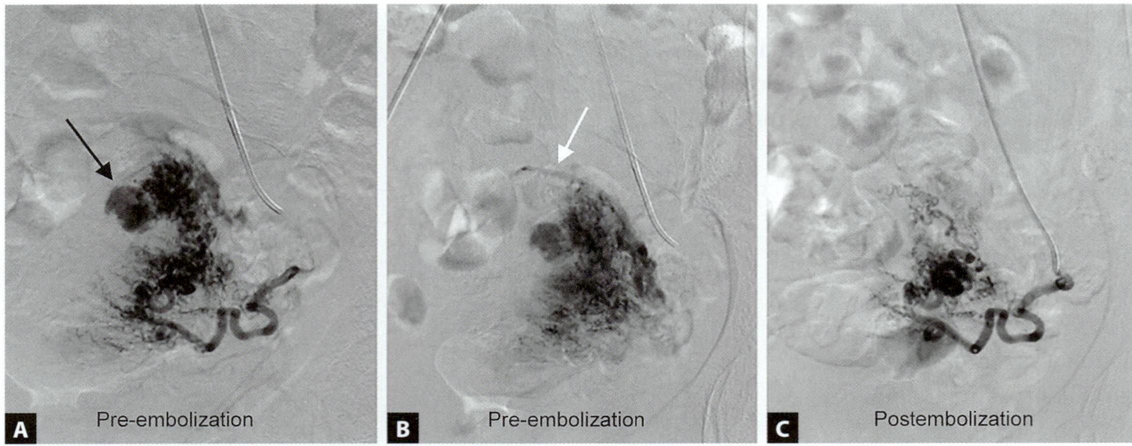

Figs. 3A to C: Angiogram of the left uterine artery showed an arteriovenous malformation (AVM) (black arrow), with an early draining vein seen at the fundus (white arrow). Postembolization run showed complete embolization of the AVM.

Angiography (Digital Subtraction Angiography)—Gold Standard[23]

Digital subtraction angiography (DSA) shows a hypervascular lesion with early venous filling. Conversely, enhanced myometrial vascularity will show a hypervascular lesion without early venous filling. Angiography has the benefit of allowing treatment (in the form of embolization) at the time of diagnosis[24] **(Figs. 3A to C)**.

Differential Diagnosis

The primary differential diagnosis on ultrasound imaging appearances is enhanced myometrial vascularity. This can be distinguished by DSA. In UAVM, serum beta-human chorionic gonadotropin (hCG) is negative.[25]

If serum beta-hCG is elevated, consider:

- GTD[26]
- *RPOC:*[27] Abnormality centered on the endometrium rather than the myometrium.

TREATMENT MODALITIES

Management of UAVM should be individualized, considering the woman's desire for future fertility and the stability of her health at presentation.

- Transcatheter uterine arterial embolization is an excellent treatment option in select cases.[28] The uterine artery is embolized with microparticles, coil, glue, or alcohol, while collateral supply maintains uterine perfusion, thus preserving fertility.[29,30]
- The effect of gonadotropin-releasing hormone agonist (GnRHa) on UAVMs is not well known. It can be used for the reduction in size of AVM, where uterine artery embolization must be postponed.[31-33]
- Oral contraceptive pills (OCPs)[34-36]
- Intramuscular (IM) and subsequent oral methylergometrine—regression of lesions based on ultrasound scan (USS).[37,38]
- Standard mode of treatment for UAVM was previously hysterectomy.[39,40]

Fertility Post AVM

Though data is limited, fertility outcomes are good after conservative management. A case series by Eling et al.[41] reported a miscarriage rate of 13.9%.

In a systematic review and metaanalysis, pregnancy rates were only 23% post embolization of AV malformations.[42]

CONCLUSION

Uterine arteriovenous malformations are on the rise, especially post retained placenta in placenta accreta spectrum. They pose a dilemma in both diagnosis and management. They not only compromise fertility and cause RPL but may also cause life-threatening hemorrhage. Restoration of fertility in these patients is a challenge. Medical management with OCP, progesterone and/or GnRH agonist, tranexamic acid, and aromatase inhibitors may reduce the amount of bleeding and buy time. Definitive treatment requires a skilled interventional radiologist to embolize all the feeding arteries. Fertility after AV malformations can be preserved but there are limited case reports on successful pregnancies post AV malformations. Hysterectomy may be required in life-threatening arterial bleeds.

REFERENCES

1. Arredondo-Soberon F, Loret de Mola JR, Shlansky-Goldberg R, Tureck RW. Uterine arteriovenous malformation in a patient with recurrent pregnancy loss and bicornuate uterus. J Reprod Med. 1997;42(4):239-43.
2. Brown JV 3rd, Asrat T, Epstein HD, Oglevie S, Goldstein BH. Contemporary diagnosis and management of a uterine arteriovenous malformation. Obstet Gynecol. 2008;112(2 Pt 2):467-70.
3. Cabero L, Saldívar D, Cabrillo E. Obstetricia y Medicina Materno-Fetal. Buenos Aires, Madrid: Editorial Médica Panamericana. 2007.
4. Stirrat GM. Recurrent miscarriage. Lancet. 1990;336(8716):673-5.
5. Rai R, Regan L. Recurrent miscarriage. Lancet. 2006;368(9535):601-11.
6. Clifford K, Rai R, Regan L. Future pregnancy outcome in unexplained recurrent first trimester miscarriage. Hum Reprod. 1997;12:387-9.
7. Lindbohm ML, Sallmén M, Taskinen H. Effects of exposure to environmental tobacco smoke on reproductive health. Scand J Work Environ Health. 2002;28(2):84-96.
8. O'Brien P, Neyastani A, Buckley A, Chang S, Legiehn G. Uterine Arteriovenous Malformations: From Diagnosis to Treatment. J Ultrasound Med. 2006;25(11):1387-92.
9. Bogic L, Brace R, Cheung C. Developmental expression of vascular endothelial growth factor (VEGF) receptors and VEGF binding in ovine placenta and fetal membranes. Placenta. 2001;22:265-75.
10. Ahmed A, Dunk C, Ahmad S, Khaliq A. Regulation of placental vascular endothelial growth factor (VEGF) and placenta growth factor (PIGF) and soluble Flt-1 by oxygen—a review. Placenta 2000;21:16-24.
11. Kingdom J, Huppertz B, Seaward G, Kaufmann P. Development of the placental villous tree and its consequences for fetal growth. Eur J Obstet Gynecol Reprod Biol. 2000;92:35-43.
12. DiSalvo J, Bayne M, Conn G, Kwok PW, Trivedi PG, Soderman DD, et al. Purification and characterization of a naturally occurring vascular endothelial growth factor.placenta growth factor heterodimer. J Biol Chem. 1995;270:7717-23.
13. Müngen E. Vascular Abnormalities of the Uterus: Have We Recently Over-Diagnosed Them? Ultrasound Obstet Gynecol. 2003;21(6):529-31.
14. Cura M, Martinez N, Cura A, Dalsaso T, Elmerhi F. Arteriovenous Malformations of the Uterus. Acta Radiol. 2009;50(7):823-9.
15. Timmerman D, Van den Bosch T, Peeraer K, Debriuwere E, Van Schoubroeck D, Stockx L, et al. Vascular malformations in the uterus: ultrasonographic diagnosis and conservative management. Eur J Obstet Gynecol Reprod Biol. 2000;92:171-8.
16. Kwon J, Kim G. Obstetric Iatrogenic Arterial Injuries of the Uterus: Diagnosis with US and Treatment with Transcatheter Arterial Embolization. Radiographics. 2002;22(1):35-46.
17. Grivell R, Reid K, Mellor A. Uterine arteriovenous malformations: a review of the current literature. Obstetrical and Gynecological Review. 2005;60(11):761-67.
18. Touhami O, Gregoire J, Noel P, Trinh XB, Plante M. Uterine arteriovenous malformations following gestational trophoblastic neoplasia: a systematic review. Eur J Obstet Gynecol Reprod Biol. 2014;181:54-9.
19. Clarke MJ, Mitchell PJ. Uterine arteriovenous malformation: a rare cause of uterine bleeding. Diagnosis and treatment. Australas Radiol. 2003;47(3):302-5.
20. Huang M, Muradali D, Thurston W, Burns P, Wilson S. Uterine Arteriovenous Malformations: Gray-Scale and Doppler US Features with MR Imaging Correlation. Radiology. 1998;206(1):115-23.
21. Przybojewski S, Sadler D. Novel image guided management of a uterine arteriovenous malformation. Cardiovasc Intervent Radiol. 2011;34:S161-6.
22. Nagayama M, Watanabe Y, Okumura A, Amoh Y, Nakashita S, Dodo Y. Fast MR Imaging in Obstetrics. Radiographics. 2002;22(3):563-80.
23. Polat P, Suna S, Kantarcy M, Alper F, Levent A. Color Doppler US in the evaluation of uterine vascular abnormalities. Radiographics. 2002;22(1):47-53.
24. Yang J, Xiang Y, Wan X, Yang X. Diagnosis and management of uterine arteriovenous fistulas with massive vaginal bleeding. Int J Gynaecol Obstet. 2004;89:114-19.
25. Timmerman D, Wauters J, Van Calenbergh S, Van Schoubroeck D, Maleux G, Van Den Bosch T, et al. Color Doppler imaging is a valuable tool for the diagnosis and management of uterine vascular malformations. Ultrasound Obstet Gynecol. 2003;21(6):570-77.
26. Chiang J, Berek J. Gestational trophoblastic disease: Epidemiology, clinical manifestations and diagnosis. In: Basow DS (Ed). Textbook of Medicine. Massachusetts Medical Society, Waltham, Massachusetts, USA, and Wolters Kluwer Publishers, Amsterdam, the Netherlands. 2010.
27. Carusi D. Retained products of conception. In: D Basow (Ed). UpToDate. Waltham, MA2012.
28. Maleux G, Timmerman D, Heye S, Wilms G. Acquired uterine vascular malformations: radiological and clinical outcome after transcatheter embolotherapy. Eur Radiol. 2006;16(2):299-306.
29. Ghai S, Rajan D, Asch M, Muradali D, Simons M, TerBrugge K. Efficacy of embolization in traumatic uterine vascular malformations. J Vase Interv Radiol. 2003;14:1401-8.

30. Patel S, Potti S, Jaspan D, Dandolu V. Embolization of uterine arteriovenous malformation for treatment of menorrhagia. Arch Gynecol Obstet. 2009;279(2):229-32.
31. Morikawa M, Yamada T, Yamada H, Minakami H. Effect of gonadotropin-releasing hormone agonist on a uterine arteriovenous malformation. Obstet Gynecol. 2006;108(3 Pt 2):751-3.
32. Tsuzuki M, Ishida T, Naitou H, Ishii R, Tomosaka M, Saga E, et al. Three different clinical courses and the conservative management of uterine arteriovenous malformation (AVM) diagnosed by color Doppler ultrasonography. J Obstet Gynaecol Res. 2018;44:1622.
33. Vilos AG, Oraif A, Machado M, Abu-Rafea B, Vilos GA. Resolution of uterine arteriovenous malformation and maintenance of reproduction in 20 women treated with a GnRH agonist concomitantly with an aromatase inhibitor and tranexamic acid. J Obstet Gynaecol Canada. 2019;41:772-81.
34. Taneja A, Chopra I, Kaur H, Naik SS, Aggarwal R, Sachdeva E, et al. Successful management of abnormal uterine bleeding from uterine arteriovenous malformations with progesterone in postabortal patients. J Obstet Gynaecol Res. 2019;45:1114-7.
35. Khatree MH, Titiz H. Medical treatment of a uterine arteriovenous malformation. Aust New Zeal J Obstet Gynaecol. 1999;39:378-80.
36. Oride A, Kanasaki H, Miyazaki K. Disappearance of a uterine arteriovenous malformation following long-term administration of oral norgestrel/ethinyl estradiol. J Obstet Gynaecol Res. 2014;40:1807-10.
37. Flynn MK, Levine D. The noninvasive diagnosis and management of a uterine arteriovenous malformation. Obstet Gynecol. 1996;88:650-2.
38. Onoyama I, Fukuhara M, Okuma A, Watanabe Y, Nakamura G. Successful pregnancy after the noninvasive management of uterine arteriovenous malformation. Acta Obstet Gynecol Scand. 2001;80:1148-9.
39. Sridhar D, Vogelzang RL. Diagnosis and treatment of uterine and pelvic arteriovenous malformations. Endovasc Today. 2018;17:1-5.
40. Karadag B, Erol O, Ozdemir O, Uysal A, Alparslan AS, Gurses C, et al. Successful treatment of uterine arteriovenous malformation due to uterine trauma. Case Rep Obstet Gynecol. 2016; 2016:3.
41. Eling R, Kent A, Robertson M. Pregnancy after uterine arteriovenous malformation-case series and literature review. Australas J Ultrasound Med. 2012;15(3):87-96. doi: 10.1002/j.2205-0140.2012.tb00012.x.
42. Ghanaati H, Avanaki MA, Ghavami N, Abbastabar H, Shakiba M, Firouznia S, et al. Pregnancy rate and outcomes following uterine artery embolization for uterine arteriovenous malformations: a systematic review and meta-analysis. J Vasc Interv Radiol. 2023;34(7):1184-91.e2. doi: 10.1016/j.jvir.2023.03.015.

CHAPTER 22

Cervical Insufficiency

Haywood L Brown

ABSTRACT

Cervical insufficiency can lead to painless mid-trimester pregnancy loss, or premature rupture of membranes due to loss of cervical mucous plug. Cerclage can be history indicated or ultrasound indicated. Mersilene tape can be placed through transvaginal route or transabdominally, which again can be via laparotomy or laparoscopy, with or without robotic assistance. Results are best achieved if it is placed close to the cervicoisthmic junction. Rescue cerclage is indicated if women present with open cervical os and bulging membranes. It is worthwhile if it can take the pregnancy to a safe period of viability.

The timing of transvaginal cerclage is soon after a normal nuchal scan, while there is a debate, whether transabdominal cerclage should be placed in early gestation (11–14 weeks) or during the interpregnancy interval. Transvaginal cerclage is best removed at 36–37 weeks or 24–48 hours after preterm premature rupture of membranes. Transabdominal cerclage requires an abdominal delivery and is often left in situ post cesarean section, if future pregnancies are desired.

Keywords: Cervical insufficiency, Cervical cerclage, Vaginal cerclage, Abdominal cerclage, Pseudocervical insufficiency, Rescue cerclage, Repeated miscarriage.

INTRODUCTION

Cervical insufficiency may be congenital or acquired due to repeated cervical dilatations in patients with recurrent pregnancy loss (RPL). It can also occur postcervical amputation, large loop excision of cervix or deep cervical tears during a difficult delivery. It can lead to mid trimester pregnancy loss or preterm birth. Hence, it is important to diagnose and manage it appropriately.

DIAGNOSIS AND MANAGEMENT

Cervical insufficiency is defined as the inability of the uterine cervix to maintain a pregnancy by shortening and/or dilating in the absence of signs or symptoms of uterine contractions in the second trimester.

There are several factors that increase the risk of cervical insufficiency. However, the first occurrence of cervical insufficiency can be unpredictable and independent of typical risk factors such as prior cervical trauma or Müllerian anomalies. In these cases, other proposed etiologies might include congenital deficiencies of collagen or elastin.

The diagnosis of cervical insufficiency or historic definition is based primarily on repeated miscarriages, in the second trimester, due to gradual yielding of the cervix, prior second trimester pregnancy loss presenting with dilation of the cervix or bulging of the amniotic membranes without contractions, or the finding of cervical shortening on ultrasound in the second trimester.[1]

More recently, routine assessment of cervical length in the second trimester can suggest a diagnosis of cervical insufficiency. However, the prior association of this finding is a marker for early-preterm delivery rather than cervical insufficiency. The finding of a short cervix prior to 18 weeks should raise suspicion for cervical insufficiency, especially if it is associated with no pain or contractions. The only other symptom may be mucous-like vaginal discharge.

Beyond vaginal ultrasound, there are no diagnostic tests predictive of cervical insufficiency. Many have been proposed historically in the nonpregnancy female who has experienced a prior second trimester pregnancy loss. These have included hysterosalpingography showing widening of the cervical canal or easy passage of Hegar or Pratt dilators through a nonpregnant cervical canal.[2,3]

Indications for cervical cerclage in the management of suspected cervical insufficiency can be based on:

- History of one or more second trimester pregnancy losses or prophylactic treatment with cerclage due to a prior history of painless second trimester cervical dilation

- Physical examination findings of a dilated cervix or bulging membranes in the second trimester and the treatment with an emergency or rescue cerclage
- Ultrasonographic findings of a shortened cervical length of <25 mm or more specifically <15 mm before 24 weeks, especially if associated with a prior history of spontaneous preterm birth before 24 completed weeks.

INDICATIONS FOR TREATMENT WITH CERVICAL CERCLAGE

Most historically indicated cerclages can be reasonably monitored by serial ultrasonographic cervical evaluation in the second trimester between 16 and 24 weeks.[4] Those individuals who should not be considered for routine prophylactic cerclage include an incidental short cervix <25 mm in the second trimester in the absence of prior preterm birth. In these cases, vaginal progesterone is an evidence-based option for those with a cervical length <20 mm before 24 weeks.[5] The exception may be twins or higher-order multiples with a significantly shortened cervix <20 mm in the second trimester with bulging membranes in the absence of contractions prior to 24 weeks, referred to as *pseudo-cervical insufficiency*. Other cases where a prophylactic cerclage is unwarranted include prior large loop electrosurgical excision procedure (LEEP) or surgical conization biopsy of cervix for dysplasia or carcinoma in situ (CIN) and Müllerian anomalies. The rare exception is prior cervical trachelectomy for cervical cancer treatment.

SURGICAL MANAGEMENT OF CERVICAL INSUFFICIENCY

Surgical management of cervical insufficiency includes transvaginal and transabdominal cerclage (TAC) placement. Standard transvaginal techniques were described by McDonald and Shirodkar.[6,7] The McDonald procedure requires no dissection and the placement of a simple stitch of nonabsorbable suture in a purse string fashion as high as possible to the cervical isthmus with adequate anterior and posterior bites. The traditional Shirodkar procedure involves dissection of the cervicovesical fold, posterior cervicorectal fold, and placement of a nonabsorbable stitch as close to the cervical internal os as possible after dissection of the bladder and rectal mucosa. The suture is placed at the internal os directly around the cervix under the cervical mucosa. The anterior and posterior mucosal incisions are then closed, burying the suture and the stump of the surgical knot. There have been modifications to the original Shirodkar procedure leaving the anterior knot exposed, which can be cut to allow for dilation of the cervix and normal labor.

Specific suture type and comparison of the two techniques for transvaginal cerclage placement has not shown superiority of one technique over the other.[8]

Suture type is typically based on surgical preference of monofilament versus braided suture. The preference toward a monofilament prolene #1 or #2 suture material is based on ease of placement and less vaginal discharge reaction postplacement. The preference is clearly in favor of a 5-mm Mersilene band for Shirodkar placement. The Mersilene band is also used in TAC placement.

One study suggested that braided suture material used for physical examination indicated cerclage had better outcomes compared to Mersilene band for the McDonald procedure.[9]

The *transabdominal placement* of a cerclage was first described by Benson and Durfee in 1965.[10] The transabdominal approach has significant advantages over transvaginal placement in that it results in higher placement of the suture at the cervicoisthmic junction of the internal cervical os, resulting in lack of slippage due to scarring, and the benefit of no foreign material in the vagina. This approach to cerclage placement has specific indications and can be performed with open laparotomy, laparoscopically or robotically. TAC placement at the cervicoisthmic junction reduces incidence of spontaneous pregnancy loss in selected patients with cervical insufficiency postcervical amputation and trachelectomy as well as failed transvaginal cerclage. The indications include:

- Failure to deliver a healthy newborn after at least one previous elective transvaginal cerclage not including rescue performed for advanced cervical dilation on physical examination
- The inability to undergo transvaginal procedure because of extreme cervical shortening or anatomical deformity or absent cervix or cervical defects making it technically impossible to perform a vaginal procedure.[11]

Transabdominal cerclage is usually performed *during pregnancy* in the late first trimester or early second trimester between 10 and 14 weeks' gestation. If the procedure is performed by laparotomy, it is best accomplished prior to 12 completed weeks for easier manipulation of the uterus to expose the cervicoisthmic junction after dissection of the bladder. A 5-mm Mersilene band is placed against the cervicoisthmic junction inside the uterine vessels so as not to take risk of hemorrhage. The suture is threaded anterior to posterior and back anteriorly and tied anteriorly, cutting the suture short. The bladder will cover the stitch, and the stitch is not disturbed at the time of cesarean delivery, leaving it in place for subsequent pregnancies.

Laparoscopic TAC has become the preferred choice for placement rather than open depending on surgical experience.[12] A prospective observational study of consecutive women who underwent TAC showed that before cerclage 76% of births occurred before 32 weeks with total neonatal survival of 27.5% and after TAC 7% of births occurred before 32 weeks with a neonatal survival of 93.5%.[13]

Preconception TAC reported by Groom in 2004 was associated with postoperative fetal survival rate of 100% in a case study of 19 women between 1994 and 2003 who reached >12 weeks of gestation.[14] A prospective observational study of consecutive women who underwent TAC from 2007 to 2017 showed a perinatal survival of viable pregnancies at 98.5% with a mean gestational age at delivery of 35.2 weeks and 79.9% delivering at 34 weeks or greater.[15] TAC may be accomplished laparoscopically **(Fig. 1)** or robotically **(Figs. 2A and B)**.

Placement can be checked by transvaginal ultrasound **(Fig. 3)**.

The disadvantage of TAC is that it requires two major surgeries: TAC and cesarean birth.

A rescue or emergency cerclage can be placed prior to viable pregnancy in women with a physical examination indicated cerclage such as those with an extremely shortened (<1.5 mm), or dilated cervix or exposed membranes. In a prospective study for Fortner et al. with rescue cerclage performed at 2 cm or greater, compared to those women <2 cm at the time of placement, gestational age at delivery was 27 weeks [confidence interval (CI) 21.9–32.0] compared to 35.6 (CI 26–38) for those <2 cm at emergency cerclage placement. The gestational age at cerclage placement was similar at 20.3 (CI 18.6–21.4) for those ≥2 versus 20.3 (CI 19.0–21.4) for those <2 cm.[16]

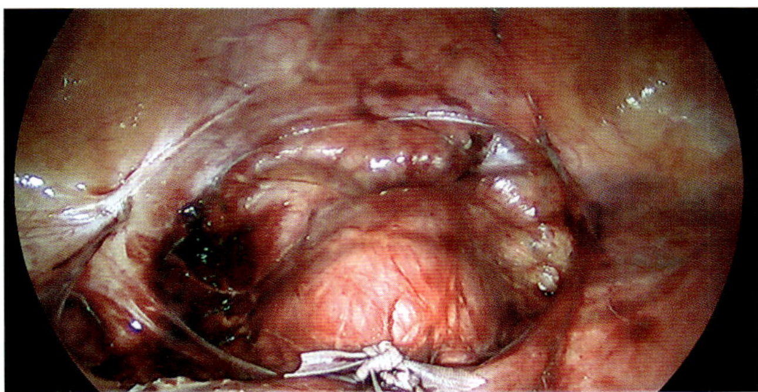

Fig. 1: Laparoscopic transabdominal cerclage.

To assist with replacement of exposed membranes at the time of cerclage placement, the exposed membranes are required to be pushed back inside the uterine cavity before placing the stitch. It is recommended to cleanse the exposed membranes with betadine solution before retracting them to reduce the incidence of chorioamnionitis. Retraction of membranes may be accomplished by using an inflated Foley bulb. This may also be accomplished by creating an artificial finger using a Haney clamp wrapped with a gauze and covered with a sterile glove **(Figs. 4A and B)**. When used properly, the artificial finger is slowly retracted from

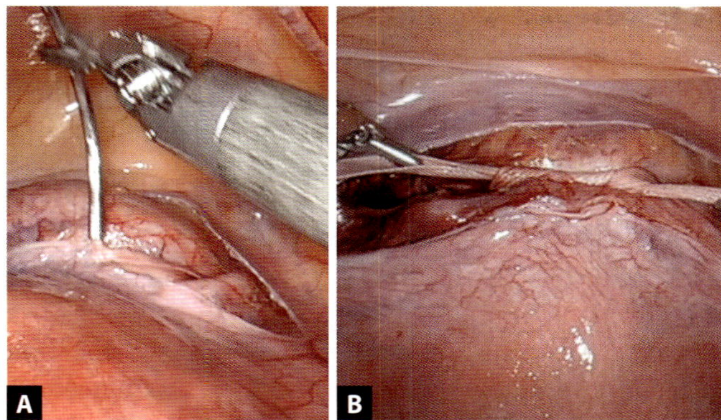

Figs. 2A and B: Robotic transabdominal cerclage.
Source: Roberts, De Assis, and Mikhail, AAGL 2022 Robotic Cerclage University, South Florida.

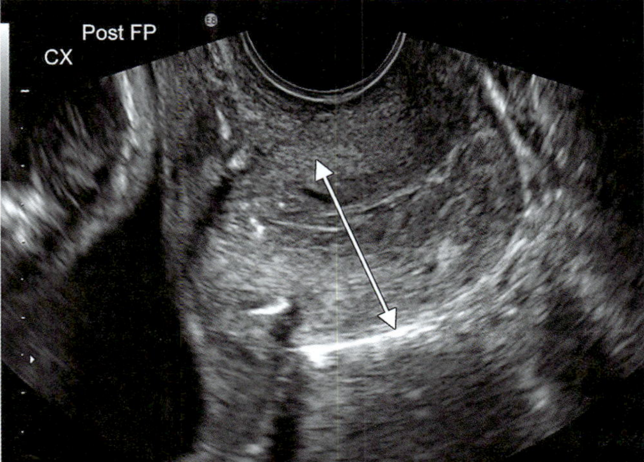

Fig. 3: Transvaginal ultrasound showing postoperative transabdominal cerclage placement.

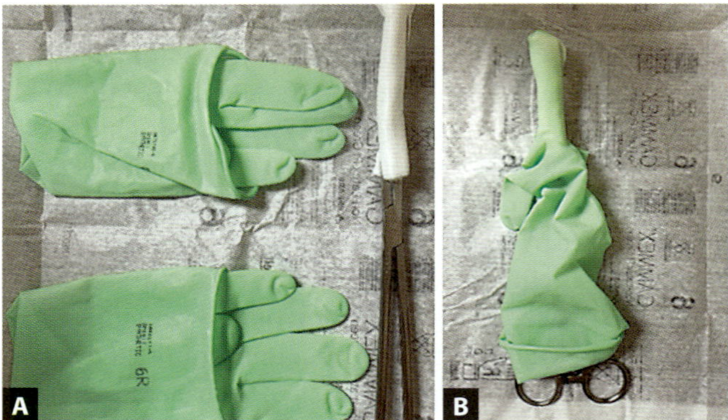

Figs. 4A and B: Artificial finger to facilitate transvaginal cerclage placement with exposed fetal membranes: (A) a sterile glove and (B) a Haney clamp wrapped with a gauze.

the cervical canal allowing the surgeon to quickly tighten the stitch around the cervix. A second stitch can be placed above the first one by retracting the knot of the first stitch downward. This is rarely if ever required and has no benefit for further maintaining the pregnancy if the transvaginal stitch is appropriately placed and tightened.

Overall, there is a low risk for *complications* after cerclage placement. The risk is greater with rescue cerclage for complications such as rupture of membranes and chorioamnionitis. TAC is associated with a greater risk for hemorrhage and might preclude uterine evacuation depending on gestational age at the time of a postprocedure pregnancy loss prior to 20–24 weeks.

Follow-up after cerclage placement whether transvaginal or transabdominal is by transvaginal ultrasound approximately every 2 weeks up to 24 weeks. Transvaginal sexual activity is typically prohibited after transvaginal McDonald procedure, which can lead to trauma to the cervix and vaginal bleeding. Physical activity is typically not limited after TAC depending on patient's history.

Prophylactic antibiotics and tocolysis have not proved to be beneficial in improving efficacy after cerclage placement.[17] However, it is typical to administer prophylactic antibiotics with emergency or rescue cerclage placement, especially if membranes are exposed. Also, prophylactic tocolysis with nonsteroidal anti-inflammatory drugs (NSAIDs) for 48 hours can be administered after rescue cerclage.

Management of women with a cerclage in place who experience preterm premature rupture of membranes (PPROM) has some controversy as to whether to remove the transvaginal McDonald stitch or leave the stitch in place. There are no randomized trials. Retention of the cerclage for >24 hour is associated with prolongation of pregnancy, but there is no greater than the usual risk of chorioamnionitis with PPROM and neonatal sepsis.[18] However, there is a significant risk for cervical trauma if active labor occurs with the cerclage in place.

There are no firm recommendations regarding the removal of a cerclage with PPROM. The decision to remove or not to remove can depend on gestational age. If PPROM occurs prior to 32–34 weeks, it is reasonable to wait for prophylaxis with maternal steroids and antibiotics and remove after 48 hours. If the rupture occurs after 34 weeks, there is no advantage in delaying cerclage removal.

Removal of a transvaginal McDonald or modified Shirodkar cerclage with an exposed knot should occur around 36–37 weeks prior to the onset of labor in the outpatient setting. Waiting for labor is not recommended because of the potential for cervical trauma with labor, effacement, and dilation of the cervix.[1] For those planning a cesarean at 39 weeks, the vaginal cerclage can be removed prior to or after the cesarean while under regional anesthesia.

CONCLUSION

Cervical insufficiency may be diagnosed by history or uncovered by physical examination on ultrasound showing a shortened cervix or exposed membranes. Cervical elastography may be added to cervical length measurement for improving diagnostic accuracy of cervical insufficiency. Transcervical cerclage is an appropriate treatment to rebuild the cervix and may be accomplished with a transvaginal or transabdominal technique for those meeting criteria. Success of cerclage placement depends on placing the stitch as close to the cervicoisthmic junction as possible and success depends on the experience of the surgeon, the history, and physical examination findings. Cerclage should be placed during pregnancy between late first trimester and prior to viability. It is best placed after the early anomaly scan between 11 and 13 completed weeks of gestation. Alternatively, transabdominal laparoscopic technique is reserved for women with vaginally inaccessible cervix, and best results are obtained when it is placed in the nonpregnant woman, post a miscarriage.

REFERENCES

1. ACOG Practice Bulletin No.142: Cerclage for the management of cervical insufficiency. Obstet Gynecol. 2014;123 (2 Pt 1):372-9. AOG0000443276.68274cc. PMID:24451674

2. Robovits FE, Cooperman NR, Lash AF. Habitual abortion: a radiographic technique to demonstrate the incompetent internal os of the cervix. Am J Obstet Gynecol. 1953;66(2):269-80.
3. Anthony GS, Calder AA, MacNaughton MC. Cervical resistance in patients with previous spontaneous mid-trimester abortion. Br J Obstet Gynaecol. 1982;89(12):1046-9.
4. Brown JA, Pearson AW, Veillon EW, Rust OA, Chauhan SP, Magann EF, et al. History- or ultrasound-based cerclage placement and adverse perinatal outcomes. J Reprod Med. 2011;56(9-10):385-92.
5. Romero R, Conde-Agudelo A, Da Fonseca E, O'Brien JM, Cetingoz E, Creasy GW, et al. Vaginal progesterone for preventing preterm birth and adverse perinatal outcomes in singleton gestations with a short cervix: a meta-analysis of individual patient data. Am J Obstet Gynecol. 2018;218(2):161-80.
6. McDonald IA. Suture of the cervix for inevitable miscarriage. J Obstet Gynaecol Br Emp. 1957;64(3):346-50.
7. Shirodkar VN. A new method of operative treatment for habitual abortions in the second trimester of pregnancy. Antiseptic. 1955;52:299-300.
8. Berghella V, Szychowski JM, Owen J, Hankins G, Iams JD, Sheffield JS, et al. Suture type and ultrasound-indicated cerclage efficacy. J Matern Fetal Neonatal Med. 2012;25(11):2287-90.
9. Bernard L, Pereira L, Berghella V, Rust OA, Mittal S, Daly S, et al. Effect of suture material on outcome of cerclage in women with a dilated cervix in the 2nd trimester: results from the expectant management compared to physical exam-indicated cerclage (EM-PEC) international cohort study. Am J Obstet Gynecol. 2006;195(6):S103.
10. Benson RC, Durfee RB. Transabdominal cervico uterine cerclage during pregnancy for the treatment of cervical incompetency. Obstet Gynecol. 1965;25:145-55.
11. Davis G, Berghella V, Talucci M, Wapner RJ. Patients with a prior failed transvaginal cerclage: a comparison of obstetric outcomes with either transabdominal or transvaginal cerclage. Am J Obstet Gynecol. 2000;183(4):836-9.
12. Burger NB, Brölmann HA, Einarsson JI, Langebrekke A, Huirne JA. Effectiveness of abdominal cerclage placed via laparotomy or laparoscopy: systematic review. J Minim Invasive Gynecol 2011;18(6):696-704.
13. Lotgering F, Gaugler-Senden IPM, Lotgering SF, Wallenburg HCS. Outcome after transabdominal cervicoisthmic cerclage. Obstet Gynecol. 2006;107(4):779-84.
14. Ades A, Parghi S, Aref-Adib M. Laparoscopic transabdominal cerclage: outcomes of 121 pregnancies. Aust N Z J Obstet Gynaecol. 2018;58(6):606-11.
15. Groom KM, Jones BA, Edmonds DK, Bennett PR. Preconception transabdominal cervicoisthmic cerclage. Am J Obstet Gynecol. 2004;191(1):230-4.
16. Fortner KB, Fitzpatrick CB, Grotegut CA, Swamy GK, Murtha AP, Heine RP, et al. Cervical dilation as a predictor of pregnancy outcome following emergency cerclage. J Matern Fetal Neonatal Med. 2012;25(10):1884-8.
17. Olatunbosun OA, al-Nuaim L, Turnell RW. Emergency cerclage compared with bed rest for advanced cervical dilation in pregnancy. Int Surg. 1995;80(2):170-4.
18. Ludmir J, Bader T, Chen L, Lindenbaum C, Wong G. Poor perinatal outcome associated with retained cerclage in patients with premature rupture of membranes Obstet Gynecol. 1994;84(5):823-6.

CHAPTER 23

Role of Laparoscopy

Nikita Trehan

ABSTRACT

Laparoscopic surgery is a valuable adjunct in the management of recurrent pregnancy loss (RPL). Removal of cavity distorting myomas, correction of certain müllerian anomalies, excision of endometrioma and deep infiltrating bowel lesions is only possible through laparoscopic surgery. Certain cases of localized adenomyosis also do very well after laparoscopic excision. Optimization of the pelvis achieved through laparoscopy improves pregnancy outcome in a variety of conditions e.g., endometriosis and pelvic inflammatory disease. Finally, transabdominal cervical cerclage is a useful technique for women who miscarry inspite of having a transvaginal cerclage.

Keywords: Laparoscopy, Myoma, Fibroid, Endometriosis, Focal adenomyosis, Abdominal cervical cerclage.

INTRODUCTION

According to American Society for Reproductive Medicine (ASRM) recurrent pregnancy loss (RPL) is defined as two or more failed clinical pregnancies.[1]

It has been postulated that uterine anomalies can frequently lead to RPL. Uterine anomalies can be classified as congenital or acquired. Congenital uterine anomalies like uterine septa can lead up to 12.6% cases of RPL,[2] and correction of this anomaly can lead to successful pregnancy outcome in 56–82% cases. Surgical correction of acquired uterine anomalies such as fibroids and adenomyosis has also shown a hugely beneficial effect on the pregnancy outcomes.

The uterine anatomical defects in women account for 3.2–6.9% of miscarriages in women with RPL.[3] Ultrasound diagnosis is quick and readily available for initial screening. Three-dimensional (3D) ultrasound and sonohysterography can recognize 95% of uterine anomalies.[4] Magnetic resonance imaging (MRI) has found to be superior in recognizing complex uterovaginal anomalies.[5] But the gold standard in evaluating uterine anomalies still remains hysterolaparoscopy.[6] **Table 1** enumerates the uterine anomalies and how beneficial is the surgical correction.

TABLE 1: Uterine defects and their corrective effect on pregnancy.

Uterine anomaly	*Effect on pregnancy outcome*
Congenital causes	
Uterine septum	Extremely beneficial
Unicornuate uterus	Lateral metroplasty found of benefit in some studies
Bicornuate uterus	Unification beneficial in some cases
Acquired causes	
Leiomyoma uterus	Extremely beneficial depending on the location
Adenomyosis uterus	Extremely beneficial
Endometriosis	Beneficial especially in deeply infiltrating endometriosis
Chronic infections like endometritis	Beneficial
Intrauterine adhesions (Asherman's syndrome)	Extremely beneficial
Cervical incompetence	Extremely beneficial in genuine cases

CONGENITAL ANOMALIES

Septate uterus is the anomaly which is most commonly associated with RPL, poor obstetric outcome, and infertility.[7,8]

Hysteroscopic metroplasty is considered the gold standard in the treatment of uterine septum. Unification of a bicornuate uterus is achieved laparoscopically by the undermentioned steps in cases of recurrent second trimester miscarriages. Steps of unification of a bicornuate uterus with hypoplastic horns is illustrated in **Figures 1 to 5**.

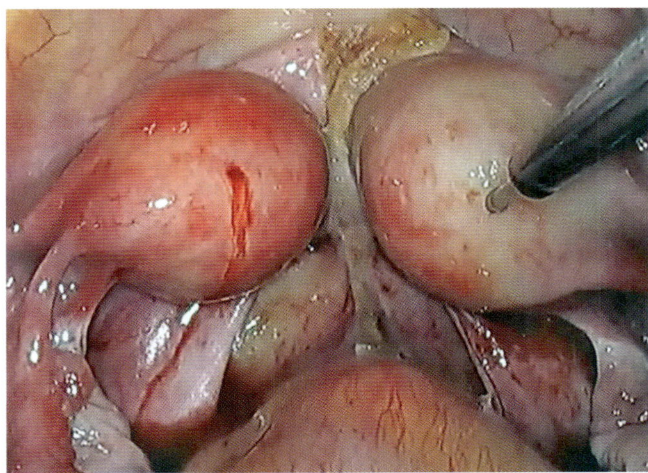

Fig. 1: Vasopressin being injected into both horns of the uterus.

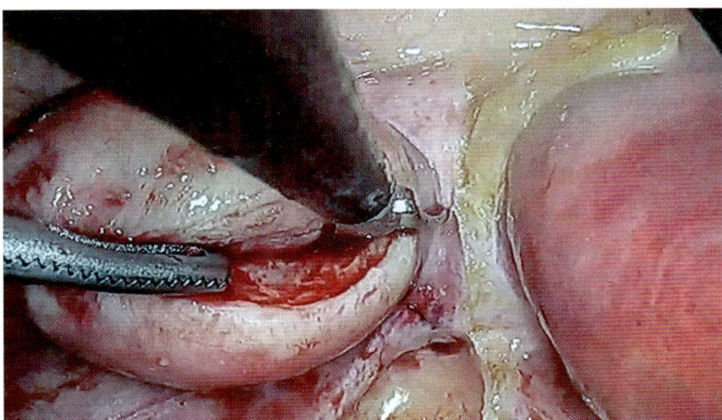

Fig. 2: Incision being given on the medial surfaces of both horns.

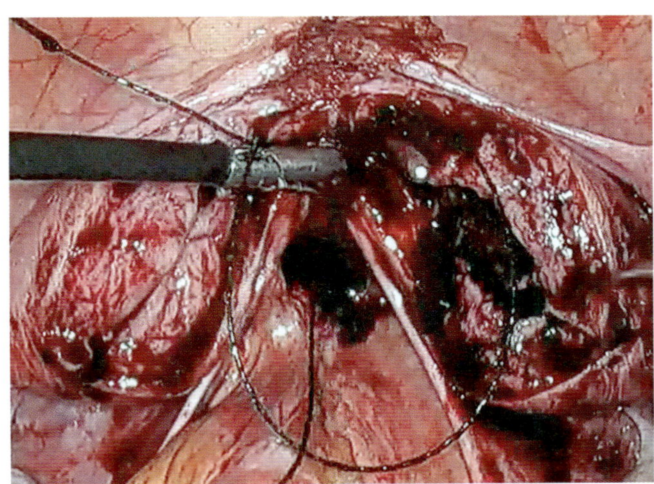

Fig. 3: Posterior seromuscular endometrium sparing stitches being taken through both horns.

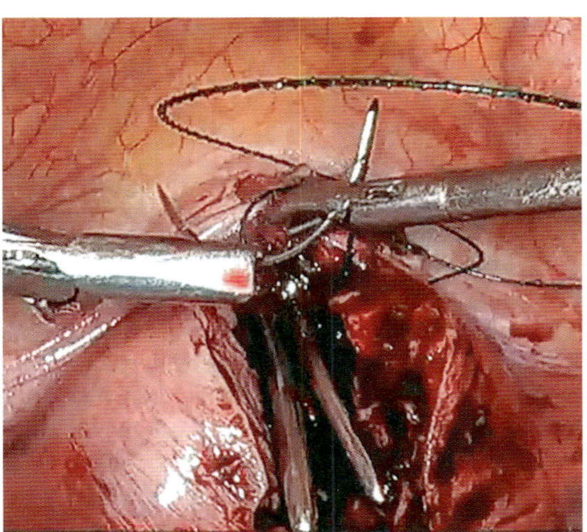

Fig. 4: Anterior seromuscular endometrium sparing stitches being taken through both horns.

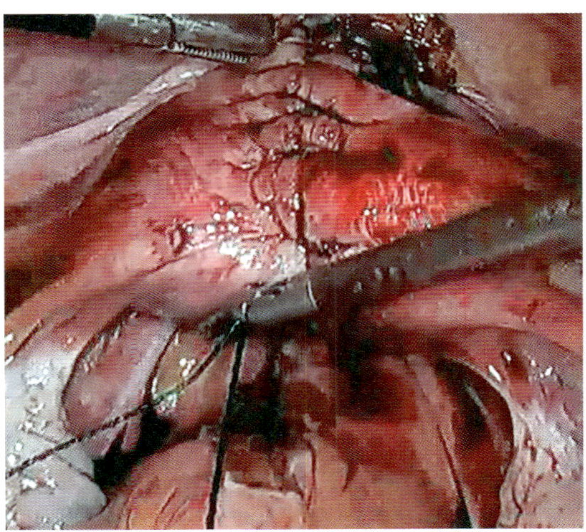

Fig. 5: Final unification of bicornuate uterus.

ACQUIRED CAUSES

Leiomyoma Uterus

Fibroids are benign monoclonal neoplasms of unclear etiology that arise from myometrial smooth muscle cells. Leiomyomas are the most common benign gynecological tumors with an estimated incidence of 70–80% in women by the age of 50 years.

Although, fibroids may be asymptomatic, they are frequently associated with a number of clinical issues including abnormal uterine bleeding especially heavy menstrual bleeding, infertility, RPL, and complaints related to the impact of the enlarged uterus on adjacent structures in the pelvis which are referred to as bulk symptoms.

BOX 1: Basic mechanisms by which fibroids lead to infertility and pregnancy loss.

Mechanism
- Distortion of the uterine cavity rendering the endometrial contour anomalous may compromise implantation potential
- An enlarged and deformed fibroid uterus may hamper sperm transport
- Cervical displacement may hinder sperm passage into the cervical canal
- Altered myometrial contractility may compromise sperm progression into the female reproductive system
- Alteration to the endometrial and myometrial blood supply may interfere with both uterine contractility and implantation
- Retained menstrual efflux due to a deformity of the uterine cavity may interfere with both sperm transport and implantation
- Deviation or obstruction of the tubal ostia may compromise tubal patency
- Alteration of the tubo-ovarian anatomic relation may impede ovum collection from the fimbria end following ovulation
- Chronic endometrial inflammation due to myomas lying adjacent to the endometrium may alter endometrial milieu
- Histologic alterations attributed to myomas lying close or in contact to the endometrial surface may impair implantation

The basic mechanisms by which fibroids lead to infertility and pregnancy loss are postulated in **Box 1**.

There are several reasons why embryo implantation may be unsuccessful in case of fibroids which leads to infertility and RPL. Firstly, abnormal peristalsis is found in the myometrium surrounding the myoma, which inhibits implantation. This abnormal peristalsis gets corrected after myomectomy also a diffuse inflammatory reaction is present surrounding a myoma which is found to get corrected following a myomectomy.[9-12] Overall, several studies, like a metaanalysis by Somigliana,[13] have shown an adverse effect of intramural fibroids on assisted reproductive technology outcomes, clinical pregnancy, and live birth rates. Another systematic review and meta-analysis by Pritts et al.[14] in 2009 showed a higher miscarriage rate in association with intramural fibroids along with decreased implantation and live birth rate. Sunkara et al. in a large study in 6,087 in vitro fertilization cycles[15] associated with intramural fibroids found that even noncavity-distorting intramural fibroids were associated with lower clinical pregnancy and live birth rates.

PREOPERATIVE PLANNING

- Myomectomy can be performed by hysteroscopic or laparoscopic routes depending on the location of the fibroids. While planning the route of myomectomy, we recommend that submucous fibroids larger than 4 cm or multiple submucous fibroids may be better approached by the laparoscopic route rather than the hysteroscopic route, as significant endometrial damage to the surrounding endometrium can occur while performing a hysteroscopic myomectomy leading to Asherman's syndrome, subsequently. The laparoscopic approach is thus preferred in these large submucous fibroids.
- Preoperative correction of anemia with total dose infusion of ferric carboxymaltose helps in avoiding/minimizing need for blood transfusion at the time of surgery and also helps in better healing and postoperative recovery of the patient.
- Preoperative gonadotropin-releasing hormone (GnRH) agonists or selective progesterone receptor modulators like ulipristal may be used to avoid menstrual bleeding and blood loss while the anemia is being corrected with iron replacement. Also, additionally these agents decrease the size of the fibroids by causing hyaline degeneration and hydropic degeneration[16] making the fibroids softer but with a loss of planes which may be advantageous in hysteroscopy but is not desirable while performing a laparoscopic myomectomy. Additionally, the GnRH agonists cause adverse effects such as menopausal hot flashes and trabecular bone loss. But ulipristal may lead to liver toxicity and acute liver injury so has to be used with extreme caution.

LAPAROSCOPIC MYOMECTOMY

Certain principles need to be adhered to while performing a laparoscopic myomectomy. The ultimate aim of these principles is to achieve a good scar after myomectomy which can withstand subsequent pregnancy.

In order to achieve a good and strong postmyomectomy scar it is important that the healing of the myoma bed should be done by primary intention and not by secondary intention (producing a big ragged scar unable to withstand subsequent pregnancy). The principles to achieve a good scar are as follows:

- *Intracapsular myomectomy:* All myomectomies should be performed keeping the pseudocapsule of the myoma intact by the intracapsular method. As the neurovascular bundles run across this pseudocapsule meticulous dissection and less use of electrocautery on the pseudocapsule is advantageous over the extracapsular approach, in terms of blood loss, operational time, and proper hysterotomy wound healing.[17]

- Meticulous hemostasis and avoidance of hematoma formation in the myomectomy scar is mandatory for a good myomectomy scar formation. Hematomas can form if some bleeders are left in the myoma bed after fibroid enucleation. Hematomas can also form if the myoma beds are not sutured adequately and dead space is left behind in the myoma bed. To avoid dead spaces being left in the myoma bed, multilayer closure of the myoma bed may be required for deep seated fibroids. Also the use of barbed sutures helps in proper approximation and adequate dispersal of uniform tension through the stitch line when used, which in turn prevents hematoma formation. Hematomas when formed can get infected easily forming micro/macro abscesses to formation of an even weaker scar.
- *Less use of electrocautery:* Whenever possible the use of electrocautery over the myoma bed should be avoided as necrosis and ischemia caused by the electrocautery can lead to the formation of a weak scar.

INTRAOPERATIVE TIPS AND TRICKS

- *Operating distance:* The primary visual port should be placed higher than usual in the Palmers or Lee-Huang point[18] in most myomectomies as the myoma screw during enucleation will pull the myoma cephalad bringing the myoma closer to the visual port and hence, will obstruct the vision if the visual port is low, especially in very large fibroids.
- Hemostasis is a major concern during myomectomy and several methods are now available to reduce bleeding at the time of myomectomy.

Impact of medical interventions on hemostasis during myomectomy.

In a study by Lisa Hickman et al.[19] an evidence-based evaluation of the various methods used to control hemostasis showed that drugs like tranexamic acid are ineffective in controlling bleeding at myomectomy. Whereas, oxytocin which were previously thought to be effective on the pregnant uterus only has been found to be effective in nonpregnant cases as well, hence, is now used effectively as a 40 units intravenous infusion during myomectomy. Vasopressin has been found to be extremely useful during myomectomy and it should be injected in a diluted dose at a single point into the uterus (and not into the fibroid) to avoid it leaking from another area. Although uncommon, several studies have reported severe cardiopulmonary complications in healthy individuals, including hypotension, bradycardia, cardiac arrest, and pulmonary edema at doses ranging from 0.2 to 0.6 units/mL. Hence, vasopressin should be diluted to a concentration of 0.05–0.3 units/mL **(Fig. 6)**.

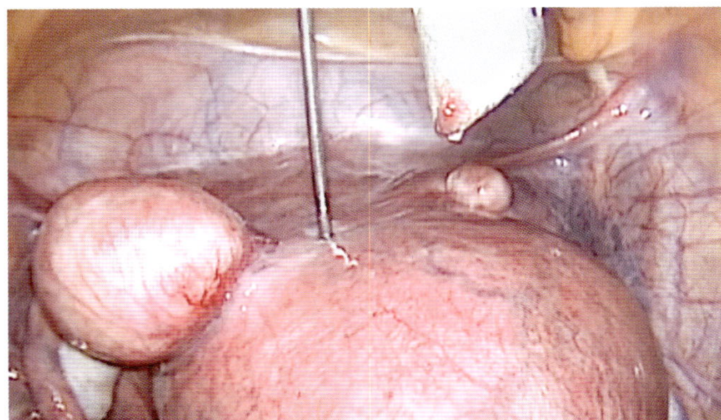

Fig. 6: Vasopressin being injected into the uterus.

Surgical methods like laparoscopic uterine artery ligation (LUAL) from origin bilaterally are extremely effective not only to control bleeding at the time of myomectomy but is also effective in preventing the recurrence of fibroids later in life. Several studies have shown that future fertility and pregnancy outcome (in terms of fetal growth restriction or placenta accreta) remain unaffected after LUAL compared to uterine artery embolization (UAE) wherein, subsequent pregnancy is not advisable as the polyvinyl alcohol particles block the complete blood supply including the collateral circulation of the uterus.

The LUAL can be performed by the lateral or posterior window technique.

In the lateral window technique, the broad ligament is opened in the avascular plane between the round ligament and the infundibulopelvic ligament and the uterine artery is clipped at its origin from the internal iliac artery, bilaterally **(Fig. 7)**.

Barbed sutures are routinely used in a baseball manner where the suture is passed inside out on both sides of the wound. Suturing in this manner has two main advantages, i.e., the myoma bed is closed with most of the suture buried inside and hence, less suture exposed minimizes the chances of bowel going and getting adherent on the barbs. Secondly, baseball suturing ensures that the dead space of the myoma bed is completely obliterated **(Fig. 8)**.

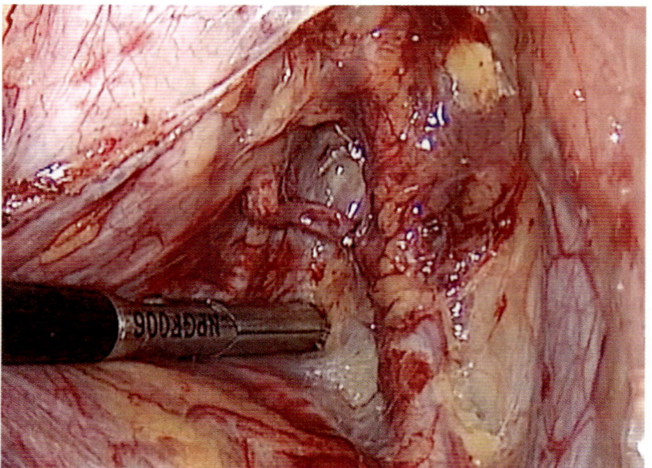

Fig. 7: Uterine artery being clipped at origin.

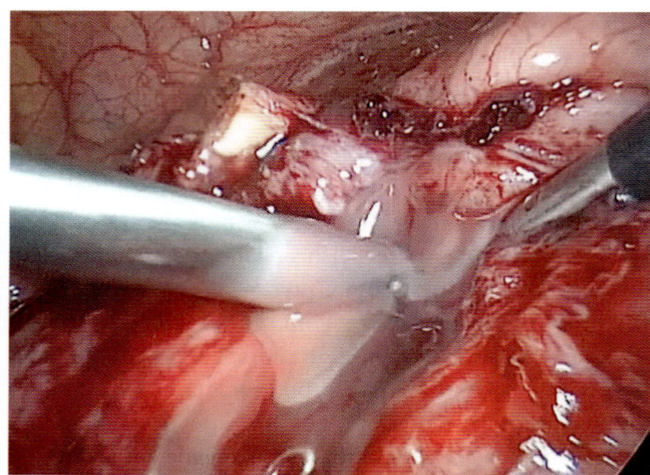

Fig. 9: Pelvic abscess being drained.

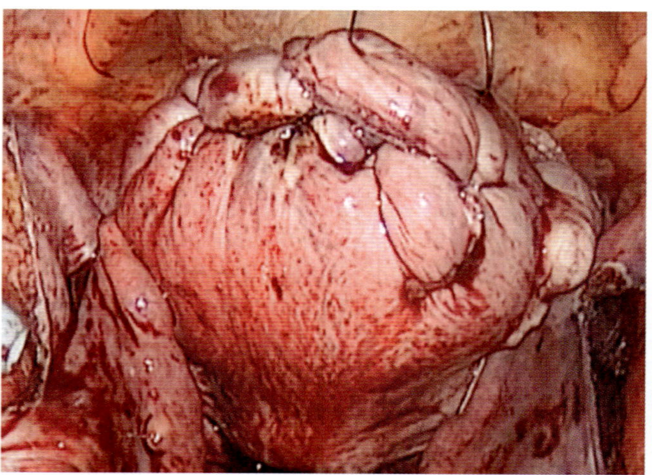

Fig. 8: Baseball suturing done with barbed sutures.

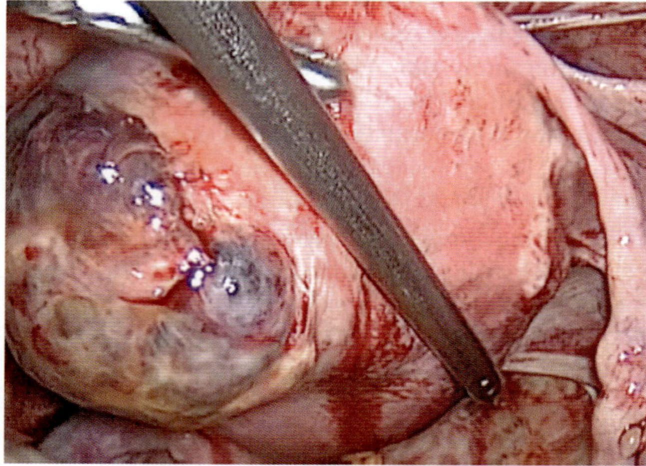

Fig. 10: Ectopic pregnancy in a myomectomy scar.

- Intra-abdominal adhesions occur more frequently after open surgery compared to after laparoscopy. Gentle tissue handling with maintenance of the peritoneal surfaces, with good hemostasis and no blood collections, less use of cautery, and minimal raw surface exposure are the usual rules to be followed to avoid postoperative adhesions. Adhesion prevention barriers such as 4% icodextrin, auto crosslinked hyaluronic acid, oxidized regenerated cellulose, and polytetrafluoroethylene have been shown to reduce adhesion development with varying results.[20-21]

Inadequately sutured myoma beds can lead to pelvic abscess formation in a hematoma which may even get infected forming a pelvic abscess, which may need laparoscopic drainage **(Fig. 9)**.

Another complication that can arise due to poor healing of a myomectomy scar is the implantation of a pregnancy in the weak myomectomy scar, leading to a scar ectopic **(Fig. 10)**.

ADENOMYOSIS AND RECURRENT PREGNANCY LOSS

Adenomyosis is identified by uterine enlargement secondary to areas of endometrium (both glands and stroma) located deep in the myometrium. These areas cause hyperplasia and hypertrophy of the surrounding myometrium which causes an enlarged uterus. Ectopic areas of the endometrium can be diffusely present throughout the myometrium or focal forming a nodular adenomyoma.[22]

Classification

The surgical/histological classification of adenomyosis was given by Grimbizis et al.[23] in 2014, describing adenomyosis into five categories.

1. Diffuse, wherein, the adenomyosis is present diffusely all over the myometrium.
2. Focal, wherein, only an adenomyotic nodule is present and rest of the myometrium is normal.
3. Cystic adenomyosis, wherein, the adenomyotic nodule has cystic content.
4. Uterine adenomyomatous polyp
5. Special categories like rectovaginal endometriosis which he classified as a form of adenomyosis as the features of rectovaginal endometriosis histologically and behaviorally are closer to adenomyosis than to endometriosis.

Mechanisms of Recurrent Pregnancy Loss in Adenomyosis

The identification of the myometrial junctional zone and of its disruption and thickening has been linked to the poor reproductive performance, mainly through the perturbed uterine peristalsis, a phenomenon that originates exclusively from the junctional zone in nonpregnant women.[24]

Additionally, a number of biochemical and functional alterations in both the eutopic and heterotopic endometrium in women with adenomyosis have now been found to lower endometrial receptivity known as "implantation marker defects." In these patients there is also altered decidualization and abnormal concentrations of intrauterine free radicals.

Also, recent evidence suggests that adenomyosis in addition to causing the symptoms of menorrhagia, dysmenorrhea, dyspareunia, dyschezia (in rectovaginal endometriosis) subfertility, and RPL is also associated with adverse pregnancy outcomes such as preterm labor, fetal growth restriction, pregnancy induced hypertension, intrauterine infections, and mysteriously, even cervical incompetence.[25-27]

Ultrasound

A transvaginal ultrasound forms a very important tool in the diagnosis of adenomyosis with the suggestive signs of an asymmetrically and diffusely enlarged uterus with increased myometrial echogenicity or linear hyperechoic bands extending deep into the myometrium and the presence of myometrial cysts. The morphological uterus sonographic assessment (MUSA) guidelines[28] have standardized the identification and reporting of adenomyosis. The new category focal adenomyosis of outer myometrium (FAOM) is a also addressed specifically in the MUSA guidelines **(Fig. 11)**.

Magnetic Resonance Imaging

On T2-weighted images a large asymmetrically enlarged uterus along with myometrial heterogenicity and presence of myometrial cysts along with enlargement of the junctional zone (the innermost myometrial layer) can be seen in adenomyosis. MRI has very high specificity and positive predictive value (>90%) and is especially useful if fibroids coexist in the same patient to differentiate between the two.

Treatment

The basic principle of medical management is by means of hormonal treatment, which only work as agents for "suppression of the disease" and surgery and excision of the lesions form the mainstay for the treatment of the disease. Hence, continuous oral contraceptive pills, Depo-Provera, levonorgestrel intrauterine contraceptive device (IUCD), danazol IUCD, and GnRH agonists all work as temporary methods for suppression of the disease (Refer to Chapter 18).

Alternative Methods

One of the new advances is the use of laparoscopic microwave ablation of adenomyosis under ultrasound guidance. Compared to laparoscopic adenomyomectomy this procedure is less invasive but is still in the early stages of development. Treatment such as high frequency ultrasound (HIFU) and UAE have been proposed for treatment of selective cases of adenomyosis their role is still controversial and data on pregnancy outcome scanty. Therefore, presently alternate treatments should be proposed in women with no desire for future pregnancy. Also, UAE for adenomyosis is technically different from when it is performed for fibroids as at angiography adenomyosis shows a reduction in arterial pattern but increase in micro vessel density making the use of polyvinyl alcohol particles less effective. Hence, the absence of a good embolic agent suited to adenomyosis currently makes this procedure less effective than when it is used for fibroid.

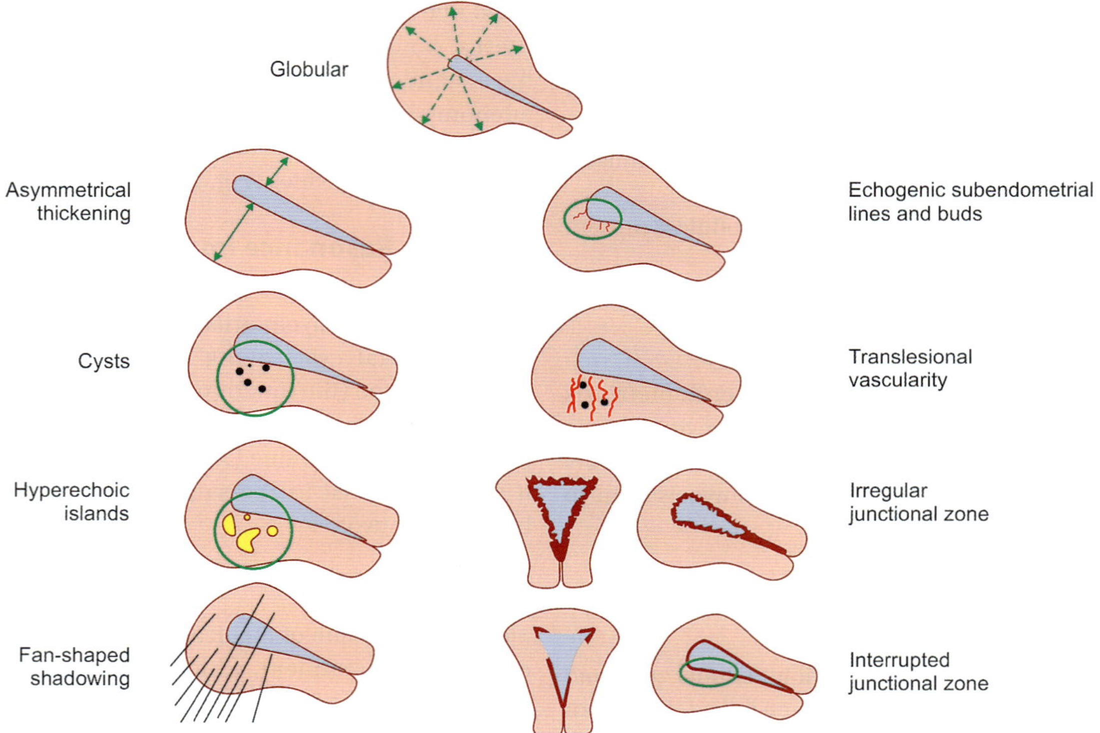

Fig. 11: Morphological uterus sonographic assessment (MUSA) guidelines for ultrasonography (USG) diagnosis of adenomyosis.

FERTILITY SPARING LAPAROSCOPIC SURGERIES

Classification of uterus sparing surgical techniques has been described in **Table 2**.

As women with adenomyosis suffer not only from an increased incidence of infertility but also from an increased incidence of recurrent miscarriages, along with menorrhagia and dysmenorrhea women desirous of future pregnancy have been treated by extensive radical adenomyomectomies for symptom relief and to achieve a good pregnancy outcome. With extensive radical adenomyomectomies the resultant scars were not strong enough to withstand subsequent pregnancy hence, several surgeons like Osada came up with special techniques like triple flap technique where after a radical adenomyomectomy the myometrium is sutured back as overlapping flaps to ensure stronger scars that can withstand subsequent pregnancy. This procedure results in >70% spontaneous conception rate. Also, along with good reproductive outcome women get a lot of relief from the dysmenorrhea and menorrhagia. It is recommended that subsequent pregnancies should be delivered by elective cesarean section only.

TABLE 2: Classification of uterus sparing surgical techniques.

Surgical category	*Technique*	*Described variant*
Complete excision	Adenomyo mectomy	*Classical technique modifications:* U-shaped adenomyomectomy, triple flap, and overlapping flaps
Partial excision	Partial adenomy mectomy	*Classical technique modifications:* Transverse H incision, asymmetric dissection

SUNRISE LAPAROSCOPIC FLAP ADENOMYOMECTOMY (FIGS. 12 TO 16)

Procedure

- The primary trocar is inserted at the modified Palmers point and then three secondary trocars are placed under vision lateral to the inferior epigastric vessels on each side and one supra pubic region.
- Dilute vasopressin is then infiltrated into the uterus.
- A vertical incision is then given over the uterus up to the endometrial cavity and 1 cm of margin of myometrium is left over the basalis layer of endometrium.

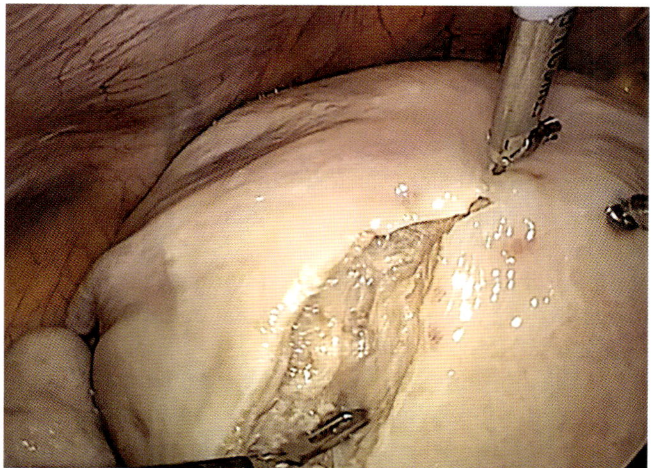

Fig. 12: Incision being given on the uterus after injecting vasopressin.

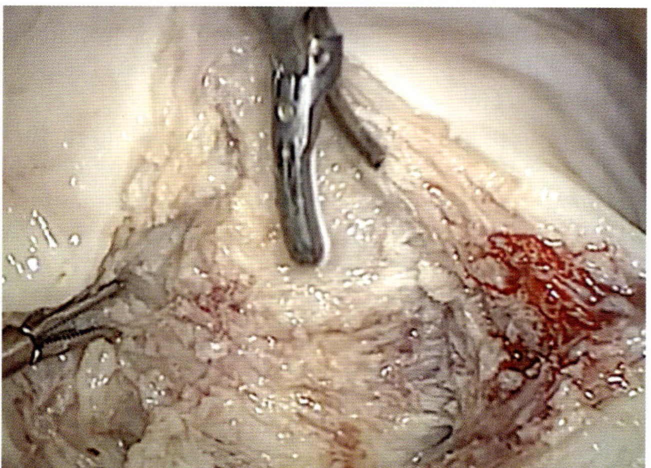

Fig. 13: 1 cm myometrium being left behind with serosa by tunneling.

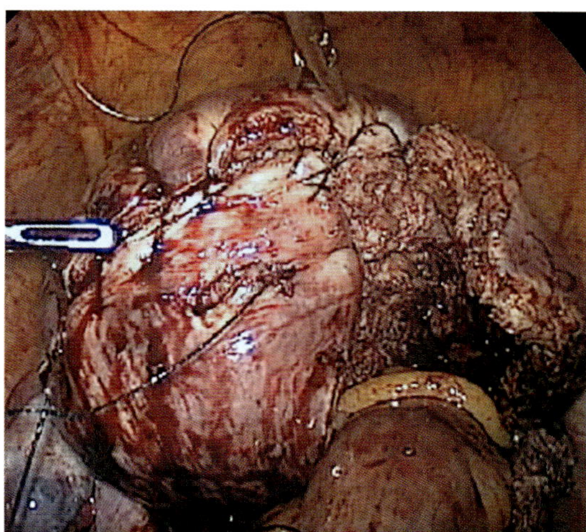

Fig. 14: Flap suturing being done.

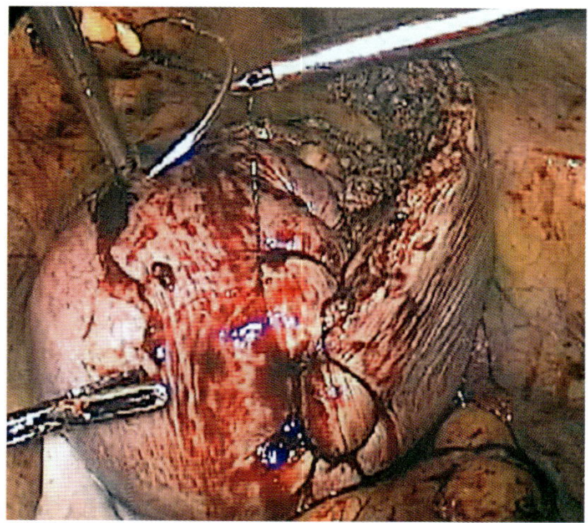

Fig. 15: Seromuscular flap being sutured one over the other.

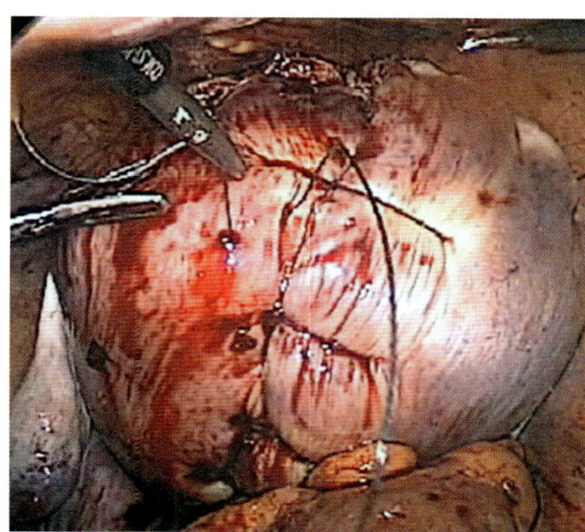

Fig. 16: Final result of a thick seromuscular overlapping flaps.

- On the serosal layer side, 1 cm of margin of myometrium is left inside by tunneling. All the in between myometrium is then excised.
- The end result is thus that the uterus is left with 1 cm myometrium over the endometrium and another 1 cm myometrium under the series.
- To make this remaining myometrium withstand subsequent pregnancy the uterus is then sutured with barbed continuous sutures as reinforcing flaps.

Technical Challenges of this Procedure

Compared to myomas there are no distinct planes/capsule hence, the excision of tissue is entirely arbitrary and left to the discretion of the surgeon. Also, the adenomyomatous tissue is difficult to hold and manipulate compared to normal myometrium.

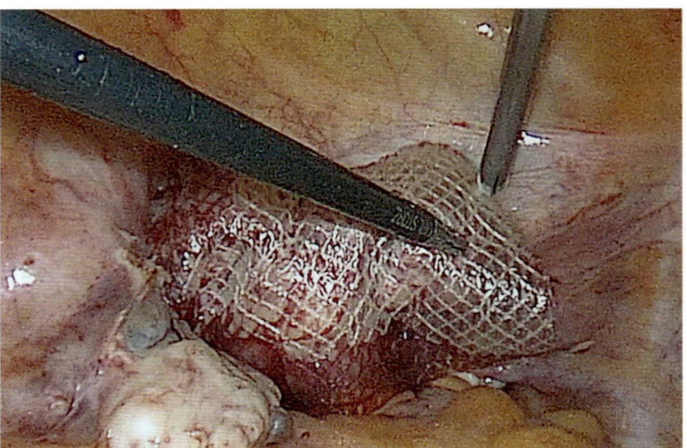

Fig. 17: Dual mesh used to cover the stitch line.

Dual Mesh being used for reinforcing the stitch line in some cases **(Fig. 17)**

The main challenge faced after adenomyomectomy is the high rate of recurrence post the procedure and hence at our center use a levonorgestrel intrauterine system (LNG IUS) device like MIRENA along with GnRH agonists for 4 months post the procedure. Mirena also helps in decreasing junctional zone abnormalities to prevent recurrence and helps with healing of the adenomyoma beds alternatively the oral GnRH antagonists such as elagolix or linzagolix can be used, in addition, for preventing recurrence. They have an additional benefit of lesser menopausal side effects like hot flashes compared to GnRH agonists.

RECTOVAGINAL ENDOMETRIOSIS

This form of adenomyosis deserves special mention as not only does it cause severe symptoms such as dyspareunia, dyschezia, and dysmenorrhea but it is also an individual cause of infertility and RPL..

DEEP INFILTRATING ENDOMETRIOSIS

The infiltration of endometriosis always happens from outside in, hence in deep infiltrating endometriosis (DIE) of bladder bowel or ureter the mucosal involvement happens at a later stage and the serosal and muscular layers are involved earlier.

The most common site of DIE is the rectovaginal septum and the rectosigmoid part of the bowel.

Retroperitoneal endometriosis is an adenomyotic disease was first proposed in 2001. They proposed that rectovaginal and rectocervical nodular endometriosis should be considered as an adenomyotic nodule lesion which consists of smooth muscle with glandular epithelium and scanty stroma. Smooth-muscle proliferation and fibrosis are responsible for the nodular appearance of endometriosis. Rectovaginal endometriosis is different from peritoneal endometriosis, in its ability to infiltrate the peritoneum and invade the neighboring structures.[29-31]

The Enzian classification[32] is used to assess and compartmentalize rectovaginal endometriosis. The basic principles of treatment of rectovaginal endometriosis are as follows:

- As these lesions are not hormone sensitive they have to be surgically excised and removed completely without compromising the functionality of the organ involved, e.g., the low anterior resection syndrome (LARS)[33] where the rectal capacity of storage is decreased leading to the patient having to defecate several times a day after resection anastomosis of rectum. "Economic Radical removal of Endometriosis" is hence practiced by most centers today.
- In endometriosis due to fibrosis and inflammation tissues are pulled in medially distorting the normal anatomy of organs. Thus in rectovaginal endometriosis the ureters and inferior hypogastric nerves are pulled in medially into the rectovaginal nodule and can be damaged during dissection of the nodule hence the surgeon should be aware of the location of the ureters and inferior hypogastric nerves at all times (bilateral damage to inferior hypogastric nerves can lead to bladder atony and sexual disturbances.)

Preoperative Assessment

A complete clinical examination with direct visualization of any vaginal nodule and elicitation of uterosacral nodularity and tenderness on pelvic vaginal (P/V) examination along with presence of a fixed retroverted uterus are the first findings of endometriosis encountered by a clinician. When clinically indicated transvaginal sonography (TVS) is used as a first line investigation to diagnose bowel endometriosis. The rectum and vagina that are adhered together by endometriosis do not slide freely as normal giving rise to the "*sliding sign*" as positive. On ultrasound bowel nodules appear hypoechoic, and in some cases a thinner section or tail is noted at one end resembling a comet hence called the "*comet sign.*" Retraction and adhesions result in the so called "*moose antler sign.*" Endometriotic implants appear as extra luminal growth from the serosa inward which helps to differentiate it from cancers that grows from mucosa toward serosa. Ultrasound mapping of nodules greatly assists in formulating the type of bowel surgery as nodules that are >3 cm in size or involve >50% of the bowel circumference and show >7 mm inward infiltration are usually planned for a segmental bowel resection. To enhance the sensitivity of the scan rectal and vaginal gel contrast is used.

Magnetic Resonance Imaging

The MRI is very commonly used for in the diagnosis of endometriotic lesions owing to its high diagnostic accuracy. MRI has a very good sensitivity and specificity. The presence of blood inside the nodule helps in exact mapping of the disease.

T1- and T2-weighted images are the most specific in identification of rectovaginal nodules especially when contrast is used as contrast helps to differentiate between the disease and the normal bowel areas.[20] The diagnosis is clinched on MRI when attachment of the rectum toward the cervix or asymmetric wall thickening of the lower third of sigmoid colon or a distinct colorectal nodule is identified. These diagnostic findings are similar to those obtained using TVS. MRI is better in differentiating and identifying multifocal lesions and for identifying higher lesions, located above the rectosigmoid junction, which cannot be visualized by TVS. MRI is hence especially useful to assess the "Depth" of endometriosis involvement.

Treatment

The digestive disturbances in bowel endometriosis are owing to the forward fixation of the bowel due to endometriosis and also due to stenosis of the bowel lumen.[34-36]

Surgery for bowel endometriosis is standardized to the following steps [(mnemonic SOSURE) (1) Sigmoid mobilization; (2) Ovarian mobilization; (3) Suspension of the ovaries and uterus; (4) Ureterolysis; (5) Rectovaginal and Pararectal space dissection; (6) Excision of all endometriosis.]

The excision of the endometriosis is decided based on the size and depth of bowel involvement.

The surgical techniques are tailored to the depth of endometriotic nodule **(Fig. 18 and Table 3)**

- *Shaving:* When endometriosis involves the serosa and muscularis layer of the bowel and the mucosa is not involved then the lesion can be shaved off the bowel without entering the mucosa this can be done by two methods (1) *The antegrade method:* Dissection is started from the bowel wall and the last part to be resected is on the torus uterinus this is the antegrade method. (2) The dissection is started from the torus uterinus and the last part to be resected is on the bowel wall this is the retrograde method which offers the advantage that the entire nodule can be lifted up with a grasper to provide counter traction and thus reduce the chance of bowel injury. Reinforcing sutures can be taken on the bowel wall where the bowel wall is found to be too thinned out.
- *Discoid resection:* This technique is used where an anterior or anterolateral full thickness bowel lesion of <3 cm is present. Herein a circular stapler is used which is angulated anteriorly.[36]
- *Segmental resection:* If >50% of the bowel lumen is involved with the endometriotic lesion or if the lesion size is >3 cm then a bowel resection is preferred over shaving or discoid resection. In order to achieve a "Tension free anastomosis" the sigmoid is mobilized to a very high level and the segment of the involved bowel is dissected in a nerve sparing technique by creating "mesocolic windows." The fat pads around the bowel are dissected and left behind to provide good vascularity to the anastomotic stapler lines. A linear stapler is

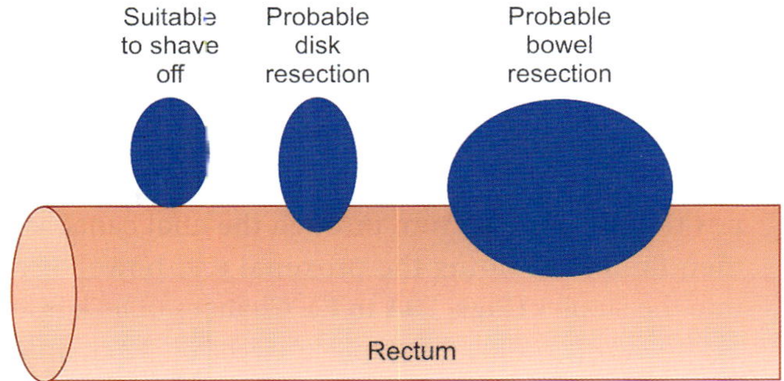

Fig. 18: Bowel involvement with endometriosis.

TABLE 3: Surgical procedure for bowel endometriosis.

Shaving/mucosal skinning	Mucosa of bowel not entered reinforcing sutures vicryl
Discoid resection	Transanal circular stapler for ant/antrolat bowel resection
Segmental resection	Full thickness with nose techniques (transanal/transvaginal)
Placement of omental patches	2 staple lines

then fired at the distal end of the involved bowel and the anvil of the circular stapler inserted above the involved part of the proximal end. The involved bowel segment is retrieved transanally or transvaginally or through a mini laparotomy. The circular stapler is then positioned in the rectum through the anal canal and then fired after fitting the proximal end bowel anvil into the stapler **(Figs. 19A to E)**. Chances of leak from the bowel increase if the staple line is low (<12 cm from the anal verge). Care should be taken when both the vagina and bowel have stitch lines close to each other as a fistula can develop. An omental patch should be placed between the two stitch lines in such cases to avoid the chance of a rectovaginal fistula formation.

Bowel integrity is always checked after any of the above procedures with the help of methylene blue injected into the rectum or air into the rectum after filling the pelvis with saline. Steps of bowel resection are shown in **Figures 20A to E**.

Postoperatively early recovery after surgery (ERAS protocols such as avoiding drains and catheters, using transversus abdominus plane (TAP) block for pain management and early feeding (as soon as bowel sounds positive) with a carbohydrate rich fluid and other fluids help the patient recover faster.

Complications

Several studies have shown that after colorectal resection complications are higher (12–22%) compared to those occurring after shaving (3–4%). Some of the complications that can be encountered are: rectovaginal fistulas, urinary fistulas, pelvic abscess, pelvic hematomas, stenosis of colorectal anastomosis, removal of rectal reservoir, risk of fecal incontinence, and urgency.

Complication of progressive endometriotic nodule can also be serious, e.g., toxic mega colon **(Fig. 21)** in a case of unoperated obstructive bowel endometriosis.

CERVICAL INSUFFICIENCY

Cervical insufficiency/incompetence is defined by the ACOG as the "inability of the cervix to retain a pregnancy in the second trimester in the absence of uterine contractions."[37-39] This entity thus results in spontaneous miscarriages in the second trimester or in preterm labor. These structural cervical abnormalities can be due to:

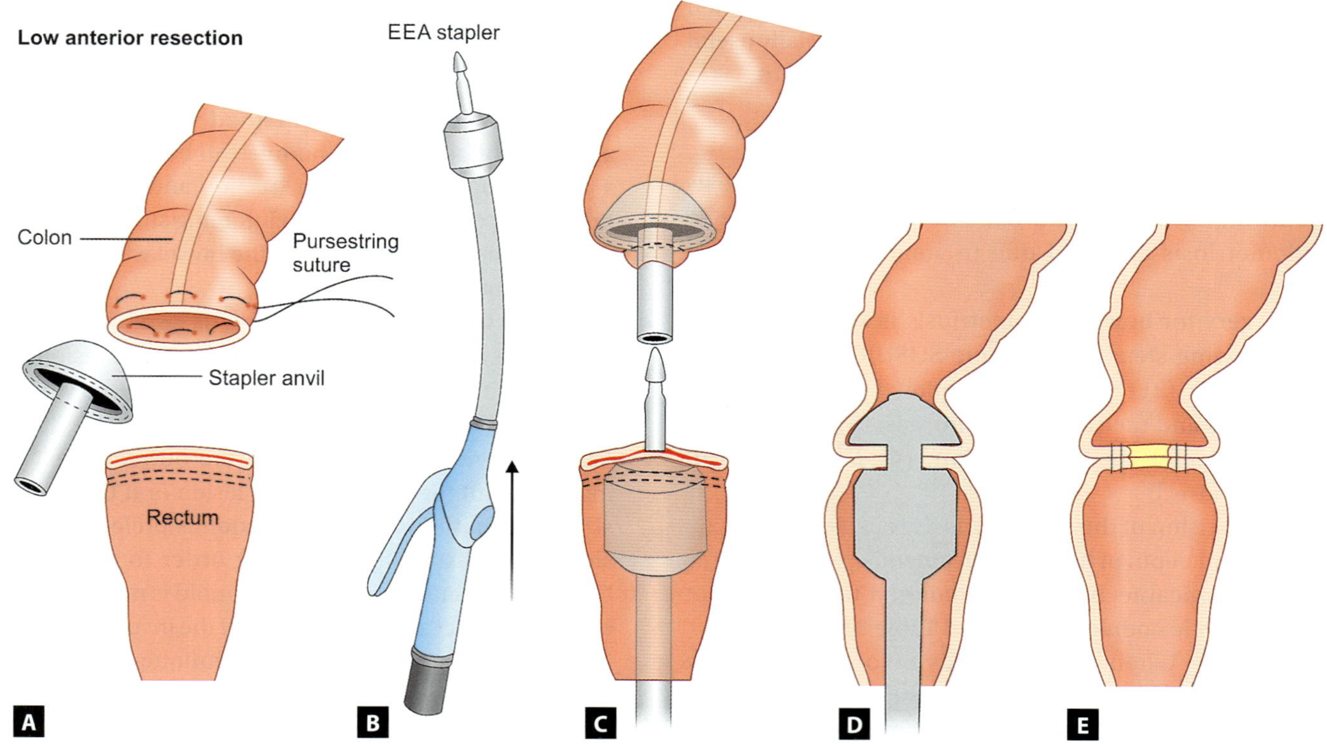

Fig. 19: Use of stapler after bowel resection.

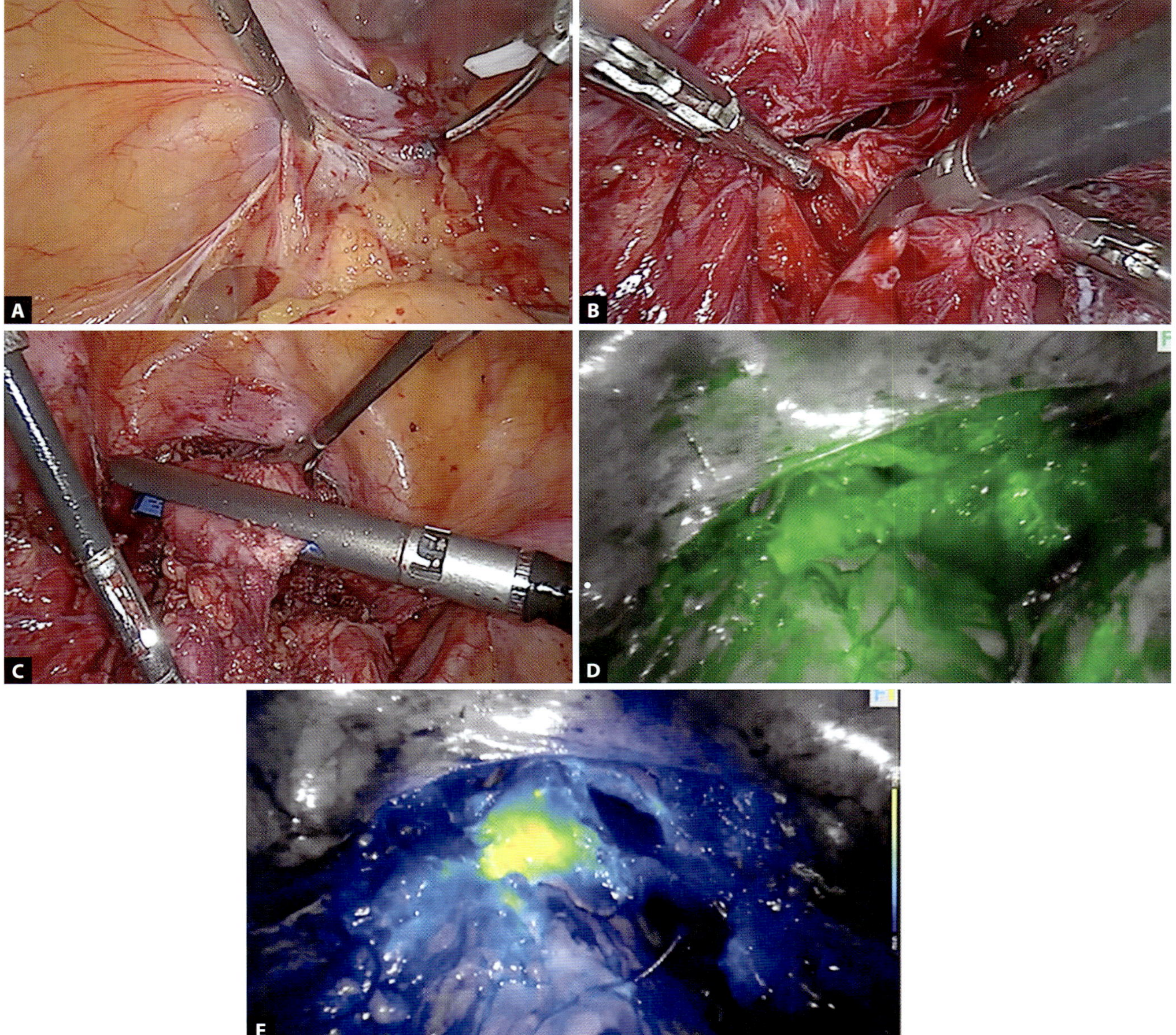

Figs. 20A to E: Steps of laparoscopic bowel resection and anastomosis for bowel endometriosis. (A) Sigmoid adhesiolysis and mobilization; (B) Ureterolysis being done for hydro nephrotic ureter; (C) Applying linear stapler proximal to affected bowel length to be resected; (D) Checking vascularity of the anastomosed bowel after Indocyanine Green dye; and (E) Checking vascularity under blue filter.
Courtesy: Sunrise Hospital, New Delhi. Operated by Dr. Nikita Trehan.

- *Congenital causes:* Mullerian anomalies like septum; collagen abnormalities like Ehler Danlos syndrome; or
- *Acquired causes:* Can happen as a result of procedures/ trauma to the cervix (previous D&C or previous cervical tear or a large loop excision of cervix for cervical intraepithelial neoplasia (CIN), or previous radical trachelectomy).

Prophylactic placement of a cervical encerclage is an effective treatment for providing structural support and for retaining the cervical mucus plug to aid the cervix in retaining the pregnancy.

Cervical cerclage is classified according to the indication for performing cerclage into the given mentioned categories:

- *History indicated encerclage:* A cervical cerclage placed prophylactically in asymptomatic women with a history of previous second trimester miscarriages [three or more as per Royal College of Obstetricians and Gynaecologists (RCOG)] or a single preterm birth. This stitch is applied either prepregnancy or during pregnancy, after first trimester anomaly screening with nuchal translucency (NT) scan and Dual marker or noninvasive prenatal testing (NIPT).
- *Ultrasound indicated cerclage:* A cervical cerclage placed prophylactically in asymptomatic women detected with having a cervical length <25 mm on ultrasound screening between 14 and 24 weeks or in high-risk women. Routine cervical length screening every 2 weeks in high-risk women (women with history of one or two previous second trimester miscarriage or preterm birth, history of cesarean section on a fully dilated cervix or history of previous cervical weakness by cervical trauma, or Mullerian defects) is recommended by NICE guidelines.
- *Emergency encerclage:* A cervical cerclage which is performed as a rescue salvage procedure in cases of premature dilatation of cervix with exposed membranes **(Fig. 22)**. This stitch is only applied after ruling out chorioamnionitis.

Cervical cerclage is also classified according to the anatomical location of the cerclage into:

- Low vaginal cerclage (Mac Donald's cerclage)
- High vaginal cerclage (after bladder mobilization like Shirodkar's stitch).
- Abdominal cerclage (at the level of internal os).
- Occlusion stitch (like Wurm's stitch).

The multicenter randomized controlled trial of transcervical versus transabdominal cervical cerclage (MAVRIC) study, demonstrated the superiority of transabdominal cerclage compared to high or low vaginal cerclage in preventing preterm birth before 32 weeks of pregnancy.

- *The fundamental principles of laparoscopic encerclage:* We are aware that the process of labor starts at the internal os, which upon commencement of dilatation further stimulates contractions and the last part to get dilated is the external os (a cerclage placed at the external os like Mac Donald's frequently fails in genuine cervical incompetence). Hence a cerclage placed abdominally at the internal os is the ideal location for placement of the encerclage.

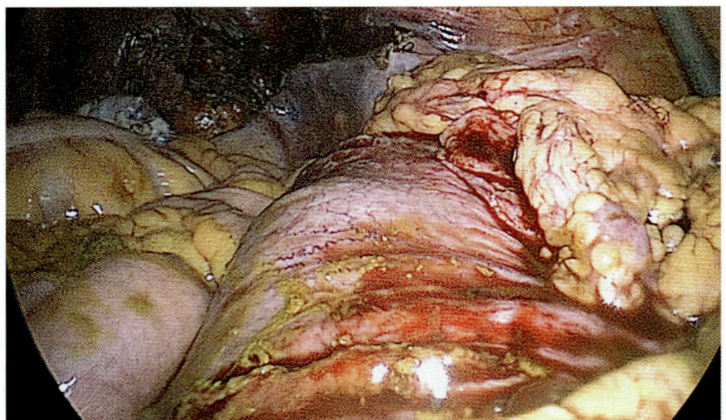

Fig. 21: Toxic megacolon seen laparoscopically.
Courtesy: Sunrise Hospital, New Delhi Operated by Dr. Nikita Trehan.

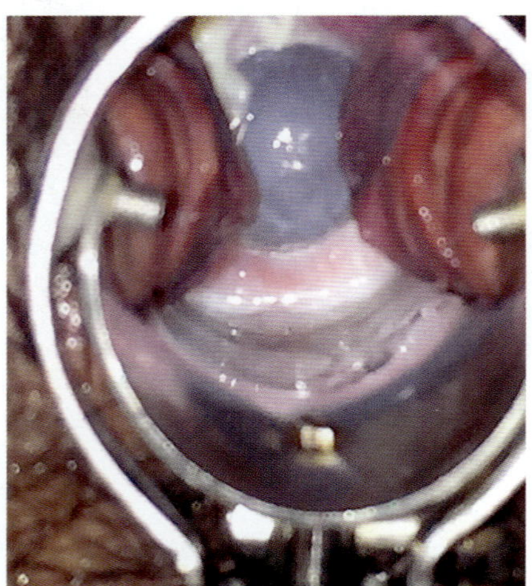

Fig. 22: Dilated os with bulging membranes.
Courtesy: Sunrise hospital, New Delhi. Operated by Dr. Nikita Trehan.

- *The sunrise method of laparoscopic encerclage:* Our method of performing a laparoscopic encerclage is designed keeping certain key points in mind:
  - The passage of the mersilene tape (the suture of choice in our method) is around the cervix and not into the matter of the cervix. This tape is passed medial to the uterine vessels as occlusion of the uterine vessels in pregnancy can lead to fetal growth restriction and placental abnormalities.
  - During pregnancy it is difficult to manipulate the pregnant uterus (as the usual uterine manipulator or myoma screw cannot be used) so creation of broad ligament windows by our method greatly aids in the passage of the needle of the mersilene tape.

- If the tape is accidentally placed at a higher level (above the internal os in the lower uterine segment) it will be useless, hence an intraoperative ultrasound to check the correct level of placement is mandatory.
- During pregnancy a low vaginal cerclage or an occlusion stitch is also placed along with the laparoscopic encerclage to prevent the loss of the cervical mucus plug as the loss of this mucus plug can lead to vaginal infections ascending during pregnancy.

Steps of Surgery

- Primary visual 10 mm trocar is entered via the Lee Huang's point. Three (5 mm) secondary working trocars are the placed under vision.
- The uterovesical fold of peritoneum is opened and bladder is pushed down **(Fig. 23)**.
- Bilateral broad ligament windows are opened and the bilateral uterine vessels identified.
- Mersilene tape is then passed medial to the uterine vessels anterior to posterior on the left side and the needle is then passed through the pouch of Douglas and posterior to anterior on the right side medial to the uterine vessels just above the level of uterosacral insertion to encircle the cervix **(Figs. 24 and 25)**.
- The needle is then cut, and 4–6 tight knots are placed **(Fig. 26)**. A check ultrasound is then performed to check the level of the stitch and the fetal heart rate is also checked.

Intraoperative Challenges While Performing a Laparoscopic Cervical Cerclage

- *Accidental injury to the pregnant uterus during primary trocar entry or secondary trocars while insertion:* In such cases we are aware that unless there is profuse bleeding which may require a stitch, a simple bipolar coagulation of the bleeding point on the surface is enough to arrest the bleeding. The gravid uterus has increased vascularity and even though the bleeding may appear greater in proportion to the injury, surface coagulation will arrest this bleeding easily. A simple stitch may also suffice in case of any doubt.
- *Accidental injury to the internal iliac and uterine vessels while creating the broad ligament windows:* Keeping

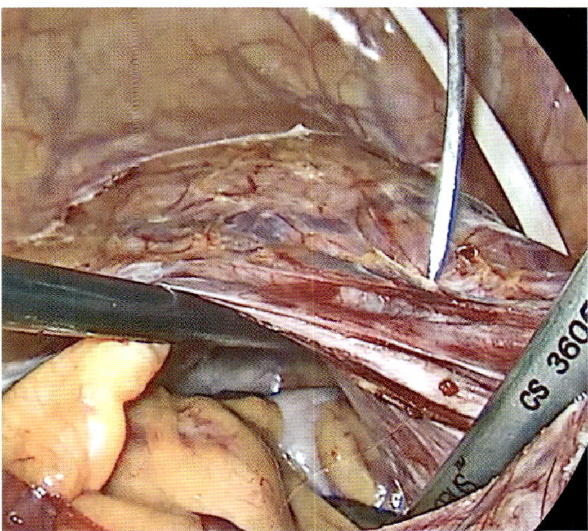

Fig. 24: Passing the tape on the right side.

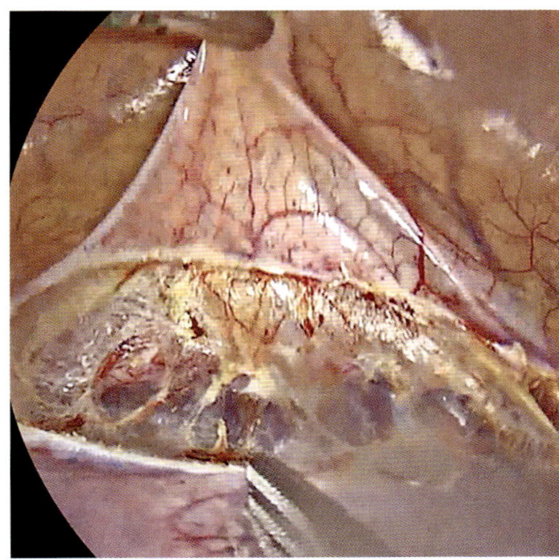

Fig. 23: Opening uterovesical (UV) fold.

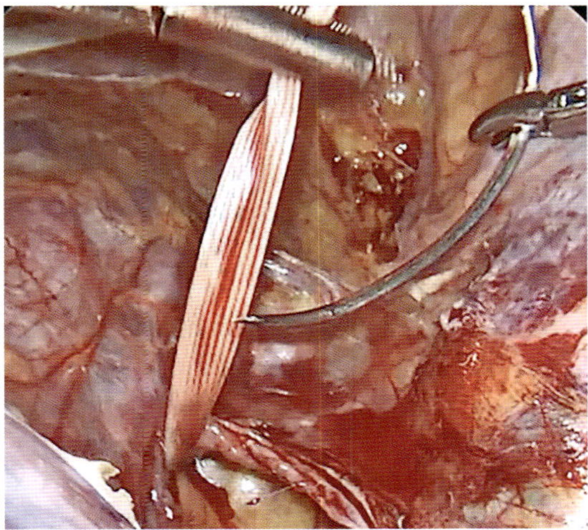

Fig. 25: Passing the tape on the left side.

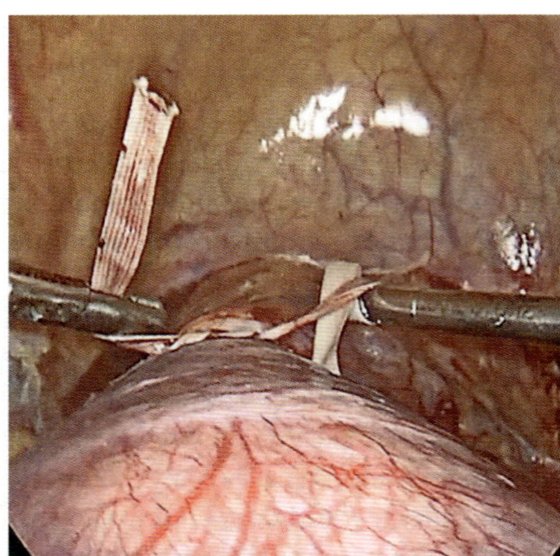

Fig. 26: 4–6 knots of tape.
Courtesy: Sunrise Hospital, New Delhi. Operated by Dr. Nikita Trehan.

vascular clips handy at such times can be extremely beneficial, as a 5 mm port can easily be converted into a 10 mm port for applying a 10 mm vascular clip on the vessel to arrest bleeding.

- *Obliterated Pouch of Douglas:* This can be one of the greatest intraoperative challenges one can face. In patients with previous history of endometriosis, pelvic inflammatory disease (PID), previous surgical adhesions, the Pouch of Douglas (POD) may be obliterated complicating the surgery to such an extent, that we may have to abandon laparoscopic approach in favor for a high vaginal cerclage like a Shirodkar, because of complete inaccessibility or completely obliterated POD or a frozen pelvis. We may also try placing the knot anteriorly by passing through the broad ligament bilaterally and pulling it down on the cervix without separating the POD adhesions (*Su technique*), however, the sequelae of this bilateral tying of uterine vessels may potentially lead to placental insufficiency and fetal growth retardation subsequently.
- *Mode of delivery after lap encerclage:* This is done by elective-cesarean route only, keeping the tape intact for the next pregnancy. In case of intrauterine death or chorioamnionitis the tape must be cut and the baby delivered without delay, instead of performing a hysterotomy.

The mersilene tape can be cut either by a laparoscopy or posterior colpotomy. It is not essential to cut the knot or remove the tape. The tape can be cut at any place in the entire encircle, following which it will become loose and the baby will deliver through open incompetent cervix.

Additionally, if an interval cerclage has been placed before this pregnancy and there is a first trimester fetal loss up 14 weeks or a termination of pregnancy for medical reasons must be performed due to a congenital anomaly, suction evacuation of the products of conception can be performed with the tape in situ.

- *Bed rest:* Post an emergency cerclage, the patient will require more bed rest compared to a patient postelective cerclage, as there are chances of a bag of membranes with amniotic fluid present between internal and external stitch (Mac Donald's or Wurm) herniating into the cervix. The effect of gravity superadded to the earlier mentioned factors can aggravate a leak from the membranes. So, bed rest is advised, so that the bag of membranes does not herniate. If the procedure is electively planned, prolonged bed rest is not warranted (as in the case of an emergency procedure) and early ambulation is not only possible but advised. To summarize, even if history indicated cerclage is not done, an ultrasound indicated elective cerclage and surveillance is better than performing a rescue cerclage.
- *Leaking:* If there is a high leak with the membranes intact and no chorioamnionitis or preterm contractions, the pregnancy can be continued with a close watch as even patients with oligohydramnios will progress and will continue quite favorably. In one such case of twin pregnancy, at our center the first twin had a high leak leading to intrauterine device (IUD), but the second twin survived and was delivered by cesarean section at 35 weeks.
- *Tape erosion:* The laparoscopic tape in rare circumstances can erode into the bladder or the cervix. In one such case at our center a lady had two successful pregnancies postlap encerclage who delivered by cesarean section at term. The mersilene tape extruded into the cervical canal a few years after her cesarean delivery and led to repeated vaginal infections and dyspareunia **(Fig. 27)**. The tape had to be removed by another laparoscopy. Thus, we now advice removal of the mersilene tape at the time of cesarean once her family is complete.

Myths Regarding Cervical Encerclage

In case of massive contractions with chorioamnionitis or otherwise/after the procedure, the tape will migrate and

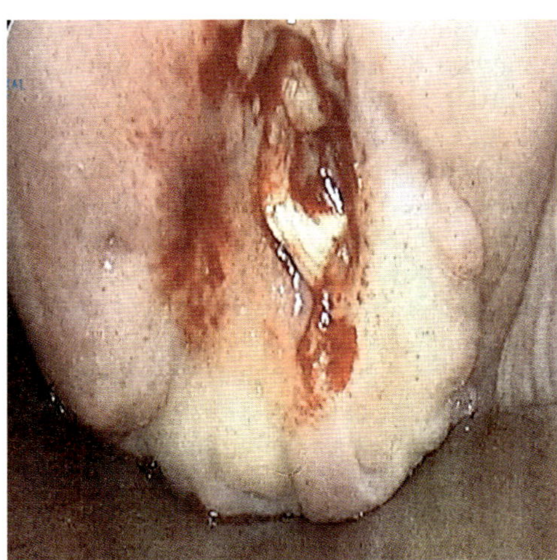

Fig. 27: Tape erosion into the cervix.
Courtesy: Sunrise Hospital, New Delhi. Operated by Dr. Nikita Trehan.

come into the cervical canal from one side. The tape will automatically become loose, hence the myth that "in case of massive contractions there can be rupture uterus" is ill founded as the tape, once it comes into the cervical canal, becomes completely free and will not lead to a bucket handle or complete rupture of the uterus.

In our vast experience of >300 cases of laparoscopic encerclage a 100% success in terms of take home baby has been achieved in cases of interval cerclage (164 cases) and a success rate of 96% has been achieved in pregnant cerclages. All the failures we have had thus far have been in cases of rescue cerclage complicated by chorioamnionitis.

CONCLUSION

Surgical removal of intramural and large submucous myomas can benefit patients suffering from RPL and recurrent implantation failure (RIF). These surgeries are complex and need meticulous preoperative planning at dedicates endoscopic centers, to minimize postoperative complications, preserve the uterine receptivity and preventing long-term pregnancy complications of scar dehiscence. Similarly, focal adenomyosis and endometriotic lesions when completely excised surgically, give better live birth rates than prolonged medical management. Laparoscopy is a good adjunct to enhance the safety of complicated hysteroscopic procedures as well. More recently cervical encerclage at the level of internal os via laparoscopy has given better results than transvaginal cerclages. Hence, laparoscopic procedures can greatly enhance the rates of achieving live births in cases of RPL.

REFERENCES

1. Practice Committee of the American Society for Reproductive Medicine. Evaluation and treatment of recurrent pregnancy loss. Fertil Steril. 2012;98:1103-11.
2. Grimbizis GF, Camus M, Tarlatzis BC, Bontis JN, Devroey P. Clinical implications of uterine malformations and hysteroscopic treatment results. Hum Reprod Update. 2001;7:161-74.
3. Jeve YB, Davies W. Evidence-based management of recurrent miscarriages. J Hum Reprod Sci. 2014;7:159-69.
4. Chandler TM, Machan LS, Cooperberg PL, Harris AC, Chang SD. Mullerian duct anomalies: from diagnosis to intervention. Br J Radiol. 2009;82:1034-42.
5. Olpin JD, Heilbrun M. Imaging of Müllerian duct anomalies. Clin Obstet Gynecol. 2009;52:40-56.
6. Taylor E, Gomel V. The uterus and fertility. Fertil Steril. 2008;89:10-16.
7. Saravelos SH, Cocksedge KA, Li TC. Prevalence and diagnosis of congenital uterine anomalies in women with reproductive failure: a critical appraisal. Hum Reprod Update. 2008;14:415-29.
8. Hamilton JA, Larson AJ, Lower AM, Hasnain S, Grudzinskas JG. Routine use of saline hysteron-sonography in 500 consecutive, unselected, infertile women. Hum Reprod. 1998;13:2463-73.
9. American Association of Gynecologic Laparoscopists (AAGL): Advancing Minimally Invasive Gynecology Worldwide. AAGL practice report: practice guidelines for the diagnosis and management of submucous leiomyomas. J Minim Invasive Gynecol. 2012;19:152-71.
10. Vlahos NF, Theodoridis TD, Partsinevelos GA. Myomas and Adenomyosis: Impact on Reproductive Outcome. Biomed Res Int. 2017;2017:5926470.
11. Yoshino O, Nishii O, Osuga Y, Asada H, Okuda S, Orisaka M, et al. Myomectomy decreases abnormal uterine peristalsis and increases pregnancy rate. J Minim Invasive Gynecol. 2012;19:63-7.
12. Yoshino O, Hayashi T, Osuga Y, Orisaka M, Asada H, Okuda S, et al. Decreased pregnancy rate is linked to abnormal uterine peristalsis caused by intramural fibroids. Hum Reprod. 2010;25:2475-9.
13. Somigliana E, Vercellini P, Daguati R, Pasin R, De Giorgi O, Crosignani PG, et al. Fibroids and female reproduction: a critical analysis of the evidence. Hum Reprod Update. 2007;13:465-76.
14. Pritts EA, Parker WH, Olive DL. Fibroids and infertility: an updated systematic review of the evidence. Fertil Steril. 2009;91:1215-23.
15. Sunkara SK, Khairy M, El-Toukhy T, Khalaf Y, Coomarasamy A. The effect of intramural fibroids without uterine cavity involvement on the outcome of IVF treatment: a systematic review and meta-analysis. Hum Reprod. 2010;25:418-29.
16. Sankaran S, Manyonda IT. Medical management of fibroids. Best Pract Res Clin Obstet Gynaecol. 2008;22:655-76.

17. Tinelli A, Malvasi A, Hurst BS, Tsin DA, Davila F, Dominguez G, et al. Surgical Management of Neurovascular Bundle in Uterine Fibroid Pseudocapsule. JSLS. 2012;16:119-29.
18. Huang KG, Lee CL. Lee-Huang point 20 years on. Gynecol Minim Invasive Ther. 2013;2:103-4.
19. Hickman LC, Kotlyar A, Shue S, et al. Hemostatic Techniques for Myomectomy: An Evidence-Based Approach. J Minim Invasive Gynecol. 2019;26(2):373.
20. Mais V, Cirronis MG, Peiretti M, Ferrucci G, Cossu E, Melis GB, et al. Efficacy of auto-cross linked hyaluronan gel for adhesion prevention in laparoscopy and hysteroscopy: a systematic review and meta-analysis of randomized controlled trials. Eur J Obstet Gynecol Reprod Biol. 2012;160:1-5.
21. Ahmad G, Duffy JM, Farquhar C, Vail A, Vandekerckhove P, Watson A, et al. Barrier agents for adhesion prevention after gynaecological surgery. Cochrane Database Syst Rev. 2008;2:CD000475.
22. Levgur M, Abadi MA, Tucker A. Adenomyosis: symptoms, histology, and pregnancy terminations. Obstet Gynecol. 2000;95:688-91.
23. Grimbizis GF, Mikos T, Tarlatzis B. Uterus sparing operative treatment for adenomyosis. Fertil Steril. 2014;101:472-87.
24. Campo S, Campo V, Benagiano G. Adenomyosis and infertility. Reprod Biomed Online. 2012;24:35-46.
25. Hashimoto A, Iriyama T, Sayama S, Nakayama T, Komatsu A, Miyauchi A, et al. Adenomyosis and adverse perinatal outcomes: increased risk of second trimester miscarriage, preeclampsia, and placental malposition. J Matern Fetal Neonatal Med. 2018;31:364-9.
26. Mochimaru A, Aoki S, Oba MS, Kurasawa K, Takahashi T, Hirahara F. Adverse pregnancy outcomes associated with adenomyosis with uterine enlargement. J Obstet Gynaecol Res. 2015;41:529-33.
27. Tamura H, Kishi H, Kitade M, Asai-Sato M, Tanaka A, Murakami T, et al. Complications and outcomes of pregnant women with adenomyosis in Japan. Reprod Med Biol. 2017;16:330-6.
28. Harmsen MJ, Van den Bosch T, de Leeuw RA, Dueholm M, Exacoustos C, Valentin L, et al. Consensus on revised definitions of Morphological Uterus Sonographic Assessment (MUSA) features of adenomyosis: results of modified Delphi procedure. Ultrasound Obstet Gynecol. 2022;60:118-31.
29. Haute Autorité de Santé. (2015). Management of endometriosis. [online] Available from https://www.has-sante.fr/jcms/c_2819733/en/management-of-endometriosis [Last accessed December, 2024].
30. Allaire C, Bedaiwy MA, Yong PJ. Diagnosis and management of endometriosis. CMAJ. 2023;195(10):E363-71.
31. Donnez J, Van Langendonckt A, Casanas-Roux F, Van Gossum JP, Pirard C, Jadoul P, et al. Current thinking on the pathogenesis of endometriosis. Gynecol Obstet Invest. 2002;54 Suppl 1:52-8; discussion 59-62.
32. Tuttlies F, Keckstein J, Ulrich U, Possover M, Schweppe KW, Wustlich M, et al. ENZIAN-score, a classification of deep infiltrating endometriosis. Zentralbl Gynakol. 2005;127(5):275-81.
33. Bokor A, Hudelist G, Dobó N, Dauser B, Farella M, Brubel R, et al. Low anterior resection syndrome following different surgical approaches for low rectal endometriosis: A retrospective multicenter study. Acta Obstet Gynecol Scand. 2021;100(5):860-7.
34. Remorgida V, Ragni N, Ferrero S, Anserini P, Torelli P, Fulcheri E. The involvement of the interstitial Cajal cells and the enteric nervous system in bowel endometriosis. Hum Reprod Oxf Engl. 2005;20(1):264-71.
35. Wolthuis AM, Meuleman C, Tomassetti C, D'Hooghe T, de Buck van Overstraeten A, D'Hoore A. Bowel endometriosis: Colorectal surgeon perspective in a multidisciplinary surgical team. World J Gastroenterol. 2014;20(42):15616-23.
36. Khazali S. Endometriosis: Causes—Symptoms—Diagnosis and Treatment. (2021). Operative techniques for Deep Endometriosis Surgery. [online] Available from https://www.endofound.org/operative-techniques-for-deep-endometriosis-surgery-shaheen-khazali-md [Last accessed December, 2024].
37. ACOG. Cerclage for the Management of Cervical Insufficiency. [online] Available from: https://www.acog.org/clinical/clinical-guidance/practice-bulletin/articles/2014/02/cerclage-for-the-management-of-cervical-insufficiency [Last accessed December, 2024].
38. Shennan A, Story L, the Royal College of Obstetricians G. Cervical Cerclage. BJOG Int J Obstet Gynaecol. 2022;129(7):1178-210.
39. NICE. (2015). Recommendations. Preterm labour and birth. [online] Available from https://www.nice.org.uk/guidance/ng25/chapter/Recommendations [Last accessed December, 2024].

SECTION

5 Imaging

CHAPTER

24

Interpregnancy Imaging

Selvaraj Ravi Lakshmy

ABSTRACT

Some Müllerian abnormalities of the uterus are associated with not only recurrent pregnancy loss (RPL) but other pregnancy complications like preterm birth and fetal growth restriction. These anomalies are difficult to diagnose in a gravid uterus and require meticulous interpregnancy ultrasound imaging to diagnose them, and take corrective measures prior to next pregnancy to avoid a miscarriage. These include unicornuate and bicornuate uterus with unequal horns. The distinction between septate uterus and bicornuate uterus on imaging is vital as the treatment modalities are entirely different and so is the pregnancy prognosis.

Keywords: Müllerian anomalies, Unicornuate uterus, Bicornuate uterus, Uterus didelphys.

INTRODUCTION

The incidence of Müllerian anomalies in women with recurrent pregnancy loss (RPL) is 5–10%. Müllerian defects are either found incidentally or during the evaluation of RPL.[1] The assessment of Müllerian anomalies in pregnancy is difficult due to alteration in the contour of uterus by the presence of the gestation sac. Hence, the interpregnancy interval is the best time period to evaluate for the presence of an existing uterine anomaly. This chapter aims at the importance of interpregnancy imaging for women with RPL.

The importance of adequate imaging during the interpregnancy period in women with recurrent abortion is that discovering a Müllerian anomaly provides a reasonable explanation for adverse pregnancy outcomes. Moreover, identification of a treatable Müllerian anomaly is crucial in the management of RPL. The prevalence of diagnosed Müllerian defects in women with RPL significantly varies in literature. These variations are due to the inaccuracy of different diagnostic tests and techniques and lack of awareness among treating clinicians.[2]

Müllerian anomalies which cause RPL are septate (35%), bicornuate (25%), and arcuate uterus (20%) followed by didelphys and unicornuate uterus.[3] Pregnancy loss can be attributed to insufficient uterine distention or abnormal implantation in a uterine septum.[4] A major life-threatening complication of an unidentified Müllerian anomaly is rupture of pregnancy in a rudimentary horn. Since Müllerian anomalies are associated with so many complications, there is a need to identify them in the prepregnancy period in women with RPL.

Detection of the type of Müllerian anomaly in women with RPL is of prime importance as the management and outcome of such patients are greatly influenced by correct diagnosis of the specific type of Müllerian anomaly.[5] Hence, there arises a need to have a classification system which improves the communication between the imaging specialists and the treating clinicians.

Of the many available classification systems of Müllerian anomaly, the most commonly used are the American Society for Reproductive Medicine and the American Fertility Society (ASRM and AFS) and the European Society of Human Reproduction and Embryology and the the European Society for Gynecological Endoscopy (ESHRE and ESGE) classification systems.

Uterine malformations are classified by ASRM into seven groups namely (1) agenesis and hypoplasia, (2) unicornuate uteri, (3) didelphys uteri, (4) bicornuate uteri, (5) septate uteri, (6) arcuate uteri, and (7) anomalies related to diethylstilbestrol exposure. This system is widely followed; however, this classification does not include vaginal anomalies and other combined anomalies of cervix and vagina.[6] However, ESHRE classification includes cervical and vaginal anomalies and they are classified in independent subclasses.

ESHRE system has three major classes namely (1) uterus (U), (2) cervix (C), and (3) vagina (V) which is further subdivided into subclasses by numericals. Uterus (U): U0—normal uterus; U1—dysmorphic uterus; U2—septate uterus; U3—bicorporeal uterus; U4—hemiuterus; U5—aplastic uterus; U6—for still unclassified cases. Cervix (C): C0—Normal; C1—Septate; C2—Double "normal"; C3—Unilateral aplasia/dysplasia; C4—Aplasia/dysplasia. Vagina (V): V0—Normal vagina; V1—Longitudinal nonobstructing vaginal septum; V2—Longitudinal obstructing vaginal septum; V3—Transverse vaginal septum/imperforate hymen; V4—Vaginal aplasia.[7] In spite of using such a good description to classify Müllerian anomalies, there is still an overlap in differentiation of dysmorphic uterus from normal and there do not exist very strict differentiation criteria to categorize the subclasses.[7-9]

Further to this, ASRM in 2021 classified Müllerian anomalies into nine categories including cervical and vaginal anomalies namely (1) Müllerian agenesis, (2) cervical agenesis, (3) unicornuate uterus, (4) uterus didelphys, (5) bicornuate uterus, (6) septate uterus, (7) longitudinal vaginal septum, (8) transverse vaginal septum, and (9) complex anomalies. The advantage of this classification system is that it is rather descriptive and does not use alphabets and numericals.[10] Though ASRM is widely used and followed, it is the ESHRE classification which gives better definition and description of the uterine anomalies as it uses three-dimensional (3D) ultrasound which is the most potential simple tool in evaluating uterine anomalies.[11]

The imaging modalities available to detect Müllerian anomalies are hysterosalpingography (HSG), two-dimensional (2D) and 3D ultrasound and MRI. The final diagnostic tools are hysteroscopy and laparoscopy. The traditional method is HSG which is an invasive procedure where a contrast dye is injected to demonstrate patent cavities and tubes. The disadvantage of HSG is that the external contour of the uterus including rudimentary segments cannot be visualized.

Moreover in routine practice, as the differentiation of a bicornuate uterus from a septate uterus is difficult with HSG, its reliability in the diagnosis of uterine anomalies is questionable.[12,13] The review of Saravelos et al. revealed that HSG had 78% sensitivity, 90% specificity, and 86% accuracy in the diagnosis of Müllerian anomalies when compared with hysteroscopy.[14]

Two-dimensional ultrasonography is the initial imaging modality in identifying Müllerian anomalies. It is better done during the secretory phase as the endometrium is better visualized in this phase. It is widely available, noninvasive, inexpensive, and serves as an initial screening tool not only to identify Müllerian anomalies but also is associated with renal anomalies if present.[15] A baseline 2D ultrasound paves the way for further diagnostic testing in RPL. Saline infusion sonohysterography has a role in assessing the nature of the uterine septum in septate uterus.[16] Vaginal and cervical septal assessment can be achieved by using gel sonovaginography.[17]

The disadvantage of 2D ultrasound is that transverse and sagittal planes are obtained and not the coronal plane which is needed for the proper classification of Müllerian anomaly. The findings that raise a suspicion of uterine anomaly on 2D ultrasound are bifid uterine cavities on transverse section **(Fig. 1)**, a broad transverse diameter of the uterus, and lateralized position of uterus in transabdominal scan.[15,18]

Three-dimensional reconstructed image provides the exact information and most often does not need any further additional imaging for categorizing the Müllerian anomaly as it provides information about both uterine cavity configuration and also the external contour of uterus.[19]

Clear demarcation of the serosal outline, tubal ostia, endometrial outline, and upper and lower uterine segments are to be clearly visualized in a coronal plane. The terminologies used in 3D ultrasound while evaluating uterine anomalies are as follows—interostial distance, uterine wall thickness, and internal and external indentation. The distance between the two tubal ostia is the interostial distance **(Fig. 2)**. The distance between the serosal outline and the midpoint on the interostial

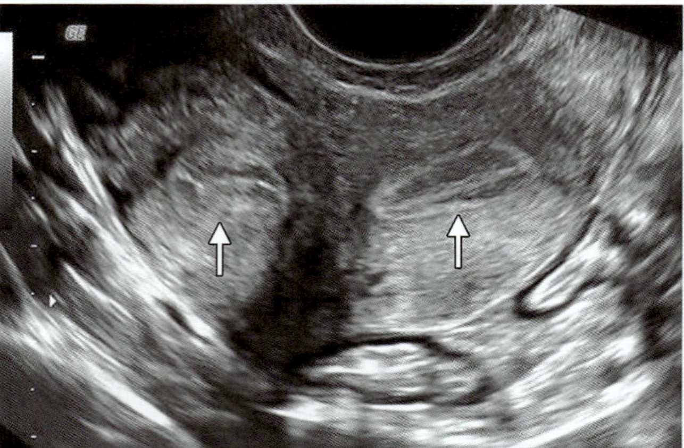

Fig. 1: Transverse view of uterus in transvaginal scan (TVS) showing broad transverse diameter of uterus with bifid endometrial cavities (arrows).

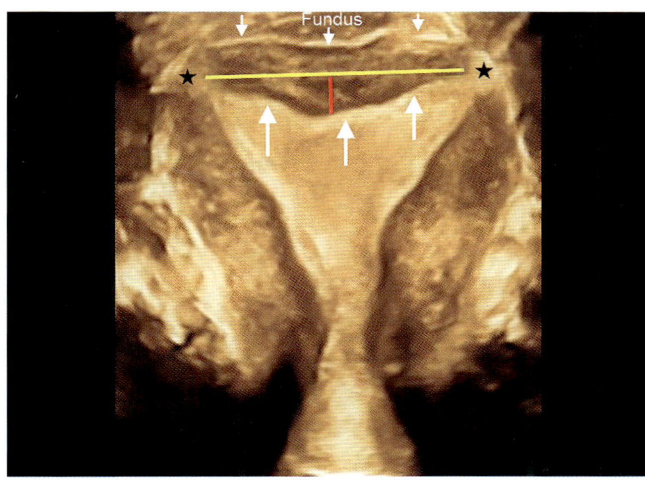

Fig. 2: Three-dimensional (3D) ultrasound rendered image of uterus, long arrows denote endometrial outline, short arrows denote serosal outline, asterix denotes tubal ostia, yellow line is the interostial distance, red line shows internal indentation—the distance between midpoint of interostial line and endometrial line.

line is the uterine wall thickness. Internal indentation is the distance between midpoint of the interostial line and endometrial line **(Fig. 2)** and external indentation is the indentation seen in the serosal outline. Interostial distance serves a screening tool for identifying common Müllerian anomalies. Interostial distance is <2 cm in hypoplastic uterus, 2–4 cm in normal/arcuate uterus and >4 cm in bicornuate uterus.[20]

On 3D ultrasound, the following steps to be followed before coming to a diagnosis.[12] Refer to **Flowchart 1**. 3D ultrasound can differentiate septate from bicornuate uterus as it can show both the external fundal indentation and duplication of the endometrial cavity. **Figures 3 and 4** shows the external fundal indentation on 2D ultrasound in a bicornuate uterus and the corresponding 3D appearance. Note that in **Figures 3 and 4** both the uterine horns are well developed.

Figures 5A to D shows a bicornuate uterus with a rudimentary horn on 2D and 3D. Note that the sagittal

Flowchart 1: Algorithmic ultrasound approach to the diagnosis of uterine anomaly.

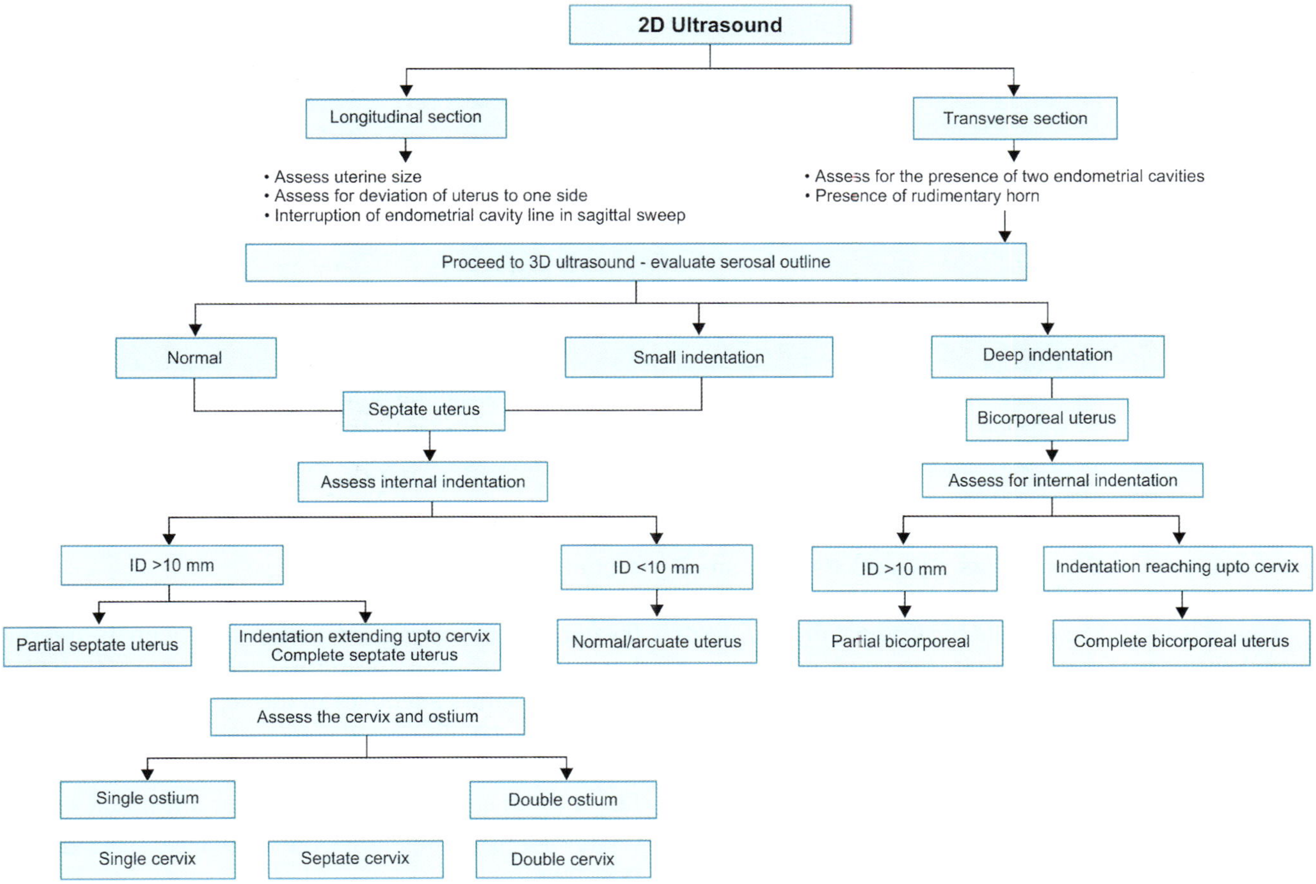

- **2D Ultrasound**
  - Longitudinal section
    - Assess uterine size
    - Assess for deviation of uterus to one side
    - Interruption of endometrial cavity line in sagittal sweep
  - Transverse section
    - Assess for the presence of two endometrial cavities
    - Presence of rudimentary horn
- Proceed to 3D ultrasound - evaluate serosal outline
  - Normal → Septate uterus
  - Small indentation → Septate uterus
    - Septate uterus → Assess internal indentation
      - ID >10 mm
        - Partial septate uterus
        - Indentation extending upto cervix Complete septate uterus
      - ID <10 mm → Normal/arcuate uterus
  - Deep indentation
    - Bicorporeal uterus → Assess for internal indentation
      - ID >10 mm → Partial bicorporeal
      - Indentation reaching upto cervix → Complete bicorporeal uterus
- Assess the cervix and ostium
  - Single ostium
  - Double ostium
  - Single cervix
  - Septate cervix
  - Double cervix

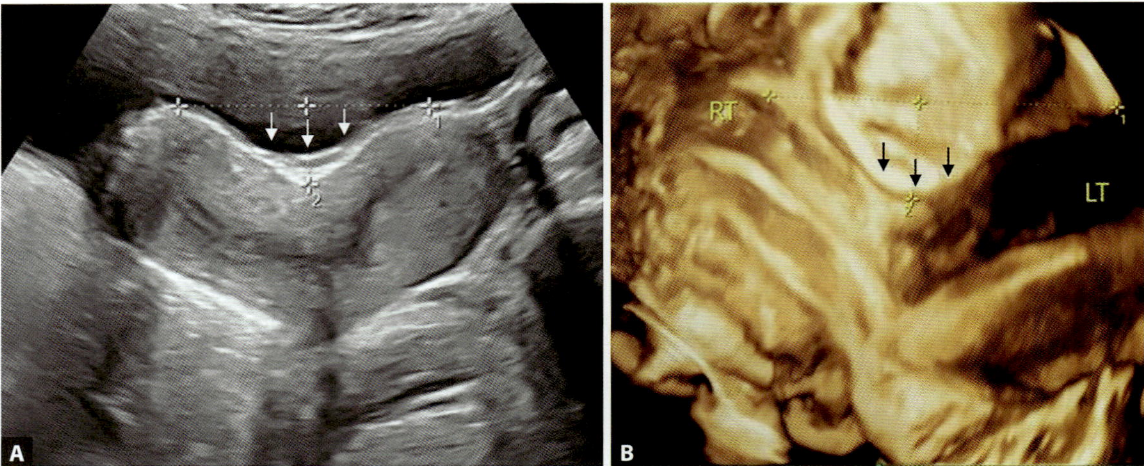

Figs. 3A and B: Bicornuate uterus two-dimensional (2D) transabdominal scan (TAS) and three-dimensional (3D) ultrasound (arrows). (A) 2D coronal section showing indentation of the serosal outline in a bicornuate/bicorporeal uterus. This section is obtained in suboptimal bladder. (B) Corresponding 3D ultrasound showing deep indentation of the external serosal surface of the uterus along with internal indentation. Class U3a—partial bicorporeal uterus in the European Society for Gynecological Endoscopy (ESHRE) classification.

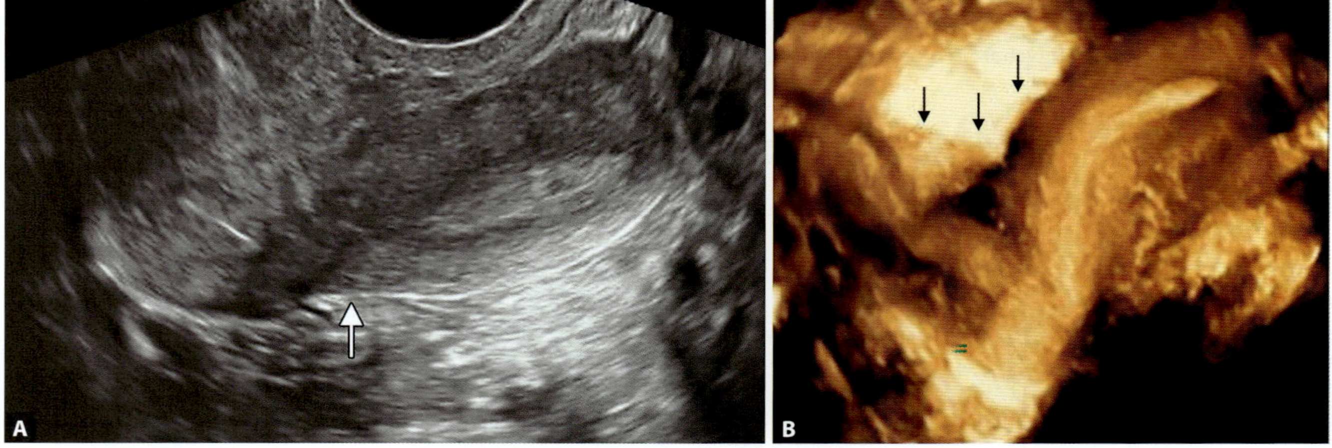

Figs. 4A and B: Bicornuate uterus two-dimensional (2D) transvaginal scan (TVS) and three-dimensional (3D) ultrasound. (A) 2D transvaginal ultrasound showing two separate endometrial cavities and wide interostial distance. Arrow points toward external indentation. (B) Corresponding 3D ultrasound showing deep external indentation in bicornuate uterus.

section of uterus in transabdominal and transvaginal section appears normal **(Figs. 5A and B)**. The small rudimentary horn is shown in **Figure 5C**.

Figure 6 shows a complete bicorporeal uterus/uterus didelphys illustrating two widely separated uterine horns with two cervices.

Figures 7A to C shows a complete septate uterus. Note that there is no suspicion of uterine anomaly in the 2D sagittal section of uterus. However, the transverse section of uterus shown in **Figure 7B** shows bifid endometrial cavities. **Figure 7C** shows the 3D image of the uterus depicting a normal serosal outline and complete septum.

Figures 8A to E shows partial septate uterus. 3D shows the normal external contour of the uterus with the internal indentation caused by the partial septum **(Fig. 8D)**. **Figure 8E** shows adequacy of the septal resection on 3D ultrasound. 3D ultrasound is invaluable in evaluating the residual septum after hysteroscopic resection **(Fig. 8E)**. Either there is no residual septum or a residual septum measuring up to 1 cm in length is considered as optimal resection.[21]

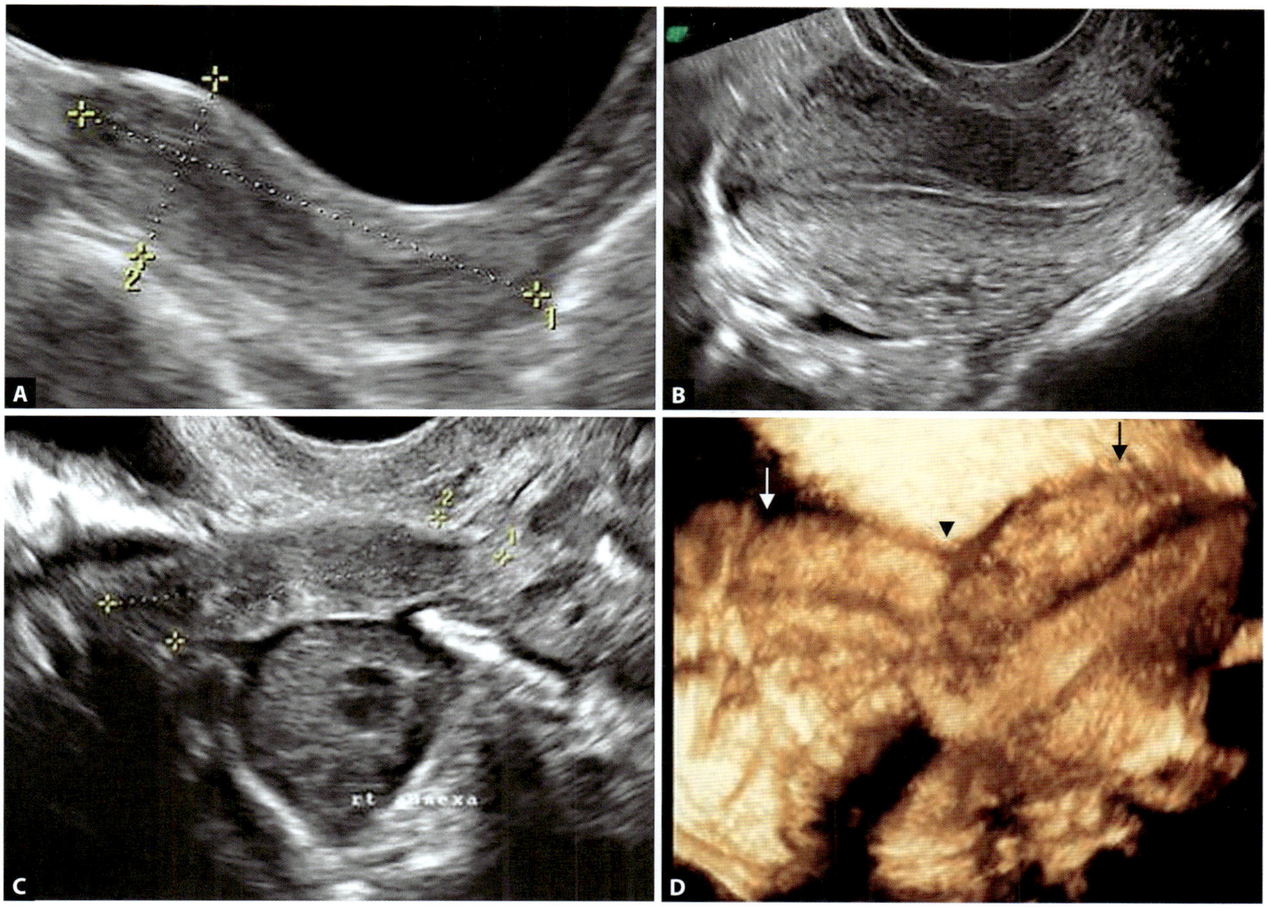

Figs. 5A to D: Bicornuate uterus with rudimentary horn. (A) Two-dimensional (2D) transabdominal scan (TAS) of uterus in sagittal section; (B) 2D transvaginal scan (TVS) of uterus in sagittal section demonstrating well developed horn; (C) 2D TVS of uterus in transverse section showing rudimentary horn; (D) 3D ultrasound image of uterus. Black arrow denotes the developed horn and white arrow denotes the rudimentary horn, arrowhead shows external indentation.

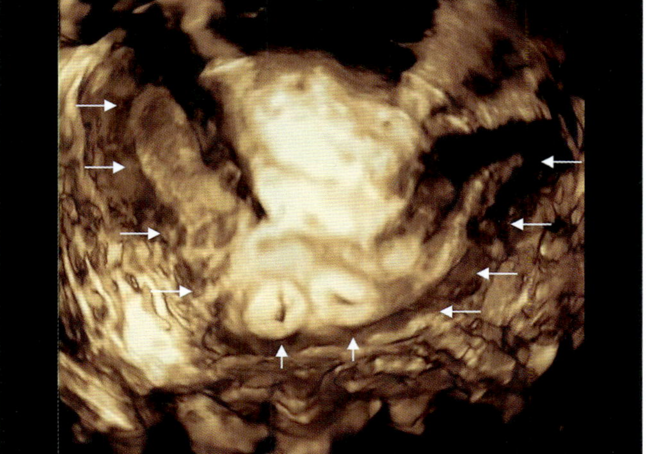

Fig. 6: Three-dimensional (3D) rendered image of uterus didelphys, short arrows show two cervices and long arrow demonstrates the widely separated uterine horns.

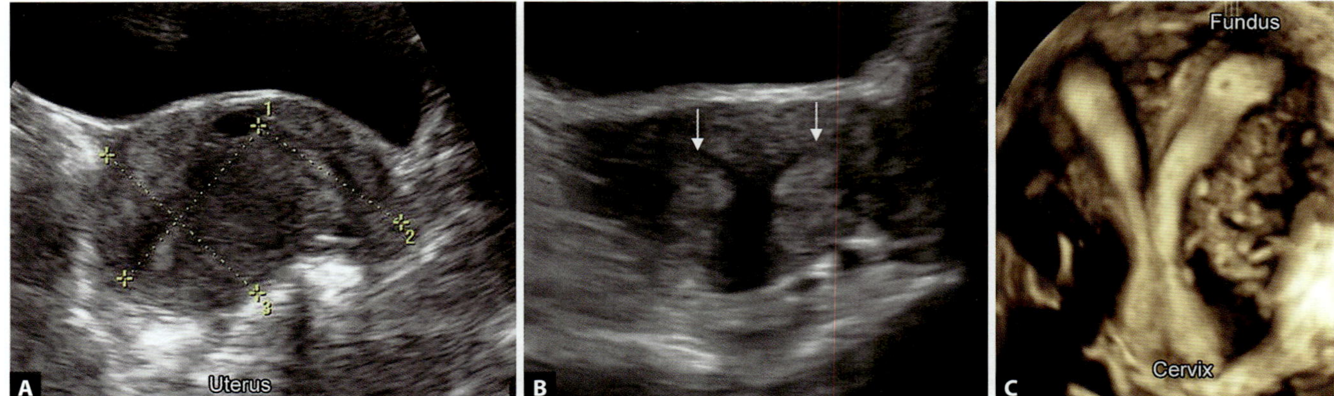

Figs. 7A to C: Complete septate uterus—Class U2B. (A) Two-dimensional (2D) transabdominal scan (TAS) of uterus in sagittal section; (B) 2D TAS of uterus in transverse section showing two separate endometrial cavities (arrows); (C) Three-dimensional (3D) section showing normal serosal outline and a complete septum dividing the endometrial cavity from fundus to cervix, Class U2B—complete septate uterus in the European Society for Gynecological Endoscopy (ESHRE) classification.

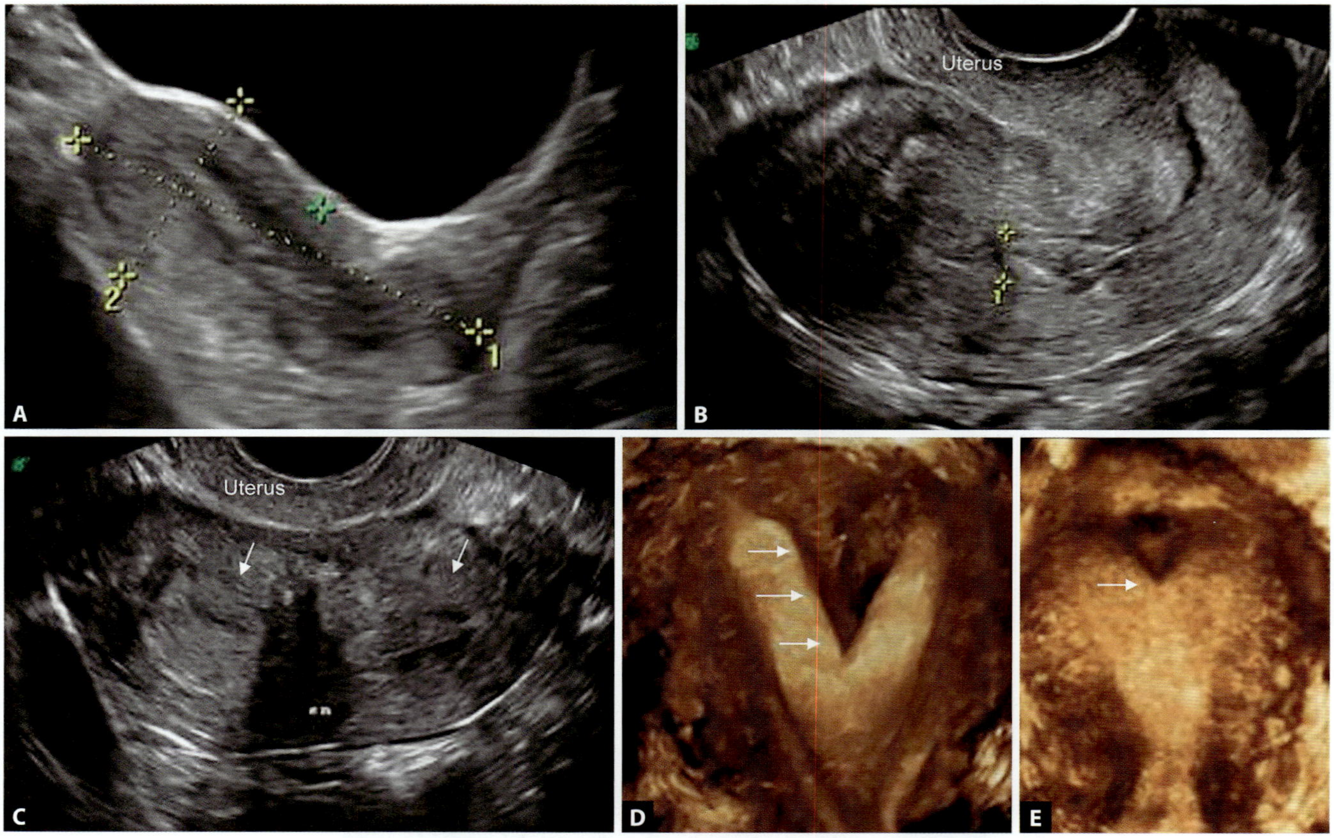

Figs. 8A to E: Partial septate uterus—Class U2A. (A) Two-dimensional (2D) transabdominal scan (TAS) of uterus in sagittal section; (B) 2D transvaginal scan (TVS) of uterus in sagittal section showing endometrial cavity line; (C) 2D transvaginal scan (TVS) of uterus in transverse section showing two separate endometrial cavities (arrows); (D) Three-dimensional (3D) ultrasound image showing normal external contour of uterus with internal fundal indentation; Class U2A—Partial septate uterus in the European Society for Gynecological Endoscopy (ESHRE) classification; (E) After septal resection (arrow points to resected septum).

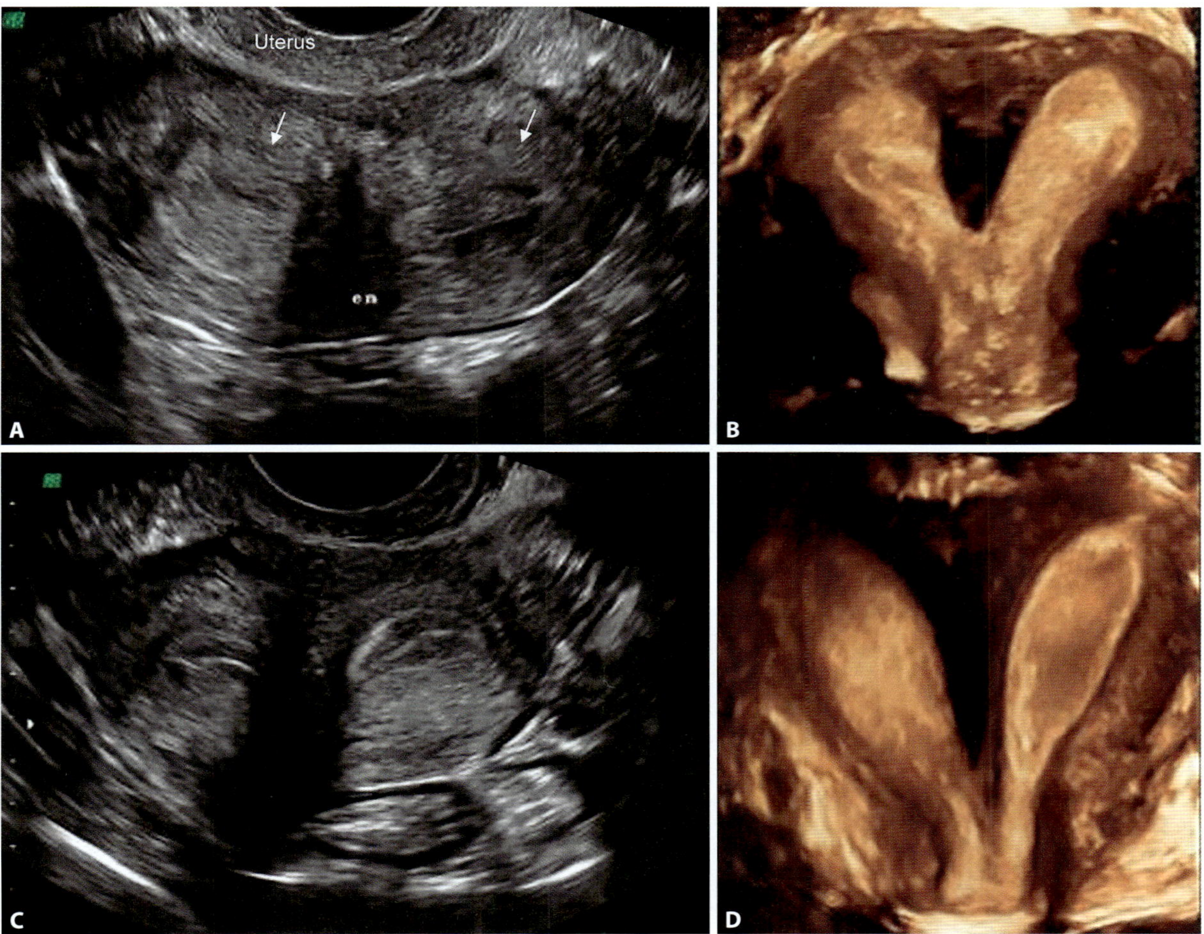

Figs. 9A to D: Partial septate versus complete septate uterus. (A) Two-dimensional (2D) transverse section of uterus showing bifid endometrial cavities; (B) Corresponding three-dimensional (3D) image showing normal serosal outline and internal indentation in partial septate uterus; (C) 2D transverse section in complete septate uterus; (D) Corresponding 3D image showing normal serosal outline and complete internal indentation in complete septate uterus.

Figures 9A to D shows comparison between partial and complete septate uterus. Note that the 2D transverse section in both partial and complete septate uterus **(Figs. 9A and C)** looks alike but the diagnosis is evident from 3D sections **(Figs. 9B and D)**.

A complete septum is easily classified but for partial septate uterus there are additional parameters described. Indentation angle, indentation depth, and indentation to wall thickness ratio are various criteria proposed to evaluate septate uterus. The best cut-offs for distinguishing septate uterus are as follows: Indentation depth of >10 mm, indentation angle <140°, indentation to wall thickness ratio >110%.[22] **Figures 10A and B** is a pictorial representation of measuring the parameters in partial septate uterus. A small indentation depth of <10 mm does not have major clinical implications and may be classified as normal or arcuate uterus.

The real reproductive impact of these small indentations is not known and the need for surgical treatment is debatable.[23]

Figures 11A to C illustrates 3D techniques to demonstrate uterine anomalies. **Figure 11A** depicts complete septate uterus using the Omniview line. **Figure 11B** is an HD live rendered image showing the internal indentation and **Figure 11C** shows the septate uterus.

Figures 12A to D shows assessment of the cervix in septate uterus. **Figures 12A and B** are a partial septate uterus with a single cervix showing single ostium. **Figures 12C and D** show complete septate uterus with double cervix. **Figures 13A and B** demonstrates 3D technique

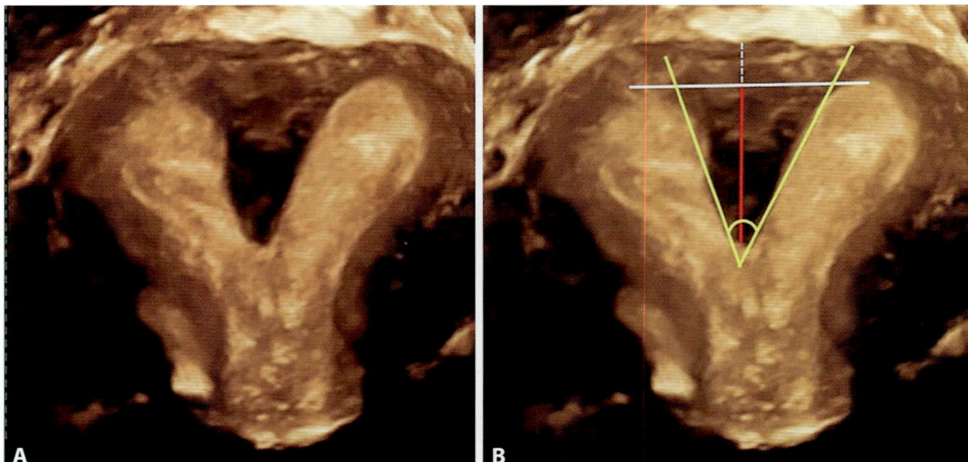

Figs. 10A and B: Measurements in partial septate uterus. White line demonstrates inter cornual line, red line shows the indentation thickness, white dashed line shows the wall thickness which is used to calculate the indentation to wall thickness ratio, yellow lines show the indentation angle.

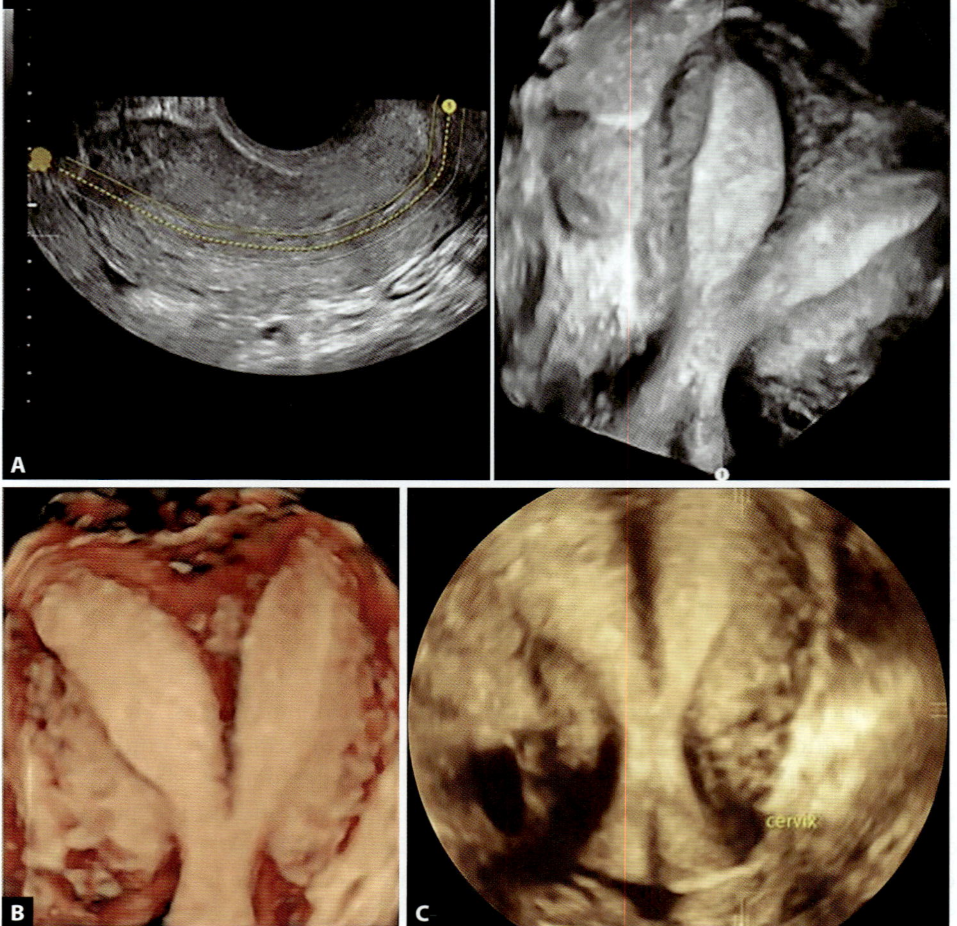

Figs. 11A to C: Three-dimensional (3D) techniques to demonstrate complete septate uterus. (A) Omniview line demonstrating coronal section of septate uterus. (B) HD live rendering of uterine cavity; (C) Complete septum dividing the cervical canal—Septate cervix.

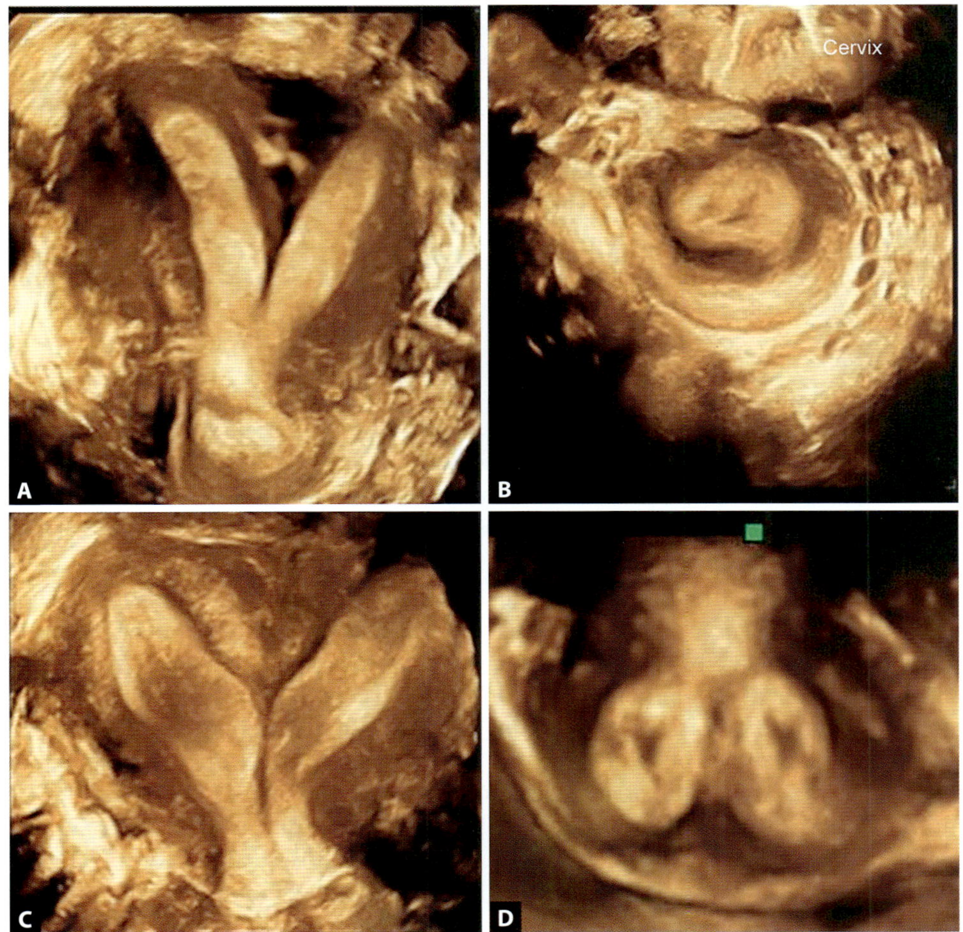

Figs. 12A to D: Assessment of cervix in septate uterus. (A and B) Partial septate uterus with single cervix—U2a C0 as per the European Society for Gynecological Endoscopy (ESHRE) classification; (C and D) Complete septate uterus with double cervix—U2b C2 as per ESHRE classification.

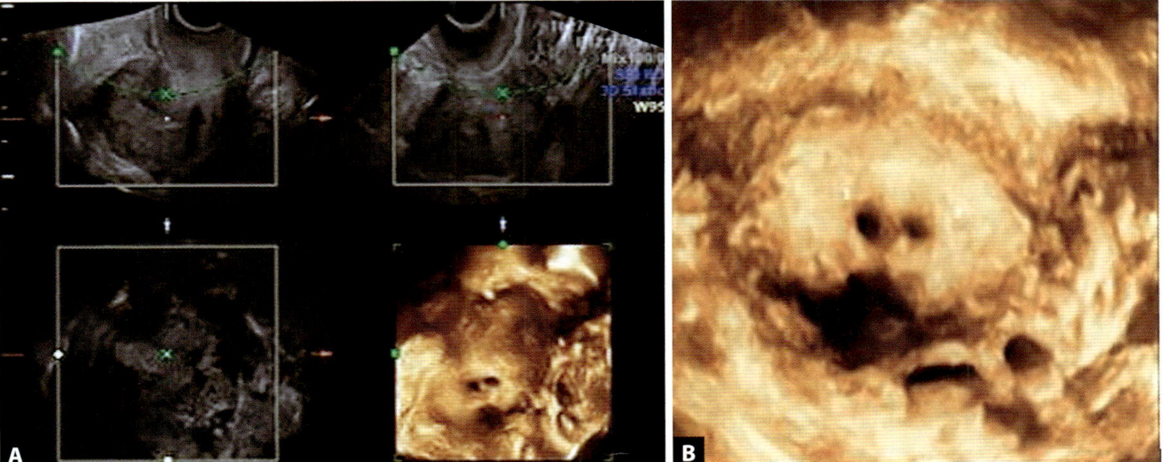

Figs. 13A and B: Three-dimensional (3D) technique to assess cervix. (A) Green line is placed in the region of cervix; (B) Shows two ostium in a septate cervix.

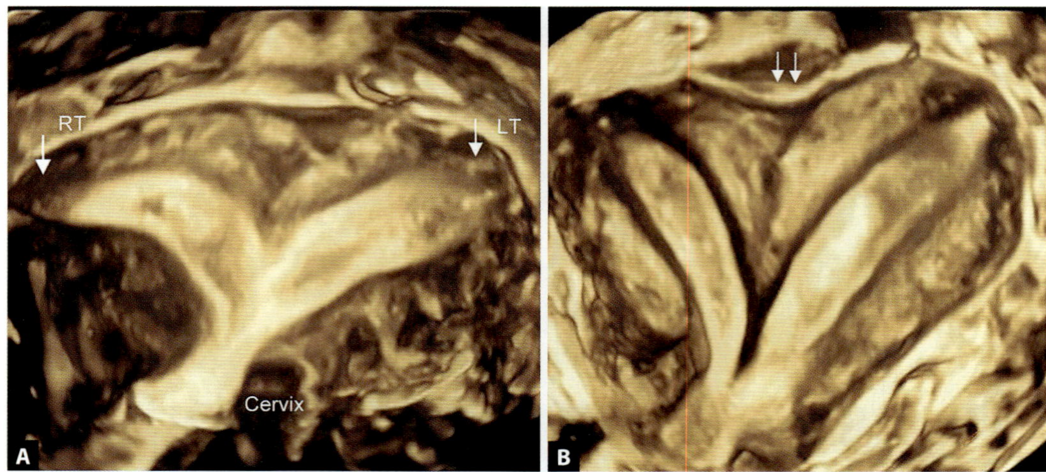

Figs. 14A and B: Overlapping features of septate and bicornuate uterus. (A) Increased intercornual distance in septate uterus; (B) Arrows show external indentation in septate uterus.

to assess cervix. **Figure 13A** shows the rendered image with green line in the region of the cervix and **Figure 13B** shows the two ostium in a septate cervix as seen through a speculum examination. The assessment of double uterine cavity is not complete without assessment of the cervix. **Figure 13** depicts the advantage of 3D ultrasound in evaluating the uterine cervix. This mode of evaluation is especially useful in cases with vaginal septum where speculum examination of the cervix is difficult.[24]

The differentiation of septate from a bicornuate uterus is important as they have different management approaches. A septate uterus needs hysteroscopic resection of the septum whereas bicornuate uteri rarely necessitate surgical intervention. However, Strassman metroplasty is done in required cases. For all practical purposes, the external contour in septate uterus is normal and smooth or with a slight indentation. In a bicornuate uterus, there is a deep external indentation and a wide interostial distance; however, there can be a significant overlap of these features **(Figs. 14A and B)**.

For those in the gray zone, the application of the 50% rule is an easy way of differentiating septate from bicornuate uterus.

If the external indentation is >50% of fundal myometrial thickness, it is categorized as bicornuate uterus. If the external indentation is <50% of myometrial thickness, it is normal/septate uterus. The advantage of having a category called bicorporeal septate uterus will allow for partial correction of the resorption anomaly.

The most common anomaly which is routinely missed on a TAS is the unicornuate uterus. During the TAS, uterus is deviated to one side and only a single cornua of the uterus is identified in a transverse sweep. 3D ultrasound clearly shows a banana-shaped uterus depicting only one cornua **(Figs. 15A and B)**. The next step is to evaluate the presence of rudimentary horn. **Figures 16A to E** shows a unicornuate uterus with a rudimentary horn. Note that the 2D sagittal TAS and TVS sections of the uterus **(Figs. 16A and B)** appear normal. The rudimentary horn is visualized in the transverse section of uterus **(Fig. 16C)**. 3D rendered images clearly demonstrate the unicornuate uterus with the rudimentary horn **(Figs. 16D and E)**.

The coronal plane visualization is the major hallmark of 3D ultrasound. Moreover, the volumes obtained can be sent for an expert opinion if necessary. Further, 3D images provide exclusive details for preoperative planning and surgical management.[19,25] The recent literature quotes an accuracy of about 90–92% for 3D ultrasound and a specificity of about 96.9–100%.[19,26-28] To summarize, when compared to many classifications, ESHRE helps in defining the Müllerian anomalies better as it is based on 3D visualization of the uterus.

Women who suffer from RPL can also have other uterine abnormalities such as intrauterine adhesions, endometrial polyps, myomas, and adenomyosis. Hysteroscopy remains the mainstay for the diagnosis of intrauterine adhesions. Submucosal myomas are known to cause RPL. About 2–3% of women with RPL are found to have uterine polyps.[29] Both uterine polyps and myomas can be identified using ultrasound. Müllerian anomalies can be present as an isolated one or can be combined with many complex syndromes. Syndromic associations

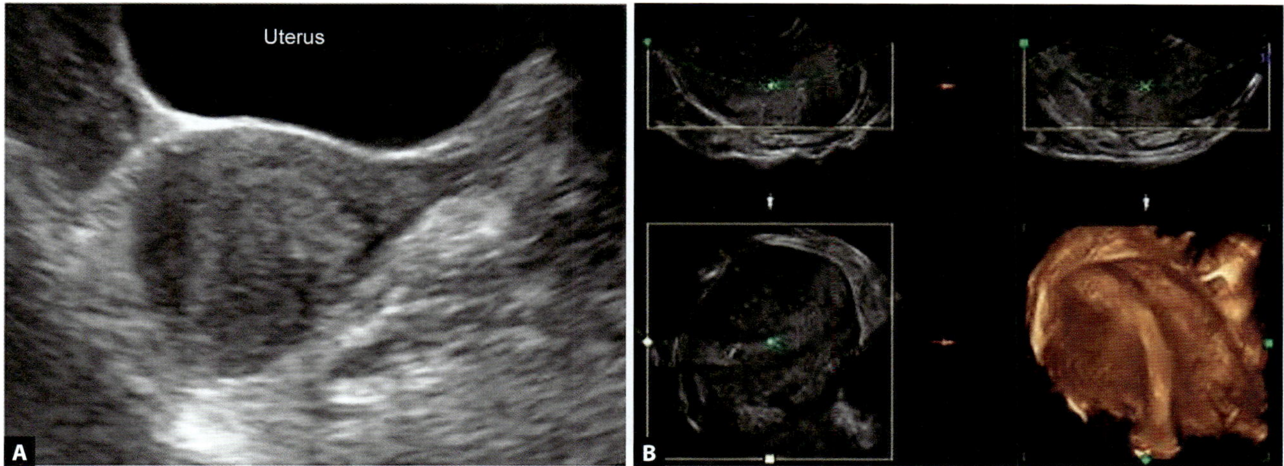

Figs. 15A and B: Unicornuate uterus. (A) Two-dimensional (2D) sagittal section of the uterus; (B) Three-dimensional (3D) rendered image showing single cornua (banana-shaped uterus) in unicornuate uterus.

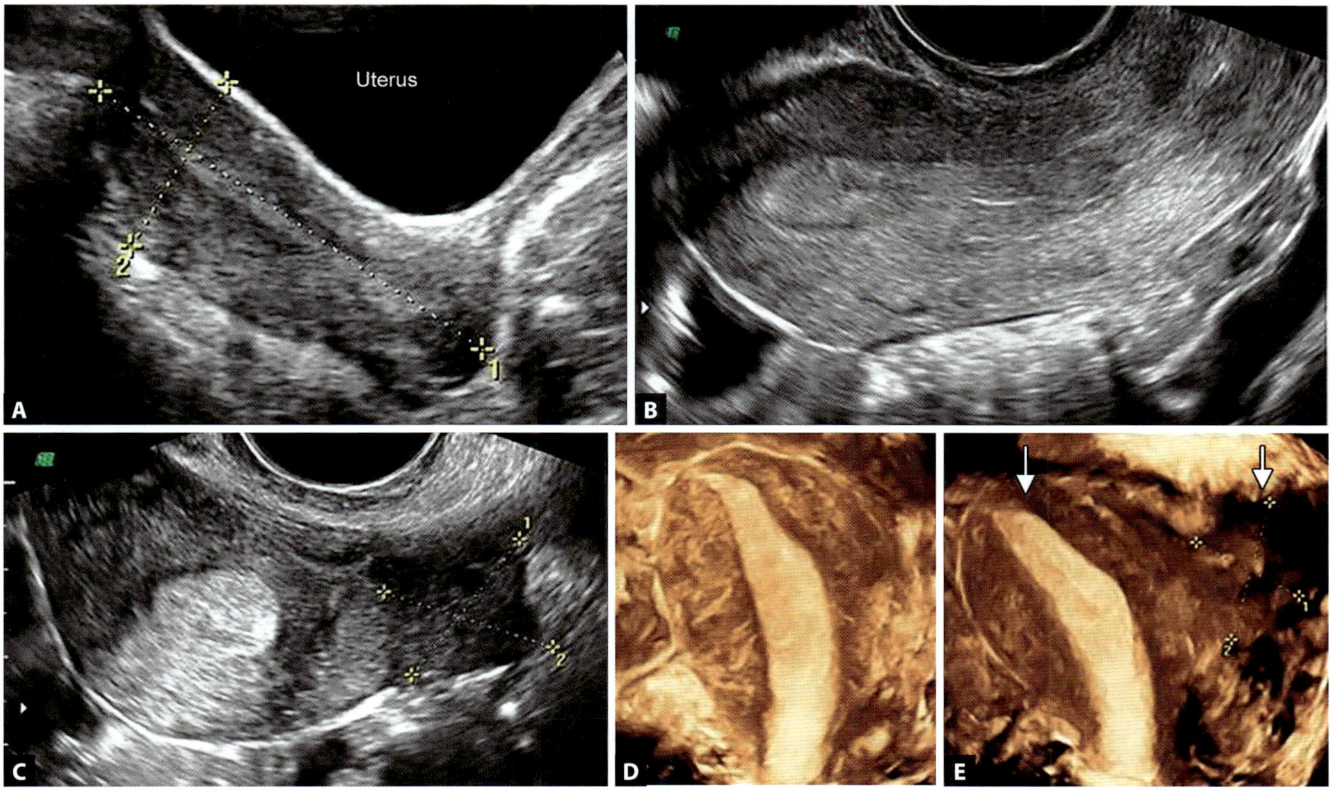

Figs. 16A to E: Unicornuate uterus with rudimentary horn. (A) Two-dimensional (2D) transabdominal scan (TAS) of uterus in sagittal section; (B) 2D transvaginal scan (TVS) of uterus in sagittal section showing endometrial cavity line; (C) 2D TVS of uterus in transverse section showing endometrial cavity on the right side and a hypoechoic lesion with absent endometrial cavity on the left side; (D) Three-dimensional (3D) ultrasound image showing banana-shaped unicornuate uterus; (E) Long arrow denotes unicornuate uterus and short arrow denotes rudimentary horn.

present early in adolescence and description of them are beyond the scope of this chapter.

Magnetic resonance imaging (MRI) though considered as gold standard is reserved for ambiguous findings in 2D and 3D ultrasound where a definitive diagnosis cannot be arrived. The accuracy of MRI for categorizing Müllerian defects is about 100%.[28,30,31] 3D US is the best alternative to MRI as it is cheaper, easily available and feasible, provides images of high resolution. Laparoscopy and hysteroscopy are essential adjuvants in evaluation of cases with complicated Müllerian anomalies. They are used as second-line tests when additional information is required to determine a diagnosis.

A simple 2D ultrasound of pelvis done during the interpregnancy period serves as a screening tool for suspecting any congenital uterine anomaly but 2D ultrasound alone would not suffice in evaluation of RPL. Since 3D ultrasound is cheap, noninvasive, and highly accurate, it is the modality of choice in evaluating Müllerian anomalies. The role of 3D ultrasound in identifying the correct type of Müllerian anomaly is illustrated in this chapter and, probably in future, it must be a sought-after tool by the clinicians in evaluating RPL.

CONCLUSION

Interpregnancy scanning by 2D and 3D imaging is a vital step to diagnose Müllerian abnormalities of the uterus as well as acquired anomalies like polyps, myomas and intrauterine synechea. T-shaped uterus with low uterine volume, is also best diagnosed in the interpregnancy interval. 2D sonography can be assisted by a sonohysterogram to delineate abnormalities in the uterine cavity.

REFERENCES

1. Speroff L, Fritz MA. Clinical gynecologic endocrinology and infertility. United States: Lippincott Williams & Wilkins; 2005.
2. Kim MA, Kim HS, Kim YH. Reproductive, obstetric and neonatal outcomes in women with congenital uterine anomalies: a systematic review and meta-analysis. J Clin Med. 2021;10(21):4797.
3. Grimbizis GF, Camus M, Tarlatzis BC, Bontis JN, Devroey P. Clinical implications of uterine malformations and hysteroscopic treatment results. Hum Reprod Update. 2001;7(2):161-74.
4. Wold AS, Pham N, Arici A. Anatomic factors in recurrent pregnancy loss. In: Hoeger KM, Piltonen TT, Giudice LC, Giacobini P, Franks S (Eds). Seminars in reproductive medicine. New York, NY: Thieme Medical Publishers, Inc.; 2006. pp. 25-32.
5. Ghi T, Casadio P, Kuleva M, Perrone AM, Savelli L, Giunchi S, et al. Accuracy of three-dimensional ultrasound in diagnosis and classification of congenital uterine anomalies. Fertil Steril. 2009;92(2):808-13.
6. Adhesions AD. The American Fertility Society classifications of adnexal adhesions, distal tubal occlusion, tubal occlusion secondary to tubal ligation, tubal pregnancies, Müllerian anomalies and intrauterine adhesions. Fertil Steril. 1988;49(6):944.
7. Di Spiezio Sardo A, Campo R, Gordts S, Spinelli M, Cosimato C, Tanos V, et al. The comprehensiveness of the ESHRE/ESGE classification of female genital tract congenital anomalies: a systematic review of cases not classified by the AFS system. Hum Reprod. 2015;30(5):1046-58.
8. Ludwin A, Coelho Neto MD, Ludwin I, Nastri CO, Costa W, Acien M, et al. Congenital Uterine Malformation by Experts (CUME): diagnostic criteria for T-shaped uterus. Ultrasound Obstet Gynecol. 2020;55(6):815-29.
9. Kaur KK, Allahbadia G, Singh M. An Update on the Advances in Classification as well as Reproductive Surgeries in Müllerian Anomalies—A Systematic Review. Am J Surg Tech Case Rep. 2020;1(1):1002.
10. Pfeifer SM, Attaran M, Goldstein J, Lindheim SR, Petrozza JC, Rackow BW, et al. ASRM müllerian anomalies classification 2021. Fertil steril. 2021;116(5):1238-52.
11. Ludwin A, Tudorache S, Martins WP. ASRM Müllerian Anomalies Classification 2021: a critical review. Ultrasound Obstet Gynecol. 2022;60(1):7-21.
12. Sugi MD, Penna R, Jha P, Pōder L, Behr SC, Courtier J, et al. Müllerian duct anomalies: role in fertility and pregnancy. Radiographics. 2021;41(6):1857-75.
13. Pellerito JS, McCarthy SM, Doyle MB, Glickman MG, DeCherney AH. Diagnosis of uterine anomalies: relative accuracy of MR imaging, endovaginal sonography, and hysterosalpingography. Radiology. 1992;183(3):795-800.
14. Saravelos SH, Cocksedge KA, Li TC. Prevalence and diagnosis of congenital uterine anomalies in women with reproductive failure: a critical appraisal. Hum Reprod Update. 2008;14(5):415-29.
15. Jayaprakasan K, Ojha K. Diagnosis of congenital uterine abnormalities: practical considerations. J Clin Med. 2022;11(5):1251.
16. Alborzi S, Dehbashi S, Parsanezhad ME. Differential diagnosis of septate and bicornuate uterus by sonohysterography eliminates the need for laparoscopy. Fertil Steril. 2002;78(1):176-8.
17. Sibal M. Gel sonovaginography: a new way of evaluating a variety of local vaginal and cervical disorders. J Ultrasound Med. 2016;35(12):2699-715.
18. Sibal M, Sibal M. Ultrasound Evaluation of Congenital Uterine Anomalies. Ultrasound Gynecol: An Atlas Guide. 2017:435-67.

19. Wu MH, Hsu CC, Huang KE. Detection of congenital müllerian duct anomalies using three-dimensional ultrasound. J Clin Ultrasound. 1997;25(9):487-92.
20. Carrington BM, Hricak H, Nuruddin RN, Secaf E, Laros Jr RK, Hill EC. Müllerian duct anomalies: MR imaging evaluation. Radiology. 1990;176(3):715-20.
21. Troiano RN, McCarthy SM. Müllerian duct anomalies: imaging and clinical issues. Radiology. 2004;233(1):19-34.
22. Ludwin A, Martins WP, Nastri CO, Ludwin I, Coelho Neto MA, Leitao VM, et al. Congenital Uterine Malformation by Experts (CUME): better criteria for distinguishing between normal/arcuate and septate uterus. Ultrasound Obstet Gynecol. 2018;51(1):101-9.
23. Russo C, Conway F, Siciliano T, Selntigia A, Martire FG, Soreca G, et al. 3D transvaginal ultrasound diagnosis of uterine septa according to different classifications: are there other measurements that correlate to reproductive outcome in small indentation length. Facts Views Vision Obs Gyn. 2022;14(2):129.
24. Lakshmy SR, Rose N, Ramachandran M. Role of three dimensional ultrasound in uterine anomalies—3D assessment of cervix in septate uteri. Int J Reprod Contracept Obstet Gynecol. 2016;5(10):3563-8.
25. Bermejo C, Martínez Ten P, Cantarero R, Diaz D, Pérez Pedregosa J, Barrón E, et al. Three-dimensional ultrasound in the diagnosis of Müllerian duct anomalies and concordance with magnetic resonance imaging. Ultrasound Obstet Gynecol. 2010;35(5):593-601.
26. Moini A, Mohammadi S, Hosseini R, Eslami B, Ahmadi F. Accuracy of 3-dimensional sonography for diagnosis and classification of congenital uterine anomalies. J Ultrasound Med. 2013;32(6):923-7.
27. Deutch TD, Abuhamad AZ. The role of 3-dimensional ultrasonography and magnetic resonance imaging in the diagnosis of Müllerian duct anomalies: a review of the literature. J Ultrasound Med. 2008;27(3):413-23.
28. Graupera B, Pascual MA, Hereter L, Browne JL, Úbeda B, Rodríguez I, et al. Accuracy of three-dimensional ultrasound compared with magnetic resonance imaging in diagnosis of Müllerian duct anomalies using ESHRE–ESGE consensus on the classification of congenital anomalies of the female genital tract. Ultrasound Obstet Gynecol. 2015;46(5):616-22.
29. Tomkiewicz J, Darmochwał-Kolarz D. The diagnostics and treatment of recurrent pregnancy loss. J Clin Med. 2023;12(14):4768.
30. Behr SC, Courtier JL, Qayyum A. Imaging of müllerian duct anomalies. Radiographics. 2012;32(6):E233-50.
31. Steinkeler JA, Woodfield CA, Lazarus E, Hillstrom MM. Female infertility: a systematic approach to radiologic imaging and diagnosis. Radiographics. 2009;29(5):1353-70.

CHAPTER 25

Ultrasound Evaluation of Endometrium

Chaitanya Nagori, Sonal Panchal

ABSTRACT

A healthy endometrium is vital for successful pregnancy implantation. Imaging of the endometrium can alert the practitioner to endometrial dysmorphology as the cause of recurrent pregnancy loss (RPL). This can then be further studied with hysteroscopy and biopsy. Various modalities have been employed to improve endometrial thickness and vascularity. These include estrogen therapy, human chorionic gonadotropin (hCG) injections, aspirin, sildenafil, pentoxifylline, L-arginine, and Granulocyte colony-stimulating factor (G-CSF). The beneficial effect of these molecules has not been proven to date. Injection of platelet-rich plasma (PRP) and stem cells has shown promise in endometrial regeneration.

Keywords: Thin endometrium, Intrauterine synechiae, Aspirin, Estrogen therapy, Sildenafil, L-arginine, pentoxifylline, G-CSF, PRP, stem cells.

INTRODUCTION

Endometrium is a tissue that ever changes its thickness and morphology being a receptor organ to estrogen and progesterone and being sensitive to other autocrine and paracrine factors. Its upper two-thirds layer, i.e., stratum compactum and spongiosum, is a functional layer and is important for implantation **(Fig. 1)** and stratum basalis, the lower one-third is for regeneration of endometrium. It is the functional layer that gives thickness to the endometrium and is regenerated from the basal layer in every cycle and is thrown off during menstruation. Normal endometrial thickness is 6–14 mm. Endometrial thickness is measured from outer margin of anterior hyperechoic line of endometrium to the outer margin of the posterior hyperechoic line of the endometrium, perpendicular to the central line of the endometrium, at its broadest part **(Fig. 2)**.

Fig. 1: Diagrammatic presentation of layers of uterus.

What is poor endometrium?

Poor endometrium and the thin endometrium are quite interchangeably used term, but it needs to be understood here that all poor endometrium are not thin, because poor endometrium also includes endometria with pathologies like polyps, hyperplasia, and fibroids. Even adenomyosis leads to inadequacy of the endometrium. Diagnosis of all these pathologies is essential for treatment and improvement of the endometrium.

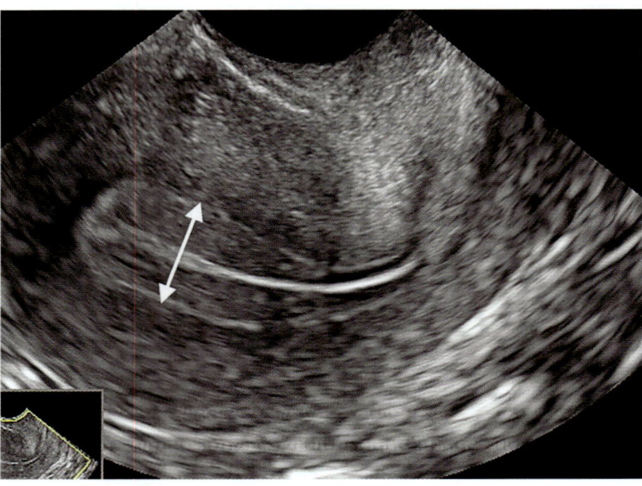

Fig. 2: Ultrasound image showing measurement of the endometrium.

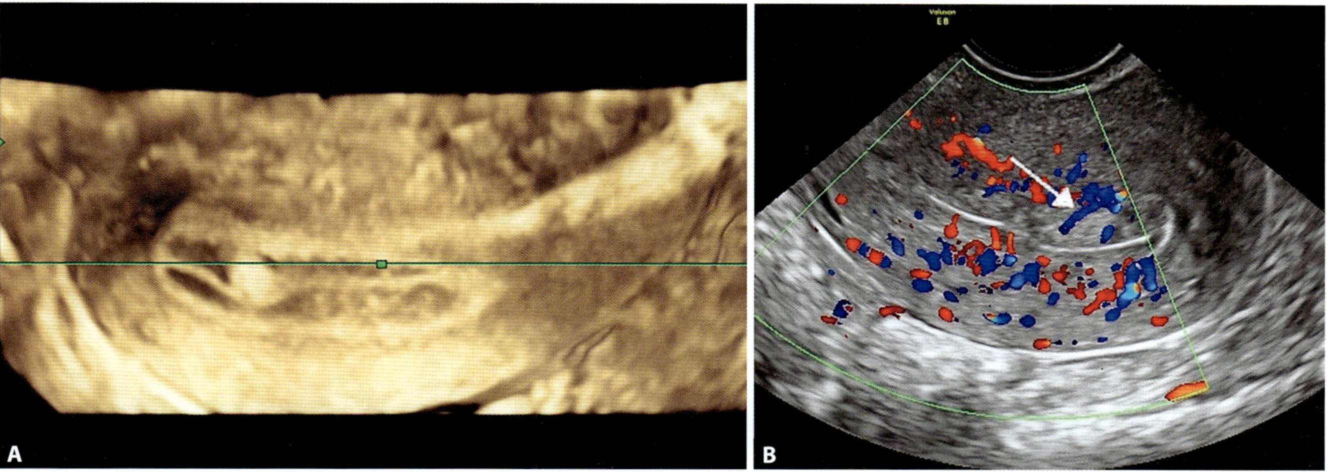

Figs. 3A and B: (A) Polyp seen as a solid round lesion in the upper half of the endometrial cavity on B-mode ultrasound; (B) Color Doppler image showing a single feeder vessel to the polyp as marked by the arrow.

As for thin endometrium, there is no unanimous consensus as to how thin is thin endometrium. 7 mm is the most accepted figure for definition by most of the workers but some also take the cut off as 8 mm. On the other hand, pregnancies have been documented between 5 and 15 mm thickness of endometrium.[1]

Endometrium is receptive or not can be judged by various measures:

- Echogenicity/morphology
- Vascularity
- Molecular technology is considered as an excellent tool to recognize receptive endometrium.[2]

Let us first discuss about the pathologies of the endometrium that affect the endometrial receptivity.

ENDOMETRIAL POLYPS

Endometrial polyps are solid lesions arising from the endometrial walls projecting into the endometrial cavity. Sonographically, these are solid echogenic lesions seen in the endometrial cavity or in between the endometrial lines with smooth margins. Polyps can be diagnosed on B-mode scan and are best visible in the periovulatory phase. Polyps may often be multiple. Moreover, many polyps have a tendency to throw off themselves on menstruation and regrow. Very small polyps may show only subtle echogenicity and are sometimes can barely be seen. The diagnostic clue to such a polyp is an abnormal curve in the central line of the endometrium. Such small polyps usually do not come in the way of implantation and do not affect endometrial receptivity.

But large polyps may fill up the endometrial cavity **(Fig. 3A)**. These need to be differentiated from endometrial hyperplasia or endometrial malignancy. Color Doppler **(Fig. 3B)** is the modality that helps in identifying and differentiating polyp from other lesions as it has a characteristic blood supply by a single feeding vessel. Infection, necrosis, or atypia shows heterogeneous echogenicity and branching of the vessels inside the polyp. Adenomyomatous polyp also shows branching of blood vessels inside the polyp mass, but has high resistance flow.

Though polyps evidently raise a concern about endometrial receptivity, there is no definite proof that these do so. Though the literature quotes that polyps larger than 1 cm and in upper half of the endometrial cavity should be surgically removed, the evidences are scarce.

ENDOMETRIAL HYPERPLASIA

This is a condition where the endometrium is thick but still the receptivity may be jeopardized. This is an overgrowth of endometrium with normal histology, presenting as thick echogenic endometrium, in part or entirety. Endometrial thickness >14 mm in premenopausal patient is considered hypertrophic, according to the literature. But it is important to understand that even normal preovulatory or secretory endometria may be 15–17 mm, so its ultrasound morphology is more important than the thickness alone. The hyperplastic endometrium may show a glandular predominance or stromal predominance and the ultrasound morphology will differ depending on the same. The endometrial–myometrial junction is well maintained.

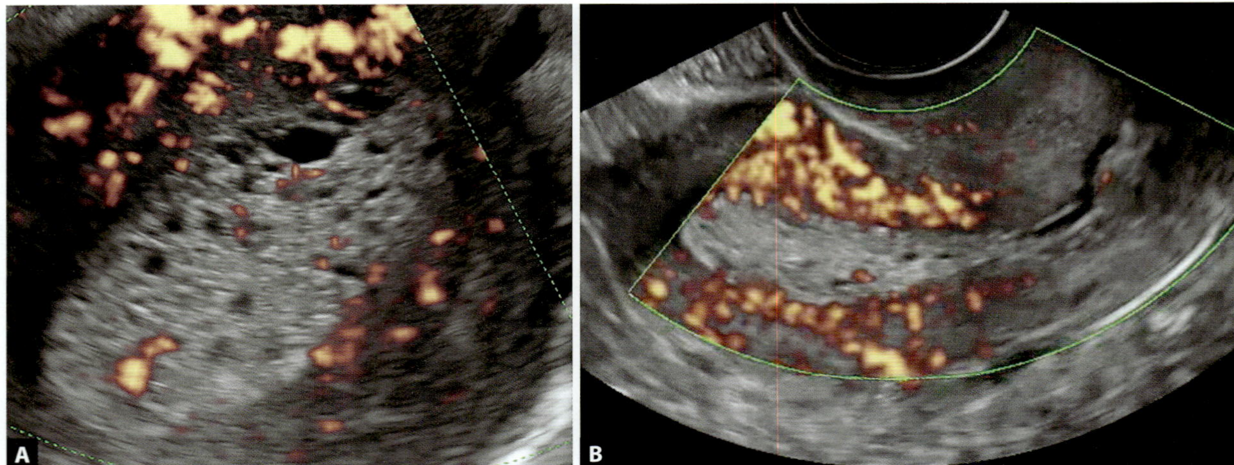

Figs. 4A and B: (A) Power Doppler image of cystic endometrial hyperplasia—thick endometrium with anechoic areas of various sizes, intact junctional zone, and scanty vascularity; (B) Thick hyperechoic endometrium with small anechoic areas—stromal endometrial hyperplasia. Power Doppler shows scanty vascularity.

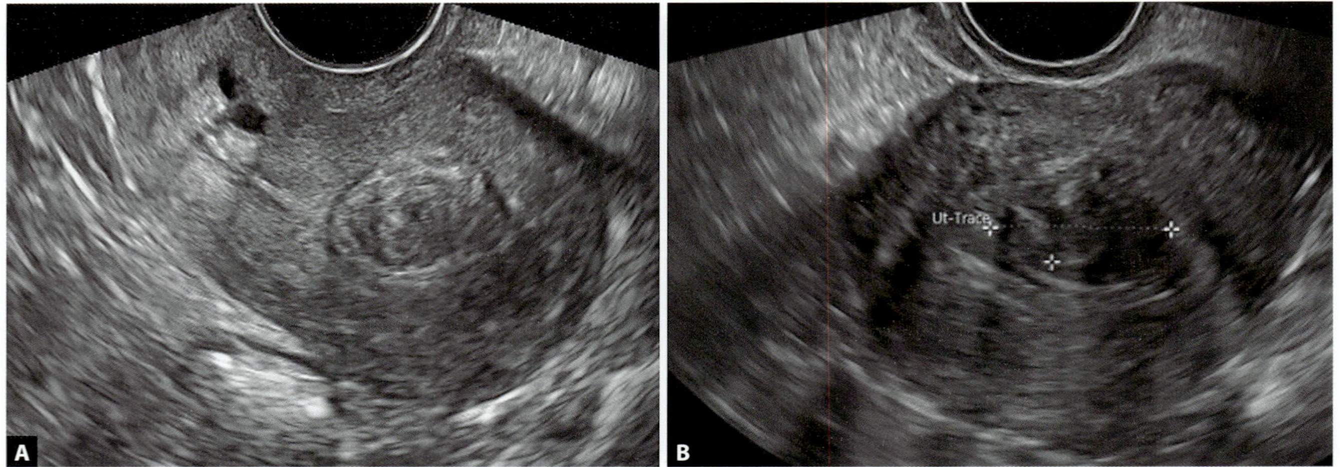

Figs. 5A and B: (A) B-mode image of type 0 fibroid; (B) B-mode image of type 2 fibroid.

Glandular/cystic endometrial hyperplasia **(Fig. 4A)** shows multiple anechoic areas of variable size in thickened endometrium. On color Doppler, it shows regularly placed vessels supplying it with normal branching pattern and mean RI of 0.55 ± 0.05. Endometrial hyperplasia **(Fig. 4B)** with stromal predominance is more solid-looking with fewer and small anechoic areas. It is quite common to see these changes in the endometrium during endometrial preparation for frozen embryo transfer. If the vascularity is scanty, it is recommended to give a withdrawal bleed and then start a fresh cycle, but in case vascularity in the endometrium is adequate, one can still take a chance and do embryo transfer in these cases.

Subendometrial fibroids (Type 0, 1, 2) **(Figs. 5A and B)** are hypoechoic to the myometrium, but isoechoic to the preovulatory endometrium (the intervening area of the preovulatory endometrium) and, therefore, are difficult to demonstrate on preovulatory scan. Often, the only clue on the preovulatory scan would be the abnormal bulge on the central line of the endometrium. But the fibroid is well demonstrated in echogenic endometrium of secretory phase as hypoechoic lesion and has peripheral vascularity typical of fibroids. This leads to compression and deshaping of the endometrium and, if in the upper half of the endometrial cavity, can affect endometrial receptivity.

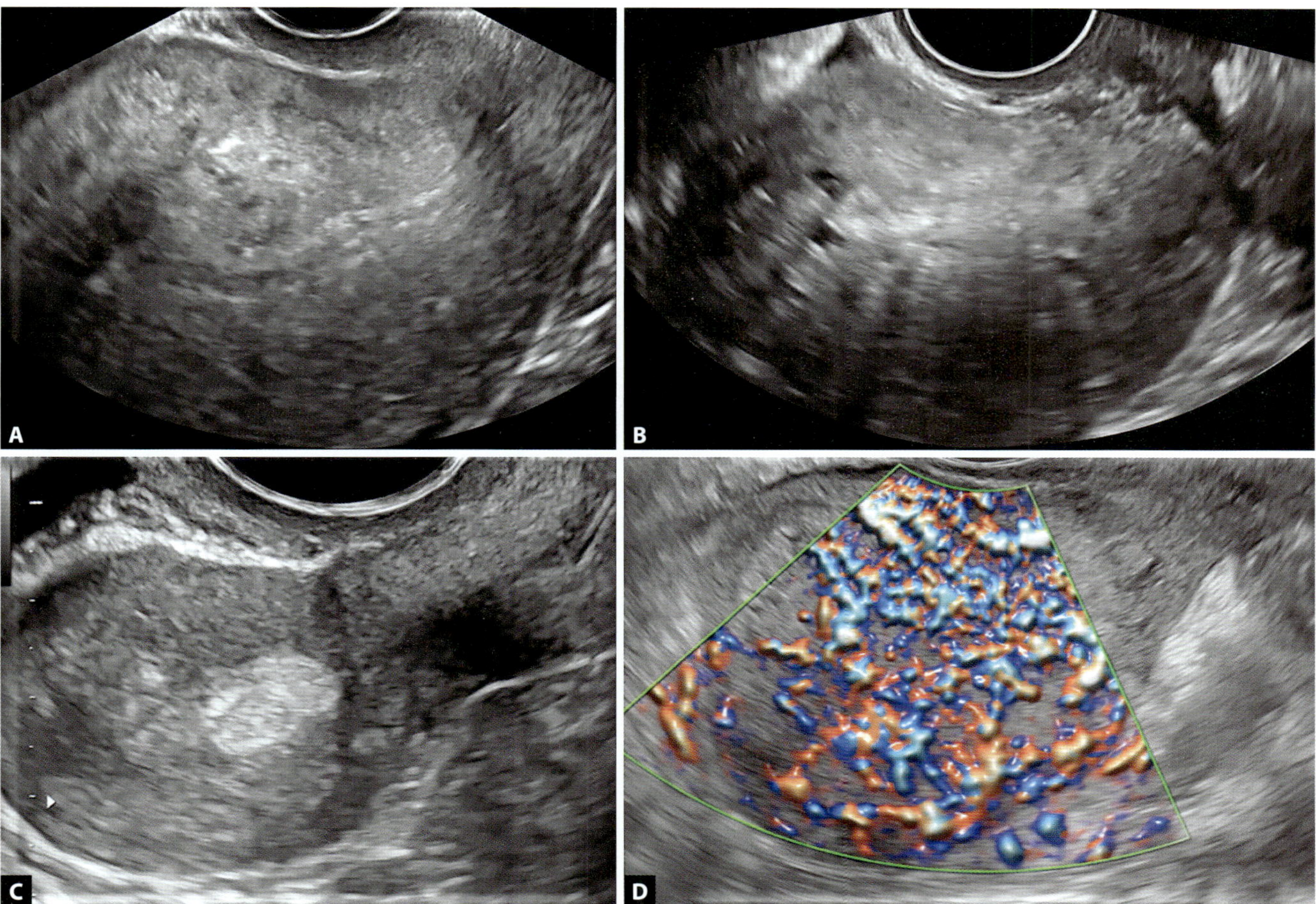

Figs. 6A to D: Adenomyosis. (A) Symmetrically enlarged uterus with heterogeneous myometrium with hyperechoic dots and lines and interrupted junctional zone; (B) Myometrial cysts (anechoic), fan shadows, and inaccessible junctional zone; (C) Hyperechoic island; and (D) Trans-lesional vessels.

Adenomyosis **(Figs. 6A to D)**, though is a myometrial pathology, does affect the endometrium significantly. This is through the mechanical effect, compression, but it is also because the junctional zone is significantly affected by adenomyosis. Affection of the junctional zone may lead to abnormal endometrial peristalsis, and also leads to abnormal endometrial vascularity, thus affecting the implantation potential of the endometrium. Adenomyosis is a very common finding in the females of reproductive age. It may present as dysmenorrhea, menorrhagia, and sometimes even dyspareunia. But since it often remains silent, especially when not severe, it may be only an incidental finding. Treating adenomyosis may require downregulation, which does not allow fertility treatment for a while and so the usual strategy is that even with adenomyosis, the endometrium develops well and shows acceptable vascularity in its inner layers, fertility treatment can be taken forward.

Adenomyosis is diagnosed on ultrasound by symmetrical/asymmetrical thickening of the myometrium, heterogeneous myometrium with hyperechoic dots, lines **(Fig. 6A)** and islands **(Fig. 6C)**, anechoic myometrial cysts, **(Fig. 6B)** irregular, interrupted, or inaccessible junctional zone, hyperechoic flecks at the junctional zone due to collapsed myometrial cysts, fan shadows (alternate hyper- and hypoechoic vertical strands), **(Fig. 6D)** question mark sign of the uterus (reverse curvature of the fundal endometrial cavity beyond the mid cavity), symmetrical/asymmetrical compression of the endometrium and vessels traversing across the lesion (trans-lesional vessels), with caliber larger than that of the normal spiral vessels.

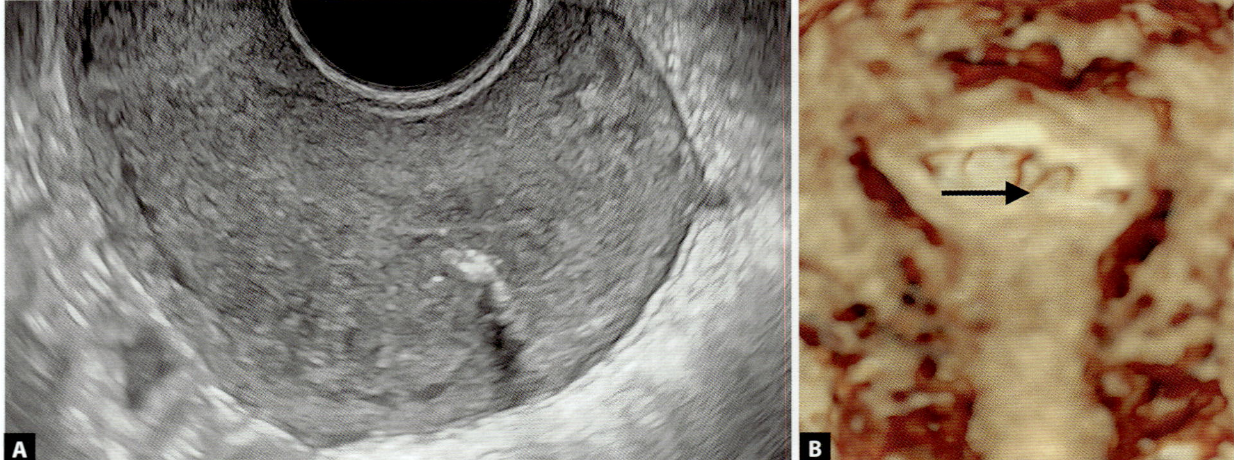

Figs. 7A and B: Thin endometrium. (A) B-mode image of thin endometrium; (B) Sonohysterography with 3D of the same uterus showing synechiae.

CAUSES OF THIN ENDOMETRIUM

- Surgical
- Radiotherapy
- Infectious
- Congenital Müllerian abnormalities
- Other causes
- Idiopathic
- *Surgical:*
  - *Dilatation and curettage:* 90% of cases of intrauterine adhesions and thin endometrium are due to cervical dilatation and postabortal curettage.[3] Adhesions interfere with implantation and sperm migration. Isthmus and cornu are the common locations. When severe adhesions occur, it is called "Asherman's syndrome". Intrauterine adhesions or synechiae are diagnosed on 2D ultrasound by persistently thin endometrium even in preovulatory and secretory phase of menstrual cycle **(Fig. 7A)**. On 3D ultrasound, especially with saline infusion sonohysterography, it is better diagnosed as echogenic strands between the endometrial layers **(Fig. 7B)**.
  - *Intrauterine surgeries:* Most common cause is hysteroscopic resection of multiple fibroids, particularly when resectoscope is used. The incidence is as high as 30–45%.[4] Bipolar resectoscope causes lesser adhesions as much as 7–8%. After hysteroscopic metroplasty, hormone replacement of IUCD insertion is not required.

    Second most common cause is septoplasty 86% and they did not find adhesions after polypectomy. So, ART is not recommended for 3 months after all these procedures or ahesiolysis.[5] But, polypectomy does not affect line of treatment.[6]
  - *Strassman operation:* Unification of uterus has been advocated in bicornuate uterus. Strassman operation is also not performed commonly these days unless there is a history of premature deliveries with complete bicornuate uterus. Because of progesterone, cervical encerclage, and good neonatal care, such operations can be avoided.
- *Radiotherapy:* Radiotherapy can damage the endometrium, and it can become atrophic and nonresponsive to hormonal therapy. Radiation-induced uterine damage is age and dose dependent. Older patients show better response to hormonal therapy. Miscarriage rates and preterm delivery rates are very high.
- *Infections:* Chronic endometritis, a very common cause of thin endometrium, hampers the uterine receptivity. It also changes endometrial peristaltic wave pattern which causes infertility.[7] Patient may have dysfunctional uterine bleeding, pelvic pain, and dyspareunia. Hysteroscopy may reveal micropolyps, adhesions, focal hyperemia, and edema with diagnostic accuracy (93%).[8]

  Tuberculosis is very common in developing countries and can be strongly suspected on ultrasound. Though most ultrasound features are not specific to tuberculosis,

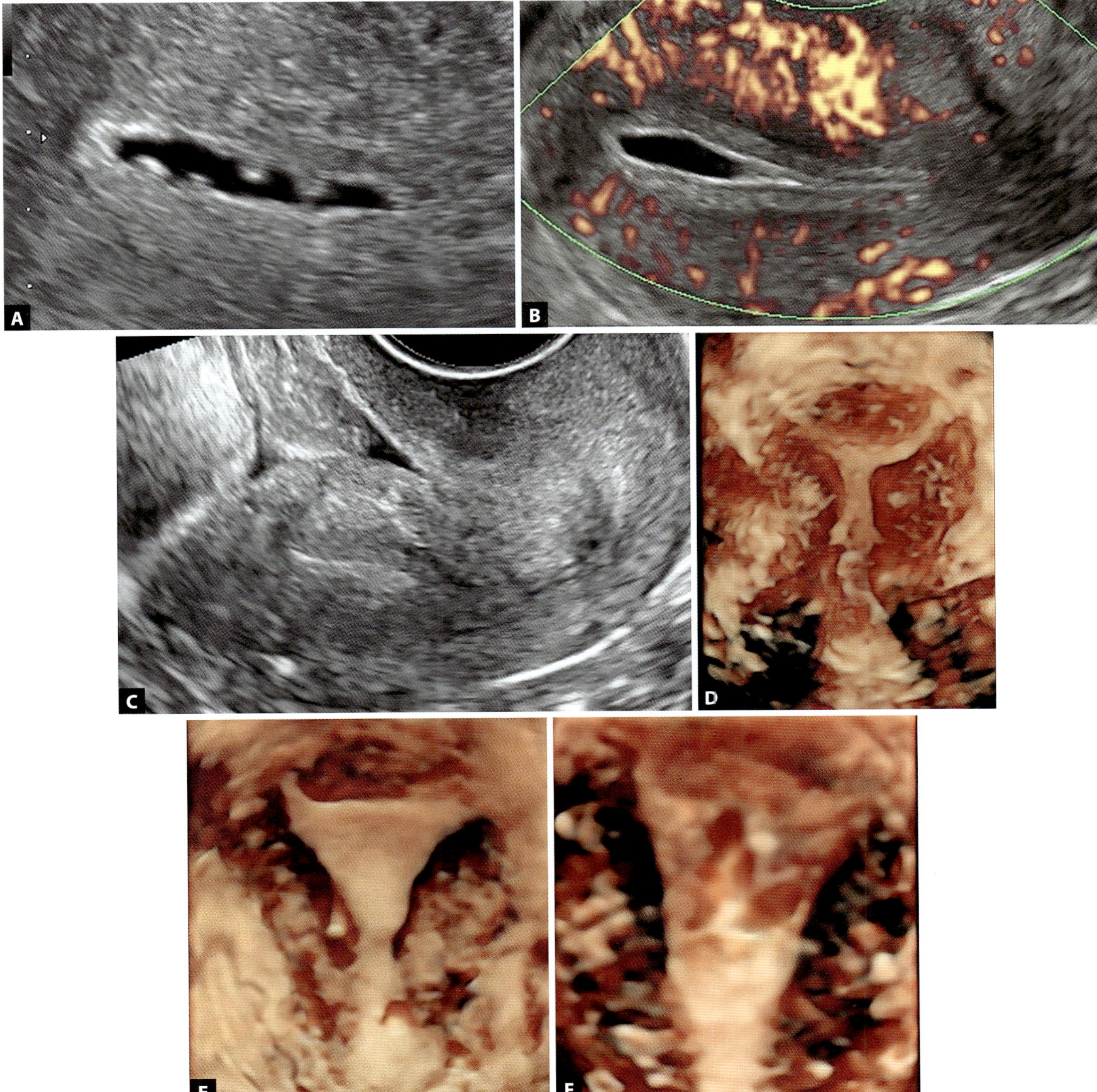

Figs. 8A to F: (A) Micropolyposis; (B) Fluid in endometrial cavity with hyperechoic margins; (C) Thin endometrium; (D) Contracted endometrial cavity; (E) Vertical orientation of interstitial part of the tube; and (F) Synechiae.

persistently thin endometrium with endometrial, subendometrial, and myometrial calcifications **(Fig. 8C)** contracted narrow endometrial cavity **(Fig. 8D)** or synechiae **(Fig. 8F)** are the signs that raise the suspicion of tuberculosis. Tuberculous endometritis may also present as fluid in the endometrial cavity in mid-proliferative phase with hyperechoic endometrial lining **(Fig. 8B)** or micropolyposis **(Fig. 8A)**. One of the most specific sign is vertical orientation of interstitial part of the tube **(Fig. 8E)**.

In patients with recurrent implantation failure, chronic endometritis is the frequent cause. Cure rate is very high after antibiotics. So, diagnosis by hysteroscopy and treatment with antibiotics improves the implantation rate.[9] For nontuberculous lesions, doxycycline 100 mg BD for 10–14 days is recommended or azithromycin is also a good option for endometritis. Otherwise, AKT (anti-Koch's therapy) is recommended.

- *Congenital Müllerian abnormalities:* Müllerian abnormalities are associated with poor reproductive outcome. The implantation failure and thin endometrium is poorly understood. There may be alteration in HOXA genes.
- *Other causes:*
  - *Estrogen deficiency:* In patients with hypogonadotropic hypogonadism, there is low estrogen level. So, the endometrium is thin. By stimulating with human menopausal gonadotropin (HMG) follicles develop, estrogen level rises and endometrium can grow to more thickness.
  - *Clomiphene citrate:* Repeated cycles of clomiphene for ovulation induction causes accumulations of zuclomiphene which causes thinning of endometrium as estrogen receptors are occupied and estrogen cannot show its effect on endometrium.
  - *Oral contraceptive (OC) pills:* Long-term use of OC pills can cause thinning of endometrium but it is regained after stopping the drug.
  - *Long-term use of progesterone:* It compacts the endometrium and decreases the thickness. But effect is reversible.

MANAGEMENT

Apart from the treatment of specific lesions/pathologies like polyps, fibroids, adenomyosis, etc., there are several drugs that have been tried empirically and some of these also have created evidences as mentioned below.

Drugs:

- Low-dose aspirin
- Sildenafil
- Tocopherol
- Pentoxifylline
- Nitroglycerin
- L-arginine
- Gonadotropin-releasing hormone (GnRH) agonist
- Estrogen
- Tamoxifen
- Human chorionic gonadotropin (hCG)
- Ovulation induction

Procedures:

- Endometrial scratching
- Granulocyte colony-stimulating factor (G-CSF)
- Platelet-rich plasma
- Stem cell therapy

Drugs

- *Low-dose aspirin:* Low-dose aspirin improves endometrial thickness and implantation by improving uterine endometrial blood flow and by reducing uterine artery resistance pulsatility index (PI). It reduces subendometrial contractility and minimizes inflammation. The recommended dose is 75–150 mg/day.

  It is widely used in IVF cycles but no beneficial effect on implantation has been documented. Weckstein et al. found improved pregnancy rates without increasing endometrial thickness due to improvement in the blood flow.[10] Cochrane review in 2010 found no benefit in endometrial preparation with aspirin.[11] A recent meta-analysis in 2017 by Wang et al. did not find any difference in implantation rate with aspirin and without aspirin group.[12] So, the current evidence to support the beneficial effect of aspirin in patients with thin endometrium is lacking and is controversial.
- *Sildenafil:* It has a vasodilator effect. It relaxes the smooth muscles of the blood vessels and increases the blood flow to the endometrium and is also claimed to increase the endometrial thickness and receptivity. The dose is 25 mg 6 hourly vaginally up to the day of trigger or embryo transfer.[13] However, Cochrane review 2014 found insufficient evidence for sildenafil to improve the thickness of the endometrium and live birth rate.[14] Clinical benefit of sildenafil in women with a recurrent thin endometrium is lacking and only few studies with small group of patients are available.
- *Tocopherol (vitamin E):* It is a vasodilator as well as antioxidant. Generally, it is used with pentoxifylline in radiation fibrosis. Significant increase in uterine diastolic blood flow and endometrial thickness was observed with 1,000 IU of vitamin E and 800 mg of pentoxifylline daily for 9 months. Increase in the endometrial thickness was also found in refractory thin endometrium in patients with premature ovarian

failure.[15] But except for radiation fibrosis, other studies are lacking for vitamin E and pentoxifylline combination to improve endometrial thickness in regular practice.

- *Pentoxifylline:* It has a vasodilating effect and reduces blood viscosity along with vitamin E. It can be used in radiation fibrosis.[16]
- *Nitroglycerin:* It releases nitric oxide (NO) and has vasodilator effect. There is no specific publication on it. Oh et al. used nitroglycerin patch on the day before embryo transfer in recurrent implantation failure patients.[17] But, no positive effect was documented. There is no current evidence to use nitroglycerin patch in women with thin endometrium.
- *L-arginine:* It is a precursor of nitric oxide. It acts as a vasodilator and also activates the immune system and inflammatory process. Takasaki et al. gave 6 mg/day of L-arginine in patients with thin endometrium. They observed endometrial thickness of >8 mm in 67%.[18] But, other evidences are not available. It is also used in radiation fibrosis by some workers.
- *Gonadotropin-releasing hormone agonist:* Patient is given luteal support by triptorelin 0.1 mg on the day of oocyte retrieval, day of embryo transfer, and 3 days later.[19] Qublan et al. found significant improvement in implantation and pregnancy rates. However, no other studies have validated these findings.
- *Estrogen:* The dose of estrogen to prepare endometrium is 6–8 mg and can be increased up to 16 mg. Minimum duration of exposure required for estrogen stimulation is 12 days and maximum is 28 days. Estrogen when given for longer duration has shown poor results. Endogenous estrogen is not required when exogenous estrogen is given. In all frozen embryo transfer (FET) cycles, it is continued up to 9 weeks of pregnancy. Estrogen can also be administered vaginally but should not be used vaginally with progesterone. Twice a week injection of 4 mg can be given when other routes fail.

  Estrogen helps endometrial preparation by causing spiral artery contraction, reduced oxygen tension in functional layer, which in turn facilitates embryo implantation.[20] Though step-up protocol of estrogen is popular, the recent studies suggest that this is not required. Estrogen can be started as 6–8 mg dose, maximum up to 16 mg per day from day one. Though only 2 mg can block the follicular development and so downregulation from luteal phase is not required.
- *Tamoxifen:* In patients having thin endometrium, tamoxifen can increase the thickness. For FET cycles, Xin Chen et al. reported tamoxifen 20 mg for 5 days and if the patient did not respond, extended regime can be tried.[21] Tamoxifen can also be used in patients having thin endometrium because of clomiphene citrate.
- *Human chorionic gonadotropin in proliferative phase*: It is produced by endometrial epithelial cells in secretory phase.[22] hCG has a local paracrine role in differentiating endometrial receptivity by regulating different cytokines and growth factors.[23] Intrauterine injection of 500 IU of hCG increases leukemia inhibitory factor (LIF) and vascular endothelial growth factor (VEGF).

  Papanikolaou et al. introduced 150 IU of hCG daily subcutaneously for 7 days from day 8 of the cycle for those who did not respond to 17-β-estradiol 8 mg/day. They found increase in endometrial thickness and clinical outcome. hCG was stopped when progesterone was started.[24] If the dose is increased or is given to the patients with normal endometrium, it can have deleterious effect on endometrial receptivity.

Procedures

- *Endometrial scratching:* Endometrial scratching causes inflammatory reaction and this injury to the endometrium may increase the chances of implantation.[25] Injury leads to favorable changes in cytokines, natural killer (NK) cells, and macrophages to improve implantation rate.

  A recent Cochrane review suggests favorable outcome with endometrial scratching.[26] Scratching causes the growth of endometrium and increases endometrial thickness. It is useful in cases with recurrent implantation failure also. Xu et al. in 2015 documented that combination of G-CSF and endometrial scratching gives favorable pregnancy rate.[27] Though more studies are required to prove its role in patients with thin endometrium. A recent study by Mackens S et al. in 2020 has documented that intentional endometrial injury in follicular phase of ovarian stimulation warrants further attention in future research as it may be harmful.[28]
- *Granulocyte colony-stimulating factor:* It is produced in various tissues in the body including vascular endothelium. It acts as a growth factor and cytokine. It causes proliferation and differentiation of endometrium

as it causes endometrial stromal cell decidualization. G-CSF may stimulate endometrial stem cells or mobilize bone marrow cells promoting growth of the endometrium. G-CSF modulates gene expression of endometrial vascular remodeling, immune regulation, and cell adhesions.[29] The first successful experience was described by Gleicher, resulted in 4 pregnancies after increasing the endometrial thickness.[30] Patients were treated with intrauterine perfusion of 30 IU of G-CSF (300 mg/mL) approximately 6–12 hours prior to hCG injection. If during egg retrieval, endometrial thickness is <7 mm, dose was repeated. The thickness was 9.3 ± 2.1 mm versus 6.4 ± 1.4 mm. But randomized controlled trial (RCT) was lacking and there was no control group for comparison. Eftekhar et al. documented improved endometrial receptivity in FET cycles when endometrial thickness was <7 mm.[31] However, Barad et al. who are pioneers of this concept were unable to demonstrate any effect of G-CSF on endometrial growth or pregnancy rate.[32]

So, even though nonrandomized studies have given good results, the published RCT failed to show any beneficial effect. So more trials are required to prove its efficacy. Present evidence is not supportive. G-CSF does not improve pregnancy outcome when endometrial thickness is normal.[33]

- *Autologous platelet-rich plasma (PRP):* Platelet-rich plasma releases cytokines and growth factors like VEGF, TGF1, and EGF. It was introduced after 10 days of estradiol valerate 12 mg in patients where endometrial thickness was <7 mm. In all five patients, endometrial thickness increased and all became pregnant after embryo transfer.[34] Shahrzad et al. did the pilot study in 2017. PRP was introduced on day 11–12 and repeated on day 13–14. Endometrial thickness increased >7 mm after the second PRP in all patients and got 5 pregnancies in 10 patients. So growth factors and cytokines from PRP may improve endometrial receptivity.[35] As PRP is autologous, there is no risk of transmission of infectious diseases and immunological reaction.

  Platelet-rich plasma infusion is done 48 hours before embryo transfer. 8 mL of venous blood is drawn, centrifuged at 1,500 g (RCF) for 10 minutes.
  - Collect blood
  - Spin at 200 g for 15 minutes
  - Then spin at 600 g for 6 minutes. The repeated reversal of the tube allows us to obtain PRP at the concentration required.
  - 0.5–6.8 mL obtained is infused with IUI cannula.
  - After 48 hours, assess endometrium, otherwise introduce second dose.

  Still the evidence is limited. Further studies are required for thin endometrium. According to Urman et al. (2019), caution is required prior to using PRP on wide scale and await the results of well-designed study.[36]
- *Stem cells:* The first case of endometrial regeneration by stem cells followed by conception was published by us in 2011.[37] Autologous bone marrow cells obtained from the iliac crest were infused into the uterus with Asherman's syndrome and thin endometrium that was unresponsive to estrogen cells was implanted on day 2 after curettage. Aspiration was done using bone marrow biopsy needle and 10-mL syringe prewashed with heparin. Total 45 mL of bone marrow was aspirated. Collection was done in CPDA (citrate–phosphate dextrose anticoagulant) medium using 1 mL of medium for 7 mL of bone marrow. It was sent to a dedicated stem cell laboratory working as per clinical GMP/GTP standard and having a working area with laminar airflow to class 100.

  Bone marrow was centrifuged using histopaque density gradient at 1,000 rpm for 10 minutes and 102 million mononuclear cells were separated. These cells were then treated by column separation technique and customized cocktail of CD9, CD90, CD133 antibodies was used for immunomagnetic isolation of endometrial angiogenic stem cells. Markers used for endometrial angiogenic stem cells were CD9, CD44, and CD90. Gene expression study for CD9, CD44, and CD90 using reverse transcription polymerase chain reaction (RT-PCR) technique was done for differentiated cells. Total 39 million marker positive endometrial angiogenic cells were supplied in 0.7 mL of PBS (phosphate buffer saline) with 2% autologous (patient's own) heat inactivated serum for transplantation on the next day for transplant.[38-42]

  Curettage was done under anesthesia. With patient in lithotomy position, Sim's speculum in place, anterior retractor was used to retract the anterior vaginal wall and vulsellum was used to hold the anterior lip of cervix. Embryo transfer cannula (Frydman classic catheter 4,5, Laboratoire CCD, France) attached with 1-mL syringe and filled with 0.7-mL stem cell suspension was advanced through cervix up to the fundal end of the endometrium under transabdominal ultrasound guidance. With the tip of the catheter 0.5 cm distal to the fundus, piston was very slowly advanced to allow slow steady flow of cell suspension in the uterine cavity. After instilling 0.3 mL of stem cell suspension at the fundus, injection was continued when cannula was gradually withdrawn out, till the tip reached mid cavity of the uterus. It was very gently and slowly withdrawn out of the internal os and then external os, continuously maintaining pressure on the piston to prevent any back flow.

This is followed by cyclical estrogen, progesterone therapy for 3–4 months, with aspirin 75 mg daily. This resulted into 7 mm + endometrium with vascularity reaching inner zones of the endometrium as confirmed on Doppler studies. Embryo transfer was done after that and resulted in conception.

Three main sources of endometrial cell reconstruction have been proposed.

1. Clonogenic cells in the endometrium
2. Epithelial progenitor cells and mesenchymal stromal stem cells from bone marrow
3. Human embryonic stem cells

These are pluripotent stem cells and are not obtained from the fibroblasts of a female with Asherman's syndrome.

Subendometrial autologous stem cell transplantation of mononuclear stem cells from iliac crest also increases endometrial thickness in patients with Asherman's syndrome. Exogenous estrogen therapy is given. This gives good results and resumption of menstruation is also observed.[43] Sentaria and colleagues infused bone marrow-derived stem cells in spiral arterioles and found increase in endometrial thickness and subsequent pregnancy.

Xavier Santamaria also did autologous stem cell therapy with CD133+ bone marrow-derived stem cells and has claimed good results.[44] According to them, some women are prone to Asherman's syndrome and these should be identified. In another study, somatic cell nuclear transfer derived HPSC5 MPCs could be advanced therapeutic strategy for specific diseases in the field of regenerative medicine.[45]

CONCLUSION

Endometrial thickness of >7 mm is associated with good implantation. The vascularity of the endometrium is more important than just the thickness. Obstetric procedures like dilatation and curettage are the most common source of endometrial damage, followed by hysteroscopic surgery for myomas and intrauterine synechiae. Chronic endometritis is treatable with good outcome. Other treatment modalities include extended estrogen therapy, low dose aspirin, and hCG injections. Other drugs employed are sildenafil, pentoxifylline, vitamin E, L arginine and G-CSF. Both PRP injections and stem cell therapy offer some hope. Endometrial scratching is not backed up with evidence.

REFERENCES

1. Cai QF, Wan F, Huang R, Zhang HW. Factors predicting the cumulative outcome of IVF/ICSI treatment: a multivariable analysis of 2450 patients. Hum Reprod. 2011;26:2532-40.
2. Cruz F, Bellver J. Live birth after embryo transfer in an unresponsive thin endometrium. Gynecol Endocrinol. 2014;30:481-4.
3. Schiper E, Valle RF, Nezhat C. Intrauterine Adhesions: Hysteroscopic evaluation and treatment, prevention and management, 3rd edition. North Miami Beach, FL: Society of Laparoscopic Surgeons; pp. 1-3.
4. Taskin O, Sadik S, Onoglu A, Gokdeniz R, Erturan E, Burak K, Wheeler JM. Role of endometrial suppression on the frequency of intrauterine adhesions after surgery resectoscope. J Am Assoc Gynecol Laparosc. 2000;7:351-4.
5. Young SL. Oestrogen and progesterone action on endometrium: a translational approach to understanding endometrial receptivity. Reprod Biomed Online. 2013;27:497-505.
6. Piereira N, Amrane S, Estes JL, Lekovich JP, Elias RT, Chung PH, et al. Does the time interval between hysteroscopic polypectomy and start of in vitro fertilization affect outcomes? Fertil Steril. 2016;105:539-44.
7. Pinto V, Matteo M, Tinelli R, Mitola P, De Ziegler D, Cicinelli E. Altered uterine contractility in women with chronic endometritis. Fertil Steril. 2015;103:1049-52.
8. Cicinelli E, Matteo M, Tinelli R, Lepera A, Alfonso R, Idraccolo U, et al. Prevalence of chronic endometritis in repeated unexplained implantation failure and the IVF success after antibiotic therapy. Hum Reprod. 2015;30:323-33.
9. Zolghadri J, Momtahan M, Aminian K, Ghaffarpasand F, Tavana Z. The value of hysteroscopy in diagnosis of chronic endometritis in patients with unexplained recurrent spontaneous abortion. Eur J Obstet Gynecol Reprod Biol. 2011;155:217-20.
10. Weckstein LN, Jacobson A, Galen D, Hampton K, Hammel J. Low dose aspirin for oocyte donation recipients with a thin endometrium: prospective, randomized study. Fertil Steril. 1997;68:927-30.
11. Glujovsky D, Pesce R, Fiszbajn G, Sueldo C, Hart RJ, Ciapponi A. Endometrial preparation for women undergoing embryo transfer with frozen embryos or embros derived from donor oocytes. Cochrane Database Syst Rev. 2010;10(10):CD006359.

12. Wang H, Huang X, Li X, Lv F, He X, Pan Y, et al. Efficacy evaluation if low dose aspirin in IVF/ICSI patients evidence from 13 RCTs: A systematic review and meta-analysis. Medicine. 2017;96:e7720.
13. Sher G, Fisch J. Vaginal Sildenafil (Viagra): a preliminary report of a novel method to improve uterine artery blood flow and endometrial development in patients undergoing IVF. Hum Reprod. 2000;15:806-9.
14. Gutarra-Vilchez RB, Urrutia G, Glujovsky D, Coscia A, Bonfill Cosp X. Vasodilators for women undergoing fertility treatment. Cochrane Database Syst Rev. 2014;10:CD010001.
15. Letur-Konirsch H, Guis F, Delanian S. Uterine restoration by radiation sequelae regression with combined pentoxifylline-tocoferol: a phase II study. Fertil Steril. 2002;77:1219-26.
16. Chiao TB, Lee AJ. Role of pentoxifylline and vitamin E in attenuation of radiation induced fibrosis. Ann Pharmacother. 2005;39:516-22.
17. Ohl J, Lefebvre-Maunoury C, Wittemer C, Nisand G, Laurent MC, Hoffman P. Nitric oxide donors for patients undergoing IVF. A prospective, double blind, randomized, placebo controlled trial. Hum Reprod. 2002;17:2615-20.
18. Takasaki A, Tamura H, Miwa I, Taketani T, Shimamura K, Sugino N. Endometrial growth and uterine blood flow: a pilot study for improving endometrial thickness in the patients with a thin endometrium. Fertil Steril. 2010;93(6):1851-8.
19. Qublan H, Amarin Z, Al-Qudah M, Diab F, Nawasreh M, Malkawi S, et al. Luteal phase support with GnRha improves implantation and pregnancy rates in IVF cycles with endometrium of < or = 7 mm on day of egg retrieval. Hum Fertil (Camb). 2008;11:43-7.
20. Casper RF. It's time to pay attention to the endometrium. Fertil Steril. 2011;96:519-21.
21. Chen X, Chen SL. Successful pregnancy in recurrent thin endometrium with new uses for an old drug. J IVF Reprod Med Genet. 2013;1:2.
22. Paiva P, Hannan NJ, Hincks C, Meehan KL, Pruysers E, Dimitriadis E, et al. Human chorionic gonadotrophin regulates FGF2 and other cytokines produced by human endometrial epithelial cells, providing a mechanism for enhancing endometrial receptivity. Hum Reprod. 2011;26:153-62.
23. Licth P, Flur H, Neuwinger J, Wallwiener D, Wildt L. Is human chorionic gonadotrophin directly involved in the regulation of human implantation? Mol Cell Endocrinol. 2007;269:85-92.
24. Papanikolaou EG, Kyrou D, Zervakakou G, Paggou E, Humaidan P. Follicular hCG endometrial priming for IVF patients experiencing resisting thin endometrium. A proof of concept study. J Assist Reprod Genet. 2013;30:1341-5.
25. Barasch A, Dekel N, Fieldust S, Segal I, Schechtman E, Granot I. Local injury to the endometrium doubles the incidence of successful pregnancies in patients undergoing in vitro fertilization. Fetil Steril. 2003;79:1317-22.
26. Nastri CO, Lensen SF, Gibreel A, Rainne-Fenning N, Ferriani RA, Bhattacharya S, et al. Endometrial injury in women undergoing assisted reproductive techniques. Cochrane Database Syst Rev. 2015;(3):CD009517.
27. Xu B, Zhang Q, Hao J, Xu D, Li Y. Two protocols to treat thin endometrium with granulocyte colony stimulating factor during frozen embryo transfer cycles. Reprod Biomed Online. 2015;30(4):349-58.
28. Mackens S, Racca A, Van De Velde H, Drakopoulos P, Tournaye H, Stoop D, et al. Follicular phase endometrial scratching: A truncated randomized controlled trial. Hum Reprod. 2020;35(5):1090-8.
29. Rahmati M, Petitbarat M, Dubanchet S, Bensussan A, Chaouat G, Ledee N. Granulocyte-colony stimulating factor related pathways tested on an endometrial ex-vivo model. PLoS One. 2014;9:e102286.
30. Gleicher N, Vidali A, Barad DH. Successful treatment of unresponsive thin endometrium. Fertil Steril. 2011;95:2123.e13-7.
31. Eftekhar M, Sayadi M, Arabjahvani F. Transvaginal perfusion of G-CSF for infertile women with thin endometrium in frozen ET program: a non-randomized clinical trial. Iran J Reprod Med. 2014;12:661-6.
32. Barad DH, Yu Y, Kushnir VA, Shohat-Tal A, Lazzaroni E, Lee HJ, et al. A randomized clinical trial of endometrial perfusion with granulocyte colony-stimulating factor in in vitro fertilization cycles: impact on endometrial thickness and clinical pregnancy rates. Fertil Steril. 2014;101:710-5.
33. Eftekhar M, Hosseinisadat R, Baradaran R, Naghshineh E. Effect of granulocyte-colony stimulating factor (G-CSF) on IVF outcomes in infertile women: A RCT. Int J Reprod Biomed. 2016;14(5):341-6.
34. Chang Y, Li J, Chen Y, Wei L, Yang X, Liang X. Autologous platelet-rich plasma promotes endometrial growth and improves pregnancy outcome during in vitro fertilization. Int J Clin Exp Med. 2015;8:1286-90.
35. Shahrzad Z, Saghar S, Nasrin S, Leila N. Treatment of thin endometrium with autologous platelets rich plasma: a pilot study. JBRA Assist Reprod. 2017;21(1):54-6.
36. Urman B, Boza A, Balaban B. Platelet rich plasma another add-on treatment getting out of hand? How can clinicians preserve the best interest of their patients? Hum Reprod. 2019;34(11):2099-2103.
37. Nagori CB, Panchal S, Patel H. Endometrial regeneration using autologous adult stem cells followed by conception by in vitro fertilization in a patient of severe Asherman's syndrome. J Hum Reprod Sci. 2011;4(1):43-8.
38. Yin AH, Miraglia S, Zanjani ED, Almeida-Porada G, Ogawa M, Leary AG, et al. AC133, a novel marker for human hematopoietic stem and progenitor cells. Blood. 1997;90:5002-12.

39. Miraglia S, Godfrey W, Yin AH, Atkins K, Warnke R, Holden JT, et al. A novel five-transmembrane hematopoietic stem cell antigen: isolation, characterization, and molecular cloning. Blood. 1997;90:5013-21.
40. Uchida N, Buck DW, He D, Reitsma MJ, Masek M, Phan TV, et al. Direct isolation of human central nervous system stem cells. Proc Natl Acad Sci USA. 2000;97:14720-5.
41. Cummings BJ, Uchida N, Tamaki SJ, Salazar DL, Hooshmand M, Summers R, et al. Human neural stem cells differentiate and promote locomotor recovery in spinal cord-injured mice. Proc Natl Acad Sci USA. 2005;102:14069-74.
42. Bussolati B, Bruno S, Grange C, Buttiglieri S, Deregibus MC, Cantino D, et al. Isolation of renal progenitor cells from adult human kidney. Am J Pathol. 2005;166:545-55.
43. Singh N, Mohanty S, Seth T, Shankar M, Bhaskaran S, Dharmendra S. Autologous stem cell transplantation in refractory Asherman's syndrome: a novel cell based therapy. J Hum Reprod Sci. 2014;7:93-8.
44. Santamaria X, Cabanillas S, Cervello I, Arbona C, Raga F, Ferro J, et al. Autologous stem cell therapy with CD 133+ bone marrow-derived stem cells for refractory Asherman's syndrome and endometrial atrophy: a pilot cohort study. Hum Reprod. 2016;31(5):1087-96.
45. Jun SM, Park M, Lee JY, Jung S, Lee JE, Shim SH, et al. Single cell-derived clonally expanded mesenchymal progenitor cell from somatic cell nuclear transfer derived pluripotent stem cells ameliorate the endometrial function in the uterus of a murine model with Asherman's syndrome. Cell Prolif. 2019;52:e12597.

SECTION

6 Maternal Systemic Causes

CHAPTER 26

Antiphospholipid Syndrome

Narinder Pal

ABSTRACT

Antiphospholipid syndrome is an acquired thrombophilia of autoimmune etiology. Screening for this disorder is based on clinical and laboratory criteria. Recurrent pregnancy loss (RPL) is one of the clinical criteria for diagnosis of APS. Laboratory testing includes anticardiolipin antibodies, lupus anticoagulant and anti-beta-2 glycoprotein 1 antibodies. Treatment is by low dose aspirin and low molecular weight heparin. Adjuvant therapies like hydroxychloroquine, intravenous immunoglobulins, and prednisolone have been used in refractory cases. Newer therapies like eculizumab, rituximab, certolizumab, and statins are being tried.

Keywords: APLA syndrome, EULAR classification, Lupus anticoagulant, Anticardiolipin antibodies, Anti-beta-2 glycoprotein 1 antibodies, Aspirin, LMWH, IVIG, HCQ, Adalimumab, Certolizumab, Eculizumab, Statins OAPS, OMAPS, NC OAPS, RPL, Rituximab.

INTRODUCTION

Antiphospholipid syndrome (APS) is an acquired, autoimmune, thrombo-inflammatory disorder with various systemic presentations. There is thrombosis of macrovessels (arterial and venous) as well as microvasculopathy along with pregnancy-related morbidities, with persistent presence of antiphospholipid antibodies (APLAs). These include lupus anticoagulant (LA), anticardiolipin (aCL) and anti-beta-2 glycoprotein 1 (aβ2GP-1) antibodies.

Historically, during the 18th century, Queen Anne Stuart of Great Britain, exhibited symptoms and signs of systemic lupus erythematosus (SLE) and suffered from repeated miscarriages and stillbirths, suggesting a diagnosis of APS. The resultant discontinuation of family lineage, marked the end of Stuart dynasty. Medically, the syndrome was first described in 1983 by Harris & Hughes, who observed features of this disorder in patients with SLE.[1,2]

In 2023, American college of Rheumatology (ACR) and European Alliance of Associations for Rheumatology (EULAR), have developed the new ACR/EULAR classification criteria, of APS. This should provide a very high level of specificity, thus laying down a very strong foundation for future APS research with uniformity.

The APS presenting with obstetric morbidities without previous thrombosis is known as obstetric antiphospholipid syndrome (OAPS), where recurrent pregnancy loss (RPL) is one of the manifestations. APS is the only autoimmune condition, where pregnancy loss is one of the criteria for its diagnosis.

In the pathophysiology of OAPS, inflammation, complement activation, and thrombosis, all play an important role.

In cases of RPL due to OAPS, treatment with low-dose aspirin (LDA) and low molecular weight heparin (LMWH), is well established. In refractory cases, hydroxychloroquine (HCQ), prednisolone, intravenous immunoglobulins (IVIG), and/or plasma exchange have been tried with variable success. HCQ has proven very effective so far, in the management of APS patients and there are several ongoing International clinical trials with HCQ. Research, with novel therapies for APS management are in progress with statins and biologics—monoclonal antibodies, tumor necrosis factor alpha antibodies (aTNF-α).

ANTIPHOSPHOLIPID SYNDROME-SUBTYPES

- *Primary APS (PAPS):* Patients of APS with the presence of APLA without any other underlying autoimmune disease.
- *Secondary APS (SAPS):* Patients with SLE or other autoimmune disorders, who are positive for APLAs and/or LA. The thrombosis risk increases by >40% in this group.

- *Obstetric APS (OAPS):* Women who fulfil the Sydney clinical criteria for APS but without any previous thrombotic event are classified as OAPS. These clinical criteria are ≥3 consecutive miscarriages before 10 weeks of gestation (RPL), at least one premature birth before 34 weeks of gestation due to preeclampsia (PE)/eclampsia, severe placental insufficiency, and unexplained still births.[3]
- *Noncriteria-obstetric APS (NC-OAPS):* These are the cases which may fulfill clinical criteria of OAPS but have low titers of APLAs or only one positive test, thus not fulfilling laboratory criteria of APS.[4] These women could test positive against other phospholipids, namely phosphatidylserine, prothrombin, annexin A5 or immunoglobulin A (IgA) aCL/β2GP-1.[5] The clinical features such as heart valve disease, livedo reticularis/racemosa, thrombocytopenia, nephropathy, and alveolar hemorrhage in association with obstetric morbidities of APS, which were previously labeled as NC-OAPS.[4] These clinical features are now included in the new 2023 ACR/EULAR classification criteria as clinical domains.[6]
- *Obstetric morbidity APS (OMAPS)* is a category of NC-OAPS patients that suffer from obstetric morbidities but do not fulfill the Sydney laboratory criteria. However, they may have good outcome if treated.
- *Catastrophic APS (CAPS):* Catastrophic APS (Asherson's syndrome) is an uncommon (<1%), potentially life-threatening form of APS involving three or more organ systems. This condition is antibody mediated, presenting with diffuse microvascular thrombosis and cytokine storm, developing in less than a week, resulting in multi organ failure.[5] According to CAPS registry, patient treated with anticoagulants, glucocorticoids, intravenous immunoglobulins (IVIG), and plasma exchange have a better prognosis.[7,8] In spite of these aggressive treatment regimens, mortality is quite high (30%). The role of complement in CAPS is suggested by successful outcome with eculizumab in some patients, who are refractory to standard treatment.[9]

ANTIPHOSPHOLIPID ANTIBODIES

Antiphospholipid antibodies are autoantibodies, directed against phosphorus-fat components of body's own cell membranes, called phospholipids.

Enzyme linked immunosorbent assay (ELISA) and functional assays are applied for their identification in the laboratory, for the diagnosis of APS.

There are three recognized APLAs, namely:

1. Lupus anticoagulant (functional clotting assay)
2. Anticardiolipin antibodies immunoglobulin G (IgG) or immunoglobulin M (IgM) (ELISA)
3. Anti-β2 glycoprotein-1 antibodies IgG or IgM (ELISA)[10]

A study by Grygiel-Gorniak et al., observed APLAs in 6% of all pregnant patients. Several viral infections are associated with elevated levels of APLAs. In a meta-analysis, about 50% of COVID-19 patients were APLA positive, mostly LA antibodies with no increased risk of thrombotic complications related to APLA positivity.[11]

PATHOPHYSIOLOGY OF OBSTETRIC ANTIPHOSPHOLIPID SYNDROME

It is important to understand the current pathophysiology of OAPS for making an accurate diagnosis as well as choosing an individualized treatment protocol, for achieving a favorable pregnancy outcome.

Recently, "two hit hypothesis" has been proposed to explain the pathophysiology of APS. 1st hit is due to autoantibodies, especially aβ2GP-1 class, which results in creating a generalized prothrombotic state, which then acts in unison with the 2nd hit, in a milieu, of subclinical vascular injury, stasis, infection or inflammation, resulting in thrombosis of vessels.

In a systematic review of literature and meta-analysis of the placental histopathology, thrombosis was rarely observed in placentae of OAPS cases. The common observations were decidual inflammation, impaired spiral artery remodeling by extravillous trophoblast, complement split product deposition of C4d class, and decreased vasculosyncytial membranes.[12]

At the cellular level APLAs, specially anti β2GP-1 antibodies, exhibit embryo-toxicity by directly targeting decidual endothelial and trophoblast cells as well as innate immune cells (neutrophils, monocytes, and platelets), due to the abundant presence of the polypeptide β2GP-1 on their cell surface.[13] β2GP-1, a plasma protein, is the main antigen identified by aβ2GP-1 and some aCL antibodies. This makes placenta a target for binding of these pathogenic anti β2GP-1, resulting in trophoblast dysfunction.[14]

At the molecular level, the expression of tissue factor (TF) in endothelial and innate immune cells, the release of proinflammatory cytokines, platelet activation, production of intracellular reactive oxygen species (ROS), and induction of complement cascade result in increased level of TNF α in decidual tissue. All above factors contribute to the development of APS.[15,16]

It is proven now that distinctive pathogenic mechanisms are operative in obstetric and vascular thrombotic APS.[17] An in vitro study, comparing the effect of purified IgG from obstetric and nonobstetric APS patients, showed inhibited trophoblast invasion with IgG from obstetric APS only, supporting the hypothesis that APLA pathogenicity is different in two APS subgroups.[18]

The pathogenesis of RPL during first trimester is due to direct inhibitory effect of APLAs on embryo development, placentation, and enhanced apoptosis of trophoblast cells.[19] Late OAPS complications such as PE, fetal growth retardation (FGR), and still births are due to thrombosis and inflammation, resulting from placental dysfunction which occurs during the second and third trimester.[20] Therefore, pathogenesis of RPL during first trimester is different from 2nd and 3rd trimester.

THE CLASSIFICATION CRITERIA FOR ANTIPHOSPHOLIPID SYNDROME

The International classification criteria for APS, first defined at Sapporo in 1999, were subsequently, updated and published in 2006 as Sydney classification criteria for APS. These modified Sydney criteria were intended for conducting multicenter research, with uniformity rather than for clinical diagnosis of APS. In practice, most of the clinicians including British Committee for Standards in Hematology guidelines for APS management used these criteria as a diagnostic tool.[21]

In October 2023, ACR/EULAR APS Classification criteria were jointly published by the ACR and EULAR.

The new ACR/EULAR classification criteria are characterized by a compulsory entry criteria of at least one positive antiphospholipid antibody (APLA) test, within 3 years of manifestation of an APLA-related clinical criteria, followed by additive weighted criteria (score range 1–7 points each), which are grouped into six clinical domains (macrovascular venous thromboembolism, macrovascular arterial thrombosis, microvasculopathy, obstetric complications, cardiac valve, and hematological manifestations) and two laboratory domains namely LA test, IgG/IgM aCL or IgG/IgM anti-β2GP-1. Patients are labeled as APS positive if they gather at least three points each, from clinical as well as laboratory domains. The EULAR classification criteria for APS, in comparison to 2006 Sydney criteria has a specificity of 99% versus 86% and sensitivity of 84% versus 99%.[6]

Tang et al., published the drawbacks of 2023 ACR/EULAR classification, as in their cohort, the number of APS patients who fulfilled new classification criteria were 367, and this number rose to 479, when Sydney classification criteria were applied. There were many patients who suffered from recurrent pregnancy losses, but could not achieve the required clinical domain score of 3, to qualify for APS diagnosis. Therefore, these patients of obstetric APS, could be denied the preventive APS treatment benefits, if not appropriately classified.[22]

The EULAR recommendations of 2019, for APS management, were based on *Classification of APLA profiles (low-risk and high-risk)* as well as their *titers*.

Following are the definitions of APLA profiles and titers:

- *Low-risk APLA profile:* Isolated aCL or anti β2GP-1 antibodies at low-medium titers, particularly if transiently positive.
- *High-risk APLA profile:* The presence (on two or more occasions at least 12 weeks apart) of LA [measured according to International Society for Thrombosis and Hemostasis (ISTH) guidelines], or of double (any combination of LA, aCL antibodies, or anti β2GP-1 antibodies) or triple (all three subtypes) APLA positivity, or the presence of persistently high APLA titers.[23]

Medium-high APLA titers: Anticardiolipin antibody of IgG and or IgM isotype in serum or plasma present in titers >40 IgG phospholipid (GPL) units or >40 IgM phospholipid (MPL) units, or > the 99th percentile, measured by a standardized ELISA. Anti β2GP-1 antibody of IgG and/or IgM isotype in serum or plasma in titer > the 99th percentile, measured by a standardized ELISA.[10]

Low-medium APLA titers: aCL or β2GP 1 antibody of IgG and IgM in serum or plasma present between 20 and 39 GPL and/or MPL.

Based on the titers and profiles of APLAs, one can even predict the risk of developing future thrombosis and obstetric events. For example, a high risk APLA profile, and presence of LA as the APLA subtype are most closely related to thrombosis risk. Similarly, presence of double and triple APLAs or persistent presence of APLAs in high titers, predisposes them to future disease.

CLINICAL PRESENTATION

The clinical manifestations of APS depend upon the underlying predominant pathology, whether, it is vascular thrombosis, or pregnancy-related morbidities or birth. Based on the presentation of the disease one can classify APS into vascular APS (VAPS) or OAPS.

Vascular Antiphospholipid Syndrome

Venous, arterial, and microvessel thrombosis, is the hallmark of VAPS.

Data from Antiphospholipid Syndrome Alliance for Clinical Trials and International Networking (APS ACTION) registries, showed that deep venous thrombosis (DVT) and/or pulmonary embolism, and cerebrovascular events [stroke and transient ischemic attack (TIA)], were the most common thrombotic manifestation of APS.[24]

Statistically, thrombosis is more common in veins than arteries, and DVT is the most frequent manifestation, affecting 30–40% of the cases.[25] Lower limb thrombosis is the common site, but any part of the venous system, including pulmonary arteries, cerebral veins, dural venous sinuses, retinal veins, renal vein, and mesenteric vein can be involved. Hepatic vein thrombosis results in Budd-Chiari syndrome.[26]

In the Euro-phospholipid Project registry, arterial thrombosis causing myocardial infarction and stroke, were the most common cause of death in (22.5%) of the VAPS cases.[27]

Sneddon's syndrome is a rare form of thrombotic arteriopathy in VAPS, characterized by cerebral vascular disease and livedo recemosa (permanent, net like reddish-blue discoloration of the skin), which can present in APS.[28] Cases of peripheral arterial disease, retinal artery occlusion, arterial thrombosis of renal, splenic, hepatic, pancreatic, and mesentery are recorded in the literature, in APS disease.[26]

Microvascular thrombosis can affect any organ system in APS patients.

In CAPS presentation, there is multisystem involvement causing thrombosis in the microvessels, whereas, in a single system involvement, kidney and skin are most frequently affected, resulting in APS nephropathy, livedo reticularis/racemosa and skin ulcers. Now, these microvascular thrombosis manifestations are included in the clinical domains of 2023 ACR/EULAR classification criteria.[6]

Obstetric Antiphospholipid Syndrome

Obstetric APS may present as:

- Recurrent early pregnancy losses at ≤10 weeks gestation;
- One or more fetal losses at ≥10 weeks gestation;
- *Still births:* OAPS is strongly associated with unexplained still birth after 22 weeks gestation, i.e., after a normal fetal anatomy scan. This was common in women that showed persistent LA positivity rather than in those with a single positivity of aCL or β2GP-1 with Elisa method.
- *Early severe preeclampsia:* The pathophysiology of early severe PE is trophoblast dysfunction which is a hallmark of APS syndrome. It is also associated with fetal loss which if repetitive may not qualify as RPL. These patients may escape the net of diagnosis and suffer repeated early neonatal losses.
- *FGR* due to placental insufficiency causing premature births and again repeated fetal losses.[3]

Recurrent pregnancy loss is very typical presentation of OAPS and is more common than late pregnancy complications such as PE, FGR, and still birth. Sheela et al. reported in their study an overall APLA positivity of 21.21% in RPL cases.[29] However, these pregnancy morbidities should be a criteria for APS testing frequently to categorize these patients. It is also mandatory to karyotype late pregnancy losses to diagnose recurrent fetal congenital anomalies and direct future genetic testing appropriately.

It should be observed that there are many patients who fail to meet Sydney clinical and laboratory criteria completely, who are classified as NC-OAPS as previously discussed in the subtype of APS. In a comparative study on 1,640 patients, representing the largest published series, OAPS (1,000 cases) and NC-OAPS (640 cases), showed OAPS patients suffered higher number of miscarriages, fetal losses, still births, early vasculopathy (PE and FGR <34 weeks) and prematurity than those in NC-OAPS groups. However, women with NC-OAPS had higher early complications such as implantation failure and late placental events (PE and FGR >34 weeks). The exact pathophysiological explanation for this difference is yet to be elucidated. In spite of differences in clinical presentations, the fetal maternal outcome was the same in these two groups, when treated with LDA and heparin.[4] Alijotas-Reig et al., observed in their cohort of 1,000 OAPS patients, that RPL was the most prevalent clinical manifestation observed (38.6%) of their cases, whereas early PE was observed in (18.1%) and fetal growth restriction due to placental insufficiency in (16.1%). Patients with recommended treatment of OAPS with (LDA and LMWH) had a good live birth rate of (85%), which dropped to (73.4%), when either LDA or heparin were used singularly, while patients with no treatment showed a poor live birth rate of (49.6%).[30]

Another nomenclature coined in this light is the *Obstetric Morbidity APS syndrome (OMAPS).* These patients present with obstetric morbidities, without having recurrent fetal loss. They then do not qualify for treatment during pregnancy but manifest as either a sporadic miscarriage followed by another pregnancy complicated by early PE or fetal growth restriction with/without PE. They thus, display varied clinical manifestations of OAPS and may not display a robust laboratory criteria. They may continue to suffer obstetric morbidities, as timely adequate treatment is not commenced.[31] We need to classify these patients to be able to institute evidence-based treatment.

MANAGEMENT OF ANTIPHOSPHOLIPID SYNDROME

The Management of OAPS patients involves close surveillance and treatment planning, before, during, and after delivery, to optimize, both maternal and fetal outcome. There should be a multidisciplinary team, including Obstetrician, Internist, and Rheumatologist, to look after these patients.

Preconception Counseling

During preconception counseling sessions in OAPS patients, a detailed history should be recorded about their previous pregnancy complications or thrombosis; presence of any noncriteria manifestations or any other autoimmune diseases, mainly SLE for the prediction of future pregnancy risk assessment. A detailed analysis of their APLA profiles/ titers should be performed, to plan their treatment, strategy during pregnancy as per the 2019 EULAR recommendations. When there is a history of RPL (three or more) at <10 weeks gestation or a pregnancy loss greater than 10 weeks-(LDA 75–100 mg) is recommended preconception.

Postpartum Care

Women on antithrombotic therapy during pregnancy need to reinstitute this during the postpartum phase. In nonthrombotic primary OAPS, it is mandatory to continue it till the mother is sedentary after a normal delivery or cesarean section. In thrombotic APS this should be continued till 6–8 weeks postpartum, till the hypercoagulable tendency of pregnancy is completely reversed.

PREGNANCY TREATMENT OF OBSTETRIC ANTIPHOSPHOLIPID SYNDROME

The current recommended treatment for OAPS patient is LDA (75–100 mg) to be started during preconception period and LMWH (prophylactic dose of 0.5 mg/kg/day), to be added once the pregnancy test is positive.[32] With this regimen, live birth rate of 70–80% could be achieved.[33] However, 20–30 % of women continue to suffer from obstetric complications despite this conventional treatment, and are labeled as refractory OAPS.[34] In these cases, HCQ, low-dose prednisolone, IVIG, and plasma exchange are given, with variable success rates. OAPS patients, who give past history of thrombosis, should receive secondary thrombo-prophylaxis, preferably with LMWH.[35]

EULAR RECOMMENDATIONS FOR ANTIPHOSPHOLIPID SYNDROME MANAGEMENT[23]

The EULAR in 2019 has set forth specific guidelines for the management of various clinical scenarios of APS.

EULAR Guidelines for Management of Obstetric Antiphospholipid Syndrome

- In women with a high-risk APLA profile but no history of thrombosis or pregnancy complications (with or without SLE), *treatment with LDA (75–100 mg/day) during pregnancy should be considered.*
- With a history of ≥3 recurrent spontaneous miscarriages <10th weeks of gestation and in those with a history of fetal loss (≥10th weeks of gestation), *combination treatment with LDA and heparin at prophylactic dosage during pregnancy is recommended.*
- With a history of delivery <34th weeks of gestation due to eclampsia or severe PE or due to recognized features of placental insufficiency, *treatment with LDA or LDA and heparin at prophylactic dosage is recommended* considering the individual's risk profile.
- With clinical, NC-OAPS *treatment with LDA alone or in combination with heparin might be considered* based on the individual's risk profile.
- With obstetric APS treated with prophylactic dose heparin during pregnancy, *continuation of heparin at prophylactic dose for 6 weeks after delivery should be considered* to reduce the risk of maternal thrombosis.

- In women with "Criteria Obstetric APS" with recurrent pregnancy complications despite combination *treatment with LDA and heparin at prophylactic dosage, increasing heparin dose to therapeutic dose or addition of HCQ or low-dose prednisolone in the first trimester may be considered.* Use of intravenous immunoglobulin (IVIG) might be considered in highly selected cases.
- In women with a history of thrombotic APS, combination *treatment of LDA and heparin at therapeutic dosage during pregnancy is recommended.*[23]
- Switching from oral antithrombotics to aspirin and therapeutic dose of LMWH and unfractionated heparin (UFH) is recommended as soon as pregnancy test is positive, and definitely before 6 weeks of pregnancy due to teratogenic effects of drugs.
  - *Primary thrombo-prophylaxis in APS:* In patients who do not give a previous history of thrombosis.
  - *Low-dose aspirin (LDA) (75–100 mg daily)* is recommended after adequate risk/benefit evaluation:
- In asymptomatic APLA carriers (not fulfilling any vascular or obstetric APS classification criteria), with a high-risk APLA profile, with or without additional risk factors.
- In patients with SLE and no history of thrombosis or pregnancy complications:
  - Patients with high-risk APLA profile, LDA is recommended.
  - Patients with low-risk APLA profile, LDA may be considered.
- In nonpregnant women, with a history of OAPS, with or without SLE.

Secondary Thrombo-prophylaxis in Antiphospholipid Syndrome

In patients with definite APS and first venous thrombosis:

- Treatment with *vitamin K antagonists (VKA), e.g., warfarin with a target international normalized ratio (INR) 2–3* is recommended.
- Direct oral anticoagulants (DOACs) could be considered in patients not able to achieve a target INR despite good adherence to VKA or those with contraindications to VKA (Rivaroxaban should not be used in patients with triple APLA positivity due to the high risk of recurrent thrombotic events).
- In patients with unprovoked first venous thrombosis, anticoagulation should be continued long term.
- In patients with provoked first venous thrombosis, therapy should be continued for a duration recommended for patients without APS according to international guidelines. Longer anticoagulation could be considered in patients with high-risk APLA profile in repeated measurements or other risk factors for recurrence.
- In patients with definite APS and recurrent venous thrombosis despite treatment with VKA with a target INR of 2–3:
  - Check compliance to VKA treatment, along with frequent INR testing.
  - If the target INR of 2–3 had been achieved, we can either add LDA, increase dose of VKA to achieve INR target of 3–4 or switch to LMWH.
- In patients with definite APS and first arterial thrombosis:
  - Treatment with VKA is recommended over treatment with LDA only.
  - Treatment with VKA with INR 2–3 or INR 3–4 is recommended, considering the individual's risk of bleeding and recurrent thrombosis. Treatment with VKA with INR 2–3 plus LDA may also be considered.
  - Based on the current evidence, rivaroxaban should not be used in patients with triple APLA positivity and arterial events, due to the high risk of recurrent thrombosis.
- In patients with recurrent arterial thrombosis despite adequate treatment with VKA, after evaluating for other potential causes, an increase of INR target to 3–4, addition of LDA or switching to LMWH can be considered. Adjunctive therapy with hydroxychloroquine or statins may prove useful.[35]

Drawbacks of the ACR/EULAR Recommendations for Obstetric Antiphospholipid Syndrome

The ACR/EULAR classification is more specific but less sensitive than the earlier Sydney criteria. This means that there is a greater potential of patients not meeting the diagnostic criteria and hence, not being treated adequately for presenting obstetric morbidities. This has been pointed out by Tang et al. in their correspondence.[22] The following drawbacks have been highlighted.

- The section on PE does not include criteria such as placental abruption, eclampsia and (hemolysis elevated liver enzymes, and low platelets (HELLP) syndrome, all of which represent severe trophoblast dysfunction and are associated with a high incidence of fetal loss.
- FGR has not been segregated from small for gestational age (SGA) which may be physiological and is not a hall mark of OAPS.
- Intrauterine fetal death is *arbitrarily* divided into early (between 10 weeks and 15 weeks 6 days) and late between 16 and 34 weeks.
- The guideline does not take into account fetal loss beyond 34 weeks as a criteria of OAPS.

We still need to improve upon the qualifying criteria for OAPS and include patients with OMPS to reach out adequately to patients with obstetric morbidities and bring them in the treatment net to be able to salvage more fetal losses.

DRUGS COMMONLY USED IN THE MANAGEMENT OF OBSTETRIC ANTIPHOSPHOLIPID SYNDROME

Aspirin

Treatment with aspirin alone is ineffective in improving the live birth rate in OAPS cases.[36] The practice of using LDA for primary thrombo-prophylaxis in OAPS patients is quite prevalent. However, in the first randomized controlled trial, where use of aspirin alone, proved ineffective in preventing thrombotic events in APLA positive patients.[37] EULAR guidelines of 2019, for treatment of OAPS patients, also support the use of aspirin for primary thrombo-prophylaxis, based on two meta-analysis that showed protective role of aspirin.[23,38,39] However, in OAPS patients LDA prophylaxis is recommended, beginning 16 weeks gestation, for the prevention of PE.[23,40]

Heparin

Heparin has been effectively used during pregnancy to avert complications of OAPS. Its potent anticomplement power was first reported by Enrique E. Ecker and Paul Gross in 1929.[41] The first randomized trial in OAPS related RPL, was a study, way back in 1992 by Cowchock et al.,[42] comparing, heparin versus prednisolone. It demonstrated the effectiveness and safety of heparin over prednisolone.

In 2020, a meta-analysis comprising of 11 studies, concluded that heparin alone or in combination with LDA was much superior to LDA alone or placebo, in OAPS cases.[36] In EULAR guideline of 2019 for treatment of OAPS, the use of heparin is highly recommended.[23] LMWH is preferred over UFH for the following reasons:

- Increased bioavailability
- Longer half-life necessitating once daily dose
- No risk of thrombocytopenia
- Lower risk of osteoporosis

Both, UFH and LMWH do not cross placenta, therefore, fetal complications have not been reported. Enoxaparin is the preferred heparin in a prophylactic dose of 0.5 mg/kg/day, and therapeutic dose of 1 mg/kg twice daily or intermediate dose 1.5 mg/kg/day of enoxaparin. The prophylactic dose of dalteparin is 100 IU/kg/day and therapeutic dose of 200 IU/kg day to be continued throughout the pregnancy and till 6–8 weeks postpartum.

Hydroxychloroquine

The remaining 20–30% women with OAPS, who are refractory to LDA and LMWH treatment have been tried with few adjunctive treatments with variable success. Sciascia et al., observed higher rate of live births, (67% vs. 57%) and a lower prevalence of APLA related pregnancy morbidities (47% vs. 63%) when HCQ was combined with standard treatment.[43] Gerde et al., showed similar successful pregnancy outcomes, in early and late pregnancy losses, and even improvement in late complications due to placental insufficiency. In a retrospective study on 87 refractory primary OAPS women, who received HCQ 400 mg with LMWH 60 mg plus LDA, were compared with women who received LMWH and LDA only. The primary and secondary outcomes were significantly better in the HCQ treated group, (97.1% vs. 62.5%). Pregnancy complications were markedly lower in HCQ group as well (8.7% vs. 37.5%) (See Appendix 1 Case 1).[44]

The HCQ has proven to be a useful adjunctive treatment so far, in the prevention of recurrent thrombosis and pregnancy complications, due to its immunomodulatory, anti-inflammatory, antithrombotic, and antiplatelet effects. With encouraging results of HCQ addition, in recent studies, the use of HCQ during pregnancy has increased. There are four ongoing prospective International clinical trials:

1. *HYPATIA:* A prospective randomized, controlled trial of HCQ to improve pregnancy outcome in women with APLA.[45]
2. *HIBISCUS:* HCQ for secondary prevention of thrombosis and obstetrical event in primary APS.[46]

3. *HYDROSAPL:* Hydroxychloroquine to achieve pregnancy without obstetrical complications in primary APL syndrome.[47]
4. *"BBQ study" trial:* Hydroxychloroquine for the prevention of recurrent miscarriages.[48]

The results of these ongoing trials are awaited to move HCQ from the list of adjuvant treatment in refractory OAPS to a drug used for primary treatment of patients with OAPS.

Corticosteroids

Steroids have been used for refractory cases of OAPS for a long time. Bramham et al., in their cohort of refractory OAPS patients, treated with low dose prednisolone, along with standard treatment (LDA plus LMWH), achieved a birth rate of 61%. Similar results were observed in another study, as there was a significant reduction in miscarriages, 38.5% versus 85.3%, between treated and untreated group.[48] High dose >20 mg/day of corticosteroids are not recommended as they cause serious side effects such as diabetes, hypertension, and preterm births, thereby jeopardizing fetal survival. Hence, steroids treatment is reserved in refractory OAPS only.[50]

Intravenous Immunoglobulins

The IVIG is known to reduce autoantibodies, decrease natural killer cell activity, and control secretion of inflammatory cytokines. Earlier studies showed its beneficial effect on the murine model. It was first used in RPL patients in 1996.[51] However, since then, human published literature has been divided on the benefits of IVIG in refractory APS patients. The published studies are all with small numbers, and varied protocols of diagnosis and treatment. Hence, a meaningful meta-analysis is not possible. Randomized controlled trial (RCT) comparing it with low dose prednisolone found IVIG to be superior.[52] Retrospective studies and case reports have also concluded that IVIG is successful in refractory OAPS. A small case series and systematic review also recommends the use of IVIG in refractory OAPS in a dose of 0.4 g/kg/day repeated every 2–3 weeks during the first trimester of pregnancy.[53] Currently, it is frequently used in CAPS, but its role in refractory OAPS still lacks robust evidence. In a recent single arm open labeled multicentric study on a small number of patients, IVIG improved obstetric outcome in a few but a combination therapy of IVIG, statins and rituximab improved obstetric outcome in more patients.[53] This proves that refractory OAPS may best be treated with a combination of drugs to target the dominant pathophysiological mechanism.

Novel Therapies in Antiphospholipid Syndrome

Anticoagulation has been the gold standard treatment so far, for the management of APS cases, with a failure rate of 20–30% in OAPS and >30% in VAPS patients. Treatment with LDA plus LMWH alone, has proven ineffective, especially in cases of CAPS, refractory APS and NC-APS. Now with the better understanding of pathogenesis of APS, novel drugs that target the immune system, are being developed and tested. Currently, the groups which are being most studied are immunomodulatory and antithrombotic drugs such as HCQ, Biologics–monoclonal antibodies (rituximab and eculizumab), anti-TNF-α antibodies therapy (adalimumab and certolizumab), and statins.

Statins

HMG-COA reductase inhibitors, known as statins, are used, primarily for hypercholesterolemia, for the prevention of primary and secondary cardiovascular diseases. Statins have shown reduction in TF expression by monocytes as well as antithrombotic and anti-inflammatory actions.[55,56] Therefore, statins can be considered as adjunctive treatment in OAPS patients, especially when patients suffer from dyslipidemia as well. Jui-Chun Chang et al.[57] in their retrospective cohort study on pregnant patients, used various statins and concluded:

- Statins can safely be used during pregnancy as there are no risks of associated congenital anomalies.
- Statins should be used cautiously, due to increased risks of low birth weight and preterm labor.

Statins were earlier classified as category X drugs and were contraindicated in pregnancy. However, in 2021 Food and drug Administration (FDA) has removed this contraindication. (For details see Chapter 58)

Tumor Necrosis Factor-alpha

In OAPS cases, increased levels of TNF-α in decidual tissue, result in placental injury, thus increasing the risk of RPL and FGR.[58]

In a prospective study, on 18 refractory OAPS cases with RPL, were treated with TNF-α blockers [adalimumab (16 cases) and certolizumab (2 cases)], with good obstetric outcome in 70%. In these cases, previous treatment with LDA, LMWH plus HCQ had proven ineffective.[59] Results are awaited for an ongoing "IMPACT study trial," where certolizumab is being evaluated along-with standard treatment (LDA plus LMWH), in pregnant women of APS with persistently positive LA.[60]

Eculizumab

Eculizumab is a humanized monoclonal antibody against complement C5, which works by interrupting the complement mediated proinflammatory events. This drug is safe during pregnancy as only small traces, cross the placenta.[61] In a study comprising 39 cases of CAPS, who were treated with eculizumab, recovery was seen in 74.4% of the patients, without recurrence of thrombosis. Eculizumab can be considered for CAPS patients, refractory to all standard therapies, especially in cases presenting with complement medicated thrombotic microangiopathy.[62]

It is also a useful adjunct in the treatment of refractory OAPS in combination with other drugs, but cost may be a limiting factor.[54]

Rituximab

Rituximab is a class of monoclonal antibodies which depletes CD-20 (B cells), which are involved in the production of APLA. In a phase II trial (RITAPS study), rituximab was tested on 19 cases of NC-APS. Maximum response was seen in thrombocytopenia and skin ulcer patients. There was no change in APLA titers after rituximab use, suggesting response is through APLA independent mechanisms.[9] Emmi et al., used rituximab in 7 cases of APS with active SLE, presenting with recurrent thrombosis. After treatment, only one (CAPS) patient developed thrombosis.[63] Other B-cell directed therapy drug used in PAPS is belimumab.

CONCLUSION

The APS syndrome is an autoimmune disorder that presents with thrombosis the VAPS and obstetric complications known as OAPS. Placental inflammation, complement activation, and thrombosis all play a major role in the pathogenesis of OAPS. Standard treatment is with LDA and LMWH, but in patient's refractory to this treatment adjuvant therapy with HCQ is effective. Low-dose prednisolone has been used as an adjuvant with variable success rates but high dose steroids (>20 mg/day) can lead to serious pregnancy complications such as gestational diabetes, hypertension, and preterm birth. Statins have also been used as adjuvant therapy. IVIG, TNF-α antagonists, complement inhibitors, and B lymphocyte directed therapy has been used as adjunctive treatment in refractory OAPS cases.[64] However, the numbers treated are small and we await more robust evidence for use of these drugs during pregnancy. Many refractory OAPS cases may respond to a combination of adjuvant drugs.

REFERENCES

1. Harris EN, Charavi AE, Boey ML, Patel BM, Mackworth-Young CG, Loizou S, et al. Anticardiolipin antibodies: Detection by radioimmunoassay and association with thrombosis in systemic lupus erythematosus. Lancet. 1983;2:1211-14.
2. Hughes GR, Harris EN, Gharavi AE. The anticardiolipin syndrome. J Rheumatol. 1985;13:486-9.
3. Miyakis S, Lockshin MD, Atsumi T, Branch DW, Brey RL, Cervera R, et al. International consensus statement on an update of the classification criteria for definite antiphospholipid syndrome (APS). J Thromb Haemost. 2006;4:295-306.
4. Alijotas-Reig J, Esteve-Valverde E, Ferrer-Oliveras R, Saez-Coment L, Lefkou E, Mekinian A, et al. Comparative study of obstetric antiphospholipid syndrome (OAPS) and non-criteria obstetric APS (NC-OAPS): report of 1640 cases from the EUROAPS registry. Rheumatology. 2019;59:1306-14.
5. Truglia S, Mancuso S, Capozzi A, Recalchi S, Riitano G, Longo A, et al. "Non-criteria antiphospholipid antibodies": Bridging the gap between seropositive and seronegative Antiphospholipid Syndrome. Rheumatology. 2021;12-17.
6. Barbhaiya M, Zuily S, Naden R, Hendry A, Manneville F, Amigo MC, et al. 2023 ACR/EULAR antiphospholipid syndrome classification criteria. Ann Rheum Dis. 2023;82:1258-70.
7. Kazzaz NM, McCune WJ, Knight JS. Treatment of catastrophic antiphospholipid syndrome. Curr Opin Rheumatol. 2016;28:2018-27.
8. Ianasi Rodriguez-Pinto, Genard Espinosa, Richard Cervera. What we know and what we don't know about catastrophic antiphospholipid syndrome. Rheumatology (Oxford) 2024;63(61):S146-S153.
9. López-Benjume B, Rodríguez-Pintó I, Amigo MC, Erkan D, Shoenfeld Y, Cervera R, et al. on behalf the CAPS Registry Project Group/European Forum on Antiphospholipid Antibodies. Eculizumab use in catastrophic antiphospholipid syndrome (CAPS): Descriptive analysis from the "CAPS Registry" Autoimmun Rev. 2022;21:103055.
10. Bustamante JG, Goyal A, Rout P, Singhal M. Antiphospholipid Syndrome. Treasure Island (FL): StatPearls Publishing; 2024.

11. Grygiel-Gorniak B, Mazurkiewicz L. Positive antiphospholipid antibodies: Observation or treatment? J Thromb Thrombolysis. 2023;56(2):301-14.
12. Viall CA, Chamley LW. Histopathology in the placentae of women with antiphospholipid antibodies; A systematic review of the literature. Autoimmun Rev. 2015;14:446-71.
13. Agostinis C, Biffi S, Garrovo C, Durigutto V, Lorenzon A, Bek A, et al. In vivo distribution of β2 glycoprotein I under various pathophysiologic conditions. Blood. 2011;118: 4231-8.
14. George J, Gilburd B, Hojnik M, Levy Y, Langevitz P, Matsuura E, et al. Target recognition of beta-2-glycoprotein I (beta2GP-I) dependent anticardiolipin antibodies: evidence for involvement of the fourth domain of beta2GP-I in antibody binding. J. Immunol. 1998;160(8):3917-23.
15. Chaturvedi S, Braunstein EM, Yuan X, Yu J, Alexander A, Chen H, et al. Complement activity and complement regulatory gene mutations are associated with thrombosis in APS and CAPS. Blood. 2020;135:239-51.
16. Chaturvedi S, Braunstein EM, Brodsky RA. Antiphospholipid syndrome: Complement activation, complement gene mutations, and therapeutic implications. J Thromb Haemost. 2021;19:607-16.
17. Bettiol A, Emmi G, Finocchi M, Silvestri E, Urban ML, Mattioli I, et al. Obstetric antiphospholipid syndrome is not associated with an increased risk of subclinical atherosclerosis. Rheumatology. 2021;59:3709-16.
18. Poulton K, Ripoll VM, Pericleous C, Meroni PL, Gerosa M, Ioannou Y, et al. Purified IgG from patients with obstetric but not IgG from non-obstetric antiphospholipid syndrome inhibit trophoblast invasion. Am J Reprod Immunol. 2015;73:390-401.
19. Di Simone N, Meroni PL, De Papa N, Raschi E, Caliandro D, De Carolis CS, et al. Antiphospholipid antibodies affect trophoblast gonadotropin secretion and invasiveness by binding directly and through adhered beta2-glycoprotein I. Arthritis Rheum. 2000;43:140-50.
20. Tong M, Viall CA, Chamley LW. Antiphospholipid antibodies and the placenta: a systematic review of their in vitro effects and modulation by treatment. Hum Reprod Update. 2015;21:97-118.
21. Keeling D, Mackie I, Moore GW, Keeling D, Mackie I, Moore GW, et al. British Committee for Standards in Haematology. Guidelines on the investigation and management of anti-phospholipid syndrome. Br J Haematol. 2012;157:47-58.
22. Tang Z, Shi H, Liu HL, Cheng X, Ye J, Su Y, et al. correspondence on 2023 ACR/EULAR antiphospholipid syndrome classification criteria: Ann Rheum Dis. 2024;83:e4.
23. Tektonidou MG, Andreoli L, Limpe M, Amoura Z, Cervera R, Costedoat-Chalumeau N, et al. EULAR recommendations for the management of antiphospholipid syndrome in adults. Ann Rheum Dis. 2019;78(10):1296-304.
24. Sevin E, Zisa D, Andrade D, Sciascia S, Pengo V, Tektonidou MG, et al.; APS ACTION Investigators. Characteristics of patients with antiphospholipid antibody positivity in the APS ACTION international clinical database and repository. Arthritis Care Res. 2022;74:324-35.
25. Pengo V, Ruffatti A, Legnani C, Gresele P, Barcellona D, Erba N, et al. Clinical course of high-risk patients diagnosed with antiphospholipid syndrome. J Thromb Haemost. 2010;8:237-42.
26. Cervera R, Piette JC, Font J, Khamashta MA, Shoenfeld Y, Camps MT, et al.; Euro-Phospholipid Project Group. Antiphospholipid syndrome: clinical and immunologic manifestations and patterns of disease expression in a cohort of 1,000 patients: clinical and Immunologic Manifestations of APS. Arthritis Rheum. 2002;46:1019-27.
27. Cervera R, Serrano R, Pons-Estel GJ, Ceberio-Hualde L, Shoenfeld Y, de Ramón E, et al.; Euro-Phospholipid Project Group (European Forum on Antiphospholipid Antibodies). Morbidity and mortality in the antiphospholipid syndrome during a 10-year period: a multicentre prospective study of 1000 patients. Ann Rheum Dis. 2015;74:1011-8.
28. Sajjan VV, Lunge S, Swamy MB, Pandit AM. Livedo reticularis: a review of the literature. Indian Dermatol Online J. 2015;6:315-21.
29. Sheela HS, Lakshmidevi M. Koganti B, Venkatesh K. The study of antiphospholipid antibodies in recurrent pregnancy loss. Int J Reprod Contracept Obstet Gynecol. 2017;6(11):5135-40.
30. Alijotas-Reig J, Esteve-Valverde E, Ferrer-Oliveras R, Saez-Comet L, Lefkou E, Mekinian A, et al. The European Registry on Obstetric Antiphospholipid Syndrome (EUROAPS): A survey of 1000 consecutive cases. Autoimmun Rev. 2019;18:406-14.
31. Alijotas Reig J, Valverde E, Oliveras RF, LLurba E, Ruffatti A, Tincani A, et al. Comparative study between obstetric antiphospholipid syndrome and obstetric morbidity related with antiphospholipid antibodies. 2018;151(6):215-22.
32. Esteve-Valverde E, Ferrer-Oliveras R, Alijotas-Reig J, Sáez-Comet L, Lefkou E, Mekinian A, et al. Obstetric antiphospholipid syndrome. Rev Clin Esp. 2016;216:135-45.
33. Mak A, Cheung MW, Cheak AA, Ho RC. Combination of heparin and aspirin is superior to aspirin alone in enhancing live births in patients with recurrent pregnancy loss and positive antiphospholipid antibodies: a meta-analysis of randomized controlled trials and metaregression. Rheumatology (Oxford). 2010;49:281-8.
34. Cervera R. Antiphospholipid syndrome. Thromb Res. 2017; 151: S43-S47.
35. Uthman I, Noureldine MHA, Ruiz-Irastorza G, Khamashta M. Management of antiphospholipid syndrome. Ann Rheum Dis. 2019;78:155-61.
36. Hamulyák EN, Scheres LJJ, Marijnen MC, Goddijn M, Middeldorp S. Aspirin or heparin or both for improving pregnancy outcomes in women with persistent

antiphospholipid antibodies and recurrent pregnancy loss. Cochrane Database Syst. Rev. 2020:5;CD012852.

37. Erkan D, Harrison MJ, Levy R, Peterson M, Petri M, Sammaritano L, et al. Aspirin for primary thrombosis prevention in the antiphospholipid syndrome: a randomized, double-blind, placebo-controlled trial in asymptomatic antiphospholipid antibody-positive individuals. Arthritis Rheum. 2007;56(7):2382-91.
38. Arnaud L, Mathian A, Ruffatti A, Erkan D, Tektonidou M, Cervera R, et al. Efficacy of aspirin for the primary prevention of thrombosis in patients with antiphospholipid antibodies: an international and collaborative metaanalysis. Autoimmun Rev. 2014;13(3):281-91.
39. Arnaud L, Mathian A, Devilliers H, Ruffatti A, Tektonidou M, Forastiero R, et al. Patient-level analysis of five international cohorts further confirms the efficacy of aspirin for the primary prevention of thrombosis in patients with antiphospholipid antibodies. Autoimmun Rev. 2015;14(3):192-200.
40. Louis JM, Parchem J, Vaught A, Tesfalul M, Kendle A, Tsigas E. Preeclampsia: a report and recommendations of the workshop of the Society for Maternal-Fetal Medicine and the Preeclampsia Foundation. Am J Obstet Gynecol. 2022;227:B2-B14.
41. Ecker E, Gross P. Anticomplementary power of heparin. J Infect Dis. 1929;44:250.
42. Cowchock FS, Reece EA, Balaban D, Branch DW, Plouffe L. Repeated fetal losses associated with antiphospholipid antibodies: a collaborative randomized trial comparing prednisone with low-dose heparin treatment. Am J Obstet Gynecol. 1992;166:1318-23.
43. Sciascia S, Branch DW, Levy RA, Middeldorp S, Pavord S, Roccatello D, et al. The efficacy of hydroxychloroquine in altering pregnancy outcome in women with antiphospholipid antibodies. Evid Clin Judgm Thromb Haemost. 2016;115:285-90.
44. Gerde M, Ibarra E, Mac Kenzie R, Suarez CF, Heer C, Alvarez R, et al. The impact of hydroxychloroquine on obstetric outcomes in refractory obstetric antiphospholipid syndrome. Thromb Res. 2021;206:104-10.
45. Schreiber K, Breen K, Cohen H, Jacobsen S, Middeldorp S, Pavord S, et al. HYdroxychloroquine to Improve Pregnancy Outcome in Women with Antiphospholipid Antibodies (HYPATIA) Protocol: A Multinational Randomized Controlled Trial of Hydroxychloroquine versus Placebo in Addition to Standard Treatment in Pregnant Women with Antiphospholipid Syndrome. Semin Thromb Hemost. 2017;43:562-71.
46. Belizna C, Pregnolato F, Abad S, Alijotas-Reig J, Amital H, Amoura Z, et al. HIBISCUS: Hydroxychloroquine for the secondary prevention of thrombotic and obstetrical events in primary antiphospholipid syndrome. Autoimmun Rev. 2018;17:1153-68.
47. Mekinian A, Vicaut E, Cohen J, Borne M, Kayem G, Fain O. Hydroxychloroquine to obtain pregnancy without adverse obstetrical events in primary antiphospholipid syndrome: French phase II multicenter randomized trial, HYDROSAPL. Gynecol Obstet Ferti Senol. 2018;46:598-604.
48. Pasquier E, De Saint-Martin L, Marhic G, Chauleur C, Bohec C, Bretelle F, et al. Hydroxychloroquine for Prevention of Recurrent Miscarriage: Study Protocol for a Multicentre Randomised Placebo-Controlled Trial BBQ Study. BMJ. 2019;9(3):e025649.
49. Bramham K, Thomas M, Nelson-Piercy C, Khamashta M, Hunt BJ. First-trimester low-dose prednisolone in refractory antiphospholipid antibody-related pregnancy loss. Blood. 2011;117:6948-51.
50. Palmsten K, Rolland M, Hebert MF, Clowse MEB, Schatz M, Xu R, et al. Patterns of prednisone use during pregnancy in women with rheumatoid arthritis: Daily and cumulative dose. Pharmaco-epidemiol. Drug Saf. 2018;27:430-8.
51. Marzusch K, Dietl J, Klein R, Hornung D, Neuer A, Berg PA. Recurrent first trimester spontaneous abortion associated with antiphospholipid antibodies: a pilot study of treatment with intravenous immunoglobulin. Acta Obstet Gynecol Scand. 1996;75(10):922-6.
52. Vaquero E, Lazzarin N, Valensise H, Menghini S, Di Pierro G, Cesa F, Romanini C. Pregnancy outcome in recurrent spontaneous abortion associated with antiphospholipid antibodies: a comparative study of intravenous immunoglobulin versus prednisone plus low-dose aspirin. Am J Reprod Immunol. 2001;45(3):174-9.
53. Urban ML, Bettiol A, Serena C, Comito C, Turrini I, Fruttuoso S, et al. Intravenous immunoglobulin for the secondary prevention of stillbirth in obstetric antiphospholipid syndrome: A case series and systematic review of literature. Autoimmun Rev. 2020;19(9):102620.
54. Kaneko K, Tsutsumi S, Fujita D, Sugiura-Ogasawara M, Mitsuda N, Matsubara K, et al. Intravenous immunoglobulin treatment for obstetric antiphospholipid syndrome refractory to conventional therapy: A single-arm, open-labelled multi-center clinical trial. Mod Rheumatol. 2024;34(3):515-22.
55. Lopez-Pedrera C, Roiz-Limon P, Aguirre MA, Barbarroja N, Pérez-Sánchez C, Buendía P, et al. Global effects of Fluvastatin on the prothrombotic status of patients with antiphospholipid syndrome. Ann Rheum Dis. 2011;70:675-82.
56. Erkan D, Willis R, Murthy VL, Basra G, Vega J, Ruiz-Limón P, et al. A prospective open label pilot study of Fluvastatin on proinflammatory and prothrombotic biomarkers in antiphospholipid antibody positive patients. Ann Rheum Dis. 2014;73:1176-80.
57. Chang J-C, Chen Y-J, Chen I-C, Lin WS, Chen YM, Lin CH. Perinatal outcomes after statin exposure during pregnancy. JAMA Network Open. 2021;4(12):e2141321.

58. Brogin Moreli J, Cirino Ruocco AM, Vernini JM, Rudge MV, Calderon IM. Interleukin 10 and tumor necrosis factor-alpha in pregnancy: aspects of interest in clinical obstetrics. ISRN Obstet Gynecol. 2012;2012:230742.
59. Alijotas-Reig J, Esteve-Valverde E, Llurba E, Gris JM. Treatment of refractory poor aPL-related obstetric outcomes with TNF-alpha blockers: Maternal-fetal outcomes in a series of 18 cases. Semin Arthritis Rheum. 2019;49(2):314-8.
60. IMPACT Study: IMProve Pregnancy in APS With Certolizumab Therapy. *This is an ongoing clinical trial which aims to evaluate the effect of certolizumab in addition to standard of care therapy (heparin and LDA) in pregnant individuals with APS and persistently positive LA. [online] Available from https://ClinicalTrials.gov/show/NCT03152058 [Last accessed December, 2024].
61. Gustavsen A, Skattum L, Bergseth G, Lorentzen B, Floisand Y, Bosnes V, et al. Effect on mother and child of eculizumab given before caesarean section in a patient with severe antiphospholipid syndrome: a case report. Medicine (Baltimore). 2017;96:e6338.
62. Erkan D, Vega J, Ramón G, Kozora E, Lockshin MD. A pilot open label phase II trial of rituximab for non-criteria manifestations of antiphospholipid syndrome. RITAPS study. Arthritis Rheum. 2013;65:464-71.
63. Emmi G, Urban ML, Scalera A, Becatti M, Fiorillo C, Silvestri E, et al. Repeated low-dose courses of rituximab in SLE-associated antiphospholipid syndrome: data from a tertiary dedicated centre. Semin Arthritis Rheum. 2017;46:e21-3.
64. Rodziewicz M, D'Cruz DP. An update on the management of antiphospholipid syndrome. Ther Adv Musculoskelet Dis. 2020;12:1759720X20910855.

CHAPTER

27

Autoimmune Diseases

Sundari N, Chandrashekara S

ABSTRACT

Maternal autoimmune diseases are associated with adverse pregnancy outcomes, including recurrent pregnancy loss (RPL). Although autoimmune diseases have a wide spectrum including thyroiditis, arthritis, systemic lupus, and others, the underlying pathological processes remain common, while the target organ differs. The mechanism of pregnancy loss is diruption of pregnancy immune tolerance, thereby, disrupting the placentation process.

Keywords: Autoimmune disease, Arthritis, Autoimmunity, Systemic lupus erythematosus, Thyroiditis, Thrombocytopenia.

INTRODUCTION

Autoimmune disease (AID) is a spectrum of disorders where the immune system initiates an attack on self-antigens, resulting in persistent inflammation leading to either tissue dysfunction or damage. It can target either a single organ or affect more than one organ. Based on the organ involved, it is classified as either organ-specific or systemic AID. Autoantibodies causing AIDs can be produced against a single cell type (such as red blood cells in autoimmune hemolytic anemia), single organ (as in autoimmune thyroiditis), or against multiple systems causing multi-organ dysfunction [as in systemic lupus erythematosus (SLE)]. It affects approximately 13% of the population at any point of time, and the prevalence is even higher if minor autoimmune disorders are considered.

Markers of autoimmunity may appear without causing the disease. Sometimes, in a significant proportion of individuals, it may not develop into a full-fledged disease in the initial stages. AID could be mediated by autoantibodies or self-reacting T cells, or both. These diseases are more predominant in women, especially in the reproductive age-group, and the risk gradually increases with age. The exact reason for this association has yet to be ascertained. The adaptability of the immune system to reproductive cycles and hormones is often considered responsible for such predilections.[1,2]

Autoimmunity can affect reproduction in various ways, and the interaction between AIDs can be bidirectional.[3] Pregnancy may trigger AIDs or exacerbate existing autoimmune problems. AIDs can directly damage reproductive structures, including the ovaries and endometrium, and disrupt various stages of implantation and fetal growth. Persisting inflammation in other organs may adversely impact the reproductive cycle, and excessive inflammation can interfere with several steps of embryonic growth. Autoantibodies may cross-react with several proteins in the placenta, triggering placental inflammation, thrombosis, and interference in fetal development.

Considering the bidirectional association, the management strategies can be approached from two different perspectives. First, by examining pregnancy in women already diagnosed with AID, and second, by exploring autoimmune factors that affect pregnancy in women not diagnosed with AIDs but who experience interference during the implantation phase. The initial part of the chapter focuses on pregnancies in women with preexisting autoimmune conditions, while the latter deals with autoimmune features in individuals who were not previously diagnosed with AID but encounter challenges during pregnancy.

PREGNANCY OUTCOME IN WOMEN DIAGNOSED WITH AUTOIMMUNE DISEASE

The course of pregnancy and fertility in a woman with preexisting AID is variable and depends on the type of disease, its status, associated autoantibodies, and the medications used prior to planning pregnancy. Diseases such as rheumatoid arthritis (RA) may remit during pregnancy while conditions such as SLE may exacerbate.

The impact of AID on pregnancy and its outcome can occur through three different mechanisms as briefed below:[1]

1. The damage caused by the disease, reduced libido, and altered sexual function may decrease fertility.
2. Active inflammation has an impact on systemic homeostasis, leading to altered hormone cycles, impairment in implantation, and sometimes abortion.
3. Autoantibodies and self-reactive cells may cross-react with antigens on the placental surface, traverse the placental barrier, and adversely affect the fetus, leading to recurrent pregnancy loss (RPL), fetal growth restriction (FGR), fetal demise, or neonatal disease.

The bidirectional effects of commonly encountered AID on pregnancy are listed in **Table 1**.

BASIC PRINCIPLES OF MANAGING PREGNANCY IN WOMEN WITH AUTOIMMUNE DISEASE

Ideally, the disease should be in remission or should exhibit the lowest possible activity to proceed with conception. However, in clinical conditions such as autoimmune thyroid disease, according to recommendations it is crucial to maintain thyroid function at optimal levels before conception. Any potentially teratogenic drugs should be discontinued, and their introduction during

TABLE 1: The effects of common AIDs on pregnancy and vice versa.

AID	*Impact on pregnancy*	*Impact on disease*
RA Psoriatic arthritis	Minimal	Conditions may improve or remain stable
Inflammatory bowel disease[4]	Increased premature delivery, FGR, LBW, and C-section	Minimal change
SLE	Increased fetal loss, PIH, LBW, FGR, and other fetal complications	Disease may adversely impact pregnancy
Scleroderma	Infertility, increased fetal loss, preeclampsia, PIH, LBW, and other fetal complications	Disease activity may either reduce or increase. Pulmonary may worsen pulmonary hypertension
Multiple sclerosis[5]	No impact on pregnancy, except drug effects	Disease may flare during postpartum period and during pregnancy
Small vessel vasculitis (GPA, MPA, and EGPA)[6]	Preterm delivery, preeclampsia, bleeding diathesis, spontaneous abortion, FGR, respiratory complications, decreased renal function	Vasculitis may worsen
Medium vessel PAN[6]	Hypertension, proteinuria, preterm birth, and intrauterine FGR	Vasculitis may worsen
Large vessel (Takayasu arteritis)[6]	Preeclampsia, LBW, and FGR	Central occult hypertension, cardiac failure, renal insufficiency or failure
Behçet's disease[6]	Preterm delivery and spontaneous abortion	Worsens oral ulceration, eye inflammation, or arthralgia
Idiopathic (immune) thrombocytopenia[7]	Bleeding into uterine cavity (peri- and postpartum bleeding), fetal thrombocytopenia is rare (5%). Does not cause RPL or other pregnancy complications	Thrombocytopenia may worsen in majority
Type 1 diabetes mellitus[5]	Preterm delivery, large birthweight babies, congenital anomalies, stillbirth, hypoglycemia in infants, neonatal death	Worsening of glycemic control
Autoimmune thyroid disease	Infertility, impaired implantation, abortion, and FGR	Needs dose escalation based on thyroid demand

(AID: autoimmune disease; EGPA: eosinophilic granulomatosis with polyangiitis; FGR: fetal growth restriction; GPA: granulomatosis with polyangiitis; LBW: low birthweight; MPA: microscopic polyangiitis; PAN: polyarteritis nodosa; PIH: pregnancy-induced hypertension; RA: rheumatoid arthritis; RPL: recurrent pregnancy loss; SLE: systemic lupus erythematosus)

pregnancy should be minimized. The patient's disease status, as well as its impact, should be such that the individual can tolerate the physiological stress associated with pregnancy. Evaluation of these patients should be a collaborative effort, coordinated with the respective specialists.

Systemic Lupus Erythematosus

Systemic lupus erythematosus is a chronic AID with multisystem involvement, predominantly impacting women of childbearing age. Despite its presence, fertility is generally unaffected; however, certain treatments, such as cyclophosphamide, may reduce ovarian reserve. In women with SLE, approximately 15–34% exhibit lupus anticoagulant antibodies, and these autoantibodies can contribute to RPL.

Preconceptional Evaluation

Preconceptional evaluation is crucial, especially for women with SLE, where avoiding unplanned pregnancies is preferable. Prepregnancy counseling and evaluation play a pivotal role in ensuring successful outcomes in terms of maternal safety and pregnancy outcome. The comprehensive assessment of SLE disease activity requires detailed clinical and laboratory evaluations of organ involvement, associated damages, and comorbidities. Immunologists and obstetricians should collaborate to outline a prospective monitoring plan, specifying the timing and mode of delivery, and the probable complications during and after pregnancy, as well as those affecting the newborn.

Laboratory Evaluation

The following comprehensive set of laboratory assessments aids in a thorough evaluation of the patient's condition:

- Antiphospholipid antibody (APLA) workup, including lupus anticoagulant (seen in 15–20% of SLE), even in the absence of prior presentations
- Anti-double-stranded deoxyribonucleic acid (DNA) antibodies (dsDNA), anti-Ro/SSA, and anti-La/SSB antibodies
- Complement levels namely CH 50, C3, and C4
- Liver function tests (LFT), renal function tests (RFT), complete blood count (CBC), urine protein and protein-creatinine ratio, uric acid levels, and coagulation profile

Preconceptional Planning

The ideal time to plan pregnancy in a woman with preexisting SLE is when the disease has been in remission for at least 6 months. A quiescent phase of SLE during the periconceptional period significantly reduces adverse maternal and pregnancy outcomes, increasing the likelihood of a live birth. A multidisciplinary approach can enhance the success rate of pregnancy outcomes in such patients.

If a woman is planning for conception and is on teratogenic drugs, it is advisable to discontinue or replace them with safer alternatives. Hydroxychloroquine (HCQ 400 mg/day), ecosprin, glucocorticoids (if required), and azathioprine are considered compatible with pregnancy. The use of cyclosporine should be considered if the benefits outweigh the risks. Tacrolimus is employed if the patient has nephritis.

In cases of preexisting hypertensive disease or hypertension developed during pregnancy, antihypertensive drugs, such as methyldopa, labetalol, and hydralazine, can be used safely. The choice of medication should be made with careful consideration of the individual's health and the potential impact on pregnancy.

Contraindications for Conception in Systemic Lupus Erythematosus Patients

Pregnancy is relatively contraindicated in subjects with conditions that increase both maternal and fetal morbidity. Conception should be deferred in women with a history of a severe lupus flare or stroke in the past 6 months, or if they have uncontrolled hypertension, cardiac failure, pulmonary hypertension, or severe valvulopathy. Conception is absolutely contraindicated in cases of active lupus nephritis and chronic renal disease, as these conditions worsen the disease and increase both maternal and fetal morbidity. Primigravidae are at a higher risk for maternal and fetal complications.

Predictors of Adverse Pregnancy Outcome

The risk assessment score, proposed by the Egyptian Rheumatology and Rehabilitation in 2022, takes into account factors such as active disease at the time of conception, the presence of antiphospholipid syndrome (APS), hypocomplementemia (C3), active lupus nephritis, and the absence of remission in the previous 6 months.[8]

If the risk score is >2 out of 5, it indicates an adverse pregnancy outcome.

COMPLICATIONS

Maternal Complications

Women with SLE experience a two- to fourfold increase in maternal complications. Preeclampsia is more common in women with SLE (16–30%) and starting aspirin therapy at 12–16 weeks of pregnancy reduces the incidence to 2–5%.[9] Other potential complications include an increased incidence of thrombosis, preterm labor, cesarean sections, infections, thrombocytopenia, development of lupus nephritis, renal failure, and cerebrovascular disorders. The maternal mortality rate is higher in patients with lupus during pregnancy.[10]

Fetal and Neonatal Complications

The incidence of both early and late pregnancy loss is higher in women with SLE, particularly when the disease is active. Approximately 10–30% of pregnancies in women with SLE experience FGR and have babies classified as small for gestational age. Neonatal lupus is reported in 3.5% of cases and manifests as congenital heart block (CHB) or rash, especially in children born to women who are positive for anti-Ro/SSA and La/SSB antibodies.

DIAGNOSIS AND MANAGEMENT OF LUPUS FLARE

Lupus flares can occur during pregnancy or the postpartum period and are classified as mild, moderate, or severe based on the severity of symptoms and organ involvement. Causes of postpartum flares include changes in hormonal milieu (estrogen and progestogens), increased prolactin levels, decreased levels of anti-inflammatory steroids, and alterations in the neuroendocrine axis. Flares are more common in primigravida, in women with nephritis, and in those who are not compliant with HCQ therapy.

General symptoms noted in patients with lupus flare include fever, rash, fatigue, and arthralgia. Further evaluation of different system involvement, such as renal, cardiac, and respiratory systems, will aid in the diagnosis and risk categorization of the woman into high, low, or intermediate risk. Investigations that assist in diagnosing the condition include rising titers of dsDNA antibody, low levels of complement C3, C4, and CH 50, and proteinuria with the presence of urinary casts.

Multidisciplinary approach involving an immunologist, nephrologist, and neonatologist is necessary for managing pregnant patients with flare. Drugs commonly used include HCQ, oral glucocorticoids, azathioprine, cyclosporine, and tacrolimus. Severe flare may require intravenous (IV) glucocorticoid pulse therapy, IV immunoglobulin (IVIG), and plasmapheresis. Inpatient treatment is essential for women experiencing a severe flare. Periodic evaluation of expectant mothers with an immunologist is paramount, along with clinical and laboratory evaluation in each trimester of pregnancy.

It is important to counsel women experiencing a lupus flare regarding the course of pregnancy, the need for frequent visits and investigations, and possible complications, as well as the importance of strict adherence to medication.

Pharmacotherapy

The American College of Rheumatology (ACR) recommends HCQ for all pregnant women who are not on therapy. If they are receiving HCQ, the ACR suggests continuing the treatment throughout pregnancy and low-dose aspirin starting from the first trimester. HCQ therapy is known to reduce the risk of congenital heart disease in the fetus and minimizes the chance of maternal flare-ups. For women with fetal echocardiography (ECHO) showing first or second-degree heart block, the ACR suggests oral dexamethasone at a dose of 4 mg daily. Furthermore, if a woman develops APS, the ACR advises initiating low molecular weight heparin.

Fetal Surveillance

An early scan should be done at 11–14 weeks for gestational age, including Down's scoring and uterine artery Doppler for the prediction of preeclampsia and FGR. The anomaly scan is recommended at 18–20 weeks, followed by growth scans every 3–4 weeks for the early detection of FGR. Fetal Doppler studies of the umbilical and middle cerebral artery from 24 weeks onwards will help optimize the time of delivery.

The presence of anti-SSA/Ro52 antibodies is strongly associated with fetal cardiac problems such as CHB, dilated cardiomyopathy, and endocardial fibroelastosis. Pregnant women who test positive for anti-Ro/SSA and/or anti-La/SSB antibodies should undergo fetal ECHO starting from 16 to 18 weeks through 26 weeks. Women with a history of a previous child diagnosed with CHB or neonatal lupus erythematosus need to have weekly fetal ECHO.[11]

Time of Delivery and Breastfeeding

The time of delivery depends on maternal and fetal conditions. If there are no further complications during pregnancy, the patient can deliver at 37–38 weeks of gestation. Patients can breastfeed the neonate if she is not receiving drugs such as azathioprine, methotrexate, cyclophosphamide, or mycophenolate.

RHEUMATOID ARTHRITIS AND PREGNANCY

Rheumatoid arthritis is more common in women of reproductive age than in men, and pregnancy has a favorable effect on the disease. The course of the disease changes during pregnancy; 50% will experience low-disease activity, 40% achieve remission, and 20% may have moderate-to-high disease activity requiring therapeutic interventions. Women who experience remission during pregnancy are more prone to postpartum flares.

Rheumatoid arthritis itself has no adverse effects on pregnancy, but disease-modifying antirheumatic drugs (DMARDs), especially methotrexate, may have lethal effects on the fetus, so medication should be stopped 3 months before conception. Patients should not conceive during therapy with DMARDs (methotrexate, leflunomide, and cyclophosphamide), and these drugs need to be stopped before conception. It is ideal for RA-positive women to have prepregnancy counseling with a rheumatologist and obstetrician, and pregnancy should be planned for 3–6 months after controlling RA. Prescriptions may need to be changed according to individual needs. Women with uncontrolled RA may face pregnancy complications such as preterm labor and FGR.

Management of Pregnancy

Rheumatoid arthritis is not a contraindication for pregnancy, and planned pregnancy after multidisciplinary counseling, selection of the time of conception, and appropriate drug alterations will result in a good pregnancy outcome.

Glucocorticoids and HCQ can be safely used during pregnancy. A slight increase in the risk of developing gestational hypertension, FGR, and preterm labor has been reported. Routine antenatal management, fetal surveillance with ultrasound, and Doppler are recommended in uncomplicated patients. The time of delivery depends on maternal and fetal conditions; vaginal delivery is not contraindicated unless the patient has pelvic girdle and spine problems. Breastfeeding is not contraindicated but may require support to handle the neonates.

AUTOIMMUNE THROMBOCYTOPENIA AND PREGNANCY

Immune thrombocytopenia (ITP) during pregnancy is an infrequent condition, with an incidence ranging from 1 to 3 in 10,000 pregnancies and 6.4 per 100,000 in children in India.[12] ITP may manifest in any trimester, with diagnosis occurring either before or during pregnancy. This autoimmune disorder involves the production of antiplatelet antibodies, which lead to platelet phagocytosis in the spleen, resulting in thrombocytopenia. Additionally, it affects platelet production in the bone marrow, leading to severe thrombocytopenia. These antibodies have the ability to cross the placenta and cause neonatal immune thrombocytopenia (NITP).

Immune thrombocytopenia is not a contraindication for pregnancy, nor associated with RPL. Furthermore, pregnancy itself does not have adverse effects on the course of ITP. However, complications may arise if the platelet count is low during pregnancy. Notably, NITP is a potential concern, with the risk of inducing fetal intracranial hemorrhage. Consequently, meticulous monitoring of the fetus is imperative to facilitate early detection and appropriate intervention.

Manamement during Pregnancy

If the platelet count is maintained at >100,000/μL, no special intervention is needed, except frequent evaluation of platelet count during pregnancy. Platelet transfusion is not required until platelet count decline <20,000/μL with spontaneous bleeding episodes, or <50,000/μL if surgery or delivery is contemplated. Administration of glucocorticoids is recommended when therapeutic intervention is warranted; prednisolone at a dosage of 1–2 mg/kg/day or betamethasone at 40 mg daily for a duration of 2 weeks is efficacious in improving the platelet count. IVIG (0.4 mg/kg/day for 3–4 days) is recommended for women who do not respond to steroids. IV anti-D immunoglobulin has yielded encouraging results in certain cases. Rituximab is not recommended during pregnancy due to its transfer across the placenta.

Neonatal Management

A newborn with neonatal alloimmune thrombocytopenia (NAIT) requires treatment to prevent intracranial and visceral hemorrhage. Matched platelet transfusion should be administered to neonates with a platelet count <10,000/μL. Additionally, IVIG at a dosage of 1 g/kg/day is effective in increasing platelet counts in neonates.

AUTOIMMUNE THYROID DISEASE

During pregnancy, the thyroid gland undergoes both anatomical and physiological changes, including an increase in volume and hormone production. Interpretation of thyroid function test results should align with pregnancy-specific values. Thyroid disorders, particularly autoimmune dysfunction, are common, affecting 10–15% of women of reproductive age and 5–20% of pregnant women. Autoimmune thyroid disorders can lead to conditions such as hyperthyroidism (Graves' disease) or hypothyroidism (Hashimoto's disease) during pregnancy. Postpartum thyroiditis, another autoimmune disorder, manifests after delivery, presenting as transient hyperthyroidism followed by hypothyroidism. Symptoms of autoimmune thyroid disease may improve during pregnancy but can worsen during postpartum period.

Work-up for Autoimmune Thyroid Disease

The diagnosis of autoimmune thyroiditis involves detecting various thyroid autoantibodies such as antithyroglobulin (TGab), antithyroid peroxidase (TPOab), and anti-TSH (thyroid stimulating hormone)-receptor autoantibodies. In pregnancy, the presence of TPOab is more common than other thyroid antibodies. First-trimester TSH testing is a standard practice, but routine thyroid autoantibody testing in unselected pregnant women is not recommended. Thyroid autoantibody testing is recommended for women with RPL or known thyroid disorders. In cases of positive TPOab and abnormal TSH values, further assessment, including T4 estimation, is advised. The presence of thyroid autoantibodies can diagnose autoimmune thyroiditis and may indicate coexistence with other AIDs.[13,14]

Pathogenesis of Rapid Pregnancy Loss

The presence of thyroid autoimmunity (TAI) can increase the risk of pregnancy wastage, leading to elevated rates of miscarriage or implantation failure. The exact mechanism by which the presence of TAI causes RPL is not clear. However, the potential mechanisms involved are classified into thyroid-dependent and thyroid-independent categories. The thyroid-dependent mechanism includes the presence of TAI causing a deficiency of thyroid hormones. The thyroid-independent mechanism acts through altered humoral and innate immunity, cross-reactivity of TAI with extra-thyroid sites, and association with other AIDs. TAI induces a pro-inflammatory T1 immune response characterized by an increased production of interleukin (IL) 2 and 7 as well as interferon gamma (INF-γ), which contributes to RPL. The presence of TAI also indicates the possible existence of other autoantibodies, such as antinuclear antibodies (ANA), or organ-specific and systemic AIDs.[14]

Management of Pregnancy in a Woman with Positive Autoantibodies with Normal Thyroid Function

Positive TAI indicates reduced thyroid reserve, causing mild thyroid hormone deficiency in pregnant women and diminishing the thyroid gland's capacity to meet pregnancy demands. For women with positive TAI and a normal TSH <2 U/mL, thyroid supplementation is unnecessary, but regular thyroid function tests are recommended in each trimester. In cases where TSH values range from 2 to 4 U/mL in early gestation with positive TAI, thyroid supplementation is advised. While screening for autoantibodies and AIDs lacks conclusive recommendations, a cross-specialist consultation is preferable if clinical symptoms are present.

Evaluation of Autoimmune Disease in Patients with Pregnancy Loss and No Clinical Features of Autoimmune Disease

Screening for autoantibodies and AIDs in a woman with a history of adverse obstetric events is inconclusive, irrespective of the available recommendations. The patient should be assessed for possible clinical symptoms and signs. If present, it is preferable to have cross-consultation with the respective specialists for a thorough evaluation and management, as per the guidelines. However, conducting ANA and antithyroid antibodies in patients without symptoms is a matter of debate.

Numerous studies have demonstrated an elevated risk of pregnancy loss in individuals with positive ANA. A major concern arises from the fact that approximately 5% of women in the reproductive age-group in the general population exhibit ANA positivity. This increases the likelihood of overtreating, otherwise normal cases with immunomodulators, including steroids, where ANA may not be the cause for pregnancy loss. Hence despite the recommendations, routine ANA testing is not conducted in women with RPL.[15] However, in situations lacking alternative explanations or in patients presenting with symptoms such as arthralgia, ANA testing may prove beneficial in identifying individuals likely to have autoimmune-related pregnancy loss.[16]

Similar controversies persist regarding thyroid autoantibodies. The European Thyroid Society recommends testing for anti-TPO and TG in the event of marginal abnormal thyroid function, even in the absence of overt dysfunction (European Thyroid Association recommendation). Literature studies support the association between positive anti-TPO and TG and an increased risk of RPL, independent of thyroid dysfunction. The role of thyroid supplementation in positive anti-TPO and TG, and the use of HCQ in management, remains uncertain.[17]

CONCLUSION

Autoimmune diseases and autoimmunity exert a bidirectional influence on pregnancy, necessitating a thorough evaluation before conception. The impact varies based on the specific autoimmune condition, with potential risks such as preterm birth and preeclampsia. A comprehensive, multispecialty approach involving rheumatologists, obstetricians, and other specialists is essential to optimize outcomes for both pregnancy and mother's health. Collaborative care ensures informed decisions about family planning, considering the disease severity, medication adjustments, and potential fluctuations in symptoms during pregnancy. Ongoing communication and coordination among healthcare professionals throughout pregnancy are crucial for monitoring and customizing treatment plans for improved outcomes.

REFERENCES

1. Merz WM, Fischer-Betz R, Hellwig K, Lamprecht G, Gembruch U. Pregnancy and autoimmune disease. Dtsch Arztebl Int. 2022;119(9):145-56.
2. Adams Waldorf KM, Nelson JL. Autoimmune disease during pregnancy and the microchimerism legacy of pregnancy. Immunol Invest. 2008;37(5):631-44.
3. Piccinni MP, Lombardelli L, Logiodice F, Kullolli O, Parronchi P, Romagnani S. How pregnancy can affect autoimmune diseases progression? Clin Mol Allergy. 2016;14:11.
4. Cornish J, Tan E, Teare J, Teoh TG, Rai R, Clark SK, et al. A meta-analysis on the influence of inflammatory bowel disease on pregnancy. Gut. 2007;56(6):830-7.
5. Vukusic S, Marignier R. Multiple sclerosis and pregnancy in the 'treatment era'. Nat Rev Neurol. 2015;11(5):280-9.
6. Murphy HR, Howgate C, O'Keefe J, Myers J, Morgan M, Coleman MA, et al. Characteristics and outcomes of pregnant women with type 1 or type 2 diabetes: a 5-year national population-based cohort study. Lancet Diabetes Endocrinol. 2021;9(3):153-64.
7. Poston JN, Gernsheimer TB. Management of immune thrombocytopenia in pregnancy. [online] Available from https://aob amegroups.org/article/view/6305/html [Last accessed December, 2024].
8. Makarm WK, Zaghlol RS, Kotb LI. Risk assessment score for adverse pregnancy outcome in systemic lupus erythematosus patients. Egyptian Rheumatol Rehab. 2022;49(1):33.
9. Schramm AM, Clowse ME. Aspirin for prevention of preeclampsia in lupus pregnancy. Autoimmune Dis. 2014;2014:920467.
10. Mehta B, Jannat-Khah D, Glaser KK, Luo Y, Sammaritanom LR, Branch DW, et al. Fetal and maternal morbidity in pregnant patients with lupus: a 10-year US nationwide analysis. RMD Open. 2023;9(1):e002752.
11. Sheng X, Song X, Xiong Y, Ren T, Chang X, Wu J, et al. Maternal and infant outcomes of pregnancy associated with anti-SSA/RO antibodies: a systematic review and meta-analysis. Pediatr Rheumatol Online J. 2023;21(1):22.
12. Anoop P. Immune thrombocytopenic purpura: historical perspective, current status, recent advances and future directions. Indian Pediatr. 2012;49(10):811-8.
13. Carp H. (Ed). Recurrent Pregnancy Loss: Causes, Controversies and Treatment, 3rd edition. Boca Raton: CRC Press; 2020.
14. ESHRE Guideline Group on RPL, Bender Atik R, Christiansen OB, Elson J, Marie Kolte A, Lewis S, et al. ESHRE guideline: recurrent pregnancy loss. Hum Reprod Open. 2018;2018(2):hoy004.
15. Papas RS, Kutteh WH. A new algorithm for the evaluation of recurrent pregnancy loss redefining unexplained miscarriage: review of current guidelines. Curr Opin Obstet Gynecol. 2020;32(5):371-9.
16. Ticconi C, Inversetti A, Logruosso E, Ghio M, Casadei L, Selmi C, et al. Antinuclear antibodies positivity in women in reproductive age: from infertility to adverse obstetrical outcomes – a meta-analysis. J Reprod Immunol. 2023;155:103794.
17. Xie J, Jiang L, Sadhukhan A, Yang S, Yao Q, Zhou P, et al. Effect of antithyroid antibodies on women with recurrent miscarriage: a meta-analysis. Am J Reprod Immunol. 2020;83(6):e13238.

CHAPTER 28

Inherited Thrombophilia

Asher Bashiri, Nave Kahana, Yona Grossman

ABSTRACT

Inherited thrombophilia is associated with late pregnancy losses. Its association with early miscarriages is controversial. In this chapter the evidence for association of each thrombophilia i.e. prothrombin gene mutation, factor V Leiden, antithrombin III, MTHFR gene mutation, protein C and protein S deficiency with recurrent pregnancy loss (RPL) has been analyzed. Some thrombophilias like factor II, factor V Leiden, MTHFR gene mutation, and protein C and S deficiency are more strongly associated with RPL than others. However, more evidence is required for their association with RPL.

Keywords: Inherited thrombophilia, Factor V Leiden, Prothrombin gene mutation, MTHFR C677T gene mutation, Antithrombin III deficiency, Protein C and Protein S deficiency.

INTRODUCTION

Hemostasis

Hemostasis is the delicate balance between vascular damage and repair. It is a tightly regulated process with the goal of limiting extensive bleeding.[1] Hemostasis comprises both primary and secondary processes that form and stabilize a blood clot.[2] Primary hemostasis occurs within minutes of vascular damage and involves platelet adhesion to a damaged endothelial wall and subsequent aggregation of the platelets to create a weak platelet plug (the primary hemostatic plug).[2] Secondary hemostasis follows to strengthen and consolidate the platelet plug via the deposition and crosslinking of fibrin.[2] Activation of fibrin requires a series of mediators known as clotting factors, which activate and amplify one another in a sequence of enzymatic conversions entitled the coagulation cascade **(Flowchart 1)**. Once the risk of hemorrhage subsides, counterregulatory mediators such as tissue plasminogen activator (tPA) are initiated to resorb the clot and repair the tissue.[2] Pro- and antithrombotic agents must be tightly regulated, as too much of either type upsets the body's balance, resulting in pathologies: excess anticoagulation leads to bleeding, whereas an overabundance of procoagulants yields thrombosis.

Thrombosis

Thrombosis is the pathological formation of blood clots.[2] Dysregulated clots have the potential to cause deep vein thrombosis (DVT) and pulmonary embolism (PE), together termed venous thromboembolism (VTE), as well as cerebral vascular attacks (CVAs).[3] Virchow's triad characterizes the three interconnected causes of thrombosis: (1) irregular blood flow (turbulent flow or stasis), (2) endothelial damage, and (3) hypercoagulable states.[2] Arterial thrombosis is commonly caused by endothelial damage due to increased shear forces, whereas venous thrombosis primarily ensues due to turbulent flow or stasis.[2,4] While the initial trigger of thrombosis may differ among arteries and veins, endothelial damage and turbulent flow augment one another, as endothelial damage can stimulate irregular flow of blood and turbulent flow can itself damage the endothelium.[2] The etiologies of VTE are thus multifactorial and include hypercoagulable states that are caused by irregularities, dysfunction, and/or mutations in one or more hemostatic mediators.[3] The various etiologies of hypercoagulable states are collectively known as thrombophilia, and they may be inherited or acquired. VTE poses a high risk to both morbidity and mortality, with a 10% mortality rate within 1 year of a VTE. Furthermore, postthrombotic syndrome (PTS) has been noted in up to 50% of patients and the associated pain, ulcers, and edema significantly diminish quality of life.[5] Therefore, patients with an increased risk of VTE or those who have suffered a prior event are often treated with anticoagulation therapy.[3]

Flowchart 1: Coagulation cascade with mechanism of action of the five primary hereditary thrombophilia.

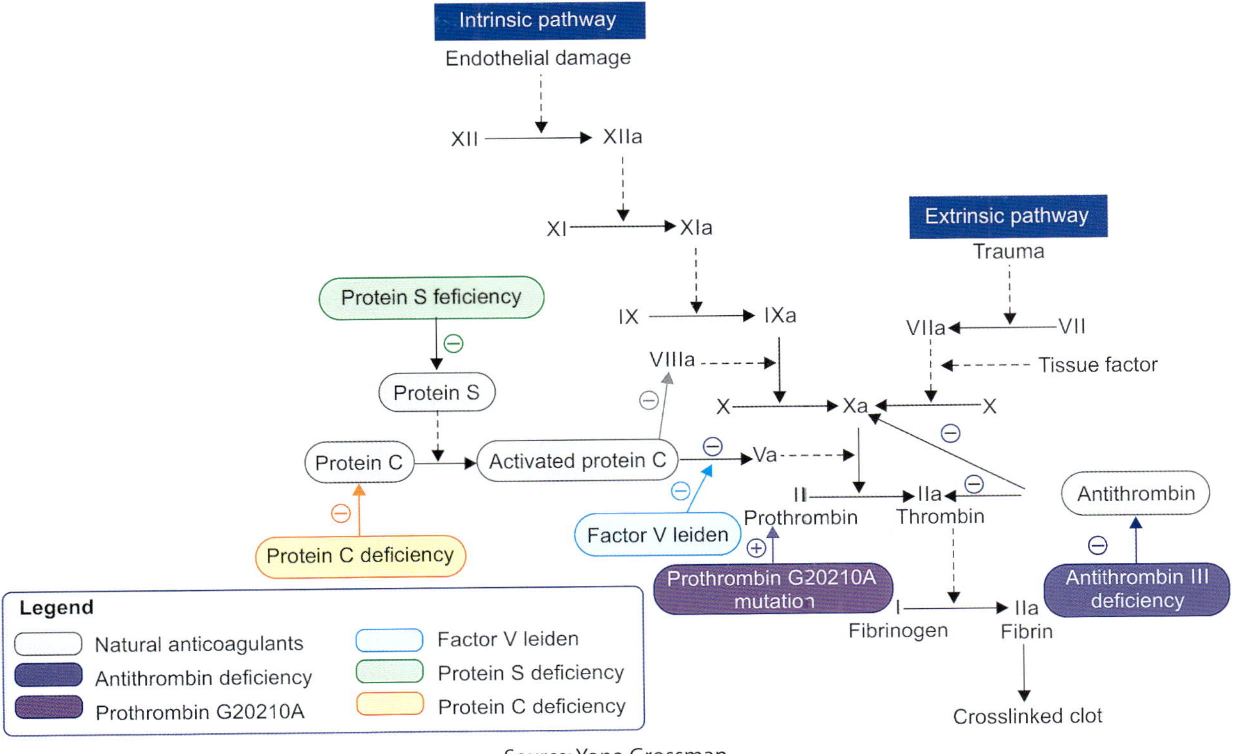

Source: Yona Grossman.

THROMBOPHILIA

Inherited Thrombophilia

Inherited thrombophilia is defined as a genetic predisposition for VTE that has an early onset (before the age of 40 years) and often recurs.[6,7] Familial clusters of VTE were first described in the early 20th century;[8,9] however, the first inherited thrombophilia, antithrombin (AT) deficiency, was only discovered in 1965.[10] This discovery provided sufficient evidence that single gene mutations may be correlated with thrombosis.[8] In the following decades an explosion of research ensued regarding various genes implicated in the coagulation system. By the 1990s, the five primary inherited thrombophilia had been elucidated, and there was significant evidence that these genetic mutations pose a significant increased relative risk (RR) of VTE.[7] Primary hereditary thrombophilia is comprised of the following diseases: factor V Leiden (FVL), prothrombin gene mutations, AT deficiency, protein C deficiency, and protein S deficiency **(Flowchart 1)**. It is important to note that there are additional rare mutations that may be associated with increased VTE.[2] Furthermore, elevated concentrations of clotting factors are heritable causes of hypercoagulable states that are not caused by single gene mutations, but rather multiple subtle changes in gene activity.[4] While not directly considered an inherited thrombophilia, methyltetrahydrofolate reductase (MTHFR) mutations are highly prevalent in certain populations and may also be implicated in VTE.[11] The following section will describe the pathophysiology and epidemiology of the five principal hereditary thrombophilia, the etiologies of increased clotting factor concentrations, and the importance of MTHFR mutations in VTE.

Factor V Leiden

Factor V Leiden is the most common inherited thrombophilia, and it exists in 50% of genetic cases and 20–25% of all VTEs.[12] Approximately 5% of the worldwide population carries this mutation.[6] However, the mutation is more common in North American and European Caucasians and is very rare among Asian and African populations.[12] FVL is caused by a point mutation of guanine to adenine at nucleotide 1601 in the gene that encodes factor V. This mutation yields the amino acid glutamine instead of arginine at factor V's cleavage site, rendering it insensitive to activated protein C (APC).[2] APC is a natural anticoagulant that breaks down factors Va and VIIIa, thereby inactivating them and halting the additional formation of fibrin **(Flowchart 1)**. Although APC levels remain unchanged, APC resistance (APCR) caused by FVL mutation decreases the efficacy of APC tenfold, disturbing the delicate balance of pro- and anticoagulation, thereby increasing the risk of thrombosis.[12] An APCR test is used to screen for FVL as it is easier and cheaper than genetic testing of FVL mutation.[13] 90% of patients with a positive APCR test possess the FVL mutation.[13] Those with heterozygosity for the FVL mutation are five times more likely to experience a VTE while homozygotes incur a 50-fold increase in VTE risk.[2]

Prothrombin G20210A Mutation

Prothrombin (factor II) is an inactive zymogen that is converted to thrombin (factor IIa) by factor Xa and the prothrombinase complex **(Flowchart 1)**. Thrombin is unique as it possesses the ability to both upregulate and depress the coagulation cascade: It converts fibrinogen to fibrin allowing for clot stabilization. However, once enough fibrin has been produced, it binds to thrombomodulin, thereby activating protein C to inhibit the clotting cascade.[14] Prothrombin G20210A mutation is a single nucleotide gain of function mutation at base pair 20210.[4] This guanine to adenine point-mutation occurs in the 3'-untranslated region of the prothrombin gene resulting in increased transcription that generates excess levels of prothrombin, precipitating a hypercoagulable state.[2] Plasma levels of prothrombin among patients heterozygous for the prothrombin G20210A mutation are approximately 30% higher than normal levels.[15] The worldwide prevalence of the prothrombin G20210A mutation is 2%, but variance between populations is high:[4] 2.5–12.5% of Middle Eastern and North African countries, 3.6% of Caucasian North Americans, and 3% of Europeans carry the prothrombin G20210A mutation. Cases of this mutation in Asian or Sub-Saharan African countries are extremely rare.[16] The prothrombin G20210A mutant allele affords a threefold increase in risk of VTE compared to the unaffected population.[4] However, prothrombin G20210A is a relatively uncommon mutation, accounting for only 6% of all VTE and 20% of inherited thrombophilia.[4]

Antithrombin Deficiency

Antithrombin is one of the most important natural anticoagulants, as it directly inhibits thrombin and factor Xa **(Flowchart 1)**. Additionally, AT is an auxiliary inhibitor of factors XIIa, XIa, and IXa. AT inhibits clotting factors by forming an irreversible bond with their active sites. While AT binding naturally occurs at a slow rate (once every 40 seconds), when heparins bind AT, they catalyze the reaction, accelerating bond formation one hundred-fold. Heparins thus optimize ATs inhibitory capabilities. AT deficiency has several subtypes each with its own etiology.[8] Type I AT deficiency is characterized by a decrease in both functional and immunological levels of AT,[8] and may be caused by gene deletions, insertions, or point mutations.[6] Type II AT deficiencies are point mutations that confer less danger, and they are defined by variant AT molecules that have a dysfunctional heparin binding site, active site, or both (pleomorphic subtype).[8] AT deficiency is an autosomal dominant disorder and most patients are heterozygotic. AT disorders are rare with a prevalence of 1:2,000–1:5,000 and they account for only 1% of all VTE events.[6]

Protein C and S Deficiencies

Protein C and its chief cofactor protein S are natural anticoagulants that downregulate the coagulation cascade via cleavage of factors Va and VIIIa to their inactivated form.[6] Free protein S binds to APC, increasing its affinity for its target clotting factors.[6] Dysfunction in either protein C or S decreases the body's ability to autoregulate clot formation and leads to hypercoagulability.[6] Both protein C and S deficiencies have two categories, where type I indicates lower plasma and activity levels of the proteins and type II indicates normal plasma levels, but decreased protein activity.[6] Multiple gene mutations have been identified in the protein C and S genes. Protein C and S deficiencies are rare mutations with a prevalence of approximately 0.3–0.5% for protein C deficiency[6] and 0.03–0.1% for protein S deficiency.[17] Protein C and S deficiencies each account for approximately 3% of VTEs.[6]

Increased Clotting Factor Concentrations

While the five aforementioned conditions are the classic causes of hereditary thrombophilia, excess clotting factors also yield hypercoagulable states and increase the risk for VTEs.[4] However, not all clotting factors incur the same risk of hypercoagulability when their levels are increased. For example, factors V, VII, and X only cause hypercoagulability when plasma levels are above the 90th percentile for their concentration. In contrast, factors II, VIII, IX, and XII exacerbate their hypercoagulable risk in a linear, dose-dependent fashion.[15] It is not common practice to routinely test for these increased clotting concentrations. Additionally, there are numerous other rare genetic mutations such as plasminogen activator inhibitor-1 (PAI-1 4G/5G) and angiotensin-converting enzyme (ACE) insertions/deletions that contribute to thrombophilia but are not commonly screened for. Although these rare mutations and increased clotting factor concentrations can increase risk of thrombosis, their prevalence is so rare that they are rendered clinically insignificant.

MTHFR Mutations

5,10-methyltetrahydrofolate reductase is an enzyme that converts tetrahydrofolate (THF) to the active 5-methyltetrahydrofolate, a crucial cofactor in the conversion of homocysteine to methionine[6] **(Fig. 1)**. Decreased production of 5-methyltetrahydrofolate diminishes the conversion capacity of homocysteine to methionine, precipitating increased plasma homocysteine levels.[18] The most frequent MTHFR mutation is a C to T point mutation at position 677 resulting in an amino acid substitution of alanine to valine. This mutation decreases the binding affinity of THF to MTHFR's active site[11] and causes a thermoinstability at 37°C, leading to decreased enzyme activity and increased homocysteine levels.[18]

While MTHFR mutations are not directly considered inherited thrombophilia, as the enzyme does not regulate hemostasis, the hyperhomocysteinemia caused by MTHFR mutations increases risk of thrombosis. Elevated homocysteine induces thrombosis by increasing endothelial damage, activating factor V, interfering with APC, and reducing thrombomodulin expression.[6] Homozygotes for the MTHFR mutation have a 70% decrease in enzyme activity[19] yielding 25% greater homocysteine levels than the general population.[11] While heterozygotes also have highly decreased MTHFR enzyme activity (up to 65%),[19] they only portray mildly increased homocysteine levels.[20] Increased folate intake helps lower these increased homocysteine levels, yet the ability of folate to lower thrombosis risk is still debated, and the association between MTHFR mutations and thrombophilia independent of homocysteine levels is inconclusive.[11]

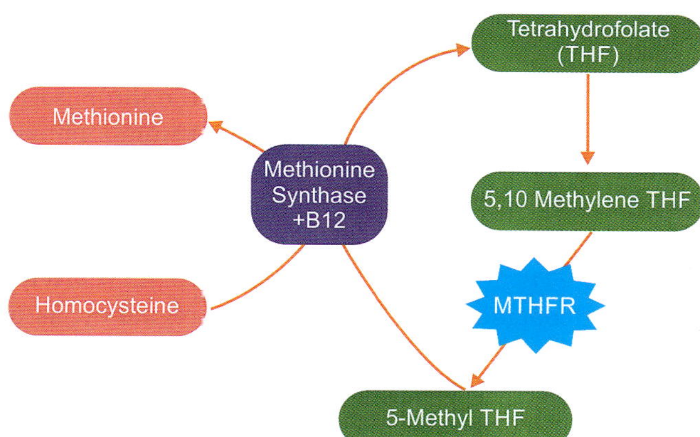

Fig. 1: The role of MTHFR in the conversion of homocysteine to methionine.

The European Society of Human Reproduction and Embryology (ESHRE) guidelines from 2022 indicate that currently MTHFR mutations without evidence of elevated homocysteine should not be screened with respect to recurrent pregnancy loss (RPL).[21]

The MTHFR C677T mutation is very common. In North America, 20–40% of Caucasian and Hispanic populations are heterozygous, while 8–20% of those populations are homozygous for the mutation.[19] This mutation is also common in Europe with approximately 13% of the population being homozygous for the mutation.[20] However, this mutation is extremely rare in sub-Saharan Africa with zero percent homozygosity.[20]

Pregnancy as an Acquired Hypercoagulable State

Normal pregnancy is associated with changes in activity levels of various hemostatic mediators, resulting in a transient, acquired, and hypercoagulable state.[22] These critical hemostatic alterations are physiological and are likely hormonally mediated.[23] Although these changes help prevent intrapartum blood loss, they augment the risk of VTE.[23] Procoagulation factors VII, VIII, X, XII, von Willebrand factor (vWF), and fibrinogen (factor I) all increase during pregnancy, whereas levels of the natural anticoagulant, protein S, decrease.[22] Factors II, V, protein C, and AT levels do not change during pregnancy and remain at normal levels.[23] Hypercoagulability increases throughout pregnancy, and by the third trimester, it reaches twice the prepregnancy state.[23] Coagulability peaks in the peripartum and immediate puerperium.[23] VTE is a leading cause of maternal death in high-income countries,[24] and the risk of VTE doubles when hereditary thrombophilia superimposes the physiological hypercoagulability of pregnancy.[6] The following data outlines the thrombosis risk of pregnant women with hereditary thrombophilia: 31–44% in AT deficiency, 10–19% in protein C and S deficiencies, and 28% in FVL.[6] Pregnant women with inherited thrombophilia are thus treated prophylactically to prevent VTE.[25] Low molecular weight heparin (LMWH) is the anticoagulant of choice during pregnancy, as it demonstrates a low teratogenic risk, it does not cross the placenta, and it has an increased safety profile relative to unfractionated heparin.[25]

Hereditary Thrombophilia and Recurrent Pregnancy Loss

The twofold increase in hypercoagulability conferred by hereditary thrombophilia during pregnancy also predisposes the pregnancy to gestational vascular complications, including RPL.[25] It thus follows that perhaps RPL is another complication of hereditary thrombophilia, just as VTE is an established sequela. In this case, RPL could be considered a thromboembolic abnormality, and it should be treated as such, in a similar manner to VTE. ESHRE guidelines from 2022 currently do not recommend screening for hereditary thrombophilia and RPL.[21] However, the evidence used to support the guideline's conclusion only include data up to 2016.[21] In recent years, research on the association of each of the five primary inherited thrombophilia as well as MTHFR mutations with RPL has increased dramatically. The following section analyzes the existing literature to elucidate new insights regarding the risk of RPL among the inherited thrombophilia to ultimately decide which conditions necessitate prepregnancy screening. Furthermore, while LMWH is used to prevent VTE in pregnant women with inherited thrombophilia,[25] its use to diminish the risk of RPL specifically in hereditary thrombophilia is controversial and will be discussed in this chapter.

SCREENING

Methods

Medline and PubMed were searched using the terms "hereditary thrombophilia" or "inherited thrombophilia" and "recurrent pregnancy loss" or "recurrent fetal loss" or "recurrent miscarriage". Studies were included in the analysis if they were published after 1990 in a reputable journal, and if they evaluate the relationship between one or more hereditary thrombophilia and RPL. A total of 20 studies were included. Conclusions as to whether screening should be conducted for each thrombophilia type in the setting of RPL were determined by type and strength of the study, as well as recency of the publication. The most important articles for each thrombophilia type will be discussed in further detail.

Factor V Leiden

The high prevalence of FVL worldwide and its frequent implication in hypercoagulability has resulted in numerous analyses on its association with RPL. Sixteen studies were included in this analysis: three meta-analyses, one systematic review and cohort study, three retrospective cohort studies, and ten case-control studies **(Table 1)**.

In 1997, Brenner et al. were the first to indicate an association between FVL and RPL.[31] This case-control study analyzed 39 cases of women with RPL and no evidence of antiphospholipid antibody (APLA) syndrome with 40 years of age and ethnicity-matched controls without RPL and with two or more successful pregnancies.[31] 19 women with RPL were positive for FVL mutations, whereas only two control-cases had FVL ($p < 0.0001$).[31] Only 19% of pregnancies resulted in live birth among women with FVL. Comparatively, women with no FVL mutation exhibited a 33% live birth rate ($p = 0.03$).[31] This study was conducted in Israel, thus its generalizability outside of the Middle East may be limited. This landmark study highlights the possible role of RPL in reducing live birth rates and the differential increase in FVL among patients with RPL.

The most recent study analyzing the correlation of FVL with RPL published in 2024 also found a positive association.[33] This study was conducted in Italy as a larger scale population study. Cernera et al. compared 468 women who experienced RPL with 430 members of the general population with no RPL and no episode of VTE.[33] This study found that 4.4% of women with RPL possess the FVL mutation compared to 2.4% of the general population ($p = 0.028$).[33]

While several studies fail to demonstrate an association between FVL and RPL, three meta-analyses have been conducted, which have all yielded a positive correlation. While Kovalevsky et al. published their analysis in 2004, the two meta-analyses conducted by Hamedi et al. and Liu et al. are more recent and were published in 2020 and 2021, respectively. Hamedi et al. analyzed 19 case-control studies conducted in Middle Eastern countries measuring

TABLE 1: Study characteristics and associations of factor V Leiden with recurrent pregnancy loss (RPL).

First author	*Study design*	*Year*	*Associated with RPL?*	*Odds ratio*	*95% CI*	*P value*
Kovalevsky[26]	Meta-analysis	2004	Yes	2.00	1.50–2.70	<0.01
Hamedi[27]	Meta-analysis	2020	Yes	2.37	1.50–3.75	0.009
Liu[28]	Meta-analysis of case controls	2021	Yes	2.44	1.96–3.03	<0.001
Turki[29]	Retrospective cohort	2016	Yes			<0.05
Iordache[30]	Retrospective cohort	2022	Yes	Homozygous: 3.66, 2.27* Heterozygous: 2.54, 1.82*		Homozygous: 0.001, 0.007* Heterozygous: 0.036, 0.049*
Brenner[31]	Case control	1997	Yes			0.03
Mitic[32]	Case control	2012	Yes	6.11	1.35–27.65	0.017
Cernera[33]	Case control	2024	Yes			0.028
Santoro[34]	Case control	2005	No			0.36
Sottilotta[35]	Case control	2006	No	3.00		0.12
Karata[36]	Case control	2012	No			>0.05
Baumann[37]	Case control	2013	No			0.86
Perés[38]	Case control	2019	No			0.72
Ahangari[39]	Case control	2019	No			0.17
Shehata[40]	Systematic review and cohort study	2022	No	1.02	0.71–1.48	0.354
Lund[41]	Retrospective cohort	2010	May be	0.48	0.23–1.01	0.05

*First trimester pregnancy loss, second trimester pregnancy.
(CI: confidence interval)

associations of FVL and RPL.[27] Using a random effects model, the pooled odds ratio (OR) of RPL for FVL carriers relative to controls is 2.37 [95% confidence interval (CI): 1.50–3.75].[27]

Liu's meta-analysis contains a larger pool of 89 studies as it analyzes all five types of hereditary thrombophilia.[28] 81 of these studies evaluated the relationship between FVL and RPL. All studies were case control except for one cohort study.[28] Additionally, studies were conducted worldwide, which increases generalizability but confers greater heterogenicity between studies. However, subgroup analysis by continent adjusts for some of this variance. This meta-analysis supports the association between FVL and RPL with an overall OR of 2.44 (95% CI: 1.96–3.03) among the 81 studies.[28] In the subgroup regional analysis, studies conducted in Africa demonstrated the highest risk of RPL among FVL carriers relative to controls (OR: 7.26, 95% CI: 3.78–13.93).[28] Studies conducted in Europe (OR: 1.75, 95% CI: 1.31–2.32), Asia (OR: 2.64, 95% CI: 1.59–4.40), and the Middle East (OR: 2.69, 95% CI: 1.86–3.90) also each yielded a positive association between FVL and RPL.[28] However, North American and Latin American studies found no significant association between FVL and RPL. Additionally, Liu's analysis highlighted the increased risk of RPL in both homozygous (OR: 2.76, 95% CI: 1.34–5.71) and heterozygous mutations (OR: 2.07, 95% CI: 1.57–2.72).[28]

It is critical to report that the 2022 systematic review and cohort study conducted by Shehata et al. found no significant association between FVL mutation and RPL.[40] Elucidating why this study yielded no association is paramount to determining the importance of screening for FVL in the case of RPL. This study argues that increased screening has resulted in overdiagnosis and overtreatment without improvement in clinical outcomes among women with RPL. Shehata et al. thus chose to conduct a large retrospective cohort study and conduct a meta-analysis to compare results.[40] It is important to note that this study defined RPL as three or more pregnancy losses while guidelines now indicate that two or more losses should warrant the RPL diagnosis. Additionally, this study only included women with recurrent first trimester pregnancy loss and had two or more losses, and second-trimester pregnancy losses been included, perhaps an association would have been found. Moreover, the cohort arm of this study was not compared with a cohort of controls, but rather a pooled control group from the literature analyzed in the meta-analysis. The meta-analysis included a total of 12 studies, 10 of which analyzed the association of hereditary thrombophilia and RPL (two measured acquired thrombophilia).[40] Only five studies evaluated the association of FVL and RPL, and no association was found (OR: 1.02, 95% CI: 0.71–1.48).[40] When prevalence of FVL among women with RPL in the cohort study (4.8%) was compared with the prevalence among controls from the meta-analysis (4.9%), no significant difference was found ($p = 0.354$), indicating no association between FVL and RPL.[40]

While only half of the 16 studies evaluating FVL indicate a positive association between FVL and RPL, the strongest research including all meta-analyses provides evidence for increased risk. Except for one systematic-review and cohort study, all studies that failed to demonstrate a correlation of FVL with RPL were case controls. The systematic review featured design weaknesses that may have confounded the data toward a negative finding. In summary, the strength of the studies that yield a positive association between FVL and RPL indicate the FVL mutations should be screened in women experiencing RPL.

Prothrombin G20210A

Like FVL, prothrombin G20210A mutations have been studied extensively. The association between prothrombin G20210A mutations and RPL was studied in 15 articles compiled in this literature review **(Table 2)**. The study designs included three meta-analyses, three retrospective cohort studies, one systematic review and cohort study, and eight case–control studies.

The three most critical studies to discuss are all meta-analyses that demonstrate a correlation between prothrombin G20210A mutation and RPL. Studies conducted by Liu et al. and Kovalevsky et al. study the relationship of various hereditary thrombophilia and RPL while Gao et al. only analyzed the prothrombin G20210A mutation. Liu's meta-analysis of 89 studies yielded 64 articles evaluating the association of prothrombin G20210A mutation with RPL.[28] A positive correlation was

TABLE 2: Studies analyzing the association of prothrombin G20210A mutation with recurrent pregnancy loss.

Author	*Study design*	*Year*	*Associated with RPL?*	*Odds ratio*	*95% CI*	*P value*
Kovalevsky[26]	Meta-analysis	2004	Yes	2.00	1.00–4.00	0.03
Gao[42]	Meta-analysis	2015	Yes	1.81	1.26–2.60	<0.05
Liu[28]	Meta-analysis	2021	Yes	2.08	1.61–2.68	<0.001
Turki[29]	Retrospective cohort	2016	Yes			<0.05
Iordache[30]	Retrospective cohort	2022	Yes	2.79, 2.81*		0.022, 0.001*
Shehata[40]	Systematic review and cohort study	2022	No			0.541
Santoro[34]	Case control	2005	No			0.13
Sottilotta[35]	Case control	2006	No	3.52		0.07
Karata[36]	Case control	2012	No			>0.05
Mitic[32]	Case control	2012	No	3.24	0.92–12.36	>0.05
Baumann[37]	Case control	2013	No			0.8
Perés[38]	Case control	2019	No	5.90		0.1
Ahangari[39]	Case control	2019	No			0.31
Cernera[33]	Case control	2024	No**			>0.99**
Lund[41]	Retrospective cohort	2010	May be	0.49	0.23–1.02	1.05

*First trimester pregnancy loss, second trimester pregnancy loss
**Associated with recurrent implantation failure ($p = 0.02$)
(CI: confidence interval)

found with an OR of 2.08 (95% CI: 1.61–2.68).[28] Subgroup analysis indicated a high degree of variance among studies conducted in Africa with respect to additional risk conferred by prothrombin gene mutation carriage (OR: 4.53, 95% CI: 0.93–22.06).[28] Since prothrombin gene mutations are more common among European and Middle Eastern populations, a higher percentage of research was conducted in these regions (28 and 15 studies, respectively).[28] Subgroup analysis of both Europe (OR: 1.93, 95% CI: 1.38–2.70) and the Middle East (OR: 2.25, 95% CI: 1.47–3.44) demonstrated a positive association between prothrombin gene mutation and RPL.[28] Studies conducted in North America (OR: 1.95, 95% CI: 0.43–8.92), Latin America (OR: 1.77, 95% CI: 0.45–6.93), and Asia (OR: 1.64, 95% CI: 0.57–4.72), however, did not establish a significant correlation.[28]

Gao et al. undertook a meta-analysis of 37 case-control trials specifically focusing on prothrombin G20210A mutation, gleaning evidence to support the association of this mutation with RPL (OR: 1.81, 95% CI: 1.26–2.60).[42] Analogously to Liu's meta-analysis, European trials compiled by Gao et al. supported the correlation of prothrombin G20210A mutation with RPL (OR: 1.80, 95% CI: 1.35–2.41).[42] However, subgroup analysis of Middle Eastern trials failed to corroborate the correlation found in Liu et al.'s regional analysis (OR: 2.39, 95% CI: 0.96–5.92).[42]

The three most recent studies examining the association of prothrombin gene mutations with RPL were conducted by Iordache et al., Shehata et al., and Cernera et al. The retrospective cohort study conducted by Iordache et al. followed 211 women with a history of pregnancy loss during the study period (2020–2022).[30] The women were stratified according to which trimester they experienced pregnancy loss, with 157 suffering first trimester loss and 54 enduring second trimester loss. Measurements including socioeconomic demographics, past medical history, obstetric characteristics (i.e., parity and gravidity), and thrombophilia assays were obtained and analyzed according to study group.[30] No significant differences were found between the first and second trimester group on any parameter except history of induced abortion, with history of medical abortion being more common among first trimester losses and surgical abortion being more common among second trimester loss. Prothrombin gene mutations were found to increase risk of RPL in both trimesters with first trimester loss conferring an OR of 2.79 (95% CI: 1.27–3.82) and second trimester loss demonstrating an OR of 2.81 (95% CI: 1.58–4.33) relative to the general population.[30]

Both Shehata et al.'s systematic review and cohort study[40] and Cernera et al.'s case-control study[33] failed to illustrate a significant difference in prothrombin G20210A mutation carriage among women with RPL relative to the general population ($p = 0.541$ and $p > 0.99$, respectively). Although the negative results from these two studies ought to influence the conclusion as to whether prothrombin mutations should be screened in RPL, two significant factors may supersede these outcomes. Shehata et al. only studied women who experienced three or more first trimester losses, which may negatively skew the results, as women who suffered from two or more losses and/or second trimester losses were excluded.[40] Additionally, while Cernera et al. did not find an increase in prothrombin mutation rates in RPL, recurrent implantation failure (RIF) was significantly higher in women with this mutation ($p = 0.02$).[33] RIF may be one specific but important cause of first trimester pregnancy loss and thus may bolster the need for screening of prothrombin mutations.

Analysis of these 15 studies illuminated the importance of screening for prothrombin G20210A mutations for RPL, as all three meta-analyses and retrospective cohort studies support the association between prothrombin G20210A and RPL. Several older case-control studies did not find increased prothrombin gene mutations in RPL relative to controls. This negative data is important to consider, however, the age and study design confer less strength relative to the more recent meta-analyses and retrospective cohort studies that yield positive outcomes. Additionally, while the systematic review and cohort study conducted by Shehata et al. does not demonstrate a positive association, the limitations in methodology may confound the outcome.

Antithrombin Deficiency

Very few studies are available that measure the association of AT deficiency with RPL. Of the 20 studies in this literature review, only two evaluated this thrombophilia: one meta-analysis and one case-control study **(Table 3)**.

The meta-analysis conducted by Liu et al. in 2021 included seven studies measuring the risk of RPL in women with AT deficiency.[28] No significant positive association between AT and RPL was found among any of the included studies, and the pooled result yielded an OR of 0.83 (95% CI: 0 29–2.36).[28] Subgroup analysis elucidated that four out of seven studies were conducted in Asia. No subgroup yielded any significant elevation in risk of RPL in AT deficiency.[28]

Mitic et al.'s case–control study included 147 women suffering from RPL and 128 controls.[32] 6.8% of women with RPL were found to have one of AT, protein C, or protein S deficiency, while no controls had any of these three conditions ($p = 0.07$).[32] Although the research conducted by Mitic et al. did yield a positive association between AT deficiency and RPL, the study population included only Serbian women and only measured second trimester losses. Thus, the generalizability of these results is limited.

Results from the available data do not currently support screening for AT deficiency in the setting of RPL. Only one study demonstrated a positive association in a limited population, while the only available meta-analysis found no increased risk of RPL in AT deficiency.

TABLE 3: Studies analyzing the association of antithrombin deficiency with recurrent pregnancy loss (RPL).

First author	*Study design*	*Year*	*Associated with RPL?*	*P value*
Liu[28]	Meta-analysis	2021	No	>0.05
Mitic[32]	Case control	2012	Yes	0.007

Protein C Deficiency

Like AT deficiency, there is limited research available regarding the association of protein C deficiency with RPL. One case–control and one retrospective cohort study found a significant correlation between protein C deficiency and RPL, while one meta-analysis did not **(Table 4)**.

Mitic et al. and Iordache et al. both found protein C to be associated with RPL.[30,32] Results and limitations of the research conducted by Mitic et al. were described above while discussing AT deficiency. The cohort study conducted by Iordache et al. following 211 women found protein C deficiency had a prevalence of 5.7% among women who experienced first trimester pregnancy loss and 14.8% of women who suffered from second trimester loss ($p = 0.034$).[30] Additionally, they found protein C deficiency to be a risk factor for RPL, presenting an OR of 2.15 (95% CI: 1.32–3.93) for first trimester loss and 2.98 (95% CI: 1.75–5.04) for second trimester loss.[30] However, they note that most clinical cases of protein C deficiency are minor and are less substantially correlated with RPL relative to severe cases.[30]

The meta-analysis conducted by Liu et al. compiled nine studies evaluating the association of protein C deficiency with RPL.[28] It is interesting to note that although this study was conducted in 2021, all available studies on protein C were published between 2005 and 2015. Each study included in this analysis had a very large CI for the demonstrated OR (i.e., 95% CI: 0.12–74.87, 0.16–70.25).[28] Only one study indicated a significant increased risk for RPL among women with protein C deficiency (OR: 17.75, 95% CI: 1.00–316.45).[28] Ultimately, the increased risk of RPL among protein C carriers was not found to be significant when the studies were pooled (OR: 1.98, 95% CI: 0.97–4.04).[28] Subgroup analysis indicated that four studies were conducted in Asia, two in Europe, and one in each of Latin America, Africa, and the Middle East.

Protein C deficiency is an incredibly rare disorder, with a prevalence of <0.5% worldwide.[4] There is therefore a limited amount of research focusing on this disorder lending to inconclusive results. While the meta-analysis did not show a significant association between protein C deficiency and RPL, the 95% CI indicated that it was almost significant. It would be interesting to elucidate how more studies would have altered the outcome of this meta-analysis. Furthermore, a more recent cohort study did find a positive association.[30] Thus, there is some reason to suggest an association between protein C deficiency and RPL exist, but more research must be conducted to ascertain a definite conclusion.

Protein S Deficiency

In the current literature review, one meta-analysis, one case–control study, and one cross-sectional study were

TABLE 4: Studies analyzing the association of protein C deficiency with recurrent pregnancy loss (RPL).

Author	*Study design*	*Year*	*Associated with RPL?*	*Odds ratio*	*95% CI*	*P value*
Liu[28]	Meta-analysis	2021	No	1.98	0.97–4.04	>0.05
Iordache[30]	Retrospective cohort	2022	Yes	2.15, 2.98*		0.009, 0.001*
Mitic[32]	Case control	2012	Yes			0.007

*First trimester pregnancy loss, second trimester pregnancy loss.
(CI: confidence interval)

found to measure the association of protein S deficiency with RPL **(Table 5)**.

Research by Mitic et al. and Liu et al. indicates that RPL is associated with protein S deficiency.[28,32] Due to the rare etiology of this deficiency, Mitic et al. grouped protein S, protein C, and AT deficiency in their research (detailed in the AT section).[32] The 10 studies collected by Liu et al. find evidence for an increased risk of RPL in women with protein S deficiency (OR: 3.45, 95% CI: 1.15–10.35).[28] However, like protein C deficiency, there is high variance surrounding the ORs as indicated by wide CIs. Distribution of studies according to region paralleled the available studies for protein C deficiency: four Asian studies, three European studies, one African study, one Latin American study, and one Middle Eastern study.[28]

Neki et al. did not find a significant association between RPL and protein C deficiency.[43] This study found that of 233 women with RPL, 1.7% had protein S deficiency with the K196E mutation compared to 1.8% of the general Japanese population who possess this mutation ($p = 0.941$).[43] However, this study researched a Japanese-specific mutation of this deficiency (K196E point mutation) that does not exist in other Asian nor Caucasian populations and thus not generalizable to other protein S deficiencies. Since the two other available studies, including one meta-analysis, illustrate an association between protein S deficiency and RPL, screening should be conducted for this thrombophilia.

MTHFR C677T Mutation

Six studies evaluate whether the MTHFR C677T mutation is associated with RPL, five of which are case-control studies and one retrospective cohort study **(Table 6)**. Five studies were conducted between 2012 and 2019, and one was published more recently in 2024. Half the studies found a significant association while the other half did not.

Cernera et al. and Ahangari et al. published the most recent studies analyzing the association between RPL and MTHFR mutation.[33,39] Similarly to the prothrombin gene mutation, Cernera et al. did not elucidate a positive association between RPL and MTHFR but did find a significant relationship between MTHFR mutation and RIF.[33] This finding is important, as RIF may be a significant etiology of RPL. The 2019 case-control study spearheaded by Ahangari et al. analyzed 245 women with more than three pregnancy losses with 250 ethnicity and age-matched controls in Iran.[39] The controls must have at least two children and no history of RPL. This Iranian study yields similar results to Karata's study in Istanbul where homozygous MTHFR C677T mutations were found in 28.5% of the study population and 14.2% of controls ($p < 0.001$) and heterozygous mutations existed in 64.3% of the study group and 38.1% of controls ($p < 0.001$).[36] In Karata et al.'s study, both homocysteine and folate levels were similar between study and control groups.[36] However, the research conducted by Ahangari et. al.

TABLE 5: Studies analyzing the association of protein S deficiency with recurrent pregnancy loss (RPL).

Author	*Study design*	*Year*	*Associated with RPL?*	*Odds ratio*	*95% CI*	*P value*
Liu[28]	Meta-analysis	2021	Yes	3.45	1.15–10.35	0.009
Mitic[32]	Case control	2012	Yes			0.007
Neki[43]	Cross sectional	2014	No			0.941

(CI: confidence interval)

TABLE 6: Studies analyzing the association of MTHFR C677T mutation with recurrent pregnancy loss (RPL).

Author	*Study design*	*Year*	*Associated with RPL?*	*Odds ratio*	*95% CI*	*P value*
Ahangari[39]	Case control	2019	Yes	5.5		<0.001
Karata[36]	Case control	2012	Yes	5.59	3.75–8.34	<0.001
Mitic[32]	Case control	2012	Yes	5.32	1.87–15.12	0.001
Cernera[33]	Case control	2024	No*			0.269
Baumann[37]	Case control	2013	No			0.68
Turki[29]	Retrospective cohort	2016	No			>0.05

*Associated with recurrent implantation failure (RIF) ($p < 0.001$)

did not describe the homocysteine and folate levels.[39] Differential levels of these chemicals between control and study groups may confound the results, as both homocysteine and folate are important mediators of successful pregnancies. The increased risk of RPL in MTHFR mutations demonstrated by these two studies elicit the hypothesis that MTHFR mutations may have greater association with RPL in the Middle East relative to other regions.[36,39]

The relationship between inherited thrombophilia and RPL has been a controversial topic with novel research lending to change in screening protocols. This literature review of 20 studies sought to synthesize the newest research to impact clinical practice and guidelines. Ultimately, it was found that both FVL and prothrombin G20210A mutation confer a significant association with RPL and should thus unequivocally be screened. Limited research existed for AT, protein C, and protein S deficiencies, yet results indicate that AT should not be screened due to limited association with RPL. Protein S deficiency did present a positive association with RPL, while protein C deficiency was more indeterminate. Screening may thus be beneficial for these two deficiencies in addition to screening for FVL and prothrombin G20210A mutation.

TREATMENT

Despite the association between inherited thrombophilia and RPL, treatment of women with RPL remains controversial. Numerous studies of various design (case-control, retrospective, prospective, RCT, and meta-analyses) have been conducted to determine the effectiveness of treating women diagnosed with hereditary thrombophilia and suffering from RPL. However, studies differ in their treatment protocols: Regimens differ by types and dose of LMWH, whether LMWH was augmented with aspirin, and trimester of treatment initiation during pregnancy. **Table 7** chronologically lists the 41 studies conducted from 1999 to the present.

This section will focus on the approach to treating women with hereditary thrombophilia experiencing RPL. The current literature review examines studies analyzing the treatment with LMWH, aspirin, or both. Studies were divided into four groups according to design: four retrospective cohort studies, three prospective cohort studies, three randomized clinical trials, and six meta-analyses **(Table 8)**. While the prior section regarding screening organized the discussion according to thrombophilia type, study design is a crucial factor in determining the impact of treatment protocols. The discussion on treatment will therefore be divided according to design. Due to the large number of studies, only the most significant studies from each category will be discussed. Each study lends a unique perspective and interpretation of how to manage and treat women with RPL and hereditary thrombophilia.

Retrospective Cohort Studies

Four retrospective studies were included in this literature review, despite their design limitations, in order to provide a comprehensive overview of the research regarding treatment of RPL in hereditary thrombophilia. All of the retrospective studies indicate that LMWH treatment with or without aspirin improves pregnancy outcomes in the setting of hereditary thrombophilia.

One of the first research on treatment of RPL in hereditary thrombophilia was a retrospective study conducted by Mutlu et al. They analyzed 204 patients with various inherited thrombophilia: MTHFR mutation, FVL heterozygous, prothrombin gene mutation, and protein C and S deficiency. 145 women were treated with 4,000 IU/day of LMWH and 80 mg/day of aspirin whereas 59 women received no treatment. Compared to the control group, the treatment group had a significantly higher rate of live births, and a reduced abortion rate [treatment group: 132 (91%), no treatment group: 35 (60%) $p < 0.01$]. Moreover, there were significantly fewer placental-mediated complications (i.e., IUGR) in the LMWH + ASA group relative to the ASA group ($p = 0.044$).[44]

Another retrospective study investigating the effect of LMWH on RPL by Aynioglu et al., included a greater number of women thereby increasing statistical power. 153 women with positive screening for inherited thrombophilia (heterozygous and homozygous—FVL, PT G202I0A, and MTHFR C677T/A1298 mutation) were divided into two groups: 89 were treated with 100 IU/kg of LMWH combined with 80 mg/day of aspirin, and 64 were not treated. 55 of the 64 women who were not treated (85.9%) with anticoagulation therapy experienced a pregnancy complication. Conversely, women treated with LMWH and aspirin had significantly lower complication rates, with 42 of the 89 treated women experiencing a pregnancy complication (47.2%) ($p = 0.003$). Additionally, the live birth rate in the treated group was significantly

TABLE 7: Studies analyzing the effect of LMWH, aspirin or both on recurrent pregnancy loss in patients with inherited thrombophilia.

Name	*Author*	*Design*	*Publication*	*Year*
Heparin for women with recurrent miscarriage and inherited thrombophilia (ALIFE2): an international open-label, randomized controlled trial (RCT)	Quenby et al.	RCT	The Lancet	2023
Recurrent miscarriage Green-top guideline No. 17	Regan et al.	Guidelines	BJOG: British Journal of Obstetrics and Gynaecology	2023
Thrombophilia thrombosis and thromboprophylaxis in pregnancy—for what and in whom?	Middeldorp et al.	Review	Hamostaseologie	2022
Treating unexplained recurrent pregnancy loss based on lessons learned from obstetric antiphospholipid syndrome and inherited thrombophilia: a propensity-score adjusted retrospective study	Scarrone et al.	A propensity-score adjusted retrospective study	Journal of Reproductive Immunology	2022
Hereditary thrombophilia and recurrent pregnancy loss: a systematic review and meta-analysis	Liu et al.	Systematic review meta-analysis	Human Reproduction	2021
Hold your needles in women with recurrent pregnancy losses with or without hereditary thrombophilia: meta-analysis and review of the literature	Intzes et al.	Meta-analysis and review	Journal of Gynecology Obstetrics and Human Reproduction	2021
The role of low molecular weight heparin on recurrent pregnancy loss: a systematic review and meta-analysis	Fangfei et al.	Meta-analysis of randomized controlled studies	Taiwanese Journal of Obstetrics and Gynecology	2020
Inherited thrombophilia and recurrent pregnancy loss: a single-center case–control study in Northwestern Algeria	Nassour-Mokhtari et al.	Case control	Egyptian Journal of Medical Human Genetics	2020
Aspirin, low molecular weight heparin, or both in preventing pregnancy complications in women with recurrent pregnancy loss and factor V Leiden mutation	Karadağ et al.	RCT	Journal of Maternal-Fetal and Neonatal Medicine	2020
The efficacy of enoxaparin for recurrent abortion: a meta-analysis of randomized controlled studies	Yangming Liu et al.	Meta-analysis of randomized controlled studies	The Journal of Maternal-Fetal and Neonatal Medicine	2019
Risk factors and role of low molecular weight heparin in obstetric complications among women with inherited thrombophilia: a cohort study	Clavijo et al.	Retrospective	Hematology, Transfusion and Cell Therapy	2019
Enoxaparin (or plus aspirin) for the prevention of recurrent miscarriage: a meta-analysis of randomized controlled studies	Tao Lin et al.	Meta-analysis of randomized controlled studies	European Journal of Obstetrics and Gynecology and Reproductive Biology	2018
Maternal thrombophilia and recurrent miscarriage: Is there evidence that heparin is indicated as prophylaxis against recurrence?	Stefanski et al.	Review	Geburtshilfe und Frauenheilkunde	2018
Obstetric outcomes of recurrent pregnancy loss patients diagnosed with inherited thrombophilia	Karadağ et al.	Case control	Irish Journal of Medical Science	2017

Contd...

Contd...

Name	Author	Design	Publication	Year
Pregnancy, thrombophilia, and the risk of a first venous thrombosis: systematic review and Bayesian meta-analysis	Croles et al.	Systematic review meta-analysis randomized controlled studies and cohort	The BMJ	2017
Hereditary thrombophilia and recurrent pregnancy loss	Pritchard et al.	Review	Clinical Obstetrics and Gynecology	2016
Guidance for the evaluation and treatment of hereditary and acquired thrombophilia	Stevens et al.	Guidelines	Journal of Thrombosis and Thrombolysis	2016
A meta-analysis of low molecular weight heparin to prevent pregnancy loss in women with inherited thrombophilia	Skieth et al.	Meta-analysis	Blood	2016
The role of low molecular weight heparin in women with hereditary thrombophilia for good perinatal outcome	Vesna Sokol et al.	Retrospective	Acta Clinica Croatica	2016
Does anticoagulant therapy improve adverse pregnancy outcomes in patients with history of recurrent pregnancy loss?	Aynioglu et al.	Retrospective	Ginekologia Polska	2016
Low molecular weight heparin plus aspirin versus aspirin alone in pregnant women with hereditary thrombophilia to improve live birth rate: meta-analysis of randomized controlled trials	Areia et al.	Meta-analysis of randomized controlled trials	Archives of Gynecology and Obstetrics	2016
Enoxaparin for prevention of unexplained recurrent miscarriage: a multicenter randomized double-blind placebo-controlled trial	Pasquier et al.	Randomized controlled trial	Blood	2015
Effects of anticoagulant therapy on pregnancy outcomes in patients with thrombophilia and previous poor obstetric history	Mutlu et al.	Retrospective	Blood Coagulation and Fibrinolysis	2015
The association between inherited thrombophilia and recurrent pregnancy loss in Turkish women	Isaoglu et al.	Case control	Clinical and Experimental Obstetrics and Gynecology	2014
Low molecular weight heparin treatment and impact of inherited thrombophilia type in pregnancies with previous adverse outcome	Aracic et al.	Prospective	The Journal of Maternal-Fetal and Neonatal Medicine	2014
Low molecular weight heparin and pregnancy outcomes in women with inherited thrombophilia: a systematic review and meta-analysis	Chen et al.	Systematic review meta-analysis randomized controlled studies and cohort	Japan Society of Obstetrics and Gynecology	2014
Aspirin and/or heparin for women with unexplained recurrent miscarriage with or without inherited thrombophilia (review)	De Jong et al. (Cochrane)	Review	Cochrane Library	2014
Anticoagulation in pregnancy complications	Middeldorp et al.	Review	Hematology (United States)	2014
Coagulation and placenta-mediated complications	Greer et al.	Review	Rambam Maimonides Medical Journal	2014

Contd...

Contd...

Name	Author	Design	Publication	Year
Monitoring of low molecular weight heparins in pregnant women with inherited thrombophilic disorders	Paskaleva et al.	Retrospective	Akusherstvo i ginekologii (Russian Journal of Obstetrics & Gynecology)	2014
Testing for inherited thrombophilia in recurrent miscarriage	De Jong et al.	Review	Seminars in Reproductive Medicine	2011
Consultative hematology: the pregnant patient pregnancy loss	Bates et al.	Review	Hematology/the Education Program of the American Society of Hematology. American Society of Hematology. Education Program	2010
SPIN (Scottish Pregnancy Intervention) study: a multicenter, randomized controlled trial of low molecular weight heparin and low-dose aspirin in women with recurrent miscarriage	Clark et al.	RCT	Blood	2010
Aspirin or anticoagulants for treating recurrent miscarriage in women without antiphospholipid syndrome	Kaandrop et al.	Meta-analysis of randomized controlled studies	Cochrane Database of Systematic Reviews	2009
Inherited thrombophilia and pregnancy complications revisited	Rodger et al.	Review	American College of Obstetricians and Gynecologists	2008
Antithrombotic prophylaxis during pregnancy in women with deficiency of natural anticoagulants	Grandone et al.	Retrospective cohort	Blood Coagulation and Fibrinolysis	2008
The association between hereditary thrombophilias and pregnancy loss	Géraldine et al.	Review	Haematologica	2005
Low molecular weight heparin versus low-dose aspirin in women with one fetal loss and a constitutional thrombophilic disorder	Gris et al.	Prospective	Blood	2004
Pregnancy outcome in patients with a history of recurrent spontaneous miscarriages and documented thrombophilias	Krabbendam et al.	Prospective cohort study	Gynecologic and Obstetric Investigation	2004
Thromboprophylaxis improves the live birth rate in women with consecutive recurrent miscarriages and hereditary thrombophilia	Carp	Prospective cohort study	Journal of Thrombosis and Haemostasis	2003
Increased risk for fetal loss in carriers of the factor V Leiden mutation	Meinardi et al.	Retrospective cohort study	Annals of Internal Medicine	1999

higher than in the untreated group ($p = 0.001$). The study results indicating that the anticoagulant therapy had a beneficial effect on women with hereditary thrombophilia and RPL.[45]

Clavijo et al. examined the effects of LMWH on pregnancy outcomes in 88 women with 250 pregnancies and hereditary thrombophilia [heterozygous FVL mutation, heterozygous II20210AG mutation, protein S and protein C deficiency, factor XII (FXII) deficiency, activated C protein resistance, antithrombin III (AT III) deficiency]. This study also found a significant correlation between recurrent miscarriages and hereditary thrombophilia ($p = 0.012$, high-risk hereditary thrombophilia (OR: 4.96, 95% CI: 1.42–17.3). LMWH showed effectiveness for reducing pregnancy complication (OR: 0.25, 95% CI: 0.12–0.54) and miscarriages (OR: 0.41, 95% CI: 0.20–0.82).[46]

TABLE 8: Studies of treatment of RPL in hereditary thrombophilia that will be described in further detail according to design.

Study type	*Author*	*Year*	*Thrombophilia type*	*n (Study group)*	*n (Control group)*	*Treatment*	*Live birth P value*	*RR/OR*	*Treatment showed benefit?*
Retrospective	Mutlu et al.	2015	MTHFR mutation FVL Heterozygous prothrombin gene mutation heterozygous Protein C deficiency Protein S deficiency	145	59	LMWH 4,000 IU/day + Aspirin 80 mg/day	$p < 0.01$	Live births 91% vs. 60%, $p < 0.01$, Perinatal complications $p = 0.044$	Yes
	Sokol et al.	2016	F II FVL PAI-1 MTHFR Antithrombin III deficiency protein C deficiency	57	13	LMWH (unspecified dosage)	$p = 0.006$	-	Yes
	Aynioglu et al.	2016	FVL PT G20210A MTHFR C677T/A1298 mutations	89	64	LMWH (100 IU/kg) + Aspirin (80 mg/day)	$p = 0.001$	-	Yes
	Clavijo et al.	2019	FVL II20210AG mutation Protein S deficiency Protein C deficiency Antithrombin III deficiency Factor XII deficiency Activated protein C resistance (APCR)	88	-	LMWH (unspecified dosage)	$p = 0.012$	High-risk hereditary thrombophilia OR: 4.96 (95% CI: 1.42–17.3); miscarriages OR: 0.41 (95% CI: 0.20–0.82), Pregnancy complication OR: 0.25 (95% CI: 0.12–0.54)	Yes

Contd...

Contd...

Study type	*Author*	*Year*	*Thrombophilia type*	*n (Study group)*	*n (Control group)*	*Treatment*	*Live birth P value*	*RR/OR*	*Treatment showed benefit?*
Prospective	Gris et al.	2004	FVL mutation Heterozygous prothrombin G20210A mutation Protein S deficiency	LMWH group = 80	Aspirin group = 80	LMWH (40 mg/day enoxaparin) or aspirin (100 mg/day)	$p = 0.0001$	OR: 15.5 (95% CI: 7–34)	Yes
	Aracic et al.	2014	FVL PT AT PC PS MTHFR PAI-1 ACE	50	50	Dalteparin (2,500–5,000 IU/day) or enoxaparin (40–80 mg/day)	$p = 0.001$	Early pregnancy loss $p = 0.001$, late pregnancy loss $p = 0.001$, term birth $p = 0.001$ Preterm births $p = 0.019$ IUFD $p = 0.0019$	Yes
	Karadağ et al.	2017	FVLM Protein C deficiency Protein S deficiency AT III heterozygous or homozygous PTGM heterozygous or homozygous	108	98	Enoxaparin (40 mg/day) + aspirin (100 mg/day)	$p < 0.05$	Live birth rate 83% vs. 68%, $p < 0.05$; miscarriage rate 13% vs. 28%, $p < 0.01$	Yes
RCT	Clark et al.	2010	FVL Prothrombin G20210A	147	143	LMWH (40 mg enoxaparin) + aspirin (75 mg)	-	OR: 0.91 (95% CI: 0.52–1.59)	No
	Karadag et al.	2020	FVL homozygous and heterozygous	61	59	Aspirin (100 mg/day) or LMWH (40 mg enoxaparin) + aspirin (100 mg/day)	$p = 0.843$	Preeclampsia: Group A 13.1%, group B 5.1%, group C 3.7%, $p = 0.042$; Preterm birth: Group A 16.4%, group B 6.8%, group C 5.5%, $p = 0.046$	No
	Quenby et al.	2023	FVL mutation Prothrombin gene mutation (G20210A) Antithrombin deficiency Protein C deficiency Protein S deficiency	164	162	LMWH (unspecified dosages and types: enoxaparin, dalteparin, tinzaparin, and nadroparin)	-	Adjusted OR: 1.08 (95% CI: 0.65–1.78)	No

Contd...

Contd...

Study type	Author	Year	Thrombophilia type	n (Study group)	n (Control group)	Treatment	Live birth P value	RR/OR	Treatment showed benefit?
Meta-analysis	Skeith et al.	2016	FVL Antithrombin deficiency MTHFR Protein C deficiency Protein S deficiency Prothrombin gene mutation	483	-	LMWH (various dosages)	$p = 0.28$	RR = 0.81 (95% CI: 0.55–1.19)	No
	Areia et al.	2016	FVL mutation Prothrombin gene mutation (G20210A) Antithrombin deficiency Protein C deficiency Protein S deficiency MTHFR	107	115	Enoxaparin/ dalteparin/ nadroparin		OR: 1.7 (95% CI: 0.72–4.0)	No
	Liu et al.	2019	Various combination	1034	-	Enoxaparin (various dosages)	$p = 0.17$	RR = 1.06 (95% CI: 0.97–1.16)	No
	Intzes et al.	2020	Various combination	301	341	LMWH (various dosages), 28 patients received LMWH + ASA	$p = 0.001$	OR: 1.65; 95% CI: 1.06–2.56; $p = 0.001$	No
	Fangfei et al.	2020		963	861	LMWH (enoxaparin, dalteparin, tinzaparin—various dosages)	$p < 0.05$	RR = 1.19 (95% CI: 1.03–1.38)	Yes
	Chen et al.	2022	Antithrombin deficiency MTHFR Protein C deficiency FVL mutation Protein S deficiency Prothrombin gene mutation	Various samples	-	LMWH (various dosages)	-	RCT: Pregnancy complications (RR = 0.76; 95% CI: 0.61–0.95; $p = 0.020$) Live birth (RR = 1.12; 95% CI: 0.93–1.34; $p = 0.230$) Cohort: live birth (RR = 1.86; 95% CI: 1.09–3.19; $p = 0.020$) Pregnancy complications (RR = 0.46; 95% CI: 0.31–0.69; $p < 0.001$)	Yes

(ACE: angiotensin-converting enzyme; AT: antithrombin; FVL: factor V Leiden; LMWH: low molecular weight heparin; OR: odds ratio; PAI-1: plasminogen activator inhibitor-1; PC: protein C; PS: protein S; PT: prothrombin; PTGM: prothrombin gene mutation G20210A; RCT: randomized controlled trial; RPL: recurrent pregnancy loss; RR: relative risk)

Prospective Cohort Studies

Several prospective studies have been conducted to determine whether LMWH treatment improves the birth rate of women with RPL and hereditary thrombophilia. Gris et al.'s 2004 landmark prospective study included 160 women with hereditary thrombophilia (FVL, factor II G20210A mutations, or protein S deficiency) who experienced one unexplained miscarriage from the 10th gestational weeks. Before conception, all patients received a daily dose of 5 mg of folic acid. From the 8th week onward, 80 women allocated blindly to aspirin or LMWH group, each group included 80 patients: 80 women received 100 mg of aspirin and 80 others received 40 mg of LMWH (enoxaparin). The results showed that 23 women from the aspirin group (28.8%) and 69 women from the LMWH allocation (86.3%) had live births (OR: 15.5, 95% CI: 7–34, $p = 0.0001$). Thus, LMWH had a superior effect on live births and fetal weight during pregnancy when compared to any group treated with aspirin.[47]

A more recent prospective study by Aracic et al. included 50 women with inherited thrombophilia (FVL, PT G20210A, MTHFR C677T mutation, PAI-1 4G/5G, and ACE insertion/deletion polymorphism) and a history of thrombotic events and/or pregnancy complications such as early and late pregnancy loss in previous pregnancies. In addition to the five major thrombophilia, this study investigated women with rare polymorphisms to understand whether they have different outcomes with respect to RPL after confirming fetal viability, the treatment began within 5–9 weeks. A total of 47 women received dalteparin at a dosage of 2,500 IU/day, while three women who started treatment at another center received enoxaparin at a dosage of 40 mg/day. Between 25 and 28 weeks of pregnancy, the dosage was doubled to 5,000 IU/day for dalteparin and 80 mg/day for enoxaparin. Relative to women with hereditary thrombophilia who are untreated during pregnancy, LMWH significantly decreased the rate of early and late pregnancy losses and improved the rate of term birth relative to prior pregnancies where these women were not treated ($p = 0.001$). LMWH-treated pregnancies resulted in fewer preterm births ($p = 0.019$) and no cases of intrauterine fetal death (IUFD) ($p = 0.0019$). The study also found that the rare thrombophilia (MTHFR, PAI-1, and ACE) did not affect pregnancy outcome differently than conventional thrombophilia (FVL, prothrombin, AT, protein C, and protein S).[48]

Karadag et al. conducted a prospective study to elucidate whether LMWH has different outcomes in women with RPL and hereditary thrombophilia relative to women with RPL without thrombophilia. This study included 108 women with RPL and hereditary thrombophilia (protein C and protein S deficiency, AT III, FVL, prothrombin mutation, and hyperhomocysteinemia) and compared them to 98 women with unexplained RPL. All participants took daily 0.4 mg folic acid until 12th weeks of gestation. The patients who were diagnosed with inherited thrombophilia were given 40 mg/day enoxaparin + 100 mg/day aspirin after determination of pregnancy, while the unexplained groups were not given any treatment. Results indicate that in the thrombophilia group, the live birth rates were significantly higher [90 (83%) vs. 67 (68%) $p < 0.05$] and also the miscarriage rates were significantly lower than in the control group [14 (13%) vs. 27 (28%) $p < 0.01$]. Additionally, even though thrombophilia prophylaxis was administered, there is an increased risk of preeclampsia in patients with RPL.[49] Therefore, LMWH may be more important for treating RPL when there is a hereditary thrombophilia. Furthermore, this study supports the hypothesis that the coagulability associated with hereditary thrombophilia directly contributes to pregnancy loss, since the anticoagulation had such a positive pregnancy outcome in these patients.

Randomized Control Trials

Several significant randomized controlled trials that have been conducted to investigate the efficacy of LMWH treatment. The SPIN study by Clark et al. is one of the first multicenter, randomized controlled trials published on 2010, compared the impact of LMWH versus low-dose aspirin in women with RPL and FVL or prothrombin G20210A mutation. The trial included 294 patients with two or more consecutive pregnancy losses at 24 or fewer weeks of gestation. 147 women were treated with 40 mg enoxaparin subcutaneously and 75 mg aspirin orally once daily and 143 women were left untreated but remained under intensive pregnancy surveillance until 36 weeks of gestation. Of the 147 participants receiving the pharmacological intervention, 32 (22%) pregnancy loss occurred, compared with 29 losses (20%) in the control group (OR: 0.91, 95% CI: 0.52–1.59). Thus, no significant improvement observed with the LMWH treatment. It should be noted, however, that only eight of 289 subjects (2.8%) were identified as heterozygous carriers of

FVL, and only five carriers were randomly assigned to pharmacological intervention. Only two of 288 subjects (0.7%) were heterozygous carriers of the prothrombin G20210A mutation, one for each arm of the study. Therefore, limited conclusions can be drawn regarding the effect of LMWH treatment among heterozygous carriers of FVL.[50]

Karadag et al. conducted a randomized controlled trial involving women with RPL and homozygous and heterozygous FVL mutations. Within a total of 2,764 RPL patients were evaluated for FVL mutation, homozygous, or heterozygous, 174 women randomly distributed to three groups; group A ($n = 61$) administered 100 mg/day aspirin orally, group B ($n = 59$) received 40 mg enoxaparin and 100 mg aspirin daily, and group C ($n = 54$) included patients using only 40 mg enoxaparin daily. Although the live birth rate and miscarriage rate did not differ significantly between the three groups ($p = 0.843$ and $p = 0.694$, respectively), the study demonstrated that the number of preeclamptic patients was significantly higher in group A [A = 8 (13.1%), B = 3 (5.1%), C = 2 (3.7%). $p = 0.042$], and the preterm birth rates were also significantly higher in the only aspirin group [A = 10 (16.4%), B = 4 (6.8%), C = 3 (5.5%), $p = 0.046$].[51] However, the lack of a fourth untreated group renders it difficult to draw any decisive conclusion about the effect of LMWH with or without aspirin on RPL women with FVL mutations.

The ALIFE2 study, a randomized control trial conducted by Quenby et al., is one of the most significant trials published in recent years. An international open-label randomized controlled trial was conducted to assess the impact of LMWH on miscarriage and adverse pregnancy outcomes in women with RPL and inherited thrombophilia. A total of 10,625 women were evaluated for eligibility between August 1, 2012, and January 30, 2021. Of those eligible, 326 conceived and were randomly assigned to two groups: 164 to LMWH and 162 to standard care. All women had an inherited thrombophilia (FVL, prothrombin gene mutation, AT III deficiency, and protein C or protein S deficiency). As part of this study, pregnant women self-administered LMWH once daily, starting as soon as possible after a positive pregnancy test and continuing until labor began. A variety of LMWHs were available, including enoxaparin, dalteparin, tinzaparin, and nadroparin, with doses that were not adjusted for body weight, and the choice of LMWH was left to the discretion of the clinician. Aspirin (150 mg daily) was allowed to pregnant women at risk of preeclampsia after 10 weeks of gestation, but no other antithrombotic medication was advised. Folic acid (400 μg daily) was recommended from before conception until 8 weeks gestation. 116 (72%) of 162 women in the LMWH group and 112 (71%) of 158 in the standard care group had livebirths (adjusted OR: 1.08, 95% CI: 0.65–1.78; absolute risk difference, 0.7%, 95% CI: 9.2–10.6%). 39 (24%) of 164 women in the LMWH group and 37 (23%) of 162 women in the standard care group reported adverse events. The author advises against the use of LMWH in women with RPL and confirmed inherited thrombophilia.[52] While this study is incredibly important to the discussion surrounding treatment for RPL in hereditary thrombophilia, there are some limitations. One important limitation is the lack of stratification based on thrombophilia type, as perhaps treatment improves outcomes in certain thrombophilia more than others.

Meta-analyses

With the introduction of meta-analyses into research, several studies have examined the effect of administering LMWH in various combinations to women with RPL. Some of the meta-analyses have found that LMWH treatment significantly improves pregnancy outcomes, lends to fewer delivery complications, and prevents thrombophilia-related complications.

Skeith et al. conducted a meta-analysis of eight RCTs on patients comparing LMWH with no treatment among women with inherited thrombophilia (FVL, AT deficiency, MTHFR, protein C and protein S deficiency, and prothrombin gene mutation), with prior late (>10 weeks) or recurrent early (<10 weeks) pregnancy loss. The studies in the meta-analysis included 483 and were comprised of various treatment regiments, including enoxaparin, dalteparin, and nadroparin, often combined with aspirin (ASA) at various dosages: Enoxaparin 40 mg or ASA 100 mg for women with one loss at ≥10 weeks, and combinations like dalteparin 5,000 IU and ASA 81 mg, or nadroparin 2,850 IU and ASA 80 mg versus aspirin alone or placebo for women with multiple losses at earlier gestational ages. There was no significant difference in live birth rate with the use of LMWH compared with no treatment (RR: 0.81, 95% CI: 0.55–1.19; $p = 0.28$). It is important to acknowledge that although this meta-analysis did not find a significant beneficial effect of LMWH in preventing pregnancy loss in thrombophilic women with RPL, the limited sample size of women who experienced RPL ($n = 66$) compared to those who experienced a single late-term loss ($n = 308$) may confound the results with respect to the benefit for RPL specifically.[53]

The meta-analysis conducted by Areia et al. explored the ability of LMWH + aspirin versus aspirin alone in pregnant women with hereditary thrombophilia to improve live birth rate. The meta-analysis included four RCTs involving a total of 222 randomized patients. Hereditary thrombophilia was defined as the presence of FVL, MTHFR, prothrombin mutations, or deficiencies of protein C, protein S, or AT III. The thrombophilia group received dalteparin 5,000 IU, nadroparin 2,850 IU or enoxaparin 40 mg with 80–100 mg aspirin. The results showed no significant differences in birth weight and other pregnancy outcomes between LMWH + aspirin versus aspirin alone [live births (OR: 1.7, 95% CI: 0.72–4.0), first trimester miscarriages [OR: 0.69 (0.22–2.16)], prematurity [OR: 0.99 (0.4–2.08)], preeclampsia [OR: 1.49 (0.63–3.5)], and small for gestational age babies [OR: 2.08 (0.96–4.47)].[54]

A systematic review and meta-analysis were conducted by Liu et al. in order to explore the effect of enoxaparin versus placebo on RPL. Searches were performed for articles published up to 2019.[55] The meta-analysis included six RCTs involving a total of 1,034 patients. The results indicated that enoxaparin did not have a significant effect compared to the control group on live birth rate (RR: 1.06; 95% CI: 0.97–1.16; $p = 0.17$) or miscarriage rate (RR: 0.71; 95% CI: 0.45–1.10; $p = 0.13$) in addition to other pregnancy outcomes that showed no significant improvement with the use of LMWH. It is worth noting that this meta-analysis included studies investigating women with both unexplained RPL and those with hereditary thrombophilia and RPL, which may affect the accuracy of the results specifically for women with hereditary thrombophilia and RPL.

The same conclusion derived from another meta-analysis by Intzes et al. examined the use of prophylactic antithrombotic therapy in women suffering from RPL. This analysis included 2,298 patients and compared RPL women with or without inherited thrombophilia who received LMWH treatment versus those who did not. The meta-analysis incorporated 12 RCTs involving 642 patients, with various inherited thrombophilia (301 in the treatment group and 341 in the control group). The treatment regimens were diverse; some studies compared treatment with enoxaparin 40 mg + 5 mg folic acid daily for 8 weeks versus control regimen of 5 mg folic acid and 100 mg aspirin for the same duration. Other studies utilized dalteparin 5,000 IU daily up to 24 weeks with controls receiving no dalteparin, and another used nadroparin 2,850 IU with 80 mg aspirin daily for <6 weeks compared to aspirin or placebo until 36 weeks. The total population analysis found that LMWH treatment was significantly effective (OR: 1.65; 95% CI: 1.06–2.56; $p = 0.001$; heterogeneity $I^2 = 77\%$, $p = 0.03$), though an OR of 1.65 does not allow for a definitive clinical recommendation. Additionally, due to high heterogeneity and significance, the statistical assessment is weakened. Quality assessments and subgroup statistical analyses indicated that LMWH treatment did not provide a benefit in live birth rates, with high heterogeneity present in the studies (OR: 2.09; 95% CI: 0.58–7.57; $p = 0.26$; $I^2 = 86\%$, $p = 0.0001$).[56]

A meta-analysis by Fangfei et al. examined the effects of LMWH treatment (enoxaparin, dalteparin, and tinzaparin) on 963 patients with RPL compared to 861 women in a control group (no treatment?). (What type of studies were included in the meta-analysis?). A higher rate of live births was observed in the LMWH group (RR: 1.19; 95% CI: 1.03–1.38; $p = 0.02$) as well as a lower rate of miscarriages (RR: 0.62; 95% CI: 0.43–0.91; $p = 0.01$). Women receiving LMWH, however, were more likely to experience adverse reactions at the injection site. No significant effects were observed on fetal weight, gestational age, thrombocytopenia, bleeding, or preeclampsia. The analyses included different LMWH products administered at different dosages, complicating the precision of treatment and dosing recommendations. Furthermore, the patients included in the studies had varying characteristics, including varying ages, treatment initiation times, and medical histories.[57]

Chen et al. conducted a meta-analysis of literature published until September 2020, encompassing 10 randomized controlled trials and 12 cohort studies, which included retrospective and prospective cohort studies, to examine women with RPL and hereditary thrombophilia. This condition includes AT III deficiency, MTHFR, protein C and protein S deficiency, FVL mutation, and prothrombin gene mutation. The analysis of RCTs included various dosages and types of LMWH with or without aspirin. Some studies investigated the effect of enoxaparin (40 mg/day) alone or combined with aspirin (75–100 mg) versus aspirin alone. Others compared dalteparin (5,000 IU) with or without aspirin (80 mg) versus no treatment or aspirin alone (80 mg). Two studies investigated nadroparin, one with 3,800 IU and no treatment for the control group, and another with 2,850 IU plus 80 mg aspirin. In the analysis of the RCTs, a statistically significant reduction in pregnancy complications was found (RR: 0.76; 95% CI: 0.61–0.95; $p = 0.020$), while no significant increase was observed in live birth rates (RR: 1.12; 95% CI: 0.93–1.34; $p = 0.230$). In the cohort studies, the treatments varied between enoxaparin 40–80 mg/day, dalteparin 2,500–5,000 IU/kg, and nadroparin. Some studies treated the groups with different combinations with or without aspirin. While most of the control groups received no treatment, some were treated with LMWH + ASA or ASA alone. A significant increase in live birth rates was detected (RR: 1.86; 95% CI: 1.09–3.19; $p = 0.020$), along with a notable decrease in pregnancy complications (RR: 0.46; 95% CI: 0.31–0.69; $p < 0.001$).[58]

Unfortunately, the literature examining treatment outcomes of women with inherited thrombophilia experiencing RPL does not provide clear, definitive answers. Some literature supports the hypothesis that treatment with LMWH lowers the risk of RPL, while other studies found no improvement in this specific parameter.

CONCLUSION

This literature review consolidates the latest research to understand the correlation between hereditary thrombophilia and RPL to elucidate the need for screening and treatment of these conditions. 20 studies analyze the relationship between hereditary thrombophilia and RPL and 41 studies explore treatment outcomes of LMWH, ASA, or both. Synthesis of these studies highlight the importance of screening for FVL and prothrombin gene mutations, as well as the possible importance of protein C and S deficiencies, as these mutations have been shown to be associated with RPL. Additionally, these conditions lend to hypercoagulability that is increased dramatically during pregnancies, elevating risk for VTEs, and cerebrovascular accidents (CVAs). Treatment of these women with LMWH is therefore advised to prevent these adverse effects. As such, screening for inherited thrombophilia to ensure timely treatment is crucial. However, the specific ability of this treatment to prevent RPL in hereditary thrombophilia has remained inconclusive.

REFERENCES

1. Versteeg HH, Heemskerk JWM, Levi M, Reitsma PH. New Fundamentals in hemostasis. Physiol Rev. 2013;93(1):327-58.
2. Kumar V, Abbas AK, Aster JC (Eds). Robbins Basic Pathology. Philadelphia, PA: Elsevier; 2013. pp. 101-9.
3. Wolberg AS, Rosendaal FR, Weitz JI, Jaffer IH, Agnelli G, Baglin T, et al. Venous thrombosis. Nat Rev Dis Primers. 2015;1:15006.
4. Rosendaal FR. Venous thrombosis: a multicausal disease. Lancet. 1999;353(9159):1167-73.
5. Kahn SR, Comerota AJ, Cushman M, Evans NS, Ginsberg JS, Goldenberg NA, et al. The postthrombotic syndrome: evidence-based prevention, diagnosis, and treatment strategies: a scientific statement from the American Heart Association. Circulation. 2014;130(18):1636-61. Erratum in: Circulation. 2015;131(8):e359.
6. De Stefano V, Finazzi G, Mannucci PM. Inherited thrombophilia: pathogenesis, clinical syndromes, and management. Blood. 1996;87(9):3531-44.
7. Middeldorp S. Inherited thrombophilia: a double-edged sword. Hematology Am Soc Hematol Educ Program. 2016;2016(1):1-9.
8. Lane DA, Mannucci PM, Bauer KA, Bertina RM, Bochkov NP, Boulyjenkov V, et al. Inherited thrombophilia: Part 1. Thromb Haemost. 1996;76(5):651-62.
9. Stevens SM, Woller SC, Bauer KA, Kasthuri R, Cushman M, Streiff M, et al. Guidance for the evaluation and treatment of hereditary and acquired thrombophilia. J Thromb Thrombolysis. 2016;41(1):154-64.
10. Egeberg O. Inherited antithrombin deficiency causing thrombophilia. Thromb Diath Haemorrh. 1965;13:516-30.
11. Den Heijer M, Lewington S, Clarke R. Homocysteine, MTHFR and risk of venous thrombosis: a meta-analysis of published epidemiological studies. Thromb Haemost. 2005;3(2):292-9.
12. Kujovich JL. Factor V Leiden thrombophilia. Genet Med. 2011;13(1):1-16.
13. Kadauke S, Khor B, Van Cott EM. Activated protein C resistance testing for factor V Leiden. Am J Hematol. 2014;89(12):1147-50.
14. Meeks SL, Abshire TC. Abnormalities of prothrombin: a review of the pathophysiology, diagnosis, and treatment. Haemophilia. 2008;14(6):1159-63.
15. Bertina RM. Elevated Clotting Factor Levels and Venous Thrombosis. Pathophysiol Haemost Thromb. 2003;33(5-6):395-400.
16. Dziadosz M, Baxi LV. Global prevalence of prothrombin gene mutation G20210A and implications in women's health: A systematic review. Blood Coagul Fibrinolysis. 2016;27(5):481-9.
17. Dykes AC, Walker ID, McMahon AD, Islam SIAM, Tait RC. A study of Protein S antigen levels in 3788 healthy volunteers: influence of age, sex and hormone use, and estimate for prevalence of deficiency state. Br J Haematol. 2001;113(3):636-41.
18. Bezemer ID, Doggen CJM, Vos HL, Rosendaal FR. No Association Between the Common MTHFR 677C→T

Polymorphism and Venous Thrombosis: Results From the MEGA Study. Arch Intern Med. 2007;167(5):497-501.
19. Moll S, Varga EA. Homocysteine and MTHFR Mutations. Circulation. 2015;132(1):e6-9.
20. Liew SC, Gupta ED. Methylenetetrahydrofolate reductase (MTHFR) C677T polymorphism: epidemiology, metabolism and the associated diseases. Eur J Med Genet. 2015;58(1):1-10.
21. ESHRE Guideline Group on RPL; Bender Atik R, Christiansen OB, Elson J, Kolte AM, Lewis S, et al. ESHRE guideline: recurrent pregnancy loss: an update in 2022. Hum Reprod Open. 2023;2023(1):hoad002.
22. Thornton P, Douglas J. Coagulation in pregnancy. Best Pract Res Clin Obstet Gynaecol. 2010;24(3):339-52.
23. Bremme KA. Haemostatic changes in pregnancy. Best Pract Res Clin Haematol. 2003;16(2):153-68.
24. Robertson L, Wu O, Langhorne P, Twaddle S, Clark P, Lowe GD, et al. Thrombophilia in pregnancy: a systematic review. Br J Haematol. 2006;132(2):171-96.
25. Sarig G, Vidergor G, Brenner B. Assessment and management of high-risk pregnancies in women with thrombophilia. Blood Rev. 2009;23(4):143-7.
26. Kovalevsky G, Gracia CR, Berlin JA, Sammel MD, Barnhart KT. Evaluation of the association between hereditary thrombophilias and recurrent pregnancy loss: a meta-analysis. Arch Intern Med. 2004;164(5):558-63.
27. Hamedi B, Feulefack J, Khan A, Sergi C. Association between factor V Leiden mutation and recurrent pregnancy loss in the middle east countries: a Newcastle-Ottawa meta-analysis. Arch Gynecol Obstet. 2020;302(2):345-54.
28. Liu X, Chen Y, Ye C, Xing D, Wu R, Li F, et al. Hereditary thrombophilia and recurrent pregnancy loss: a systematic review and meta-analysis. Hum Reprod. 2021;36(5):1213-29.
29. Turki RF, Assidi M, Banni HA, Zahed HA, Karim S, Schulten HJ, et al. Associations of recurrent miscarriages with chromosomal abnormalities, thrombophilia allelic polymorphisms and/or consanguinity in Saudi Arabia. BMC Med Genet. 2016;17(Suppl 1):69.
30. Iordache O, Anastasiu-Popov DM, Anastasiu DM, Craina M, Dahma G, Sacarin G, et al. A Retrospective Assessment of Thrombophilia in Pregnant Women with First and Second Trimester Pregnancy Loss. Int J Environ Res Public Health. 2022;19(24):16500.
31. Brenner B, Mandel H, Lanir N, Younis J, Rothbart H, Ohel G, et al. Activated protein C resistance can be associated with recurrent fetal loss. Br J Haematol. 1997;97(3):551-4.
32. Mitic G, Kovac M, Povazan L, Magic Z, Djordjevic V, Salatic I, et al. Inherited thrombophilia is associated with pregnancy losses that occur after 12th gestational week in Serbian population. Clin Appl Thromb Hemost. 2010;16(4):435-9.
33. Cernera G, Liguori R, Bruzzese D, Castaldo G, De Placido G, Conforti A, et al. The relevance of prothrombotic genetic variants in women who experienced pregnancy loss or embryo implantation failure: A retrospective analysis of 1922 cases. Int J Gynaecol Obstet. 2024;165(1):148-54.
34. Santoro R, Iannaccaro P, Sottilotta G. Mutazioni protrombotiche in donne con aborto ricorrente e morte fetale intrauterina [Prothrombotic gene mutations in women with recurrent abortions and intrauterine fetal death]. Minerva Ginecol. 2005;57(4):447-50.
35. Sottilotta G, Oriana V, Latella C, Luise F, Piromalli A, Ramirez F, et al. Genetic prothrombotic risk factors in women with unexplained pregnancy loss. Thromb Res. 2006;117(6):681-4.
36. Karata S, Aydin Y, Ocer F, Buyru A, Balci H. Hereditary Thrombophilia, Anti-Beta2 Glycoprotein 1 IgM, and Anti-Annexin V Antibodies in Recurrent Pregnancy Loss. Am J Reprod Immunol. 2012;67(3):251-5.
37. Baumann K, Beuter-Winkler P, Hackethal A, Strowitzki T, Toth B, Bohlmann MK. Maternal Factor V Leiden and Prothrombin Mutations Do Not Seem to Contribute to the Occurrence of Two or More Than Two Consecutive Miscarriages in Caucasian patients. Am J Reprod Immunol. 2013;70(6):518-21.
38. Perés Wingeyer S, Aranda F, Udry S, Latino J, de Larrañaga G. Inherited thrombophilia and pregnancy loss. Study of an Argentinian cohort. Med Clin (Barc). 2019;152(7):249-54.
39. Ahangari N, Doosti M, Mousavifar N, Attaran M, Shahrokhzadeh S, Memarpour S, et al. Hereditary thrombophilia genetic variants in recurrent pregnancy loss. Arch Gynecol Obstet. 2019;300(3):777-82.
40. Shehata H, Ali A, Silva-Edge M, Haroon S, Elfituri A, Viswanatha R, et al. Thrombophilia screening in women with recurrent first trimester miscarriage: is it time to stop testing? - a cohort study and systematic review of the literature. BMJ Open. 2022;12(7):e059519.
41. Lund M, Nielsen HS, Hviid TV, Steffensen R, Nyboe Andersen A, Christiansen OB. Hereditary thrombophilia and recurrent pregnancy loss: a retrospective cohort study of pregnancy outcome and obstetric complications. Hum Reprod. 2010;25(12):2978-84.
42. Gao H, Tao FB. Prothrombin G20210A mutation is associated with recurrent pregnancy loss: A systematic review and meta-analysis update. Thromb Res. 2015;135(2):339-46.
43. Neki R, Miyata T, Fujita T, Kokame K, Fujita D, Isaka S, et al. Nonsynonymous mutations in three anticoagulant genes in Japanese patients with adverse pregnancy outcomes. Thromb Res. 2014;133(5):914-8.
44. Mutlu I, Mutlu MF, Biri A, Bulut B, Erdem M, Erdem A. Effects of anticoagulant therapy on pregnancy outcomes in patients with thrombophilia and previous poor obstetric history. Blood Coagul Fibrinolysis. 2015;26(3):267-73.
45. Aynioglu O, Işik H, Sahbaz A, Alptekin H, Bayar U. Does anticoagulant therapy improve adverse pregnancy outcomes in patients with history of recurrent pregnancy loss? Ginekol Pol. 2016;87(8):585-90.
46. Clavijo MM, Mahuad CV, Reparaz M de los AV, Aizpurua MF, Ventura A, Casali CE. Risk factors and role of low molecular

weight heparin in obstetric complications among women with inherited thrombophilia—a cohort study. Hematol Transfus Cell Ther. 2019;41(4):303-9.

47. Gris JC, Mercier E, Quéré I, Lavigne-Lissalde G, Cochery-Nouvellon E, Hoffet M, et al. Low-molecular-weight heparin versus low-dose aspirin in women with one fetal loss and a constitutional thrombophilic disorder. Blood. 2004;103(10):3695-9.
48. Aracic N, Roje D, Drmic Hofman I, Capkun V, Stefanovic V. Low molecular weight heparin treatment and impact of inherited thrombophilia type in pregnancies with previous adverse outcome. J Matern Fetal Neonatal Med. 2015;28(3):306-10.
49. Karadağ C, Yoldemir T, Karadağ SD, İnan C, Dolgun ZN, Aslanova L. Obstetric outcomes of recurrent pregnancy loss patients diagnosed with inherited thrombophilia. Ir J Med Sci. 2017;186(3):707-13.
50. Clark P, Walker ID, Langhorne P, Crichton L, Thomson A, Greaves M, et al. SPIN (Scottish Pregnancy Intervention) study: a multicenter, randomized controlled trial of low-molecular-weight heparin and low-dose aspirin in women with recurrent miscarriage. Blood. 2010;115(21): 4162-7.
51. Karadağ C, Akar B, Gönenç G, Aslancan R, Yılmaz N, Çalışkan E. Aspirin, low molecular weight heparin, or both in preventing pregnancy complications in women with recurrent pregnancy loss and factor V Leiden mutation. J Matern Fetal Neonatal Med. 2020;33(11):1934-9.
52. Quenby S, Booth K, Hiller L, Coomarasamy A, de Jong PG, Hamulyák EN, et al. Heparin for women with recurrent miscarriage and inherited thrombophilia (ALIFE2): an international open-label, randomised controlled trial. Lancet. 2023;402(10395):54-61.
53. Skeith L, Carrier M, Kaaja R, Martinelli I, Petroff D, Schleußner E, et al. A meta-analysis of low-molecular-weight heparin to prevent pregnancy loss in women with inherited thrombophilia. Blood. 2016;127(13):1650-5.
54. Areia AL, Fonseca E, Areia M, Moura P. Low-molecular-weight heparin plus aspirin versus aspirin alone in pregnant women with hereditary thrombophilia to improve live birth rate: meta-analysis of randomized controlled trials. Arch Gynecol Obstet. 2016;293(1):81-6.
55. Liu Y, Shan N, Yuan Y, Tan B, Che P, Qi H. The efficacy of enoxaparin for recurrent abortion: a meta-analysis of randomized controlled studies. J Matern Fetal Neonatal Med. 2021;34(3):473-8.
56. Intzes S, Symeonidou M, Zagoridis K, Stamou M, Spanoudaki A, Spanoudakis E. Hold your needles in women with recurrent pregnancy losses with or without hereditary thrombophilia: Meta-analysis and review of the literature. J Gynecol Obstet Hum Reprod. 2021;50(4):101935.
57. Jiang F, Hu X, Jiang K, Pi H, He Q, Chen X. The role of low molecular weight heparin on recurrent pregnancy loss: A systematic review and meta-analysis. Taiwan J Obstet Gynecol. 2021;60(1):1-8.
58. Chen Y, Wang T, Liu X, Ye C, Xing D, Wu R, et al. Low molecular weight heparin and pregnancy outcomes in women with inherited thrombophilia: A systematic review and meta-analysis. J Obstet Gynaecol Res. 2022;48(8):2134-50.

CHAPTER

29

Thromboelastography

Manju Puri, Jyoti Mishra

ABSTRACT

Thromboelastography is a bedside test that will measure the time taken for a clot to form, the tensile strength of the clot formed and the clot lysis time. It can detect subtle disorders of the coagulation cascade that can result from gene polymorphism in thrombophilia genes and also plasminogen activator inhibitor genes. It is a very economical bedside test. Performing this test in unexplained recurrent pregnancy loss (RPL) may help us decide which patients will benefit with low molecular weight heparin therapy.

Keywords: Thromboelastography, Unexplained RPL, Plasminogen activator inhibitor, Clot lysis, Clot tensile strength, ROTEM.

INTRODUCTION

Thromboelastography (TEG) is a noninvasive test that quantitatively estimates the dynamic changes during clot formation. It is a viscoelastic test for global assessment of hemostasis. It is an efficient method of assessing thrombosis and overcomes the limitation of conventional methods by providing information on both cellular (platelets) and plasmatic (coagulation factors) components. It basically measures the viscoelastic properties of whole blood as it clots providing comprehensive information on the process of clot formation including clot strength and fibrinolysis. It is a bedside, point of care test that can provide rapid results within 30–60 minutes.[1,2] Meaningful information can be obtained within 10 minutes of initiating the test when maximum clot firmness is reached.[3] Many patients of hitherto unexplained recurrent pregnancy loss (uRPL) may have subtle clotting defects and/or clot lysis defects that are not diagnosed with conventional coagulation test panels. It is proposed that including TEG in their workup will be useful in identifying women that may benefit with anticoagulant therapy.

HISTORY

Thromboelastography was developed by Dr Hellmut Hartert at the University of Heidelberg in Germany in 1948.[4] TEG was first used clinically in Vietnam war in 1980s to guide blood transfusions in wounded soldiers.[2] Later, its application was found beneficial in patients undergoing liver transplant and cardiac surgery.[3,5] It is now used in patients undergoing major blood loss due to trauma, surgery, or childbirth to optimize replacement of blood and blood components.[2,6-8] Recently, a modified version rapid TEG (rTEG) is proposed which is said to be a more refined version of TEG to guide blood transfusion.[9] It is performed on noncitrated whole fresh blood samples within 4 minutes of sampling. TEG has proven to be a robust method and is cost-effective as compared to other conventional blood tests.[5] However, it requires daily standardization.

PROCEDURE

The protocol of TEG involves simple steps that start with placing the blood sample into an oscillating cup at 37°C followed with suspending a pin from the torsion wire into the sample cup. Further, the motion of the cup is coupled to the pin because of fibrin strand formation. This coupling is directly proportional to the clot strength. There is an electromagnetic transducer which detects the increased tension in the wire and generates an electrical signal that is amplified to create a trace, which is displayed on the computer screen and is proportional to the clot strength. The coagulation pathway is depicted in **Figure 1**.[10]

As the blood coagulates, it begins to adhere to the cup and the pin. The movement of the cup induces motion on the pin. The gradually increasing viscoelastic mechanical properties of the blood reflect the development of the three-dimensional fibrin mesh and platelet components of the clot. The greater the viscoelasticity of the clot, the

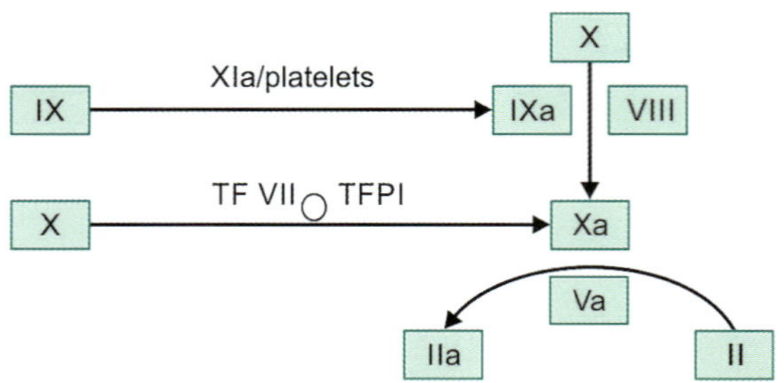

Fig. 1: Coagulation Pathway. (TF: tissue factor (factor III); TFPI: tissue factor pathway inhibitor; II: prothrombin; IIa: thrombin; VII: clotting factor 7; VIII: clotting factor 8; IX: clotting factor 9; X: clotting factor 10 prothrombin; Xa: thrombin; XIa: activated clotting factor 11)

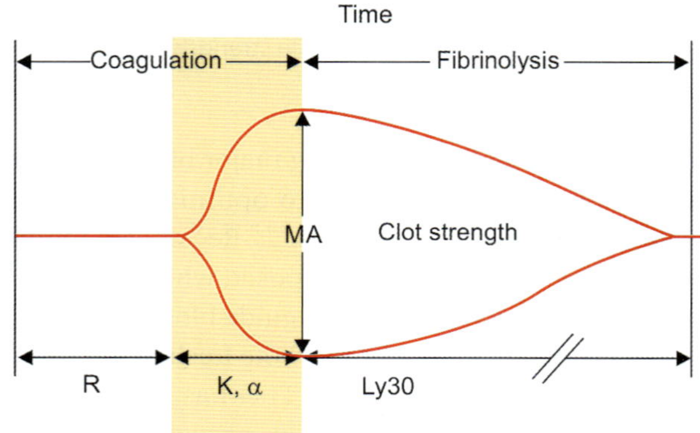

Fig. 2: Normal waveforms obtained in thromboelastography (TEG).

higher the amplitude of the pin motion. As fibrinolysis starts, the clot begins to dissolve gradually, and the clot loses its contact with the detection pin, which has less induced motion. The graphical image of the amplitude of movement of the pin as a function of time is recorded as a thromboelastogram. These changes are then quantified by software. The various measurements recorded in TEG are as follows **(Fig. 2)**.

- R is the reaction time that is time of start to formation of clot to 2 mm clot. It reflects clot initiation that is the time from activation of coagulation cascade to generate thrombin and fibrin.
- K and α angle reflect kinetics of clot formation, K is the time from clot initiation 2 mm to maximum amplitude (MA) 20 mm and α angle is a tangent line joining the R (2 mm) to MA (20 mm). The maximum amplitude (MA) reflects the maximum clot strength.
- LY30 is the percentage of clot lysis 30 minutes after MA is reached and reflects clot stability and breakdown.

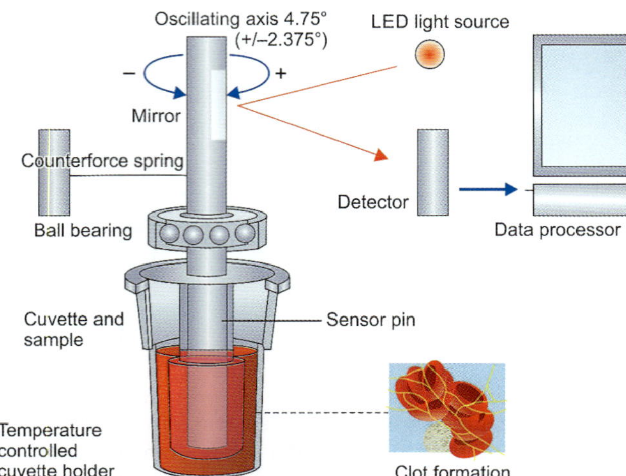

Fig. 3: Rotational thromboelastography (ROTEM).

An adaptation of TEG is rotational thromboelastography (ROTEM) **(Fig. 3)**. In this, the cup remains stationary but the pin rotates. The results are like TEG. In hypercoagulable states, the R time shortens and viscoelasticity of the clot increases.

ROLE OF THROMBOELASTOGRAPHY IN RECURRENT PREGNANCY LOSS

The etiology of recurrent pregnancy loss remains unexplained in >50% of cases. A modest association of recurrent pregnancy loss with inherited thrombophilia has been suggested in literature but is contradictory due to heterogeneity in the studies as regards definition of RPL, types of RPL, and geographic variations.[11]

Prothrombotic state is associated with an increased trophoblast apoptosis and impaired trophoblast invasion.

Hypercoagulation affects the blood flow to the uterus and placenta and may lead to the formation of microthrombi, or even placental infarction, resulting in insufficient blood supply to the placenta, ischemia, and hypoxia of the embryo or fetus, embryo- or fetal dysplasia, and abortion.[11]

There is lack of evidence of a causal association between inherited thrombophilia and RPL and the beneficial effect of administration of anticoagulants to such patients for improving pregnancy outcomes. The role of screening and treatment of RPL patients with anticoagulants like low-molecular-weight heparin (LMWH) has been controversial.[12] Logically, there could be a subset of prothrombotic patients with decidual vasculopathy and placental thrombosis who may benefit

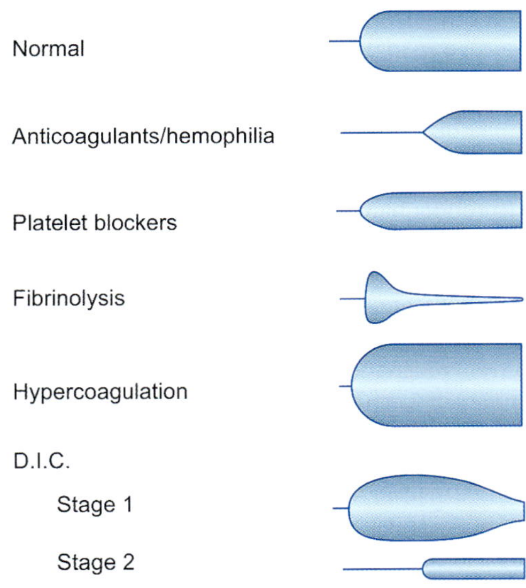

Fig. 4: Pathological waveforms.

from anticoagulant therapy. The challenge is to identify those. Thromboelastogram can identify abnormalities in coagulation by monitoring the whole process of coagulation and fibrinolysis **(Fig. 4)**.[5]

Many workers have studied the role of TEG in the assessment of prothrombotic tendency in women with uRPL **(Fig. 3)**[13] Rai et al.,[14] in his study, estimated the maximum amplitude, i.e., the measure of clot strength which reflects the degree of fibrinolysis in women who had three or more consecutive miscarriages at <12 weeks gestation. The maximum amplitude (MA) was found to be 66 mm versus 61.5 mm among cases and controls, respectively. The rate of clot lysis, i.e., LY30 determining the percentage decrease in amplitude at 30 minutes was found to be 2.5% versus 4.9% among cases and controls, respectively. Further, the study revealed that an MA value of 64 or above (via TEG) was found to be a predictor of miscarriage. The study also revealed a prepregnancy MA of >64 mm having a sensitivity of 68% and specificity of 82% to predict miscarriage.

Another study by Yao H et al. reported that MA and α values were significantly increased in women with RPL compared to controls while R and K were significantly lower. Further, MA and α values increased with the number of abortions. α value reflects the rate of blood clot formation and reinforcement in vivo, while MA value reflects the function of platelet aggregation hence suggesting prothrombotic tendency.[15]

The advantage of TEG over conventional tests for hemostasis is that conventional tests do not consider the dynamic in vivo process of hemostasis involving the interaction between the coagulation and fibrinolytic factors with platelets. TEG is a test for whole blood hemostasis and possibly has the potential of identifying women with hemostatic abnormalities not detected by conventional tests with resultant prothrombotic state. This can then help selection of a subset of women with unexplained RPL likely to benefit from anticoagulant treatment in the form of aspirin or LMWH by facilitating implantation and placentation.[16,17] TEG has proven to be useful for predicting risk of morbidity and in differentiation of physiologic hypercoagulable state (pregnancy) from pathological.[18]

Abnormalities of the clot lysing system may also lead to RPL by allowing the persistence of microthrombi that may routinely form in the placental microcirculation. The clot lysing enzyme is plasmin which is derived from the inactive proenzyme plasminogen. Plasmin breaks down the fibrin clot to fibrinogen degradation products (FDPs). Plasminogen activator inhibitor 1 (PAI-1) inhibits the conversion of plasminogen to plasmin. Mutations or aberrant expression of *PAI-1* genes may alter the clot lysis dynamics and is associated with RPL.[19] A recent meta-analysis has concluded that PAI-1 4G/5G polymorphism with an [odds ratio (OR): 2.57; 95% confidential interval (CI): 1.69–3.90).[20] PAI-1 levels can be assayed in maternal blood by an enzyme-linked immunosorbent assay (ELISA) assay. However, TEG has been found useful in diagnosis and management of cases with PAI-1 polymorphism and deficiency.[21]

There are few limitations to TEG as it requires daily calibration as compared to other conventional tests and needs to be done by trained personnel. Moreover, many technical variations have been reported about this procedure and the results obtained.[22] The results of TEG are also affected by age, gender, and alcohol consumption. More studies are required to explore the place of TEG in evaluation of patients with recurrent pregnancy loss.

CONCLUSION

Thromboelastography has not received due attention in the field of obstetrics & gynecology. Pregnancy being a thrombogenic environment, we encounter adverse pregnancy outcomes, which could be thrombogenic in etiology, but are not diagnosed by standard thrombophilia screening. A simple clot assay will guide the practitioner if thrombolytic therapy will be indicated during pregnancy.

REFERENCES

1. Vig S, Chitolie A, Bevan DH, Halliday A, Dormandy J. Thromboelastography: a reliable test? Blood Coagul Fibrinolysis. 2001;12(7):555-61.
2. Perry DJ, Fitzmaurice DA, Kitchen S, Mackie IJ, Mallett S. Point-of-care testing in haemostasis. Br J Haematol. 2010;150(5):501-14.
3. Doran CM, Woolley T, Midwinter MJ. Feasibility of using rotational thromboelastometry to assess coagulation status of combat casualties in a deployed setting. J Trauma. 2010;69(1):40-8.
4. HARTERT H. Blood clotting studies with Thrombus stressography; a new Investigation procedure. Klin Wochenschr. 1948;26(37-38):577-83.
5. Salooja N, Perry DJ. Thrombelastography. Blood Coagul Fibrinolysis. 2001;12(5):327-37.
6. Plotkin AJ, Wade CE, Jenkins DH, Smith KA, Noe JC, Park MS, et al. A reduction in clot formation rate and strength assessed by thrombelastography is indicative of transfusion requirements in patients with penetrating injuries. J Trauma. 2008;64(2 Suppl):S64-8.
7. Schöchl H, Frietsch T, Pavelka M, Jámbor C. Hyperfibrinolysis after major trauma: differential diagnosis of lysis patterns and prognostic value of thrombelastometry. J Trauma. 2009;67(1):125-31.
8. Ganter MT, Hofer CK. Coagulation monitoring: current techniques and clinical use of viscoelastic point-of-care coagulation devices. Anesth Analg. 2008;106(5):1366-75.
9. Kashuk JL, Moore EE, Le T, Lawrence J, Pezold M, Johnson JL, et al. Noncitrated whole blood is optimal for evaluation of postinjury coagulopathy with point-of-care rapid thrombelastography. J Surg Res. 2009;156(1):133-8.
10. Thakur M, Ahmed AB. A Review of Thromboelastography. Int J Periop Ultrasound Appl Technol. 2012;1(1): 25-9.
11. Liu X, Chen Y, Ye C, Xing D, Wu R, Li F, et al. Hereditary thrombophilia, and recurrent pregnancy loss: a systematic review and meta-analysis. Hum Reprod. 2021;36(5):1213-29.
12. Quenby S, Booth K, Hiller L, Coomarasamy A, de Jong PG, Hamulyák EN, et al. Heparin for women with recurrent miscarriage and inherited thrombophilia (ALIFE2): an international open-label, randomised controlled trial. Lancet. 2023;402(10395):54-61.
13. Rai R, Shlebak A, Cohen H, Backos M, Holmes Z, Marriott K, et al. Factor V Leiden and acquired activated protein C resistance among 1000 women with recurrent miscarriage. Hum Reprod. 2001;16(5):961-5.
14. Rai R, Tuddenham E, Backos M, Jivraj S, El'Gaddal S, Choy S, et al. Thromboelastography, whole-blood haemostasis and recurrent miscarriage. Hum Reprod. 2003;18(12):2540-3.
15. Yao H, Ji Y, Zhou Y. Analysis of blood coagulation indexes, thromboelastogram and autoantibodies in patients with recurrent pregnancy loss. Pak J Med Sci. 2022;38(7):2005-10.
16. Oberkersch R, Attorresi AI, Calabrese GC. Low-molecular-weight heparin inhibition in classical complement activation pathway during pregnancy. Thromb Res. 2010;125(5):e240-5.
17. Di Simone N, Di Nicuolo F, Sanguinetti M, Ferrazzani S, D'Alessio MC, Castellani R, et al. Low-molecular weight heparin induces in vitro trophoblast invasiveness: role of matrix metalloproteinases and tissue inhibitors. Placenta. 2007;28(4):298-304.
18. Hobson AR, Agarwala RA, Swallow RA, Dawkins KD, Curzen NP. Thrombelastography: current clinical applications and its potential role in interventional cardiology. Platelets. 2006;17(8):509-18.
19. Zhai J, Li Z, Zhou Y, Yang X. The role of plasminogen activator inhibitor-1 in gynecological and obstetrical diseases: An update review. J Reprod Immunol. 2022;150:103490.
20. Maghsudlu M, Noroozi Z, Zokaei E, Motevaseli E. Systematic review and meta-analysis of association between plasminogen activator inhibitor-1 4G/5G polymorphism and recurrent pregnancy loss: an update. Thromb J. 2024;22(1):44.
21. Prabhakaran N, Laziuk K, Hammer RD. The utility of thromboelastography and tranexamic acid in plasminogen activator inhibitor deficiency during pregnancy: a rare case report. Blood Coagul Fibrinolysis. 2020;31(1):87-91.
22. Scarpelini S, Rhind SG, Nascimento B, Tien H, Shek PN, Peng HT, et al. Normal range values for thromboelastography in healthy adult volunteers. Braz J Med Biol Res. 2009;42(12):1210-7.

CHAPTER 30

Thyroid Disorders

Matthew George Apostolou, Vageesh Ayyar D, Ahmed Shelbaia

ABSTRACT

Thyroid dysfunction is associated with poor pregnancy outcome and fetal neurodevelopmental issues. Screening for thyroid disorders is preferable in the prepregnancy period or at first antenatal visit. In patients of recurrent pregnancy loss (RPL), it is mandatory to screen for both thyroid function test as well as antithyroid antibodies. Treatment of both clinical and subclinical hypothyroidism is recommended in the reproductive age group. Monitoring of thyroid function is recommended in each trimester of pregnancy for good outcome. Hyperthyroidism, though rare, is also associated with poor pregnancy outcome and requires treatment.

Keywords: Thyroid dysfunction, Subclinical hypothyroidism, Thyroid autoimmunity TPOAb, Hyperthyroidism, Universal screening of thyroid function test.

INTRODUCTION

A miscarriage is the spontaneous loss of a pregnancy in utero before the fetus reaches viability. This definition is valid in the UK up until 23 weeks and 6 days of pregnancy, keeping in mind that with the recent advances in neonatal care, more babies can survive before 24 weeks of gestation. Sporadic and recurrent miscarriages are the two main groups; the former usually happen during the first trimester.[1] Approximately half of miscarriages in the first 10 weeks of pregnancy are caused by random numerical chromosomal errors, such as trisomy, monosomy, or polypoidy.[2,3] Its incidence increases with age and may affect between 10 and 50% of women aged 20–45 years, respectively.[1,3] On the other hand, recurrent miscarriage or recurrent pregnancy loss (RPL) has been traditionally defined as three or more miscarriages and it affects only 1–3% of women.[4] For women who miscarry in the second trimester, where random fetal chromosomal abnormalities are far less common, the frequency is likewise around 1%.[5]

There are significant differences in terms and definitions used in reference to recurrent miscarriage. The American Society for Reproductive Medicine (ASRM) defines RPL as two or more clinical pregnancy losses.[6] The European Society of Human Reproduction and Embryology (ESHRE) defines RPL as two or more pregnancy losses at any gestational age with the exclusion of ectopic and molar pregnancies.[4] While the Royal College of Obstetricians and Gynaecologists (RCOG), in their previous Green-top Guideline published in 2011, defines RPL as the three or more consecutive first trimester miscarriages, the latest RCOG guideline published in 2023 states the miscarriages do not necessarily have to be consecutive to be defined as recurrent miscarriage, owing to the fact that the incidence of certain diagnoses does not appear to differ between women with consecutive versus nonconsecutive losses.[1]

Thyroid hormones are important for reproduction, maintaining successful pregnancy and normal fetal development, especially the neurological development. Thyroid disorders are common worldwide in the childbearing period, and pregnancy puts additional strain on the hypothalamic-pituitary-thyroid axis. Consequently, these disorders are frequent in pregnancy, and in particular, the borderline abnormalities. Correction of both overt hypothyroidism and hyperthyroidism is crucial for reduction of several adverse obstetric outcomes including fetal loss.[7]

Thyroid autoimmunity, which is defined by positive titers of thyroid peroxidase antibodies (TPOAbs) and/or thyroglobulin antibodies, was found to be independently associated with the incidence of miscarriage in 1990.[8] Additional research has shown that pregnancy loss can be attributed to subclinical hypothyroidism (SCH), which is defined as elevated thyroid-stimulating hormone (TSH) levels and normal free thyroxine (FT4), as well as overt hypothyroidism, which is defined by low FT4 and elevated TSH.[9-12] Furthermore, there is now debate on what constitutes an increased TSH level; recent guidelines recommend an upper limit of 4.0 mIU/L as diagnostic, as opposed to the earlier recommendation of 2.5 mIU/L.[13]

Thyroid disorders, particularly SCH and autoimmune thyroid disease (AITD), are increasingly recognized as significant factors influencing fertility treatment outcomes.[14,15] This is especially important in the context of assisted reproductive technologies (ARTs), where even subtle thyroid imbalances can disrupt the delicate hormonal balance necessary for success.[16,17]

Subclinical hypothyroidism, characterized by elevated TSH levels with normal FT4 levels, can have a profound impact on fertility. Even mild elevations in TSH concentrations, within the upper normal range, have been linked to fertilization failure in women undergoing in vitro fertilization (IVF).[2] This suggests that SCH may influence oocyte physiology, potentially affecting egg quality and the likelihood of successful fertilization.

The presence of TPOAbs, a hallmark of AITD, may directly interfere with normal ovarian function. Studies have shown that women with female factor infertility are more likely to be TPOAb-positive than age-matched controls, even in the presence of normal thyroid function.[18-20] This highlights a potential direct impact of TPOAb on ovarian processes, independent of thyroid hormone levels. It is important to note that the impact of AITD extends beyond natural conception and influences ART outcomes. A systematic review of 12 studies investigating the effects of AITD on IVF and intracytoplasmic sperm injection (ICSI) outcomes revealed slightly lower live birth rates and slightly higher miscarriage rates in TPOAb-positive women.[21] This suggests that TPOAb, regardless of thyroid function, can negatively impact the success of ART procedures.

Adding to the complexity, TPOAb-positive women undergoing ovarian stimulation for ART often experience a rise in TSH levels, even if initially euthyroid. This TSH elevation, typically remaining within the upper normal range, underscores the sensitivity of the thyroid gland to the hormonal fluctuations inherent in ART and the potential need for closer monitoring and management in these women.

THYROID PHYSIOLOGY AND ASSESSMENT IN PREGNANCY

It is crucial to understand the thyroid physiology in pregnancy, as this forms the basis for interpretation of the thyroid function test in pregnancy and the possible adverse obstetric outcomes with the different thyroid disorders. The demand on the maternal thyroid is increased in pregnancy for several reasons, such as augmented urinary excretion of the iodine, elevated thyroxine-binding globulin (TBG) levels, a rise in thyroid hormone degradation by placental type III deiodinase, and the fetal consumption of the maternal thyroid. As a consequence, the maternal production of the thyroid rises through compensatory mechanisms as the increased thyroidal production of FT4 and free triiodothyronine (FT3) triggered by the placental secretion of human chorionic gonadotropin (hCG).[7,22]

- Reduced iodine concentration secondary to the increased urinary excretion can precipitate iodine deficiency, causing enlargement of the thyroid gland (goiter) and low maternal thyroxine (T4), particularly in cretinism-endemic areas.[23] In regions that are not endemic but have mild-to-moderate iodine deficiencies, goiter has also been found. This is particularly relevant to the UK, which is iodine deficient, and children with lower IQ have complicated pregnancies with mild-to-moderate iodine deficiency.[24] Therefore, iodine supplements are required during pregnancy in iodine-deficient areas. Ideally, the deficiency should be addressed before conception by either universal salt iodization or focusing on women who are of reproductive age.
- Increase in TBG levels brought on by increased hepatic synthesis can lead to a rise in overall T4 and T3 levels.
- Human chorionic gonadotropin is a glycoprotein hormone secreted by the placenta in the first trimester. It shares a common α-subunit with TSH but has a unique β-subunit, which confers specificity. In the first trimester, hCG may function as a TSH agonist, increasing free T4 and decreasing TSH levels,[25] leading to gestational hyperthyroidism, a biochemical condition rather than a clinically evident problem. There is enough evidence to show an association between hyperemesis gravidarum and hyperthyroidism due to excessive hCG stimulation. Additionally, there is evidence that women who have positive autoantibodies to thyroid peroxidase (TPOAb) may also have a reduced ability to respond to hCG, which means they will not be able to handle the extra strain on their thyroid. This could help to explain the link between thyroid autoimmunity and unfavorable pregnancy outcomes.[26]
- FT4 rises transiently in the first trimester as an effect of the increased hCG, but it falls slightly in the second and third trimesters. FT3 follows the same pattern.[27] The normal ranges for free T4 and T3 are reduced.

Compared to outside pregnancy, free T4 has a narrower and lower range.[25]

- TSH level decreases in the first trimester affected by rise in FT4, and then increases in the second and third trimesters.

The diagnosis of maternal thyroid disorders is crucial for maternal and fetal well-being. The importance of the availability of reliable, accurate tests for thyroid functions in pregnancy comes from the fact that many of the normal symptoms and signs of pregnancy as a hypermetabolic state overlap with those due to thyroid dysfunction. The physiological changes that occur during pregnancy, however, present a legitimate difficulty for the interpretation of thyroid function tests.

Whenever possible, the current American Thyroid Association guidelines suggest using local population-based reference values that are specific to pregnancy.[13] Furthermore, the use of trimester-specific reference intervals is required since normal thyroid status varies throughout pregnancy **(Table 1)**.[7,28,29]

The use of TSH solely is unreliable, as it should be combined with measurement of T4 levels to differentiate between overt and subclinical thyroid diseases.[25]

There is equilibrium between the free and protein-bound fractions, and approximately 99% of T3 and T4 are bound to plasma transport proteins, primarily to the TBG and less frequently to the albumin. The protein-bound part serves as a reservoir, whereas the free component is the active form. Although it is considerably simpler to detect total thyroid hormone, some laboratories choose to assess FT4 because of the physiological changes that have been discussed in relation to pregnancy.[7,28]

TABLE 1: Pregnancy specific normal range of thyroid function test results.

	TSH (mU/L)	*Thyroxine (T4) (pmol/L)*	*Triiodothyronine (T3) (ng/mL)*
Non-pregnant	0.27–4.2	12–22	3.1–6.8
First trimester	0–5.5	10–16	3–7
Second trimester	0.5–3.5	9–15.5	3–5.5
Third trimester	0.5–4	8–14.5	2.5–5.5

(TSH: thyroid-stimulating hormone)

Source: Adapted from Cotzias C, Wong SJ, Taylor E, Seed P, Girling J. A study to establish gestation-specific reference intervals for thyroid function tests in normal singleton pregnancy. Eur J Obstet Gynecol Reprod Biol. 2008;137(1):61-6, with permission.

Depending on the clinical situation, TPOAb and thyroid-stimulating hormone receptor antibody (TRAb) may be advantageous. Low TSH levels during pregnancy are associated with TRAb in 60–70% of cases, and they should be monitored since they may result in fetal and neonatal hyperthyroidism. TPOAb can predict the risk of hypothyroidism.[13]

EFFECTS OF THYROID DYSFUNCTIONS

While overt maternal hypothyroidism, referred to as elevated TSH and low maternal FT4 concentrations, occurs in approximately 0.2–0.6% of pregnant women.[30,31] SCH, defined as elevated TSH and normal FT4 concentrations, can occur in up to 18% of pregnancies according to the precise criteria and TSH cut-point used.[13,21]

Graves' disease is usually the cause of pathological overt hyperthyroidism, which occurs in about 0.2% of pregnancies. However, 1% of pregnancies may be preceded by maternal Graves' disease that has already been treated. Gestational thyrotoxicosis (suppressed TSH and elevated FT4), which is mostly brought on by excess hCG and usually accompanied by hyperemesis gravidarum, occurs in up to 3% of pregnancies. It is thought to be a nonpathological cause of subclinical hyperthyroidism and typically accounts for the majority of cases detected during pregnancy.[20]

Graves' disease is the cause of hyperthyroidism in pregnancy in over 95% of cases. Rarely, it could be the result of toxic adenoma or toxic multinodular goiter. Preterm labor, perinatal death, fetal growth restriction (FGR), and miscarriage are all more likely to occur in untreated during pregnancy. Thyroid-stimulating antibodies may cause fetal or neonatal thyrotoxicosis.[25]

The European Society of Human Reproduction and Embryology has ruled out a causal relation between hyperthyroidism and RPL.

Atrophic thyroiditis and Hashimoto disease are the two main reasons of hypothyroidism, keeping in mind that it can be iatrogenic after thyroidectomy or radioactive iodine treatment. Subacute (de Quervain's) thyroiditis and postpartum thyroiditis can cause transient hypothyroidism. Uncontrolled cases are at increased risk of miscarriage, preterm labor, low birth weight, and preeclampsia. Untreated cases have been also linked to neurodevelopmental delay in the offsprings. By contrast, no studies have proven the benefit of universal screening in pregnancy with thyroxine replacement to improve the intelligent quotient. Severe iodine deficiency in pregnancy may cause permanent brain damage—neurological cretinism (deaf mutism, spastic motor disorder, and hypothyroidism)—in the child.[25]

Subclinical hypothyroidism has milder adverse obstetric consequences than overt hypothyroidism, yet they are still quite similar. A small observational study has noted the incidence of SCH to be raised in women with recurrent miscarriage.[1,32] Also, data from a meta-analysis on sporadic miscarriages suggests an association.[1,33] A higher risk of miscarriage, placental abruption, and premature delivery is linked to SCH.[18,34] But, it has not been linked to raising the likelihood of the child's development being impaired.[35,36] Thyroid antibodies were linked to an increased risk of recurrent miscarriages according to two systematic reviews and meta-analyses.[37,38]

Overt hypothyroidism has consistently been shown to be the cause of the RPL, and hence, it should be treated. There are conflicting opinions about SCH and/or thyroid autoimmunity. Part of this uncertainty comes from newer guidelines suggesting a new upper limit of normal for TSH of 4.0 mIU/L rather than the previous 2.5 mIU/L.[13]

MANAGEMENT

The management of SCH and TPOAb in women undergoing fertility treatment, especially ART, is a subject of ongoing debate. Some clinicians advocate for levothyroxine (LT4) treatment to normalize TSH levels in women with SCH, particularly those with TPOAb, before and during ART. The goal is to optimize thyroid hormone levels, potentially improving egg quality, fertilization rates, and pregnancy outcomes. However, the evidence supporting LT4 treatment is not conclusive. While some studies have shown potential benefits, others report no significant differences in pregnancy outcomes based on TSH levels or TPOAb status.[23,24] This highlights the need for a personalized approach to managing thyroid disorders in women seeking fertility treatment, which should include a thorough assessment of thyroid function, consideration of TPOAb status, and careful monitoring of TSH levels during ovarian stimulation. The decision to initiate LT4 treatment should be made on a case-by-case basis, considering individual patient factors and the potential risks and benefits.

There is a significant association between TPOAbs, thyroid dysfunction, and recurrent miscarriage, as evidenced by the meta-analyses.[37,38] There is an agreement between most of the guidelines not to treat isolated positive TPOAb cases. Nevertheless, the antibody status can be utilized to identify pregnant women who require thyroid function monitoring during the pregnancy. The RCOG Scientific Impact Paper No. 70 on Subclinical Hypothyroidism and Antithyroid Autoantibodies in Women with Subfertility or Recurrent Pregnancy Loss reported that performing routine antenatal TPOAb testing (in addition to thyroid function tests) for women with recurrent miscarriage versus regular thyroid function tests starting in early pregnancy are both viable options until clinical and cost-effectiveness analyses are available.[39]

Accordingly, women with a history of recurrent miscarriages should be offered thyroid function tests and assessment for TPOAbs according to the most recent Green-top Guideline recommendation on recurrent miscarriage from the RCOG.[1]

There was no difference between the two groups in the TABLET study, a double-blind placebo-controlled trial that compared the live birth rates of euthyroid women with TPOAbs and a history of miscarriage who received LT4 versus a placebo. This included subgroup analysis of women who experienced recurrent miscarriages.[39] This study was the rational for the RCOG recommendation not to offer LT4 treatment for euthyroid women with TPOAb-positive test and history of recurrent miscarriage.[1]

In the context of SCH, RCOG Scientific Impact Paper No. 70 found that while there is not enough evidence to warrant treatment for mild SCH (TSH >2.5 mIU/L), there is low quality evidence for treating women with moderate SCH (TSH >4.0 mIU/L). They recommend TSH testing in cases of TPO euthyroid antibody status at 7–9 weeks of gestation and in every subsequent trimester due to the possibility of progression to hypothyroidism.[40]

The American Thyroid Association has used the TSH level and the TPOAb status to stratify the recommendation for LT4 treatment. They give a strong recommendation for thyroxine use with a TSH >4 mIU/L and autoimmunity, a weak recommendation for thyroxine with a TSH >2.5 mIU/L and autoimmunity, and a weak recommendation for thyroxine in cases of TSH >4 mIU/L without autoimmunity.[13]

For management of overt hypothyroidism, most women do not typically need to change their thyroxine dosage during pregnancy or the puerperium if they are euthyroid at the start of the pregnancy. Any increase in dosage should be determined by interpreting thyroid function tests using the pregnancy-specific reference.[25]

For management of overt hyperthyroidism, antithyroid drugs (ATDs) are the preferred line of treatment with the carbimazole (CBZ) and propylthiouracil (PTU) being the most common of this group to be used in the pregnancy. Both can cross the placenta and may cause fetal hypothyroidism and goiter in high doses. It is therefore recommended to use the lowest therapeutic dose. The choice of the ATD to be used is based on its side effect, while CBZ has been claimed for many years to cause aplasia cutis if used in the first trimester; PTU is known to increase the risk of maternal hepatotoxicity. Consequently, most of the guidelines advise to use PTU in the first trimester, and then switch to CBZ. More recent data, however, indicates that there are no advantages to switching from CBZ to PTU during the first trimester and that the rates of malformations are comparable with both CBZ and PTU, but slightly lower with PTU.[7,25]

Management of Thyroid Disorders during Assisted Reproduction

Professional guidelines recommend thyroid function screening for women undergoing assisted reproduction, although the specific tests and timing may vary depending on the guideline and individual patient factors.[14,41-43] TSH is the initial screening test for thyroid dysfunction, as it is sensitive to subtle changes in thyroid hormone levels. Women should ideally have a TSH measurement within 12 months preceding conception. TPOAb testing is recommended for women with risk factors for thyroid autoimmunity, including a personal or family history of thyroid disease, other autoimmune disorders, or RPL. Some guidelines recommend TPOAb testing when TSH values are repeatedly above 2.5 mIU/L. FT4 is usually measured if the TSH is abnormal to confirm a diagnosis of hypothyroidism or hyperthyroidism.

The aim is to optimize thyroid function and mitigate potential adverse effects on treatment outcomes.[17] For SCH, the decision to treat with LT4 is individualized, considering TSH levels, TPOAb status, and patient preferences. The primary goal of LT4 therapy in SCH is to normalize TSH levels. Many clinicians aim for a TSH below 2.5 mIU/L before and during ART, as some studies have shown that achieving this target is associated with improved pregnancy outcomes. LT4 replacement can improve oocyte quality, increase fertilization rates, and potentially reduce the risk of miscarriage and other pregnancy complications.

The evidence supporting LT4 treatment in euthyroid TPOAb-positive women is less clear-cut. Some studies have shown that LT4 treatment reduces miscarriage rates and improves live birth rates, while others, such as the TABLET trial,[44] have not demonstrated a significant benefit. More recently, the T4LIFE trial[40] investigated LT4 for RPL in euthyroid women with TPOAb. This randomized, placebo-controlled trial included 187 women but was stopped prematurely due to slow recruitment. No significant difference in live birth rates was found between the LT4 and placebo groups (50% vs. 48%, respectively). From this, the authors did not recommend routine LT4 use in this population. This conflicting evidence, along with the paucity of data, highlights the need for further research into alternative interventions for RPL in women with TPOAb. The decision to treat euthyroid TPOAb-positive women with LT4 is often made on a case-by-case basis, considering factors such as TSH levels, previous pregnancy history, and patient preferences.[16,45]

Regular monitoring of thyroid function is critical, particularly for women with SCH or TPOAb positivity.[17,46] Women with SCH already on LT4 therapy require an empirical dose increase upon pregnancy confirmation, achieved by weekend dose doubling or a daily dose increase. TSH levels should be checked at 7–9 weeks of gestation and monitored regularly throughout pregnancy. Those with prepregnancy clinical hypothyroidism should have thyroid blood tests checked every 4–6 weeks during pregnancy, and with a further test a few weeks after delivery. However, it may not be necessary to test this frequently in later pregnancy if the thyroid levels have remained stable.[1]

Ethical Considerations in the Management of Thyroid Disease in Women with Recurrent Pregnancy Loss

Given the complexities of thyroid disease and its impact on RPL, particularly in the context of assisted reproduction, careful consideration of ethical implications is essential. Managing thyroid dysfunction in women with RPL requires a nuanced approach that balances the desire to optimize pregnancy outcomes with the paramount importance of respecting patient autonomy and informed choice.

Informed consent forms the bedrock of this ethical framework. Women must be provided with clear, comprehensive, and accessible information about the nature of thyroid disease and its potential influence on pregnancy, encompassing the spectrum of thyroid disorders and their potential adverse effects on both maternal and fetal health. This should include a detailed explanation of the purpose and limitations of thyroid function tests, ensuring women understand the rationale for testing, the interpretation of results (including the significance of thyroid autoantibodies), and the potential for inaccuracies. Furthermore, a thorough discussion of treatment options, including LT4, is essential, encompassing the mechanisms of action, potential side effects, long-term implications, and the potential consequences of both pursuing and forgoing treatment. It is equally important to acknowledge the uncertainties inherent in managing SCH and the role of thyroid autoantibodies in RPL, emphasizing the evolving nature of the evidence and ensuring women understand that treatment decisions may not always be straightforward (See Appendix 1 Case 10).

UNIVERSAL THYROID SCREENING IN PREGNANCY: A CONTINUING DEBATE

Building upon the discussion of thyroid disease and its implications for RPL, this section delves into the contentious issue of universal thyroid screening in pregnancy. As previously highlighted, thyroid disorders, particularly SCH, can have subtle yet potentially significant effects on both maternal and fetal health. The potential for undiagnosed or inadequately managed thyroid dysfunction to contribute to adverse pregnancy outcomes has fueled a debate regarding the merits of universal thyroid screening during pregnancy. We will aim to critically examine the arguments for and against this approach, highlighting the ethical considerations and the need for further research to inform evidence-based practice.

The concept of universal thyroid screening in pregnancy represents a significant point of contention within the medical community, with arguments both for and against its implementation. At the heart of this debate lie questions of efficacy, evidence-based practice, and the potential benefits and risks associated with early detection and treatment of thyroid disorders in pregnant women.

Arguments in Favor of Universal Screening

Proponents of universal screening highlight several key points to support their stance.[13,14,16,22,44,46] First, they argue that universal screening facilitates the identification of a greater number of women with thyroid dysfunction compared to targeted screening approaches. This is particularly relevant for SCH, a condition characterized by mildly elevated TSH levels but normal FT4 concentrations. Given the often subtle or absent symptoms of SCH, many cases might go undetected without universal screening. Additionally, it is worth mentioning evidence recommending gestation-specific reference ranges for TSH and free T4 measurements.[10]

Second, advocate point to the potential benefits of early treatment for SCH. While the evidence is not entirely conclusive, some studies suggest a link between SCH and adverse pregnancy outcomes such as miscarriage, preterm delivery, and preeclampsia.[11,12,32] Furthermore, there is an association between SCH and neurointellectual impairment of the child. Early detection and intervention with LT4 therapy could potentially mitigate these risks.[8,26]

Third, economic arguments are also put forward, with studies indicating that universal screening for AITD during the first trimester may prove cost-effective compared to no screening. This perspective considers not only the direct costs of treatment but also the potential long-term healthcare expenses associated with managing the consequences of untreated thyroid dysfunction in both mothers and their offspring.

Finally, universal screening allows for the identification of women at risk of postpartum thyroiditis. This condition, characterized by transient thyroid dysfunction following delivery, can have significant implications for maternal well-being and may require appropriate management.[7,47,48]

Arguments Against Universal Screening

Despite these compelling arguments, opposition to universal screening persists, rooted primarily in concerns regarding the current lack of robust, high-quality evidence to conclusively demonstrate the benefits of this approach.[11] While some studies suggest positive outcomes associated with early treatment of SCH, these findings are often countered by other research indicating no significant impact on pregnancy outcomes or child development. The only prospective randomized trial specifically designed to assess the value of screening in relation to childhood cognitive function failed to show any benefit.[8] The TABLET trial's findings suggest that simply supplementing thyroid hormone in euthyroid women with thyroid autoimmunity does not improve pregnancy outcomes. This implies that a deficiency in thyroid hormone is not the primary driver of pregnancy loss in these women. Instead, the results support the hypothesis that an underlying immune system dysfunction, characterized by the presence of thyroid autoantibodies, may be the key contributor to adverse pregnancy outcomes. This "hostile immune environment", rather than a relative thyroid hormone deficiency, could potentially disrupt the delicate balance necessary for successful implantation and placental development, leading to pregnancy loss.[3,4] The recent discovery of thyroid peroxidase (TPO) expression on mature granulosa cells provides further support for the hypothesis that immune mechanisms play a significant role in pregnancy loss among euthyroid women with thyroid autoimmunity.[49]

Another significant concern relates to the uncertainty surrounding the optimal treatment thresholds for SCH. The definition of SCH itself is evolving, with ongoing debate regarding the appropriate TSH cutoff values for diagnosis, particularly in pregnancy. This uncertainty complicates treatment decisions, potentially leading to the unnecessary medicalization of women with mild thyroid abnormalities who might not derive any clinical benefit from treatment. Furthermore, some studies raise concerns about the potential risks associated with LT4 treatment in certain subgroups of pregnant women, such as those with upper normal TSH concentrations. These risks include possible increases in preterm birth, gestational hypertension, and preeclampsia.[50,51]

CURRENT RECOMMENDATIONS AND CLINICAL PRACTICE

Given the current state of evidence, most professional societies, particularly in iodine-sufficient countries, advocate a targeted case-finding approach rather than universal screening.[6,11] This involves selectively testing pregnant women who present with specific symptoms suggestive of thyroid dysfunction, have a personal or family history of thyroid disease, or reside in areas known for moderate-to-severe iodine deficiency. However, this approach inevitably misses a significant proportion of women with thyroid dysfunction, as highlighted by studies reporting that targeted screening fails to identify between 33 and 81% of cases.

It is important to note that there is significant variation in clinical practice, with many clinicians already incorporating routine TSH testing in pregnant women, despite the lack of clear consensus from professional guidelines. A European survey revealed that 42% of respondents routinely screened all pregnant women for thyroid dysfunction.[5] This discrepancy between evidence-based recommendations and actual clinical practice underscores the complexity of the debate and the need for further research to inform clinical decision-making.

FUTURE DIRECTIONS: ONGOING RESEARCH AND THE NEED FOR CLARITY

The debate surrounding universal thyroid screening in pregnancy remains unresolved with significant implications for public health policy and clinical practice. The medical community eagerly awaits the findings of robust, well-designed studies that will definitively clarify the benefits and risks of screening and treatment for various forms of thyroid dysfunction in pregnancy. These studies should address the limitations of previous research, moving beyond simply identifying women with thyroid antibodies to ensuring that they are accurately classified and truly represent those with thyroid disorders. This involves carefully selecting and categorizing participants to minimize the inclusion of women without genuine thyroid conditions. Furthermore, to determine the true effectiveness of LT4, future studies must utilize dosing regimens that achieve meaningful differences in thyroid function parameters between treatment and placebo groups. This may involve individualizing dosages based on factors such as TSH levels, antibody titers, and gestational age. Standardizing and implementing reliable methods for measuring thyroid antibodies across different studies will also be crucial for improving the accuracy of diagnoses and ensuring consistency. Finally, focusing on the effects of LT4 treatment in specific subgroups of women, such as those with RPL, specific causes of infertility, or those undergoing assisted reproduction, will provide more targeted insights into the potential benefits and risks of intervention. By addressing these crucial areas, future research can provide the clarity needed to inform evidence-based guidelines and clinical decision-making regarding thyroid screening and treatment in pregnancy. This will ultimately lead to improved care and outcomes for women with thyroid disorders who are planning pregnancy or experiencing pregnancy complications.

CONCLUSION

Investigating thyroid dysfunction and thyroid autoimmunity, as well as optimizing thyroid function test is vital in women with RPL and those undergoing assisted reproduction. It will maximize their chances of a healthy pregnancy and normal fetal outcome. Effective management requires a patient-centered approach with individualized treatment strategies based on a thorough assessment of thyroid function, TPOAb status, and close monitoring of TSH levels. Collaboration between fertility specialists and endocrinologists is essential to navigate the complexities of thyroid disease in this population and optimize reproductive outcomes.

REFERENCES

1. British Thyroid Foundation. (2024). Thyroid disorders in pregnancy. [online] Available from https://www.btf-thyroid.org/thyroid-disorders-in-pregnancy [Last accessed December, 2024].
2. Repelaer van Driel-Delprat CC, van Dam EWCM, van de Ven PM, Aissa K, Ter Haar MK, Feenstra Y, et al. Thyroid function and IVF outcome for different indications of subfertility. Reprod Fertil. 2021;2(4):280-91.
3. Dosiou C, Stagnaro-Green A. The TABLET trial: Limitations and implications. BMC Med. 2019;126(17).
4. Stagnaro-Green A, Roman SH, Cobin RH, el-Harazy E, Alvarez-Marfany M, Davies TF. Detection of at-risk pregnancy by means of highly sensitive assays for thyroid autoantibodies. JAMA. 1990;264(11):1422-5.
5. Vaidya B, Hubalewska-Dydejczyk A, Laurberg P, Negro R, Vermiglio F, Poppe K. Treatment and screening of hypothyroidism in pregnancy: results of a European survey. Eur J Endocrinol. 2012;166(1):49-54.
6. Maraka S, Mwangi R, McCoy RG, Yao X, Sangaralingham LR, Singh Ospina NM, et al. Thyroid hormone treatment among pregnant women with subclinical hypothyroidism: US national assessment. BMJ. 2017;356:i6865.
7. Lazarus JH, Bestwick JP, Channon S, Paradice R, Maina A, Rees R, et al. Antenatal thyroid screening and childhood cognitive function. N Engl J Med. 2012;366(6):493-501.
8. Abalovich M, Alcaraz G, Kleiman-Rubinsztein J, Pavlove MM, Cornelio C, Levalle O, et al. The relationship of preconception thyrotropin levels to requirements for increasing the levothyroxine dose during pregnancy in women with primary hypothyroidism. Thyroid. 2010;20(10):1175-8.
9. Lambert-Messerlian G, McClain M, Haddow JE, Palomaki GE, Canick JA, Cleary-Goldman J, et al. First- and second-trimester thyroid hormone reference data in pregnant women: a FaSTER (First- and Second-Trimester Evaluation of Risk for aneuploidy) Research Consortium study. Am J Obstet Gynecol. 2008;199(1):62.e1-6.
10. De Groot L, Abalovich M, Alexander EK, Amino N, Barbour L, Cobin RH, et al. Management of thyroid dysfunction during pregnancy and postpartum: an Endocrine Society clinical practice guideline. J Clin Endocrinol Metab. 2012;97(8):2543-65. Erratum in: J Clin Endocrinol Metab. 2021;106(6):e2461.
11. Lepoutre T, Debiève F, Gruson D, Daumerie C. Reduction of miscarriages through universal screening and treatment of thyroid autoimmune diseases. Gynecol Obstet Invest. 2012;74(4):265-73.
12. Dosiou C, Barnes J, Schwartz A, Negro R, Crapo L, Stagnaro-Green A. Cost-effectiveness of universal and risk-based screening for autoimmune thyroid disease in pregnant women. J Clin Endocrinol Metab. 2012;97(5):1536-46.
13. Thung SF, Funai EF, Grobman WA. The cost-effectiveness of universal screening in pregnancy for subclinical hypothyroidism. Am J Obstet Gynecol. 2009;200(3):267.e1-7.
14. Lazarus J, Brown RS, Daumerie C, Hubalewska-Dydejczyk A, Negro R, Vaidya B. 2014 European thyroid association guidelines for the management of subclinical hypothyroidism in pregnancy and in children. Eur Thyroid J. 2014;3(2):76-94.
15. Krassas GE, Poppe K, Glinoer D. Thyroid function and human reproductive health. Endocr Rev. 2010;31(5):702-55.
16. Regan L, Rai R, Saravelos S, Li TC; Royal College of Obstetricians and Gynaecologists. Recurrent MiscarriageGreen-top Guideline No. 17. BJOG. 2023;130(12):e9-e39.
17. Dhillon-Smith RK, Boelaert K, Jeve YB, Maheshwari A, Coomarasamy A; Royal College of Obstetricians and Gynaecologists. Subclinical hypothyroidism and antithyroid autoantibodies in women with subfertility or recurrent pregnancy loss: Scientific Impact Paper No. 70 June 2022: Scientific Impact Paper No. 70 June 2022. BJOG. 2022;129(12):e75-e88.
18. Gill S, Cheed V, Morton VAH, Gill D, Boelaert K, Chan S, et al. Evaluating the Progression to Hypothyroidism in Preconception Euthyroid Thyroid Peroxidase Antibody-Positive Women. J Clin Endocrinol Metab. 2022;108(1):124-34.
19. Abalovich M, Mitelberg L, Allami C, Gutierrez S, Alcaraz G, Otero P, et al. Subclinical hypothyroidism and thyroid autoimmunity in women with infertility. Gynecol Endocrinol. 2007;23(5):279-83.
20. Al-Hussein K, Al-Mukhalafi Z, Bertilsson PA, Jaroudi K, Shoukri M, Hollander J. Value of flow cytometric assay for the detection of antisperm antibodies in women with a history of recurrent abortion. Am J Reprod Immunol. 2002;47(1):31-7.
21. Robinson L, Gallos ID, Conner SJ, Rajkhowa M, Miller D, Lewis S, et al. The effect of sperm DNA fragmentation on miscarriage rates: a systematic review and meta-analysis. Hum Reprod. 2012;27(10):2908-17.
22. Taylor PN, Minassian C, Rehman A, Iqbal A, Draman MS, Hamilton W, et al. TSH levels and risk of miscarriage in women on long-term levothyroxine: a community-based study. J Clin Endocrinol Metab. 2014;99(10):3895-902.
23. Seungdamrong A, Steiner AZ, Gracia CR, Legro RS, Diamond MP, Coutifaris C, et al. Preconceptional antithyroid peroxidase antibodies, but not thyroid-stimulating hormone, are associated with decreased live birth rates in infertile women. Fertil Steril. 2017;108(5):843-50.
24. Busnelli A, Paffoni A, Fedele L, Somigliana E. The impact of thyroid autoimmunity on IVF/ICSI outcome: a systematic review and meta-analysis. Hum Reprod Update.

2016;22(6):775-90. Erratum in: Hum Reprod Update. 2016;22(6):793-4.

25. Chen CW, Huang YL, Tzeng CR, Huang RL, Chen CH. Idiopathic Low Ovarian Reserve Is Associated with More Frequent Positive Thyroid Peroxidase Antibodies. Thyroid. 2017;27(9):1194-1200.
26. Agarwal A, Cho CL, Esteves SC. Should we evaluate and treat sperm DNA fragmentation? Curr Opin Obstet Gynecol. 2016;28(3):164-71.
27. Carlini T, Paoli D, Pelloni M, Faja F, Dal Lago A, Lombardo F, et al. Sperm DNA fragmentation in Italian couples with recurrent pregnancy loss. Reprod Biomed Online. 2017;34(1):58-65.
28. Ramasamy R, Scovell JM, Kovac JR, Cook PJ, Lamb DJ, Lipshultz LI. Fluorescence in situ hybridization detects increased sperm aneuploidy in men with recurrent pregnancy loss. Fertil Steril. 2015;103(4):906-909.e1.
29. Bareh GM, Jacoby E, Binkley P, Chang TC, Schenken RS, Robinson RD. Sperm deoxyribonucleic acid fragmentation assessment in normozoospermic male partners of couples with unexplained recurrent pregnancy loss: a prospective study. Fertil Steril. 2016;105(2):329-36.e1.
30. Zidi-Jrah I, Hajlaoui A, Mougou-Zerelli S, Kammoun M, Meniaoui I, Sallem A, et al. Relationship between sperm aneuploidy, sperm DNA integrity, chromatin packaging, traditional semen parameters, and recurrent pregnancy loss. Fertil Steril. 2016;105(1):58-64.
31. Zhao J, Zhang Q, Wang Y, Li Y. Whether sperm deoxyribonucleic acid fragmentation has an effect on pregnancy and miscarriage after in vitro fertilization/intracytoplasmic sperm injection: a systematic review and meta-analysis. Fertil Steril. 2014;102(4):998-1005.e8.
32. Bajoria R, Fisk NM. Permeability of human placenta and fetal membranes to thyrotropin-stimulating hormone in vitro. Pediatr Res. 1998;43(5):621-8.
33. Imam SN, Shamsi MB, Kumar K, Deka D, Dada R. Idiopathic recurrent pregnancy loss: role of paternal factors; a pilot study. J Reprod Infertil. 2011;12(4):267-76.
34. Motak-Pochrzest H, Malinowski A. The occurrence of immunological disturbances in patients with recurrent miscarriage (RM) of unknown etiology. Neuro Endocrinol Lett. 2013;34(7):701-7.
35. American College of Obstetricians and Gynecologists. ACOG Practice Bulletin. Clinical management guidelines for obstetrician-gynecologists. Number 37, August 2002. (Replaces Practice Bulletin Number 32, November 2001). Thyroid disease in pregnancy. Obstet Gynecol. 2002;100(2):387-96.
36. Fan J, Zhang Y, Zhang C, Barjaktarovic M, Yang X, Peeters RP, et al. Persistency of Thyroid Dysfunction from Early to Late Pregnancy. Thyroid. 2019;29(10):1475-84.
37. Saxena P, Misro MM, Chaki SP, Chopra K, Roy S, Nandan D. Is abnormal sperm function an indicator among couples with recurrent pregnancy loss? Fertil Steril. 2008;90(5):1854-8.
38. Ruixue W, Hongli Z, Zhihong Z, Rulin D, Dongfeng G, Ruizhi L. The impact of semen quality, occupational exposure to environmental factors and lifestyle on recurrent pregnancy loss. J Assist Reprod Genet. 2013;30(11):1513-8.
39. Dhillon-Smith RK, Middleton LJ, Sunner KK, Cheed V, Baker K, Farrell-Carver S, et al. Levothyroxine in Women with Thyroid Peroxidase Antibodies before Conception. N Engl J Med. 2019;380(14):1316-25.
40. Nazarpour S, Ramezani Tehrani F, Simbar M, Tohidi M, Alavi Majd H, et al. Effects of levothyroxine treatment on pregnancy outcomes in pregnant women with autoimmune thyroid disease. Eur J Endocrinol. 2017;176(2):253-65.
41. Salvi M, How J. Pregnancy and autoimmune thyroid disease. Endocrinol Metab Clin North Am. 1987;16(2):431-44.
42. Kung AW, Lau KS, Kohn LD. Epitope mapping of tsh receptor-blocking antibodies in Graves' disease that appear during pregnancy. J Clin Endocrinol Metab. 2001;86(8):3647-53.
43. Vos XG, Smit N, Endert E, Tijssen JG, Wiersinga WM. Frequency and characteristics of TBII-seronegative patients in a population with untreated Graves' hyperthyroidism: a prospective study. Clin Endocrinol (Oxf). 2008;69(2):311-7.
44. Negro R, Mangieri T, Coppola L, Presicce G, Casavola EC, Gismondi R, et al. Levothyroxine treatment in thyroid peroxidase antibody-positive women undergoing assisted reproduction technologies: a prospective study. Hum Reprod. 2005;20(6):1529-33.
45. Ota H, Amino N, Morita S, Kobayashi K, Kubota S, Fukata S, et al. Quantitative measurement of thyroid blood flow for differentiation of painless thyroiditis from Graves' disease. Clin Endocrinol (Oxf). 2007;67(1):41-5.
46. Horacek J, Spitalnikova S, Dlabalova B, Malirova E, Vizda J, Svilias I, et al. Universal screening detects two-times more thyroid disorders in early pregnancy than targeted high-risk case finding. Eur J Endocrinol. 2010;163(4):645-50.
47. Benvenga S. Targeted Antenatal Screening for Predicting Postpartum Thyroiditis and Its Evolution Into Permanent Hypothyroidism. Front Endocrinol (Lausanne). 2020;11:220.
48. Premawardhana LD, Parkes AB, John R, Harris B, Lazarus JH. Thyroid peroxidase antibodies in early pregnancy: utility for prediction of postpartum thyroid dysfunction and implications for screening. Thyroid. 2004;14(8):610-5.
49. Monteleone P, Faviana P, Artini PG. Thyroid peroxidase identified in human granulosa cells: another piece to the thyroid-ovary puzzle? Gynecol Endocrinol. 2017;33(7):574-6.
50. Maraka S, Singh Ospina NM, O'Keeffe DT, Rodriguez-Gutierrez R, Espinosa De Ycaza AE, Wi CI, et al. Effects of Levothyroxine Therapy on Pregnancy Outcomes in Women with Subclinical Hypothyroidism. Thyroid. 2016;26(7):980-6.
51. Amino N, Tada H, Hidaka Y, Crapo LM, Stagnaro-Green A. Therapeutic controversy: Screening for postpartum thyroiditis. J Clin Endocrinol Metab. 1999;84(6):1813-21.

CHAPTER 31

Polycystic Ovarian Syndrome

Duru Shah, Padma Rekha Jirge

ABSTRACT

Polycystic ovarian syndrome is associated with recurrent pregnancy loss (RPL) and underlying etiology can be multifactorial. Hyperandrogenemia, insulin resistance, obesity, hyperhomocysteinemia, and gene polymorphism are some known contributors to RPL. Proven therapies are lifestyle modifications, weight loss, metformin therapy and in select cases low molecular weight heparin is recommended. Most pregnancy losses associated with polycystic ovary syndrome are preventable with adequate work up and management.

Keywords: Polycystic ovarian syndrome, Hyperinsulinemia, Hyperandrogenemia, Hyperhomocysteinemia, Metformin.

INTRODUCTION

Recurrent pregnancy loss (RPL) is a multifactorial condition with spontaneous loss of conceptus before 24 weeks of gestation. 0.3–1% of women experience two or more consecutive miscarriages during the reproductive lifespan. Endocrinopathies are considered as an important cause of RPL.[1] Polycystic ovary syndrome (PCOS) is the most common endocrinopathy seen in women of reproductive age group. There is an international consensus for utilizing Rotterdam criteria for the diagnosis of PCOS. It necessitates the presence of any two of the following three criteria: (1) Chronic anovulation, (2) clinical hyperandrogenism or biochemical hyperandrogenemia, and (3) polycystic ovarian morphology (PCOM) on transvaginal sonography.[2] Recently, it is recommended that serum anti-Müllerian hormone (AMH) values can be used in place of PCOM as a diagnostic criterion for PCOS.[3]

Various criteria have been used for the classification of PCOS. These include the National Institutes of Health (NIH) criteria, proposed in 1992; the Rotterdam criteria, jointly proposed by the European Society of Human Reproduction and Embryology (ESHRE) and the American Society for Reproductive Medicine (ASRM) during a meeting at Rotterdam in 2002; and the more recent position statement issued by the Androgen Excess PCOS (AE-PCOS) society in 2006. Which criterion is best applied is a matter of debate.[4] The use of well-accepted Rotterdam criteria is mandatory for the diagnosis of PCOS, as such a diagnosis has important systemic, metabolic, and reproductive implications throughout a woman's lifetime. Even though infertility is the most common reproductive disorder seen in women with PCOS, 10% of women with PCOS experience RPL.[5] This chapter addresses the mechanisms involved in the occurrence of RPL in women with PCOS, followed by a section on the management strategies.

FACTORS CONTRIBUTING TO RECURRENT PREGNANCY LOSS IN POLYCYSTIC OVARY SYNDROME

Hyperandrogenemia and insulin resistance (IR) are the two important etiological factors that contribute toward all the clinical consequences of PCOS. In addition, hyperhomocysteinemia, obesity, and thrombophilia are implicated in the occurrence of RPL in women with PCOS. Elevated AMH levels also influence reproductive outcomes.[6]

Hyperandrogenism and Hyperandrogenemia

Hyperandrogenism refers to excessive production of androgens along with clinical features of hirsutism and acne or frontal alopecia. However, hyperandrogenemia refers to increased blood levels of androgens only. Three of the four recognized phenotypes of PCOS have either clinical hyperandrogenism or biochemical hyperandrogenemia. This endocrine abnormality is commonly detected during the evaluation of women with RPL and PCOS. The underlying mechanisms for RPL due to hyperandrogenemia are considered to be hyperhomocysteinemia and altered endometrial receptivity.[7]

Insulin Resistance and Hyperinsulinemia

Insulin resistance is associated with an increased risk of pregnancy loss in women with PCOS. Current evidence suggests that elevated triglycerides and altered immune responses due to IR may lead to RPL in these women. In addition, hyperhomocysteinemia as a consequence of IR may also result in RPL.[8]

Hyperhomocysteinemia

Women with PCOS have IR that interferes with amino acid metabolism and results in the accumulation of homocysteine (Hcy). Hyperhomocysteinemia may impair implantation by affecting endometrial blood flow and vascular integrity. It has been associated with RPL in women with PCOS.[8-10] Significantly elevated levels of Hcy may also occur due to hyperandrogenemia.[6]

Thrombophilia

Studies have shown an association between RPL in PCOS with hypofibrinolysis, factor V Leiden mutations,[4] and protein C deficiency.[11] Impaired fibrinolysis has also been reported in PCOS.[12] Impaired fibrinolytic activity has been reported in RPL as well.[13] However, a recent systematic review and meta-analysis could not identify an association between inherited thrombophilia and RPL in women with PCOS but identified that women with PCOS and RPL have a high risk of thromboembolism.[14]

Obesity

Obesity is commonly seen in women with PCOS. Women with PCOS and obesity experience similar endocrine and metabolic disturbances. A recent systematic review and meta-analysis show that obese women have a 24–47% increased risk of RPL.[15] However, this meta-analysis did not analyze whether PCOS is independently associated with an increased risk of RPL. The increased risk in obese women is attributed to altered endometrial receptivity.[16]

Gene Polymorphisms

Gene polymorphisms continue to be investigated as a cause of RPL in PCOS. M2 haplotype of annexin 5 gene, methylenetetrahydrofolate reductase polymorphism, and IL-6-174G/C GG genotype have all been implicated in the RPL associated with PCOS.[17]

MANAGEMENT

Management of RPL in PCOS involves establishing a firm diagnosis of PCOS as the first step. This involves clinical evaluation for signs of hyperandrogenism such as hirsutism, acne vulgaris, and female pattern of balding. In addition, the presence of acanthosis nigricans and skin tags alert to the presence of IR. A transvaginal ultrasound for diagnosing PCOM using appropriate criteria is important.[3] In the absence of clinical hyperandrogenism, biochemical evaluation for total testosterone and free androgen index may be performed to confirm hyperandrogenemia. In addition, a lipid profile and oral glucose tolerance test with a 75-g sugar load should be performed once the diagnosis of PCOS is confirmed.[3] It is also necessary to rule out other well-established causes of RPL while implicating PCOS as the cause of RPL. Screening for inherited/acquired thrombophilia is a part of such evaluation and may show abnormalities commonly reported in women with PCOS.

Lifestyle modification, metformin, and low-molecular-weight heparin have been used in the management of RPL in PCOS. Lifestyle modification and weight management are of proven benefit in reducing the endocrine and metabolic abnormalities associated with PCOS. However, its beneficial role in the subset of women with RPL has not been studied hitherto. Considering its positive role in alleviating various signs and symptoms of PCOS, appropriate counseling for lifestyle management should be incorporated into the management of RPL.

Lifestyle Modifications

Diet and exercise have been the mainstays of lifestyle modifications. Various diets have been recommended, and the most favorable is the diet low in carbohydrates and fats and high in protein and fiber. Exercise programs that can be integrated comfortably within the work schedule and are sustainable are recommended. Promoting a hobby like sports or dance is a good way of incorporating exercise.[5] A combination of diet and exercise works much better than either intervention alone. Although there is published evidence for lifestyle modification and PCOS,[18] there is a paucity of data on lifestyle modification and RPL in PCOS.

Metformin

Metformin has been used successfully in women with PCOS and RPL to reduce the risk of further miscarriage.[19]

Another study in women with RPL and PCOS with evidence of IR has shown that metformin therapy reduces further miscarriage.[20] The daily dose of metformin varies from 1 to 2.55 g/day in divided doses.[21] It can be safely continued during pregnancy.[22]

Low-molecular-weight Heparin

A combination of metformin (1.5–2.55 g/day) and enoxaparin (60 mg/day) or enoxaparin alone has been found to reduce the risk of further miscarriage and increase the probability of live birth in women with PCOS and RPL with coagulation disorders.[23] A combination of low-dose aspirin (75 mg/day) and low-molecular-weight heparin has been used successfully in those with hyperhomocysteinemia.[10] In these patients, vitamin supplementation with folic acid, vitamin B_6, and B_{12} has also been successfully used to lower Hcy levels both prepregnancy and during pregnancy. (See Chapter 34)

Ovarian drilling is known to reduce the hormonal abnormalities of PCOS and improve ovulation and pregnancy. Ovarian drilling with laparoscopic monopolar cautery or laser was advocated as it resulted in shorter time to pregnancy and less side effects of gonadotropins, including multiple pregnancies through assisted reproductive technology (ART).[24] Its use has fallen into disrepute after a Cochrane review in 2020,[25] which could not confirm its superiority over gonadotropin use and also reported complications such as risk of anesthesia, infections, adhesions, and some cases of poor ovarian reserve following the procedure. However, its role in the prevention of RPL in PCOS has never been studied. Hence, it is not advocated in women with RPL.

CONCLUSION

Recurrent pregnancy loss is a multifactorial condition, and a detailed evaluation for all the known causes is important. PCOS with inherent hyperandrogenemia and IR is understood to contribute to RPL. In addition, the presence of obesity or thrombophilia is of further prognostic value. An empathetic approach, a systematic assessment, and appropriately planned therapy all contribute toward a successful outcome in subsequent pregnancies. The treatment strategy may include metformin and low-dose aspirin with low-molecular-weight heparin as stand alone or combination therapy. Appropriate lifestyle management is an integral part of the management strategy as well.

REFERENCES

1. Smith ML, Schust DJ. Endocrinology and recurrent early pregnancy loss. Semin Reprod Med. 2011;29(6):482-90.
2. Rotterdam ESHRE/ASRM-Sponsored PCOS consensus workshop group. Revised 2003 consensus on diagnostic criteria and long-term health risks related to polycystic ovary syndrome (PCOS). Hum Reprod. 2004;19(1):41-7.
3. Teede HJ, Tay CT, Laven J, Dokras A, Moran LJ, Piltonen TT, et al. Recommendations from the 2023 International Evidence-based Guideline for the Assessment and Management of Polycystic Ovary Syndrome. Fertil Steril. 2023;189(2):G43-G64.
4. Chang S, Dunaif A. Diagnosis of Polycystic Ovary Syndrome: Which Criteria to Use and When? Endocrinol Metab Clin North Am. 2021;50(1):11-23.
5. Glueck CJ, Awadalla SG, Phillips H, Cameron D, Wang P, Fontaine RN. Polycystic ovary syndrome, infertility, familial thrombophilia, familial hypofibrinolysis, recurrent loss of in vitro fertilized embryos, and miscarriage. Fertil Steril. 2000;74(2):394-7.
6. Liu S, Hong L, Mo M, Xiao S, Wang X, Fan X, et al. Association of antimüllerian hormone with polycystic ovarian syndrome phenotypes and pregnancy outcomes of in vitro fertilization cycles with fresh embryo transfer. BMC Pregnancy Childbirth. 2022;22(1):171.
7. Kondapaneni V, Gutlapalli SD, Poudel S, Zeb M, Toulassi IA, Cancarevic I. Significance of Homocysteine Levels in the Management of Polycystic Ovarian Syndrome: A Literature Review. Cureus. 2020;12(10):e11110.
8. Chakraborty P, Goswami SK, Rajani S, Sharma S, Kabir SN, Chakravarty B, et al. Recurrent pregnancy loss in polycystic ovary syndrome: role of hyperhomocysteinemia and insulin resistance. PLoS One. 2013;8(5):e64446.
9. Nelen WL, Blom HJ, Steegers EA, den Heijer M, Eskes TK. Hyperhomocysteinemia and recurrent early pregnancy loss: a meta-analysis. Fertil Steril. 2000;74(6):1196-9.
10. Asanidze E, Kristesashvili J, Parunashvili N, Urjumelashvili M, Tsetskhladze Z, Asanidze A. Hyperhomocysteinemia and pregnancy outcomes in women with polycystic ovary syndrome: A case-control study. Int J Reprod Biomed. 2023;21(2):167-74.
11. Moini A, Tadayon S, Tehranian A, Yeganeh LM, Akhoond MR, Yazdi RS. Association of thrombophilia and polycystic ovarian syndrome in women with history of recurrent pregnancy loss. Gynecol Endocrinol. 2012;28(8):590-3.
12. Yildiz BO, Haznedaroğlu IC, Kirazli S, Bayraktar M. Global fibrinolytic capacity is decreased in polycystic ovary syndrome, suggesting a prothrombotic state. J Clin Endocrinol Metab. 2002;87(8):3871-5.
13. Maghsudlu M, Noroozi Z, Zokaei E, Elahe Motevaseli. Systematic review and meta-analysis of association between plasminogen activator inhibitor-1 4G/5G polymorphism and recurrent pregnancy loss: an update. Thrombosis J. 2024;22:44.

14. Cavalcante MB, Sarno M, Cavalcante CT de MB, Júnior EA, Barini R. Coagulation Biomarkers in Women with Recurrent Miscarriage and Polycystic Ovarian Syndrome: Systematic Review and Meta-Analysis. Geburtshilfe und Frauenheilkunde. 2019;79(7):697.
15. Cavalcante MB, Sarno M, Peixoto AB, Araujo Júnior E, Barini R. Obesity and recurrent miscarriage: A systematic review and meta-analysis. J Obstet Gynaecol Res. 2019;45(1): 30-8.
16. Cozzolino M, García-Velasco JA, Meseguer M, Pellicer A, Bellver J. Female obesity increases the risk of miscarriage of euploid embryos. Fertil Steril. 2021;115(6):1495-502.
17. Wartena R, Matjila M. Polycystic ovary syndrome and recurrent pregnancy loss, a review of literature. Front Endocrinol. 2023;14:1183060.
18. Gu Y, Zhou G, Zhou F, Wu Q, Ma C, Zhang Y, et al. Life Modifications and PCOS: Old Story But New Tales. Front Endocrinol. 2022;13:808898.
19. Nawaz FH, Rizvi J. Continuation of metformin reduces early pregnancy loss in obese Pakistani women with polycystic ovarian syndrome. Gynecol Obstet Invest. 2010;69(3):184-9.
20. Zolghadri J, Tavana Z, Kazerooni T, Soveid M, Taghieh M. Relationship between abnormal glucose tolerance test and history of previous recurrent miscarriages, and beneficial effect of metformin in these patients: a prospective clinical study. Fertil Steril. 2008;90(3):727-30.
21. McCarthy EA, Walker SP, McLachlan K, Boyle J, Permezel M. Metformin in obstetric and gynecologic practice: a review. Obstet Gynecol Surv. 2004;59(2):118-27.
22. Hyer S, Balani J, Shehata H. Metformin in Pregnancy: Mechanisms and Clinical Applications. Int J Mol Sci. 2018;19(7):1954.
23. Ramidi G, Khan N, Glueck CJ, Wang P, Goldenberg N. Enoxaparin-metformin and enoxaparin alone may safely reduce pregnancy loss. Transl Res. 2009;153(1):33-43.
24. Lebbi I, Ben Temime R, Fadhlaoui A, Feki A. Ovarian Drilling in PCOS: Is it Really Useful? Front Surg. 2015;2:30.
25. Bordewijk EM, Ng KYB, Rakic L, Mol BWJ, Brown J, Crawford TJ, et al. Laparoscopic ovarian drilling for ovulation induction in women with anovulatory polycystic ovary syndrome. Cochrane Database Syst Rev. 2020;2(2):CD001122.

CHAPTER 32

Insulin Resistance and Metabolic Syndrome

Uma Ram, Mathangi T

ABSTRACT

Insulin resistance as seen in polycystic ovarian syndrome and diabetes mellitus is associated with recurrent pregnancy loss (RPL). Yet checking for insulin resistance is not a recommendation of any RPL guideline. Women with insulin resistance which can be simply diagnosed by altered waist hip ratio may also be at a risk of RPL. Meta-analysis has shown that women with RPL have lower fasting glucose to fasting insulin ratio as compared to controls. It is a well-known fact that metformin therapy reduces the incidence of miscarriage in women with diabetes mellitus and polycystic ovaries, but will it be justified to treat women with metabolic syndrome and RPL with metformin therapy is an unanswered question. Do high levels of triglycerides that often accompany metabolic syndrome also play a role in the pathophysiology of RPL is also an unanswered question.

Keywords: Metformin, Insulin resistance, Hyperhomocysteinemia, RPL, HOMA-IR, Fasting insulin, Fasting glucose/insulin ratio, Hypertriglyceridemia.

INTRODUCTION

Recurrent pregnancy loss (RPL) is defined as the loss of three or more consecutive pregnancies and is estimated to occur in 1% of reproductive-age couples.[1] Causes can be multifactorial, starting from uterine factors, immunologic factors such as antiphospholipid syndrome, endocrine factors such as diabetes mellitus (DM), polycystic ovary syndrome (PCOS), thyroid disease and antibodies, hyperprolactinemia, genetic factors such as aneuploidy, and many others. 30–40% of RPL cases remain unexplained, despite the recent advances in testing and diagnosis. Impaired glucose tolerance and overt diabetes are potential risk factors for RPL. Increased insulin resistance (IR) and higher fasting insulins (FIs) are seen in women with RPL. There is also some data that women with RPL[2] have a higher risk of subsequently having a stroke or developing metabolic syndrome.[3] Therefore, there may be underlying genetic, thrombogenic, metabolic, or immune defects that contribute to both RPL and cardiovascular disease. Obesity itself is associated with an increase in IR and other metabolic abnormalities. Additionally, there is evidence of benefit from metabolic interventions from weight loss and metformin use on pregnancy loss. While clear guidelines do not yet exist, this is an area of potential benefit where larger studies are needed.

EVALUATION OF INSULIN METABOLISM DYSFUNCTION

The effect of insulin to promote absorption and utilization of glucose by cells, organs, and tissues is lower in women with IR when compared to the normal. Markers that are used to assess insulin metabolism dysfunction in women with RPL are FIs, fasting blood glucose (FBG), fasting glucose to fasting insulin (FG:FI) ratio, and IR. The homeostatic model assessment insulin resistance (HOMA-IR) is an indirect method to quantify IR and pancreatic β-cell function. Quantitative insulin sensitivity check index (QUICKI) is another tool to assess IR, but their clinical use is still controversial.[4] Although there are studies that look at association of RPL and IR, the greatest limitation that remains is the lack of universal IR/insulin assay.

PATHOPHYSIOLOGY

The exact mechanism that causes RPL in women with IR is not clear, though multiple hypotheses have been made.

- The first one is that an uncontrolled diabetic-like state is created in the fetal environment when there is IR, causing early pregnancy loss. In vitro tests have shown increased transport of glucose by first-trimester cytotrophoblasts when there are high insulin levels, independent of the glucose levels, probably because of upregulation of the glucose transporter type 1 (GLUT1) system.

- The second possibility is higher plasminogen activator (PA) inhibitor levels, which is a major fibrinolysis inhibitor. In women with PCOS, increasing PA inhibitor levels are seen with increasing levels of insulin, and the levels also reduce when treated with insulin-sensitizing agents. It is possible that high PA inhibitor levels and their increased activity cause recurrent miscarriage through thrombotic induction of placental insufficiency. High levels of PA inhibitor activity are found in women with RPL with unknown etiology.[5]

EVIDENCE FROM LITERATURE

Insulin resistance was seen to be more prevalent in women with RPL, and Craig et al. showed that IR was more common in nondiabetic women with RPL when compared to controls [odds ratio (OR): 3.55, 95% confidence interval (CI): 1.40–9.01] using FG and FG:FI.[5] Fasting glucose, FI, and IR were seen to be higher in women with idiopathic RPL.[6] A meta analysis done by Cai et al. has shown higher fasting blood glucose, FI and HOMA IR levels as well as a lower FG/FI ratio in women with RPL.[7]

Elevation in total homocysteine (tHcy) levels, hyperhomocysteinemia (HHcy), or combinations of these conditions have been described as playing a role in the pathogenesis of RPL.[8] There is a role for IR and homocysteine (Hcy) abnormalities noted in women with PCOS and obesity with pregnancy loss. It is important to remember that smoking, vitamin B, and folic acid levels also impact Hcy levels.

High Hcy was significantly associated with RPL in both PCOS and non-PCOS populations.[9] Hcy increases inflammatory responses, inhibits proliferation, and impairs endothelial function, thereby causing vascular injury and increasing hypercoagulability. Hcy also seems to be associated with defective chorionic villus vascularization. Therefore, this possibly explains the association of IR, RPL, and Hcy.

The peripheral IR status increases during pregnancy, and this results in high levels of maternal amino acids and lipids, thereby enhancing placental transfer of glucose and other nutrients. The placenta is responsive to high concentrations of maternal insulin, especially in obese women in early pregnancy, and this is probably due to altered gene expression caused by modulated mitochondrial steroid hormone production and energy metabolism.[7]

It is known that remodeling of the uterine decidual spiral arterioles for a high-velocity and low-resistance blood flow is essential for placental function throughout pregnancy. Insulin is a vasoactive substance, and IR can be associated with endothelial dysfunction and disrupting vessel function, leading to pregnancy loss. Therefore, IR status may play a role in placental dysfunction and thereby pregnancy loss.

In small studies, elevated triglycerides (TGs) are seen in a subgroup of women with RPL who do not have PCOS or obesity. In these women, the increased TG was positively associated with the ratio of $CD3^{+}CD4^{+}/CD3^{+}CD8^{+}$ and reduced insulin sensitivity and hyperinsulinemia.[9] Considering the higher prevalence of dyslipidemia and its newfound association with inflammatory markers and RPL, this may be something to explore further in addressing unexplained RPL.[10]

POLYCYSTIC OVARY SYNDROME AND INSULIN RESISTANCE

Polycystic ovary syndrome is associated with an increased risk of miscarriage of 20–40% when compared to 10–20% among the general population.[11] PCOS is more prevalent in women with RPL (82% vs. 18%). Pregnancy loss in PCOS is largely attributed to IR, hyperinsulinemia, elevated luteinizing hormone (LH) levels, and hyperandrogenemia (both testosterone and androstenedione concentrations), which are thought to have adverse effects on the endometrial receptivity. However, the exact mechanism is still unclear.

A higher risk of miscarriage (OR: 1.41, 95% CI: 1.04–1.91) was seen in women with PCOS in a recent meta-analysis, including 29 studies.[12] High body mass index (BMI) and IR are associated with an increased risk of miscarriage in women with PCOS undergoing assisted reproductive treatment (ART),[13] suggesting that there is a compounding impact of the metabolic problems in these women.

When compared to fertile women, the prevalence of IR is higher in women with RPL whether PCOS is present or not. A case-control study showed the highest FI levels in women with PCOS and RPL and lower levels in other groups.[11] Though some studies showed that there was a reduction in miscarriage rates when women with PCOS were treated with metformin for IR, another trial showed no reduction in miscarriage rates when treated with metformin compared to clomiphene.[11]

Increased androgen index appeared to be a prognostic factor for subsequent miscarriage for women with RPL but is not recommended yet as routine testing for women with RPL due to a lack of strong evidence.[4] The European Society of Human Reproduction and Embryology (ESHRE) does not recommend testing of FI and fasting blood sugar/ assessment of PCOS to improve pregnancy outcome in subsequent pregnancies in women with RPL.

DIABETES MELLITUS

Prevalence of DM is similar to general population in women with RPL, and women with poorly controlled DM are at high risk for early pregnancy loss. On the other hand, well-controlled DM is not considered a cause for RPL.[1,11] Women whose glycosylated hemoglobin (HbA1c) level was >4 SD above the mean had higher pregnancy loss rates when compared with women with lower HbA1c levels, said a collaborative study by the National Institute of Child Health and Human Development (NICHD). Neither the Royal College of Obstetricians and Gynaecologists (RCOG) nor the American College of Obstetricians and Gynecologists (ACOG) recommend testing for occult DM. However, in a country like India, where the prevalence of DM is high, where often women access care only in pregnancy and may not have been tested before, it is good practice to screen for diabetes and IGT by checking HbA1c levels at the first point of contact if there is a family history of diabetes (See Appendix 1 Case 6).

METFORMIN THERAPY

In women with DM or IR, metformin therapy will improve glycemic control. The question is whether metformin therapy will lower miscarriage rates in women with metabolic syndrome and IR and impaired glucose tolerance. A single prospective cohort study compared pregnancy outcomes in women who continued metformin therapy during pregnancy and found that the miscarriage rate was 8.9% in metformin group and 36% in the control group, with a p value of <0.001.[14] However, larger studies are needed on this subject. Whether lowering TG levels reduces the risk of miscarriage is a question that needs to be answered. A systematic review on this subject has been initiated, and we shall await the results.[15]

CONCLUSION

Women with RPL were associated with IR, impaired FBG, HOMA-IR, and lower glycemic index (GI) ratios. There is a need for more research in this area to guide as to which are the most important biomarkers to check in women with RPL. Early screening and the management of IR can help pregnancy outcomes in women with RPL. Logical thinking suggests that lowering IR in these women will help improve pregnancy outcomes. Lifestyle[5] modification with a healthy, low-carbohydrate, and fiber-rich diet coupled with a moderate exercise program should be advised. However, there is a definite need for studies to understand, whether interventions such as lifestyle changes and insulin-sensitizing drugs improve pregnancy outcomes in women with IR and RPL.

REFERENCES

1. Regan L, Rai R, Saravelos S, Li T-C; on behalf of the Royal College of Obstetricians and Gynaecologists. Recurrent Miscarriage: Green-top Guideline No. 17. BJOG. 2023;130(12):e9-e39.
2. Liang C, Chung H-F, Dobson AJ, Hayashi K, van der Schouw YT, Kuh D, et al. Infertility, recurrent pregnancy loss, and risk of stroke: pooled analysis of individual patient data of 618 851 women. BMJ. 2022;377:e070603.
3. Bae JH, Jung YM, Lee J, Shivakumar M, Park CW, Park JS, et al. Future risk of metabolic syndrome after recurrent pregnancy loss: a cohort study using UK Biobank. Fertil Steril. 2023;120(6):1227-33.
4. Bender Atik R, Christiansen OB, Elson J, Kolte AM, Lewis S, Middeldorp S, et al.; ESHRE Guideline Group on RPL. ESHRE guideline: recurrent pregnancy loss: an update in 2022. Hum Reprod Open. 2023;2023(1):hoad002.
5. Craig LB, Ke RW, Kutteh WH. Increased prevalence of insulin resistance in women with a history of recurrent pregnancy loss. Fertil Steril. 2002;78(3):487-90.
6. Ispasoiu CA, Chicea R, Stamatian FV, Ispasoiu F. High fasting insulin levels and insulin resistance may be linked to idiopathic recurrent pregnancy loss: a case-control study. Int J Endocrinol. 2013;2013:576926.
7. Cai WY, Luo X, Lv HY, Fu KY, Xu J. Insulin resistance in women with recurrent miscarriage: a systematic review and meta-analysis. BMC Pregnancy Childbirth. 2022; 22(1):916.
8. Qublan HS, Eid SS, Ababneh HA, Amarin ZO, Smadi AZ, Al-Khafaji FF, et al. Acquired and inherited thrombophilia: implication in recurrent IVF and embryo transfer failure. Hum Reprod. 2006; 21(10):2694-98.
9. Chakraborty P, Goswami SK, Rajani S, Sharma S, Kabir SN, Chakravarty B, et al. Recurrent Pregnancy Loss in Polycystic

Ovary Syndrome: Role of Hyperhomocysteinemia and Insulin Resistance. PLoS One. 2013;8(5):e64446.

10. Liu Y, Du M, Gan Y, Bao S, Feng L, Zhang J. Triglyceride Induced Metabolic Inflammation: Potential Connection of Insulin Resistance and Recurrent Pregnancy Loss. Front Endocrinol. 2021;12:621845.
11. Togas Tulandi, Haya M Al-Fozan. (2024). Recurrent pregnancy loss: Definition and etiology. [online] Available from https://www.uptodate.com/contents/recurrent-pregnancy-loss-definition-and-etiology [Last accessed December, 2024].
12. Sha T, Wang X, Cheng W, Yan Y. A Meta-Analysis of Pregnancy-Related Outcomes and Complications in Women With Polycystic Ovary Syndrome Undergoing IVF. Reprod BioMed Online. 2019;39(2):281-93.
13. Sun Y-F, Zhang J, Xu Y-M, Cao Z-Y, Wang Y-Z, Hao G-M, et al. High BMI and Insulin Resistance Are Risk Factors for Spontaneous Abortion in Patients With Polycystic Ovary Syndrome Undergoing Assisted Reproductive Treatment: A Systematic Review and Meta-Analysis. Front Endocrinol (Lausanne). 2020;11:592495.
14. Al-Biate MA. Effect of metformin on early pregnancy loss in women with polycystic ovary syndrome. Taiwan J Obstet Gynecol. 2015;54(3):266-9.
15. Nassif DS, Januário BL, Sousa BA, Thabane L, Abbade JF. Effectiveness of metformin to pregnant women with PCOS to reduce spontaneous abortion and gestational diabetes mellitus: a protocol for an overview of reviews. BMJ Open. 2024;14(3):e078217.

CHAPTER 33

Diminished Ovarian Reserve

Krishna Deepti Mogili, Chaitanya Shembekar

ABSTRACT

Diminished ovarian reserve (DOR) is checked by serum anti-Müllerian hormone (AMH) levels as well as the antral follicle count. Currently none of the guidelines recommend testing for DOR in patients with recurrent pregnancy loss (RPL). With the changing canvass of RPL, elderly women can present with recurrent early aneuploid losses or even biochemical pregnancies. It has been shown that DOR is more common in women with RPL. Then again women with DOR more often require assisted reproductive technology (ART) procedures to achieve a pregnancy than women with normal ovarian reserve. In the context of advanced maternal age, it may worthwhile testing for ovarian reserve and to shorten time to pregnancy whether by spontaneous conception or through ART.

Keywords: Diminished ovarian reserve, Time to pregnancy, Recurrent miscarriage, Anti-Müllerian hormone, AFC, ART.

INTRODUCTION

Ovarian reserve can be defined as the number of oocytes left in the ovary at any given point in time.[1] It implies oocyte quantity and not quality. The number of oocytes in a female fetus peaks at 20 weeks of gestation and is reported to be about 6–7 million. At birth, this number is decreased to around 1 million, and by the age of 7 years, only 300,000 oocytes survive.[2] With age, due to ovulation and further follicular atresia, the number of oocytes naturally decline, leading to a decrease in ovarian reserve and menopause. In addition to advancing age, there are various other established risk factors, which can lead to a decrease in ovarian reserve, like extensive ovarian surgery, endometriosis, smoking, chemoradiation, and genetic factors (*FMR1* genetic mutation). Women of the same age are also reported to show significant variations in ovarian reserve.[3]

MEASURES OF OVARIAN RESERVE

Ovarian reserve can be determined by both biochemical and ultrasonographic measures.

However, it is important to note that there have not been universally accepted reference ranges for these tests till date.

Biochemical measures include:

- Early follicular phase serum follicle-stimulating hormone (FSH), estradiol (E2), and inhibin B
- Serum anti-Müllerian hormone (AMH)
- Clomiphene citrate challenge test
- Ultrasonographic measures include early follicular phase measurement of the antral follicular count and ovarian volume.[4]

Biochemical Tests

Serum FSH, E2, and inhibin B are measured in the early follicular phase. E2 and inhibin B are secreted by the granulosa cells, and their negative feedback leads to low FSH levels in the early follicular phase. High levels of serum FSH on days 2–5 is suggestive of decreased ovarian reserve (DOR). When the oocyte pool is reducing, due to insufficient secretion of E2 and inhibin B, FSH levels are not fully suppressed, which leads to an increase in basal FSH and increase in E2 (60–80 pg/mL).[5] This high E2 levels will go on to suppress the FSH levels to normal. Therefore, raised E2 levels with normal FSH needs to be approached with caution. FSH is known to exhibit intercycle variability. Therefore, a cutoff of 10–20 IU/L[5] is said to be specific of DOR.

Serum AMH is another biochemical marker, which is cycle-independent. It is released by the granulosa cells in preantral and small antral follicles. Some studies have reported a cutoff of 1.0 ng/mL or less[5]; however, due to a nonuniformity in the AMH assays, a generalized cutoff has not been reported.

Clomiphene citrate challenge test is a dynamic biochemical test, which measures serum FSH levels before and after stimulation with clomiphene citrate. The American Society of Reproductive Medicine (ASRM) recommends that this test is of no clinical importance; therefore, it should not be done anymore in today's practice.[4]

Ultrasound Measures

Ultrasound measurement of ovarian volume is not commonly used for diagnosis of DOR due to lack of standardization and sensitivity. Transvaginal ultrasonographic measurement of antral follicles (follicles 2–0 mm in diameter) is shown to be a reliable marker for DOR. There is no standardized cutoff for this as well; however, studies have used a cutoff of 5 follicles in both ovaries to predict poor ovarian response to in vitro fertilization (IVF) stimulation.[6]

POOR OVARIAN RESERVE AND RECURRENT PREGNANCY LOSS

Recurrent pregnancy loss (RPL) affects about 1% of the population, and in almost 50% of these couples, the cause remains unknown.[7] Female age is an independent risk factor for RPL and diminished ovarian reserve due to a decline in the quality and quantity of oocytes, respectively.[8] With advancing maternal age, the risk of aneuploid fetus increases, which is one of the important causes of RPL.[9] The role of DOR in RPL and whether tests of ovarian measure should routinely be carried out in women with RPL are debatable. To date, neither the ASRM nor the Royal College of Obstetricians and Gynaecologists (RCOG) recommend testing of ovarian reserve in women with RPL.[10,11] However, there is new and upcoming evidence to suggest that DOR can be a causative factor in RPL.[12]

DIMINISHED OVARIAN RESERVE IN RECURRENT PREGNANCY LOSS COMPARED TO NON-RECURRENT PREGNANCY LOSS FERTILE WOMEN

In a cross-sectional study conducted by Atasevir et al.,[1] comparing women with RPL with age-matched fertile women seeking contraception, the percentage of women with FSH ≥11 U/L was significantly greater in RPL group compared to the control group (18.3% vs. 4.3%). Similarly, the percentage of women with serum AMH levels ≤1 ng/mL was greater in the RPL group (19.7%) compared to the control group (5.7%). This difference was also statistically significant.

This was further reinforced by a meta-analysis by Bunnewell et al.[3] comparing RPL with non-RPL fertile women with an odds ratio (OR) of 2.45; 95% confidence interval (CI): 1.16–5.19, suggesting a possibility of an association between DOR and RPL.

DIMINISHED OVARIAN RESERVE IN RECURRENT PREGNANCY LOSS COMPARED TO NON-RECURRENT PREGNANCY LOSS IN SUBFERTILE WOMEN

In a retrospective study conducted by Hoffmann et al.[8] in couples attending fertility clinic, it was found that DOR (assessed by clomiphene citrate challenge test) was equal as observed (18% in both the groups) in women with RPL and in subfertile women without RPL. Reproductive outcome following treatment was poorer in women with DOR whether they had a history of RPL or not. This study did not find a greater incidence of DOR in RPL population compared to the general infertile population.

DIMINISHED OVARIAN RESERVE IN WOMEN WITH UNEXPLAINED RECURRENT PREGNANCY LOSS COMPARED TO EXPLAINED RECURRENT PREGNANCY LOSS

In a study conducted by Wald et al.,[13] day-3 serum FSH and AMH levels were compared in patients with a known cause of RPL and in unexplained RPL. It was found that DOR was significantly higher in women with unexplained RPL compared to explained RPL (48% vs. 29%, $p = 0.005$). Another interesting finding in this study is that they found this association higher in patients <38 years of age compared to patients ≥38 years.

A cohort study by Bliddal et al.[2] in women with a background of unexplained RPL, serum AMH levels were correlated with live birth in the next pregnancy. This study did not find any association between DOR (as measured by serum AMH levels) and RPL (as measured by a prospective live birth). Live birth was lower with an increase in the number of previous pregnancy losses. Therefore, Bliddal et al. do not recommend AMH screening in women with unexplained RPL.

A meta-analysis by Bunnewell et al.[3] supports the association of DOR in women with unexplained RPL compared to explained RPL with an OR of 3.23; 95% CI: 1.81–5.76; and $p < 0.0001$.

WHICH ONE OF THE OVARIAN RESERVE TESTS TO BE USED?

Each of the ovarian reserve test described earlier has its own limitations. There is a lack of consensus on which ovarian reserve test accurately predicts DOR, and there is also no standardization of the reference values. Most of the literature so far has assessed ovarian reserve tests in the subfertile population to predict the response to ovarian stimulation, and none of these tests can accurately predict a live birth in the general population or in women undergoing fertility treatment.[4] The ASRM recommends AMH to be a more sensitive marker compared to FSH, and AMH and antral follicle count (AFC) are also equally reliable if AFC is done in an experienced center. Again, these recommendations are in the background of subfertility.

In a systematic review of 15 studies by Bunnewell et al.,[3] evaluating six ovarian reserve markers, namely serum AMH, FSH, luteinizing hormone (LH), E2, FSH:LH ratio, and AFC, to look at the relation between DOR and RPL, it was found that AFC and AMH had the best prognostic value to predict DOR in the background of RPL. Levels of FSH, LH, and E2 did not show any significant variations in women with and without RPL. The limitations of this systematic review include a smaller number of studies included and smaller sample size in each of these studies.

In a retrospective study on a small cohort of 79 patients,[14] the authors corelated AMH levels to the gestational age at the time of miscarriage. Women who had an anembryonic fetal loss had a median AMH level of 0.7 ng/mL compared to 1.8 ng/mL in women who had an embryonic fetal loss ($p = 0.044$). The same data showed that the miscarriage rate was 62% in women with AMH <1 ng/mL compared to 19% in women with AMH >1 ng/mL ($p = 0.001$).

In another retrospective analysis, women with three miscarriages had a lower AMH level than women with no history of miscarriage ($p = 0.05$) even after age stratification.[15] Also, the number of women with diminished ovarian reserve was higher in women with three miscarriages compared to those with no miscarriage ($p = 0.001$).

In a recent prospective study, it was concluded that low AMH levels (<1 ng/mL) are associated with lower spontaneous pregnancy rates and increased time to pregnancy.[16] In women with RPL, practitioners often perform AMH assays, in a clinic setting. This is relevant in patients with recurrent biochemical pregnancies and early losses, to prevent repeated aneuploid embryo losses. AMH also prognosticates the time to pregnancy. It will also help to decide which patients can try to conceive naturally and the patients that may require ART procedures or genetic evaluation of the embryo prior to implantation. Hence it is a useful test in women with advanced maternal age and repeated early aneuploid losses. There is mounting evidence DOR is higher in RPL group, yet none of the guidelines recommend testing for DOR in RPL patients to date.

TREATMENT

The treatment of RPL involves treating the cause if known; otherwise, expectant management is still the treatment of choice in unexplained RPL,[7] with a reported successful future pregnancy of 50–60%. IVF/intracytoplasmic sperm injection (ICSI) with preimplantation genetic testing for aneuploidies (PGT-A) is not recommended for couples with unexplained RPL.[8] The RCOG only recommends preimplantation genetic testing for structural rearrangement (PGT-SR) as an option for couples with chromosomal rearrangements. The treatment for DOR is assisted reproductive technology (ART) i.e., IVF/ICSI. Whether this would be suitable for women with a background of RPL or unexplained RPL is something that requires further investigation.

CONCLUSION

Recurrent pregnancy loss is a very challenging condition to treat. This is further aggravated, as most of the times the cause remains unknown. An informed decision making and individualized approach are crucial in the management of RPL. Currently, evaluation for DOR is not routinely recommended in patients with RPL. However, it can be considered in women with unexplained RPL, depending on other risk factors such as age and smoking. Serum AMH and AFC are shown to be reliable predictors of DOR. However, further studies with a larger study population are needed to put down robust recommendations.

REFERENCES

1. Atasevir M, Soyman Z, Demirel E, Gencdal S, Kelekci S. Diminished ovarian reserve: Is it a neglected cause in the assessment of recurrent miscarriage? A cohort study. Fertil Steril. 2016;105(5):1236-40.
2. Bliddal S, Feldt-Rasmussen U, Forman JL, Hilsted LM, Larsen EC, Christiansen OB, et al. Anti-Müllerian hormone and live birth in unexplained recurrent pregnancy loss. Reprod Biomed Online. 2023;46(6):995-1003.

3. Bunnewell SJ, Honess ER, Karia AM, Keay SD, Al Wattar BH, Quenby S. Diminished ovarian reserve in recurrent pregnancy loss: a systematic review and meta-analysis. Fertil Steril. 2020;113(4):818-27.
4. Chang HJ, Han SH, Lee JR, Jee BC, Lee BI, Suh CS, et al. Impact of laparoscopic cystectomy on ovarian reserve: serial changes of serum anti-Mullerian hormone levels. Fertil Steril. 2010;94(1):343-9.
5. Daney de Marcillac F, Pinton A, Guillaume A, Sagot P, Pirrello O, Rongieres C. What are the likely IVF/ICSI outcomes if there is a discrepancy between serum AMH and FSH levels? A multicenter retrospective study. J Gynecol Obstet Hum Reprod. 2017;46(8):629-35.
6. Practice Committee of the American Society for Reproductive Medicine. Evaluation and treatment of recurrent pregnancy loss: a committee opinion. Fertil Steril. 2012;98(5):1103-11.
7. Hansen KR, Knowlton NS, Thyer AC, Charleston JS, Soules MR, Klein NA. A new model of reproductive aging: the decline in ovarian non-growing follicle number from birth to menopause. Hum Reprod. 2008;23(3):699-708.
8. Hoffman GE, Khoury J, Thie J. Recurrent pregnancy loss and diminished ovarian reserve. Fertil Steril. 2000;74(6): 1192-5.
9. Klinkert ER, Broekmans FJ, Looman CW, Habbema JD, te Velde ER. The antral follicle count is a better marker then basal follicle-stimulating hormone for the selection of older patients with acceptable pregnancy prospects after in vitro fertilization. Fertil Steril. 2005;83(3):811-4.
10. Regan L, Rai R, Saravelos S, Li TC. Recurrent Miscarriage Green-top Guideline No.17. BJOG. 2023;130(12):e9-e39.
11. Practice Committee of the American Society for Reproductive Medicine. Testing and interpreting measures of ovarian reserve: a committee opinion. Fertil Steril. 2012;98(6):1407-15.
12. TG Baker. A quantitative and cytological study of germ cells in human ovaries. Proc R Soc Lond B Biol Sci. 1963;158:417-33.
13. Wald KA, Shahine LK, Lamb JD, Marshall LA, Hickok LR. High incidence of diminished ovarian reserve in young unexplained recurrent pregnancy loss patients. Gynecol Endocrinol. 2020;36(12):1079-81.
14. Pils S, Stepien N, Kurz C, Nouri K, Promberger R, Ott J. Anti-Mullerian hormone is linked to the type of early pregnancy loss in idiopathic recurrent miscarriage: a retrospective cohort study. Reprod Biol Endocrinol. 2017;15(1):60.
15. Tan J, Luo L, Jiang J, Yan N, Wang Q. Decreased Ovarian Reserves with an Increasing Number of Previous Early Miscarriages: A Retrospective Analysis. Front Endocrinol (Lausanne). 2022;13:859332.
16. Nelson SM, Shaw M, Ewing BJ, McLean K, Vechery A, Briggs SF. Antimüllerian hormone levels are associated with time to pregnancy in a cohort study of 3,150 women. Fertil Steril. 2024;122(6):1114-23.

CHAPTER 34

Hyperhomocysteinemia

Ritu Jain, Mala Arora

ABSTRACT

Hyperhomocysteinemia (Hhcy) is associated with many conditions, including genetic mutations, nutritional deficiencies, insulin resistance, polycystic ovarian syndrome, and certain medications. High homocysteine levels can affect multiple organs and their function. It affects embryo quality in assisted reproduction. During pregnancy it may cause endothelial and trophoblastic dysfunction, formation of platelet rich thrombi and attenuation of plasminogen activator binding sites. This results in intravascular thrombi in both the arterial and venous system, which leads to pregnancy complications. It can be easily treated by nutritional supplements of folic acid, vitamin B_6 and B_{12}. In certain situations of Hhcy, anticoagulation may also be required to improve pregnancy outcomes.

Keywords: Hyperhomocysteinemia, RPL, DNA methylation, Pregnancy complications, MTHFR gene mutation, Folic acid, Vitamin B_6, Vitamin B_{12}.

INTRODUCTION

Homocysteine is a fundamental intermediary metabolite and the decomposition product of methionine metabolism, first identified 90 years ago by *Butz and du Vigneaud.*[1]

Homocysteine, an intermediary product in methionine and one carbon metabolism, is important in cellular metabolism and *protein synthesis.*[2] Homocysteine levels vary between men and women, with a normal range between 5 and 15 μmol/L. Hyperhomocysteinemia (Hhcy) is when levels exceed 15 μmol/L.[3]

The clinical manifestation of Hhcy is diverse; it affects every process of reproduction like spermatogenesis, folliculogenesis and embryo formation, implantation, and growth. It is an established cause for congenital malformations like neural tube defects, and cardiac malformations, miscarriages, placental abruption, hypertension, and preeclampsia (PE). It is also a predisposing factor for cardiovascular, cerebrovascular, thromboembolic diseases, Alzheimer's and dementia.

UNDERSTANDING PATHOPHYSIOLOGY

Homocysteine is a sulfur-containing amino acid consisting of a glycine core with a 2-mercaptoethyl side-chains **(Fig. 1)**. Homocysteine is biosynthesized in vivo from essential amino acid methionine via a multistep process involving vitamin B_6, B_{12}, and folic acid. Methionine is first converted to *S*-adenosyl methionine (SAM-e) by a reaction catalyzed by S-adenosylmethionine synthetase. The adenosine is then hydrolyzed to yield L-homocysteine which is metabolized to cystathionine by cystathionine β-synthase, using pyridoxine (vitamin B_6) as a cofactor. Homocysteine is also recycled to L-methionine via N5-methyl tetrahydrofolate as the methyl donor and cobalamin (vitamin B_{12})-related enzymes, hence completing the cycle[4] **(Fig. 2)**.

ETIOLOGY

Hyperhomocysteinemia may occur due to:

- Increased production of methionine (transmethylation)
- Decreased synthesis of cysteine (transsulfuration)
- Decreased conversion of homocysteine to methionine (remethylation)

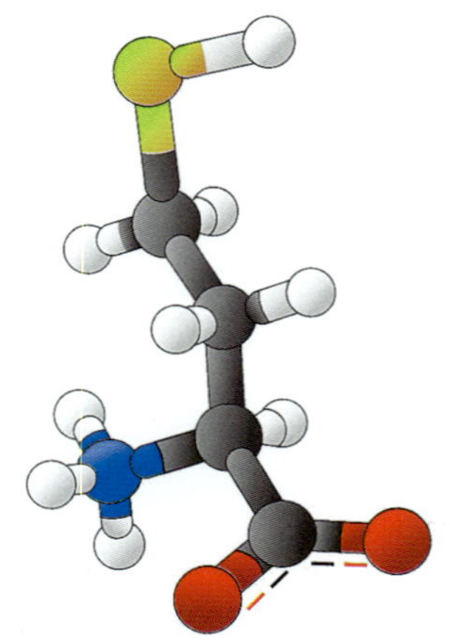

Fig. 1: Structure of homocysteine.

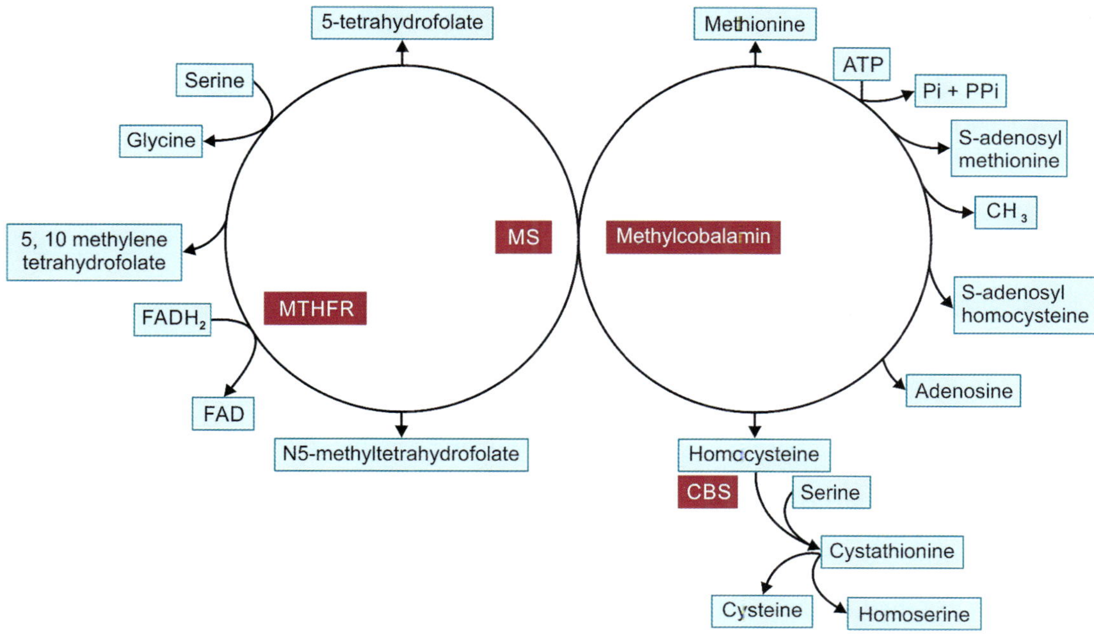

Fig. 2: Homocysteine metabolism. (CBS: cystathionine β-synthase; MTHFR: methylene tetrahydrofolate reductase; MS: methionine synthase; FAD and FADH2: flavin adenine dinucleotide; ATP: adenosine triphosphate; Pi: phosphate; PPi: pyrophosphate)

- Decreased metabolism or decreased renal excretion of homocysteine, renal insufficiency, or malabsorption

Some of the known causes of Hhcy include:

- *Nutritional deficiencies:* Up to two-thirds of all Hhcy cases are due to nutritional deficiencies. These are folate, B_{12}, and B_6, all vitamins that act as cofactors and help control levels of homocysteine.
- *Genetic mutations:* The methylene tetrahydrofolate reductase (MTHFR) gene can show mutations of various kinds. The most significant is MTHFR 1793 G>A polymorphism. It is over represented in the recurrent miscarriage (RM) group 15.38% versus 4.14% in controls. Other mutations like the 677 C>T and 1298 A>C do not show a significant preponderance in the RM group.[5] Mutation in the cystathionine β synthase (CBS) gene results in severe Hhcy, with levels in the range of 50–100 µg/mL. This is a rare metabolic disorder and presents with homocystinuria.[6]
- Polycystic Ovarian disease and insulin resistance. Insulin resistance is associated with hyperhomocysteinemia which may be responsible for RPL in this population.[7]
- *Medications:* Some people acquire Hhcy by taking certain medications, including anticonvulsants, cyclosporine, methotrexate, proton pump inhibitors, and theophylline.
- *Medical conditions:* Liver disease, kidney disease, hypothyroidism, and some cancers can increase HC to dangerous levels.
- *MTHFR gene mutation:* Levels of homocysteine are lower in pregnant state due to hemodilution and some fetal absorption. Its level being lowest in 2nd trimester.

DIAGNOSIS

Homocysteine levels are checked in the fasting state with an overnight fast of >8 hours. The blood should be centrifuged immediately after collection and cooled for accurate results.

Methionine loading test is recommended to unmask the tendency to Hhcy. After an 8 hour fast, the patient is administered methionine capsules 100 mg/kg body weight (for a 60 kg women, it would be 6 gm, i.e., 12 capsules of 500 mg taken together). Blood is drawn for homocysteine levels after 4 hours. Elevated homocysteine levels are classified in **Box 1**.

Incidence

Both the authors screened all recurrent pregnancy loss (RPL) patients for Hhcy. Pooled data from two clinics is presented here. Total number of RPL patients screened were 306. Hhcy was documented in 33% of patients of

BOX 1: Classification of hyperhomocysteinemia.

- 5–15 mmol/L: Normal levels
- 15–30 mmol/L: Mild hyperhomocysteinemia
- 30–100 mmol/L: Moderate hyperhomocysteinemia
- >100 mmol/L: Severe hyperhomocysteinemia

TABLE 1: RPL patients with Hhcy.

	Numbers (percentage %)
Number of RPL screened	306
Normal homocysteine	203
Patients with Hhcy	103 (103/306—33.66%)
Mild Hhcy	69 (69/103—66.99%)
Moderate Hhcy	26 (26/103—25.24%)
Severe Hhcy	8 (8/103—7.76%)

(Hhcy: Hyperhomocysteinemia; RPL: Recurrent pregnancy loss)

which 67% had mild, 26% had moderate, and only 7.7% had severe Hhcy **(Table 1)**. All patients were treated with supplementing folic acid 5 mg, along with vitamin B_6, i.e., pyridoxine 40–100 mg and vitamin B_{12} 500 μg daily throughout pregnancy. In addition, they received low-dose aspirin 75 mg daily and some received low-molecular weight heparin 40 IU daily subcutaneously. Two patients with severe Hhcy had birth defects, one had spina bifida and the other had a ventricular septal defect. >80% of these patients developed gestational hypertension and/or PE as well as fetal growth restriction (FGR) when pregnancy continued to the third trimester. APLA syndrome was coexistent in four cases.

PATHOGENESIS

Hyperhomocysteinemia causes trophoblastic and placental dysfunction by increased production of free radicals like hydrogen peroxide and superoxide which causes oxidative injury of endothelial cells, initiates cascade of thrombosis, diminished blood vessels in chorionic villi, and compromised blood circulation at the maternal-fetal interface. Hhcy also reduces nitric oxide (NO) release by endothelial cells and increases endothelial dysfunction. **(Box 2)**.

Hyperhomocysteinemia is associated with a large spectrum of pregnancy complications, including neural tube defects, cardiac malformations, RPL, PE, preterm delivery placental abruption, FGR, and gestational diabetes mellitus (GDM). It is also implicated in restenosis of coronary grafts, stroke, and Alzheimer 's disease. Moderate

BOX 2: Impact of hyperhomocysteinemia on vascular system.

- Hyperhomocysteinemia
- Intimal thickening
- Endothelial dysfunction
- Smooth muscle hypertrophy
- Platelet accumulation
- Formation of platelet rich accumulative thrombi
- Attenuation of plasminogen activator binding sites

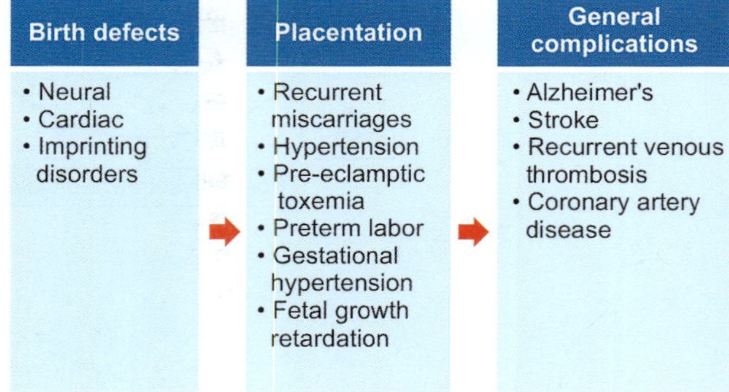

Fig. 3: Complications of hyperhomocysteinemia.

Hhcy (15–30 μmol/L) may predispose to recurrent venous thrombosis. These effects are potentiated if there is coexisting hereditary thrombophilia or antiphospholipid syndrome[8,9] **(Fig. 3)**.

Folliculogenesis

Follicular fluid contains homocysteine.[10] Systemic homocysteine levels reflect the follicular fluid homocysteine levels. High homocysteine concentration (>14.7 μmol/L) in the follicular fluid affects follicular development and decreases embryo quality.[11]

Szymanski and Kazdepka-Zieminska[12] found that that there is a relationship between homocysteine levels and oocyte maturity. Oocytes with low homocysteine levels are higher quality and better maturity. Prospective cohort study by Y Razi et al.[13] has shown significant association between follicular fluid homocysteine and oocyte maturation.

In human oocytes and in the early preimplantation embryo, homocysteine is preferentially recycled by folate pathway as cysteine beta synthase, is poorly expressed or absent. Follicular homocysteine levels are higher after ovarian stimulation and affect oocyte maturity. High homocysteine levels may adversely affect embryo cleavage and development by remodulation of early embryonic methylation pattern.[14] It causes decreased division and increased fragmentation of cells and hence affects embryo quality. During folliculogenesis, Hhcy may also promote apoptosis, leading to follicular atresia.

Hyperhomocysteinemia in Male Reproduction

Hyperhomocysteinemia affects spermatogenesis especially sperm quality and DNA methylation. DNA methylation is an epigenetic modification integral to chromosome structure, X chromosome inactivation, and gene imprinting. Disruption of spermatogenesis process is detrimental to spermatogenesis and embryo quality.[15] It has been speculated that aberrant sperm DNA[16] methylation may lead to epigenetic defects that adversely affect the first and subsequent generations of offspring.[16]

Recurrent Miscarriages

25% of women with a recurrent loss have Hhcy or at least a pathological methionine loading test. In a study Del Bianco et al.[17] showed that 33% women with recurrent miscarriages have elevated homocysteine levels.

A meta-analysis published in 2000 concluded that the risk of recurrent miscarriage is increased in patients with either pre or after load Hhcy, as well as MTHFR gene 677C to T mutation.[18] They show trophoblast dysfunction, diminished blood flow in microvilli along with faulty gametogenesis, and embryogenesis, that leads to miscarriages **(Fig. 4)**. Pregnancy loss may range from implantation failure to second trimester miscarriages. The incidence of miscarriage is increased and pregnancy outcome is poor if there is associated congenital or acquired thrombophilia, and/or antiphospholipid syndrome. Fetal congenital heart defects and neural tube defects are common with Hhcy and may lead to induced termination of pregnancy. Recurrent early miscarriage relates to both remethylation and transsulfuration defects and functional Hhcy due to B_{12}, B_6, and folic acid deficiency. Supplementation of folic acid and vitamins B_{12} and B_6 decreases homocysteine levels and improves pregnancy outcome.[19] A recent review confirms the association of Hhcy and pregnancy complications.[9]

MTHFR Gene Mutation

Methylene tetrahydrofolate reductase is an enzyme that helps to convert homocysteine to methionine. Mutations in the MTHFR gene will lead to high homocysteine levels. Two types of mutations have been documented, C677T (cytosine to thiamine nucleotide mutation at nucleotide 677) and A1298C (adenosine to cytosine mutation at nucleotide 1298), both can cause amino acid substitution and render the enzyme MTHFR less stable. Individuals harboring these mutations can have elevated homocysteine levels.

The MTHFR T/T genotype has been shown to be a significant risk factor for recurrent implantation failure.[18] Females with the MTHFR 677TT genotype have RPL, as it shows Hhcy, increased natural killer cells, and decreased expressions of 25(OH) vitamin D, which could all be responsible for RPL.[20] The MTHFR 677C to T genotype can raise the morbidity of RPL by two to three times. Low-dose aspirin, enoxaparin, and folic acid were the most effective therapy in women with RM who carried a C677T *MTHFR* mutation as compared to only folic acid and low-dose aspirin (See Appendix 1 Case 3).[21]

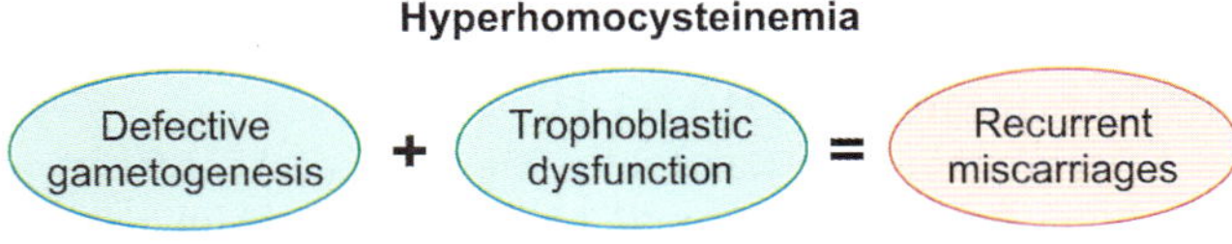

Fig. 4: Mechanism of recurrent pregnancy loss.

Congenital Abnormalities

Maternal Hhcy is associated with cardiac and neural tube defects. There is a stronger association of ventricular septal defect, transposition of great vessels, and tetralogy of Fallot with maternal Hhcy.[22] Functional Hhcy due to deficiency of folate and B_{12} can lead to neural tube defects.[23] This has been documented with Hhcy in the mother but recent studies suggest that males with Hhcy can also father children with neural tube defects.[24]

Hypertension

Hyperhomocysteinemia is more common in pregnancies complicated by hypertensive disorders of pregnancy. White WM concluded in his study that in comparison to normal pregnancies, a record of pregnancy-induced hypertension (PIH) was related to a 4.5% higher serum homocysteine level ($p < 0.05$) and 1.6-fold elevated odds of displaying an elevated homocysteine.[25]

Another case-control study by Serrano NC reflected that high maternal serum homocysteine level was a risk factor for PE.[26] The increased homocysteine expression is also an indicator of cardiovascular disease later.

Preterm Labor

Hyperhomocysteinemia induces preterm labor in many ways. It is an important and crucial marker of placental vascular disease. It potentiates inflammation and increases the cellular gap links, hence causing premature delivery.[27]

Homocysteine could independently promote idiopathic contraction of the myometrium.[28] Hhcy leads to more frequent and high amplitude uterine contractions by inhibiting activation of methyltransferase. Hhcy is also associated with preterm premature rupture of membranes.[29]

Placental Abruption

Hyperhomocysteinemia is a significant risk factor in abruption of placentae and pregnancy loss as shown in a systematic review.[30]

Fetal Growth Retardation

Hyperhomocysteinemia is associated with fetal growth retardation as it restrains the transfer of endogenous amino acids in the placenta. Also, the activity and protein expression of Na^+/K^+ ATPase are reduced in microvillous syncytiotrophoblast plasma membranes in pregnancies of intrauterine growth restriction. The association was first published in 2003[31] and has been validated more recently.[32] Supplementation of folic acid, vitamin B_6, and B_{12} appears to improve fetal growth in such cases.[33]

Gestational Diabetes Mellitus

There is a variable correlation between high homocysteine levels and gestational diabetes. Hhcy relates to reduced fasting and 2-hour glucose numbers and decreased odds of GDM.[34] A case-controlled study from China has shown an association of gestational diabetes risk with increased homocysteine levels in their pregnant population. The GDM risk was 1.79 times higher in patients with increased total homocysteine (≥7.29 µmol/L) relative to females with lower total homocysteine expression (<5.75 µmol/L).[35]

CONCLUSION

High homocysteine levels are associated with risks to both the mother and fetus during reproduction. Its association with poor outcome in ART cycles and recurrent implantation failure is established. However, its association with neural tube defects in the fetus is most widely studied. Identification of this risk led many nations to fortify their grain with folic acid to reduce homocysteine levels and prevent neural tube defects in the population. Similarly, the association of Hhcy with pregnancy-induced hypertension, abruptio placentae, and gestational diabetes is well established. There is evidence for its association with RPL, but the evidence is not very robust. In many western countries where the grain is fortified, this data is not available. But in India, Hhcy is common and in our data presented, it has an association with RPL and other pregnancy complications. Correcting nutritional deficiencies is important in this population and anticoagulation may be required to improve pregnancy outcomes. It becomes especially important in patients with underlying inherited thrombophilia or other coagulation disorders.

REFERENCES

1. Butz L, du Vigneaud V. The formation of a homologue of cystine by the decompensation of methionine with sulfuric acid. J Biol Chem. 1932;99:135-42.
2. Miller JW. (2005). Homocysteine. Encyclopedia of Human Nutrition, 2nd edition. Introduction. [online] Available from https://shop.elsevier.com/books/encyclopedia-of-human-nutrition/allen/978-0-08-045428-3. [Last accessed December, 2024]
3. Veeranki S, Gandhapudi SK, Tyagi SC. Interactions of hyperhomocysteinemia and T cell immunity in causation of hypertension. Can J Physiol Pharmacol. 2017;95(3):239-46.
4. Kumar A, Palfrey HA, Pathak R, Kadowitz PJ, Gettys TW, Subramanyam NM. The metabolism and significance of homocysteine in nutrition and health. Nutr Metab (Lond). 2017;14:78.
5. Seremak-Mrozikiewicz A, Drews K, Kurzawinska G, Bogacz A, Grzeskowiak E, Mrozikiewicz PM. The significance of 1793G>A polymorphism in MTHFR gene in women with first trimester recurrent miscarriages. Neuro Endocrinol Lett. 2010;31(5):717-23.
6. Arora M. Hyperhomocysteinemia and Pregnancy. ECAB Series Elsevier. Gurgaon: Elsevier India; 2014.
7. Maleedhu P, M V, S S B S, Kodumuri PK, Devi D V. Status of Homocysteine in Polycystic Ovary Syndrome (PCOS). J Clin Diagn Res. 2014;8(2):31-3.
8. Thakur P, Bhalerao A. High Homocysteine Levels During Pregnancy and Its Association With Placenta-Mediated Complications: A Scoping Review. Cureus. 2023;15(2):e35244.
9. Dai C, Fei Y, Li J, Shi Y, Yang X. A Novel Review of Homocysteine and Pregnancy Complications. Biomed Res Int. 2021;2021:6652231.
10. Steegers-Theunissen RP, Steegers EA, Thomas CMG, Hollanders HM, Peereboom-Stegeman JH, Trijbels FJ, et al. Study on the presence of homocysteine in ovarian follicular fluid. Fertil Steril. 1993;60:1006-10.
11. Ebisch IMW, Peters WH, Thomas CM, Wetzels AM, Peer PG, Steegers RP. Homocysteine, glutathione and related thiols affect fertility parameters in the (sub) fertile couple. Hum Reprod. 2006;21:1725-33.
12. Szymanski W, Kazdepka-Zieminska A. Effect of homocysteine concentration in follicular fluid on a degree of oocyte maturity. Gynekol Pol. 2003;74:1392-6.

13. Razi Y, Eftekhar M, Fesahat F, Dehghani Firouzabadi R, Razi N, Sabour M, et al. Concentrations of homocysteine in follicular fluid and embryo quality and oocyte maturity in infertile women: a prospective cohort. J Obstet Gynaecol. 2021;41(4):588-93.
14. Melissa R, Wayne J. Epigenetics in fertilization and preimplantation embryo development. Prog Biophys Mol Biol. 2013;113(3):423-32.
15. Aitken RJ, De Iuliis GN. Origins and consequences of DNA damage in male germ cells. Reprod Biomed Online. 2007;14:727-33.
16. Barroso M, Handy DE, Castro R. The link between hyperhomocysteinemia and hypomethylation: Implications for cardiovascular disease. J. Inborn Errors Metab Screen. 2017;5:1-15. https://doi.org/10.1177/2326409817698994
17. Del Bianco A, Maruotti G, Fulgieri AM, Celeste T, Lombardi L, Amato NA, et al. Aborti spontanei ricorrenti e iperomocisteinemia [Recurrent spontaneous miscarriages and hyperhomocysteinemia]. Minerva Ginecol. 2004;56(5):379-83.
18. Nelen WL, Blom HJ, Steegers EA, den Heijer M, Eskes TK. Hyperhomocysteinemia and recurrent early pregnancy loss: a meta-analysis. Fertil Steril. 2000;74(6):1196-9.
19. Mukhopadhyay I, Pruthviraj V, Rao PS, Biswas M. Hyperhomocysteinemia in recurrent pregnancy loss and the effect of folic acid and vitamin B12 on homocysteine levels: a prospective analysis. Int J Reprod Contracept Obstet Gynecol. 2017;6(6):2258-61.
20. Ota K, Takahashi T, Han A, Damvaeba S, Mizunuma H, Kwak-Kim J. Effects of MTHFR C677T polymorphism on vitamin D, homocysteine and natural killer cell cytotoxicity in women with recurrent pregnancy losses. Hum Reprod. 2020;35(6):1276-87.
21. Merviel P, Cabry R, Lourdel E, Lanta S, Amant C, Copin H, et al. Comparison of two preventive treatments for patients with recurrent miscarriages carrying a C677T methylenetetrahydrofolate reductase mutation: 5-year experience. J Int Med Res. 2017;45(6):1720-30.
22. Malik RA, Lone MR, Ahmed A, Koul KA, Malla RR. Maternal hyperhomocysteinemia and congenital heart defects: A prospective case control study in Indian population. Indian Heart J. 2017;69(1):17-9.
23. Kucha W, Seifu D, Tirsit A, Yigeremu M, Abebe M, Hailu D, et al. Folate, Vitamin B12, and Homocysteine Levels in Women with Neural Tube Defect-Affected Pregnancy in Addis Ababa, Ethiopia. Front Nutr. 2022;9:873900.
24. Yu Y, Jia C, Shi Q, Zhu Y, Liu Y. Hyperhomocysteinemia in men with a reproductive history of fetal neural tube defects. Medicine (Baltimore). 2019;98(2):e13998.
25. White WM, Turner ST, Bailey KR, Mosley TH Jr, Kardia SL, Wiste HJ, et al. Hypertension in pregnancy is associated with elevated homocysteine levels later in life. Am J Obstet Gynecol. 2013;209(5):454.e1-e7.
26. Serrano NC, Quintero-Lesmes DC, Becerra-Bayona S, Guio E, Beltran M, Paez MC, et al. Association of pre-eclampsia risk with maternal levels of folate, homocysteine and vitamin B12 in Colombia: a case-control study. PLoS One. 2018;13(12):e0208137.
27. Kramer MS, Kahn SR, Rozen R, Evans R, Platt RW, Chen MF, et al. Vasculopathic and thrombophilic risk factors for spontaneous preterm birth. Int J Epidemiol. 2009;38(3):715-723.
28. Ayar A, Celik H, Ozcelik O, Kelestimur H. Homocysteine-induced enhancement of spontaneous contractions of myometrium isolated from pregnant women. Acta Obstet Gynecol Scand. 2003;82(9):789-93.
29. Ferguson SE, Smith GN, Walker MC. Maternal plasma homocysteine levels in women with preterm premature rupture of membranes. Medical Hypotheses. 2001;56(1):85-90.
30. Ray JG, Laskin CA. Folic acid and homocyst(e)ine metabolic defects and the risk of placental abruption, pre-eclampsia and spontaneous pregnancy loss: a systematic review. Placenta. 1999;20(7):519-29.
31. Infante-Rivard C, Rivard GE, Gauthier R, Théorêt Y. Unexpected Relationship between Plasma Homocysteine and Intrauterine Growth Restriction. Clin Chem. 2003;49(9):1476-82.
32. Gaiday A, Balash L, Tussupkaliyev A. The Role of High Concentrations of Homocysteine for the Development of Fetal Growth Restriction. Rev Bras Ginecol Obstet. 2022;44(4): 352-9.
33. Leeda M, Riyazi N, de Vries JIP, Jakobs C, van Geijn HP, Dekker GA. Effects of folic acid and vitamin B6 supplementation on women with hyperhomocysteinemia and a history of preeclampsia or fetal growth restriction. Am J Obstet Gynecol. 1998;179(1):135-9.
34. López-Quesada E, Antònia Vilaseca M, Gómez E, Lailla JM. Are plasma total homocysteine and other amino acids associated with glucose intolerance in uncomplicated pregnancies and preeclampsia? Eur J Obstet Gynecol Reprod Biol. 2005;119(1):36-41.
35. Deng M, Zhou J, Tang Z, Xiang J, Yi J, Peng Y, et al. The correlation between plasma total homocysteine level and gestational diabetes mellitus in a Chinese Han population. Sci Rep. 2020;10(1):18679.

CHAPTER 35

Role of Vitamin D

Jayati Dureja, BS Susheela Rani

ABSTRACT

Vitamin D is not only essential for bone health, but plays important roles in pregnancy immune modulation, placental development and angiogenesis. It could be responsible for epigenetic changes as well. There is a silent epidemic of vitamin D deficiency that may be responsible for unexplained recurrent pregnancy loss (RPL). The supplementation of vitamin D, in the recommended daily dosage, should start from the preconception period and continued throughout the pregnancy.

Keywords: Vitamin D deficiency, RPL, Immune dysregulation, Epigenetic causes.

INTRODUCTION

The sunshine vitamin, ideally available in abundance, has surprisingly been reported deficient in up to 88.6% of adolescent girls and 84% of pregnant women in Northern India.[1]

Alarming, because vitamin D has an increasing repertoire of nonclassical actions coming to light over the last decade, ranging from immune modulation to placental maturation via trophoblast invasion and placental spiral artery remodeling which can have long-term maternal–fetal consequences, starting from early pregnancy. The lack of sufficient vitamin D is thus being increasingly linked with aberrant endometrial receptivity, dysregulated placentation, and proinflammatory immune processes—all also identified as processes responsible for recurrent pregnancy loss (RPL).[2,3] Its association with recurrent miscarriages is well established, a systematic review and meta-analysis published in 2022 involving 7,663 women in both observational studies and randomized controlled trials concluded that low vitamin D levels were associated with recurrent miscarriage.[4]

In this chapter, we will explore the underlying mechanisms by which the role of vitamin D in immune regulation, angiogenesis at placental level and epigenetics is being increasingly associated with RPL. Elucidating the link between vitamin D deficiency and miscarriage risk may pave the way for targeted screening and intervention strategies aimed at reducing the burden of RPL.

MECHANISM OF ACTION OF VITAMIN D IN RECURRENT PREGNANCY LOSS

Placental Development

Historically, the human placenta was one of the first extrarenal tissues shown to be capable of synthesizing 1,25(OH)2D, with CYP27B1 activity detectable in both maternal decidua and fetal trophoblast. The placenta is a "Barrier Site" which expresses a high concentration of many components of the vitamin D signal transduction pathway, including vitamin D receptor (VDR), and cytochrome P450 genes, CYP27B1, CYP24A, etc. allowing for active vitamin D synthesis to regulate localized responses. Vitamin D upregulates M2 macrophages and Th2 innate immunity that help improve endometrial receptivity through immune regulation locally. Adequate vitamin D levels may ensure proper intracrine immune system regulations along with angiogenesis that allows for trophoblastic invasion and placental spiral artery remodeling leading to the development of a healthy placenta and decidua.[2-5]

Hormone Balance

Vitamin D levels influence the synthesis and secretion of placental prolactin and human chorionic gonadotropin (hCG), which is beneficial to the nutrition of endometrium and the maintenance of corpus luteum function. Thus, low vitamin D levels potentially result in a hostile environment for the growing fetus, with inadequate nutrition, which presents clinically anywhere between recurrent miscarriage to preeclampsia.[3,5]

Immune Regulation

Vitamin D participates in both innate and adaptive immune responses. In normal pregnancy, the adaptive immune responses are known to be downregulated while innate immunity is upregulated in an attempt to benefit the fetus as an allograft. Vitamin D promotes a shift from Th1 to Th2 cell phenotype by both downregulating IFN-γ and upregulating IL-4 to produce immune tolerance at the maternal-fetal interface of the placenta, helping in embryo implantation. Decidual M2 macrophages promote fetal-maternal immune tolerance, tissue remodeling, and clearance of apoptotic cell, and vitamin D helps in conversion of M1 macrophages to M2 type in the decidua. The placenta is probably the most prominent site for extrarenal activation of vitamin D during pregnancy, serving as an important basis of its immunomodulatory function.

In RPL, about 50% cases have no clearly defined pathology and are associated with immune system dysregulation to some degree. In women with recurrent miscarriage, reduced CYP27B1 at the fetal-maternal interface has been noted, which can be responsible for reduced rates of implantation and the decreased local immunological protection for embryo. Women with insufficient levels of serum vitamin D have also reported higher number of pregnancy loss compared to those with normal levels.[5]

Women with recurrent miscarriages who have low levels of serum vitamin D also have abnormally high levels of $CD19^+$ B cells and $CD56^+$ NK cells, indicating a predominantly Th1- type response (IFN-γ and TNF-α), and an elevated NK cell cytotoxicity in their peripheral blood samples. Studies show that vitamin D supplementation results in a sharp decline in these peripheral Th1 cell types, supporting the immunomodulatory role of 1,25(OH)2D.[6]

Vitamin D deficiency indirectly may also exacerbate known autoimmune causes of RPL like antiphospholipid antibody (APA) syndrome. A low vitamin D level has been associated with increased odds of positive APA, antinuclear antigen antibody, anti-ssDNA and thyroid peroxidase (TPO) antibody in women with RPL. The severity and susceptibility for autoimmune diseases increase in women with vitamin D deficiency and its supplementation has beneficial effects. For instance, correction of vitamin D deficiency in patients with APS is shown to have a suppressive effect on anti-β2 glycoprotein expression, thus decreasing the risk of thrombosis.[7]

Epigenetics

The HOXA-10 (homeobox A10) gene expression is very important for development of the uterus and essential for endometrial development, allowing uterine receptivity to implantation of the embryo. The HOXA-10 is regulated by progestins and estrogens, acting via the estrogen response elements, and by 1,25(OH)2D, exerting its influence through VDRE (vitamin D response element). An orchestrated symphony between all these factors results in normal decidualization. HOXA-10 expression is known to be upregulated by 1,25-(OH)2D3 in human endometrial stromal cells, highlighting the epigenetic role of vitamin D levels in transcriptional activation of the homeobox gene. Low levels of vitamin D can impact the expression of the gene, and in turn the functional differentiation of the endometrium. The quality of implantation processes is potentially epigenetically modifiable by vitamin D supplementation in cases with RPL.[5,6,8]

INVESTIGATIONS AND DIAGNOSIS

As vitamin D deficiency is largely subclinical and silent, the only way to screen is to draw a blood sample for plasma 25(OH)D. It is the major circulating form of vitamin D which represents both oral sources and vitamin D produced from sun exposure. It has a half-life of approximately 2–3 weeks, compared to the biologically active form 1,25(OH) D3 which has a half-life of only 4–6 hours.

Estimation of plasma 25(OH)D levels is the most reliable marker of vitamin D status. High-performance liquid chromatography (HPLC) is the gold standard method to measure this but owing to its cumbersome methodology. Immunoassays such as radioimmunoassay (RIA), enzyme-linked immunosorbent assay (ELISA), chemiluminescence immunoassay, and protein binding assays are used in routine testing of 25(OH)D in clinical laboratories. Advances in liquid chromatography tandem mass spectroscopy (LC-MS) also allow for the direct measurement of 25(OH)D in human serum.[9]

The following levels based on immunoassay tests are recommended by most laboratories:

- *Vitamin D deficiency:* Plasma 25(OH)D levels <20 ng/mL

- *Vitamin D insufficiency:* Plasma 25(OH)D = 21–29 ng/mL
- *Vitamin D sufficiency:* Plasma 25(OH)D >30 ng/mL

MANAGEMENT

Vitamin D3 supplements are available in capsule, tablet, and liquid forms, as well as depo injection for patients with poor compliance. It is safe to administer the depo form during early/late pregnancy in deficient women to expeditely bring the vitamin D levels to normal. The recommended dose of vitamin D in women with vitamin D deficiency is 2,000–4,000 units daily.[10,11] The recommended daily intake of vitamin D during pregnancy and lactation was over 1,000 units per day.[12] Doses <1,000 units per day were inadequate during pregnancy. As per guidelines of the endocrine society, a routine daily supplementation is superior to intermittent high-dose supplementation.[13] However, women with severe deficiency in early pregnancy will definitely be benefitted with high-dose supplementation, even though it is parenteral.

Recommended daily dose of vitamin D is depicted in **Table 1**.

While multiple studies have established an association between vitamin D deficiency and miscarriages, there is currently no evidence that supplementation of vitamin D in such women helps reduce recurrent miscarriages. A systematic review published by Tamblyn et al. included 4 highly heterogeneous studies with variable treatment dose of vitamin D in women with recurrent miscarriages. Though these women had fewer miscarriages than controls, the difference was not statistically significant.[4] Vitamin D supplementation (20 IU/day) for 2 months in women with recurrent miscarriage significantly reduced the percentage of peripheral blood $CD19^+$ B cells, the percentage of TNF-α-producing Th cells, and NK cytotoxicity at all effector-to-target ratios in a study conducted by Chen et al., supporting the hypothesis that vitamin D plays an immunomodulatory role in RPL.[6]

TABLE 1: Recommended daily dose of vitamin D.

Condition	*Dosage*
Vitamin D deficiency/insufficiency in pregnancy	2,000–4,000 IU/day
Vitamin D deficiency/insufficiency in postpartum period	4,000–6,400 IU/day
Vitamin D sufficient levels in preconception, pregnancy, and postpartum	1,000–2,000 IU/day

The National Academy of Medicine (NAM) recommends that vitamin D supplementation dose in nonpregnant women and women in preconceptional period with vitamin D deficiency, should be 60,000 IU/month or 2,000 IU/day.[14] The recommended daily allowance has progressively increased over the last decade, with the emerging role of vitamin D in immune-modulation. Another recent review[15] emphasizes the role of vitamin D in early immune adaptation to pregnancy.

In a recent meta-analysis, it was observed that women with RPL had lower vitamin D levels than controls.[16] It is also speculated that women with RPL had a paucity of vitamin D receptors and a decreased expression of CYP27B1 in the villous and decidual tissue, thereby causing vitamin D deficiency at the cellular level and leading to immune dysregulation and pregnancy loss. Another recent study looked at genetic variation of maternal vitamin D receptor (VDR) Fok1 gene and found that it was associated with RPL. It is thus postulated that not only deficient vitamin D levels will contribute to RPL but vitamin D receptor polymorphism, which may be genetic or epigenetic, is also associated with RPL. Further studies will be required to prove this hypothesis. However, for current practice, it is mandatory to optimize vitamin D levels in patients with RPL. The association of vitamin D with autoimmunity is examined in a study that compared vitamin D levels in nonpregnant state among three groups i.e., healthy controls and women with RPL with or without autoantibodies.[15] It was observed that women with RPL had lower vitamin D levels than controls, but RPL women with autoantibodies like antiphospholipid and antinuclear antibodies had even lower levels of vitamin D, thereby proving that vitamin D deficiency is associated with autoimmunity.

CONCLUSION

Vitamin D deficiency is a silent modern day pandemic with far reaching consequences on reproductive and maternal health. Women with unexplained RPL with underlying vitamin D deficiency could benefit from vitamin D supplementation and its potential effects on immune modulation, endometrial receptivity, angiogenesis, and placentation during early pregnancy. The role of vitamin D in epigenetics could impact the next generation significantly. Further research is needed to establish the impact of vitamin D supplementation in the prepregnancy state as well as during each trimester of pregnancy to prevent immune complications like recurrent miscarriages.

REFERENCES

1. Sahu M, Bhatia V, Aggarwal A, Rawat V, Saxena P, Pandey A, et al. Vitamin D deficiency in rural girls and pregnant women despite abundant sunshine in northern India. Clin Endocrinol. 2009;70(5):680-4.
2. Jones G, Prosser DE, Kaufmann M. Cytochrome P450-mediated metabolism of vitamin D. J Lipid Res. 2014;55(1):13-31.
3. Ganguly A, Tamblyn JA, Finn-Sell S, Chan SY, Westwood M, Gupta J, et al. Vitamin D, the placenta and early pregnancy: effects on trophoblast function. J Endocrinol. 2018;236(2):R93-103.
4. Tamblyn JA, Pilarski NS, Markland AD, Marson EJ, Devall A, Hewison M, et al. Vitamin D and miscarriage: a systematic review and meta-analysis. Fertil Steril. 2022;118(1):111-22.
5. Ji JL, Muyayalo KP, Zhang YH, Hu XH, Liao AH. Immunological function of vitamin D during human pregnancy. Am J Reprod Immunol. 2017;78(2):e12716.
6. Chen X, Yin B, Lian RC, Zhang T, Zhang HZ, Diao LH, et al. Modulatory effects of vitamin D on peripheral cellular immunity in patients with recurrent miscarriage. Am J Reprod Immunol. 2016;76(6):432-8.
7. Zhao H, Wei X, Yang X. A novel update on vitamin D in recurrent pregnancy loss. Mol Med Rep. 2021;23(5):1-8.
8. Du H, Daftary GS, Lalwani SI, Taylor HS. Direct regulation of HOXA10 by 1, 25-(OH) 2D3 in human myelomonocytic cells and human endometrial stromal cells. Mol Endocrinol. 2005;19(9):2222-33.
9. Holick MF. Vitamin D status: measurement, interpretation, and clinical application. Ann Epidemiol. 2009;19(2):73-8.
10. Dawodu A, Saadi HF, Bekdache G, Javed Y, Altaye M, Hollis BW. Randomized controlled trial (RCT) of vitamin D supplementation in pregnancy in a population with endemic vitamin D deficiency. J Clin Endocrinol Metab. 2013;98(6):2337-46.
11. Mithal A, Kalra S. Vitamin D supplementation in pregnancy. Indian J Endocrinol Metab. 2014;18(5):593-6.
12. Hollis BW, Wagner CL. Assessment of dietary vitamin D requirements during pregnancy and lactation. Am J Clin Nutr. 2004;79(5):717-26.
13. Lazaretti-Castro M, Lips P, Mitchell DM, Murad MH, Powers S, Rao SD, et al. Vitamin D for the Prevention of Disease: An Endocrine Society Clinical Practice Guideline. J Clin Endocrinol Metab. 2024;109(8):1907-47.
14. Gonçalves DR, Braga A, Braga J, Marinho A. Recurrent pregnancy loss and vitamin D: A review of the literature. Am J Reprod Immunol. 2018;80(5):e13022.
15. Farazmand T, Rahbarian R, Jalali M, Ghahremani A, Razi A, Namdar Ahmadabad H. Vitamin D levels in non-pregnant women with a history of recurrent pregnancy loss with and without autoantibodies. Caspian J Intern Med. 2024;15(2):266-72.
16. Sharif K, Sharif Y, Watad A, Yavne Y, Lichtbroun B, Bragazzi NL, et al. Vitamin D, autoimmunity and recurrent pregnancy loss: More than an association. Am J Reprod Immunol. 2018;80(3):e12991.

SECTION 7

Life Style Factors

CHAPTER

36

Obesity

Naama Steiner, Lindsey Ann Choi, Gary Levy, Asher Bashiri

ABSTRACT

Obesity is an independent risk factor for recurrent pregnancy loss (RPL). Many studies and meta-analysis have shown an increased risk of RPL in obese as compared to overweight and normal weight women. The mechanism of pregnancy loss is multifactorial. Obesity negatively influences the oocyte quality as seen in the donor oocyte model. The endometrium may also be nonreceptive and there is an increased production of inflammatory and prothrombotic agents. Hence, women in the prepregnancy period should be sensitized to maintain a healthy body mass index (BMI). There is a paucity of studies to show that weight loss will reverse above changes.

Keywords: Obesity, RPL, Oocyte quality, Donor oocyte, PCOS, BMI, PAI-1.

INTRODUCTION

General

Obesity has become a major health problem worldwide. "Globesity" could be defined as a new global epidemic of obesity and being overweight. It is associated with complications and chronic conditions such as type 2 diabetes, cardiovascular diseases, hypertension, dyslipidemia, hyper-cholesterolemia, cancer, and various psychosocial and psychopathological disorders.[1-5] The etiology of obesity is universally recognized as multifactorial with complex interactions between genetic, behavioral, and environmental factors.[6] Genetics plays an important role but behavioral factors, such as dysfunctional eating habits and low levels of physical activity, are the modifiable causes strictly connected to obesity and obesity-related complications.[7]

Definitions

The World Health Organization defines:

- Normal weight as body mass index (BMI) of 18.5–24.9 kg/m^2
- Overweight as BMI of 25–29.9 kg/m^2, and
- Obesity as a BMI over 30 kg/m^2

Obesity was further divided into three classes:

1. Body mass index 30.0–34.9 kg/m^2 (class 1)
2. Body mass index 35.0–39.9 kg/m^2 (class 2), and
3. Body mass index 40 kg/m^2 and over (class 3 or morbid obesity)

Obesity in pregnancy is defined as a BMI of 30 kg/m^2 or more at the first antenatal consultation.[8]

OBESITY AND ADVERSE PREGNANCY OUTCOMES

Many studies were published in recent years discussing the association of obesity with adverse pregnancy outcomes. In 2015, a systematic review of multiple review articles compared pregnant women of healthy weight with obese women and evaluated health outcomes for the mother and/or the infant. Analysis of the 22 reviews demonstrates gestational diabetes, preeclampsia, gestational hypertension, depression, instrumental and cesarean birth, and surgical site infections are more likely to occur in obese pregnant women compared with women with a healthy weight. Maternal obesity is also linked to greater risk of preterm birth, large for gestational age infants, postpartum hemorrhage, congenital anomalies, and perinatal death. It is also linked to subfertility and an increase in time to conception.[9,10]

OBESITY AND OFFSPRING OUTCOMES

The well-being of the next generation is also compromised. Maternal obesity is a significant risk factor for obesity, cardiovascular, and metabolic sequelae in the offspring resulting in lifelong consequences. A meta-analysis of four studies demonstrated that maternal prepregnancy obesity was linked to a threefold higher risk of childhood obesity in the offspring.[11] Both maternal prepregnancy obesity and excessive gestational weight gain are associated with hypertension, dyslipidemia, insulin resistance, and elevated inflammatory markers in childhood.[12] Excessive maternal BMI is also associated with an increased risk for autism spectrum disorders (ASDs) in the offspring. A recent meta-analysis showed a linear dose-response relationship for each 5 kg/m^2 increase in maternal BMI, pooled relative risk (RR) 1.16 (1.01, 1.33).[13] Maternal obesity is also a risk factor for cancer in the offspring. A population-based study conducted in California observed that children born to overweight mothers (prior to pregnancy), were at increased risk of leukemia.[14]

OBESITY AND SPORADIC PREGNANCY LOSS

Obesity is associated with an increased risk of 1st trimester pregnancy loss. A meta-analysis of 16 studies concluded that women with BMI more than 25 kg/m^2 had significantly higher odds of pregnancy loss, regardless of the method of conception.[15] There is a dose response connection between the BMI and the RR for pregnancy loss. On the other side, the risk of pregnancy loss is also increased in underweight women [RR 1.08; 95% confidence interval (CI) 1.05–1.11] **(Fig. 1)**.[16]

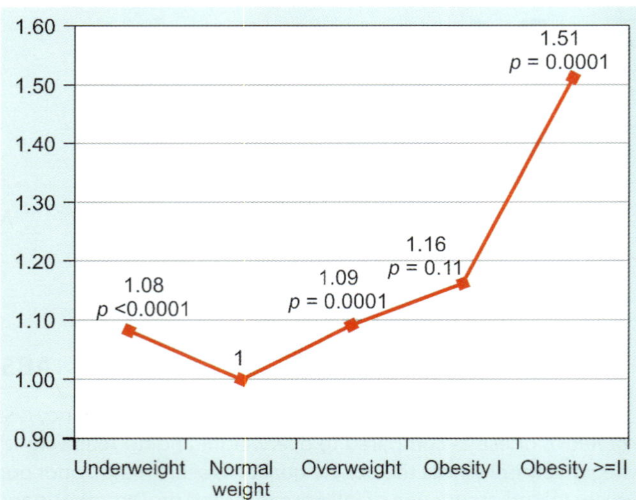

Fig. 1: Risk of miscarriage according to maternal prepregnancy body mass index category.[16]

Source: Reprinted with permission from (Elsevier) Balsells M, Garcia-Patterson A, Corcoy R. Systematic review and meta-analysis on the association of prepregnancy underweight and miscarriage. Eur J Obstet Gynecol Reprod Biol. 2016;207:73-9.

ASSOCIATION BETWEEN OBESITY AND RECURRENT PREGNANCY LOSS

A case control study of 1,644 obese (BMI >30 kg/m^2) women compared to 3,288 age-matched normal weight controls (BMI 19–24.9 kg/m^2) found that the risks of early pregnancy loss and recurrent early pregnancy losses (three or more pregnancy losses between 6 and 12 weeks) were significantly higher in the obese patients (OR 1.2 and 3.5, 95% CI 1.01–1.46 and 1.03–12.01, respectively; $p = 0.04$, for both).[17]

Metwally et al. conducted a prospective study of 844 pregnancies from 491 patients with recurrent pregnancy loss to investigate the effects of obesity on the risk of pregnancy loss in subsequent pregnancies. They found that obese patients had significantly higher odds of pregnancy loss (OR 1.71; 95% CI 1.05–2.8); however, no significant association was found between overweight women and recurrent pregnancy loss (RPL) (OR 1.02; 95% CI 0.72–1.45). They concluded that in women with recurrent pregnancy loss, a mild increase in the BMI does not increase the risk of pregnancy loss, whereas obese patients have a small but significant increased risk of pregnancy loss in subsequent pregnancies. The risk of pregnancy loss was highest for underweight and obese patients, whereas the risk was similar for women with normal and overweight BMIs.[18] In 2012, a systematic review compared pregnancy loss rates in obese (BMI ≥28 or 30 kg/m^2), overweight (BMI 25–29 kg/m^2), and normal weight (BMI <25 kg/m^2) women. Six studies met the criteria with a cohort of 28,538 women. Pooled analysis revealed a higher pregnancy loss rate of 13.6% in 3,800 obese versus 10.7% in 17,146 normal BMI women (OR 1.31; 95% CI 1.18–1.46). Although, the cohort was small, there was a higher prevalence of recurrent early pregnancy loss in obese versus normal BMI women (0.4% vs. 0.1%; OR 3.51; 95% CI 1.03–12.01). In women with recurrent pregnancy loss, there was a higher pregnancy loss rate in the obese versus overweight and normal weight women (46% vs. 43%; OR 1.71).[19] Lo et al. determined the relationship between maternal BMI and the primary outcome of pregnancy in 696 couples with unexplained recurrent pregnancy loss. Logistic regression demonstrated that maternal obesity (BMI ≥30 kg/m^2) significantly increased the risk of pregnancy loss (OR 1.73; 95% CI 1.06–2.83). No difference in the pregnancy loss rate was found among those who were overweight (OR 1.27; 95% CI 0.89–1.83).[20]

Sugiura-Ogasawara summarized those four studies in recent review on RPL and obesity, published in 2015 **(Table 1)**.[21]

TABLE 1: Studies concerning the association between obesity and recurrent pregnancy loss.[21]

	Study design	Number of patients	Definition of obese	Definition of RM	OR (95% CI)
Lashen et al. 2004[17]	Case–control study	*1,644 obese women:* 3,288 age-matched with normal BMI	• Obese BMI >30 kg/m^2 • *Normal BMI:* 19–24.9 kg/m^2	Early (6–12 weeks) three or more	• *Early miscarriage:* 1.2 (1.01–1.46) • *Early RM:* 3.5 (1.03–12.0)
Metwally et al. 2010[18]	Prospective cohort	844 subsequent pregnancies in 491 patients with RM	First subsequent pregnancy in 696 patients with unexplained RM		• *Obese:* 1.71 (1.05–2.8) • *Underweight:* 3.98 (1.06–14.92)
Lo et al. 2012[20]	Prospective cohort	First subsequent pregnancy in 696 patients with unexplained RM	• *Obese BMI:* 30 kg/m^2 • *Overweight BMI:* 25.0–29.99 kg/m^2 • *Normal BMI:* 18.5–24.99 kg/m^2 • Underweight BMI	Three or more	• *Obese:* 1.73 (1.06–2.83) • *Asian:* 2.87 (1.52–5.39) • *Age:* 1.99 (1.45–2.73) • *Number of previous miscarriages:* 2.08 (1.42–3.06)
Boots et al. 2014[24]	Prospective cohort	117 aborted conceptuses of subsequent miscarriage	• *Obese BMI:* 30 kg/m^2 • Nonobese BMI	Two or more RPL	*Relative risk of euploid rate:* 1.63 (1.08–2.47)

(BMI: body mass index; CI: confidence interval; OR: odds ratio; RPL: recurrent pregnancy loss)
Source: Reprinted with permission from (Elsevier) Sugiura-Ogasawara M. Recurrent pregnancy loss and obesity. Best Pract Res Clin Obstet Gynaecol. 2015;29(4):489-97.

Recently, a retrospective analysis of 592 patients, in tertiary level of RPL clinic in South Africa concluded that BMI seems to have a substantial impact on RPL.[22]

MECHANISMS

It is well known that aneuploidy is a direct cause of sporadic and RPL.[23] However, most pregnancy losses among obese women are euploid. In an observational, prospective cohort study, Boots et al. demonstrated that the frequency of euploid pregnancy loss is increased in obese women. Conventional cytogenetic analysis, microsatellite analysis, and/or comparative genomic hybridization, when indicated, were performed in aborted conceptuses of a total of 372 women with recurrent early pregnancy loss (defined as ≥2 pregnancy losses <10 weeks), and at least one ultrasound documented pregnancy loss with chromosome results. Of the 117 subsequent pregnancy losses with chromosome results, the frequency of a euploid pregnancy loss among obese (BMI ≥30 kg/m^2) women was 58% compared with 37% in nonobese (BMI <30 kg/m^2) women (RR = 1.63; 95% CI 1.08–2.47) **(Table 2)**.[24] In 2010, a retrospective, case control study of 204 pregnancy losses also reported a significant increase in euploid (46,XX or 46,XY) pregnancy losses in overweight or obese women compared with women of normal weight.[25]

While the exact mechanism of obesity on pregnancy loss is not well understood, several factors are involved. Hypotheses include:

- Detrimental effect on ovaries, affecting oocyte quality and thus, embryo viability
- Adverse impact of obesity on endometrial development
- Increased production of inflammatory and prothrombotic agents by adipose tissue and/or release from the endothelium secondary to stimulation by adipocyte-derived factors.

Oocyte

One hypothesis assumes that obesity has detrimental effect on ovaries, affecting oocyte quality and ultimately embryo viability. The most effective way of separating the influence of obesity on the ovary and endometrium in humans is the donor oocyte model. In this model, good quality oocytes from healthy, nonobese young women are employed. This would isolate the influence of obesity on pregnancy outcome that would be mediated by the endometrium and/or its environment. Luke et al. used a database of 45,163 in vitro fertilization (IVF) cycles to evaluate the odds of failure to achieve a clinical intrauterine pregnancy and failure to achieve a live birth (equal to pregnancy loss) stratified by a woman's age, BMI, and oocyte source (autologous vs.

TABLE 2: Miscarriages with chromosome results (*n* = 578), before and subsequent to recurrent early pregnancy loss evaluation.[24]

	Prior miscarriages (n = 461)			*Subsequent miscarriages (n = 117)*		
	Obese	*Nonobese*	*Total*	*Obese*	*Nonobese*	*Total*
Euploid	42	226	268	18	32	50
Euploid female (46,XX or balanced translocation)	28	143	171	6	18	24
Confirmed by microsatellite analysis (MSA)	4	23	27	5	15	20
Unconfirmed	24	120	144	1	3	4
Euploid male (46,XY or balanced translocation)	14	83	97	12	14	26
Noneuploid	31	162	193	13	54	67
Trisomy	23	11	34	11	39	50
Trisomy with polyploidy	5	15	20	1	0	1
Monosomy	5	15	20	1	3	4
Monosomy with trisomy	0	1	1	0	1	1
Monosomy with polyploidy	0	5	5	0	4	4
Polyploidy	2	23	25	0	7	7
Unbalanced translocation	1	4	5	0	0	0

Source: Reprinted with permission from (Elsevier) Boots CE, Bernardi LA, Stephenson MD. Frequency of euploid miscarriage is increased in obese women with recurrent early pregnancy loss. Fertil Steril. 2014;102(2):455-9.

donor). They found that an increased BMI is a risk factor for pregnancy loss in pregnancies achieved with autologous oocytes but not with donor oocytes. Based on these results, it can be concluded that obesity mediates an endocrine and metabolic environment that may negatively influence oocyte quality, and therefore embryo development, subsequent implantation, and pregnancy outcome.[26] In 2013, a systematic review and meta-analysis addressed the association between BMI and outcomes of donor oocyte recipients. The data suggests that obesity does not affect IVF outcomes in women using donor oocytes. One conclusion is that oocyte quality rather than endometrial receptivity may be the more important factor influencing IVF outcomes in obese women using autologous oocytes.[27]

Endometrium

In contrast to the previous oocyte theory, endometrial receptivity is another possible explanation for impaired implantation and pregnancy loss in obese patients. In a retrospective study of 712 donor ovum recipients with known BMI, obesity was associated with a significant increase in early pregnancy losses. Specifically in the obese group, there was a statistically significant, fourfold increase in the risk of abortion compared with patients with a normal BMI (38.1% vs. 13.3%).[28] A systematic review and meta-analysis of 3,000 patients from 16 studies investigated the association between obesity and pregnancy loss. The primary outcome of pregnancy loss was compared in obese and overweight individuals and normal weight women. Similar to the results obtained in the trial evaluating pregnancies conceived with donor oocytes, this meta-analysis demonstrated a significantly higher odds of pregnancy loss in the overweight or obese group (OR 1.52; 95% CI 1.10–2.09).[15]

Inflammatory and Prothrombotic Agents

Another proposed mechanism is an increased production of inflammatory and prothrombotic agents. Plasminogen activator inhibitor-1 (PAI-1) is a prothrombotic agent produced by adipose tissue or released from the endothelium secondary to stimulation by adipocyte-derived factors. Its activity is directly related to BMI and has been associated with increased rates of pregnancy loss in women that are obese or have polycystic ovarian syndrome (PCOS).[29,30] It has been suggested that plasminogen activators and their inhibitors play an important role in facilitating trophoblasts invasion of the uterus and maintenance of blood fluidity within placental intervillous spaces.[31] Similarly, Glueck et al. have reported that PAI-1 activity is associated with RPL without correlation to PCOS.[29,30] Leptin is a hormone secreted by an adipocyte that regulates energy homeostasis with stimulatory effects at the hypothalamus and pituitary, as well as inhibitory actions at the gonads. Leptin production has been shown to have an important role in the early maintenance of pregnancy. Plasma levels have been shown to correlate with the BMI. Laird et al. performed a study aimed to correlate leptin levels with pregnancy outcomes in women with RPL. In this study, serum leptin and leptin-binding activity were measured in women who had a history of recurrent pregnancy loss during weeks 5–6 and 7–8 of pregnancy. The serum concentrations correlated with subsequent pregnancy outcome. Women who subsequently miscarried had significantly lower plasma leptin concentrations than women who had term births.[32]

It can be concluded that obesity is associated with high leptin levels while low leptin levels are associated with pregnancy loss. With further increase in the BMI, a state of leptin *resistance* and *relative deficiency* may exist. This may explain the poor reproductive performance, such as pregnancy loss, in these women. Conditions with excess energy stores or metabolic disturbances, such as obesity and PCOS, often have elevated serum or follicular fluid leptin levels. It seems that relative leptin deficiency or resistance may be at least partly responsible for the reproductive abnormalities that occur with these conditions.[33]

OBESITY AND POLYCYSTIC OVARIAN SYNDROME

Although, women with PCOS may have a greater risk of spontaneous abortion, there is a close link between obesity and PCOS. It appears that obesity may act as an independent risk factor for spontaneous pregnancy loss, regardless of the presence or absence of PCOS.[28] For example, Wang et al. suggested that the higher risk of spontaneous abortion observed in women with PCOS was likely due to their high prevalence of obesity and the type of treatment they received. After adjusting for these two factors, the risk of spontaneous abortion in women with PCOS compared with the women without PCOS was no longer statistically significant.[34]

WEIGHT LOSS

Can all these health issues be avoided by prevention of obesity? Clark et al. reported that weight loss among women with elevated BMI is associated with decreased pregnancy loss rate in anovulatory obese women.[35] This potential effects of weight loss on the RPL should be assessed in future studies. Not only that, any women that pursue preconception, counseling should be advised, weight reduction prior to pregnancy to optimize pregnancy outcomes.

CONCLUSION

Obesity is a major risk factor for noncommunicable diseases, adverse pregnancy outcomes, sporadic pregnancy loss, and RPL. While the mechanism of obesity on pregnancy losses is not clear, hypotheses include the oocyte quality, the endometrium, or other inflammatory and prothrombotic agents produced by adipose tissue released from endothelium. Regardless, weight loss has been shown to decrease pregnancy loss and should be taken into consideration during preconception counseling.

REFERENCES

1. Wadden TA, Brownell KD, Foster GD. Obesity: responding to the global epidemic. J Consult Clin Psychol. 2002; 70(3):510-25.
2. Byrne SM, Cooper Z, Fairburn CG. Psychological predictors of weight regain in obesity. Behav Res Ther. 2004;42(11):1341-56.
3. Flegal KM, Graubard BI, Williamson DF, Gail MH. Excess deaths associated with underweight, overweight, and obesity. JAMA. 2005;293(15):1861-7.
4. Prospective Studies Collaboration, Whitlock G, Lewington S, Sherliker P, Clarke R, Emberson J, et al. Body-mass index and cause-specific mortality in 900,000 adults: collaborative analyses of 57 prospective studies. Lancet. 2009;373(9669):1083-96.
5. Castelnuovo G, Manzoni GM, Pietrabissa G, Corti S, Giusti EM, Molinari E, et al. Obesity and outpatient rehabilitation using mobile technologies: the potential mHealth approach. Front Psychol. 2014;5:559.
6. Marcus MD, Wildes JE. Obesity: is it a mental disorder? Int J Eat Disord. 2009;42(8):739-53.
7. Dombrowski SU, Sniehotta FF, Avenell A, Johnston M, Maclennan G, V Araújo-Soares, et al. Identifying active ingredients in complex behavioural interventions for obese adults with obesity-related co-morbidities or additional risk factors for co-morbidities: a systematic review. Health Psychol Rev. 2012;6(1):7-32.
8. Centre for Public Health Excellence at NICE (UK), National Collaborating Centre for Primary Care (UK). Obesity: The Prevention, Identification, Assessment and Management of Overweight and Obesity in Adults and Children. London: National Institute for Health and Clinical Excellence; 2006.
9. Marchi J, Berg M, Dencker A, Begley C. Risks associated with obesity in pregnancy, for the mother and baby: a systematic review of reviews. Obes Rev. 2015;16(8):621-38.

10. Poston L, Caleyachetty R, Cnattingius S, Corvalán C, Uauy R, Herring S, et al. Preconceptional and maternal obesity: epidemiology and health consequences. Lancet Diabetes Endocrinol. 2016;4(12):1025-36.
11. Yu Z, Han S, Zhu J, Sun X, Ji C, Guo X. Pre-pregnancy body mass index in relation to infant birth weight and offspring overweight/obesity: a systematic review and meta-analysis. PLoS One. 2013;8(4):e61627.
12. Gaillard R, Steegers EA, Duijts L, Felix JF, Hofman A, Franco OH, et al. Childhood cardiometabolic outcomes of maternal obesity during pregnancy: The Generation R Study. Hypertension. 2014;63(4):683-91.
13. Wang Y, Tang S, Xu S, Weng S, Liu Z. Maternal Body Mass Index and Risk of Autism Spectrum Disorders in Offspring: A Meta-analysis. Sci Rep. 2016;6(6):34248.
14. Contreras ZA, Ritz B, Virk J, Cockburn M, Heck JE. Maternal pre-pregnancy and gestational diabetes, obesity, gestational weight gain, and risk of cancer in young children: a population-based study in California. Cancer Causes Control. 2016;27(10):1273-85.
15. Metwally M, Ong KJ, Ledger WL, Li TC. Does high body mass index increase the risk of miscarriage after spontaneous and assisted conception? A meta-analysis of the evidence. Fertil Steril. 2008;90(3):714-26.
16. Balsells M, Garcia-Patterson A, Corcoy R. Systematic review and meta-analysis on the association of prepregnancy under- weight and miscarriage. Eur J Obstet Gynecol Reprod Biol. 2016;207:73-9.
17. Lashen H, Fear K, Sturdee DW. Obesity is associated with increased risk of first trimester and recurrent miscarriage: matched case-control study. Hum Reprod. 2004;19(7):1644-6.
18. Metwally M, Saravelos SH, Ledger WL, Li TC. Body mass index and risk of miscarriage in women with recurrent miscarriage. Fertil Steril. 2010;94(1):290-5.
19. Boots C, Stephenson MD. Does obesity increase the risk of miscarriage in spontaneous conception: a systematic review. Semin Reprod Med. 2011;29(6):507-13.
20. Lo W, Rai R, Hameed A, Brailsford SR, Al-Ghamdi AA, Regan L. The effect of body mass index on the outcome of pregnancy in women with recurrent miscarriage. J Family Community Med. 2012;19(3):167-71.
21. Sugiura-Ogasawara M. Recurrent pregnancy loss and obesity. Best Pract Res Clin Obstet Gynaecol. 2015; 29(4): 489-97.
22. Matjila MJ, Hoffman A, van der Spuy ZM. Medical conditions associated with recurrent miscarriage-Is BMI the tip of the iceberg? Eur J Obstet Gynecol Reprod Biol. 2017;214:91-6.
23. Rai R, Regan L. Recurrent miscarriage. Lancet. 2006; 368(9535): 601-11.
24. Boots CE, Bernardi LA, Stephenson MD. Frequency of euploid miscarriage is increased in obese women with recurrent early pregnancy loss. Fertil Steril. 2014;102(2):455-9.
25. Landres IV, Milki AA, Lathi RB. Karyotype of miscarriages in relation to maternal weight. Hum Reprod. 2010;25(5): 1123-6.
26. Luke B, Brown MB, Stern JE, Missmer SA, Fujimoto VY, Leach R; SART Writing Group. Female obesity adversely affects assisted reproductive technology (ART) pregnancy and live birth rates. Hum Reprod. 2011;26(1):245-52.
27. Jungheim ES, Schon SB, Schulte MB, DeUgarte DA, Fowler SA, Tuuli MG. IVF outcomes in obese donor oocyte recipients: a systematic review and meta-analysis. Hum Reprod. 2013;28(10):2720-7.
28. Bellver J, Rossal LP, Bosch E, Zúñiga A, Corona JT, Meléndez F, et al. Obesity and the risk of spontaneous abortion after oocyte donation. Fertil Steril. 2003;79(5):1136-40.
29. Glueck CJ, Sieve L, Zhu B, Wang P. Plasminogen activator inhibitor activity, 4G5G polymorphism of the plasminogen activator inhibitor 1 gene, and first-trimester miscarriage in women with polycystic ovary syndrome. Metabolism. 2006;55(3):345-52.
30. Glueck CJ, Wang P, Fontaine RN, Sieve-Smith L, Tracy T, Moore SK. Plasminogen activator inhibitor activity: an independent risk factor for the high miscarriage rate during pregnancy in women with polycystic ovary syndrome. Metabolism. 1999;48(12):1589-95.
31. Graham CH. Effect of transforming growth factor-beta on the plasminogen activator system in cultured first trimester human cytotrophoblasts. Placenta. 1997;18(2-3): 137-43.
32. Laird SM, Quinton ND, Anstie B, Li TC, Blakemore AI. Leptin and leptin-binding activity in women with recurrent miscarriage: correlation with pregnancy outcome. Hum Reprod. 2001;16(9):2008-13.
33. Moschos S, Chan JL, Mantzoros CS. Leptin and reproduction: a review. Fertil Steril. 2002;77(3):433-44.
34. Wang JX, Davies MJ, Norman RJ. Polycystic ovarian syndrome and the risk of spontaneous abortion following assisted reproductive technology treatment. Hum Reprod. 2001;16(12):2606-9.
35. Clark AM, Ledger W, Galletly C, Tomlinson L, Blaney F, Wang X, et al. Weight loss results in significantly improvement in pregnancy and ovulation rates in anovulatory obese women. Hum Reprod. 1995;10(10):2705-12.

CHAPTER 37

Environmental Factors

Isha Wadhawan, Mala Arora, Namrata Singh

ABSTRACT

The effect of air pollution on the developing fetus has not been studied in detail. Presence of particulate matter of 2.5 μm has been shown to induce an inflammatory response in the body and generate reactive oxygen species (ROS) that may alter the redox potential at the site of implantation. Other harmful air pollutants like nitrogen dioxide (NO_2), nitrogen oxide (NO), sulfur dioxide (SO_2), and polycyclic aromatic hydrocarbons (PAH), present in vehicular smoke, have not been studied so well. Another major threat to health is posed by chemical pollutants like pesticides, microplastics, and endocrine disrupting chemicals, which are so ubiquitously present in our environment today. The effects of maternal use of tobacco, alcohol, recreational drugs and caffeine are known to be harmful, but we do not have robust data on their safe lower limits of exposure.

Keywords: RPL, Environmental pollutants, Tobacco, Alcohol, Caffeine, Particulate matter, Pesticides, Microplastics, Endocrine disrupting chemicals, ROS.

INTRODUCTION

Our environment impacts almost all aspects of health including our ability to procreate, that is, our fertility as well as the health of our pregnancies.[1] While there is strong evidence for association of certain environmental factors like cigarette smoking[2] with recurrent pregnancy loss (RPL), some others such as pesticides and endocrine-disrupting chemicals[3,4] may also increase the risk of repeated miscarriage. However, there is significant room for research as evidence based and accurate information continues to limited on the subject. Therefore, providers often find it challenging to counsel distraught couples with RPL who quiz them on the impact their environment may have had on pregnancy loss.

Recurrent pregnancy loss continues to be an enigma for care providers and patients alike. Understanding possible risks of environmental factors and their contribution toward pregnancy loss may be helpful in tailoring a clinician's advice and care in an attempt to decrease the physical and emotional morbidity of RPL.

The environmental factors or pollutants may be categorized in three broad categories:

- Air pollutants (that may be inhaled)
- Chemical pollutants (that may be ingested from food, water, etc.)
- *Others:* Tobacco, alcohol, and recreational drugs

AIR POLLUTANTS

Air pollution, as defined by the World Health Organization (WHO)[5] (2019) is the contamination of internal or external environment by any chemical, physical, or biological agent that modifies natural atmosphere characteristic. In the changing world of dynamics, where we are witnessing an increase in number of pollutants on a daily basis, their effects on human biology cannot be overseen. There are many studies revolving around the effect of air pollution on morbidity and mortality of humans—most evaluate the effects on the respiratory system. Fortunately, many recent studies have tried to find link between environmental pollutants and fertility and reproduction with a special emphasis on recurrent pregnancy losses.

Pollutants most commonly studied are carbon monoxide (CO), particulate matter 2.5 and 10 ($PM_{2.5}$ and PM_{10}), nitrogen dioxide (NO_2), nitrogen monoxide (NO), ozone gas (O_3), carbon dioxide (CO_2), polycyclic aromatic hydrocarbons (PAH), and sulfur dioxide (SO_2). Among these, particulate matter 2.5 was most extensively studied and has shown to have a positive association with pregnancy loss in multiple studies.[6,7]

It should be understood that the effect of these pollutants with RPL is not a linear one, instead it involves many variables such as duration of exposure, gestational age during exposure and a susceptible subpopulation.

Furthermore, finding the exact correlation can be difficult since many a times a pregnancy failure occurs even before the pregnancy is detected.

Pathophysiology

Various studies had already been done on how exposure to pollutants can initiate inflammatory response in the body. Recent studies have tried to find out if the underlying principle holds true even in case of in utero exposure.

The fundamental principle attributes the production of "reactive oxygen species" (ROS) as an initiator to the cascade of inflammatory process.[8,9] ROS causes an increase of oxidiative stress, which in turn leads to endothelial disruption resulting in an increase in permeability and hence increase in platelet adhesion and aggregation leading to thrombogenicity.[8,10]

Few biochemicals have been studied as the marker of inflammatory process. One of them is myeloperoxidase (MPO).[8] MPO is stored in inflammatory cells like neutrophils, monocyte, and macrophages. A rise in levels of this enzyme has been noted in ischemia and reperfusion injury. Surprisingly, their levels were found to be raised in the pollutants exposed group of one study, signifying inflammatory response to pollutants.

Similarly, another study measured elevated levels of C-reactive protein (CRP), in response to exposure to particulate matter, as a marker of acute inflammation.[11,12]

Hence, it is safe to conclude that exposure to pollutants does initiate acute inflammatory processes in the body. To identify any similar effect in-utero, such markers were studied in cord blood sample of the fetus in exposed mothers.[11] One study suggested that in-utero exposure to particulate matter, particularly during 2nd trimester was associated with rise in lipo-oxygenase pathway metabolites (primary pathway for generation of leukotrienes from arachidonic acid) in cord blood sample.[9]

Few other studies have concluded that oxidative stress interferes with placental development, implantation, and can even result in chromosomal anomalies in early gestation, all of which can cause recurrent pregnancy losses.[13] This serves as indirect evidence of pollutants leading to recurrent miscarriages.

Studies done on animal models correlating exposure to pollutants and pregnancy losses have presented some interesting outcomes. One such study, to know the effects of benzo-a-pyrene (BaP) on mice, suggested that the pollutants resulted in more miscarriages, implantation failure, and fetal resorption in a dose-dependent manner.[9] It is important to emphasize here that BaP is the most abundant pollutant among polycyclic aromatic hydrocarbons (PAH), the common sources of which are air and water pollutants, barbecued and fried fish, and cigarettes. The active metabolite of BaP is benzopyrene-7,8-diol-9,10 epoxide (BPDE) which accumulates in placenta and crosses the placental barrier. It activates the apoptosis pathway in trophoblast thus resulting in early pregnancy failure.[14]

Duration of Exposure

Most studies, including one prospective cohort study, found positive correlation of RPL with average chronic exposure of ozone (O_3) and particulate matter ($PM_{2.5}$), whereas acute exposure was found unrelated to miscarriages (except for carbon particles, which showed positive relation even with acute exposure). The strong association with $PM_{2.5}$ is mainly due to its sulfate component. The population of attributable risks in this study was found to be 12% with O_3 and 13% with $PM_{2.5}$.[6]

Prevention

While the evidence for short-term and long-term exposure of pollutants on pregnancy is mounting, further trials on preconception exposure are awaited. Still a multidisciplinary approach can be implemented like alerts from health authorities on the days of poorer air quality for high-risk groups such as asthmatics and pregnant women. Behavioral changes like reducing outdoor activities, mask wearing on a day of poor air quality can also be encouraged.

CHEMICAL POLLUTANTS

Among all the chemical pollutants in food and water, the most studied for their association with repeated pregnancy loss are heavy metals. Low levels of certain metals such as iron, copper, magnesium, chromium, selenium, and vitamin E were associated with RPL, while high levels of cadmium and lead were associated with RPL as reported by Aborisade et al. in 2013.[15] A similar correlation of exposures to lead, calcium, and selenium to unexplained recurrent miscarriage was also noted 10 years later by Zhang et al.[16]

A small case control study done in Lucknow, India, with 70 participants in the RPL and control group each noted statistically significant raised levels of pesticides namely—β-hexachlorocyclohexane, malathion, chlorpyrifos, and fenvalerate in the cases compared to the controls.[17] A more recent news blog also commented on correlation between pesticides and RPL. (*https://beyondpesticides.org/dailynewsblog/Dec 2014*)

As early as 1990, Guirguis et al. recommended decreasing exposure to waste anesthetic gases based on their study wherein over 10,000 hospital staff. Higher pregnancy loss was seen in personnel working in operating and recovery rooms who were exposed to anesthetic gases.[18]

Limited studies on *video displays units (VDU)* and electromagnetic field exposure had inconclusive results.[19] The same review reported multiple poor quality studies associating exposure to organic solvents (like those found in paints, varnishes, certain perfumes, agricultural products, etc.) with pregnancy loss, though association with RPL was not evaluated.[19]

Plastics pollution is rapidly increasing and causing major concern globally. Plastics byproducts may enter our bodies through ingestion, inhalation, or dermal contacts. Microplastics and nanoplastics have been detected in various parts of the human body, the female reproductive system, the placenta, amniotic fluid, and breast milk.[20] This has raised major concern and interest in the scientific community. Mice models and in-vitro studies of human trophoblasts have demonstrated toxic effects on reproductive function by causing apoptosis of cells and inducing miscarriage.[21,22]

Endocrine disruptive chemicals (EDCs) are a group of almost 800 chemicals defined by the WHO as "an exogenous substance or mixture that alters function(s) of endocrine systems and consequently causes adverse health affects in an organism, its progeny, and/or populations."[23] These include chemicals such as bisphenols, phthalates, pesticides, polycyclic aromatic hydrocarbons (PAHs), perfluorinated compounds (PFCs), parabens, phytoestrogens, and others that are commonly found in food packaging, bottles, cans, dinnerware, nonstick cookware, dental sealants, medical equipment, pharmaceutical-coating printing papers, personal care products, toys, textiles, building materials, natural sources such as soy products and legumes (for phytoestrogens).[24] One may be exposed to these through ingestion, inhalation, or skin contact. In the last decade, a number of animal and observational studies have suggested an association between exposure to EDCs. Their impact on fertility and pregnancy has been reviewed by a Spanish group in November, 2023.[24] The focus of these studies has been assessment of infertility;[25] teratogenicity[26] and obstetric complications,[27-30] though some have also noted increased incidence of pregnancy loss.[31,32] The maximum data is available for bisphenols and phthalates.[33] The exact mechanisms of action of these products need to be delineated. However, this definitely raises a concern on regulation of these products that are produced on multiple occasions on a daily basis.

To conclude, direct evidence demonstrating a causal relationship between chemical pollutants and RPL in humans is awaited. However, multiple studies—both poor and good quality in animals and observations in humans suggest a strong possibility of causality especially for heavy metals, and chemicals such as bisphenols, phthalates, and pesticides. The scientific community needs to buck up and gather larger and stronger data, generate awareness while simultaneously considering pushing policy makers and major players like governments to restrict use of some of these chemicals which are increasingly present in the environment. Major shift in policy, backed by strong data, akin the Montreal Protocol for the ozone hole (and restriction of chloro-flouro-carbons) is the need of the hour if we wish to protect the reproductive and overall well-being of our population at large.

OTHERS

Certain substances in our environment that are often part of routine exposure and ingestion may have toxic impact on pregnancies—like tobacco (in various forms), caffeine, and alcohol.

Tobacco Exposure

A strong association between smoking in the mother, her partner or both with poor obstetric, neonatal, and childhood outcomes is established. The association with RPL has been unclear. However, new data have compelled modification of recommendations.[34]

More than a decade ago, Zhang et al., in a retrospective study, reported that though direct consumption of tobacco, alcohol, or caffeine was not associated with pregnancy loss, passive smoking significantly increased risk of RPL with >1 hour of exposure increasing the risk almost five times.[35]

Older studies reported conflicting results, however, du Fosse et al. in 2021, undertook a meta-analysis of eight studies wherein the incidence of pregnancy loss increased with paternal smoking of >10 cigarettes/day prior to conception after adjusting for maternal age.[36] As a result, assessing environmental factors in the male partner including smoking and alcohol exposure has been upgraded from good practice point to an evidence-based recommendation in the most recent ESHRE guidelines.[34]

Noncigarette tobacco product use among men and women is prevalent in low to middle income countries like India as they are less expensive.[37] While their impact or oral health is well known, we have almost no data or research on their association with reproductive health—a major gap in knowledge.

Caffeine

Caffeine appears to be associated with loss late in pregnancy. Furthermore, the association seems to be dose dependent based on observational and retrospective data. Some women with a certain genotype of *CYP1A2* (*1F alleles) may be genetically predisposed to greater impact of caffeine on their systems and, therefore, their pregnancies due to reduced ability to assimilate caffeine.[38] For a rough reference point, a teaspoon of ground coffee may have up to 60 mg of caffeine, and about 63 mg caffeine is present in one shot of espresso. Instant coffee (e.g., Nescafe sachets) may have 50–90 mg of caffeine in a 2-g sachet.

Observational studies have noted that caffeine was associated with late pregnancy loss and still birth; however, results were confounded by the symptom of nausea (women with nausea did not drink coffee).[39]

Similarly, retrospective studies have demonstrated between 3- and 16-fold increase in incidence of RPL for moderate (150–300 mg/day) and high caffeine (>300 mg/day) ingesting women during the periconception period compared to women who were exposed to mild caffeine intake.[40]

Alcohol Exposure

Women are advised to avoid alcohol during the periconception and antenatal period due to an established risk of fetal alcohol syndrome. Evidence on incidence of pregnancy loss is limited but does demonstrate a dose-dependent risk of loss with maternal and paternal alcohol intake. Studies by Anderson and Avalos noted and increased risk of pregnancy loss for women who drank as less as 2 to 4 drinks/week.[41,42] Additionally, for couples undergoing fertility treatments, poor outcomes and sperm parameters were seen with paternal alcohol intake of five drinks/week.[43,44] However, there are no studies on the impact of alcohol and chances of live births in couples with RPL.

As a result of emerging new evidence in couples with RPL, alcohol intake and other lifestyle factors of the male partner are to be assessed per ESHRE 2022 recommendations development group. This is an upgradation, as previously this was listed only as a "good practice point."[34]

Recreational Drugs

Investigating marijuana and its impact on various aspects of human reproduction has garnered a lot of interest in recent years as its use has increased and has been legalized in certain parts of the world. With respect to spontaneous or recurrent miscarriages, data evaluating over 500 women over almost 10 years reported an increased risk of nonlive births in marijuana users versus nonusers.[45] Another study evaluating HIV infected women over close to 25 years noted similar results with increased incidence of spontaneous miscarriages in those using marijuana.[46] These studies though large and spanning many years are confounded by various characteristics of study population including ethnicity, concomitant smoking, poor compliance to HIV therapy and high viral load. Cocaine abuse in any form is a well-established risk factor for pregnancy loss especially when used with tobacco.[47]

Ways to Reduce Exposure

The authors stress on promotion of preconception counseling. Among couples in the reproductive age group, smoking, alcohol, and recreational drug use and caffeine consumption seem to be on the rise. A preconception session preferably with both partners is advisable, where caffeine intake, recreational tobacco, alcohol, and drug intake can be reviewed in a sensitive manner. Associated risks explained and formal assistance offered to those who meet criteria and are willing to quit the same. Additional research to gather more evidence on risks to pregnancy, the dose at which risk increases and proof of improved outcomes when intake is held or decreased would be greatly helpful for care providers and couples.

CONCLUSION

The rising trends in environmental pollution, both air and chemical pollutants, are a threat to the reproductive outcomes and need to be researched in depth. This will alert policy makers to take steps to curb pollution.

Prepregnancy counseling is important for lifestyle modification of both partners that should be maintained not only during pregnancy but also after childbirth as well to reduce the risk of neonatal complications. Cessation of smoking, tobacco exposure in other forms, alcohol, and recreational drugs is beneficial to reproductive health.

REFERENCES

1. Dimitriadis E, Menkhorst E, Saito S, Kutteh WH, Brosens JJ. Recurrent pregnancy loss. Nat Rev Dis Prim. 2020;6(1):98.
2. ESHRE Guideline Group on RPL; Bender Atik R, Christiansen OB, Elson J, Kolte AM, Lewis S, et al. ESHRE guideline: recurrent pregnancy loss. Hum Reprod Open. 2018;2018(2):hoy004.
3. Krieg SA, Shahine LK, Lathi RB. Environmental exposure to endocrine-disrupting chemicals and miscarriage. Fertil Steril. 2016;106:941-7.
4. Zhang L, Liu W, Hou K, Lin J, Zhou C, Tong X, et al. Air pollution-induced missed abortion risk for pregnancies. Nat Sustain. 2019;2(11):1011-7.
5. https://www.who.int/health-topics/air-pollution#tab=tab
6. Ha S, Ghimire S, Martinez V. Outdoor Air Pollution and Pregnancy Loss: a Review of Recent Literature. Curr Epidemiol Rep. 2022;9:387-405.
7. Ha S, Sundaram R, Buck Louis GM, Nobles C, Seeni I, Sherman S, et al. Ambient air pollution and the risk of pregnancy loss: a prospective cohort study. Fertil Steril. 2018;109:148-53.
8. Li W, Wilker EH, Dorans KS, Rice MB, Schwartz J, Coull BA, et al. Short-Term Exposure to Air Pollution and Biomarkers of Oxidative Stress: The Framingham Heart Study. J Am Heart Assoc. 2016;5(5):e002742.
9. Ye Y, Jiang S, Zhang C, Cheng Y, Zhong H, Du T, et al. Environmental Pollutant Benzo[a]pyrene Induces Recurrent Pregnancy Loss through Promoting Apoptosis and Suppressing Migration of Extravillous Trophoblast. Biomed Res Int. 2020;2020:8983494.
10. Patel MM, Chillrud SN, Deepti KC, Ross JM, Kinney PL. Traffic-related air pollutants and exhaled markers of airway inflammation and oxidative stress in New York City adolescents. Environ Res. 2013;121:71-8.
11. Lanki T, Hampel R, Tiittanen P, Andrich S, Beelen R, Brunekreef B, et al. Air Pollution from Road Traffic and Systemic Inflammation in Adults: A Cross-Sectional Analysis in the European ESCAPE Project. Environ Health Perspect. 2015;123(8):785-91.
12. Viehmann A, Hertel S, Fuks K, Eisele L, Moebus S, Möhlenkamp S, et al. Long-term residential exposure to urban air pollution, and repeated measures of systemic blood markers of inflammation and coagulation. Occup Environ Med. 2015;72(9):656-63.
13. Slama R, Darrow L, Parker J, Woodruff TJ, Strickland M, Nieuwenhuijsen M, et al. Meeting Report: Atmospheric Pollution and Human Reproduction. Environ Health Perspect. 2008;116(6):791-8.
14. Sultana Z, Maiti K, Aitken J, Morris J, Dedman L, Smith R. Oxidative stress, placental ageing-related pathologies and adverse pregnancy outcomes. Am J Reprod Immunol. 2017;77:e12653.
15. Aborisade OB, Charles-Davies MA, Okunlola MA. Environmental Influences in Normal Weight Women with History of Recurrent Pregnancy Loss. Int J Trop Dis Health. 2013;3(3):257-66.
16. Zhang Y, Yan X, Tan J, Tan J, Liu C, Yang P, et al. Exposure of Reproductive-Aged Women to Multiple Metals and Its Associations with Unexplained Recurrent Miscarriage. Toxics. 2023;11(10):830.
17. Pandey A, Jaiswar SP, Ansari NG, Deo S, Sankhwar P, Pant S, et al. Pesticide Risk and Recurrent Pregnancy Loss in Females of Subhumid Region of India. Niger Med J. 2020;61(2):55-9.
18. Guirguis SS, Pelmear PL, Roy ML, Wong L. Health effects associated with exposure to anaesthetic gases in Ontario hospital personnel. Br J Indus Med. 1990;47:490-7.
19. Gold EB, Tomich E. Occupational hazards to fertility and pregnancy outcome. Occup Med (Philadelphia, PA). 1994;9:435-69.
20. Paul I, Mondal P, Haldar D, Halder G. Beyond the cradle-Amidst microplastics and the ongoing peril during pregnancy and neonatal stages: A holistic review. J Hazard Mater. 2024;469:133963.
21. Hu J, Qin X, Zhang J, Zhu Y, Zeng W, Lin Y, et al. Polystyrene microplastics disturb maternal-fetal immune balance and cause reproductive toxicity in pregnant mice. Reprod Toxicol. 2021;106:42-50.
22. Wan S, Wang X, Chen W, Wang M, Zhao J, Xu Z, et al. Exposure to high dose of polystyrene nanoplastics causes trophoblast cell apoptosis and induces miscarriage. Part Fibre Toxicol. 2024;21(1):13.
23. Rolfo A, Nuzzo AM, De Amicis R, Moretti L, Bertoli S, Leone A. Fetal-Maternal Exposure to Endocrine Disruptors: Correlation with Diet Intake and Pregnancy Outcomes. Nutrients. 2020;12:1744.
24. Puche-Juarez M, Toledano JM, Moreno-Fernandez J, Gálvez-Ontiveros Y, Rivas A, Diaz-Castro J, et al. The Role of Endocrine Disrupting Chemicals in Gestation and Pregnancy Outcomes. Nutrients. 2023;15(21):4657.
25. Liu X, Wang Z, Liu F. Chronic exposure of BPA impairs male germ cell proliferation and induces lower sperm quality in male mice. Chemosphere. 2021;262:127880.
26. Harnett KG, Moore LG, Chin A, Cohen IC, Lautrup RR, Schuh SM. Teratogenicity and toxicity of the new BPA alternative TMBPF, and BPA, BPS, and BPAF in chick embryonic development. Curr Res Toxicol. 2021;2:399-410.

27. Ye Y, Tang Y, Xiong Y, Feng L, Li X. Bisphenol A exposure alters placentation and causes preeclampsia-like features in pregnant mice involved in reprogramming of DNA methylation of WNT2. FASEB J. 2019;33:2732-42.
28. Ticiani E, Gingrich J, Pu Y, Vettathu M, Davis J, Martin D, et al. Bisphenol S and Epidermal Growth Factor Receptor Signaling in Human Placental Cytotrophoblasts. Environ Health Perspect. 2021;129:27005.
29. Huang S, Li J, Xu S, Zhao H, Li Y, Zhou Y, et al. Bisphenol A and bisphenol S exposures during pregnancy and gestational age—A longitudinal study in China. Chemosphere. 2019;237:124426.
30. Kim S, Park E, Park EK, Lee S, Kwon JA, Shin BH, et al. Urinary Concentrations of Bisphenol Mixtures during Pregnancy and Birth Outcomes: The MAKE Study. Int J Environ Res Public Health. 2021;18:10098.
31. Song W, Puttabyatappa M, Zeng L, Vazquez D, Pennathur S, Padmanabhan V. Developmental programming: Prenatal bisphenol A treatment disrupts mediators of placental function in sheep. Chemosphere. 2020;243:125301.
32. Kaimal A, Al Mansi MH, Dagher JB, Pope C, Varghese MG, Rudi TB, et al. Prenatal exposure to bisphenols affects pregnancy outcomes and offspring development in rats. Chemosphere. 2021;276:130118.
33. Yan D, Jiao Y, Yan H, Liu T, Yan H, Yuan J. Endocrine-disrupting chemicals and the risk of gestational diabetes mellitus: A systematic review and meta-analysis. Environ Health. 2022;21:53.
34. ESHRE Guideline Group on RPL; Bender Atik R, Christiansen OB, Elson J, Kolte AM, Lewis S, et al. ESHRE guideline: recurrent pregnancy loss: an update in 2022. Hum Reprod Open. 2023;2023(1):hoad002.
35. Zhang BY, Wei YS, Niu JM, Li Y, Miao ZL, Wang ZN. Risk factors for unexplained recurrent spontaneous abortion in a population from southern China. Int J Gynaecol Obstet. 2010;108:135-8.
36. du Fossé NA, Van der Hoorn ML, Buisman NH, Van Lith JMM, Le Cessie S, Lashley E. Paternal smoking is associated with an increased risk of pregnancy loss in a dose-dependent manner: a systematic review and meta-analysis. Fertil Steril. 2021;2:227-38.
37. England LJ, Kim SY, Tomar SL, Ray CS, Gupta PC, Eissenberg T, et al. Non-cigarette tobacco use among women and adverse pregnancy outcomes. Acta Obstet Gynecol Scand. 2010;89(4):454-64.
38. Sata F, Yamada H, Suzuki K, Saijo Y, Kato EH, Morikawa M, et al. Caffeine intake, CYP1A2 polymorphism and the risk of recurrent pregnancy loss. Mol Hum Reprod. 2005;11:357-60.
39. Maconochie N, Doyle P, Prior S, Simmons R. Risk factors for first trimester miscarriage—results from a UK-population-based case-control study. BJOG: Int J Obstet Gynaecol. 2007;114:170-86.
40. Stefanidou EM, Caramellino L, Patriarca A, Menato G. Maternal caffeine consumption and sine causa recurrent miscarriage. Eur J Obstet Gynecol Reprod Biol. 2011;158:220-4.
41. Andersen AM, Andersen PK, Olsen J, Gronbaek M, Strandberg-Larsen K. Moderate alcohol intake during pregnancy and risk of fetal death. Int J Epidemiol. 2012;41:405-13.
42. Avalos LA, Roberts SC, Kaskutas LA, Block G, Li DK. Volume and type of alcohol during early pregnancy and the risk of miscarriage. Subst Use Misuse. 2014;49:1437-45.
43. Brandes M, Verzijden JC, Hamilton CJ, de Weys NP, de Bruin JP, Bots RS, et al. Is the fertility treatment itself a risk factor for early pregnancy loss? Reprod Biomed Online. 2011;22:192-9.
44. Jensen TK, Gottschau M, Madsen JO, Andersson AM, Lassen TH, Skakkebaek NE, et al. Habitual alcohol consumption associated with reduced semen quality and changes in reproductive hormones; a cross-sectional study among 1221 young Danish men. BMJ Open. 2014;4:e005462.
45. Coleman-Cowger VH, Schauer GL, Peters EN. Marijuana and tobacco co-use among a nationally representative sample of US pregnant and non-pregnant women: 2005-2014 National Survey on Drug Use and Health findings. Drug Alcohol Depend. 2017;177:130-5.
46. Wall KM, Haddad LB, Mehta CC, Golub ET, Rahangdale L, Dionne-Odom J, et al. Miscarriage among women in the United States women's interagency HIV study, 1994-2017. Am J Obstet Gynecol. 2019;221(4):347.e1-347.e13.
47. Ness RB, Grisso JA, Hirschinger N, Markovic N, Shaw LM, Day NL, et al. Cocaine and tobacco use and the risk of spontaneous abortion. N Engl J Med. 1999;340(5):333-9.

SECTION

8 Miscellaneous

CHAPTER 38

Recurrent Biochemical Pregnancy

Ameet Patki, Mrinmayi Dharmadhikari

ABSTRACT

Biochemical pregnancies are common to both recurrent implantation failure and recurrent pregnancy loss (RPL). The incidence is fairly high, and they pose a diagnostic dilemma as no pregnancy tissue is available for genetic testing. Advanced maternal age, assisted reproductive technology (ART) pregnancies, autoimmune disorders and genetically abnormal embryos are the most common cause of biochemical pregnancies. A complete RPL work up is warranted in these cases as well.

Keywords: Biochemical pregnancies, RPL, RIF, Autoimmunity, hCG.

INTRODUCTION

Biochemical pregnancy (BP), also known as chemical pregnancy, nonvisualized pregnancy, or pregnancy of unknown location in simple terms, is a positive β-human chorionic gonadotropin (hCG) test with no pregnancy on ultrasound. The Society for Assisted Reproductive Technology (SART) defines this as "when a woman's pregnancy test is initially positive but becomes negative before a gestational sac is visible on ultrasound." A number of questions arise by reading this definition, but there is still a lack of adequate data and large studies that would adequately help in diagnosing, defining, and understanding the implications of this medical phenomenon before we can appropriately manage these pregnancies, especially with respect to future recurrence. Pregnancy loss before viability is quite common, and there are numerous scientific studies around this. Unfortunately, however, there is a need for consistent terminology defining each of these early pregnancy losses, including BPs.

The European Society of Human Reproduction and Embryology (ESHRE) in 2015 has published the nomenclature and classification of early pregnancy losses, including BPs, in order to correctly diagnose this entity and differentiate it from other similar clinical situations for a more universal and standardized approach and for comparisons of scientific results related to this elusive entity[1] **(Table 1)**.

TABLE 1: Terminology for classifying pregnancy failure prior to viability.[1]

Pregnancy loss	*Spontaneous pregnancy demise*
Early pregnancy loss	Spontaneous pregnancy demise before 10 weeks of gestational age (before 8th developmental week)
Nonvisualized pregnancy loss	Spontaneous pregnancy demise based on decreasing serum or urinary β-hCG levels and nonlocalization on ultrasound, if performed[2]
Biochemical pregnancy loss	Spontaneous pregnancy demise based on decreasing serum or urinary β-hCG levels without an ultrasound evaluation[3]
Miscarriage	Intrauterine pregnancy demise confirmed by ultrasound or histology[4,5]

(hCG: human chorionic gonadotropin)

INCIDENCE

The reported incidence of BPs in the fertile population is between 13 and 22% of pregnancies.[6-8] This, however, may be confounded, because pregnancy test sensitivity has increased and may be able to detect other sources of hCG such as endometrial, pituitary, or phantom hCG. Additionally, a false positive result may be due to extraneous hCG administered in an assisted reproductive technology (ART) cycle. Laboratory variations may also lead to false positive results, and getting the repeat test done in the same laboratory minimizes interlaboratory differences and errors while interpreting the reports. These low levels of hCG, which are detected due to high test sensitivity, that is, isolated raised hCGs, may be falsely interpreted as BPs. Hence, it has been suggested that the presence of rising hCG levels seen on two consecutive tests should be considered significant, and one raised level should be described as isolated raised hCG.[9] It is important to bear in mind that a number of pregnancies diagnosed as BPs are actually early ectopic pregnancies, which fail to develop further and resolve spontaneously. In the infertile population, the reported incidence of BPs is reported to be 14–18%.[10,11] A higher incidence has been reported in patients undergoing in vitro fertilization (IVF) (22–31%) when compared with the general infertile population.[12-14]

CAUSES

The cause of BPs may be varied. These may be related to the embryo, maternal causes, or even paternal causes related to the sperm. Though there is adequate data implicating male factors in recurrent pregnancy loss and recurrent implantation failure, there is no information associating these with recurrent BPs, and this aspect needs to be studied further.

Age is an important factor leading to pregnancy losses. Women should be sensitively informed that the risk of pregnancy loss rapidly increases after the age of 40 years.[15,16] Delayed implantation can occur due to pregnancy loss because of several reasons, including aneuploidies. Also, poor endometrial receptivity can lead to hindrance in implantation, thus resulting in a pregnancy loss.

The use of gonadotropins in IVF cycles for controlled ovarian hyperstimulation affects the endometrial expression of certain genes and proteins. This is also true in frozen embryo transfer cycles due to the use of high-dose progesterone and estrogen. These may lead to alterations in the endometrium, affecting implantation as well as proper embryo growth and development. This has been implicated as one of the causes of BPs encountered during IVF treatment cycles.[11] The incidence of BPs may be higher during fresh embryo transfer cycles compared to frozen embryo cycles, reflecting alterations in the endometrial receptivity as a probable cause.[17] Keeping this in mind, it has been suggested that changes in ovarian stimulation protocols, the use of frozen and thawed embryo cycles, and the use of endometrial stimulation prior to transferring embryos could help prevent BPs.

It is the hyperglycosylated form of hCG (hCG-H), which is produced at the beginning of pregnancy.[18,19] It is produced by the cytotrophoblast of the developing embryo and is autocrine in nature. It plays an important role in the invasiveness of the syncytiotrophoblast. Low levels of this hormone were seen in BPs. In a study by Sasaki et al.,[20] only 8 out of 36 BPs produced hCG-H levels >40% on the day of implantation. On the other hand, all of the normal term pregnancies produced levels of hCG-H >40%. A thin endometrium due to various causes, like a T-shaped uterus, may not allow proper invasion by the syncytiotrophoblast, leading to inappropriate placentation. This is known to be an important cause for recurrent implantation failure in IVF cycles and can also lead to BPs due to poor endometrial receptivity.[21] Hysteroscopic metroplasty has been shown to improve clinical pregnancy rates as well as live birth rates in these patients in numerous studies, especially in those with recurrent implantation failure.[22,23]

A luteal dose of hCG administered in IVF practice aims to support implantation. Though hCG-H is patented and not available for commercial use, commercially available hCG is used. hCG is known to prevent further miscarriages in women with recurrent pregnancy loss as per the Cochrane Database Systematic Review, 2013.[24]

In a study by Lee et al.,[25] the authors compared the etiologies of 44 couples with recurrent BPs (more than two BPs) following IVF with etiologies associated with recurrent pregnancy losses in 43 couples, which served as the control group.

Their study results showed that the rate of immune factors like elevated natural killer cell activity and the rate of autoimmune biomarkers, antinuclear antibody (ANA), rheumatoid arthritis (RA) factor, antithyroglobulin antibody (TgAb), lupus anticoagulant (LA), anticardiolipin immunoglobulin G (IgG), IgM, anti-DNA, antimicrosomal Ab, and thrombophilia did not significantly differ between the two groups ($p = 0.361$). These pathogenic autoantibodies affect the blood circulation at the placental level and are also implicated in altered immune responses, which can lead to miscarriages and BPs. The authors suggest offering variable immunomodulation treatment to patients with recurrent BPs after IVF cycles similar to the treatment offered to those with recurrent pregnancy loss in those suspected to have abnormal immune responses. The differences in diminished ovarian reserve ($p = 0.552$), incidence of uterine factors ($p = 0.206$), and unknown causes ($p = 0.161$) also were not statistically significant.

The incidence of parental chromosome abnormality was similar between the two groups, though higher than in the general population (0.7%).[26] When a parental chromosomal anomaly like a balanced translocation or inversion is suspected to be the cause of recurrent BPs, then a preimplantation genetic diagnosis can be done to choose euploid embryos for transfer with the aim of preventing a BP.

IMPLICATIONS

The emotional turmoil and uncertainty of the future associated with BPs when couples encounter a positive pregnancy test after a convoluted IVF procedure but without it developing into a clinical pregnancy is one of the reasons why some leave the IVF program in disappointment. Besides the psychological implications on the couple, recurrent BPs are important clinically as predictors of future pregnancy outcome. A BP increases the chances of future IVF pregnancies, being a positive predictor of the same.[27,28] On the other hand, they are a negative predictor of pregnancy outcomes due to their association with higher recurrent BPs and miscarriage rates.[29] Each additional BP decreases the chances of subsequent live births, similar to the relative risk conferred by miscarriages. ESHRE considers BPs as pregnancy losses; hence, ≥2 BPs can be regarded as pregnancy losses and therefore can be assumed to warrant treatment in order to prevent recurrence.[9]

There is insufficient data in literature to formulate evidence-based guidelines for the management of these patients with recurrent BPs. There are, however, suggestions based on smaller studies on a theoretical basis and based on the experience of authors that are available. This calls for larger randomized controlled trials and more research in this field, given its implications.

CONCLUSION

The advancements in the field of ART have made parenthood a reality for numerous couples. The emotional, physical, and financial burden, however, still has to be borne by these couples. The time period while waiting for the pregnancy test can be one of the most anxious periods for these couples who are eagerly awaiting the result. A positive test for pregnancy can lead to a BP where the initial positive test fails to develop into a healthy pregnancy and subsequent childbirth. This can be a cause of psychological as well as physical morbidity for many such couples. Keeping this in mind, efforts should be made to define the cause of recurrent BPs, and appropriate strategies based on evidence should be followed for a positive outcome in future pregnancies. Appropriate counseling and support go a long way for these couples during this time of emotional lability and anxiety. Clinicians and caregivers play a pivotal role in modeling the emotional constitution and providing optimum information and support to these couples with respect to this entity. Therefore, it is paramount to keep abreast of the research and recommendations as well as implications of recurrent BPs, so that these couples receive optimum care and support in these trying times.

REFERENCES

1. Bender Atik R, Christiansen OB, Elson J, Kolte AM, Lewis S, Middeldorp S, et al.; ESHRE Guideline Group on RPL. ESHRE guideline: recurrent pregnancy loss. Hum Reprod Open. 2018;2018(2):hoy004.
2. Kolte AM, van Oppenraaij RH, Quenby S, Farquharson RG, Stephenson M, Goddijn M, et al.; ESHRE Special Interest Group Early Pregnancy. Non-visualized pregnancy losses are prognostically important for unexplained recurrent miscarriage. Hum Reprod. 2014;29:931-37.
3. Farquharson RG, Stephenson MD (Ed). Early Pregnancy. New York: Cambridge University Press; 2010.
4. ASRM Practice Committee. Definitions of infertility and recurrent pregnancy loss: a committee opinion. Fertil Steril. 2013;99:63.
5. Stephenson M, Kutteh W. Evaluation and management of recurrent early pregnancy loss. Clin Obstet Gynecol. 2007;50:132-45.
6. Zinaman MJ, Clegg ED, Brown CC, O'Connor J, Selevan SG. Estimates of human fertility and pregnancy loss. Fertil Steril. 1996;65:503-9.
7. Coulam CB, Chapman C, Rinehart JS. What is a preclinical pregnancy loss? J Assist Reprod Genet. 1998;15:184-7.
8. Hakim RB, Gray RH, Zacur H. Infertility and early-pregnancy loss. Amer J Obstet Gynecol. 1995;172:1510-7.
9. Carp H. Biochemical Pregnancies: How Should They Be Interpreted? Gynecol Reprod Endocrinol Metabol. 2020;01:04-07.
10. Salumets A, Suikkari AM, Mäkinen S, Karro H, Roos A, Tuuri T. Frozen embryo transfers: implications of clinical and embryological factors on the pregnancy outcome. Hum Reprod. 2006;21:2368-74.
11. Zeadna A, Son WY, Moon JH, Dahan MH. A comparison of biochemical pregnancy rates between women who underwent IVF and fertile controls who conceived spontaneously. Hum Reprod. 2015;30:783-8.
12. Liu HC, Jones GS, Jones HW Jr, Rosenwaks Z. Mechanisms and factors of early pregnancy wastage in in vitro

fertilization-embryo transfer patients. Fertil Steril. 1988;50:95-101.
13. Bjercke S, Tanbo T, Dale PO, Mørkrid L, Abyholm T. Human chorionic gonadotrophin concentrations in early pregnancy after in-vitro fertilization. Hum Reprod. 1999;14:1642-6.
14. Hourvitz A, Lerner-Geva L, Elizur SE, Baum M, Levron J, David B, et al. Role of embryo quality in predicting early pregnancy loss following assisted reproductive technology. Reprod Biomed Online. 2006;13:504-9.
15. Grande M, Borrell A, Garcia-Posada R, Borobio V, Munoz M, Creus M, et al. The effect of maternal age on chromosomal anomaly rate and spectrum in recurrent miscarriage. Hum Reprod. 2012;27:3109-17.
16. Lund M, Kamper-Jorgensen M, Nielsen HS, Lidegaard O, Andersen AM, Christiansen OB. Prognosis for live birth in women with recurrent miscarriage: what is the best measure of success? Obstet Gynecol. 2012;119:37-43.
17. Shapiro BS, Daneshmand ST, Garner FC, Aguirre M, Hudson C, Thomas S. Evidence of impaired endometrial receptivity after ovarian stimulation for in vitro fertilization: a prospective randomized trial comparing fresh and frozen-thawed embryo transfers in high responders. Fertil Steril. 2011;96:516-8.
18. Cole LA. hCG and hyperglycosylated hCG in the establishment and evolution of hemochorial placentation. J Reprod Immunol. 2009;82:112-8.
19. Evans J. Hyperglycosylated hCG: a Unique Human Implantation and Invasion Factor. Am J Reprod Immunol. 2016;75(3):333-40.
20. Sasaki Y, Ladner DG, Cole LA. Hyperglycosylated human chorionic gonadotropin and the source of pregnancy failures. Fertil Steril. 2008;89:1781-6.
21. Dickey RP, Olar TT, Taylor SN, Curole DN, Harrigill K. Relationship of biochemical pregnancy to pre-ovulatory endometrial thickness and pattern in patients undergoing ovulation induction. Hum Reprod. 1993;8:327-30.
22. Uyar E, Usal D, Selam B, Cincik M, Bagis T. IVF outcomes after hysteroscopic metroplasty in patients with T-shaped uterus. Fertil Res Pract. 2019;5:15.
23. Zhang Y, Zhu Y, Ge B, Sui M, Zheng Z, Sun J. Reproductive outcome of hysteroscopic metroplasty for women with T-shaped uterus: a retrospective study. Reprod Health. 2022;19(1):78.
24. Morley LC, Simpson N, Tang T. Human chorionic gonadotrophin (hCG) for preventing miscarriage. Cochrane Database Syst Rev. 2013:CD008611.
25. Lee HM, Lee HJ, Yang KM, Cha SH, Ahn HK, Kim YJ. Etiological evaluation of repeated biochemical pregnancy in infertile couples who have undergone in vitro fertilization. Obstet Gynecol Sci. 2017;60(6):565-70.
26. Franssen MT, Korevaar JC, Leschot NJ, Bossuyt PM, Knegt AC, Gerssen-Schoorl KB, et al. Selective chromosome analysis in couples with two or more miscarriages: case-control study. BMJ. 2005;331:137-41.
27. De Neubourg D, Gerris J, Mangelschots K, Van Royen E, Vercruyssen M, Elseviers M. Single top quality embryo transfer as a model for prediction of early pregnancy outcome. Hum Reprod. 2004;19:1476-9.
28. Haas J, Lerner-Geva L, Yerushalmi GM, Maman E, Yinon Y, Baum M, et al. Previous abortion is a positive predictor for ongoing pregnancy in the next cycle in women with repeated IVF failures. Reprod Biomed Online. 2012;25:339-44.
29. Yang R, Yang S, Li R, Chen X, Wang H, Ma C, et al. Biochemical pregnancy and spontaneous abortion in first IVF cycles are negative predictors for subsequent cycles: an over 10,000 cases cohort study. Arch Gynecol Obstet. 2015;292:453-8.

CHAPTER

39 Recurrent Molar Pregnancies

Rosemary A Fisher, Neil J Sebire

ABSTRACT

Recurrent molar pregnancies are the result of genetic mutations in *NLRP7* or *KHDC3L* genes. Familial recurrent hydatidiform mole requires identification of mutations in the above genes in the villous tissue, after a woman gives a history of three consecutive molar pregnancies. Women with positive mutations run the risk of persistent trophoblastic disease after each molar pregnancy and will require ovum donation for a successful pregnancy outcome.

Keywords: Familial recurrent hydatidiform mole, Recurrent hydatidiform mole, *NLRP7*, *KHDC3L* gene mutation.

INTRODUCTION

Hydatidiform mole (HM), or molar pregnancy, is a type of abnormal pregnancy characterized by overgrowth of the placenta and poor fetal development. While, most molar pregnancies are sporadic, any woman who has a HM is at increased risk of a subsequent molar pregnancy.[1-4] While the risk of a further HM is approximately 1% after a single molar pregnancy, increasing to 13% after two or more HM,[5] the most likely outcome of a future pregnancy for most women with a HM is still a full-term normal delivery. However, among women with recurrent hydatidiform mole (RHM), there is a small subset of women with an inherited predisposition to molar pregnancies for whom a future successful pregnancy is unlikely. For appropriate management of women with RHM, it is important to identify those women who have an inherited predisposition to these pregnancies. This first requires accurate pathological diagnosis to reliably differentiate HM from other types of pregnancy loss.

PATHOLOGY OF HYDATIDIFORM MOLES

On the basis of histopathological features, HM can be classified into two major categories that reflect their unusual genetic origin: (1) complete hydatidiform mole (CHM) and (2) partial hydatidiform mole (PHM).[6,7] The majority of CHM and PHM are currently evacuated in the 1st or early 2nd trimester, at which time the histopathological diagnostic criteria may be different from those classically described at later gestations.[8] Recognition of these specific features allows a confident histopathological diagnosis to be made in most cases. The use of ancillary techniques, such as flow cytometry,[9] immunohistochemistry,[10] and molecular studies,[11,12] will usually facilitate the diagnosis in cases where the morphological features are inconclusive. However, the basis for the diagnosis of CHM and PHM remains detailed examination of tissue morphology on routine hematoxylin and eosin (H&E) stained sections **(Figs. 1A to C)**.

In the 1st trimester, CHM demonstrates chorionic villi with scattered larger, hydropic villi, but hydrops is usually not marked in early pregnancy. Similarly, some villi may exhibit early cistern formation but again this is not a constant feature. At low power, the villi show a highly characteristic "budding" architecture, with focally marked mucoid/myxoid degeneration of the villous stroma and abundant nuclear karyorrhectic stromal debris. It should be noted that villi from cases of CHM may contain blood vessels in early pregnancy, usually collapsed, but very occasionally containing fetal red blood cells.[13] Finally, and most importantly, the diagnosis of CHM requires the presence of abnormal villous trophoblast proliferation, recognized as more than two layers of trophoblast, often with nuclear pleomorphism, forming circumferential masses. Sheets of pleomorphic extravillous trophoblast may also be present. Extravillous trophoblast invasion is also abnormal in pregnancies affected by CHM, showing

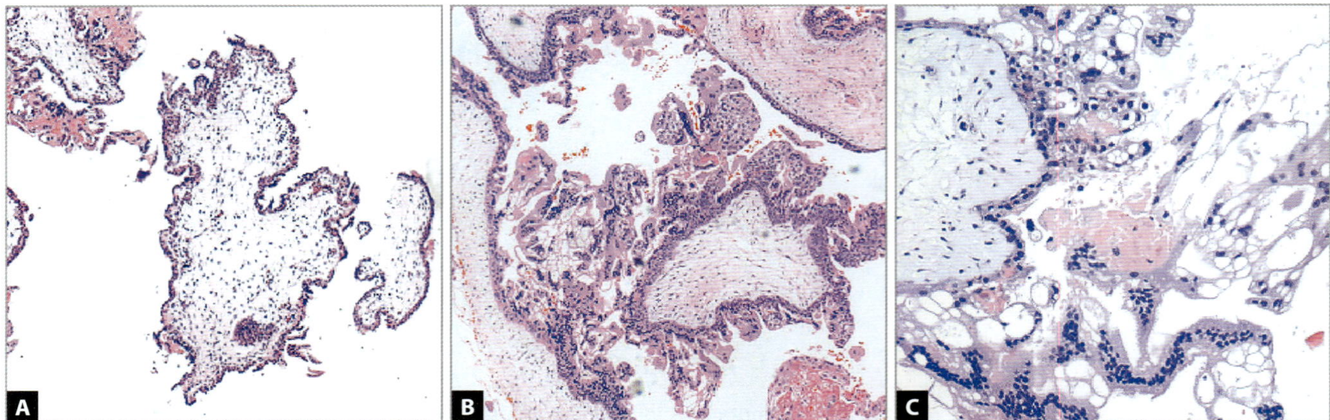

Figs. 1A to C: Photomicrographs showing characteristic morphological features of (A) PHM; (B) AnCHM; and (C) BiCHM. (H&E original magnifications (A) 40×; (B) 100×; and (C) 250×). (AnCHM: androgenetic complete hydatidiform mole; BiCHM: biparental complete hydatidiform mole; H&E: hematoxylin and eosin; PHM: partial hydatidiform mole)

prominent implantation site reaction with absence of normal endovascular trophoblast plugging.[14]

First trimester PHM also demonstrates characteristic histological features including chorionic villi of varying sizes, patchy mild villous hydrops with occasional scattered cisterns, and larger villi exhibiting an abnormal, irregular "dentate" outline with cleft formation and round or oval pseudoinclusions. Villi usually demonstrate blood vessels often containing nucleated fetal red blood cells, sometimes with angiomatoid change. Diagnostic abnormal, nonpolar trophoblast hyperplasia is present, but this is almost always focal and less marked than in CHM. The villous stroma shows a mixture of hydropic change and stromal fibrosis in different villi, without stromal karyorrhectic debris. Although abnormal trophoblast hyperplasia is a requirement for the diagnosis of HM, the extent of such hyperplasia appears to have no prognostic importance.

In women who have a second molar pregnancy, this is most likely to be of the same type as the first, although some women may have a combination of CHM and PHM. In women with an inherited predisposition to RHM, subsequent molar pregnancies are likely to be CHM.[5] While the CHM in these women may occasionally show atypical features, they are often pathologically indistinguishable from CHM that occurs sporadically **(Figs. 1A to C)**.[15] A differential diagnosis between women who have two or more HM by chance and those that have an inherited predisposition to molar pregnancies relies on genetic analysis of the molar tissue.

GENETICS OF HYDATIDIFORM MOLES

Both the shared pathological features that distinguish HM from other types of reproductive loss and the characteristics that enable a differential diagnosis between CHM and PHM reflect their genetic origin. Despite CHM having a normal diploid number of chromosomes, like PHM, which are triploid,[6] they have an excess of paternal chromosomes. PHMs have two sets of chromosome from the father, most resulting from fertilization of an ovum by two sperms **(Figs. 2A to C)**[16-18] with occasional PHM reported to arise by fertilization of an ovum by a diploid sperm.[19,20]

The majority of CHMs are diploid but are androgenetic having no maternal contribution to the nuclear genome.[21,22] Most arise following fertilization of an ovum by a single sperm that then undergoes reduplication to restore the diploid chromosome number,[23-26] while approximately 20% arise by dispermic fertilization of an ovum **(Figs. 2A to C)**.[27-29] Thus, both CHM and PHM have two paternal contributions to the genome. However, CHMs have no maternal contribution to the nuclear genome. The fate of the maternal chromosomes in CHM is uncertain. Although abnormal segregation of chromosomal material to the polar bodies during meiosis would theoretically result in an anucleate ovum, it has been suggested that androgenetic conceptions are more likely to arise following postzygotic diploidization of a triploid conceptus.[30] In other respects, the ovum in CHM appears to be genetically normal with the mitochondrial deoxyribonucleic acid

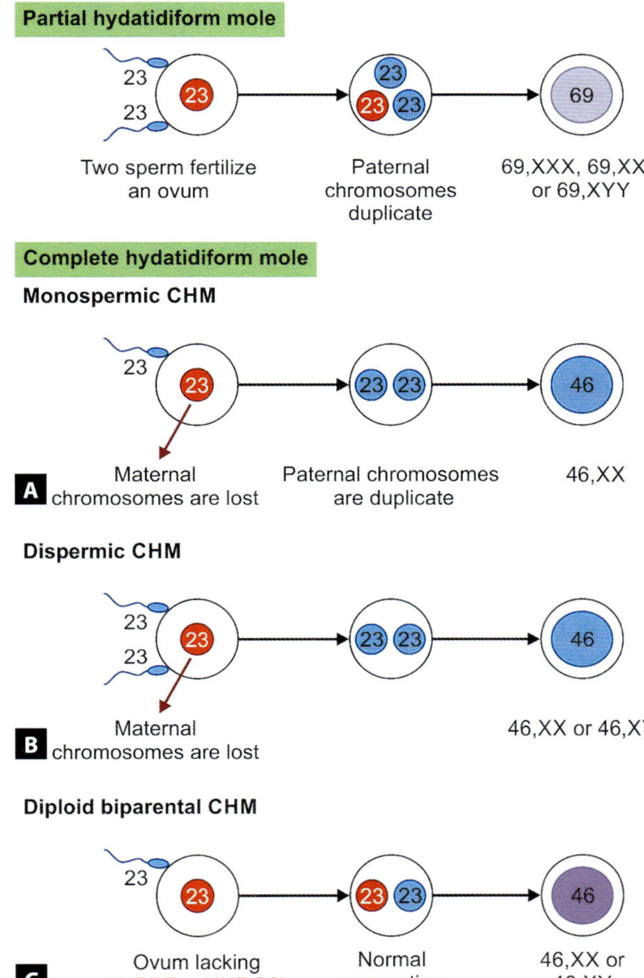

Figs. 2A to C: Origin of partial and complete hydatidiform moles. PHMs are triploid and almost all arise by dispermy. The majority of CHMs are androgenetic and arise from (A) fertilization of an ovum from which maternal chromosomes are lost and in which paternal chromosomes undergo duplication, or (B) fertilization of an ovum, from which maternal chromosomes are lost, by two sperm, and (C) a BiCHM arising following normal fertilization of an ovum from a woman with mutations in *NLRP7* or *KHDC3L*. (BiCHM: biparental complete hydatidiform mole; PHM: partial hydatidiform mole)

(DNA) being maternally inherited in the same way as that of a normal conception.[31,32]

FAMILIAL RECURRENT HYDATIDIFORM MOLES

The incidence of HM varies considerably among different ethnic groups with the highest rates reported in Southeast Asia.[33] Recent studies in the UK suggest an incidence of approximately 1 in 600 conceptions[34] with a significantly higher incidence in the Asian population.[35] Therefore, sporadic HM might occasionally occur in more than one member of a family by chance. However, the occurrence of RHM in more than one member of a family by chance should be extremely rare. The first report of familial recurrent hydatidiform mole (FRHM) described three unrelated Indian kindreds in which two or more individuals presented with molar pregnancies.[36] Subsequent reports described affected families of Italian, Lebanese, German, and Irish origin[37-40] with affected family members being sisters or cousins.

Genetic studies of the CHMs in these families showed that, rather than being androgenetic with two paternal contributions to the genome, they were in fact biparental in origin with a chromosomal complement from each parent **(Figs. 2A to C)**.[40-42] This observation together with the pattern of inheritance seen in these families suggested that FRHM is an autosomal recessive condition in which chromosomally normal conceptions develop as CHM.[43] In addition to these family studies, a number of individual women with RHM were also been shown to have diploid biparental complete hydatidiform mole (BiCHM) consistent with an autosomal recessive condition in which only a single individual might be affected in a small sibship.[44,45] However, it is important for clinical management to be aware that not all women with RHM have FRHM and that some individuals with RHM have been shown to have CHM of typical androgenetic origin.[46]

While most women with FRHM have only CHM, some may present with other types of pregnancy including PHM, nonmolar miscarriage, stillbirth, or very occasionally normal pregnancy, in addition to RHM.[41,43,47,48] Where PHMs in these families have been investigated these have also been found to be diploid and biparental, rather than triploid[40,49] and are, therefore, likely to represent BiCHM as opposed to androgenetic complete hydatidiform mole (AnCHM). In addition, a diagnosis of BiCHM cannot be excluded where tissue from a spontaneous miscarriage has not been examined. Thus, the proportion of CHM in women with FRHM is likely to be much higher than the 75% reported.[43]

Familial Recurrent Hydatidiform Moles are the Result of Mutations in *NLRP7* or *KHDC3L*

Two genes have now been found to be associated with FRHM. Mutations in *NLRP7* (*NALP7*) were initially identified as the cause of FRHM in four families from different ethnic backgrounds.[50] Since then, over 100 families with FRHM have been investigated for mutations in *NLRP7* and approximately, 90% of these women found to be homozygous or compound heterozygotes for point mutations, splice site mutations, insertions, small deletions, duplications, or large *Alu*-mediated deletions[47,50-58] **(Fig. 3)**. While some mutations identified occur in several families, many in particular the protein truncating mutations currently appear to be exclusive to a single family. Occasional individuals with BiCHM have been found to have no mutations in *NLRP7*.[53,54,59] Further investigation of these cases led to the identification of a second gene associated with FRHM, *KHDC3L* (c6orf221).[60] To date, eight families in which FRHMs are a result of mutations in *KHDC3L* have been reported, five being homozygous for small deletions, one having a variant in the initiation codon, one with a splice site mutation, and a single case heterozygous for a small deletion and a variant in the initiation codon.[60-62] A recent publication also confirms that the above two mutations are the most important ones in familial RHM.[63]

Differential Diagnosis of Familial Recurrent Hydatidiform Moles

Approximately, one in four women with two CHM will go on to have a third CHM. However, only about 60% will have FRHM.[5] The remainder will have recurrent AnCHM. While these women clearly have poor obstetric histories, recurrent AnCHM does not appear to be familial and is not associated with mutations in *NLRP7* or *KHDC3L*.[55,63-66] These women often have normal live births in addition to CHM, whereas, for women with FRHM, the most likely outcome in any pregnancy is a CHM with live births extremely rare.[43,48] A diagnosis of FRHM should be considered in women with RHM but this should be supported by genetic analysis of the molar tissue.

Since both AnCHM and BiCHM are diploid, the differential diagnosis relies on techniques such as fluorescent microsatellite genotyping which can determine the parental origin of the molar tissue. Following polymerase chain reaction amplification of DNA, from parental blood and formalin-fixed paraffin-embedded sections of molar tissue, with a panel of primers for short tandem repeat loci on different chromosomes, the products are resolved by capillary electrophoresis and sizes of the different alleles calculated using specialist software.[11,67] AnCHM will have only one, or occasionally both, paternal alleles present, while the rare BiCHM will usually have both a maternal and paternal contribution to the genome **(Figs. 4A and B)**. While these are usually diploid, occasional CHMs in women with FRHM are found to be digynic with one paternal and two maternal contributions to the genome. This would normally result in

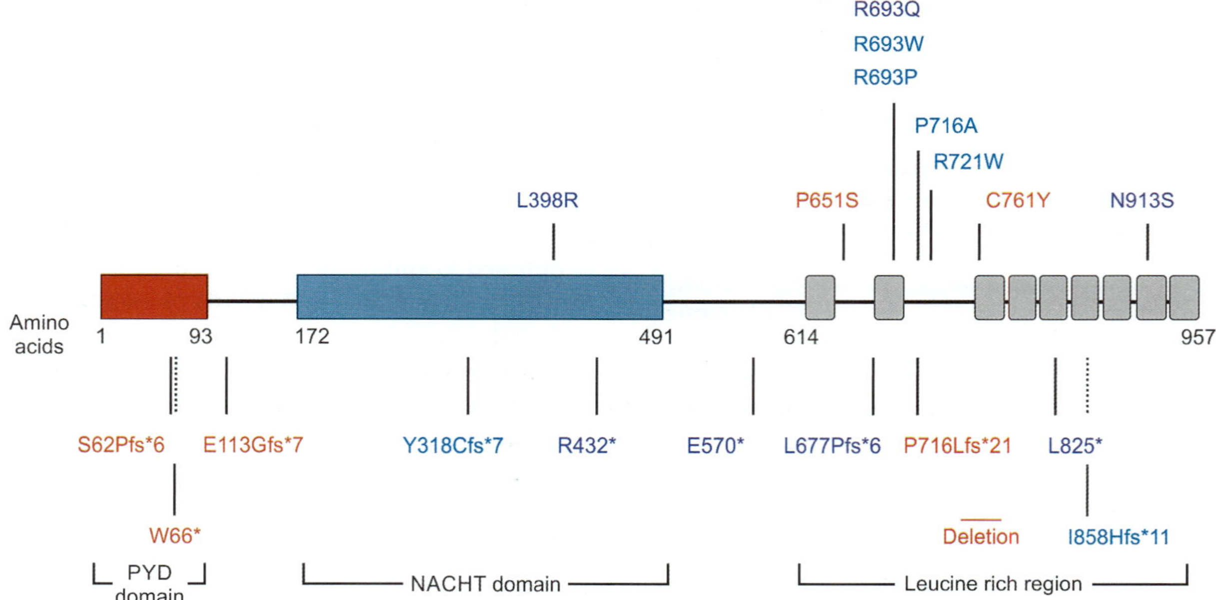

Fig. 3: Schematic representation of *NLRP7* showing examples of protein truncating (bottom panel) and missense (upper panel) mutations, in cases of familial recurrent hydatidiform mole (FRHM).[53,55,57,58] Mutations found in more than one family are shown in blue, those reported in other series in purple, and those currently reported in only a single family in red.

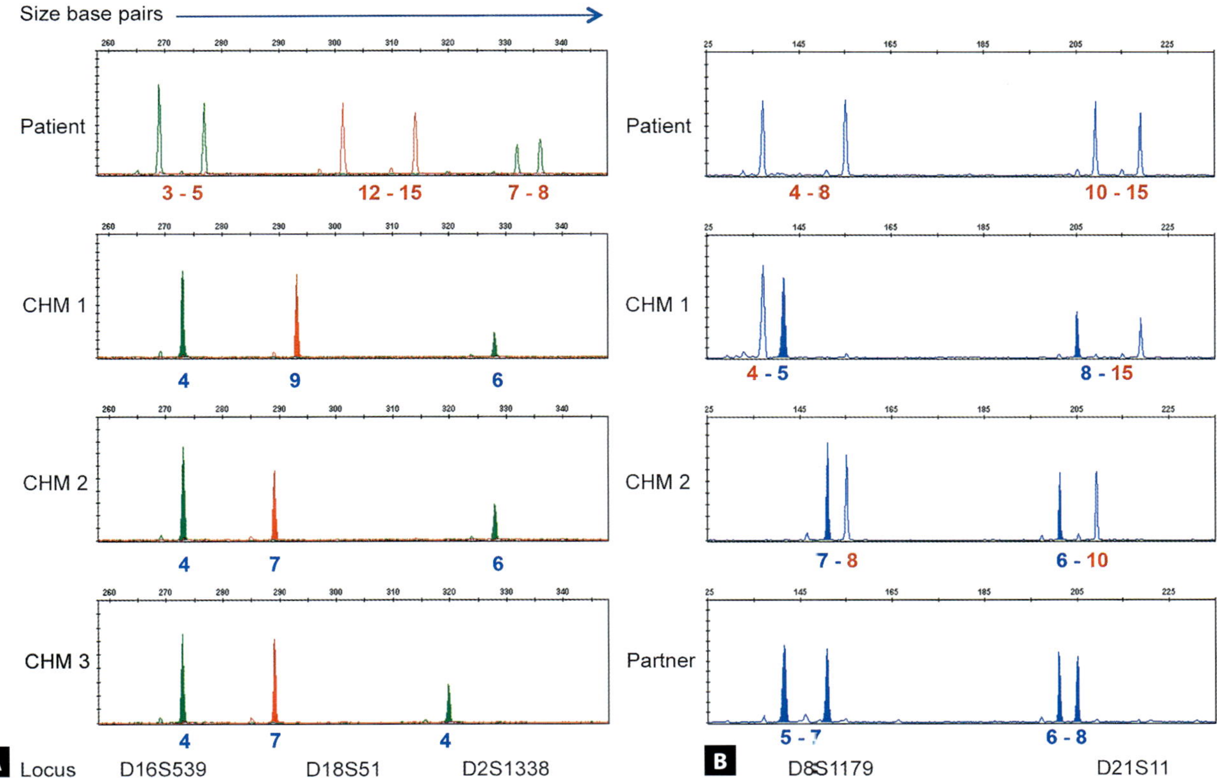

Figs. 4A and B: Representative electropherograms showing polymorphic microsatellite markers in DNA from cases of RHM. (A) Three CHMs all of which are homozygous for alleles not found in the patient at several loci (D16S539, D18S51, and D2S1338 shown) indicating that they are paternally derived and that all three CHMs are, therefore, AnCHM; and (B) Two BiCHM having a single maternal and a single paternal allele at each locus (D8S1179 and D21S11 shown) indicating that they are B CHM, thereby confirming a diagnosis of FRHM. (AnCHM: androgenetic complete hydatidiform mole; BiCHM: biparental complete hydatidiform mole; DNA: deoxyribonucleic acid; FRHM: familial recurrent hydatidiform mole; RHM: recurrent hydatidiform mole)

a pregnancy with a very different pathology.[68,69] However, in the presence of mutations in *NLRP7* or *KHDC3L*, these pregnancies will also develop as CHM despite the presence of two maternal genomes.[70]

A pathological diagnosis of FRHM can be confirmed by sequencing *NLRP7* and *KHDC3L* and demonstrating mutations in either gene. While mutations will be identified in almost all cases, occasional women have been described in which no mutations were found in either gene.[53,55,60] These individuals may have mutations in regulatory elements or intragenic duplications, not detected by conventional sequencing. However, it is tempting to speculate that there might be additional genes associated with FRHM. Identifying mutations in individuals with FRHM not only confirms a diagnosis but enables counseling and screening of other family members to determine affected or carrier status **(Fig. 5)**. This is particularly important for nulliparous women in affected families who are considering pregnancy.

Familial Recurrent Hydatidiform Moles are Associated with Abnormal Genomic Imprinting

For a small number of genes, only the copy of the gene inherited from the mother or the copy inherited from the father is transcriptionally active while the second allele remains silent or "imprinted".[71] In both typical AnCHM and PHM, the presence of two paternal chromosome complements is likely to give rise to overexpression of paternally expressed genes and the trophoblastic proliferation of the placenta seen in both. The presence of embryonic development in PHM, virtually absent in CHM, is thought to be due to the additional presence of maternally transcribed genes in PHM.

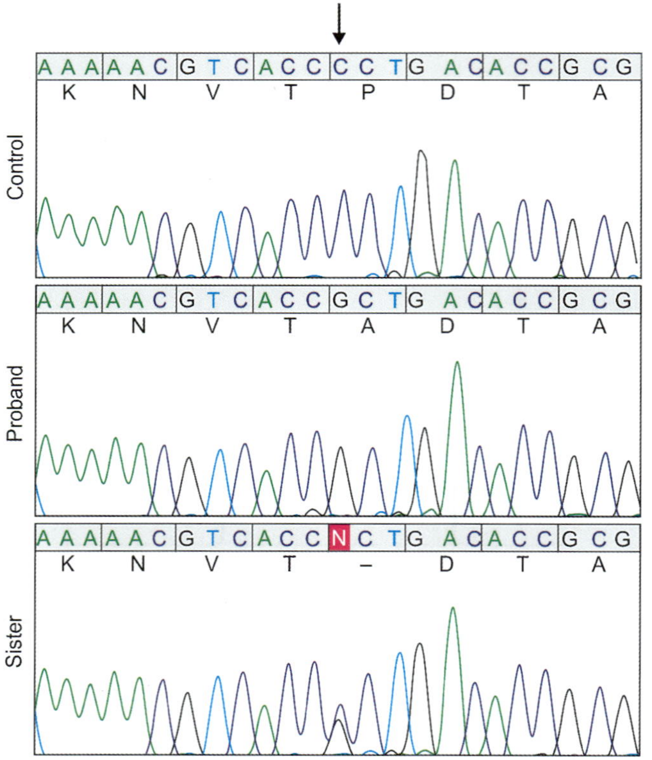

Fig. 5: Partial sequence of exon 6 of *NLRP7* in a patient with familial recurrent hydatidiform mole (FRHM) and her nulliparous sister. While the patient is homozygous for a C to G base change (c.2146C>G; p.P716A) (arrowed), her sister is heterozygous for the base change indicating that she is a carrier who would be expected to have normal reproductive outcomes.

Since the pathology of BiCHM parallels that of AnCHM, dysregulation of genomic imprinting is likely to be the underlying defect in FRHM. Abnormal expression of imprinted genes has now been confirmed in both AnCHM and BiCHM. At the protein level $p57^{KIP2}$, the product of the maternally transcribed, paternally imprinted, cyclin-dependent kinase inhibitor *CDKN1C,* absent from the cytotrophoblast and villous mesenchyme of AnCHM, is also absent from these cells in BiCHM from women with FRHM **(Figs. 6A to C).**[45] Imprinted genes are typically marked by differentially methylated regions, dependent on the parent of origin.[72] Several studies have now shown a number of maternally imprinted genes in BiCHM from women with *NLRP7*[51,73,74] or *KHDC3L* mutations[75] to have a paternal methylation pattern similar to that of AnCHM.

Functions of *NLRP7/KHDC3L*

NLRP7 is a maternal effect gene in that the products of the maternal gene are needed for early embryonic development. Its product, *NLRP7,* is a member of the NACHT, leucine-rich repeat, and PYD containing (NLRP) protein family, a family of proteins implicated in the activation of proinflammatory caspases through multiprotein complexes called inflammasomes.[76] *NLRP7* itself has been reported to act as a feedback regulator of caspase-1-dependent interleukin-1-beta secretion and effect cytokine production[77,78] and it has been suggested that women with defective *NLRP7* might, therefore,

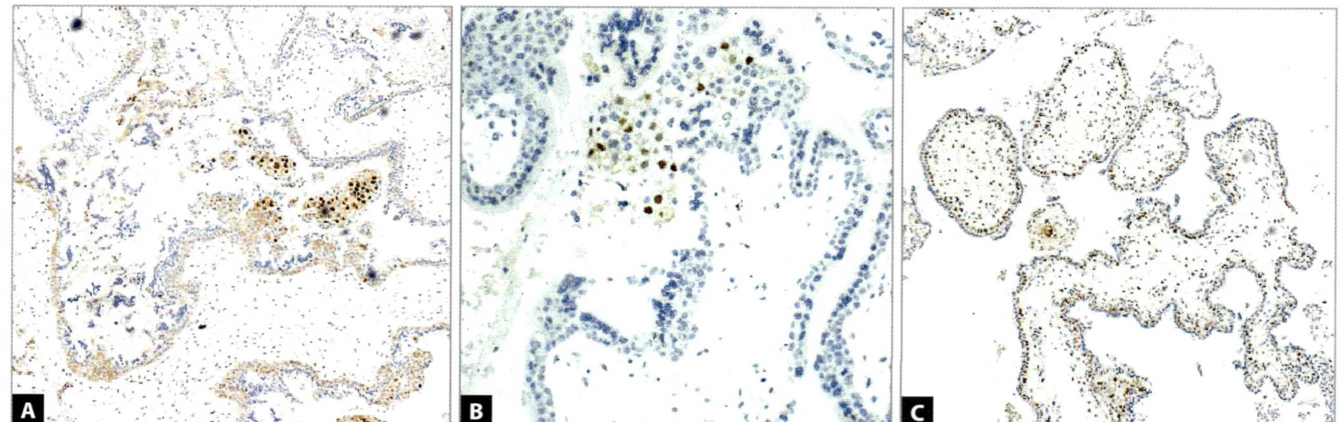

Figs. 6A to C: Photomicrographs demonstrating an absence of $p57^{KIP2}$ immunostaining in the villus cytotrophoblast and stroma of an AnCHM (A) and a BiCHM (B). While a typical triploid PHM demonstrates extensive positive nuclear staining of both villous cytotrophoblast and stroma (C). Positively staining nonvillus trophoblast acts as a control, in both cases of CHM. (Original magnifications A, 100×; B, 100×; and C, 40×). (AnCHM: androgenetic complete hydatidiform mole; BiCHM: biparental complete hydatidiform mole; PHM: partial hydatidiform mole)

fail to mount an appropriate immune response during pregnancy.[79]

A different role for *NLRP7*, that of establishing or maintaining the maternal imprint, is suggested by the similar aberrant expression of imprinted genes observed in BiCHM and AnCHM and the demonstration that *NLRP7* is expressed in human oocytes and preimplantation embryos.[53,80] In both males and females, methylation marks are removed in the primordial germ cells and reestablished during gametogenesis. Following fertilization, a wave of demethylation takes place but does not include imprinted genes that retain allele-specific methylation enabling normal embryonic development.[81] Lack of methylation at maternally methylated regions in BiCHM, without the gain of methylation at paternally methylated regions seen in AnCHM, with two paternal genomes, suggests that *NLRP7* is important for acquisition or maintenance of the maternal imprint. Further evidence that *NLRP7* is important in enabling correct maternal imprinting and normal embryonic development comes from the demonstration that donation of an ovum from an unaffected donor resulted in a normal full-term delivery in a patient with FRHM.[82]

KHDC3L, the second maternal effect gene associated with FRHM, is an established member of the maternal subcortical maternal complex (SCMC), made up of at least four proteins encoded by maternal effect genes and essential for zygote development.[83] Since *NLRP7* and *KHDC3L* have been shown to colocalize to the oocyte cytoskeleton,[84] *NLRP7* may also be a member of the SCMC.[85] However, it remains to be established how the SCMC, with an essentially cytoplasmic location, plays a role in methylation of the nuclear genome.

Clinical Significance of Recurrent Hydatidiform Moles

Women who have a HM are concerned that they may experience another HM in subsequent pregnancies, and that, if the molar tissue does not resolve spontaneously following evacuation, they might need chemotherapy for gestational trophoblastic neoplasia (GTN). While women with PHM may experience a second HM, this is rare and may occur in any subsequent pregnancy.[5] However, women with a CHM have approximately 1% chance of another CHM in the next pregnancy with 20% of these women experiencing a third CHM. It is observed that 40% of women who go on to have a third CHM will have AnCHM. While these women may have intervening normal pregnancies and could potentially go on and have future normal pregnancies, they may wish to avoid the risk of another CHM by undergoing *in vitro* fertilization (IVF) with preimplantation genetic diagnosis (PGD) to exclude AnCHM.[86]

More than 80% of women with two CHMs go on to have normal pregnancies, genotyping to exclude FHRM, is recommended after three CHMs. However, it might be considered after two consecutive CHMs in a woman with no normal pregnancies as the chance of having FRHM for these women is 25%.[5] While the possibility of a normal pregnancy cannot be entirely excluded in women with FRHM, these rare pregnancies may be restricted to women with missense mutations in *NLRP7* or *KHDC3L* rather than the more severe truncating mutations[48] (unpublished observations). Different types of mutations may also account for the different reproductive outcomes in women with FRHM, some individuals experiencing only CHM while others may also experience miscarriages and occasional stillbirths.[87] A history of other pregnancies in addition to RHM should not exclude a diagnosis of FRHM.

Conventional IVF is not an option for women with FRHM since PGD would be unable to differentiate between a normal diploid conception and a chromosomally normal conception that was going to develop as a BiCHM. For women with FRHM, normal pregnancy can be achieved by using a donor ovum.[81] To date, at least seven successful pregnancies with ovum donation have been achieved[48] (unpublished observations) confirming the success of this approach.

Having established a diagnosis of FRHM, sequencing of *NLRP7* and *KHDC3L* in women with RHM may also be useful in establishing a diagnosis in cases where tissue from the molar pregnancy is not available, with the caveat that mutations have not been identified in all cases of FRHM and absence of mutations in these genes does not exclude a diagnosis of FRHM. Establishing the mutation(s) involved is also important for counseling other family members.

All women should be screened, using serial serum human chorionic gonadotropin measurements, following a molar pregnancy to identify the development of GTN.[88] The incidence of GTN is very much higher after CHM than any other type of pregnancy and in the UK approximately 13.6% of women with CHM require subsequent chemotherapy for GTN,[33,34] that following a molar pregnancy is usually invasive mole. Despite the different ways in which they arise, the incidence of GTN following BiCHM is similar to that of AnCHM.[5] Women with FRHM are, therefore, at a high risk of GTN due to the number of molar pregnancies they experience making it important that these women are identified as early as possible. The management of GTN has been updated and summarized by the Society of Obstetricians and Gynecologists of Canada (SOGC).[89]

CONCLUSION

Familial recurrent hydatidiform mole is a rare autosomal recessive condition characterized by CHM of biparental, rather than androgenetic, origin. It is important to recognize this condition both for the women themselves and for their families. Affected individuals are unlikely to achieve a normal pregnancy naturally and with each molar pregnancy there is a risk of developing persistent disease requiring chemotherapy. Two genes, *NLRP7* and *KHDC3L*, are known to be associated with this condition both showing a variety of different mutations in affected individuals. Identification of these mutations then enables screening and counseling of other family members. However, not all women with recurrent CHM have FRHM. A minority have recurrent CHM of typical androgenetic origin and may benefit from conventional IVF with PGD. However, for women with mutations in *NLRP7* or *KHDC3L*, who consequently display aberrant imprinting within the ovum, IVF with a donor ovum may be the only way to achieve a successful pregnancy. This distinction between FRHM and RHM of androgenetic origin can be made by genotyping villous tissue from the molar pregnancies and showing whether they are androgenetic or diploid with a maternal contribution to the genome.

ACKNOWLEDGMENT

The authors gratefully acknowledge infrastructure support from the Cancer Research UK Imperial Centre, the Imperial Experimental Cancer Medicine Centre, and the National Institute for Health Research Imperial Biomedical Research Centre.

REFERENCES

1. Bagshawe KD, Dent J, Webb J. Hydatidiform mole in England and Wales 1973-83. Lancet. 1986;2:673-7.
2. Lorigan PC, Sharma S, Bright N, Coleman RE, Hancock BW. Characteristics of women with recurrent molar pregnancies. Gynecol Oncol. 2000;78:288-92.
3. Matsui H, Iitsuka Y, Suzuka K, Seki K, Sekiya S. Subsequent pregnancy outcome in patients with spontaneous resolution of HCG after evacuation of hydatidiform mole: comparison between complete and partial mole. Hum Reprod. 2001;16:1274-7.
4. Sebire NJ, Fisher RA, Foskett M, Rees H, Seckl MJ, Newlands ES. Risk of recurrent hydatidiform mole and subsequent pregnancy outcome following complete or partial hydatidiform molar pregnancy. BJOG. 2003;110:22-6.
5. Eagles N, Sebire NJ, Short D, Savage PM, Seckl MJ, Fisher RA. Risk of recurrent molar pregnancies following complete and partial hydatidiform moles. Hum Reprod. 2015;30:2055-63.
6. Szulman AE, Surti U. The syndromes of hydatidiform mole. I. Cytogenetic and morphological correlations. Am J Obstet Gynecol. 1978;131:665-71.
7. Szulman AE, Surti U. The syndromes of hydatidiform mole. II. Morphologic evolution of the complete and partial mole. Am J Obstet Gynecol. 1978;132:20-7.
8. Sebire NJ, Fisher RA, Rees HC. Histopathological diagnosis of partial and complete hydatidiform mole in the first trimester of pregnancy. Pediatr Dev Pathol. 2003;6:69-77.
9. Paradinas FJ, Browne P, Fisher RA, Foskett M, Bagshawe KD, Newlands E. A clinical, histopathological and flow cytometric study of 149 complete moles, 146 partial moles and 107 non-molar hydropic abortions. Histopathology. 1996;28:101-10.
10. Castrillon DH, Sun D, Weremowicz S, Fisher RA, Crum CP, Genest DR. Discrimination of complete hydatidiform mole from its mimics by immunohistochemistry of the paternally imprinted gene product p57KIP2. Am J Surg Pathol. 2001;25:1225-30.
11. Fisher RA, Tommasi A, Short D, Kaur B, Seckl MJ, Sebire NJ. Clinical utility of selective molecular genotyping for diagnosis of partial hydatidiform mole; retrospective study from a regional trophoblastic disease unit. J Clin Pathol. 2014;67:980-4.
12. Hui P, Buza N, Murphy KM, Ronnett BM. Hydatidiform moles: genetic basis and precision diagnosis. Annu Rev Pathol. 2017;12:449-85.
13. Paradinas FJ, Fisher RA, Browne P, Newlands ES. Diploid hydatidiform moles with fetal red blood cells in molar villi. 1—Pathology, incidence, and prognosis. J Pathol. 1997;181:183-8.
14. Sebire NJ, Rees H, Paradinas F, Fisher R, Foskett M, Seckl M, et al. Extravillus endovascular implantation site trophoblast invasion is abnormal in complete versus partial molar pregnancies. Placenta. 2001;22:725-8.
15. Sebire NJ, Savage PM, Seckl MJ, Fisher RA. Histopathological features of biparental complete hydatidiform moles in women with NLRP7 mutations. Placenta. 2013;34:50-6.
16. Lawler SD, Fisher RA, Pickthall VJ, Povey S, Evans MW. Genetic studies on hydatidiform moles. I. The origin of partial moles. Cancer Genet Cytogenet. 1982;5:309-20.

17. Jacobs PA, Szulman AE, Funkhouser J, Matsuura JS, Wilson CC. Human triploidy: relationship between parental origin of the additional haploid complement and development of partial hydatidiform mole. Ann Hum Genet. 1982;46: 223-31.
18. Lawler SD, Fisher RA, Dent J. A prospective study of hydatidiform mole. Am J Obstet Gynecol. 1991;164:1270-7.
19. Zaragoza MV, Surti U, Redline RW, Millie E, Chakravarti A, Hassold TJ. Parental origin and phenotype of triploidy in spontaneous abortions: predominance of diandry and association with the partial hydatidiform mole. Am J Hum Genet. 2000;66:1807-20.
20. Savage P, Sebire N, Dalton T, Carby A, Seckl MJ, Fisher RA. Partial molar pregnancy after intracytoplasmic sperm injection occurring as a result of diploid sperm usage. J Assist Reprod Genet. 2013;30:761-4.
21. Kajii, T, Ohama K. Androgenetic origin of hydatidiform mole. Nature. 1977;268:633-4.
22. Wake N, Takagi N, Sasaki M. Androgenesis as a cause of hydatidiform mole. J Natl Cancer Inst. 1978;60:51-7.
23. Lawler SD, Pickthall VJ, Fisher RA, Povey S, Evans MW, Szulman AE. Genetic studies of complete and partial hydatidiform moles. Lancet. 1979;2(8142):580. doi: 10.1016/s0140-6736(79)91632-5. PMID: 89576.
24. Jacobs PA, Wilson CM, Sprenkle JA, Rosenshein NB, Migeon BR. Mechanism of origin of complete hydatidiform moles. Nature. 1980;286:714-6.
25. Lawler SD, Povey S, Fisher RA, Pickthall VJ. Genetic studies on hydatidiform moles. II. The origin of complete moles. Ann Hum Genet. 1982;46:209-22.
26. Jacobs PA, Hunt PA, Matsuura JS, Wilson CC, Szulman AE. Complete and hydatidiform mole in Hawaii: cytogenetics, morphology and epidemiology. Br J Obstet Gynaecol. 1982;89:258-66.
27. Ohama K, Kajii T, Okamoto E, Fukuda Y, Imaizumi K, Tsukahara M, et al. Dispermic origin of XY hydatidiform moles. Nature. 1981;29:551-2.
28. Fisher RA, Povey S, Jeffreys AJ, Martin CA, Patel I, Lawler SD. Frequency of heterozygous complete hydatidiform moles, estimated by locus-specific minisatellite and Y chromosome-specific probes. Hum Genet. 1989;8:259-63.
29. Kovaks BW, Shahbahrami B, Tast DE, Curtin JP. Molecular genetic analysis of complete hydatidiform moles. Cancer Genet Cytogenet. 1991;54:143-52.
30. Golubovsky MD. Postzygotic diploidization of triploids as a source of unusual cases of mosaicism, chimerism and twinning. Hum Reprod. 2003;8:36-42.
31. Wallace DC, Surti U, Adams CW, Szulman AE. Complete moles have paternal chromosomes but maternal mitochondrial DNA. Hum Genet. 1982;61:145-7.
32. Edwards YH, Jeremiah SJ, McMillan SL, Povey S, Fisher RA, Lawler SD. Complete hydatidiform moles combine maternal mitochondria with a paternal nuclear genome. Ann Hum Genet. 1984;48:119-27.
33. Steigrad SJ. Epidemiology of gestational trophoblastic diseases. Best Pract Res Clin Obstet Gynaecol. 2003;17:837-47.
34. Savage PM, Sita-Lumsden A, Dickson S, Iyer R, Everard J, Coleman R, et al. The relationship of maternal age to molar pregnancy incidence, risks for chemotherapy and subsequent pregnancy outcome. J Obstet Gynaecol. 2013;33:406-11.
35. Tham BW, Everard JE, Tidy JA, Drew D, Hancock BW. Gestational trophoblastic disease in the Asian population of Northern England and North Wales. BJOG. 2003;110:555-9.
36. Ambani LM, Vaidya RA, Rao CS, Daftary SD, Motashaw ND. Familial occurrence of trophoblastic disease—report of recurrent molar pregnancies in sisters in three families. Clin Genet. 1980;18:27-9.
37. Parazzini F, La Vecchia C, Franceschi S, Mangili G. Familial trophoblastic disease: case report. Am J Obstet Gynecol. 1984;149:382-3.
38. Kircheisen R, Ried T. Hydatidiform moles. Hum Reprod. 1994;9:1783-5.
39. Seoud M, Khalil A, Frangieh A, Zahed L, Azar G, Nuwayri-Salti N. Recurrent molar pregnancies in a family with extensive intermarriage: report of a family and review of the literature. Obstet Gynecol. 1995;86:692-5.
40. Hodges MD, Rees HC, Seckl MJ, Newlands ES, Fisher RA. Genetic refinement and physical mapping of a biparental complete hydatidiform mole locus on chromosome 19q13.4. J Med Genet. 2003;40:e95.
41. Helwani MN, Seoud M, Zahed L, Zaatari G, Khalil A, Slim R. A familial case of recurrent hydatidiform molar pregnancies with biparental genomic contribution. Hum Genet. 1999;105:112-5.
42. Sensi A, Gualandi F, Pittalis MC, Calabrese O, Falciano F, Maestri I, et al. Mole maker phenotype: possible narrowing of the candidate region. Eur J Hum Genet. 2000;8:641-4.
43. Fisher RA, Hodges MD, Newlands ES. Familial recurrent hydatidiform mole: a review. J Reprod Med. 2004;49:595-601.
44. Fisher RA, Khatoon R, Paradinas FJ, Roberts AP, Newlands ES. Repetitive complete hydatidiform mole can be biparental in origin and either male or female. Hum Reprod. 2000;15:594-8.
45. Fisher RA, Hodges MD, Rees HC, Sebire NJ, Seckl MJ, Newlands ES, et al. The maternally transcribed gene p57(KIP2) (CDNK1C) is abnormally expressed in both androgenetic and biparental complete hydatidiform moles. Hum Mol Genet. 2002;11:3267-72.
46. van der Smagt JJ, Scheenjes E, Kremer JA, Hennekam FA, Fisher RA. Heterogeneity in the origin of recurrent complete hydatidiform moles: not all women with multiple molar pregnancies have biparental moles. BJOG. 2006;113:725-8.
47. Nguyen NM, Slim R. Genetics and epigenetics of recurrent hydatidiform moles: basic science and genetic counselling. Curr Obstet Gynecol Rep. 2014;3:55-64.

48. Akoury E, Gupta N, Bagga R, Brown S, Déry C, Kabra M, et al. Live births in women with recurrent hydatidiform mole and two NLRP7 mutations. Reprod Biomed Online. 2015;31:120-4.
49. Sunde L, Vejerslev LO, Jensen MP, Pedersen S, Hertz JM, Bolund L. Genetic analysis of repeated, biparental, diploid, hydatidiform moles. Cancer Genet Cytogenet. 1993;66:16-22.
50. Murdoch S, Djuric U, Mazhar B, Seoud M, Khan R, Kuick R, et al. Mutations in NALP7 cause recurrent hydatidiform moles and reproductive wastage in humans. Nat Genet. 2006;38:300-2.
51. Kou YC, Shao L, Peng HH, Rosetta R, del Gaudio D, Wagner AF, et al. A recurrent intragenic genomic duplication, other novel mutations in NLRP7 and imprinting defects in recurrent biparental hydatidiform moles. Mol Hum Reprod. 2008;14:33-40.
52. Milhavet F, Cuisset L, Hoffman HM, Slim R, El-Shanti H, Aksentijevich I, et al. The infevers autoinflammatory mutation online registry: update with new genes and functions. Hum Mutat. 2008;29:803-8.
53. Wang CM, Dixon PH, Decordova S, Hodges MD, Sebire NJ, Ozalp S, et al. Identification of 13 novel NLRP7 mutations in 20 families with recurrent hydatidiform mole; missense mutations cluster in the leucine-rich region. J Med Genet. 2009;46:569-75.
54. Hayward BE, De Vos M, Talati N, Abdollahi MR, Taylor GR, Meyer E, et al. Genetic and epigenetic analysis of recurrent hydatidiform mole. Hum Mutat. 2009;30:E629-39.
55. Dixon PH, Trongwongsa P, Abu-Hayyah S, Ng SH, Akbar SA, Khawaja NP, et al. Mutations in NLRP7 are associated with diploid biparental hydatidiform moles, but not androgenetic complete moles. J Med Genet. 2012;49:206-11.
56. Reddy R, Nguyen NM, Sarrabay G, Rezaei M, Rivas MC, Kavasoglu A, et al. The genomic architecture of *NLRP7* is Alu rich and predisposes to disease-associated large deletions. Eur J Hum Genet. 2016;24:1445-52.
57. Buyukkurt S, Fisher RA, Vardar MA, Evruke C. Heterogeneity in recurrent complete hydatidiform mole: presentation of two new Turkish families with different genetic characteristics. Placenta. 2010;31:1023-5.
58. Hemida R, van Doorn H, Fisher R. A novel genetic mutation in a patient with recurrent biparental complete hydatidiform mole: a brief report. Int J Gynecol Cancer. 2016;26:1351-3.
59. Landolsi H, Rittore C, Philibert L, Missaoui N, Hmissa S, Touitou I, et al. Screening for NLRP7 mutations in familial and sporadic recurrent hydatidiform moles: report of 2 Tunisian families. Int J Gynecol Pathol. 2011;30:348-53.
60. Parry DA, Logan CV, Hayward BE, Shires M, Landolsi H, Diggle C, et al. Mutations causing familial biparental hydatidiform mole implicate c6orf221 as a possible regulator of genomic imprinting in the human oocyte. Am J Hum Genet. 2011;89:451-8.
61. Reddy R, Akoury E, Phuong Nguyen NM, Abdul-Rahman OA, Dery C, Gupta N, et al. Report of four new patients with protein-truncating mutations in C6orf221/KHDC3L and colocalization with NLRP7. Eur J Hum Genet. 2013;21:957-64.
62. Rezaei M, Nguyen NM, Foroughinia L, Dash P, Ahmadpour F, Verma IC, et al. Two novel mutations in the KHDC3L gene in Asian patients with recurrent hydatidiform mole. Hum Genome Var. 2016;3:16027.
63. Florea A, Caba L, Grigore AM, Antoci LM, Grigore M, Gramescu MI, et al. Hydatidiform Mole-Between Chromosomal Abnormality, Uniparental Disomy and Monogenic Variants: A Narrative Review. Life (Basel). 2023;13(12):2314.
64. Manokhina I, Hanna CW, Stephenson MD, McFadden DE, Robinson WP. Maternal NLRP7 and C6orf221 variants are not a common risk factor for androgenetic moles, triploidy and recurrent miscarriage. Mol Hum Reprod. 2013;19:539-44.
65. Andreasen L, Christiansen OB, Niemann I, Bolund L, Sunde L. NLRP7 or KHDC3L genes and the etiology of molar pregnancies and recurrent miscarriage. Mol Hum Reprod. 2013;19:773-81.
66. Mahadevan S, Wen S, Balasa A, Fruhman G, Mateus J, Wagner A, et al. No evidence for mutations in NLRP7 and KHDC3L in women with androgenetic hydatidiform moles. Prenat Diagn. 2013;33:1242-7.
67. Banet N, DeScipio C, Murphy KM, Beierl K, Adams E, Vang R, et al. Characteristics of hydatidiform moles: analysis of a prospective series with p57 immunohistochemistry and molecular genotyping. Mod Pathol. 2014;27:238-54.
68. McFadden DE, Kwong LC, Yam IY, Langlois S. Parental origin of triploidy in human fetuses: evidence for genomic imprinting. Hum Genet. 1993;92:465-9.
69. McFadden DE, Robinson WP. Phenotype of triploid embryos. J Med Genet. 2006;43:609-12.
70. Fallahian M, Sebire NJ, Savage PM, Seckl MJ, Fisher RA. Mutations in NLRP7 and KHDC3L confer a complete hydatidiform mole phenotype on digynic triploid conceptions. Hum Mutat. 2013;34:301-8.
71. Morison IM, Reeve AE. A catalogue of imprinted genes and parent-of-origin effects in humans and animals. Hum Mol Genet. 1998;7:1599-609.
72. Reik W, Walter J. Genomic imprinting: parental influence on the genome. Nat Rev Genet. 2001;2:21-32.
73. El-Maarri O, Seoud M, Coullin P, Herbiniaux U, Oldenburg J, Rouleau G, et al. Maternal alleles acquiring paternal methylation patterns in biparental complete hydatidiform moles. Hum Mol Genet. 2003;12:1405-13.
74. Sanchez-Delgado M, Martin-Trujillo A, Tayama C, Vidal E, Esteller M, Iglesias-Platas I, et al. Absence of maternal methylation in biparental hydatidiform moles from women with NLRP7 maternal-effect mutations reveals widespread placenta-specific imprinting. PLoS Genet. 2015;11:e1005644.

75. Judson H, Hayward BE, Sheridan E, Bonthron DT. A global disorder of imprinting in the human female germ line. Nature. 2002;416:539-42.
76. Martinon F, Gaide O, Pétrilli V, Mayor A, Tschopp J. NALP inflammasomes: a central role in innate immunity. Semin Immunopathol. 2007;29:213-29.
77. Kinoshita T, Wang Y, Hasegawa M, Imamura R, Suda T. PYPAF3, a PYRIN- containing APAF-1-like protein, is a feedback regulator of caspase-1-dependent interleukin-1 beta secretion. J Biol Chem. 2005;280:21720-5.
78. Messaed C, Akoury E, Djuric U, Zeng J, Saleh M, Gilbert L, et al. NLRP7, a nucleotide oligomerization domain-like receptor protein, is required for normal cytokine secretion and co-localizes with Golgi and the microtubule-organizing center. J Biol Chem. 2011;286: 43313-23.
79. Slim R, Wallace EP. NLRP7 and the genetics of hydatidiform moles: recent advances and new challenges. Front Immunol. 2013;4:242.
80. Zhang P, Dixon M, Zucchelli M, Hambiliki F, Levkov L, Hovatta O, et al. Expression analysis of the NLRP gene family suggests a role in human preimplantation development. PLoS One. 2008;3:e2755.
81. Smallwood SA, Kelsey G. De novo DNA methylation: a germ cell perspective. Trends Genet. 2012;28:33-42.
82. Fisher RA, Lavery SA, Carby A, Abu-Hayyeh S, Swingler R, Sebire NJ, et al. What a difference an egg makes. Lancet. 2011;378:1974.
83. Bebbere D, Masala L, Albertini DF, Ledda S. The subcortical maternal complex: multiple functions for one biological structure? J Assist Reprod Genet. 2016;33:1431-8.
84. Akoury E, Zhang L, Ao A, Slim R. NLRP7 and KHDC3L, the two maternal-effect proteins responsible for recurrent hydatidiform moles, co-localize to the oocyte cytoskeleton. Hum Reprod. 2015;30:159-69.
85. Monk D, Sanchez-Delgado M, Fisher RA. NLRPs, the subcortical maternal complex and genomic imprinting. Reproduction. 2017;154:R161-70.
86. Ogilvie CM, Renwick PJ, Khalaf Y, Braude PR. First use of preimplantation genotyping in prevention of recurrent diandric complete hydatidiform mole. Reprod Biomed Online. 2009;19:224-7.
87. Nguyen NM, Zhang L, Reddy R, Déry C, Arseneau J, Cheung A, et al. Comprehensive genotype-phenotype correlations between NLRP7 mutations and the balance between embryonic tissue differentiation and trophoblastic proliferation. J Med Genet. 2014;51:623-34.
88. Seckl MJ, Sebire NJ, Fisher RA, Golfier F, Massuger L, Sessa C, et al. Gestational trophoblastic disease: ESMO Clinical Practice Guidelines for diagnosis, treatment and follow-up. Ann Oncol. 2013;24:vi39-50.
89. Eiriksson L, Dean E, Sebastianelli A, Salvador S, Comeau R, Jang JH, et al. Guideline No. 408: Management of Gestational Trophoblastic Diseases. J Obstet Gynaecol Can. 2021;43(1):91-105.e1.

CHAPTER 40

Recurrent Ectopic Pregnancy

Latha Venkatram, Srimathy Raman

ABSTRACT

Ectopic pregnancy happens in approximately 11 in 1,000 pregnancies and is a potentially life-threatening condition. Recurrent ectopic pregnancy (REP) can happen in 11–27% of patients and presents dilemmas in diagnosis and management. Recurrence rates depend on the cause of the primary ectopic pregnancy and its management. Prior infection and surgery are the most important factors that influence the recurrence rates. Knowledge of the etiology behind the primary ectopic pregnancy helps the physician in counseling the patients about recurrence rates.

Keywords: Ectopic pregnancy, Recurrent ectopic pregnancy, Risk factors, Tubal surgery, Management of ectopic pregnancy.

INTRODUCTION

Ectopic pregnancy occurs when implantation of the pregnancy happens outside the endometrial cavity.[1] This happens roughly in about 11 in 1,000 pregnancies.[2] The most common site of an ectopic pregnancy is the fallopian tube, and it accounts for 96% of all ectopic pregnancies. It is important to diagnose and manage ectopic pregnancies appropriately as they can be associated with sudden, severe hemorrhage which can cause significant morbidity and mortality. There are various risk factors which increase the chances of a primary ectopic pregnancy. The physical and psychological morbidity associated with ectopic pregnancy can be substantial especially if it is diagnosed late and this impact is greater if there is a recurrence. Recent evidence points out that women who have suffered ectopic pregnancies are at increased risk of adverse pregnancy outcomes in the subsequent intrauterine pregnancy as well. This could be because of additional risk factors like advanced age, use of ART, presence of endometriosis, etc. It is important to understand the factors that increase the occurrence of a recurrent ectopic pregnancy (REP) as this will influence the treatment options.

CASE SCENARIOS

We present few case scenarios to highlight the dilemmas in deciding the optimal treatment.

- Primary ectopic pregnancy in the left tube treated with expectant management and subsequent ectopic on the same side
- Primary ectopic pregnancy in the left tube treated with methotrexate and subsequent ectopic on the same side
- Primary ectopic pregnancy in the right tube treated with salpingotomy and subsequent ectopic on the same side
- Primary ectopic in the left tube, treated with salpingotomy, recurrence on the same side and right tube noted to have peritubal adhesions during laparoscopy
- Primary ectopic pregnancy in the left tube treated with salpingectomy and now recurrence on the right side
- Primary ectopic pregnancy in the left tube treated with methotrexate and subsequent ectopic in the right side treated with methotrexate and now recurrence again
- Failed medical treatment for left tubal primary ectopic and salpingectomy performed. Right tubal ectopic gestation subsequently
- Left salpingectomy for primary ectopic, 2nd ectopic on the right. Salpingotomy performed. Now repeat ectopic on the right side. Patient keen on conserving the right tube
- Left salpingectomy for primary ectopic, 2nd ectopic on the right. Salpingotomy performed. Now stump ectopic on the left side

PRIMARY ECTOPIC PREGNANCY

1–2% of all pregnancies can be an ectopic pregnancy. It can happen in any pregnant woman with or without identified risk factors. Specific risk factors include damage to fallopian tubes—postinfection/surgery, smoking, infertility, lower annual income, lack of contraceptive use, in vitro fertilization (IVF) conception, etc.[3] Damage to fallopian tubes can be manifested as adhesions, fimbrial agglutination, beading, etc. However, both sexually transmitted infections (STIs) and their impact on tubes can be occult without any obvious abnormalities. There are also other risk factors identified like in utero exposure to diethylstilbestrol (DES), use of intrauterine contraceptive device (IUCD), history of infertility, alcohol use, and use of oral contraceptive pills (OCPs).

RECURRENT ECTOPIC PREGNANCY

The major risk factor for an REP is the occurrence of the first ectopic pregnancy. As infertility is a main risk factor of ectopic pregnancy, this will impact the subsequent ectopic and intrauterine pregnancy rates. The quoted chance of a successful intrauterine pregnancy following an ectopic pregnancy is 38–89%.[2] The quoted chances of REP are variable with reported 10–27% recurrence rates.[4,5] Studies have also found that the chances of a third ectopic could be as high as 40%.[6] 35 and 58% of patients after two and three ectopic pregnancies respectively remained infertile. Many women after REP may not choose to conceive and hence these figures may be lower than the actual incidences.

There is no major randomized controlled trial on the causes and management of REP. Some of the risk factors like pelvic infections and tubal surgeries increase the risk of recurrence.[7] It is important to remember the recurrence risks whenever we counsel and manage women with any ectopic pregnancy. The question of whether recurrence risk can be mitigated is still debatable. The interventions performed at the time of first ectopic pregnancy can influence the recurrence rates. Hence, for secondary prevention of a recurrence, it is important to understand what the modifiable risk factors are.

Etiology of Recurrent Ectopic Pregnancy

The exact etiology of REP largely remains unknown. The most consistent risk factors for REP were prior pelvic surgery and pelvic pathology such as tubal adhesions, fimbrial agglutination or tubal damage with evidence of hydrosalpinx recognized at the time of surgery for the primary ectopic pregnancy.[7] This is because generally tubal damage due to infection tends to be bilateral and so even if they have had a salpingectomy, recurrences can happen in the other tube. There are some studies suggesting that pre-existing tubal damage as in pelvic inflammatory disease (PID) could be severe enough to prevents any future pregnancies and hence the recurrences.

It has been noted that women with REP are more likely to be elderly and have had previous miscarriages and surgeries like evacuation of retained products of conception (ERPC). Other risk factors noted have been the presence of psychiatric illness and lower education level.[8] An interim successful intrauterine pregnancy and delivery seems to be protective against the development of an REP.[9]

It is still not clear how the recurrences will be affected if the previous ectopic was in association with specific risk factors like the presence of IUCD and/or conception after IVF or with no previous tubal factors. If the primary ectopic pregnancy was in a woman with an IUCD in situ, it has been noted that her chances of recurrent ectopic were lowered by almost a third.[7]

Recurrence and Interpregnancy Interval

There is no strong evidence on the time interval needed before women can conceive after an ectopic pregnancy and its effect on recurrences. However, if women have been treated with methotrexate, then the recommended interval before conception is 3 months, because of the effect of medication on fetal structural development.[2]

Impact of Previous Management Methods

Ectopic pregnancy can be managed by:

- Conservative management
- Medical treatment with methotrexate
- Surgical treatment in the form of salpingotomy or salpingectomy[2]

An important point to reflect on is whether the recurrence is determined by the management of the first ectopic pregnancy. The quoted recurrence rates for the different management strategies are variable. However, it has been noted that having a prior expectant management, laparotomy and salpingotomy are associated with higher recurrence rates.

Surgical management: Most tubal ectopic pregnancies are managed surgically—either laparoscopically or by laparotomy. There is no strong evidence that either option has any difference on the outcome of subsequent pregnancy, though some studies have found better outcomes after laparoscopy.[10,11] The surgical techniques in the management of ectopic pregnancy include either salpingotomy or salpingectomy. As discussed earlier, as abnormalities of the fallopian tubes are generally bilateral, even salpingectomy can be associated with REP in the other tube.

Intrauterine pregnancy rates after salpingotomy have been noted to be slightly higher 60.7% versus 56.2% after salpingectomy.[2] However, recurrence also has been noted to be slightly higher in the salpingotomy group (8% vs. 5%). Hence, the recommendation is that women should be offered salpingectomy, if the contralateral tube is healthy, as salpingotomy is not associated with significantly better fertility outcomes. However, if there are concerns about the presence of contralateral tube damage, salpingotomy is preferred over salpingectomy as this might lead to higher intrauterine pregnancy rates.[2]

Medical management: Medical management with systemic methotrexate is a successful management option for select ectopic pregnancies and can be considered if they fulfil the criteria for the same. Successful medical treatment with methotrexate seems to be associated with decreased chances, and even protects against recurrences.[12] Hence, secondary prevention of recurrence is possible by appropriate medical management of primary ectopic pregnancy. The impact of the methotrexate dose on recurrence is not clear. It has been noted that the need for a second dose of methotrexate can increase the chance of recurrences. Also, failure of primary medical management followed by subsequent surgery was associated with higher recurrence rates than administering a repeat dose.

Expectant management: Expectant management can be offered to carefully selected cases of ectopic pregnancy. It is a less invasive option and some studies have noted that it is associated with better future fertility outcomes and a shorter time to the next pregnancy.[13] However, expectant management for recurrences is not favored as evidence points to a possible halving of the recurrence rates with surgical management and a twofold to threefold increased risk of recurrence when expectant management is done for the second time, especially when the first two were in the same tube.

Comparison of the methods: There have been several studies that have compared the different methods of management and no statistical differences have been noted on the recurrent ectopic rates. There also have been no notable differences in the tubal patency rates when the tubes have been checked with hysterosalpingography of the ipsilateral or the contralateral tube.

The best approach of the first ectopic pregnancy should be tailored to the specific circumstances of the patient but it is important to remember that this may impact the future fertility and recurrence rates. But currently, there is no clear evidence on the best form of management with regards to these factors as the management is dependent on different aspects like the size of the mass, beta-hCG values, symptoms, and patient preferences.[12,13]

Diagnosis

Symptoms and diagnosis of REP are generally like primary ectopic pregnancy. However, studies have shown that women with REP may have lower chances of presenting with vaginal bleeding.[7] It is important to maintain a high degree of suspicion to enable early diagnosis and management of REP. It is also important that patients are counseled of this and asked to report early in their next pregnancy for an early viability scan as well as to seek care early if they develop any symptoms of ectopic pregnancy. Serial measurements of beta-hCG values in early pregnancy may not give a reliable clue to the location of the pregnancy and should be combined with transvaginal scan.

Management of Recurrent Ectopic Pregnancy

The general principles of management are like the management of the first ectopic pregnancy. But as discussed earlier, if the recurrence is in the same tube, caution must be exercised if a repeat expectant management is planned as it is associated with a higher recurrence of a third ectopic pregnancy.[14] Few studies have found that the success of medical management (where applicable) especially a single-dose regime was slightly lower in REP.[15] A multiple dose regimen may be needed in REP. The evidence for optimal management, medical or surgical, to reduce the chances of third ectopic is limited.

Before performing surgical management of REP, counseling and consent should be done regards the need for possible salpingectomy/clipping of the contralateral tube if there is obvious tubal damage and the need for subsequent IVF.

RARE RECURRENCES

Stump Ectopic Pregnancy

Ectopic pregnancy in the tubal stump after salpingectomy is rare and accounts for 0.4–1.2% of ectopic pregnancies.[16,17]

Salpingectomy as a treatment for primary ectopic pregnancy usually obviates recurrences on the ipsilateral side. However, recurrences have been noted on the stump after both partial and total salpingectomy. The exact mechanism for this recurrence is not clear though there are different explanations proposed. Spermatozoa could be passing through the patent tube on the other side and then fertilizing the ovum on the remnant stump or the fertilized ovum from the normal tube via intrauterine migration could implant on the stump. There is also a possibility that the remnant stump could recanalize and establish a connection between the uterus and peritoneal cavity. Hence, to prevent recurrences after a salpingectomy, it is important not to leave any remnant portion of the tube.

Rarer Forms of REP in Nontubal Locations—Cornual Recurrences

Cornual pregnancy is when the implantation happens in a congenitally abnormal uterus and interstitial pregnancy occurs when the implantation happens in the interstitial part of the fallopian tube. However, the terms cornual pregnancy and interstitial pregnancy have been used synonymously by various authors.[2] Primary ectopic pregnancy in these locations is rare but recurrences of interstitial pregnancy have also been reported. The etiology for recurrences is not clear though it is thought to be like recurrent tubal ectopic and possibly to some anatomical abnormality of the utero tubal junction. The preferred management of the recurrence is surgical, with wedge resection and reconstruction of the myometrium. This still can result in rupture in subsequent pregnancies and hence caution must be exercised during the subsequent pregnancy.[18]

Recurrent Cesarean Scar Pregnancy

The incidence of cesarean scar pregnancy (CSP) has been steadily increasing. Recurrent CSP though rare has been reported with varying rates, being quoted in literature. Recurrences have been linked to the size of the niche, the treatment modality of the primary CSP. Available data is sparse, but it is felt that recurrences are more common than previously thought and hence this should be incorporated in the counseling of women with primary CSP, who are keen on future fertility.[19]

Recurrent Ovarian Ectopic Pregnancy

Ovarian ectopic pregnancy is a rare and possibly random event. Subsequent reproductive outcomes have been noted to be favorable with little data on the recurrence rates.[20]

ROLE OF MUC1

MUC1 is a transmembrane glycoprotein that is found in female reproductive organs like the vagina, cervix, endometrium, and tubes. In vitro studies have shown it to prevent early implantation because of its antiadhesive properties. It has been noted with immunohistochemical and monoclonal antibodies that MUC1 is lower in women with ectopic pregnancy. It is proposed that analysis of MUC1 expression in the tubes could be used as a marker in predicting possible recurrence and so in these women, surgical management of salpingectomy could be performed to avoid recurrences. However, further studies are needed to identify such markers that could guide the management of first ectopic pregnancy to prevent recurrences.[21]

The technique of salpingoscopy[22] was developed to visualize intratubal adhesions thereby performing salpingectomy of diseased tubes. However, it has a steep learning curve and is not widely practiced.

CASE SCENARIOS: MANAGEMENT APPROACH

- Primary ectopic pregnancy in the left tube treated with expectant management and subsequent ectopic on the same side.
  Management: Prefer surgical approach—salpingectomy if other tube is normal. May also consider medical management.
- Primary ectopic pregnancy in the left tube treated with methotrexate and subsequent ectopic on the same side.
  Management: Prefer surgical management—salpingectomy
- Primary ectopic pregnancy in the right tube treated with salpingotomy and subsequent ectopic on the same side.
  Management: Recommend surgical management—salpingectomy.
- Primary ectopic in the left tube, treated with salpingotomy, recurrence on the same side and right tube noted to have peritubal adhesions during laparoscopy.
  Management: Consider bilateral salpingectomy with prior consent. If not, recommend ipsilateral salpingectomy.

- Primary ectopic pregnancy in the left tube treated with salpingectomy and now recurrence on the right side.
  Management: Can consider any suitable treatment but counsel regards the possibility of bilateral tubal damage and hence recurrences.
- Primary ectopic pregnancy in the left tube treated with methotrexate and subsequent ectopic in the right side treated with methotrexate and now recurrence again.
  Management: Difficult decision about fertility preservation versus bilateral salpingectomy as possible bilateral tubal damage—needs individualized shared decision-making. Alternatively, consider ipsilateral salpingectomy.
- Failed medical treatment for left tubal primary ectopic and salpingectomy performed. Right tubal ectopic gestation subsequently.
  Management: Can consider medical management; can consider salpingotomy if no obvious peritubal adhesions/pelvic pathology; can also consider salpingectomy if opting for IVF.
- Left salpingectomy for primary ectopic, 2nd ectopic on the right. Salpingotomy performed. Now repeat ectopic on the right side. Patient keen on conserving the right tube.
  Management: Counsel regarding high risk of recurrences in all treatment options apart from salpingectomy; discuss IVF and recommend salpingectomy.
- Left salpingectomy for primary ectopic, 2nd ectopic on the right. Salpingotomy performed. Now stump ectopic on the left side.
  Management: Completion of left salpingectomy and if right tube is obviously damaged, counsel for salpingectomy and IVF.

CONCLUSION

Recurrent ectopic pregnancy can occur in 10–20% of patients who had a previous ectopic pregnancy. There is no consensus opinion on the etiology, prevention, and management of REP. Evidence points to prior pelvic infections and surgery to be strongly associated with the recurrence of ectopic pregnancy. The occurrence of intrauterine pregnancy after an ectopic pregnancy is protective against REP. Management of primary ectopic pregnancy can impact the recurrence rates. Understanding the recurrence rates helps the physician and the patient maintain a high index of suspicion, and helps in early diagnosis, and management. Medical management with methotrexate where possible seems to have advantages in improving pregnancy outcomes and preventing recurrences. Patient preferences for future fertility options are important while considering the management methods. Individualized combined decision making, counseling of different fertility options, and outcomes prior to choosing the treatment methods are important.

REFERENCES

1. American College of Obstetricians and Gynecologists. ACOG practice bulletin: tubal ectopic pregnancy. Obstet Gynecol. 2018;131(3):e91-e103.2.
2. Elson CJ, Salim R, Potdar N, Chetty M, Ross JA, Kirk EJ; Royal College of Obstetricians and Gynaecologists. Diagnosis and management of ectopic pregnancy. BJOG. 2016;123:e15-e55.
3. Tonick S, Conageski C. Ectopic Pregnancy. Obstet Gynecol Clin N Am. 2022;49:537-49.
4. Skjeldestad, Hadgu A, Eriksson N. Epidemiology of repeat ectopic pregnancy: a population-based prospective Cohort Study. Obstet Gynecol. 1998;91(1):129-135.
5. Butts S, Sammel M, Hummel A, Chittams J, Barnhart K. Risk factors and clinical features of recurrent ectopic pregnancy: a case control study. Fertil Steril. 2003;80(6):1340-4.
6. Uotila J, Heinonen PK, Punnonen R. Reproductive outcome after multiple ectopic pregnancies. Int J Fertil. 1989;34(2):102-5.
7. Petrini A, Spandorfer S. Recurrent Ectopic Pregnancy: Current Perspectives. Int J Womens Health. 2020;12:597-600.
8. Wang X, Huang L, Yu Y, Xu S, Lai Y, Zeng W. Risk factors and clinical characteristics of recurrent ectopic pregnancy: a case-control study. J Obstet Gynaecol Res. 2020;46(7):1098-103.
9. Zhang D, Shi W, Li C, Yuan JJ, Xia W, Xue RH, et al. Risk factors for recurrent ectopic pregnancy: a case-control study. Br J Obstet Gynaecol. 2016;123(S3):82-9.
10. Ellaithy M, Asiri M, Rateb A, Altraigey A, Abdallah K. Prediction of recurrent ectopic pregnancy: a five-year follow-up cohort study. Eur J Obstet Gynecol Reprod Biol. 2018;225:70-8.
11. Cheng X, Tian X, Yan Z, Jia M, Deng J, Wang Y, et al. Comparison of the fertility outcome of salpingotomy and salpingectomy in women with tubal pregnancy: a systematic review and meta-analysis. PLoS One. 2016;11(3):e0152343.
12. Hao H-J, Feng L, Dong L-F, Zhang W, Zhao X-L. Reproductive outcomes of ectopic pregnancy with conservative and surgical treatment: A systematic review and meta-analysis. Medicine. 2023;102(17):e33621.
13. Baggio S, Garzon S, Russo A, Ianniciello CQ, Santi L, Laganà AS, et al. Fertility and reproductive outcome after tubal ectopic pregnancy: comparison among methotrexate,

surgery, and expectant management. Arch Gynecol Obstet. 2021;303:259-68.
14. Karavani G, Gutman-Ido E, Herzberg S, Chill HH, Cohen A, Dior UP. Recurrent tubal ectopic pregnancy management and the risk of a third ectopic pregnancy. J Minim Invasive Gynecol. 2021;28(8):1497-1502.e1.
15. Levin G, Dior UP, Shushan A, Gilad R, Benshushan A, Rottenstreich A. Success rate of methotrexate treatment for recurrent vs. primary ectopic pregnancy: a case-control study. J Obstet Gynaecol. 2020;40(4):507-11.
16. Ismail SIMF. REP after partial salpingectomy, distal and proximal, therapeutic, and prophylactic. Gynecol Surg. 2009;6:281-2.
17. Ko PC, Liang CC, Lo TS, Huang HY. Six cases of tubal stump pregnancy: complication of assisted reproductive technology? Fertil Steril. 2011;95(7):2432.e1-4.
18. Siow A, Ng S. Laparoscopic management of 4 cases of recurrent cornual ectopic pregnancy and review of literature. J Minim Invasive Gynecol. 2011;18(3):296-302.
19. Timor-Tritsch IE, Horwitz G, D'Antonio F, Monteagudo A, Bornstein E, Chervenak J, et al. Recurrent Cesarean scar pregnancy: case series and literature review. Ultrasound Obstet Gynecol. 2021;58:121-6.
20. Wong CH, Wang YL, Huang JP. Postoperative reproductive outcomes in women with ovarian pregnancy: A retrospective analysis. Taiwan J Obstet Gynecol. 2021;60(2):295-8.
21. Bozdag G, Atak ZG, Yapici Z, Demirol A, Usubutun A, Gurgan T. Five recurrent ectopic pregnancies in a patient with MUC1 expression deficiency. J Obstet Gynaecol. 2011;31(7):666-7.
22. Marana R, Catalano GF, Muzii L. Salpingoscopy. Curr Opin Obstet Gynecol. 2003;15(4):333-6.

SECTION

9 Treatment

CHAPTER 41

Role of Natural Micronized Progesterone

Adam J Devall, Arri Coomarasamy

ABSTRACT

Progesterone is known to be a pregnancy supporting hormone. Two large randomised clinical trials, PROMISE and PRISM, failed to show a beneficial effect of natural micronized progesterone therapy over placebo. Currently, micronized progesterone therapy is recommended in patients that present with vaginal bleeding and give a history of one or more miscarriages.

Keywords: Natural micronized progesterone, Vaginal bleeding, Recurrent miscarriage, LPD.

INTRODUCTION

Progesterone is an endogenous hormone derived from cholesterol steroids, which is primarily produced by the corpus luteum in the ovaries during the menstrual cycle. Its principal role is to regulate maturation of the oocytes, ovulation, myometrial quiescence, mammary gland growth, and endometrial enzymes.[1-5] Progesterone is also vital to establish and maintain a pregnancy, modulating the endometrial structure and function to enable implantation of the early embryo.[6] The aim of this chapter is to discuss the role and use of progesterone in early pregnancy.

Researchers, physicians, and patients have been prompted to consider progesterone supplementation during early pregnancy to prevent miscarriages due to its significant physiological importance. This topic has been a subject of research for over 70 years and has been extensively debated in medical literature. The significance of the corpus luteum in maintaining a successful pregnancy was first identified in rabbits during the 1910s.[7,8] Further experiments showed that lutectomy in rabbits prevented pregnancy,[9] while supplementation of estradiol and progesterone in lutectomised rabbits prolonged pregnancy.[10-12] Similar effects have been observed in humans, where withdrawal of progesterone in early pregnancy leads to miscarriage, and antiprogesterone drugs are potent inducers of abortion.[13]

LUTEAL PHASE DEFECT

The consideration of progesterone supplementation in cases of a progesterone-related issue, commonly referred to as "luteal phase defect" (LPD), has been prompted by the significant physiological importance of progesterone. LPD is recognized as one of the contributing factors to a genetically normal "euploid" miscarriage.[14] Progesterone plays a crucial role in maintaining the decidua, and it is hypothesized that a malfunction in the corpus luteum's function can lead to decreased progesterone levels, thereby increasing the risk of miscarriage.[15] However, there is currently no precise definition for LPD, and reliable tests to identify individuals with this condition are lacking. Although serum and salivary progesterone have been utilized, the diagnostic and prognostic value of progesterone levels remains uncertain.[16,17] Moreover, the interpretation of a progesterone result is complicated by the direction of causality, as it is impossible to determine whether low progesterone levels in early pregnancy are the cause or the effect of a miscarriage. Hence, the clinical usefulness of both individual and consecutive serum progesterone measurements is restricted when it comes to accurately distinguishing between a healthy and a faulty luteal phase.

BIOLOGICAL RATIONALE FOR PROGESTERONE SUPPLEMENTATION

A history of previous miscarriages and vaginal bleeding are two significant clinical risk factors for miscarriage. A meta-analysis revealed that the risk of miscarriage increases along a biological gradient, with women who have no history of miscarriage having an 11% risk of miscarriage, and those with six or more previous miscarriages having a 64% risk **(Fig. 1)**.[18] Progesterone supplementation has been attempted in these contexts to prevent miscarriages in asymptomatic women with a history of recurrent miscarriages[19] and to rescue a pregnancy in women who have started to bleed in early pregnancy.[20] However, the biological rationale for progesterone supplementation and its limitations must be considered. Numeric chromosome errors are responsible for approximately half of all miscarriages, with trisomy being the most common.[15] Aneuploid miscarriages occur randomly, therefore, the risk of an aneuploid miscarriage is not increased according to the number of previous miscarriages. Conversely, "euploid" miscarriages are more frequently diagnosed as the number of previous miscarriages increases **(Fig. 2)**.[21] Therefore, the potential therapeutic opportunity for progesterone is greatest in women with a large number of previous miscarriages. These findings are important in the context of the latest clinical trial data on the effectiveness of progesterone to prevent miscarriage in both recurrent and threatened miscarriage.

NATURAL MICRONIZED PROGESTERONE AND SYNTHETIC PROGESTOGENS

In the 1930s, Russell Marker successfully synthesized progesterone through the process of "Marker Degradation" using a type of Mexican yam as the starting material.[22] It is important to note that the natural micronized progesterone produced through this process is structurally identical to progesterone synthesized in the human body. This achievement led to the commencement of clinical

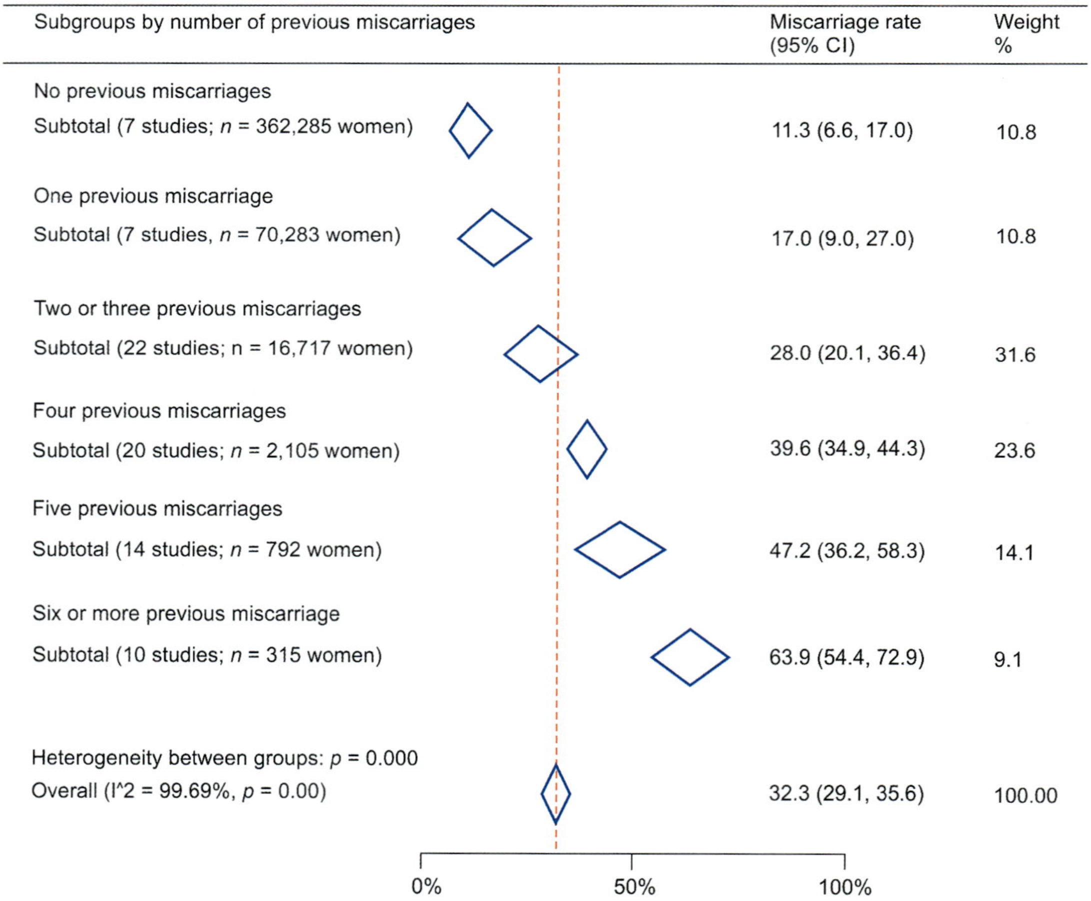

Subgroups by number of previous miscarriages	Miscarriage rate (95% CI)	Weight %
No previous miscarriages		
Subtotal (7 studies; *n* = 362,285 women)	11.3 (6.6, 17.0)	10.8
One previous miscarriage		
Subtotal (7 studies, *n* = 70,283 women)	17.0 (9.0, 27.0)	10.8
Two or three previous miscarriages		
Subtotal (22 studies; n = 16,717 women)	28.0 (20.1, 36.4)	31.6
Four previous miscarriages		
Subtotal (20 studies; *n* = 2,105 women)	39.6 (34.9, 44.3)	23.6
Five previous miscarriages		
Subtotal (14 studies; *n* = 792 women)	47.2 (36.2, 58.3)	14.1
Six or more previous miscarriage		
Subtotal (10 studies; *n* = 315 women)	63.9 (54.4, 72.9)	9.1
Heterogeneity between groups: *p* = 0.000		
Overall (I^2 = 99.69%, *p* = 0.00)	32.3 (29.1, 35.6)	100.00

0% 50% 100%

Fig. 1: A meta-analysis to assess the risk of miscarriage by the number of previous miscarriages.
Systematic review methods: Databases: MEDLINE, EMBASE, CCTR, CDSR, DARE; Search period: From respective database inception to June 2019; Search terms (MESH): Recurrent miscarriage (habitual abortion, pregnancy loss, fetal demise, fetal loss) AND prediction and prognosis (significance, score, marker, role, index, indicator, nomogram, forecast, goal, calculate, estimate, project, likelihood, extrapolate, implication or prototype); Review Outcome: Miscarriage categorized by previous number of pregnancy losses.

trials for progesterone supplementation in the 1950s.[23] Since then, various synthetic progestogen analogs have been developed[24] and subsequently evaluated for their effectiveness in preventing miscarriages.

EFFECTIVENESS OF NATURAL MICRONIZED PROGESTERONE TREATMENT IN RECURRENT AND THREATENED MISCARRIAGE

Given the crucial function of progesterone in human reproduction, it is unsurprising that the administration of exogenous supplemental progesterone is considered for pregnancy treatment protocols. A recent Cochrane meta-analysis examined the use of progesterone in preventing miscarriage for both women with a history of three or more miscarriages (recurrent miscarriage) and women presenting with early pregnancy bleeding (threatened miscarriage). The analysis considered all available evidence on the use of different progestogens to treat threatened miscarriage, focusing only on high-quality and reliable trial data.[25]

Based on the findings of a single trial involving 826 women,[26] the evidence indicates that vaginal micronized progesterone administered up to 12 weeks gestation has minimal or no impact on the live birth rate in women with recurrent miscarriage when compared to a placebo [risk ratio (RR) 1.04, 95% CI: 0.95–1.15, high-certainty evidence]. This study conducted a prespecified subgroup analysis based on the number of previous miscarriages. The study population was divided into two subgroups, one consisting of women with three previous miscarriages and the other consisting of women with four or more miscarriages. Additionally, a subgroup analysis was performed for women with three, four, five, and six or more previous miscarriages to generate hypotheses and assess the existence of a biological gradient within these subgroups. The results indicated a potential trend for greater benefit with an increasing number of previous miscarriages **(Fig. 3)**. However, the small sample sizes in the subgroups and the large p value for the test of subgroup interaction ($p = 0.41$) suggested an inconclusive subgroup effect. Nonetheless, the findings generated a hypothesis that a subgroup effect existed with a biological gradient related to the increasing number of previous miscarriages.

In women with no previous miscarriages and early pregnancy bleeding, the meta-analysis found that vaginal

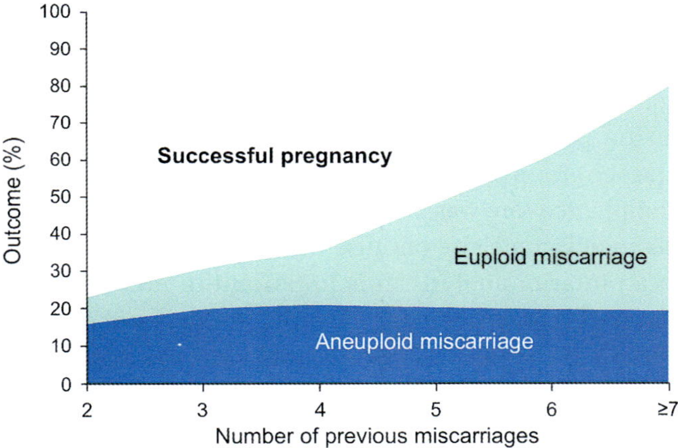

Fig. 2: Risk of aneuploid and euploid miscarriages by the number of previous miscarriages.
Source: Redrawn from Ogasawara M, et al., 2000.[21]

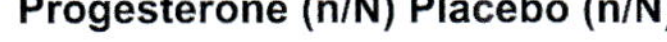

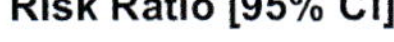

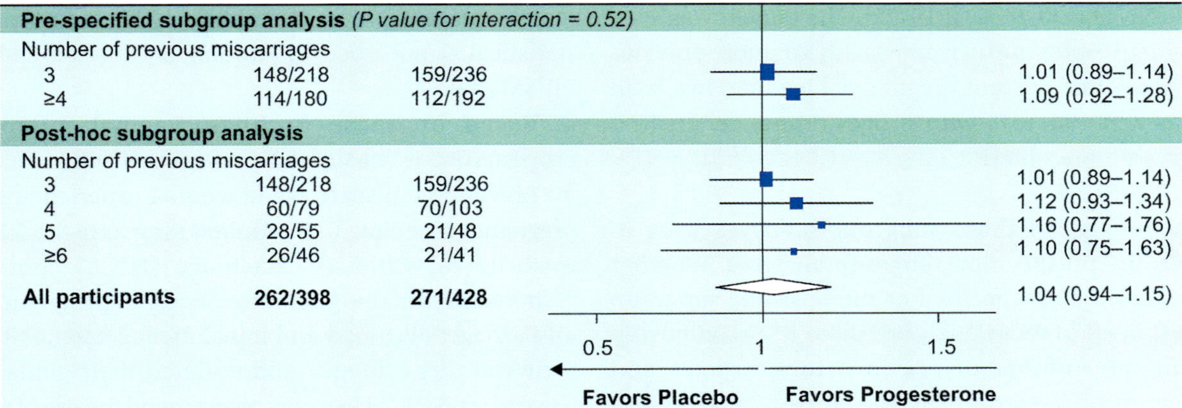

Fig. 3: PROMISE Trial subgroup analysis by number of previous miscarriages on the outcome of live birth >24 weeks.

micronized progesterone administered up to 16 weeks gestation likely does not significantly improve the live birth rate compared to a placebo (RR 0.99, 95% CI 0.95–1.04, high-certainty evidence). However, for women with one or more previous miscarriages and early pregnancy bleeding, vaginal micronized progesterone was found to increase the live birth rate compared to a placebo (RR 1.08, 95% CI 1.02–1.15, high-certainty evidence). Importantly, the use of vaginal micronized progesterone did not increase the risk of congenital anomalies or adverse drug events. The risk ratios for congenital abnormalities and adverse drug events were 1.00 (95% CI 0.68–1.46) and 1.07 (95% CI 0.81–1.39), respectively. These conclusions are supported by moderate-certainty evidence.

The trial that provided the majority of the data for this analysis was the *PR*ogesterone *I*n *S*pontaneous *M*iscarriage (PRISM) trial.[27] In this trial, there was a prespecified subgroup analysis by the number of previous miscarriages, with the study population was split into three subgroups: women without a history of miscarriage; women with 1 or 2 previous miscarriages; and women with 3 or more previous miscarriages. There were two other relevant subgroup analyses: the first grouping women into those who had no previous miscarriage or those who had any number of previous miscarriages; and the second grouping women by 0, 1, 2, ≥3 previous miscarriages, to explore in detail for a possible biological gradient. The *p* values for “subgroup by treatment” interactions were consistent with differential subgroup effects. The live birth rate was 75% (689/914) with progesterone, versus 70% (619/886) with placebo (RR 1.09, 95% CI 1.03–1.15) for the subgroup of women with 1 or more previous miscarriage(s) and bleeding in the current pregnancy [number needed to treat (NNT) = 20, 95% CI 19–22]. The benefit was even greater for the subgroup of women with 3 or more previous miscarriages and current pregnancy bleeding; live birth rate was 72% (98/137) with progesterone, versus 57% (85/148) with placebo (RR 1.28, 95% CI 1.08–1.51; NNT = 8, 95% CI 7–10).

The findings of these subgroup analyses were in line with the prespecified subgroup analyses. Whether we consider the prespecified or the post-hoc subgroup analyses, in all of these analyses, there is a relationship between the number of previous miscarriages and the effect of progesterone, as was already observed in the PROMISE trial.[26] A history of previous miscarriage identifies those at risk of a future miscarriage, and the risk of a future miscarriage increases with the increasing number of previous miscarriages **(Fig. 1)**. Specifically, it is the risk of euploid miscarriages that increase with increasing number of previous miscarriages, meanwhile the risk of miscarriage from sporadic aneuploidies remains broadly constant **(Fig. 2)**. The observed biological gradient in clinical effect increases our confidence that the history of previous miscarriage is a valid prognostic marker for future miscarriage. If one of the causes of miscarriage is LPD, then the prevalence of LPD can be expected to increase with the increasing number of previous miscarriages, and consequently greater treatment effect from progesterone can be expected.

Since the publication of this meta-analysis, two further trials assessing vaginal micronized progesterone for threatened miscarriage have been published. The STOP study[28] was a single-center, double-blind, placebo-controlled trial that found a live birth rate of 82% (112/136) in the progesterone group and 84% (112/133) in the placebo group (RR 0.98; 95% CI 0.88–1.09). The overall drug compliance rate was 55%, and the trial did not reach the planned sample size because it was stopped prematurely at an interim analysis. It is important to note the high live birth rate observed in this trial in the placebo group (84%), which indicates that this was a low-risk population of women that were included in trial. These women who have a good prognosis are unlikely to need any treatment including progesterone. The PREEMPT trial[29] was a multicenter, double-blind, placebo-controlled trial that found a live birth rate of 75% (197/264) in the progesterone group and 71% (190/269) in the placebo group. The live birth rate in this trial was 4% higher in absolute terms that the placebo group, and although this did not achieve statistical significance, the finding is consistent with the PRISM trial.

Based on these findings, vaginal micronized progesterone is considered a safe and effective treatment for preventing miscarriage in women experiencing early pregnancy bleeding. In the United Kingdom, the National Institute for Clinical Excellence (NICE) committee responsible for the guideline “Ectopic pregnancy and miscarriage: diagnosis and initial management (NG126)” reviewed this evidence and updated their guidance in November 2021.[30] They now recommend the use of vaginal micronized progesterone for women who have a history of one or more previous miscarriages and early pregnancy bleeding, as they are considered to be at dual risk.

CONCLUSION

The available evidence suggests a slight yet positive impact of vaginal progesterone supplementation during early pregnancy, which appears to be influenced by the number of previous miscarriages. The data indicates that progesterone therapy does not provide any benefits for women experiencing early pregnancy bleeding without a history of miscarriages. However, for high-risk women who have both early pregnancy bleeding and a history of one or more previous miscarriages, progesterone treatment is beneficial. Therefore, we recommend sharing this information with women at a high risk of miscarriages to facilitate shared decision-making. Our recommendation is to offer women who have vaginal bleeding and a history of one or more previous miscarriages a treatment regimen of vaginal micronized progesterone, with a dosage of 400 mg twice daily. This treatment should be initiated upon the onset of vaginal bleeding and continued until 16 completed weeks of gestation.

REFERENCES

1. Conneely OM, Mulac-Jericevic B, DeMayo F, Lydon JP, O'Malley BW. Reproductive functions of progesterone receptors. Recent Prog Horm Res. 2002;57:339-55.
2. Gellersen B, Fernandes MS, Brosens JJ. Non-genomic progesterone actions in female reproduction. Hum Reprod Update. 2009;15(1):119-38.
3. Mulac-Jericevic B, Mullinax RA, DeMayo FJ, Lydon JP, Conneely OM. Subgroup of reproductive functions of progesterone mediated by progesterone receptor-B isoform. Science (New York, N.Y.). 2000;289(5485):1751-4.
4. Zakar T, Hertelendy F. Progesterone withdrawal: key to parturition. Am J Obstet Gynecol. 2007;196:289-96.
5. Zakar T, Mesiano S. How does progesterone relax the uterus in pregnancy? N Engl J Med. 2011;364(10):972-3.
6. Di Renzo GC, Giardina I, Clerici G, Mattei A, Alajmi AH, Gerli S. The role of progesterone in maternal and fetal medicine. Gynecol Endocrinol. 2012;28:925-32.
7. Fraenkel L. Neue Experimente zur Function des Corpus luteum. Arch Gynaekol. 1910;91:705-61.
8. Hammond J. On the causes responsible for the developmental progress of the mammary glands in the rabbit during the latter part of pregnancy. Proc R Soc Lond B Biol Sci. 1917;89:534-46.
9. Corner GW. Physiology of the corpus luteum. I. The effect of very early ablation of the corpus luteum upon the embryos and uterus. Am J Physiol. 1928;86:74-81.
10. Allen WM. Physiology of the corpus luteum. VIII. Interrelationship of oestrin and the corpus luteum as determined by their effects in the adult rabbit. Am J Physiol. 1932;100:650-63.
11. Allen WM, Heckel GP. Prolongation of the corpus luteum in the pseudopregnant rabbit. Science. 1936;84:161-2.
12. Allen WM. Some effects of estrin and progestin in the rabbit. Cold Spring Harbor Symp Quant Biol. 1937;5:66-83.
13. Csapo AI, Pulkkinen MO, Wiest WG. Effects of luteectomy and progesterone replacement therapy in early pregnant patients. Am J Obstet Gynecol. 1973;115:759-65.
14. Palomba S, Santagni S, La Sala GB. Progesterone administration for luteal phase deficiency in human reproduction: an old or new issue? J Ovarian Res. 2015;8:77.
15. Stephenson MD, Awartani KA, Robinson WP. Cytogenetic analysis of miscarriages from couples with recurrent miscarriage: a case-control study. Hum Reprod. 2002;17:446-51.
16. Pillai RN, Konje JC, Tincello DG, Potdar N. Role of serum biomarkers in the prediction of outcome in women with threatened miscarriage: a systematic review and diagnostic accuracy meta-analysis. Hum Reprod Update. 2016;22:228-39.
17. Tulppala M, Björses UM, Stenman UH, Wahlström T, Ylikorkala O. Luteal phase defect in habitual abortion: progesterone in saliva. Fertil Steril. 1991;56:41-4.
18. Coomarasamy A, Devall AJ, Brosens JJ, Quenby S, Stephenson MD, Sierra S, et al. Micronised vaginal progesterone to prevent miscarriage: a critical evaluation of randomized evidence. Am J Obstet Gynecol. 2020;223(2):167-76.
19. Haas DM, Hathaway TJ, Ramsey PS. Progestogen for preventing miscarriage in women with recurrent miscarriage of unclear etiology. Cochrane Database Syst Rev. 2018;10(10):CD003511.
20. Wahabi HA, Fayed AA, Esmaeil SA, Bahkali KH. Progestogen for treating threatened miscarriage. Cochrane Database Syst Rev. 2018;(8):CD005943.
21. Ogasawara M, Aoki K, Okada S, Suzumori K. Embryonic karyotype of abortuses in relation to the number of previous miscarriages. Fertil Steril. 2000;73:300-4.
22. Lehmann PA, Bolivar A, Quintero R. Russell E. Marker. Pioneer of the Mexican steroid industry. J Chem Educ. 1973; 50:195-9.
23. Swyer GI, Daley D. Progesterone implantation in habitual abortion. Br Med J. 1953;1:1073-7.
24. García-Sáenz M, Ibarra-Salce R, Pozos-Varela FJ, Mena-Ureta TS, Flores-Villagómez S, Santana-Mata M, et al. Understanding progestins: from basics to clinical applicability. J Clin Med. 2023;12(10):3388.

25. Devall AJ, Papadopoulou A, Podesek M, Haas DM, Price MJ, Coomarasamy A, et al. Progestogens for preventing miscarriage: a network meta-analysis. Cochrane Database Syst Rev. 2021;4(4):CD013792.
26. Coomarasamy A, Williams H, Truchanowicz E, Seed PT, Small R, Quenby S, et al. A randomized trial of progesterone in women with recurrent miscarriages. N Engl J Med. 2015;373(22):2141-8.
27. Coomarasamy A, Devall AJ, Cheed V, Harb H, Middleton LJ, Gallos ID, et al. A randomized trial of progesterone in women with bleeding in early pregnancy. N Engl J Med. 2019;380:1815-24.
28. McLindon LA, James G, Beckmann MM, Bertolone J, Mahomed K, Vane M, et al. Progesterone for women with threatened miscarriage (STOP trial): a placebo-controlled randomized clinical trial. Hum Reprod. 2023;38(4):560-8.
29. Abenhaim HA, Audibert F, Gagnon R, Girard I, Kellow Z, Klam S. Progesterone for Prevention of Miscarriage and Preterm Birth in Women With First-Trimester Bleeding: PREEMPT Trial [A260]. Obstet Gynecol. 2022;44(5):599.
30. NICE Guideline [NG126]. Ectopic pregnancy and miscarriage: diagnosis and initial management. [online] Available from https://www.nice.org.uk/guidance/ng126. [Last accessed December, 2024]

CHAPTER 42

Role of Dydrogesterone

Sreeba Balakrishanan, Ashok Kumar

ABSTRACT

Dydrogesterone is a synthetic analog of progesterone, whose molecular structure closely resembles natural progesterone. However, it is orally available and is more potent than natural micronized progesterone. It has been shown to be an immune modulator by maintaining Th2 dominance in early pregnancy. This helps to prevent pregnancy loss. Evidence of dydrogesterone use in pregnancy is presented.

Keywords: Dydrogesterone, Unexplained RPL, Immune modulation.

INTRODUCTION

Recurrent pregnancy loss (RPL), a heartbreaking and perplexing condition, refers to the occurrence of three or more consecutive pregnancy losses before the 20th week of gestation as defined by Royal College of Obstetricians and Gynaecologist[1] and as two or more pregnancy losses as defined by the American Society of Reproductive Medicine.[2] It is a distressing experience that can lead to physical and emotional strain for couples longing to start or expand their families. Approximately 50% of RPL have no clearly defined etiology.[3] RPL can be categorized into primary and secondary; primary RPL refers to pregnancy loss in women who never had a live birth and secondary RPL is defined as pregnancy loss in women who had a previous live birth.[4] The etiology of RPL can be classified as genetic, anatomic, endocrine, antiphospholipid antibody syndrome, immunological and environmental factors. Balanced, reciprocal, and Robertsonian translocations in the fetus can predispose to spontaneous miscarriages. Diabetes[5] and thyroid dysfunction[2,6] can cause RPL. If left untreated, an APLS results in a pregnancy loss in 50–90% of the cases.[7] APLS causes an increased risk of thrombosis and placental insufficiency, causing RPL.[8]

In the quest to address this complex issue, medical science has explored various interventions, one of which is dydrogesterone—a synthetic progestin.

Progesterone plays a crucial role in the maintenance of pregnancy. It is secreted by the corpus luteum that provides early pregnancy support until placental production takes over at 10–12 weeks of gestation which is called the luteo-placental shift, which is a highly vulnerable period. Low levels of circulating progesterone have been linked to impending miscarriage.[9]

PHARMACOLOGY OF DYDROGESTERONE

Dydrogesterone, chemically designated as 6-dehydro-9β,10α-progesterone, is an orally active progestogen with a unique profile. Unlike other synthetic progestins, dydrogesterone's molecular structure closely resembles that of natural progesterone, a hormone pivotal for the establishment and maintenance of pregnancy. This structural similarity is thought to contribute to its efficacy and tolerability in pregnancy-related conditions, including RPL.

It has 1.5 times higher affinity for progesterone receptor and the oral bioavailability is 5–6 times more as compared to vaginal route.[10] Dydrogesterone can be safely given to mother owing to absence of antiandrogenic effect. There are no evidences suggestive of masculinization of a female fetus[11] and it does not affect normal secretory transformation of endometrium.[12]

One of the primary roles of dydrogesterone in RPL is to provide hormonal support to the endometrial lining during the crucial early stages of pregnancy.[13] After conception, the fertilized egg attaches itself to the uterine lining, and a healthy endometrial environment is essential for successful implantation. Dydrogesterone exerts its influence by stimulating the endometrium, making it receptive to embryo implantation. By maintaining an optimal endometrial milieu, dydrogesterone enhances the chances of successful embryo attachment and subsequent development. Furthermore, dydrogesterone's progestational activity extends beyond the endometrial realm. It helps maintain the uterine environment by promoting vascular stability and reducing uterine contractions. These mechanisms collectively contribute to a nurturing environment for the developing embryo, reducing the risk of miscarriage often associated with uterine contractility issues.

IMMUNOLOGY OF PREGNANCY: A FINE BALANCE

It is worth noting that dydrogesterone's use in RPL is not limited to its gestational effects alone. The immunology of pregnancy is a very unique, highly controlled system, which allows for survival of a fetus (semi-allograft) and also protecting a pregnant woman.[14] There are immune shifts in pregnancy, which facilitate maternal-fetal tolerance. There is Th1/Th2 shift wherein Th1 is proinflammatory and Th2 is anti-inflammatory.[15] Healthy pregnancy is said to be Th2 biased whereas unexplained RPL is Th1 biased leading to increase in the level of IL 12 and IFN gamma. Now, the Th1/Th2 paradigm has been expanded into the Th1/Th2/Th17 and regulatory T (Treg) cells paradigm.[16] Th17 cells, which produce the proinflammatory cytokine, IL-17, play important roles for the initiation of inflammation[17] Treg cells are known to inhibit proliferation and cytokine production in both $CD4^+$ and $CD8^+$ T cells, immunoglobulin production by B cells, cytotoxic activity of natural killer (NK) cells, and maturation of dendritic cells (DCs), resulting in induction of tolerance.[18,19]

Another factor involved is PIBF (progesterone-induced blocking factor) which prevents inflammatory and thrombotic reaction to fetus and also promotes Th2 shift.[20] Natural killer cells present in the decidua control trophoblastic invasion and allow for adequate feto-maternal perfusion and in some cases of idiopathic RPL these cells can attack the trophoblast. PIBF has been proposed to have blocking effects on NK cells degranulation. The hormone also plays a role in immune modulation, potentially influencing the delicate balance between maternal immune response and embryo recognition. Imbalanced immune responses have been implicated in some cases of RPL, and dydrogesterone's immunomodulatory properties could potentially contribute to reducing the risk of immune-related pregnancy losses, thus PIBF contributes to successful implantation by regulating the maternal immune response.

It has been proposed that cell-mediated immunological mechanisms may account for a proportion of the cases of "unexplained" RPL and it is likely that Th1-mediated maternal reactivity may be an important cause of RPL. Studies on human pregnancy failure conducted in four laboratories, support the concept that successful pregnancy occurs in a Th2-biased situation, while Th1-type immunity may lead to pregnancy failure. Raghupathy et al.[21] concluded that dydrogesterone suppresses the production of the pro-inflammatory cytokines IFN-γ and TNF-α and upregulates the production of the anti-inflammatory cytokine IL-4. The objective of this study was to compare the concentrations of Th1 and Th2 cytokines produced by peripheral blood mononuclear cells from women undergoing unexplained recurrent spontaneous abortion (RSA) with those produced during normal pregnancy at a similar gestational stage. Significantly higher concentrations of Th2 cytokines were produced by the first trimester normal group than by the RSA group, while significantly higher concentrations of Th1 cytokines were produced by the abortion group as compared to first trimester normal pregnancy, indicating a distinct Th2-bias in normal pregnancy and a Th1-bias in unexplained RSA. Thus, progesterone clearly has immunomodulatory (i.e., suppressive or inhibitory) effects on several immune responses Piccinni et al.[22] demonstrated significantly higher concentrations of IL-4- and IL-10-producing T cell clones from the decidua of women with normal pregnancy than from women with recurrent abortions.

TWO SIDES OF COIN

It is crucial to approach any medical treatment, including dydrogesterone, with a comprehensive understanding of its potential benefits and drawbacks.

El-Zibdeh[23] conducted a three-arm study wherein 180 women of <35 years of age with three or more pregnancy losses were recruited. They compared dydrogesterone treatment with human chorionic gonadotrophin, with supportive care and supportive care alone. Miscarriage was significantly ($p \leq 0.05$) more common in the control group (29%; 14/48 women) than in the dydrogesterone group (13.4%; 11/82 women). In contrast, there were no significant differences between the human chorionic gonadotropin (hCG) group (18%; 9/50 women) and the control group. No significant differences were seen between the two active treatment groups. No adverse effects were reported during treatment with dydrogesterone or hCG. In conclusion, hormonal support with dydrogesterone in early pregnancy can reduce the chances of spontaneous pregnancy loss in women with recurrent abortion due to is immunomodulatory effect.

A study conducted by Kale et al.[24] conducted a study in which a total of 200 patients were randomized to vaginal progesterone 600 mg/day (n = 100) or oral dydrogesterone 30 mg/day (n = 100). While 74 patients had two miscarriages in the progesterone group, 68 patients had two miscarriages in the dydrogesterone group. The time required for complete cessation of bleeding was significantly lesser among patients who received oral dydrogesterone compared to those who received intravaginal progesterone [53.90 ± 9.09 vs. 94.60 ± 7.29 h, $p < 0.0001$]. Numerically higher number of patients receiving oral dydrogesterone had a successful continuation of pregnancy up to 24 weeks of gestation, as well as till full term compared to progesterone group (70 vs. 75).

Progesterone influences structural and functional modification of the endometrial vasculature, which further improves endometrial receptivity during the window of implantation. Progesterone upregulates endothelial nitric oxide synthase (eNOS) expression in uterine and spiral arteries necessary for implantation. A study conducted in India evaluated the differences in uteroplacental blood flow and pregnancy outcome in women with unexplained recurrent pregnancy loss (uRPL) following administration of micronized vaginal progesterone and oral dydrogesterone. Oral dydrogesterone appears to be equally effective in improving endometrial blood flow as compared with micronized progesterone but dydrogesterone salvaged pregnancy more (92%) as compared to micronized progesterone (82%).[25]

Another meta-analysis conducted by Saccone et al. in 2017 analyzed 10 trials including 1,586 women with recurrent miscarriage.[26] Eight studies used placebo as control and were double-blind. Two RCTs used natural progesterone, whereas the other eight studies used progestins: medroxyprogesterone, cyclopentylenol ether of progesterone (PCPE), i.e., quingestrone, dydrogesterone, or 17-hydroxyprogesterone caproate. It was seen that women in progestogens group in the first trimester and before 16 weeks had a lower risk of recurrent miscarriage (RR 0.72, 95% CI 0.53–0.97) and higher live birth rate (RR 1.07, 95% CI 1.02–1.15) compared with those who did not take any progesterone. No significant differences were found in other secondary outcomes, including preterm birth (RR 1.09, 95% CI 0.71–1.66), neonatal mortality (RR 1.80, 95% CI 0.44–7.34), and fetal genital abnormalities (RR 1.68, 95% CI 0.22–12.62).[26]

A meta-analysis conducted by Guo H[27] included 2,454 RSA patients: 1,216 were in the experimental group (dydrogesterone) and 1,238 in the control group (progesterone, hCG, placebo, or active immunotherapy). Meta-analysis showed that the pregnancy success rate of the experimental group was higher than the control group, and the adverse reaction rate was lower than the control group. In addition, subgroup analysis also revealed that the experimental group had a higher pregnancy success rate than the control group and a lower adverse reaction rate. Levels of progesterone and hCG in the experimental group were dramatically higher than the control group after treatment. The experimental group also had higher levels of interleukin 4 (IL-4) and interleukin 10 (IL-10) than the control group, while levels of interferon-gamma (IFN-γ) were lower.

A 2019 Cochrane review suggested that progesterone supplementation for RPL may reduce the rate of pregnancy loss in further pregnancies.[28]

There is some evidence that oral dydrogesterone is initiated when fetal heart action can be confirmed. Furthermore, as progesterone is important during implantation of the embryo, benefit from supplementation may be realized if progesterone is administered from the luteal phase, rather than after a positive pregnancy test.[29]

Dydrogesterone is probably recommended for luteal phase support. When compared to progesterone, oral dydrogesterone has similar ongoing pregnancy rate.[30] The scope of progesterone use has been studied in peri ovulatory phase also. Effects of dydrogesterone and progesterone for luteal-phase support (LPS) in women undergoing assisted reproductive techniques (ART) were studied. A total of 3,809 women undergoing ART from eight centers were included: 1,523 were allocated to use dydrogesterone for LPS, 1,388 were allocated to use vaginal progesterone capsules and 898 were allocated to use vaginal progesterone gel. Oral dydrogesterone seems to be as effective as vaginal progesterone for LPS in ART cycles, and appears to be better tolerated.[31] Another randomized, double-blind, double-dummy phase III trial on the use of daily 30 mg oral dydrogesterone versus daily 600 mg micronized vaginal progesterone for LPS in IVF confirms that despite oral administration and first pass through the liver, dydrogesterone was as well tolerated as vaginal progesterone in safety analyses.[32]

In a study conducted by Bashiri et al., the impact of dydrogesterone on the live birth rate in patients with RPL regardless of other concurrent treatments was explored. Oral administration of dydrogestrone,10 mg twice daily was found to be independently linked to a higher live birth rate compared to the control group.[33] A study by Patki et al.[34] comparing 30 mg/day oral dydrogesterone with 600 mg/day micronized vaginal progesterone in 675 randomized patients suggested superiority of oral dydrogesterone in terms of clinical pregnancy achievement (RR 1.39, 95% CI 1.13–1.72).

A structured psychological support is vital to protect the patient's well-being because pregnancy loss can take an immense toll on the mental health of the women. Such support not only reassures her that she is taking all possible steps to support her pregnancy, but also helps her and her partner cope with the emotional challenges of pregnancy loss and navigate the stressful waiting period in subsequent pregnancies. A study by Tetruashvili et al. highlights the importance of considering psychological health as part of the treatment strategy for women experiencing RPL, in addition to standard medical interventions such as progestogen therapy.[35]

CONCLUSION

Dydrogesterone emerges as a valuable drug in the management of RPL. Its ability to mimic natural progesterone's actions, support endometrial receptivity, reduce uterine contractility, and potentially modulate immune responses showcases its multifaceted role in enhancing pregnancy outcomes. However, its administration should be tailored to individual cases, accounting for other underlying causes of RPL. It is beneficial in the treatment of threatened miscarriage in women with RPL and otherwise.

REFERENCES

1. Royal College of Obstetricians and Gynaecologists. Recurrent Miscarriage: Green-top Guideline No. 17. BJOG. 2023;00:1-31.
2. Practice Committee of the American Society for Reproductive Medicine. Evaluation and treatment of recurrent pregnancy loss: A committee opinion. Fertil Steril. 2012;98(5):1103-11.
3. Daya S, Stephenson MD. Frequency of factors associated with habitual abortion in 197 couples. Fertil Steril. 1996;66(1):24-9.
4. Ansari AH, Kirkpatrick B. Recurrent pregnancy loss. An update. J Reprod Med. 1998;43(9):806-14.
5. Hantoushzadeh S, Kohandel Gargari O, Shafiee A, Seighali N, Ghaemi M. Glucose metabolism tests and recurrent pregnancy loss: Evidence from a systematic review and meta-analysis. Diabetol Metabol Syndrome. 2023;15(1).
6. Ticconi C, Rotondi F, Veglia M, Pietropolli A, Bernardini S, Ria F, et al. Antinuclear autoantibodies in women with recurrent pregnancy loss. Am J Reprod Immunol. 2010;64(6):384-92.
7. Christiansen OB. Evidence-based investigations and treatments of recurrent pregnancy loss. Curr Opini Obstetr Gynecol. 2006;18(3):304-12.
8. Yetman DL, Kutteh WH. Antiphospholipid antibody panels and recurrent pregnancy loss: Prevalence of anticardiolipin antibodies compared with other antiphospholipid antibodies. Fertil Steril. 1996;66(4):540-6.
9. Shah D, Nagarajan N. Luteal insufficiency in first trimester. Ind J Endocrinol Metabol. 2013;17(1):44.
10. Gruber CJ, Huber JC. The role of Dydrogesterone in recurrent (habitual) abortion. J Steroid Biochem Molecul Biol. 2005;97(5):426-30.
11. Wang M-H, Baskin LS. Endocrine disruptors, genital development, and hypospadias. J Androl. 2008;29(5): 499-505.
12. Nagy B, Szekeres-Barthó J, Kovács GL, Sulyok E, Farkas B, Várnagy Á, et al. Key to life: Physiological role and clinical implications of progesterone. Intern J Molecul Sci. 2021;22(20):11039.
13. Griesinger G, Tournaye H, Macklon N, Petraglia F, Arck P, Blockeel C, et al. Dydrogesterone: Pharmacological profile and mechanism of action as luteal phase support in assisted reproduction. Reproductive Bio Med Online. 2019;38(2):249-59.
14. Orefice R. Immunology and the immunological response in pregnancy. Best Pract Res Clin Obstetr Gynaecol. 2021;76:3-12.
15. Park JC, Han JW, Lee SK. T helper cell pathology and recurrent pregnancy losses; Th1/Th2, Treg/Th17, and other T cell responses. In: Kwak-Kim J (Ed). Immunology of Recurrent Pregnancy Loss and Implantation Failure. Academic Press Inc.; 2022. pp. 27-53.
16. Peck A, Mellins ED: Plasticity of T-cell phenotype and function: The T helper type 17 example. Immunology. 2009;129:147-53.
17. Crome SQ, Wang AY, Levings MK. Translational mini-review series on Th17 cells: function and regulation of human T helper 17 cells in health and disease. Clin Exp Immunol. 2010;159:109-19.

18. Sakaguchi S. Naturally arising Foxp3-expressing CD25+ CD4+ regulatory T cells in immunological tolerance to self and non-self. Nat Immunol. 2005;6:345-52.
19. Akbar AN, Vukmanovic-Stejic M, Taams LS, Macallan DC. The dynamic co-evolution of memory and regulatory CD4+ T cells in the periphery. Nat Rev Immunol. 2007;7:231-7.
20. Miko E, Halasz M, Jericevic-Mulac B, Wicherek L, Arck P, Arató G, et al. Progesterone-induced blocking factor (PIBF) and trophoblast invasiveness. J Reprod Immunol. 2011;90(1):50-7.
21. Raghupathy R, Al-Azemi M. Modulation of Cytokine Production by the Dydrogesterone Metabolite Dihydro-dydrogesterone. Am J Reprod Immunol. 2015;74(5):419-26.
22. Piccinni M-P, Beloni L, Livi C, Maggi E, Scarselli G, Romagnani S. et al. Defective production of both leukemia inhibitory factor and type 2 T-helper cytokines by decidual T cells in unexplained recurrent abortions. Nature Med. 2018;4:1020-4.
23. El-Zibdeh MY. Dydrogesterone in the reduction of recurrent spontaneous abortion. J Steroid Biochem Mol Biol. 2005;97(5):431-4.
24. Kale AR, Kale AA, Yelikar K. A Comparative, Randomized Control Trial in Patients of Per Vaginal Bleeding Comparing Efficacy of Oral Dydrogesterone Versus Vaginal Progesterone in Successful Pregnancy Outcome for Patients with Recurrent Pregnancy Loss. J Obstet Gynecol India. 2021;71:591-95.
25. Ghosh S, Chattopadhyay R, Goswami S, Chaudhury K, Chakravarty B, Ganesh A. Assessment of sub-endometrial blood flow parameters following dydrogesterone and micronized vaginal progesterone administration in women with idiopathic recurrent miscarriage: A pilot study. J Obstetr Gynaecol Res. 2014;40(7):1871-6.
26. Saccone G, Schoen C, Franasiak JM, Scott RT Jr, Berghella V. Supplementation with progestogens in the first trimester of pregnancy to prevent miscarriage in women with unexplained recurrent miscarriage: a systematic review and meta-analysis of randomized, controlled trials. Fertil Steril. 2017;107(2):430-38.
27. Guo H, Lu Q. Efficacy of dydrogesterone on treating recurrent miscarriage and its influence on immune factors: a systematic review and meta-analysis. Ann Palliat Med. 2021;10(10):10971-85.
28. Haas DM, Hathaway TJ, Ramsey PS. Progestogen for preventing miscarriage in women with recurrent miscarriage of unclear etiology. Cochrane Database Syst Rev. 2018;10(10):CD003511.
29. ESHRE Guideline Group on RPL; Bender Atik R, Christiansen OB, Elson J, Kolte AM, Lewis S, et al. ESHRE guideline: recurrent pregnancy loss: an update in 2022. Hum Reprod Open. 2023;2023(1):hoad002.
30. Ovarian Stimulation TEGGO, Bosch E, Broer S, Griesinger G, Grynberg M, Humaidan ESHRE guideline: ovarian stimulation for IVF/ICSI. Hum Reprod Open. 2020;2020(2):hoaa009.
31. Barbosa MW, Silva LR, Navarro PA, Ferriani RA, Nastri CO, Martins WP. Dydrogesterone vs progesterone for luteal-phase support: systematic review and meta-analysis of randomized controlled trials. Ultrasound Obstet Gynecol. 2016;48(2):161-70.
32. Griesinger G, Blockeel C, Tournaye H. Oral dydrogesterone for luteal phase support in fresh in vitro fertilization cycles: a new standard? Fertil Steril. 2018;109(5):756-62.
33. Bashiri A, Galperin G, Zeadna A, Baumfeld Y, Wainstock T. Increased Live Birth Rate with Dydrogesterone among Patients with Recurrent Pregnancy Loss Regardless of Other Treatments. J Clin Med. 2023;12(5):1967.
34. Patki A, Pawar VC. Modulating fertility outcome in assisted reproductive technologies by the use of dydrogesterone. Gynecol Endocrinol. 2007;23 Suppl 1:68-72.
35. Tetruashvili N, Domar A, Bashiri A. Prevention of Pregnancy Loss: Combining Progestogen Treatment and Psychological Support. J Clin Med. 2023;12(5):1827.

CHAPTER 43

Assisted Reproductive Technology

Partha Sarathi Das

ABSTRACT

The role of assisted reproductive technology (ART) is expanding in recurrent pregnancy loss (RPL). These procedures help to shorten the time to pregnancy, which may be important in advanced maternal age and patients with diminished ovarian reserve.

The ability to perform genetic testing on blastocyst stage embryos and replace only euploid embryos reduces miscarriage rates. In recurrent aneuploidy. The option of using donor gametes/embryos can also be considered through ART.

Keywords: Recurrent pregnancy loss, DNA fragmentation index, Assisted reproductive technologies, ART, IVF-ICSI, blastocyst culture, BCL 6 assay, PGT-A.

"Hope is beautiful", we strive to make your hope a reality.

Recurrent pregnancy loss (RPL) presents a difficult scenario for clinicians struggling to help patients and couples anxiously seeking a solution. RPL takes the couple on an emotional roller coaster ride and a breakdown of hope with each devastating loss. The etiology of RPL remains enigmatic and multifaceted, and there could be multiple reasons for one loss. This chapter delves into the management of RPL cases from an assisted reproductive technology (ART) point of view and how in vitro fertilization (IVF) and its adjunct treatment can sometimes help these subsets of patients toward a successful outcome. The aim is to shed light on this condition and underscore the importance of continued research and compassionate care in helping couples navigate this challenging journey.

Prevalence for RPL is underreported.

- 5% of women of reproductive age experience ≥2 consecutive miscarriages
- <1% experience three or more miscarriages consecutively.
- Data reporting on 1st-trimester pregnancy loss is still scarce as many losses are unreported or inconclusive due to recall or reporting bias.
- Prevalence varies due to demographic profiles and the lack of a standardized definition of RPL.[1]

Recurrent miscarriage breeds apprehensions and concerns, often leading patients to doubt themselves and their ability to have a baby successfully. These are the groups of women who are falling pregnant but unable to continue the pregnancy to term. A subset of these women can benefit with advanced ART procedures. Studies show that most patients have a successful outcome with a step-by-step meticulous approach and supportive care.

HOW ASSISTED REPRODUCTIVE TECHNOLOGY–IN VITRO FERTILIZATION CAN HELP PATIENTS WITH REPEATED MISCARRIAGES?

The emotional impact of RPL and its burden affects the patient, the couple, and the family. There is a need to explore and treat the underlying cause, and accordingly plan treatment. The objectives are:

- Reduction in time to pregnancy (TTP) helps to alleviate stress. The need of the hour is to conceive at the earliest and complete the pregnancy journey without any complications.
- As "everything matters in reproduction", many aspects of reproduction are laid bare, tested, and evaluated to ensure that the embryo implants and a healthy pregnancy continues to term.
- It aids in establishing a diagnosis in hitherto unexplained RPL

Assisted reproductive technology techniques have advanced tremendously in the past decades, with improved results of vitrification and preimplantation genetic testing for aneuploidy (PGT-A). As a nascent procedure, >35 years ago, IVF catered to the treatment of infertile couples. New techniques have evolved, and better understanding has improved in the field of reproductive endocrinology, ovarian function, oocyte quality, ovarian reserve, fertilization, preimplantation embryology, endometrial factors in implantation, immune dysfunction, sperm health and the recent trends of microbiome in implantation and early pregnancy. Each of these components has a significant role to play in a successful outcome. Precision medicine is an integral component of healthcare, and there is an increasing focus on a personalized or individualized approach during ART in RPL patients. IVF with PGT-A is an excellent option that patients experiencing aneuploid recurrent miscarriages can opt for, to reduce TTP. Sequential frozen embryo transfer (FET) is preferred as it would allow PGT-A on the trophectoderm of the blastocyst and also optimize the window of implantation. Hence for RPL, better results are obtained with a frozen rather than a fresh embryo transfer.

Most patients with RPL are fertile, so the scientific rationale for IVF in these patients is debatable. IVF can be a good solution for elderly women with RPL as all parameters are checked in one, and all events required in establishing a successful pregnancy are corrected before replacing the embryo. Improving egg, sperm, and embryo quality and ensuring euploid status, enhancing endometrial receptivity, and using supportive treatment ensures a successful outcome in most cases. The best predictor for a successful fertility outcome is maternal age; hence early intervention in the form of assisted reproductive technology-intracytoplasmic sperm injection (ART-ICSI) could result in successful outcomes. Establishing pregnancy and ensuring a live birth outcome requires a strong interplay of many factors. The notable ones are sperm, eggs, embryo, uterus, endometrial lining, immune tolerance of the mother, hormonal milieu, and genetics. The couple undergoes a detailed evaluation before embarking on the IVF program. Lifestyle changes are encouraged, and supplements and antioxidants are advised. Every case is individualized and personalized to cater to the couple's needs.

IMPROVING SPERM HEALTH BEFORE ASSISTED REPRODUCTIVE TECHNOLOGY–INTRACYTOPLASMIC SPERM INJECTION

Before starting IVF, especially in patients with RPL, a comprehensive semen test is done, including semen analysis, semen culture and sensitivity, and DNA fragmentation index (DFI). Vitamins and supplements are advised to ensure sperm health, hoping to produce healthy, good-quality embryos. Studies have shown that the sperm of men with RPL have reduced viability with increased DNA damage compared to fertile controls.[2,3]

SPERM SELECTION TECHNIQUES TO SELECT THE BEST SPERM FOR INTRACYTOPLASMIC SPERM INJECTION: SEMEN MICROFLUIDIC ASSESSMENT

It is crucial to assess the sperm integrity and double strand deoxynucleic acid (dsDNA) breaks, which can eventually contribute to embryo chromosomal abnormalities. Given the inverse relationship between sperm chromatin fragmentation (SCF), and motility, a selection of the most motile sperm by microfluidic sperm selection (MFSS) enhances the chances of obtaining spermatozoa with an intact genome, thus contributing to the generation of more euploid embryos that are capable of implanting and yielding term pregnancies.[4] MFSS is commercially available as Zymot, can be used to select the best healthy sperm for ICSI. Studies have shown that Zymot prepared sperms can pick up sperms with less DNA damage and higher motility.[5]

In case of poor semen morphology, testicular scan can be done to rule out varicocele. Varicocelectomy can be considered in severe cases of varicocele and in men with high DFI. Varicocelectomy improves semen quality, increases pregnancy rate, and decreases the miscarriage rate significantly. Each case has to be individualized and treated accordingly for the best outcome.[6]

Table 1 mentions the efficacy of both available and emerging techniques that aim to improve the quality of the sperm pool available for use in ART.[7]

IMPROVING OOCYTE HEALTH BEFORE ASSISTED REPRODUCTIVE TECHNOLOGY, CONTROLLED OVARIAN HYPERSTIMULATION

Women with RPL, before embarking on the IVF program, are advised to start antioxidants and supplements, including folate, Vitamin D, Co-enzyme Q10, and multivitamins, to ensure a healthy competent oocyte for fertilization. Lifestyle changes, including exercise and avoidance of alcohol and smoking, are encouraged for both partners. Holistic care and support by providing psychological counseling is an ongoing part of the treatment process.

TABLE 1: Sperm selection techniques.

Summary of sperm analysis and selection modalities currently being adopted in clinical research and trial settings.

Selection mechanism	*Method*	*Sperm analysis*	*Sperm selection*
Density	Gradient separation	✓	✓
Surface charge	Electrophoresis zeta method	✓	×
Morphological characteristics	Motile sperm organelle morphology examination	✓	✓
	Intracytoplasmic sperm injection	×	✓
	Intracytoplasmic morphologically selected sperm	✓	✓
Motility characteristics	Microfluidics	✓	✓
Membrane integrity	Hypo-osmotic swelling test	✓	×
Membrane proteins	Hyaluronic acid	✓	✓
	Magnetic activated cell sorting	✓	×
DNA chromatin integrity	DNA fragmentation	✓	×

CONTROLLED OVARIAN HYPERSTIMULATION

In vitro fertilization success depends on obtaining good quality matured eggs to obtain healthy embryos. That is why a good cycle of controlled ovarian stimulation, controlled ovarian hyperstimulation (COH), is needed to harvest healthy mature oocytes to generate good-quality embryos. After a thorough baseline scan check and estradiol E2, FSH, and LH monitoring, ovarian stimulation is started on day two or three of the menstrual cycle. Appropriate doses of gonadotropins are used to ensure optimum folliculogenesis. Initial dose of gonadotropins is based on the patient's age, body mass index (BMI), anti-Müllerian hormone (AMH), and antral follicle count (AFC) count. If prior ovarian stimulations were done, then the way the patient responded, whether it was a sluggish response or a hyper response, is also considered, and based on that, gonadotropin dose is decided. These are the small steps taken to obtain a healthy mature egg for fertilization. The aim is to ensure optimal outcomes without risks of ovarian hyperstimulation syndrome (OHSS), a dreaded complication usually seen in hyper responders.

The choice of IVF protocol depends on the physician's evaluation and patients' compliance. Agonist protocol or antagonist protocol can both be used during COH. Studies have shown that the outcome between these two protocols is the same. Recent advances favor using antagonist cycles as it only lasts 10–13 days of injections, and the patient's compliance is maximum. Growth hormone can be added as an adjunct treatment if the previous IVF cycle has not resulted in good-quality eggs and embryos. GH has no untoward side effects and can only maximize the chances of obtaining good-quality eggs.[8]

The chances of obtaining good-quality oocytes are compromised in women diagnosed with diminished ovarian reserve and low AMH. Adding testosterone supplements such as dehydro-epi-androsterone (DHEA) can provide marginal benefit in obtaining healthy gametes. Diminished ovarian reserve (DOR) directly or indirectly also plays a critical role in the causation of RPL.[9] The matured oocytes obtained will finally predict the number of available blastocysts.

The final step in COH is the trigger injection which can be given either in the form of HCG alone, dual trigger with agonist injection, or agonist injection alone. The final trigger injection is to ensure the optimum yield of matured eggs and at the same time to avoid OHSS. The egg harvesting procedure is done under short anesthesia approximately 36 hours post-trigger injection. ICSI is preferably done for all mature eggs obtained using the sperms selected by the microfluidic assessment, Zymot.

USING TIME LAPSE TECHNOLOGY TO CHECK EMBRYO KINETICS

Time Lapse System Embryoscope

Time-lapse embryo scope is an incubator equipped with an inbuilt camera that captures images of embryos undergoing cell division at regular intervals without disturbing the embryo growth. It takes digital images of embryos from the fertilization stage till the blastocyst stage. These time-lapse images can assess the embryo kinetics, and a clear understanding of exact cellular embryo division can be ascertained without removing the embryo from the incubator. The continuous recording of these images creates a time-lapse video to observe embryo development from a single cell to the blastocyst stage in real time. Traditional methods involving removing embryos from the incubator for assessment at specific intervals, are now replaced with time lapse technology, which avoids disruption to embryo environment and hence quality. Embryologists can closely monitor every critical stage of embryo growth on time lapse videos and thus better select viable embryos.

The obvious advantages of time lapse embryoscopes are:

- Maintaining stable culture conditions and limiting the exposure of embryos to changes in gas composition, temperature, and movement, which can influence and compromise embryo viability. Along with PGT-A, time-lapse monitoring can be an added tool for deciding the best embryo to transfer.[10]
- Time-lapse embryo scope monitoring offers a deeper understanding of embryo development. The ability to check the embryo from its inception up until the stage of a blastocyst just before implantation has given a wealth of information on how an embryo behaves and divides. Any abnormal division is noted and the best embryo with the best embryo kinetics is selected for transfer.

It is noteworthy that sometimes the excellent morphologically graded embryos turn out to be aneuploid, and therefore, subjecting these embryos for comprehensive chromosome screening and corelating with the preimplantation genetic screening (PGS) report is the new trend. Studies done in different parts of the world demonstrated improved clinical pregnancy and live birth rates (LBR) when using the embryoscope for embryo selection.[11]

One of the foremost causes of recurrent miscarriage is a chromosomal abnormality of the embryo. Time-lapse helps select morphologically viable embryos and provides additional information about embryo kinetics and division patterns. Abnormal cell division in slow-growing embryos may indicate abnormal genetics, which may predict the viability and likelihood of successful implantation. A lot can be understood with a time-lapse monitoring of the embryos, and data gathered from these images can be correlated with other parameters, and the right personalized intervention can be implemented to increase the chances of a successful pregnancy.

USING THE NEXT GENERATION SEQUENCING TECHNIQUE TO SELECT THE EUPLOID EMBRYO FOR IMPLANTATION

Preimplantation Genetic Testing for Aneuploidy

Preimplantation genetic screening, PGT, and PGT-A are the acronyms for 24 chromosome screening of embryos. The test is to screen the embryos for 24 chromosomes to ensure that the embryo has equal distribution of chromosomes to form a healthy embryo.

Understanding the underlying genetic causes of recurrent miscarriages is crucial for effective management and improved pregnancy outcomes. Half of all miscarriages are due to chromosomal abnormalities; they either lack or gain a chromosome copy, making it aneuploid. As we understand that RPL is a diverse syndrome with many causes, the most common being embryonic aneuploidy. The only way to ascertain whether an egg is chromosomally normal is to fertilize it, culture the embryo to day 5 blastocyst, and then do PGT-A on the trophectoderm cells of the embryo.

Preimplantation genetic testing for aneuploidy use in RPL patients significantly raises clinical pregnancy rates (CPRs) while reducing loss rates and provides a 50% relative increase in delivery rates. PGT-A is a useful adjunct in the care of patients with RPL.[12] The European Society of Human Reproduction and Embryology (ESHRE) has published guidelines in which PGT-M for monogenic disorders and PGT-SR for structural rearrangements were described as established alternatives to invasive prenatal diagnosis. PGT-A should be included in the treatment of repeated miscarriages.[13]

Advantages of Preimplantation Genetic Testing for Aneuploidy

- *Identifying chromosomal and genetic errors:* Genetic or chromosomal errors in the embryo are the foremost causes of repeated pregnancy loss. The presence of a strong family history of genetic mutations or repeated miscarriages, necessitates PGT-M. In case of absent family history of genetic abnormality, PGT-A can be done to screen the normal from the abnormal embryos. The prevalence of chromosomal abnormalities is higher in embryos from women with RPL than in those with no history of loss.[14] By identifying the genetically normal embryos through PGT-A, the risk of implanting abnormal embryos is reduced, thus leading to higher chances of a healthy take-home baby. PGT-A increases CPRs and reduces miscarriage rates.[15] In case of a positive family history of abnormal genetics, PGT-M can be considered to screen the embryos from the heritable condition and transfer the unaffected and normal ones. In that way, the heritable condition is severed, and the disease transmission is halted in future generations.

- *Recent advances in embryo screening:* Traditional methods of chromosome testing such as fluorescent in situ hybridization (FISH), involved screening of only five chromosomes 13,18,21,X, and Y, while PGT-A either standard or noninvasive uses advanced techniques such as next generation sequencing (NGS) to screen the entire 24 chromosomal complement. This comprehensive chromosome screening provides more accurate and reliable results and helps to select the normal embryo for transfer.[16]
- The euploid status of the embryo results in higher chances of implantation and sustenance of pregnancy. PGS is crucial in IVF treatment, especially in women with RPL. PGS has demonstrated its role in pregnancy outcomes, reduction in miscarriage, and alleviating emotional burden.

Disadvantages

- It adds to the cost of IVF treatment cycle
- Debates still exist about the mosaic embryos and whether to transfer or not to transfer these embryos. It has been shown that some mosaic embryos have the capability of correcting the mosaicism during the process of cell division.
- Sometimes many embryos are discarded being aneuploid and abnormal leaving the patient with no embryos to transfer.

ENSURING A HEALTHY FAVORABLE ENDOMETRIUM AND STRATEGIES TO MAXIMIZE IMPLANTATION

Endometrial Evaluation and Testing

Endometrial preparation is started for the implantation phase, only once we have euploid embryo/s cryopreserved. The relevance of the endometrial factor in reproductive medicine is currently poorly researched and understood. Numerous endometrial factors can cause recurrent miscarriage and or implantation failure after IVF. The major ones are—anatomical distortion or irregularity of the endometrial cavity caused by polyps, fibroid, adenomyosis, septum, scars, fibrosis, and adhesions. A thin endometrial lining of <7 mm can result in suboptimal outcomes. An inflammatory environment due to endometriosis, adenomyosis, hydrosalphinges, or autoimmune disorders hampers implantation. Surgical management of previous pregnancy losses or any kind of surgical evacuation procedure may cause underlying scar, fibrosis, or inflammation as well as traumatic cervical incompetence. Endometrial inflammation may be the root cause of many unexplained pregnancy mishaps.[17,18]

BCL6 analysis (CiceroDx, Huntington Beach, CA) has been developed to detect endometrial BCL6 overexpression in women with repeated pregnancy loss or implantation failure. Excessive endometrial expression of BCL6 alters endometrial receptivity.[19] This could be due to inflammation caused by molecular-level endometriosis or hydrosalpinges. In a single endometrial biopsy sample, BCL6 expression is the only test to identify endometriosis, progesterone resistance, and endometritis. BCL6 is found in over 50% of women with unexplained infertility and 65% with two or more IVF failures. Progesterone resistance is a condition that causes unfavorable changes in the uterine lining blocking the important hormone progesterone from carrying out its vital role in preparing the endometrium for embryo survival. The addition of the CD138 marker can help detect endometritis which is a chronic inflammation of the endometrial lining mostly due to bacterial infection. A high level of BCL6 marker >1.4 suggests inflammation due to endometriosis, adenomyosis, or hydrosalpinges. A thorough pelvic scan is warranted to rule out pelvic deposits of endometriosis and adenomyosis. Laparoscopy is indicated to optimize the pelvis by fulguration of endometriotic lesions and/or adenomyotic lesions. The presence of hydrosalpinges warrants its removal followed by two cycles of down-regulation with GnRH agonists 3.75 mg, before planning for FET. Receptive Dx testing can be done in women with recurrent miscarriage, unexplained infertility, recurrent implantation failure, women with limited embryo reserve who want the best outcome per embryo transferred. Women with suspected or molecular endometriosis and aberrant BCL6 expression have worse reproductive outcomes following embryo transfer, including a high miscarriage rate, poor implantation rate, low LBR and low CPR, compared to cycles pretreated with medical and surgical management.[20]

Receptiva Dx BCL6 is tested by a simple endometrial biopsy done during a mock hormone replacement therapy (HRT) cycle or a normal cycle during the window of implantation. In a mock HRT cycle, pipelle biopsy of the endometrium is done after 5 days of progesterone start and in a natural cycle, 7 days post LH surge or 10 days post ovulation. The sample is collected, placed in a preservative (10% formalin vial), and shipped to the molecular facility for testing. Turnaround time (TAT) is usually 7 days.

The question frequently asked is whether this biopsy can be done in the same cycle as egg retrieval. Ideally, it would not be right to do a biopsy in the same cycle as the IVF stimulation, because the high hormone levels could impact the results as well as the molecular transcriptomics of the endometrial lining. It is better to do the biopsy in a subsequent mock HRT cycle that mimics the FET cycle.

ENDOMETRIAL TRIO: ENDOMETRIAL RECEPTIVITY ASSAY, ANALYSIS OF INFECTIOUS CHRONIC ENDOMETRITIS, AND ENDOMETRIAL MICROBIOME METAGENOMIC ANALYSIS

Endometrial receptivity assay (ERA) is designed to evaluate endometrial receptivity. It is the first diagnostic test that determines each woman's unique personalized embryo transfer timing, therefore synchronizing the embryo transfer with an individualized window of implantation. The ERA predictor algorithm is based on artificial intelligence (AI), allowing for continual refinements and achieving personalized embryo transfer recommendations with the highest accuracy. This molecular diagnostic tool uses NGS to analyze the expression level of 248 genes related to the status of endometrial receptivity. ERA is indicated for patients with implantation failure of endometrial origin or in patients with recurrent euploid miscarriages, women with limited embryo reserve who wish to maximize their chances of successful implantation and LBR per embryo transfer. ERA results could be interpreted based on receptive, pre-receptive, or post-receptive, and accordingly, the timing of embryo transfer procedure can be personalized based on the report.

Limitations of the Test

Inconclusive reports are seen in <5% of cases, which means the biopsy sample has failed to obtain a sufficient tissue quantity and quality to make a diagnosis. In this regard, a new biopsy will be advised. Pregnancy is not guaranteed even if the ERA test is receptive. Poor embryo quality, genetic abnormalities, and previous pathologies can also reduce the likelihood of becoming pregnant. ERA tests only the receptivity status of the endometrium and cannot provide a prediction for the ongoing pregnancy health.[21,22]

ENDOMETRIAL MICROBIOME METAGENOMIC ANALYSIS

Vaginal microbiome in healthy women is dominated by *Lactobacillus iners*, *Lactobacillus crispatus*, *Lactobacillus gasseri*, and *Lactobacillus jensenni*. Alteration of any of these florae may alter the physiological conditions resulting in dysbiosis, and negative outcomes. The vaginal microbiome is lactic acid-producing, which lowers the vaginal pH, and this low pH prevents the growth of other pathogenetic bacteria such as *Gardnerella vaginalis*, *Chlamydia trachomatis*, and other microbes. Sexual practices, hygiene, vaginal douching, and other personal habits may influence instability among vaginal microbiotas.[23-26]

A total of 30% of infertile women have pathogenic bacteria detected in their endometrium. Endometrial microbiome metagenomic analysis (EMMA) analyzes the endometrial microbiome to detect the presence of dominant good bacteria and abnormal pathogenic bacteria. It uses reverse transcription-polymerase chain reaction (RT-PCR) technology to provide endometrial microbiome information by analyzing the presence and quantity of the most common and relevant bacterial pathogens of the reproductive tract. It also detects the abundance of *Lactobacillus* in the endometrium that will favor implantation. EMMA determines whether the endometrial microbiome environment is optimal for embryo implantation. If the endometrial microbiome environment is not optimal for embryo implantation, a recommendation for a probiotic is advised. Probiotics should be started at least 2 months before embryo transfer and continued in the first trimester.

Analysis of infectious chronic endometritis (ALICE) analyzes pathogenic bacteria responsible for causing endometritis. If ALICE shows the presence of abnormal pathogenic organisms, then a specifically targeted antibiotic is used before transfer. ALICE only detects the presence of pathogens associated with chronic endometritis. A negative result does not rule out the presence of other endometrial pathogens. It is a diagnostic test to detect and quantify the most common pathogenic bacteria causing chronic endometritis, recommending appropriate antibiotic and probiotic treatment.

Indications for EMMA/ALICE test

- Patients with recurrent miscarriage
- Patients with repeated implantation failures

The test can benefit any patient wishing to conceive by assessing the microbiological environment that the embryo will encounter after implantation.[27]

Next generation sequencing allows the identification of culturable and nonculturable endometrial pathogens associated with chronic endometritis. The most appropriate antibiotic is recommended based on the bacteria detected.[28]

STRATEGIES TO IMPROVE IMPLANTATION AND LIVE BIRTH RATE

Gut Microbiome and Recurrent Pregnancy Loss

Microbiome refers to the diverse community of organisms in our body. It includes bacteria, fungi, viruses, and archaea, forming a complex biosystem that interacts with the host and plays an important role in various physiological pathways in our day-to-day living. The gut microbiome and vaginal microbiome are the two big ecosystems that play a significant role in reproduction and pregnancy sustenance.

So How is a Leaky Gut Leading to Recurrent Pregnancy Loss?

A leaky gut, occurring for reasons we cannot explain yet, allows the passage of inflammatory mediators, through the intestinal barrier, which might elicit immune dysfunction in endometrial tissue. Hence, when increased intestinal permeability and higher circulating levels of lipopolysaccharides (LPS) are detected, there might be a higher risk of endometrial inflammation and reproductive disorders. Immune dysregulation, hormonal imbalances, inflammation, and oxidative stress with the release of pro-inflammatory molecules disrupt safe pregnancy outcomes. Studies and research are being done globally, focusing on the role of microbiome and human reproduction. Studies have shown that women with a history of RPL had different gut microbiota profiles than healthy volunteers. This was due to an alteration in the immune response and inflammation. Studies have also found that patients with RPL had altered microbial diversity in the gut compared to healthy controls. The low diversity was found more in women with repeated losses. Probiotics and prebiotic supplementation as therapeutic strategies is gaining widespread attention in improving pregnancy outcome. More clinical trials must be conducted to establish these supplementations efficacy and understand the in-depth causal relationship between gut microbiome and pregnancy loss. This will help to personalize interventions for patients with recurrent miscarriages. Probiotic supplementation at the start of IVF, during IVF, and continuation till pregnancy does go a long way to benefit women, especially with RPL.[29,30]

ROLE OF ENDOSCOPY PROCEDURES—LAPAROSCOPY/ HYSTEROSCOPE

Hysteroscopy is an endoscopy procedure that involves the insertion of a thin caliber hysteroscope with a channel for free fluid flow. A hysteroscope is inserted through the vaginal orifice inside the cervix and into the uterus, which is distended with a free jet of water. It allows for a real-time assessment of the vagina (vaginoscopy), cervix, and endometrial cavity with the tubal ostial opening. Hysteroscopy can be performed in an outpatient setting called office hysteroscopy or under anesthesia if it needs surgical correction or if the patient is apprehensive. It is through the hysteroscopy procedure that all the corrective surgical interventions of the uterine cavity are done, rectifying any cervical stenosis, diagnosing chronic endometritis, and sampling it for histopathological analysis and also hysteroscopy-directed removal of products of conception, which can be subjected to karyotype in case of RPL. This allows the unnecessary, blind dilatation and curettage (D&C) procedure, which can sometimes damage the endometrial lining, thus preventing pregnancy or causing endometritis, Asherman's syndrome or thin lining due to vigorous curettage.

Therapeutic advantages of hysteroscopy in RPL are:

- Diagnosis and removing endometrial or cervical polyp
- Removal of a fibroid indenting the endometrial cavity
- Diagnosis of adenomyosis and removal of adenomyotic gland indenting the endometrial cavity
- Corrective surgery for septum and septoplasty
- Metroplasty if needed in case of thin endometrial lining
- Adhesiolysis in the presence of adhesions, scar, and fibrosis

- Understanding the cervical canal shape integrity and deciding the possible role of cervical stitch if diagnosed with a patulous cervix, especially in cases of RPL.

Hysteroscopy should be considered before embryo transfer for its therapeutic advantages in maximizing the chances of implantation. 3D and 4D ultrasound scans can show brilliant ultrasound-rendered pictures but, a hysteroscope can visualize the cavity in real time and rectify any problem in the same sitting. The latest hysteroscopes available nowadays are easy-to-handle and maneuver and that is why hysteroscopy is finding its role more and more in the armamentarium of reproductive medicine, especially in women with RPL. Laparoscopy is necessary to delink the fallopian tubes in the presence of hydrosalpinx, myomectomy in the presence of myoma indenting the cavity, or endometriotic deposit and cyst fulguration.

ELECTIVE SINGLE EMBRYO TRANSFER

Endometrial preparation for FET is done in a natural or hormone replacement cycle with estradiol valerate tablets. Progesterone is added with the appearance of a triple-line endometrium pattern. Elective embryo transfer is done in the most atraumatic manner under ultrasound guidance.

ROLE OF IMMUNE MODULATION

Immune modulation during implantation is a highly enigmatic and complex phenomenon. The maternal body's innate defense system prepares for the embryo to be shielded from attack by her immune cells. Pregnancy is unique in that the growing fetus is foreign to the mother. The maternal immune system modulates to tolerate the embryo as self rather than foreign, thus, allowing successful implantation and propagation of pregnancy to live birth. The recognition of proteins as self is directed by immune lymphocytes known as T-regulatory (Treg) cells. These cells modulate the maternal immune response in favor of acceptance and sustenance of pregnancy. Immune dysfunction may be alloimmune or autoimmune. An appropriate balance between T helper cell 1 (TH1) and T helper cell 2 (TH2) needs to be maintained. The dominance of TH1 activates the cytotoxic immune system causing flooding of inflammatory mediators resulting in negative outcomes. Immune dysfunction in RPL cannot be disregarded. Appropriate treatment should be offered in the form of steroids, intralipids, and immunoglobulins, as immune cells and molecules play an important role in nurturing placental development, maintaining tolerance, and promoting fetal growth. Autoimmune conditions such as systemic lupus erythematosus (SLE) and antiphospholipid antibody syndrome can contribute to RPL by generating immune response that can attack the dividing pregnancy cells.

Therapeutic Strategies

Glucocorticoids: Prednisolone or dexamethasone can modulate the immune response favoring pregnancy.

Intralipids: Intravenous therapy with intralipids which is a fat emulsion containing soy and essential fatty acid extract regulates immune response and favors maternal immune tolerance. It creates an environment favoring implantation. Elevated levels of CD56, CD19, CD 5, natural killer cells, and elevated cytokines (TNF-a, IFN) have been observed in women with RPL. Intralipid infusion helps reduce these elevated cytokines favoring pregnancy outcomes. The infusion lasts for 1–2 hours and is offered every fortnightly. Headache and allergic reactions are the side effects sometimes seen during infusion.

Intravenous immunoglobulin (IVIG): IVIG promotes and regulates a tolerant maternal environment favoring implantation and sustenance of pregnancy.

Hydroxychloroquine (HCQ): HCQ has anti-inflammatory and anti-thrombotic effects and thus may improve pregnancy outcomes in patients with autoimmunity and RPL. HCQ decreases the circulating levels of Interleukin 1, 2, 6, TNF-a, and interferon-gamma promoting the TH2 processes that normally prevail in a normal pregnancy.[31-33]

ROLE OF ARTIFICIAL INTELLIGENCE IN RECURRENT PREGNANCY LOSS

Assisted reproduction technique is a breakthrough in medical science, and we all know that it is barely 40 years old. Even with ART, we have tackled just a few of the challenges of infertility and recurrent miscarriage. The number of variables to monitor and analyze in an IVF cycle poses a challenge. Taking help of AI protocols minimizes the human error in analyzing all the variables involved.

Artificial intelligence can be integrated in ART at multiple steps, such as:

- Artificial intelligence can be used in COH which is a complex procedure involving hormonal injections to ensure follicle growth and retrieving a healthy oocyte. AI can help determine the correct gonadotropin, doses, and timing of injections. It can track the follicular progress by interpreting data obtained from ultrasound scans, helping decide the type of trigger, its dosage, and timing of oocyte retrieval process to increase the likelihood of success.

- Artificial intelligence in the assessment of oocyte quality via a software called Violet
- *Artificial intelligence in sperm selection (spermbot):* AI helps in sperm selection. It is a daunting task that embryologists face to select a single sperm from the millions in the sample provided for ICSI.
- Robotic ICSI can remove the human error during ICSI.
- *Artificial intelligence in embryo selection:* In the laboratory, AI can aid in embryo morphology assessment. IVF relies highly on visual assessments prone to error and impaired decision-making. AI implementation in the laboratory allows for reliable, objective, and integrated data of embryo kinetics, morphology, and genetics. The software is called ERICA (endometrial receptivity international classification algorithm).
- Artificial intelligence tools can also be used in techniques such as laser-assisted hatching (LAH) and PGT-A biopsy, reducing human error to some extent.
- Artificial intelligence is useful in analyzing vast amounts of medical and embryology data. Integrating them based on outcomes and present patterns beyond human perception and capabilities. In short, AI can help to select the best sperm, egg, and finally select the best embryo for transfer.
- Artificial intelligence can integrate with an electronic medical records system (EMR) and can work up a new patient for IVF.
- Artificial intelligence can assess oocyte quality, sperm selection, fertilization assessment, embryo assessment, aneuploid prediction, embryo transfer selection, embryo witnessing, and overall quality management.
- Artificial intelligence provides excellent potential and promises to improve clinical outcomes and laboratory efficiency. The latter is a crucial focus because of increased IVF clinical volumes.
- Artificial intelligence can process large amounts of data, especially images, and based on this extensive, diverse data, different AI algorithms can be produced to improve pregnancy outcomes.

Artificial intelligence-related ongoing clinical trials as on May 2023 are given in **Table 2**.[34]

TABLE 2: Artificial intelligence (AI)-related ongoing clinical trials.

AI system	*Ongoing clinical trial*
Magenta AI	Correlation of oxidative stress and oocyte quality in fertility preservation
CHLOE	Evaluate to study the performance of CHLOE algorithm on the prediction of blastocyst formation in women undergoing IVF
Hera Score	*A life Hera system:* Adjunctive tool for prioritizing embryos deemed suitable for transfer

The human touch can never be replaced, but we can work with AI closely to improve outcomes in ART.

CONCLUSION

Patients with RPL need support, guidance, and education from their healthcare providers. It is prudent to adopt IVF treatment in a subset of RPL patients that do not conceive easily. However, these IVF cycles have to be personalized to the patients' needs. The following step-by-step approach results in favorable outcomes as summarized below:

- Careful planning of COH protocol for obtaining good quality eggs.
- Using the microfluidic sperm sorting (Zymot) to select sperms for ICSI.
- Preimplantation genetic screening for aneuploidy PGT-A to select euploid embryos.
- Endometrial biopsy for BCL6, ERA, EMMA, and ALICE
- Downregulation for a cycle or two helps to reset the hormonal profile favoring implantation and pregnancy.
- Office hysteroscopy evaluation to check for endometrium. This not only evaluates the endometrial cavity in real time but also aids in mapping and opening up the cervical canal for easy, atraumatic embryo transfer.
- Frozen elective single embryo transfer cycle with HRT or natural cycle protocol to ensure a healthy endometrial lining. Progesterone and adjuvants for luteal support. The dosage may need to be personalized.
- Embryo transfer to be done under ultrasound guidance in the most atraumatic way. Care should be taken to measure the cavity length before the actual transfer. It should be done under ultrasound guidance. In the case of a retroverted uterus wherein abdominal ultrasound does not show the endometrial cavity in its entirety, TVS-guided embryo transfer should be done to see the exact placement of the embryo. Transferring

the embryo 1 cm below the fundus has a better chance of implantation.

- Thromboprophylaxis in the form of blood thinners such as low-molecular-weight heparin (LMWH) and baby aspirin if indicated. This can be continued until the first trimester or the complete duration of pregnancy.
- Immunoprophylaxis by offering HCQ, steroids, intralipids, IVIG, or a combination of therapies if indicated.
- Achieving a favorable uterine microbiome by offering probiotics, either oral or vaginal.
- Acupuncture helps in destressing and improves blood flow.[35]
- Psychological support and counseling through the course of treatment.[36]

Applying above principles to the IVF program and individualizing every case is the key to achieving success in RPL couples.

REFERENCES

1. Stirrat GM. Recurrent miscarriages. Lancet. 1990;336:673-5.
2. Ruixue W, Hongli Z, Zhihong Z, Rulin D, Dongfeng G, Ruizhi L. The impact of semen quality, occupational exposure to environmental factors, and lifestyle on recurrent pregnancy loss. J Assist Reprod Genet. 2013;30:1513-18.
3. Brahem S, Mehdi M, Landolsi H, Mougou S, Elghezal H, Saad A. Semen parameters and some DNA fragmentation as causes of recurrent pregnancy loss. Urology. 2011;78:792-6.
4. Kocur OM, Xie P, Cheung S, Souness S, McKnight M, Rosenwaks Z, et al. Can a sperm selection technique improve embryo ploidy? Andrology. 2023;11(8):1605-12.
5. Pardinas Garcia ML, de los Santos JM, Vilora T, Jaen DO, Martin A, De Los Santos MJ. Microfluidic-based device selects sperm with less DNA damage and higher motility. What else? Human Reprod. 2022;37(Supplement 1).
6. Mansour Ghanaie M, Asgari SA, Dadrass N, Allahkhah A, Iran-Pour E, Safarinejad MR. Effects of varicocele repair on spontaneous first trimester miscarriage: a randomized clinical trial. Urol J. 2012;9(2):505-13.
7. Vaughan DA, Sakkas D. Sperm selection methods in the 21st century. Biol Reprod. 2019;101(6):1076-82.
8. Quaas AM, Penzias AS, Adashi EY. The role of growth hormone in assisted reproduction. Front Endocrinol (Lausanne). 2022;13:1055097.
9. Bunnewell SJ, Honess ER, Karia AM, Keay SD, Al Wattar BH, Quenby S. Diminished ovarian reserve in recurrent pregnancy loss: a systematic review and meta-analysis. Fertil Steril. 2020;113:818-27.
10. Harper J, Jackson E, Sermon K, Aitken RJ, Harbottle S, Mocanu E, et al. Adjuncts in the IVF laboratory: where is the evidence for "add-on" interventions? Hum Reprod. 2017;32:485-91.
11. Rubio C, Bellver J, Rodrigo L, Castillón G, Guillén A, Vidal C, et al. In vitro fertilization with preimplantation genetic diagnosis for aneuploidies in advanced maternal age: a randomized, controlled study. Fertil Steril. 2017;107(5):1122-9.
12. Kim JG, Murugappan G, Lathi RB, Osman EK, Neal SA, Scott RT. Preimplantation genetic testing for aneuploidy (PGT-A) reduces miscarriage and improves live birth rates in recurrent pregnancy loss patients. Fertil Steril. 2019;112(3) Supplement:E401.
13. ESHRE Guideline Group on RPL; Bender Atik R, Christiansen OB, Elson J, Kolte AM, Lewis S, et al. ESHRE guideline: recurrent pregnancy loss. Hum Reprod Open. 2018;2018(2):hoy004.
14. Munné S, Chen S, Fischer J, Colls P, Zheng X, Stevens J. Preimplantation genetic diagnosis reduces pregnancy loss in women aged 35 and older with recurrent miscarriages. Fertil Steril. 2005;84(2):331-5.
15. Mumusoglu S, Telek SB, Ata B. Preimplantation genetic testing for aneuploidy in unexplained recurrent pregnancy loss: a systematic review and meta-analysis. Fertil Steril. 2024:S0015-0282(24)01957-5. PMID: 39151684.
16. Forman EJ, Upham KM, Cheng M, Zhao T, Hong KH, Treff NR, et al. Comprehensive chromosome screening alters traditional morphology-based embryo selection: a prospective study of 100 consecutive cycles of planned fresh euploid blastocyst transfer. Fertil Steril. 2013;100(3):718-24.
17. Lessey BA, Lebovic DI, Taylor RN. Eutopic endometrium in women with endometriosis: ground zero for the study of implantation defects. Semin Reprod Med. 2013;31(2):109-24.
18. Bruner-Tran KL, Herington JL, Duleba AJ, Taylor HS, Osteen KG. Medical management of endometriosis: emerging evidence linking inflammation to disease pathophysiology. Minerva Ginecol. 2013;65(2):199-213.
19. Lessey BA, Castelbaum AJ, Sawin SW, Buck CA, Schinnar R, Bilker W, et al. Aberrant integrin expression in the endometrium of women with endometriosis. J Clin Endocrinol Metab. 1994;79:643-9.
20. Likes CE, Cooper LJ, Efird J, Forstein DA, Miller PB, Savaris R, et al. Medical or surgical treatment before embryo transfer improves outcomes in women with abnormal endometrial BCL6 expression. J Assist Reprod Genet. 2019;36(3):483-90.
21. Simon C, Gomez C, Cabanillas S, Pellicer A, Mol BW, Valbuena D, et al. in vitro fertilization with personalized blastocyst transfer versus fresh or frozen blastocyst transfer: a multicenter randomized clinical trial. Fertil Steril. 2019;112.
22. Ruiz-Alonso M, Blesa D, Díaz-Gimeno P, Gómez E, Fernández-Sánchez M, Carranza F, et al., the endometrial receptivity array for diagnosis and personalized embryo

transfer as a treatment for patients with repeated implantation failure. Fertil Steril. 2013;100(3):818-24.
23. Zariffard MR, Saifuddin M, Sha BE, Spear GT. Detection of bacterial vaginosis-related organisms by real-time PCR for Lactobacilli, Gardnerella vaginalis and Mycoplasma hominis. FEMS Immunol Med Microbiol. 2002;34(4):277-81.
24. Wiesenfeld HC, Hillier SL, Krohn MA, Landers DV, Sweet RL. Bacterial vaginosis is a strong predictor of Neisseria gonorrhoeae and Chlamydia trachomatis infection. Clin Infect Dis. 2003;36(5):663-8.
25. Srinivasan S, Liu C, Mitchell CM, Fiedler TL, Thomas KK, Agnew KJ, et al. Temporal variability of human vaginal bacteria and relationship with bacterial vaginosis. PLoS One. 2010;5(4):e10197.
26. Brotman RM, Bradford LL, Conrad M, Gajer P, Ault K, Peralta L, et al. Association between Trichomonas vaginalis and vaginal bacterial community composition among reproductive-age women. Sex Transm Dis. 2012;39(10):807-12.
27. Moreno I, Codoner FM, Vilella F, Valbuena D, Martinez-Blanch JF, Jiminez-Almazan J, et al. Evidence that the endometrial microbiota has an effect on implantation success or failure. Am J Obstet Gynecol. 2016;215:684-703.
28. Moreno I, Garcia-Grau I, Perez-Villaroya D, Gonzalez-Monfort M, Bahçeci M, Barrionuevo MJ, et al. endometrial microbiota composition is associated with reproductive outcomes in infertile patients. Microbiome. 2022;10(1):1.
29. Punzón-Jiménez P, Labarta E. The impact of the female genital tract microbiome in women health and reproduction: a review. J Assist Reprod Genet. 2021;38(10):2519-41.
30. Garmendia JV, De Sanctis CV, Hajdúch M, De Sanctis JB. Microbiota and recurrent pregnancy loss (RPL); More than a Simple Connection. Microorganisms. 2024;12(8):1641.
31. Van den Borne BE, Dijkmans ba, de Rooij HH, le Cessie S, Verweij CL. Chloroquine and hydroxychloroquine equally affect tumor necrosis factor alpha, IL6, and interferon-gamma production by peripheral blood mononuclear cells. J Rheumatol. 1997;24:55-60.
32. Kwak-Kim J, Gilman-Sachs A. Clinical implication of natural killer cells and reproduction. Am J Reprod Immunol. 2015;73(3):232-40.
33. Kumar A. Immunomodulation in recurrent miscarriage. J Obstet Gynaecol India. 2014;64(3):165-8.
34. Letterie G. Artificial intelligence and assisted reproductive technologies: 2023. Ready for prime time? Or not. Fertil Steril. 2023;120(1);32-7.
35. Guven PG, Cayir Y, Borekci B. Effectiveness of acupuncture on pregnancy success rates for women undergoing in vitro fertilization: a randomized controlled trial. Taiwan J Obstet Gynecol. 2020;59(2):282-6.
36. The ESHRE Guideline Group on RPL, Atik RB, Christiansen OB, Elson J, Kolte AM, Lewis S, et al. ESHRE Guideline on the management of recurrent pregnancy loss. Human Reprod Open. 2023;1:hoad002.

CHAPTER 44

Intravenous Immunoglobulins

Wael Saab, Srividya Seshadri, Wiam Saab

ABSTRACT

Intravenous immunoglobulin (IVIG) is purified immunoglobulin G isolated from whole blood. It is used to treat a variety of medical conditions. It was first used successfully in a patient of Lupus and recurrent pregnancy loss (RPL) in 1988. It is beneficial in cases of refractory antiphospholipid syndrome, RPL with autoimmunity, recurrent implantation failure, and some cases of unexplained euploid pregnancy losses. It is best given prior to embryo transfer in assisted reproductive technology (ART) pregnancies and continued at periodic intervals in the first trimester.

Keywords: Intravenous immunoglobulin, RPL.

INTRODUCTION

Intravenous immunoglobulin (IVIG) is successfully used in many autoimmune conditions. Its use in recurrent pregnancy loss (RPL) is promising especially when RPL is related to autoimmunity. Clear indications for its use in RPL need to be defined by robust evidence which is so far sparse.

HISTORY OF INTRAVENOUS IMMUNOGLOBULIN

Production

Immunoglobulin G (IgG) is procured from a large meticulously screened donor pool encompassing between a 1,000 and 100,000 healthy blood or plasma donors.[1,2] The plasma source is primarily composed of contributions from plasma donors (approximately 80%), with the remaining 20% derived from whole blood donations.[3] The isolation of immunoglobulins from plasma has an unique history, dating back to the development of the fractionation process, known as the "Cohn-Oncley procedure", by Edwin Cohen and colleagues during World War II.[4] IgG isolation techniques have undergone significant advancements over time. Initially, cold alcohol fractionation served as the primary method, followed by additional purification steps to eliminate non-IgG proteins.

To ensure patient safety, most intravenous immunoglobulin (IVIG) preparations undergo a series of treatments designed to inactivate or remove potential bloodborne pathogens.[5] These treatments encompass low pH exposure, fatty acid/alcohol or solvent/detergent combinations, and heat treatment (pasteurization). Additionally, nanofiltration or depth filtration methods are employed to eliminate potential prions.

The final product is a highly purified IgG, typically exceeding 95% purity. However, trace quantities of other proteins, sugars, salts, and stabilizing agents, such as glycine or proline, may be present depending on the manufacturer and their specific purification process.[5] These additives can influence the in vivo tolerance of the preparation.

The World Health Organization (WHO) has established some standards for the manufacturing of IVIG preparations.[6,7] These guidelines stipulate that IVIG be sourced from a large donor pool (at least 1,000 individuals), exhibit minimal IgA content, be devoid of preservatives or stabilizers with the potential for in vivo accumulation, and undergo minimal biochemical modifications while retaining opsonizing and complement-fixing activities.

Modern technological advancements and meticulous formulation strategies employed in IVIG preparation ensure improved in vivo tolerance, reduced side effects, particularly regarding infectious agent transmission, and ultimately contribute to enhanced patient recovery.[8]

CLINICAL APPLICATIONS OF INTRAVENOUS IMMUNOGLOBULIN

Intravenous immunoglobulin serves as a cornerstone therapy for both primary and secondary immunodeficiency states. Its efficacy extends to a broad spectrum

BOX 1: Intravenous immunoglobulin (IVIG) use in the treatment of primary and secondary immune deficiency states and a variety of autoimmune and inflammatory disorders.

Immunodeficiency states:
- Primary (congenital/hereditary) immunodeficiencies
- Severe protein loss (e.g., through malnutrition or gastrointestinal or renal losses)
- Post-hematopoietic cell transplantation (HCT)
- Chronic lymphocytic leukemia (CLL)
- Multiple myeloma
- Therapies that suppress immunoglobulin production

Infections:
- CLL with recurrent infections requiring intravenous antibiotics or hospitalization
- Chronic parvovirus infection complicated by anemia
- Relapsing or severe *Clostridioides* (formerly *Clostridium*) *difficile* infection
- Toxic shock syndrome
- Measles post-exposure prophylaxis (if the patient is immunocompromised or nonimmune)
- Some enteroviral infections

Autoimmune/inflammatory conditions:
- Immune thrombocytopenia (ITP)
- Neonatal alloimmune thrombocytopenia
- Acquired von Willebrand disease (vWD) in the setting of lymphoproliferative or other immunologic disorders
- Autoimmune hemolytic anemia (AIHA)
- Autoimmune neutropenia
- Acquired factor VIII inhibitor
- Guillain-Barré syndrome
- Myasthenia gravis
- Kawasaki disease
- Chronic inflammatory demyelinating polyneuropathy (CIDP)
- Multifocal motor neuropathy
- Some HIV-associated neuropathies

Alloimmune processes:
- Hemolytic disease of the fetus and newborn (HDFN)
- Post-transfusion purpura
- Platelet alloimmunization with bleeding (as a temporizing measure) antibody-mediated organ transplant rejection)
- Hyperhemolytic crisis (a form of delayed hemolytic transfusion reaction) in individuals with sickle cell disease (SCD)

of autoimmune and inflammatory disorders, as detailed in **Box 1**. However, national guidelines for IVIG use exhibit some variations.

The National Health Service (NHS) in the United Kingdom advocates for IVIG in various immunodeficiencies but advises against its use for sepsis (except in cases with identified specific toxins), multiple sclerosis, neonatal sepsis, and pediatric human immunodeficiency virus (HIV).[9] Conversely, the American Academy of Allergy, Asthma, and Immunology acknowledges that primary immunodeficiency represents a minority of IVIG applications.[10] The academy emphasizes the appropriateness of IVIG for other conditions, citing a six-fold mortality reduction in neonatal sepsis and its utility in both adult and pediatric HIV cases. Additionally, it considers IVIG as a potential second-line therapy for relapsing-remitting multiple sclerosis.[10]

Beyond these established applications, global clinical practice frequently utilizes IVIG for diverse autoimmune and alloimmune conditions, including women experiencing recurrent implantation failure (RIF) or RPL. However, the academy discourages its use in chronic fatigue syndrome and pediatric autoimmune neuropsychiatric disorders associated with streptococcal infection (PANDAS).[11]

MECHANISM OF ACTION

Intravenous immunoglobulin exhibits both anti-inflammatory and pro-inflammatory effects.[12] Its immunomodulatory actions are mediated through various mechanisms, including F(ab')2-, Fc-, and SIGNR1-dependent pathways, among others. F(ab')2-dependent mechanisms include preventing target cell depletion by antibody-dependent cytotoxicity of monocytes and natural killer (NK) cells, interfering with cellular interactions via receptors such as Fas/Fas ligand (CD95L) on lymphocytes and monocytes, neutralizing cytokines and autoantibodies, and eliminating anaphylatoxins such as C3a and C5a.[13] Fc-dependent mechanisms involve competing for the neonatal Fc receptor, expanding and activating natural regulatory T cells,[14-16] limiting immune complex binding to activating Fcγ receptors (FcγRs), regulating dendritic cell activation, modulating innate immune effector cells, and inducing B cell apoptosis.[13,17] The SIGNR1-dependent mechanism occurs on macrophages, where IVIG upregulates inhibitory FcγRs, downregulates activating FcγRs, and ultimately induces anti-inflammatory effects[13] FcγRs are expressed on most innate immune cells, including basophils, eosinophils, neutrophils, mast cells, monocytes, macrophages, dendritic cells, and B cells. Additional immunological functions of IVIG include inducing T cell apoptosis,[18] suppressing T-cell priming,[19] decreasing NK cell levels and cytotoxicity,[20] inhibiting B cell autoantibody production,[21] binding to $CD5^+$ B cells,[22] and altering Th1/Th2 gene expression towards a Th2 pattern.[23] In women with RPL, IVIG has been shown to suppress Th1/Th2 and Th17/Treg cell ratios. Interestingly, in women with the lowest quartile of Th17/Treg cell ratios, IVIG normalized the ratio.[24] This demonstrates that IVIG functions as an immunomodulant rather than a simple immunosuppressant.

IMMUNE ASPECT OF RECURRENT PREGNANCY LOSS

Recurrent pregnancy loss is defined as two or more pregnancy losses.[25,26] It is categorized as primary RPL, referring to a series of pregnancy losses without a previous birth, and secondary RPL, indicating pregnancy losses following a previous live birth or stillbirth. Embryonic aneuploidy is considered a major cause of RPL, accounting for 55% of primary RPL and 35% of secondary RPL.[27] The incidence of RPL is reported to be 0.05% among reproductive-age women (18–42 years old) and 0.65% among women who became pregnant during the same period.[28] Despite these statistics, progress in developing diagnostic approaches to uncover underlying etiologies has been slow, leading to the empirical use of multiple treatment regimens. Immune abnormalities, including cellular and autoimmune disorders, have been associated with RPL, RIF, intrauterine embryonic death (IUE), and other obstetrical complications such as preeclampsia.[29] Studies have shown that women experiencing recurrent reproductive failures often exhibit dysregulated cellular immunity, including increased NK cell levels and cytotoxicity, propensities to T helper (Th)1 over Th2, and Th17 over regulatory T (Treg) immunities.[30,31] Approximately 30.5% of women with RPL have elevated NK cell levels, 31.6% have abnormal NK cell cytotoxicity, and 34.7% have shifted Th1/Th2 cell ratios.[30] Autoimmune abnormalities such as antiphospholipid antibody syndrome (APS) and autoimmune thyroiditis have also been linked to reproductive failures.[32,33] The prevalence of antiphospholipid antibodies (APAs) is estimated to be up to 20% in women with RPL and 30% in women with RIF.[34] Given these findings, immunomodulatory treatments for cellular and autoimmune abnormalities may improve reproductive outcomes in women with immune-related reproductive failures. The first reported case of treatment for RPL was by Carreras et al.,[35] where a woman with nine RPLs successfully delivered a live-born infant after IVIG treatment. Subsequently, additional cases of successful IVIG treatment in women with RPL and various complications were reported.[36] Since then, numerous IVIG clinical trials have been conducted in women with RPL, and its application has expanded to other reproductive failures. As per ESHRE 2022 recommendations, administering repeated high doses of IVIG very early in pregnancy might enhance the live birth rate (LBR) for women experiencing four or more cases of unexplained RPL.

META-ANALYSES OF INTRAVENOUS IMMUNOGLOBULIN FOR RECURRENT PREGNANCY LOSS

Nine randomized placebo-controlled trials and five randomized treatment as usual controlled trials (RCTs) investigating IVIG efficacy in women with RPL have been published with conflicting results.[37] A 2014 Cochrane systematic review with meta-analysis found no significant beneficial effect of IVIG over placebo in improving the LBR after RPL.[37] Egerup et al.'s systematic review of 11 RCTs showed no significant difference in the no LBR with IVIG in RPL compared with placebo or treatment as usual (RR 0.92, 95% CI 0.75–1.12, $p = 0.42$).[38] Wang et al.'s meta-analysis of 11 studies showed a marginally significant difference in LBR between IVIG treatment and placebo groups with unexplained RPL (RR =1.25, 95% CI 1.00 to 1.56, $p = 0.05$).[39] Achilli et al.'s meta-analysis including seven RCTs concluded no role for immunotherapy in improving LBR in women undergoing IVF treatment or in preventing idiopathic RPL.[40] The most recent meta-analysis by Christiansen et al., including 13 studies, demonstrated a significant difference in LBR with IVIG treatment using the fixed-effect method (RR 1.20, 95% CI 1.0–1.37, $p = 0.004$), but not with the random-effects model (RR 1.17, 95% CI 0.95–1.44, $p = 0.14$).[41] Sensitivity analyses showed that preconception IVIG treatment significantly increased LBR (RR 1.69, 95% CI 1.33–2.14, $p < 0.0001$), and a borderline significant therapeutic effect was noticed in secondary aborters (RR 1.24, 95% CI 0.96–1.59, $p = 0.06$).[41] Higher dose and presence of autoimmunity tended to increase the success rate after IVIG treatment.[41-42] These factors should be considered for patient selection and IVIG treatment planning. **Table 1** lists the meta-analysis published so far on IVIG.

EFFICACY OF INTRAVENOUS IMMUNOGLOBULIN IN RECURRENT PREGNANCY LOSS WITH IMMUNE ABNORMALITIES

The effectiveness of IVIG therapy is influenced by the timing of administration and patient-specific factors, such as idiopathic versus immune etiologies. Clark et al. found that idiopathic (immune test-negative) controls

TABLE 1: Meta-analysis summary for intravenous immunoglobulin (IVIG) and recurrent pregnancy loss.

No.	Year author country	No. of studies included	Type of studies included	Outcomes	Event/total		Risk ratio (95% CI)	Overall p-value
					Experiment	Control		
1.	2020 Woon et al. UK	3	2 prospective + 1 retrospective cohort studies	LBR	140/152	35/91	2.31 (1.66, 3.21)	<0.00001
				Miscarriage rate	12/152	56/91	0.15 (0.06, 0.37)	<0.00001
2.	2019 Christiansen et al. Denmark	13	RCT	LBR	219/325	173/312	1.20 (1.0, 1.37) *Fixed effects method*	0.004
				LBR	219/325	173/312	1.17 (0.95, 1.44) *Random-effects method*	0.14
3.	2018 Achilli et al. UK	2	RCT	Primary RPL pre-ovulatory IVIG LBR	29/79	21/78	1.56 (0.79, 3.09)	0.20
		3	RCT	Primary RPL post-conception IVIG LBR	46/60	49/63	0.92 (0.39, 2.17)	0.85
		3	RCT	Secondary RPL	40/70	32/67	1.45 (0.73, 2.90)	0.29
4.	2016 Wang et al. China	11	RCT	Total LBR	202/297	151/285	1.25 (1.00, 1.56)	0.05
				Primary RPL LBR	57/93	63/90	0.88 (0.71, 1.07)	0.20
				Secondary RPL LBR	69/112	53/108	1.26 (0.99, 1.61)	0.06
				Primary + Secondary RPL LBR	126/205	116/198	1.05 (0.90, 1.23)	0.53 (0.02)
				Preconception IVIG LBR	80/107	47/106	1.67 (1.3, 2.14)	<0.0001
				Post-implantation IVIG LBR	122/190	104/179	1.10 (0.93, 1.29)	0.27
				Preconception + Post-implantation IVIG LBR	202/297	151/285	1.27 (1.11, 1.46)	0.0005 (0.005)
5.	2015 Egerup et al. Denmark	11	RCT	Total no LBR	107/265	113/266	0.92 (0.75, 1.12)	0.42
				Primary RPL no LBR	35/91	23/90	1.32 (0.88, 1.98)	0.18
				Secondary RPL no LBR	46/111	58/110	0.77 (0.58, 1.02)	0.06
				Primary + Secondary RPL no LBR	81/202	83/200	0.91 (0.73, 1.15)	0.44 (0.03)

Contd...

Contd...

No.	Year author country	No. of studies included	Type of studies included	Outcomes	Event/total		Risk ratio (95% CI)	Overall p-value
					Experiment	Control		
6.	2011 Ata et al. Canada	6	RCT	Total LBR	107/139	133/266	0.92 (0.55, 1.54)	Z = 0.3
				Primary RPL LBR	49/74	54/73	0.67 (0.32, 1.39)	Z = 1.08
				Secondary RPL LBR	29/44	26/41	1.15 (0.47, 2.84)	Z = 0.31
				Preconception LBR	35/62	31/59	1.21 (0.58, 2.51)	Z = 0.51
				Postconception LBR	53/77	56/74	0.71 (0.34, 1.47)	Z = 0.93
7.	2007 Hutton et al. Canada	7	RCT	Total LBR	105/172	95/173	1.28 (0.78, 2.1)	0.33
				Primary RPL LBR	57/93	63/90	0.66 (0.35, 1.26)	0.21
				Secondary RPL LBR	30/47	17/44	2.71 (1.09, 6.73)	0.03
				Preconception LBR	30/49	21/53	2.39 (1.08, 5.33)	0.03
				Postconception LBR	75/123	72/130	0.96 (0.55, 1.65)	0.87
				Primary RPL, Preconception LBR	5/10	4/10	1.50 (0.26, 8.82)	0.65
				Primary RPL, Postconception LBR	52/83	59/80	0.58 (0.29, 1.16)	0.94
				Secondary RPL, Preconception LBR	7/10	6/11	1.94 (0.32, 11.76)	0.47
				Secondary RPL, Postconception LBR	23/37	12/33	3.04 (1.06, 8.73)	0.04
8.	2006 Practice Committee ASRM USA	5	RCT	Primary RPL LBR	75/121	56/125	0.98 (0.45, 2.13)	
				Secondary RPL LBR			2.19 (0.65, 7.39)	
9.	1999 Daya et al. Canada	6	RCT	Successful pregnancy (progressed to at least 20 WOG)	78/125	71/115	1.08 (0.63, 1.86)	0.43
				LBR	76/125	68/115	1.14 (0.66, 1.95)	0.60
10.	1998 Daya et al. Canada	4	RCT	LBR	57/99	47/99	1.48 (0.84, 2.60)	0.17

had significantly higher success rates than immune test-positive controls (62.2% vs. 21.7%, $p < 0.005$). IVIG treatment significantly improved success rates in immune test-positive patients compared to controls (57.6% vs. 21.7%, $p < 0.05$).[43] A meta-analysis of nonrandomized controlled trials on IVIG in women with elevated NK cell levels showed a LBR favoring the intervention (RR 2.57, 95% CI 1.79–3.69, $p < 0.05$),[44] suggesting potential benefits of immunotherapy despite significant heterogeneity ($I^2 = 62\%$).

Intravenous immunoglobulin has also been used in patients with RPL and autoantibodies. In Jeremic et al.'s trial with 40 RPL women with positive APA,[45] half received aspirin plus heparin, and the other half received IVIG, aspirin, and heparin. There was no significant difference in gestational success rates between the groups (85% vs. 90%; $p > 0.05$), but fewer obstetrical complications were observed in the IVIG group. In contrast, a trial by Dendrinos et al. found that low-molecular-weight heparin (LMWH) plus low-dose aspirin (LDA) had a higher LBR than IVIG in 85 RPL women with APS (72.5% vs. 39.5%; $p = 0.007$). Triolo et al. found similar results, with LMWH plus LDA having a marginally higher LBR than IVIG (84% vs. 57%; $p = 0.06$). These studies indicate that heparin and aspirin treatment is at least as effective as IVIG in RPL patients with APS, noting the lack of blinding in these trials.

Nyborg et al. studied 52 women with RPL following IVF/ICSI treatment who received IVIG and prednisone. The cumulative LBR was 61.5%, suggesting a promising treatment for RPL post-assisted reproductive therapies.[46] Patients with positive autoantibody tests had a 40.6% LBR compared to 59.4% in autoantibody-negative patients ($p = 0.44$), showing effectiveness in both groups.[46]

Tenti et al.'s review on IVIG in APS reported benefits in selected cases such as conventional treatment failure, anticoagulation contraindications, and concurrent autoimmune manifestations or infections.[47] IVIG is crucial in combination therapy for catastrophic antiphospholipid syndrome (CAPS).[47-49] Further studies are needed to identify which subgroups of autoantibodies in RPL patients benefit most from IVIG therapy.

Elevated NK cell counts and cytotoxicity are linked with RPL. IVIG therapy reduces NK cell-related parameters,[50] improving LBR.[51] Kwak et al. reported that 86.3% of women with elevated NK cell counts had successful pregnancies after IVIG and anticoagulation treatment.[51] Spanish cohort studies also showed increased pregnancy rates and LB with IVIG use in RPL patients with elevated NK cell levels.[52-53] Lee et al. demonstrated higher LBRs in idiopathic RPL cases with cellular immune abnormalities treated with IVIG (82% vs. 42%).[54] Additionally, altered T-cell immunity, including elevated Th1/Th2 cell ratios, increased Th17 cells, and suppressed Tregs, is implicated in RPL9, 12, 13. IVIG treatment significantly decreased $CD3^+$ $CD16^+$ $CD56^+$ NKT and $CD4^+$ $CD25^+$ T cell frequencies, with varying in vitro suppression of NK cell activity by different IVIG sources.[55]

PROTOCOL FOR INTRAVENOUS IMMUNOGLOBULIN TREATMENT IN WOMEN WITH RECURRENT IMPLANTATION FAILURE AND RECURRENT PREGNANCY LOSS

Currently, there is no standardized protocol for the optimal dosage or frequency of IVIG administration in women with RIF and RPL. Most studies have administered IVIG at 1- to 4-week intervals. Given the IgG half-life of 21–25 days in healthy individuals and 17.7–37.6 days in immunodeficient patients,[56] the maximum interval should not exceed 3–4 weeks. The Korean Society of Reproductive Immunology recommends IVIG administration at 400 mg/kg every 3–4 weeks, starting from early pregnancy for RPL patients or at the beginning of the in vitro fertilization cycle for RIF patients.[57] While one group has reported using massive IVIG therapy (100 g over 5 days after gestational sac detection),[58] additional data are needed to confirm its efficacy and safety during pregnancy.

Recent meta-analyses have shown significantly increased LBRs with preconceptional IVIG treatment[41] suggesting that this approach should be considered for women with reproductive failure of immune etiology. Advances in laboratory testing now allow for personalized treatment based on individual laboratory, radiological, and clinical findings. For example, IVIG dosage and interval can be tailored and adjusted according to baseline NK cell levels and cytotoxicities, Th1/Th2 ratios, and autoimmune status, with subsequent monitoring. This personalized approach may help reduce unnecessary medication during conception cycles and pregnancy.

The decision-making process regarding treatment intervals, when to discontinue treatment, and the selection of follow-up laboratory tests is left to the clinician's discretion. This allows for monitoring of IVIG's effectiveness in controlling immune pathology and the patient's clinical progress. Such a personalized approach aims to optimize treatment outcomes while minimizing potential risks and unnecessary interventions.

SIDE EFFECTS OF INTRAVENOUS IMMUNOGLOBULIN

Side effects of IVIG treatment include adverse reactions in 20–50% of recipients, though severe side effects are rare. Common reactions include headache, fever, and rash. Severe adverse events, such as hospitalization due to infusion-related symptoms, premature rupture of membranes before 28 weeks gestation, and cesarean section rates, are comparable to placebo. Risk factors for reactions include hyperviscosity states, organ dysfunction, and prothrombotic stimuli.

Adverse reactions are most likely during the first infusion and depend on the dose and infusion rate. Mitigation strategies include ensuring adequate hydration, treating pre-existing infections, starting with a low infusion rate, and maintaining a consistent IVIG brand. Anaphylactic reactions, though very rare, can occur in IgA-deficient patients. Renal insufficiency, potentially caused by sugar stabilizers in high-dose treatments, requires monitoring of renal function tests.

There is a theoretical risk of transmitting infectious agents, but this is extremely unlikely. IVIG can cause transient abnormalities in laboratory blood tests, including false-positive results for certain autoantibodies. No significant side effects have been reported in mothers or babies exposed to IVIG prior to conception and during pregnancy.

CONCLUSION

Intravenous immunoglobulin shows promise for patients with RIF and RPL, particularly those with immune abnormalities such as elevated natural killer cell levels and cytotoxicity, shifted Th1/Th2 cell ratios, and positive autoantibodies. Preconception treatment appears more effective than postconception treatment. Recent meta-analyses generally support IVIG treatment, though significant heterogeneity in study populations limits strong recommendations.

The impact of embryonic aneuploidies on pregnancy outcomes should not be overlooked, as they may contribute significantly to implantation failures and miscarriages. IVIG treatment for RPL and RIF currently has Level II evidence for medical application, based on meta-analyses of randomized controlled trials.

Further large randomized controlled trials are needed to identify which subcategories of patients benefit most from IVIG treatment. Additional studies are also required to establish optimal timing for infusions and to refine treatment protocols.

REFERENCES

1. Durandy A, Kaveri SV, Kuijpers TW, Basta M, Miescher S, Ravetch JV, et al. Intravenous immunoglobulins–understanding properties and mechanisms. Clin Exp Immunol. 2009;158(Suppl 1):2-13.
2. World Health Organization. (2004). WHO Guidelines on viral inactivation and removal procedures intended to assure the viral safety of human blood plasma products. [online] Available from https://www.who.int/publications/m/item/WHO-TRS924-Annex4. [Last accessed December, 2024].
3. Knezevic-Maramica I, Kruskall MS. Intravenous immune globulins: an update for clinicians. Transfusion. 2003;43(10):1460-80.
4. Cohn EJ, Strong LE, et al. Preparation and properties of serum and plasma proteins; a system for the separation into fractions of the protein and lipoprotein components of biological tissues and fluids. J Am Chem Soc. 1946;68:459-75.
5. Prins C, Gelfand EW, French LE. Intravenous immunoglobulin: properties, mode of action and practical use in dermatology. Acta Derm Venereol. 2007;87(3):206-18.
6. Bulletin of the World Health Organization. Appropriate uses of human immunoglobulin in clinical practice: memorandum from an IUIS/WHO meeting. Bull World Health Organ. 1982;60(1):43-7.
7. World Health Organization. (1994). Requirements for the collection, processing, and quality control of blood, blood components, and plasma derivatives. [online] Available from https://www.who.int/bloodproducts/publications/WHO_TRS_840_A2.pdf. [Last accessed December, 2024].
8. Radosevich M, Burnouf T. Intravenous immunoglobulin G: trends in production methods, quality control and quality assurance. Vox Sang. 2010;98(1):12-28.
9. National Health Service. (2011). Clinical guidelines for immunoglobulin use (second edition update). [online] Available from https://assets.publishing.service.gov.uk/government/uploads/system/uploads/attachment_data/file/216671/dh_131107.pdf. [Last accessed December, 2024].
10. American Academy of Allergy Asthma and Immunology. (2011). Eight Guiding Principles for Effective Use of IVIG for Patients with Primary Immunodeficiency. [online] Available from https://www.aaaai.org/Aaaai/media/MediaLibrary/PDF%20Documents/Practice%20Resources/IVIG-guiding-principles.pdf. [Last accessed December, 2024].
11. Orange J, Hossny E, Weiler C, Ballow M, Berger M, Bonilla FA, et al. Use of intravenous immunoglobulin in human

disease: a review of evidence by members of the Primary Immunodeficiency Committee of the American Academy of Allergy, Asthma and Immunology. J Allergy Clin Immunol. 2006;117(4 Suppl): S525-53.

12. Ermakov EA, Nevinsky GA, Buneva VN. Immunoglobulins with non-canonical functions in inflammatory and autoimmune disease states. Int J Mol Sci. 2020;21(15):5392.
13. Schwab I, Nimmerjahn F. Intravenous immunoglobulin therapy: how does IgG modulate the immune system? Nat Rev Immunol. 2013;13(3):176-89.
14. De Groot AS, Moise L, McMurry JA, Wambre E, Van Overtvelt L, Moingeon P, et al. Activation of natural regulatory T cells by IgG Fc-derived peptide "Tregitopes". Blood. 2008;112(8):3303-11.
15. Ephrem A, Chamat S, Miquel C, Fisson S, Mouthon L, Caligiuri G, et al. Expansion of CD4+CD25+ regulatory T cells by intravenous immunoglobulin: a critical factor in controlling experimental autoimmune encephalomyelitis. Blood. 2008;111(2):715-22.
16. Kessel A, Ammuri H, Peri R, Pavlotzky ER, Blank M, Shoenfeld Y, et al. Intravenous immunoglobulin therapy affects T regulatory cells by increasing their suppressive function. J Immunol. 2007;179(8):5571-75.
17. Seite JF, Cornec D, Renaudineau Y, Youinou P, Mageed RA, Hillion S. IVIg modulates BCR signaling through CD22 and promotes apoptosis in mature human B lymphocytes. Blood. 2010;116(10):1698-1704.
18. Prasad NK, Papoff G, Zeuner A, Bonnin E, Kazatchkine MD, Ruberti G, et al. Therapeutic preparations of normal polyspecific IgG (IVIg) induce apoptosis in human lymphocytes and monocytes: a novel mechanism of action of IVIg involving the Fas apoptotic pathway. J Immunol. 1998;161(7):3781-90.
19. Tha-In T, Metselaar HJ, Tilanus HW, et al. Intravenous immunoglobulins suppress T-cell priming by modulating the bidirectional interaction between dendritic cells and natural killer cells. Blood. 2007;110(9):3253-62.
20. Jacobi C, Claus M, Wildemann B, Wingert S, Korporal M, Römisch J, et al. Exposure of NK cells to intravenous immunoglobulin induces IFN gamma release and degranulation but inhibits their cytotoxic activity. Clin Immunol. 2009;133(3):393-401.
21. Tsubakio T, Kurata Y, Katagiri S, Kanakura Y, Tamaki T, Kuyama J, et al. Alteration of T cell subsets and immunoglobulin synthesis in vitro during high dose gamma-globulin therapy in patients with idiopathic thrombocytopenic purpura. Clin Exp Immunol. 1983;53(3):697-702.
22. Vassilev T, Gelin C, Kaveri SV, Zilber MT, Boumsell L, Kazatchkine MD. Antibodies to the CD5 molecule in normal human immunoglobulins for therapeutic use (intravenous immunoglobulins, IVIg). Clin Exp Immunol. 1993;92(3):369-72.
23. Mouzaki A, Theodoropoulou M, Gianakopoulos I, Vlaha V, Kyrtsonis MC, Maniatis A. Expression patterns of Th1 and Th2 cytokine genes in childhood idiopathic thrombocytopenic purpura (ITP) at presentation and their modulation by intravenous immunoglobulin G (IVIg) treatment: their role in prognosis. Blood. 2002;100(5):1774-9.
24. Kim DJ, Lee SK, Kim JY, Na BJ, Hur SE, Lee M, et al. Intravenous immunoglobulin G modulates peripheral blood Th17 and Foxp3(+) regulatory T cells in pregnant women with recurrent pregnancy loss. Am J Reprod Immunol. 2014;71(5):441-50.
25. ESHRE Guideline Group on RPL; Bender Atik R, Christiansen OB, Elson J, Kolte AM, Lewis S, et al. ESHRE guideline: recurrent pregnancy loss. Hum Reprod Open. 2018;2018(2):hoy004.
26. Practice Committee of the American Society for Reproductive Medicine. Definitions of infertility and recurrent pregnancy loss: a committee opinion. Fertil Steril. 2013;99(1):63.
27. Coulam CB, Stephenson M, Stern JJ, Clark DA. Immunotherapy for recurrent pregnancy loss: analysis of results from clinical trials. Am J Reprod Immunol. 1996;35(4):352-9.
28. Rasmark Roepke E, Matthiesen L, Rylance R, Christiansen OB. Is the incidence of recurrent pregnancy loss increasing? A retrospective register-based study in Sweden. Acta Obstet Gynecol Scand. 2017;96(11):1365-72.
29. Aoki K, Kajiura S, Matsumoto Y, Ogasawara M, Okada S, Yagami Y, et al. Preconceptional natural-killer-cell activity as a predictor of miscarriage. Lancet. 1995; 345(8961):1340-42.
30. Lee SK, Na BJ, Kim JY, Hur SE, Lee M, Gilman-Sachs A, et al. Determination of clinical cellular immune markers in women with recurrent pregnancy loss. Am J Reprod Immunol. 2013;70(5):398-411.
31. Lee SK, Kim JY, Hur SE, Kim CJ, Na BJ, Lee M, et al. An imbalance in interleukin-17-producing T and Foxp3(+) regulatory T cells in women with idiopathic recurrent pregnancy loss. Hum Reprod. 2011;26(11):2964-71.
32. Kim NY, Cho HJ, Kim HY, Yang KM, Ahn HK, Thornton S, et al. Thyroid autoimmunity and its association with cellular and humoral immunity in women with reproductive failures. Am J Reprod Immunol. 2011;65(1):78-87.
33. Jaslow CR, Carney JL, Kutteh WH. Diagnostic factors identified in 1020 women with two versus three or more recurrent pregnancy losses. Fertil Steril. 2010;93(4):1234-43.
34. Buckingham KL, Chamley LW. A critical assessment of the role of antiphospholipid antibodies in infertility. J Reprod Immunol. 2009;80(1-2):132-45.
35. Carreras LD, Perez GN, Vega HR, Casavilla F. Lupus anticoagulant and recurrent fetal loss: successful treatment with gammaglobulin. Lancet. 1988;2(8607):393-94.
36. Scott JR, Branch DW, Kochenour NK, Ward K. Intravenous immunoglobulin treatment of pregnant patients with recurrent pregnancy loss caused by antiphospholipid

antibodies and Rh immunization. Am J Obstet Gynecol. 1988;159(5):1055-6.

37. Group TGRI. Intravenous immunoglobulin in the prevention of recurrent miscarriage. The German RSA/IVIG Group. Br J Obstet Gynaecol. 1994;101(12):1072-7.
38. Egerup P, Lindschou J, Gluud C, Christiansen OB, ImmuReM IPD Study Group. The Effects of intravenous immunoglobulins in women with recurrent miscarriages: a systematic review of randomised trials with meta-analyses and trial sequential analyses including individual patient data. PLoS One. 2015;10(10):e0141588.
39. Wang SW, Zhong SY, Lou LJ, Hu ZF, Sun HY, Zhu HY. The effect of intravenous immunoglobulin passive immunotherapy on unexplained recurrent spontaneous abortion: a meta-analysis. Reprod Biomed Online. 2016;33(6): 720-36.
40. Achilli C, Duran-Retamal M, Saab W, Serhal P, Seshadri S. The role of immunotherapy in in vitro fertilization and recurrent pregnancy loss: a systematic review and meta-analysis. Fertil Steril. 2018;110(6):1089-1100.
41. Christiansen OB, Kolte AM, Krog MC, Nielsen HS, Egerup P. Treatment with intravenous immunoglobulin in patients with recurrent pregnancy loss: an update. J Reprod Immunol. 2019;133:37-42.
42. Higgins J, Thomas J, Chandler J, Cumpston M, Tianjing Li, Page MJ, et al. Cochrane Handbook for Systematic Reviews of Interventions version 6.1 (updated September 2020). Cochrane. 2020.
43. Clark DA. The power of observation. Am J Reprod Immunol. 2011;66(2):71-5.
44. Woon EV, Day A, Bracewell-Milnes T, Male V, Johnson M. Immunotherapy to improve pregnancy outcome in women with abnormal natural killer cell levels/activity and recurrent miscarriage or implantation failure: a systematic review and meta-analysis. J Reprod Immunol. 2020;142:103189.
45. Jeremic K, Pervulov M, Gojnic M, Dukanac J, Ljubic A, Stojnic J. Comparison of two therapeutic protocols in patients with antiphospholipid antibodies and recurrent miscarriages. Vojnosanit Pregl. 2005;62(6):435-9.
46. Nyborg KM, Kolte AM, Larsen EC, Christiansen OB. Immunomodulatory treatment with intravenous immunoglobulin and prednisone in patients with recurrent miscarriage and implantation failure after in vitro fertilization/intracytoplasmic sperm injection. Fertil Steril, 2014;102(6):1650-5.e1.
47. Tenti S, Cheleschi S, Guidelli GM, Galeazzi M, Fioravanti A. Intravenous immunoglobulins and antiphospholipid syndrome: How, when and why? A review of the literature. Autoimmun Rev. 2016;15(3):226-35.
48. Kwak JY, Beaman KD, Gilman-Sachs A, Ruiz JE, Schewitz D, Beer AE. Up-regulated expression of CD56+, CD56+/CD16+, and CD19+ cells in peripheral blood lymphocytes in pregnant women with recurrent pregnancy losses. Am J Reprod Immunol. 1995;34(2):93-9.
49. Roussev RG, Ng SC, Coulam CB. Natural killer cell functional activity suppression by intravenous immunoglobulin, intralipid and soluble human leukocyte antigen-G. Am J Reprod Immunol. 2007;57(4):262-9.
50. Heilmann L, Schorsch M, Hahn T. CD3-CD56+CD16+ natural killer cells and improvement of pregnancy outcome in IVF/ICSI failure after additional IVIG-treatment. Am J Reprod Immunol. 2010;63(3):263-5.
51. Kwak JY, Kwak FM, Ainbinder SW, Ruiz AM, Beer AE. Elevated peripheral blood natural killer cells are effectively downregulated by immunoglobulin G infusion in women with recurrent spontaneous abortions. Am J Reprod Immunol. 1996;35(4):363-9.
52. Ramos-Medina R, García-Segovia A, Gil J, Carbone J, Aguarón de la Cruz A, Seyfferth A, et al. Experience in IVIg therapy for selected women with recurrent reproductive failure and NK cell expansion. Am J Reprod Immunol. 2014;71(5):458-66.
53. Moraru M, Carbone J, Alecsandru D, Castillo-Rama M, García-Segovia A, Gil J, et al. Intravenous immunoglobulin treatment increased live birth rate in a Spanish cohort of women with recurrent reproductive failure and expanded CD56(+) cells. Am J Reprod Immunol. 2012;68(1):75-84.
54. Lee SK, Kim JY, Han AR, Hur SE, Kim CJ, Kim TH, et al. Intravenous immunoglobulin G improves pregnancy outcome in women with recurrent pregnancy losses with cellular immune abnormalities. Am J Reprod Immunol. 2016;75(1):59-68.
55. Clark DA, Coulam CB, Stricker RB. Is intravenous immunoglobulins (IVIG) efficacious in early pregnancy failure? A critical review and meta-analysis for patients who fail in vitro fertilization and embryo transfer (IVF). J Assist Reprod Genet. 2006;23(1):1-13.
56. Baxter HealthCare Corp. (2019). Gammagard Liquid. [online] Available from https://www.fda.gov/media/78185/download. [Last accessed December, 2024].
57. Sung N, Han AR, Park CW, Park DW, Park JC, Kim NY, et al. Intravenous immunoglobulin G in women with reproductive failure: The Korean Society for Reproductive Immunology practice guidelines. Clin Exp Reprod Med. 2017;44(1):1-7.
58. Yamada H, Takeda M, Maezawa Y, Ebina Y, Hazama R, Tanimura K, et al. A high dose intravenous immunoglobulin therapy for women with four or more recurrent spontaneous abortions. ISRN Obstet Gynecol. 2012;2012:512732.

CHAPTER 45

Evidence for Intravenous Immunoglobulin Use in Recurrent Pregnancy Loss

Ole Bjarne Christiansen

ABSTRACT

Intravenous immunoglobulins (IVIG) are most comprehensively studied in the setting of autoimmunity and recurrent pregnancy loss (RPL). Several studies have measured the immunological markers like Th17, Natural killer (NK) cells and T regulatory (Treg) cells before and after IVIG administration and confirmed that these markers improved. Current evidence suggests that women with high number of euploid secondary miscarriages should be treated with preconception IVIG and this should be followed up during pregnancy with high dose IVIG i.e., 0.4 g/kg body weight given every 3 weeks. IVIG is more effective in women with a higher number of previous miscarriages and those with positive biomarkers for autoimmunity e.g., high uterine natural killer cell count.

Keywords: Intravenous immunoglobulins, IVIG, RPL, Secondary miscarriages, Natural Killer cells.

INTRODUCTION

Recurrent pregnancy loss (RPL) has traditionally been defined as three or more consecutive pregnancy losses (miscarriages before gestational week 23 and biochemical pregnancies) and this definition is still supported by some specialist societies; whereas, other societies of reproductive medicine define RPL as two or more pregnancy losses.[1-4] RPL affects 1–5% of all women trying to conceive depending on the definition. Primary RPL refers to a series of pregnancy losses without a previous birth whereas secondary RPL is defined as a series of pregnancy losses subsequent to a previous live birth or stillbirth. In some patients, the condition is associated with parental chromosomal abnormalities, uterine malformations, and endocrine, infectious, or thrombophilic disturbances. Sometimes the condition can be explained by repeated de novo chromosomal abnormalities, which have occurred in the embryos.

Immunological disturbances are hypothesized to play an important role in RPL. This is supported by animal studies, e.g., finding natural killer (NK) cells or T regulatory (Treg) cells in the uterus being of importance for implantation and fetal growth.[5,6] In humans, many immunological biomarkers can be found with increased prevalence in women with RPL and display a negative prognostic impact.[7-10] However, the exact pathophysiological mechanisms behind immune disturbances and RPL are still unclear.

Various types of immune-based therapies have been tested in women experiencing RPL including glucocorticoids, allogeneic lymphocyte immunization, hydroxychloroquine, tacrolimus, and intravenous immunoglobulin (IVIG).[11-16] In this review, the focus will be on IVIG since, in my view, it is the most comprehensively tested immunomodulatory intervention in RPL.

INTRAVENOUS IMMUNOGLOBULIN

Intravenous immunoglobulin formulations are made by extracting the immunoglobulin G (IgG) fractions from plasma from normal blood donors. Because of preventive virus screening and inactivation procedures, transmission of infections [e.g., human immunodeficiency virus (HIV) and hepatitis] by IVIG transfusion has not been reported for decades.[17]

High-dose IVIG (e.g., 0.4 g/kg for 5 days) is an established treatment in many autoimmune and inflammatory diseases. Suggested mechanisms of action are: interaction with Fc-receptors, inhibition of formation of/or elimination of immune complexes, suppression and neutralization of autoantibodies, interference with antigen presentation, neutralization of inflammatory cytokines, effects on apoptosis, attenuation of NK cells, and expansion of regulatory T lymphocytes.[18-22]

AIMS OF THE REVIEW

In this survey, I review the evidence from relevant studies for a possible treatment effect of IVIG in RPL. The focus will be to identify subsets of women with RPL who will benefit most from IVIG treatment and identify treatment protocols, which seem most efficient.

INTRAVENOUS IMMUNOGLOBULIN AND RECURRENT PREGNANCY LOSS OUTCOME

So far by July 2024, 10 genuine randomized placebo-controlled trials (RCTs) investigating IVIG in women with RPL have been published.[23-32] Results of systematic reviews and meta-analyses of the therapeutic effect of IVIG in RPL based on the majority of the trials have been conflicting. Wong et al. found no significant beneficial effect of IVIG over placebo in improving the live birth rate after RPL whereas Egerup et al., found that IVIG had a borderline ($p = 0.06$) significant therapeutic effect in patients with secondary RPL.[33,34] The most recent meta-analysis of 15 studies found a significant benefit of IVIG [odds ratio (OR) = 3.06, 95% confidence interval (CI): 1.23–7.64] in all RPL patients but the results must be considered cautiously since several of the included studies were not placebo-controlled.[35] Since this meta-analysis was published, a large RCT finding a significant effect of high dose IVIG in patients with more than equal to four consecutive pregnancy loss was published by Yamada et al.[32] This trial has for the first time been included in a systematic review and meta-analysis performed by my group.[36] The study showed a significant therapeutic effect of IVIG in some of the subanalyses and subsets of patients (see underneath).

IMMUNOLOGICAL CHANGES IN RECURRENT PREGNANCY LOSS PATIENTS AFTER INTRAVENOUS IMMUNOGLOBULIN

Several studies have measured relevant immunological biomarkers in RPL patients before and after IVIG treatment: T-helper (Th-)1 and Th17 cell frequency and NK cell number and NK cytotoxicity significantly decreased after IVIG and Treg cells increased and these changes were claimed to be associated with subsequent pregnancy success.[37-42] Yamada et al. in a study based on their placebo-controlled RCT of IVIG in patients with four or more pregnancy losses also found that IVIG increased Treg cell percentages and decreased NK cell activity significantly in patients with subsequent live birth.[43] However, no randomized placebo-controlled RCT of IVIG has so far been performed in RPL patients selected due to the presence of specific immunological biomarkers suggested to indicate an increased risk of pregnancy loss.[44]

SUBSETS OF RECURRENT PREGNANCY LOSS PATIENTS THAT BENEFIT MOST FROM INTRAVENOUS IMMUNOGLOBULIN

Several RCTs, cohort studies, and previous systematic reviews have suggested that particular subsets of RPL women benefit from IVIG treatment: secondary RPL patients and patients with selected immune disturbances.[34,39,45]

PRIMARY VERSUS SECONDARY RECURRENT PREGNANCY LOSS

There is evidence that the immunological disturbances characterizing primary and secondary RPL are different. Increased numbers and activity of peripheral blood NK cells have been reported in primary RPL compared with secondary RPL, whereas increased plasma levels of inflammatory cytokines and immunity against male-specific minor histocompatibility (HY) antigens characterize secondary RPL.[46-49] Different effects of IVIG in the two RPL subsets are therefore expected.

The systematic review and meta-analysis by Hutton et al. found that the treatment effect of IVIG was significant in secondary RPL but not in primary RPL.[45] In the systematic review and meta-analysis Egerup et al., 11 relevant RCTs involving RPL patients were identified. In all patients, a relative risk (RR) of 0.92 (95% CI: 0.75–1.12) for *no live birth* [corresponding to an RR of 1.02 (95% CI: 0.70–1.48) for *live birth* in all RPL patients was found after IVIG].[34] In contrast, in patients with secondary RPL, the RR for *live birth* after IVIG was 1.24 (0.96–1.59; $p = 0.06$), which can be translated into a borderline significant benefit of IVIG in secondary RPL.[34]

Wang et al. published a similar systematic review and meta-analysis on the effect of IVIG in RPL including two RCTs only published in Chinese, which were not included in the analysis by Egerup et al.[34,50] The meta-analysis found that IVIG treatment was associated with a RR for the birth of 1.26 (95% CI: 0.99–1.60; $p = 0.06$) in secondary RPL versus RR = 0.88 (95% CI: 0.71–1.08; $p = 0.20$) in primary RPL. The difference between the effect in the two subgroups was significantly different ($p = 0.02$). Both meta-analyses thus agree that IVIG has a borderline significant therapeutic effect in secondary RPL. In contrast, a systematic review and meta-analysis by Kofod et al. including the most recent RCTs of IVIG in the treatment of RPL was not able to find any better outcome in IVIG-treated secondary RPL patients compared with primary RPL patients.[32,36]

PATIENTS WITH FEW VERSUS MULTIPLE PREGNANCY LOSSES

The review by Kofod et al. based on individual patient data retrieved either directly from the original articles or from contacting the authors of the studies, found for the first time that IVIG significantly increased the livebirth rate in IVIG-treated patients with multiple previous pregnancy losses (≥6) compared with placebo.[36]

PATIENTS WITH IMMUNOLOGICAL ABNORMALITIES VERSUS NO ABNORMALITIES

Intravenous immunoglobulin has a documented effect in a series of diseases with an autoimmune background such as idiopathic thrombocytopenic purpura, Guillain-Barré syndrome, and myasthenia gravis often characterized by the presence of autoantibodies. It is therefore natural to suggest that it will exhibit higher efficiency in women with RPL positive for autoantibodies or other immune disturbances compared to those without. In addition to autoantibodies, it would be of particular interest to study whether patients with high NK cell count or NK cytotoxicity in the blood or endometrium constitute a target group for IVIG therapy since numerous studies have shown that IVIG treatment of women with RPL reduces these NK-cell related parameters and the reduction of NKT or NK cell numbers after IVIG may increase the live birth rate.[37-39] Several cohort studies have found higher live birth rates in IVIG-treated RPL patients with, e.g., increased numbers of NK cells or Th1/Th2 bias than in patients with similar disturbances not getting IVIG (often due to the high costs) but the studies were not randomized and therefore the results must be considered with care.[40-42] In a systematic review and meta-analysis, statistically significant increased risk ratios for live births were found in RPL and recurrent implantation failure patients with immune disturbances treated with IVIG (2.57, 95% CI: 1.79–3.69) compared with those not IVIG treated.[44] In a not yet published RCT from my group, RPL patients undergoing IVF/ICSI were randomly allocated to IVIG/prednisolone or placebo and a series of relevant immunological analyses were undertaken before IVIG infusion at the time of embryo transfer, and after 4 weeks of immunotherapy in patients being pregnant or not pregnant.[51] This study will hopefully provide information about which immune biomarkers can identify RPL patients who will in particular benefit from IVIG/prednisolone.

INTRAVENOUS IMMUNOGLOBULIN TREATMENT PROTOCOLS THAT SEEM TO BE MOST EFFICIENT IN RECURRENT PREGNANCY LOSS

High Dose Intravenous Immunoglobulin versus Lower Doses Intravenous Immunoglobulin

In the treatment of several autoimmune diseases, IVIG protocols providing 0.4 g/kg body weight for 5 consecutive days are standard doses with documented clinical effects.[18] None of the RCTs of IVIG in RPL except for one trial has administered dosages approaching these doses.[32] In almost all published trials, the protocol prescribed 0.4 g/kg body weight with 2–3 weeks intervals. In our former meta-analysis, we looked at the efficiency of IVIG in RCTs providing dosages above versus below the median dosage of 84 g IVIG until gestational week 10 in all RCTs.[34] The RR for miscarriage in the high dosage group was 0.85 (95% CI: 0.64–1.12) compared with RR 1.19 (95% CI: 0.81–1.75) in the low dosage group, the difference between RRs was, however, not significant ($p = 0.17$). The trend for higher treatment efficiency with the higher doses was explored in a recent meta-analysis by Kofod et al. where it was confirmed that RCTs of IVIG using the highest amounts of IVIG (above median 77.5 g) resulted in significantly better therapeutic effect in terms of live birth rate than RCTs providing lower doses (below median).[36]

Preconception versus Postconception Intravenous Immunoglobulin Treatment

Implementation of some of the effects of IVIG on immunological interactions takes time and therefore starting infusions only when the pregnancy test is positive may, in principle, be too late to prevent a new pregnancy loss in women with RPL with a history of early first trimester losses. Hutton et al. in their meta-analysis did several subanalyses and found that in RCTs of IVIG in RPL where infusions were started before conception, the outcome in the treated patients was significantly better than in those who received a placebo whereas no treatment effect could be found in RCTs starting infusions after conception.[45] In the meta-analysis by Wang et al. including a higher number of RCTs, similar findings were reported.[50] The RR for live birth in patients who received IVIG before conception versus those who received placebo was 1.69 (95% CI: 1.33-2.14; $p < 0.0001$).[50] However, it should be noticed that there was substantial overlap between the RCTs analyzed in the two meta-analyses. In contrast, in the meta-analysis of Egerup et al., no benefit was found in patients who received IVIG before versus after conception.[34]

CONCLUSION

In systematic reviews and meta-analyses of all RCTs with no subgroup analyses, the therapeutic benefit of IVIG in the prevention of RPL is nonsignificant but should be noted that the number of RCTs included in the recent analyses has varied between 10 and 15 due to different inclusion criteria. Previous subgroup analyses showed that women with secondary RPL were borderline statistically more responsive to IVIG than women with primary RPL, but recent meta-analyses cannot confirm this. A recent meta-analysis suggests that the benefit of IVIG treatment in terms of livebirth rate is strong and statistically significant in patients with ≥6 previous pregnancy losses. In a previous meta-analysis, initiating IVIG before conception increases the live birth rate compared with starting infusions during pregnancy; however, recent meta-analyses could not confirm this. A novel meta-analysis of RCTs indicates that IVIG dosages closer to those used in autoimmune/inflammatory diseases might be more efficient than lower dosages in reducing the risk of pregnancy loss.

Cohort studies suggest that IVIG treatment might be more efficient in patients positive for biomarkers associated with dysregulated immunity than in those without such biomarkers, but evidence from RCTs, which have selected patients due to the presence or absence of immune biomarkers is needed. **Figure 1** is an attempt to synthesize the aforementioned evidence presented. The figure represents evidence generated from systematic reviews regarding treatment protocols and patient characteristics, but is also influenced by the authors conviction.

In the planning of future RCTs investigating the efficiency of IVIG in RPL treatment, the lessons learned in the trials undertaken so far should be incorporated.

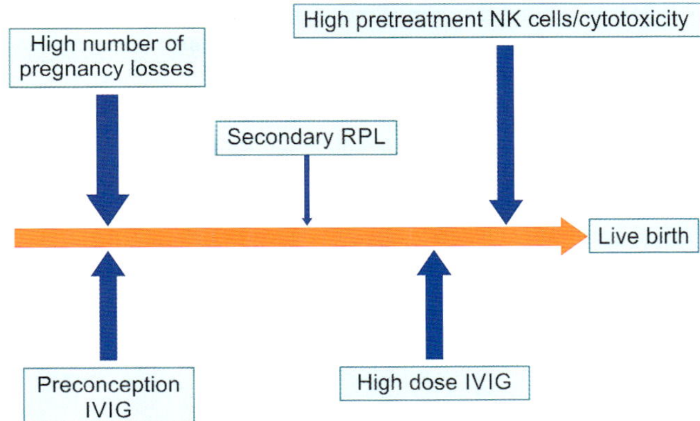

Fig. 1: The estimated relative contribution of patient-related and treatment protocol-related factors for the chance of livebirth in RPL patients receiving IVIG. The width of the arrows reflects the suggested impact of each factor. (IVIG: intravenous immunoglobulin; NK: natural killer; RPL: recurrent pregnancy loss)

Overall, IVIG seems to be a promising treatment for patients with RPL selected due to specific criteria and treated according to validated protocols as reviewed in this chapter.

REFERENCES

1. Toth B, Würfel W, Bohlmann M, Zschocke J, Rudnik-Schöneborn S, et al. Recurrent Miscarriage: Diagnostic and Therapeutic Procedures. Guideline of the DGGG, OEGGG, and SGGG (S2k-Level, AWMF Registry Number 015/050). Geburtshilfe Frauenheilkd. 2018;78(4):364-81.
2. Royal College of Obstetricians and Gynecologists. (2011). The investigation and treatment of couples with recurrent first-trimester and second-trimester miscarriage. [online] Available from https://rcog.org.uk/media/3cbgonl0/gtg_17.pdf [Last accessed December, 2024].
3. Practice Committee of American Society for Reproductive Medicine. Definitions of infertility and recurrent pregnancy loss: a committee opinion. Fertil Steril. 2013;99(1):63.
4. ESHRE Guideline Group on RPL; Bender Atik R, Christiansen OB, Elson J, Kolte AM, Lewis S, et al. ESHRE guideline: recurrent pregnancy loss: an update in 2022. Hum Reprod Open. 2023;(1):hoad002.
5. Guimond MJ, Wang B, Croy BA. Engraftment of bone marrow from severe combined immunodeficient (SCID) mice reverses the reproductive deficits in natural killer cell-deficient tg epsilon 26 mice. J Exp Med. 1998;187(2):217-23.
6. Aluvihare VR, Kallikourdis M, Betz AG. Regulatory T cells mediate maternal tolerance to the fetus. Nat Immunol. 2004;5(3):266-71.
7. Kruse C, Rosgaard A, Steffensen R, Varming K, Jensenius JC, Christiansen OB. Low serum level of mannan-binding

lectin is a determinant for pregnancy outcome in women with recurrent spontaneous abortion. Am J Obstet Gynecol. 2002;187(5):1313-20.

8. Hiby SE, Regan L, Lo W, Carrington M, Moffett A. Association of maternal killer-cell immunoglobulin-like receptors and parental HLA-C genotypes with recurrent miscarriage. Hum Reprod. 2008;23(4):972-6.
9. King K, Smith S, Chapman M, Sacks G. Detailed analysis of peripheral blood natural killer (NK) cells in women with recurrent miscarriage. Hum Reprod. 2010;25(1):52-8.
10. Thangaratinam S, Tan A, Knox E, Kilby MD, Franklyn J, Coomarasamy A. Association between thyroid autoantibodies and miscarriage and preterm birth: meta-analysis of evidence. BMJ. 2011;342:d2616:
11. Tang A, Alfirevic Z, Turner MA, Drury JA, Small R, Quenby S. A feasibility trial of screening women with idiopathic recurrent miscarriage for high uterine natural killer cell density and randomizing to prednisolone or placebo when pregnant. Hum Reprod. 2013;28(7):1743-52.
12. Recurrent Miscarriage Trialists Group (RMITG). Worldwide collaborative observational study and meta-analysis on allogenic leukocyte immunotherapy for recurrent spontaneous abortion. Recurrent Miscarriage Immunotherapy Trialists Group. Am J Reprod Immunol. 1994;32(2):55-72.
13. Hooper A, Bacal V, Bedaiwy MA. Does adding hydroxychloroquine to empiric treatment improve the live birth rate in refractory obstetrical antiphospholipid syndrome? A systematic review. Am J Reprod Immunol. 2023;90(3): e13761.
14. Liu J, Li M, Fu J, Yuan G, Li N, Fu Y, et al. Tacrolimus improved the pregnancy outcomes of patients with refractory recurrent spontaneous abortion and immune bias disorders: a randomized controlled trial. Eur J Clin Pharmacol. 2023;79(5):627-34.
15. Mueller-Eckhardt G, Heine O, Neppert J, Künzel W, Mueller-Eckhardt C. Prevention of recurrent spontaneous abortion by intravenous immunoglobulin. Vox Sang. 1989; 56(3):151-4.
16. Christiansen OB, Mathiesen O, Lauritsen JG, Grunnet N. Intravenous immunoglobulin treatment of women with multiple miscarriages. Hum Reprod. 1992;7(5):718-22.
17. Späth PJ, Kempf C. Challenges and achievements in pathogen safety of intravenous immunoglobulin. In: Dalakis MC, Späth PJ (Eds). Intravenous immunoglobulins in the third millennium. London: Parthenon Publishing Group; 2004. pp. 9-20.
18. Imbach P. 2004. Immunomodulation by intravenous immunoglobulin: idiopathic thrombocytopenic purpura as a model. In: Dalakas MC, Späth PJ. Intravenous immunoglobulins in the third millennium. Parthenon Publishing Group, London. pp. 29-35.
19. Negi V-S, Elluru S, Sibéril S, Graff-Dubois S, Mouthon L, Kazatchkine MD, et al. Intravenous immunoglobulin: An update on the clinical use and mechanisms of action. J Clin Immunol. 2007;27(3):233-45.
20. Baerenwaldt A, Biburger M, Nimmerjahn F. Mechanisms of action of intravenous immunoglobulins. Exp Rev Clin Immunol. 2010;6(3):425-34.
21. Schwab I, Nimmerjahn F. Intravenous immunoglobulin therapy: how does IgG modulate the immune system? Nat Reviews Immunol. 2013;13(3):176-89.
22. Trinath J, Hegde P, Sharma M, Maddur MS, Rabin M, Vallat JM, et al. Intravenous immunoglobulin expands regulatory T cells via induction of cyclooxygenase-2-dependent prostaglandin E2 in human dendritic cells. Blood. 2013;122(8):1419-27.
23. The German RSA/IVIG Group. Intravenous immunoglobulin in the prevention of recurrent miscarriage. BJOG. 1994;101(12):1072-7.
24. Christiansen OB, Mathiesen O, Husth M, Rasmussen KL, Ingerslev HJ, Lauritsen JG, et al. Placebo-controlled trial of treatment of unexplained secondary recurrent spontaneous abortions and recurrent late spontaneous abortions with i.v. immunoglobulin. Hum Reprod. 1995;10(10):2690-5.
25. Coulam C, Krysa L, Stern J, Bustillo M. Intravenous immunoglobulin for treatment of recurrent pregnancy loss. Am J Reprod Immunol. 1995;34(6):333-7.
26. Perino A, Vassiliadis A, Vucetich A, Colacurci N, Menato G, Cignitti M, et al. 1997. Short-term therapy for recurrent abortion using intravenous immunoglobulins: results of a double-blind placebo-controlled Italian study. Hum Reprod. 1997;12(11):2388-92.
27. Stephenson MD, Dreher K, Houlihan E, Wu V. Prevention of unexplained recurrent spontaneous abortion using intravenous immunoglobulin: a prospective, randomized, double-blinded, placebo-controlled trial. Am J Reprod Immunol. 1998;39(2):82-8.
28. Jablonowska B, Selbing, A, Palfi M, Ernerudh J, Kjellberg S, Lindton B. Prevention of recurrent spontaneous abortion by intravenous immunoglobulin: a double-blind placebo-controlled study. Hum Reprod. 1999;14(3):838-41.
29. Christiansen OB, Pedersen B, Rosgaard A, Husth M. A randomized, double-blind, placebo-controlled trial of intravenous immunoglobulin in the prevention of recurrent miscarriage: evidence for a therapeutic effect in women with secondary recurrent miscarriage. Hum Reprod. 2002;17(3):809-16.
30. Stephenson MD, Kutteh WH, Purkis S, Librach C, Schultz P, Houlihan E, et al. Intravenous immunoglobulin and idiopathic secondary recurrent miscarriage: a multicentered randomized placebo-controlled trial. Hum Reprod. 2010;25(9):2203-9.
31. Christiansen OB, Larsen EC, Egerup P, Lunoee L, Egestad L, Nielsen HS. Intravenous immunoglobulin treatment for secondary recurrent miscarriage: a randomised, double-blind, placebo-controlled trial. BJOG. 2015;122(4):500-8.

32. Yamada H, Deguchi M, Saito S, Takeshita T, Mitsui M, Saito T, et al. Intravenous immunoglobulin treatment in women with four or more recurrent pregnancy losses: a double-blind, randomised, placebo-controlled trial. EClinicalMedicine. 2022;50:101527.
33. Wong LF, Porter TF, Scott JR. Immunotherapy for recurrent miscarriage. Cochrane Database Syst Rev. 2014;2014(10): CD000112.
34. Egerup P, Lindschou J, Gluud C, Christiansen OB, ImmunoReM IPD study group. The effects of intravenous immunoglobulins in women with recurrent miscarriages: A systematic review of randomised trials with meta-analyses and trial sequential analyses including individual patient data. PLoS ONE. 2015;10(10):e141588.
35. Shi Y, Tan D, Hao B, Zhang X, Geng W, Wang Y, et al. Efficacy of intravenous immunoglobulin in the treatment of recurrent spontaneous abortion: A systematic review and meta-analysis. Am J Reprod Immunol. 2022;88(5):e13615.
36. Kofod LM, Pedersen M, Andersen M, Christensen E, Pedersen P, Egerup P, et al. The effect of intravenous immunoglobulin versus placebo in patients with recurrent pregnancy loss: a systematic review and meta-analysis of randomized trials. Hum Reprod. 2024;39(Suppl 1):3175.
37. Van den Heuvel MJ, Peralta CG, Hatta K, Han VK, Clark DA. Decline in number of elevated blood CD3(+) CD56(+) NKT cells in response to intravenous immunoglobulin treatment correlates with successful pregnancy. Am J Reprod Immunol. 2007;58(5):447-59.
38. Heilmann L, Schorsch M, Hahn T. CD3-CD56+CD16+ natural killer cells and improvement of pregnancy outcome in IVF/ICSI failure after additional IVIG-treatment. Am J Reprod Immunol. 2010;63(3):263-65.
39. Moraru M, Carbone J, Alecsandru D, Castillo-Rama M, García-Segovia A, Gil J, et al. Intravenous immunoglobulin treatment increased live birth rate in a Spanish cohort of women with recurrent reproductive failure and expanded CD56(+) cells. Am J Reprod Immunol. 2012;68(1):75-84.
40. Ramos-Medina R, García-Segovia A, Gil J, Carbone J, Aguarón de la Cruz A, Seyfferth A, et al. Experience in IVIg therapy for selected women with recurrent reproductive failure and NK cell expansion. Am J Reprod Immunol. 2014;71(5):458-66.
41. Ahmadi M, Aghdam SA, Nouri M, Babaloo Z, Farzadi L, Ghasemzadeh A, et al. Intravenous immunoglobulin (IVIG) treatment modulates peripheral blood Th17 and regulatory T cells in recurrent miscarriage patients: Non randomized, open-label clinical trial. Immunol Letters. 2017;192:12-9.
42. Ahmadi M, Ghaebi M, Abdolmohammadi-Vahid S, Abbaspour-Aghdam S, Hamdi K, Abdollahi-Fard S, et al. NK cell frequency and cytotoxicity in correlation to pregnancy outcome and response to IVIG therapy among women with recurrent pregnancy loss. J Cell Physiol. 2019;234(6):9428-37.
43. Yamada H, Deguchi M, Saito S, Takeshita T, Mitsui M, Saito T, et al. High doses of intravenous immunoglobulin stimulate regulatory T cell and suppress natural killer cell in women with recurrent pregnancy loss. J Reprod Immunol. 2023;158:103977.
44. Woon EV, Day A, Bracewell-Milnes T, Male V, Johnson M. Immunotherapy to improve pregnancy outcome in women with abnormal natural killer cell levels/activity and recurrent miscarriage or implantation failure: A systematic review and meta-analysis. J Reprod Immunol. 2020;142:103189.
45. Hutton B, Sharma R, Fergusson D, Tinmouth A, Hebert P, Jamieson J, et al. Use of intravenous immunoglobulin for treatment of recurrent miscarriage: a systematic review. BJOG. 2007;114(2):134-42.
46. Shakhar K, Ben-Eliyahu S, Loewenthal R, Rosenne E, Carp H. Differences in number and activity of peripheral natural killer cells in primary versus secondary recurrent miscarriage. Fertil Steril. 2003;80(2):368-75.
47. Kuon RJ, Vomstein K, Weber M, Müller F, Seitz C, Wallwiener S, et al. The "killer cell story" in recurrent miscarriage: association between activated peripheral lymphocytes and uterine natural killer cells. J Reprod Immunol. 2017;119:9-14.
48. Piosik ZM, Goegebeur Y, Klitkou L, Steffensen R, Christiansen OB. Plasma TNF-α levels are higher in early pregnancy in patients with secondary compared with primary recurrent miscarriage. Am J Reprod Immunol. 2013;70(5):347-58.
49. Nielsen HS, Steffensen R, Varming K, Van Halteren AG, Spierings E, Ryder LP, et al. Association of HY-restricting HLA class II alleles with pregnancy outcome in patients with recurrent miscarriage subsequent to a firstborn boy. Hum Mol Genet. 2009;18(9):1684-91.
50. Wang SW, Zhong SY, Lou LJ, Hu ZF, Sun HY, Zhu HY. The effect of intravenous immunoglobulin passive immunotherapy on unexplained recurrent spontaneous abortion: a meta-analysis. Reprod Biomed Online. 2016;33(6):720-36.
51. Nørgaard-Pedersen C, Nielsen K, Steffensen R, Eriksen L, Jørgensen MM, Kesmodel US, et al. Intravenous immunoglobulin and prednisolone to women with unexplained recurrent pregnancy loss after assisted reproductive technology treatment: a protocol for a randomised, double-blind, placebo-controlled trial. BMJ Open. 2022;12(9):e64780.

CHAPTER 46

Lipid Emulsion Therapy

Hrishikesh D Pai, Meenu Handa

ABSTRACT

Lipid emulsion is composed of soy oil and is rich in polyunsaturated fatty acids (PUFA) and medium-chain unsaturated fatty acids (MUFA) as well as medium-chain triglycerides (MCT). It is used for parenteral nutrition but is also indicated in recurrent pregnancy loss due to autoimmune disorders. Increased natural killer cell population in the endometrium may be an indication for administration of intralipids. A recent meta-analysis confirms that intralipid therapy will benefit patients with increased uterine natural killer cell population in the mid luteal phase endometrial biopsy.

Keywords: Lipid emulsion therapy, Intralipid, Natural killer cells, Autoimmunity RPL, RIF.

INTRODUCTION

The etiology of recurrent pregnancy loss (RPL) can be multifactorial.[1-4] It can be due to genetic cause, anatomic, endocrine, antiphospholipid antibody syndrome, immunological, or environmental.[5] Up to 50% of patients with RPL have no clearly defined etiology. RPL is commonly categorized into primary, which refers to pregnancy loss in women who never had a live birth, and secondary, in women who had a previous pregnancy that proceeded beyond viability, i.e., 28 weeks.[6]

Recent studies have suggested a strong role of immunological abnormalities both in RPL and recurrent implantation failures (RIF). Increased number of natural killer (NK) cells and proinflammatory cytokines have been described.[7] Various immunomodulatory factors have been studied to unravel the mystery of maternal tolerance to the fetal allograft and its failure in RIF and RPL.[8]

Various immunomodulatory treatments have been attempted, e.g., paternal leukocyte therapy, intravenous immunoglobulin (IVIG), granulocyte colony-stimulating factor, and intralipid.[8-11] Among these, the lipid emulsion therapy (LET) has shown some positive response in patients with RIF and RPL.

ROLE OF NATURAL KILLER CELLS IN RECURRENT PREGNANCY LOSS AND RECURRENT IMPLANTATION FAILURES

Natural killer cells are a part of the innate immune system and typically function as cytotoxic lymphocytes responsible for innate immunity in infections as well as pregnancy. NK cell activity does not require prior sensitization and is responsible for the secretion of tumor necrosis factor (TNF)-alpha and interferon gamma (IFN). The main function of NK cells is lysis of cells with foreign antigens via apoptosis.[9] The growing embryo does not express major human leukocyte antigens (HLA) and only expresses HLA-G on the trophoblast. HLA-G prevents NK cell activity and allows the maternal immune system to recognize fetal antigens as self. Hence, abnormal expression of HLA gene may be involved in RPL. NK cells also undergo interaction with the *HLA-G* gene, which is highly expressed in the trophoblast to prevent the activity of NK cells and the self-recognition of fetal antigens by the maternal immune system, suggesting that the *HLA-G* gene promoter single nucleotide polymorphism (SNP) is involved in RPL.[10]

Natural killer cells are classified according to their cell differentiation (CD) antigen and are numbered CD3–CD56 lymphocytes. CD56+ expression is classically divided into CD56^{bright}, also known as high-intensity CD56, and CD56^{dim}, also known as low-intensity NK cells. The CD56^{dim} NK cell subset is characterized by its cytotoxicity and high expression of CD16 receptor involved in antibody-dependent cell cytotoxicity (ADCC). In contrast, CD56^{bright} NK cells are characterized by a high proliferative activity and the production of immune-regulatory cytokines. The different expressions of CD56 and CD16, along with other surface receptors, modulate the cytolytic or immunoregulatory capacity of these cells.

It was also noted that peripheral natural killer (pNK) and uterine natural killer (uNK) cells (CD16-/56+^{bright}) have very different phenotypes and functions, leading to much confusion over their role in RPL.[11] It has been seen that pNK cells comprise about 10–15% of the total lymphocytes in the blood. CD56^{dim} subset constitutes about 90% and the minor CD56^{bright} subset comprises about 10% of total NK cells in peripheral blood. But so far, reliable reproductive reference ranges have not been established, and there is no agreement on their upper threshold value in pregnancy. pNK cells ≥12% have been associated with poor reproductive outcome.[12] On the other hand, uNK cells are mostly comprising CD56^{bright} and CD16– cells. Although uNK cells play an important role in the maternal immune response to pathogens, they are primarily involved in trophoblastic invasion and angiogenesis.[13]

Natural killer cells are characterized as uNK cells present in the endometrium and pNK cells present in the peripheral blood. The counts of pNK and uNK cells do not always correlate. There is more data on pNK cells due to the ease of sampling, and their count ranges from 5% to 29% in healthy individuals. Their counts vary among different ethnicities and ages and also show different ranges for different genders and exposure to stress and are increased in RIF and RPL.[14,15] Abnormal expression of NK cells in the endometrium during the luteal phase of the menstrual cycle is more closely linked to RPL. uNK cells can be studied in a noninvasive, pipelle endometrial biopsy. This is best performed in the mid-luteal phase of the menstrual cycle (day 21), as this is when the uNK cell concentration peaks.

INTRALIPIDS

Lipid emulsions (LEs) are a fat emulsion containing a mixture of unsaturated fatty acids (FAs) such as linoleic and α-linolenic acid. LEs were first used for parenteral nutrition in 1945 and commercially used from 1950s. At present, commercial LEs are a fat emulsion containing medium- and long-chain triglycerides.[16]

The composition of LE has been evolving.

- The first generation exclusively had soy oil (SO), which has a high percentage of polyunsaturated fatty acids (PUFA).
- The second generation had coconut oil, which has medium-chain triglycerides (MCT).
- The third generation has olive oil along with soy, having a composition of 65% medium-chain unsaturated fatty acids (MUFA) and 20% PUFA.
- Lately, even fish oil containing omega-3 fatty acids, *eicosapentaenoic acid (EPA) and docosahexaenoic acid (DHA)*, has been added to the above composition.[17]
- Present-day formulations contain 20% soybean oil, 1.2% egg yolk phospholipids, 2.25% glycerin, and water for injection.

Lipid emulsion therapy is contraindicated in the presence of allergy to egg, soybean, and peanut protein.

At the cellular level, intralipid restores abnormal NK cell activity in the endometrium to normal levels. By propagating its anti-inflammatory property, intralipids may improve embryo implantation. The earliest studies on immune modulatory effect of intralipids were published in 2008 by Roussev.[18] The suppression of uNK cell activity occurs within 1 week of administration in 80%, but the rest may need a second infusion after 2–3 weeks, and a small number require a third infusion to normalize NK activity. Although an association exists between increased uNK cell activity and RPL/RIF, there is still a paucity of data on whether suppressing uNK cell activity by intralipids will improve pregnancy outcomes. Further randomized trials on outcomes after intralipid administration and the exact pathophysiological mechanisms still need to be worked out.[19]

Side effects after administration are rare but may include acute kidney injury, acute lung injury, pancreatitis, and an increased susceptibility to infections. However, these are most often observed with dosages employed for parenteral nutrition rather than the spaced-out dosage of immune modulation.

INTRALIPIDS AND CLINICAL APPLICATION

A recent double-blind, randomized, controlled trial for women undergoing in vitro fertilization (IVF) and suffering from unexplained infertility and increased NK cell activity showed a significant increase in ongoing pregnancy and live birth rates. Women in intralipid group received intralipid infusion 20% in 250 mL of saline on the day of the embryo transfer and repeated every 2 weeks after positive pregnancy test until 12 weeks.[8] They are infused at a rate of 1 mL/min to start with, which can later be increased to 2–3 mL/min. The total infusion time could vary from 30 minutes to 2 hours.

In a meta-analysis published in 2021, 12 studies with 2,676 participants were evaluated, and there was strong evidence that intralipid infusion can improve implantation and live birth rate in women suffering from recurrent miscarriages with immunological reasons.[20]

Though intralipids are not recommended as a routine intervention for unexplained RPLs or RIFs, but they can be considered when there is failure of standard treatment and in the presence of identifiable risk factors like mild autoimmunity.[21]

There is no consensus as to when to start intralipid infusions. Some start it on the third day of menstrual cycle, others in mid-follicular phase, and still others on the day of oocyte retrieval or up to 8 days post embryo transfer. The rationale is to administer it prior to the implantation window. Infusions are repeated every 2 weeks, and a total of 3–12 infusions may be required per patient. Post positive pregnancy test result, infusion frequency may vary, ranging from 2 to 4 weeks. What is needed are large-scale, double-blind studies to test LE before recommending it for routine use.[22]

In a recent publication, it was used successfully in a patient with RPL on the day of oocyte retrieval and another infusion a week later, i.e., 3 days postembryo transfer. Whether to continue the infusions during pregnancy at 3-weekly intervals is left to the clinicians' discretion, as the most crucial time is the peri-implantation period.[23]

CONCLUSION

The role of intralipid therapy in RPL is limited to the subset of patients who demonstrate a high uNK cell activity on a mid-luteal phase endometrial biopsy. Also, women with RPL who undergo assisted reproductive technology (ART) cycles for various indications may benefit from intralipid therapy prior to the implantation window and soon after implantation, when routine workup is unremarkable, standard treatments have failed, and autoimmune pregnancy loss is suspected. Although the uNK cell profile shows improvement after LET, there are as yet no randomized controlled trials to prove that pregnancy outcomes are improved after LET as compared to placebo. Since the two doses of intralipid currently recommended in the ART treatment cycle are easy to administer, cost-effective, and devoid of major side effects, it has gained favor among ART practitioners doing ART cycles for RPL patients and dealing with RIF. However, further studies are urgently warranted on this subject.

REFERENCES

1. RCOG. (2023). Green Top Guideline No.17. [online] Available from https://www.rcog.org.uk/guidance/browse-all-guidance/green-top-guidelines/recurrent-miscarriage-green-top-guideline-no-17/ [Last accessed December, 2024].
2. Zegers-Hochschild F, Adamson GD, Dyer S, Racowsky C, de Mouzon J, Sokol R, et al. The international glossary on infertility and fertility care, 2017. Fertil Steril. 2017; 108(3):393-406.
3. ASRM. Evaluation and treatment of recurrent pregnancy loss: a committee opinion. Fertil Steril. 2012;98(5): 1103-11.
4. Bender Atik R, Christiansen OB, Elson J, Kolte AM, Lewis S, Middeldorp S; ESHRE Guideline Group on RPL. Hum Reprod Open. 2018;2018(2):hoy004.
5. Stephenson MD. Frequency of factors associated with habitual abortion in 197 couples. Fertil Steril. 1996; 66(1):24-9.
6. Ansari AH, Kirkpatrick B. Recurrent pregnancy loss. An update. J Reprod Med. 1998;43(9):806-14.
7. Martini AE, Jasulaitis S, Fogg LF, Uhler ML, Hirshfeld-Cytron JE. Evaluating the utility of intralipid infusion to improve live birth rates in patients with recurrent pregnancy loss or recurrent implantation failure. J Hum Reprod Sci. 2018; 11(3):261-8.
8. Dakhly DMR, Bayoumi YA, Sharkawy M, Gad Allah SH, Hassan MA, Gouda HM, et al. Intralipid supplementation in women with recurrent spontaneous abortion and elevated levels of natural killer cells. Int J Gynaecol Obstet. 2016;135(3):324-7.
9. Geller MA, Miller JS. Use of allogeneic NK cells for cancer immunotherapy. Immunotherapy. 2011;3(12): 1445-59.
10. Yazdani N, Shekari Khaniani M, Bastami M, Ghasemnejad T, Afkhami F, Mansoori DS. HLA-G regulatory variants and haplotypes with susceptibility to recurrent pregnancy loss. Int J Immunogenet. 2018;45(4):181-9.
11. Horowitz A, Strauss-Albee DM, Leipold M, Kubo J, Nemat-Gorgani N, Dogan OC, et al. Genetic and environmental determinants of human NK cell diversity revealed by mass cytometry. Sci Transl Med. 2013;5(208):208ra145.
12. Thum MY, Bhaskaran S, Abdalla HI, Ford B, Sumar N, Shehata H, et al. An increase in the absolute count of CD56dimCD16+CD69+ NK cells in the peripheral blood is associated with a poorer IVF treatment and pregnancy outcome. Hum Reprod. 2004;19(10):2395-400.
13. Montaldo E, Del Zotto G, Della Chiesa M, Mingari MC, Moretta A, De Maria A, et al. Human NK cell receptors/markers: a tool to analyze NK cell development, subsets and function. Cytometry A. 2013;83(8):702-13.
14. Lédée N, Vasseur C, Petitbarat M, Chevrier L, Vezmar K, Dray G, et al. Intralipid may represent a new hope for patients with reproductive failures and simultaneously an over-immune endometrial activation. J Reprod Immunol. 2018;130:18-22.
15. Santillán I, Lozano I, Illán J, Verdú V, Coca S, Bajo-Arenas JM, et al. Where and when should natural killer cells be

tested in women with repeated implantation failure? J Reprod Immunol. 2015;108:142-8.
16. Ferreira IK. Terapia nutricional em Unidade de Terapia Intensiva [Nutritional therapy in Intensive Care Unit]. Rev Bras Ter Intensiva. 2007;19(1):90-7.
17. Calder PC, Adolph M, Deutz NE, Grau T, Innes JK, Klek S, et al. Lipids in the intensive care unit: recommendations from the ESPEN Expert Group. Clin Nutr. 2018;37(1):1-18.
18. Roussev RG, Acacio B, Ng SC, Coulam CB. Duration of intralipid's suppressive effect on NK cell's functional activity. Am J Reprod Immunol. 2008;60:258-63.
19. Sfakianoudis K, Rapani A, Grigoriadis S, Pantou A, Maziotis E, Kokkini G, Tsirligkani C, et al. The Role of Uterine Natural Killer Cells on Recurrent Miscarriage and Recurrent Implantation Failure: From Pathophysiology to Treatment. Biomedicines. 2021;9(10):1425.
20. Kumar P, Marron K, Harrity C. Intralipid therapy and adverse reproductive outcome: is there any evidence? Reproduction and Fertility. 2021;(2):173-86.
21. Rimmer MP, Black N, Keay S, Quenby S, Al Wattar BH. Intralipid infusion at time of embryo transfer in women with history of recurrent implantation failure: A systematic review and meta-analysis. J Obstet Gynaecol Res. 2021;47:2149-56.
22. Paula Renata Bueno Campos Canella, Barini R, Patrícia de Oliveira Carvalho. Lipid emulsion therapy in women with recurrent pregnancy loss and repeated implantation failure: The role of abnormal natural killer cell activity. J Cell Mol Med. 2021;25:2290-96.
23. Anya OC, Ajayi ER, Solanke HR, Ohanaka AI, Ubana KD. The Use of Intralipid Infusions in the Prevention of Embryo Implantation Failure. Cureus. 2024;16(2):e53368.

CHAPTER 47

Role of Human Chorionic Gonadotropin

Jonathan Cohen

ABSTRACT

Human chorionic gonadotropin (hCG) stimulates the corpus luteum to secrete not only progesterone but many other growth factors like relaxin, inhibin, prostaglandins, and many more. It also acts on the endometrium to secrete cytokines that facilitate implantation. There is mounting evidence that mid-luteal administration of hCG will improve implantation and reduce the incidence of recurrent pregnancy loss (RPL). Continued administration is recommended by some till 12 weeks, but it should be used with caution, as it may lead to ovarian hyperstimulation syndrome.

Keywords: Human chorionic gonadotropin, hCG, Corpus luteum, hyperglycosylated hCG (hCG-H).

ROLE OF HUMAN CHORIONIC GONADOTROPIN IN PHYSIOLOGICAL CONDITION

The human chorionic gonadotropin (hCG) hormone is secreted by the trophoblast, starting from the first day of the pregnancy. The main role of hCG secretion is to maintain and enhance the corpus luteum (CL) activity, which is mainly progesterone secretion. Nevertheless, hCG has different isoforms and different roles, following endocrine and autocrine ways.[1] The regular form of hCG is secreted by the syncytiotrophoblast, whereas the hyperglycosylated hCG (hCG-H) is secreted by the cytotrophoblast. The syncytiotrophoblast is the outer layer of the trophoblast that invades into the maternal endometrium; it is acellular and does not expand mitotically. The cytotrophoblast is the inner layer of the trophoblast; it expands mitotically to mature into the syncytiotrophoblast in order to form primary chorionic villi. hCG-H acts primarily through transforming growth factor-beta (TGF-β) receptors on cytotrophoblast. The comparison of the two hCG molecules is presented in **Table 1**.

TABLE 1: Human chorionic gonadotropin (hCG) versus hyperglycosylated human chorionic gonadotropin (hCG-H).

hCG	*hCG-H*
Endocrine—acts on corpus luteum	Autocrine—acts on cytotrophoblast
Produced by syncytiotrophoblast	Produced by cytotrophoblast
Promotes progesterone production	Invasion promoter—proliferation of cytotrophoblast
Important for corpus luteum rescue	Promotes implantation, prevents miscarriage
Plays a role mainly in first trimester	Plays a role in mid trimester for hemochorial implantation
Angiogenic role in the uterus	Better predictor of pregnancy outcome and predicts pre-eclampsia

Action on the Corpus Luteum

Human chorionic gonadotropin targets the CL cells that produce:

- Progesterone
- Prostaglandin E2 (PGE2)
- Inhibin
- Relaxin
- Many more hitherto unidentified molecules

Human chorionic gonadotropin also stimulates estradiol production in human granulosa lutein cells. hCG secretion is hence responsible for the CL rescue, and its role is fundamental to allow the CL to secrete all the proimplantation molecules.[2]

Action on the Uterus

Human chorionic gonadotropin has also a direct effect on the uterus. hCG is secreted by the blastocyst, and it can inhibit insulin-like growth factor B1 (IGFB1) and therefore enhance the time period available for potential implantation. hCG stimulates endometrial cells to secrete leukemia inhibitory factor (LIF) and decreases the secretion of interleukin-6 (IL-6).

Human chorionic gonadotropin plays a role in the immunotolerance of the endometrium vis-à-vis the embryo. It modifies the balance between inflammatory [T helper 1 (Th1)/Th17] and anti-inflammatory [Th2/T regulatory (Treg)] cells, favoring the Th1 to Th2 shift and thus allowing the implantation of the semiallogenic embryo.[3]

Stromal cells will undergo decidualization under hCG influence, and it will also induce the trophoblast invasion by promoting the differentiation of cytotrophoblast into syncytiotrophoblast. The angiogenic effect of hCG on the uterus is powerful and necessary for implantation.[2]

It therefore appears that hCG has a crucial role in implantation and early pregnancy development, allowing effective maintenance of CL and preparation for implantation and endometrial support.

LUTEAL INSUFFICIENCY AND MISCARRIAGE RISK

The idea of hCG supplementation in recurrent miscarriage derives from the luteal insufficiency concept. It has been suggested that some women suffer from luteal insufficiency and that this could lead to miscarriages.[4]

LUTEAL INSUFFICIENCY DEFINITION AND CONSEQUENCES ON PREGNANCY LOSS

Following Fraenkel's discovery that CL was indispensable to maintain gestation in rabbits, Corner and Allen discovered in 1929 that the administration of the hormone extracted from CL into rabbit females that were mated the day before castration allowed a normal implantation and gestation of the embryos until normal parturition. This hormone was later defined and called progesterone. The presence of an active CL is mandatory to maintain the pregnancy in humans until a certain week of gestation.[5]

Although luteal deficiency is described in the literature since 1949, there is no precise definition. Since the progesterone level alone is not diagnostic of luteal insufficiency, as its action depends on the number of progesterone receptors induced in the endometrium during the follicular phase. Since the secretion of progesterone is pulsatile and a single measurement in mid-luteal phase is not enough to diagnose luteal insufficiency, it is opined to use the term luteal phase insufficiency when the luteal phase duration is less than 10 days.[4] Balasch et al.[6] defined luteal deficiency based on histological features of endometrial biopsy. They showed a higher rate of abnormal biopsies in women with recurrent pregnancy loss (RPL) than in fertile and infertile patients. On the other hand, Ogasawara et al.[7] showed no difference in mid-luteal progesterone levels in women with RPL than in control patients. Consequently, the European Society of Human Reproduction and Embryology (ESHRE) 2023 guidelines on RPL did not recommend any luteal phase insufficiency testing in women with RPL.[8]

Since hCG promotes the secretion of not only progesterone but also many other growth molecules from the CL as well as angiogenic factors in the endometrium, it is a fair candidate in the prevention of early miscarriages, disregarding the presence or absence of any luteal phase insufficiency. Let us examine the evidence for the above hypothesis. Most of the randomized controlled trials (RCTs) have been exhaustively reported in the 2013 Cochrane Review.[9]

EFFECT OF HUMAN CHORIONIC GONADOTROPIN SUPPLEMENTATION TO PREVENT MISCARRIAGE IN WOMEN WITH RECURRENT PREGNANCY LOSS

There are a few studies on the effect of hCG supplementation in the first trimester of pregnancy to reduce the miscarriage risks. A meta-analysis of Morley et al. was published in 2013.[9] The meta-analysis includes five studies, and we will examine them. The studies included in the meta-analysis were RCTs that compared hCG versus placebo or no treatment in preventing the onset of a miscarriage.

The first study was published in 1982 by Svigos in Australia.[10] It was an RCT conducted on 32 women with a history of two or more consecutive miscarriages. Treatment given was hCG 9,000 units three times per week. Treatment was initiated after diagnosis of pregnancy by ultrasound at 6–7 weeks and was continued until 12 weeks. They reported 1 miscarriage out of 13 patients under treatment and 9 miscarriages out of 15 patients in the placebo group [risk ratio (RR) = 0.13 (0.02, 0.88)].

The second study was published by Harrisson in 1985 in Ireland.[11] It was an RCT conducted on 20 women with a history of three or more consecutive miscarriages.

Treatment was initiated after the diagnosis of pregnancy by ultrasound. Treatment given was hCG 10,000 IU loading dose and then 5,000 IU twice weekly to week 12 and then 5,000 IU twice weekly to week 16. They reported no miscarriage out of 10 patients under treatment and 7 miscarriages out of 10 patients in the placebo group [RR = 0.07 (0, 1.03)].

The third study was also published by Harrison in 1992.[12] It was an RCT conducted on 75 women with a history of recurrent miscarriages. Treatment was initiated after the diagnosis of pregnancy by ultrasound. Treatment given was hCG 10,000 IU loading dose and then 5,000 IU twice weekly to week 12 and then 5,000 IU twice weekly to week 16. As a result, 83% of the pregnancies on hCG were successful (6 miscarriages out of 36 patients) compared with 79% on placebo (8 miscarriages out of 39 patients) [RR = 0.81 (0.31, 2.11)].

The fourth study was published by Quenby in 1994.[13] It was an RCT conducted on 81 women with a history of two or more consecutive miscarriages. Treatment was initiated after the diagnosis of pregnancy by ultrasound prior to 6 weeks' gestation. Treatment given was hCG 10,000 IU loading dose and then 5,000 IU twice weekly to week 14. In women with regular menstrual cycles, it was found that hCG had no beneficial effect, the pregnancy success rate being 86% in both groups (6 miscarriages out of 42 patients under treatment and 6 miscarriages out of 39 patients in the placebo group) [RR = 0.93 (0.33, 2.64)]. However, women with oligomenorrhea had a pregnancy success rate of 40% in the placebo group but a statistically significant improvement to 86% if hCG was given.

The fifth study was published by El-Zibdeh in 2005.[14] It was an RCT conducted on 98 women with a history of three or more consecutive miscarriages. Treatment was started as soon as possible after the confirmation of pregnancy and continued until the 12th gestational week. Treatment given was hCG 5,000 IU once every 4 days until 12 weeks. They reported 9 miscarriages out of 50 patients (18%) under treatment and 14 miscarriages out of 48 patients (29%) in the placebo group [RR = 0.62 (0.3, 1.29)].

In total, when combining the five studies, there were 22 miscarriages out of 151 patients in the hCG group (14.6%) and 44 miscarriages out of 151 patients in the placebo group (29%). hCG was significantly reducing the number of miscarriages compared to placebo with RR = 0.51 (0.32-0.81). Among these five studies, the two that present significant results are the studies of Harrison in 1985 and Svigos in 1982, and they are the studies with the fewest number of participants (respectively 20 and 28 patients).

Fox et al. published a retrospective study in 2017 that evaluated the role of mid-luteal hCG injection on women with RPL.[15] RPL was defined as two or more consecutive first-trimester losses. Among 98 women, 53 received hCG injection 1 week after ovulation, and 45 women did not. In the treated group, there were 44 pregnancies, including 10 miscarriages, and in the nontreated group, there were 38 pregnancies, including 25 miscarriages (38% reduction risk of miscarriage, $p = 0.003$).

Based on these results, ESHRE 2023 guidelines on RPL management concluded that there was insufficient evidence to recommend the use of hCG to improve live birth rate "in women with RPL and luteal phase insufficiency." They considered that studies were too limited to recommend hCG treatment in such patients.[8]

DISCUSSION

In our opinion, there is a clear physiological inaccuracy in the strategy followed by the majority of the studies, except in Fox et al.'s retrospective study. In the hypothesis of hCG deficiency, the lack of hCG production by the embryo itself shall lead to a deficit in the CL secretions and have direct consequences in the endometrial preparation for implantation. If we want the treatment to be efficient, we formulate the hypothesis that hCG administration should replace the hCG that is not enough secreted by the embryo. When delivering 10,000 IU of hCG subcutaneously, hCG concentration in the maternal blood will never exceed 337.9 IU/mL on the day of higher concentration and then decrease progressively.[16] In the studies that we reported here, the treatment was always initiated when the pregnancy was diagnosed by ultrasound. We can suppose that hCG was already high at this time, and we can challenge the idea of hCG supplementation at this moment. According to us, if the objective is to correct a hypothetic luteal phase insufficiency, we shall administer hCG during the luteal phase, which means immediately after ovulation. When administrating hCG at the moment of the ovulation, the molecule will directly target the follicle and hypothetically the endometrium and mimic the luteinizing hormone (LH) activity but with a stronger and longer action. In the hypothesis of a successful implantation, hCG level in the blood will progressively increase and overcome the maximum level of hCG levels following subcutaneous hCG concentration approximately 2 weeks after ovulation.

Consequently, if we aimed to prove the positive impact on pregnancy evolution of hCG administration, I suggest that we start after ovulation with a trigger dose and that we continue with smaller doses in order to provide a high hCG level in the blood until the day that the trophoblast will take over the secretion of hCG and provoke hCG blood level much higher than the level obtained following hCG subcutaneous administration.

A clinical trial—the Heart Outcomes Prevention Evaluation (HOPE) trial[17]—is recruiting patients for a prospective randomized study to compare the administration of progesterone versus a single shot of hCG in mid-luteal phase. It is an interesting study, which has yet to start recruitment. We strongly need a study like this and other new RCTs with robust methodology to provide evidence to support the use of mid-luteal hCG in patients with RPL who undergo follicular monitoring. The concept is physiologically supported but needs more evidence to support its recommendation in guidelines.

REFERENCES

1. d'Hauterive SP, Close R, Gridelet V, Mawet M, Nisolle M, Geenen V. Human Chorionic Gonadotropin and Early Embryogenesis: Review. Int J Mol Sci. 2022;23(3): 1380.
2. Gridelet V, Perrier d'Hauterive S, Polese B, Foidart JM, Nisolle M, Geenen V. Human Chorionic Gonadotrophin: New Pleiotropic Functions for an "Old" Hormone During Pregnancy. Front Immunol. 2020;11:343.
3. Clark DA, Chaouat G, Arck PC, Mittruecker HW, Levy GA. Cytokine-dependent abortion in CBA × DBA/2 mice is mediated by the procoagulant fgl2 prothrombinase [correction of prothombinase]. J Immunol. 1998;160(2): 545-9.
4. Practice Committees of the American Society for Reproductive Medicine and the Society for Reproductive Endocrinology and Infertility. Diagnosis and treatment of luteal phase deficiency: a committee opinion. Fertil Steril. 2021;115(6):1416-23.
5. Corner GW, Allen WM. Physiology of the corpus luteum. 1929. Am J Obstet Gynecol. 2005;193(4):1574.
6. Balasch J, Creus M, Márquez M, Burzaco I, Vanrell JA. The significance of luteal phase deficiency on fertility: a diagnostic and therapeutic approach. Hum Reprod. 1986; 1(3):145-7.
7. Ogasawara M, Kajiura S, Katano K, Aoyama T, Aoki K. Are serum progesterone levels predictive of recurrent miscarriage in future pregnancies? Fertil Steril. 1997;68(5): 806-9.
8. Bender Atik R, Christiansen OB, Elson J, Kolte AM, Lewis S, Middeldorp S, et al.; ESHRE Guideline Group on RPL. ESHRE guideline: recurrent pregnancy loss: an update in 2022. Hum Reprod Open. 2023;2023(1):hoad002.
9. Morley LC, Simpson N, Tang T. Human chorionic gonadotrophin (hCG) for preventing miscarriage. Cochrane Database Syst Rev. 2013;(1):CD008611.
10. Svigos J. Preliminary experience with the use of human chorionic gonadotrophin therapy in women with repeated abortion. Clin Reprod Fertil. 1982;1(2):131-5.
11. Harrison RF. Treatment of habitual abortion with human chorionic gonadotropin: results of open and placebo-controlled studies. Eur J Obstet Gynecol Reprod Biol. 1985; 20(3):159-68.
12. Harrison RF. Human chorionic gonadotrophin (hCG) in the management of recurrent abortion; results of a multi-centre placebo-controlled study. Eur J Obstet Gynecol Reprod Biol. 1992;47(3):175-9.
13. Quenby S, Farquharson RG. Human chorionic gonadotropin supplementation in recurring pregnancy loss: a controlled trial. Fertil Steril. 1994;62(4):708-10.
14. El-Zibdeh MY. Dydrogesterone in the reduction of recurrent spontaneous abortion. J Steroid Biochem Mol Biol. 2005;97(5):431-4.
15 Fox C, Azores-Gococo D, Swart L, Holoch K, Savaris RF, Likes CE, et al. Luteal phase HCG support for unexplained recurrent pregnancy loss - a low hanging fruit? Reprod Biomed Online. 2017;34(3):319-24.
16. Radicioni M, Leuratti C, Cometti B. Randomized Pharmacokinetic Study of a Highly Purified Human Chorionic Gonadotropin and of a Recombinant Human Chorionic Gonadotropin Following Single Subcutaneous Administration in Healthy Women. Clin Drug Investig. 2022;42(3):199-206.
17. HOPE Trial Randomised Control Trial comparing Progesterone and HCG supplementation in RPL NCT05365464.

CHAPTER 48

Role of Granulocyte Colony-stimulating Factor

Fabio Scarpellini, Marco Sbracia

ABSTRACT

Granulocyte colony stimulating factor is a cytokine that has been used successfully in patients with thin endometrium and recurrent implantation failure prior to embryo transfer. In an initial randomized control trial in patients with unexplained euploid recurrent pregnancy loss (RPL) it improved live birth rates, but subsequently other studies have shown inconsistent results. We currently need more scientific evidence to prove or disprove its role in RPL.

Keywords: Granulocyte colony stimulating factor, Unexplained RPL, RIF, Thin endometrium.

INTRODUCTION

Cytokines seems to have a fundamental role in embryo implantation, embryo development, trophoblast invasion, placental growth though all pregnancy, and some of them have been thoroughly investigated, such as colony-stimulating factors (CSFs), macrophage colony-stimulating factor (M-CSF or CSF1), granulocyte-macrophage colony-stimulating factor (GM-CSF or CSF2), and granulocyte colony-stimulating factor (G-CSF or CSF3).[1-3] They have gained particular interest due to their possible use for the treatment of reproductive affections.

The CSFs are a group of glycoproteins binding to specific receptors on hematopoietic stem cells, promoting cell proliferation and differentiation into macrophages and granulocytes.[3] They show different structures and gene location, also have different receptors.

Macrophage colony-stimulating factor is a cytokine of 554 amino acids with a molecular weight of 60,179 kDa, the gene is located on the short arm of chromosome 1, region 1p13.3.[4] It binds to a specific receptor, the M-CSFR or CD115, encoded by a gene located on the long arm of chromosome 5, region 5q32; this gene codes for a protein of 972 amino acids and is 107,984 kDa in molecular weight, a receptor related to the tyrosine kinase protein family.[3-5]

Granulocyte-macrophage colony-stimulating factor is a protein of 14,435 kDa in molecular weight, consisting of 144 amino acids, encoded by a gene located on the long arm of chromosome 5, region 5q31, in a cluster of genes associated with the 5q-syndrome and acute myelogenous leukemia.[6] GM-CSF binds to a specific receptor, the GM-CSFR or CD116, whose gene is located in the Xp22.32 and Yp11.3 regions encoding for a protein of 46,207 kDa in molecular weight.[7]

Granulocyte colony-stimulating factor is a glycoprotein of 174–180 amino acids long and with a molecular weight of 19,600 kDa. Its gene is located on the long arm of chromosome 17, region 17q11.2-q12. It binds to a specific receptor, the G-CSFR or CD114, encoded by a gene on the short arm of chromosome 1, region 1p35-34.3, a protein of 92,156 in molecular weight.[8] Granulocyte-CSFR is associated with signal transduction through the JAK-STAT3 pathways.

G-CSF stimulates bone marrow to produce granulocytes and stem cells released into the bloodstream. G-CSF and its receptor have been found on trophoblasts and in the decidua of several mammals including human placenta.[9-11] An antiabortive role was demonstrated for G-CSF in the animal model, and its depletion was indirectly involved in miscarriages.[12,13] It has also been shown that G-CSF has a positive effect on trophoblast metabolism.[14] Furthermore, G-CSF is secreted in follicular fluid and its levels correlated with oocyte competence and implantation potential of corresponding embryos.[15]

GRANULOCYTE COLONY-STIMULATING FACTOR AND RECURRENT PREGNANCY LOSS

Several studies have been published in the recent years reporting the data of large series of analysis for aneuploidy by molecular genetic testing on deoxyribonucleic acid (DNA) samples obtained in case both in case of sporadic miscarriages and recurrent pregnancy loss (RPL) miscarriages.[16-18] These data showed that in both cases the rate of product of conceptions aneuploidy was similar, ranging from 56 to 60% of cases.[16-19] It has been reported in these study that numerical chromosome abnormality was more likely to occur in cases with advanced maternal age, an earlier gestational age, fewer previous pregnancy losses, and pregnancy with a female fetus.[18,19] Furthermore, also in case of preimplantation genetic testing for aneuploidy (PGT-A) on embryos obtained in women with RPL or infertility undergoing in vitro fertilization (IVF) the rate was similar for aneuploidy in both groups.[20,21]

These results showed that in RPL women with 4–5 consecutive miscarriages their outcome is worse than in patients with a lower number of miscarriages, since they have euploid embryos that will be miscarried without known reasons.[18-20]

Recurrent miscarriage is defined as the occurrence of three or more early consecutive losses or two late pregnancy losses prior to the 20th week of gestation according to the European Society of Human Reproduction and Embryology (ESHRE).[22] The American Society for Reproductive Medicine (ASRM) instead defined the occurrence of two or more pregnancy failures as RPL.[23] Recurrent implantation failure is still not well-defined condition, and in the literature can be found many definitions. The ESHRE Working Group on Recurrent Implantation Failure published in 2023 the ESHRE good practice recommendations paper providing the following definition for recurrent implantation failure (RIF): "RIF describes the scenario in which the transfer of embryos considered to be viable has failed to result in a positive pregnancy test sufficiently often in a specific patient to warrant consideration of further investigations and/or interventions," without reporting a cutoff number for transferred embryos.[24]

Recognized causes for RPL are generally considered parental chromosomal defects, infections, endocrinological causes (thyroid defects, diabetes, and polycystic ovaries), uterine abnormalities, antiphospholipid antibody syndrome, or other autoimmune conditions.[25] However, >40% of RPL cases remain unexplained[25] and for them several causes have been proposed, including the alloimmune response. RPL could be due to an imbalance in the Th1/Th2 systems, with a prevalence during pregnancy of Th1 cytokine production with a cytotoxic role, instead of Th2 cytokine production with an immunosuppression role.[26] Several treatments have been proposed for RPL, but all these treatments showed controversial results.[27]

We evaluated the role of G-CSF in early pregnancy and its use in the treatment of recurrent pregnancy loss (RPL),[28] as well as other authors studied its effect on RIF.[29] We started use G-CSF in RPL in 1997, successfully treating a woman after five consecutive miscarriages. We used this treatment in several other women with encouraging results (the pilot study was presented in 1998 at the Annual ASRM meeting). We conducted a controlled randomized study published in 2009.[28] We selected a group of patients fulfilling these inclusion criteria: woman's age <39 years, more than four previous miscarriages, failure of previous treatments for RPL, and they had to be negative for all the known causes of RPL. The patients had to have normal karyotyping of embryonic tissues in their last miscarriage. Sixty-eight patients were included in the study: 35 women underwent daily administration of filgrastim, the recombinant G-CSF, 1 µg (100,000 IU)/kg/day from the 6th day after ovulation until the occurrence of menstruation or to the end of the 9th week of gestation. Instead, 33 subjects were treated with saline solution in the same way. The live births in women treated with G-CSF were 82.8%, whereas in the controls they were 48.5% ($p = 0.0061$). The number of patients needed to treat for one additional live birth was 2.9. None of the newborns showed any major or minor abnormalities. This study showed that G-CSF is a promising tool for the treatment of selected cases of RPL. We increased the number of patients in our randomized controlled trial, confirming the early results. In patients treated with G-CSF the delivery rate observed was 83.3% whereas in the placebo group it was 44.4% ($p < 0.0001$). Subsequently we treated a total of 270 women with RPL, from three up to six abortions (age from 29 up to 43 years old) with G-CSF at the same dosage previously reported. In these women we observed a delivery rate of 81.1%. In this group of patients when the data were stratified for the woman's age and number of previous abortions, we observed that patients that take more advantages from the treatment were patients with four or more previous miscarriages and with an age <40 years old. G-CSF has been also tried in the treatment of RIF such as showed by the studies published in literature. Subsequently to a paper of Wurfel et al. in 2010[29] on the role of G-CSF treatment in RIF women showing lack of killer cell immunoglobulin-like receptors, several other authors reported data on this issue with inconsistent results. A recent multicenter randomized controlled trial of a single dose of G-CSF used subcutaneously before embryo transfer in 112 patients with RIF showed an improved clinical pregnancy rate in the intervention group.[30] However, in 2021 a meta-analysis has been published on the efficacy of therapies and interventions RIF, showing that subcutaneous G-CSF administration resulted the most promising therapeutic options for RIF patients.[31] In our opinion, G-CSF treatment in RIF patients should be used only after PGT-A, to exclude from the embryo transfer, embryos with chromosomal aneuploidy. It has been estimated that >50% IVF embryos show a chromosomal abnormality determining implantation failure. Consequently, future studies on any treatment for RIF should include only patients undergoing PGT-A and subsequent transfer of only chromosomally normal embryos, to obtain consistent results.

Recently, G-CSF has been used in the treatment of "thin endometrium" in IVF cycles prior to embryo transfer to increase the endometrium thickness. An early paper by Gleicher et el.[32] reported that the intrauterine instillation of G-CSF promoted the growth of "thin endometrium" (<7 mm) before embryo transfer; several other papers were published after the first report showing inconsistent results. Meta-analysis published on this issue has shown inconclusive results, since there is a lack of controlled studies on this issue, whereas there are several reviews and meta-analysis. Probably there would be some patients that can take advantage of this treatment, but the paucity of data does not justify its use routinely.

Side effects commonly reported by patients are mild fever and occasionally bony pains. Leukocytosis may be observed on a full blood count. Concerns may be raised on the safety of this treatment during pregnancy. G-CSF treatment during pregnancy seems to be healthy and devoid of adverse and side effects for the mothers and the fetuses, such as showed by several surveys conducted on pregnant women with chronic neutropenia treated with high dose of G-CSF, as well as in the studies conducted on RPL women, where G-CSF is used with much lower dosage. The use of G-CSF during pregnancy is safe since in our experience as well as in the literature no serious adverse effects have been reported.[33-35]

To date there is no evidence about the mechanism of action of G-CSF on pregnancy, even though there is circumstantial evidence about how this cytokine may interact with the trophoblast and immune system. G-CSF activates and mobilizes stem cells, it is used to increase the number of stem cells after their transplant, or to activate the reconstruction of the vascular bed after heart ischemia, and in neurology to treat patients with severe degenerative diseases. In our study we observed a significant increase of human chorionic gonadotropin (β-hCG) levels in the ongoing pregnancies from the fifth through the ninth gestational week of gestation in G-CSF treated pregnancies compared to normal pregnancies.[28] These data show a direct effect of this cytokine on the trophoblast, with the mobilization and activation of placental stem cells. Another mechanism of action may be the effect of G-CSF on lymphocytes, several studies evidenced that G-CSF promotes the mobilization and proliferation of several lymphocytic and dendritic cells, in particular regulatory T (Treg) and CD2 cells.[36,37] Our unpublished data showed that women with RPL treated with G-CSF had a remarkable increase of peripheral blood levels of Treg cells compared to normal pregnancy. Furthermore, in a selected group of RIF patients that failed to be pregnant after egg donation cycles, the treatment with GM-CSF significantly increased the peripheral Treg cells in the treated women compared to controls treated with saline infusion.[38] In women with RPL treated with G-CSF who miscarried again (due to chromosomal abnormalities) an increase of Treg cells in the decidua compared to the controls we observed, as well as for c-kit, vascular endothelial growth factor receptor-2 (VEGFR-2), and VEGF (antigens expressed in stem cells) showed a significant increase in G-CSF treated group.[39] These data suggest that G-CSF may mobilize stem cells and immune cells enhancing trophoblast function. On the other hand, in the 2019 the results of the RESPONSE study were published showing no differences for pregnancy outcome in patients with unexplained RPL treated with G-CSF or not.[40] However, this study was poorly conducted, since they put to in the same different kind of RPL patients, woman's age, number of previous miscarriages, associated pathologies, etc., looking for a "magic bullet" that may resolve all problems, such as was evidenced by several authors.[41]

CONCLUSION

In the evaluation of the effectiveness of any treatment in RPL there are several difficulties. Several factors play a confounding role such as maternal age, number of previous miscarriages, causes of miscarriages, especially chromosomal embryo abnormalities occurring at high rate, and rising with maternal age.[25] Furthermore, it has been shown that the spontaneous resolution of RPL occurs in 40–60% of cases, depending on the number of previous miscarriages.[25] Considering of all these covariates, a controlled randomized study should include a large number of patients, that only with more randomized placebo-controlled multicentric trials the problem can be solved. Nowadays, several centers are using G-CSF for RPL and/or RIF. However, data published has a heterogeneous population and is not randomized or placebo controlled. There are effective treatments for RPL with clear immunologic origin, such as in antiphospholipid syndrome where heparin plus aspirin gives good pregnancy rates.[25] For idiopathic RPL there is currently no evidence of an effective treatment apart from tender loving care.[27] G-CSF may be effective in patients with unexplained RPL <40 years old, with at least four previous miscarriages, and proved absence of chromosomal abnormalities in the last embryo aborted, or in RIF after PGT-A.

REFERENCES

1. Armstrong DT, Chaouat G. Effects of lymphokines and immune complexes on murine placental cell growth in vitro. Biol Reprod. 1989;40:466-74.
2. Oreshkova T, Dimitrov R, Mourdjeva M. A cross-talk of decidual stromal cells, trophoblast, and immune cells: a prerequisite for the success of pregnancy. Am J Reprod Immunol. 2012;68:366-73.
3. Stanley ER, Berg KL, Einstein DB, Lee PS, Pixley FJ, Wang Y, et al. Biology and action of colony—stimulating factor-1. Mol Reprod Dev. 1997;46:4-10.
4. Saltman DL, Dolganov GM, Hinton LM, Sublett JE, Deaven LL, Foust JT, et al. Reassignment of the human macrophage colony stimulating factor gene to chromosome 1p13-21. Biochem Biophys Res Commun. 1992;182:1139-43.
5. Galland F, Stefanova M, Lafage M, Birnbaum D. Localization of the 5'end of the MCF2 oncogene to human chromosome 15q15→q23. Cytogenet Cell Genet. 1992;60:114-6.
6. Cantrell MA, Anderson D, Cerretti DP, Price V, McKereghan K, Tushinski RJ, et al. Cloning, sequence, and expression of a human granulocyte/macrophage colonystimulating factor. Proc Natl Acad Sci U S A. 1985;82:6250-4.
7. Rappold G, Willson TA, Henke A, Gough NM. Arrangement and localization of the human GM-CSF receptor alpha chain geneCSF2RA within the X-Y pseudoautosomal region. Genomics. 1992;14:455-61.
8. Tweardy DJ, Anderson K, Cannizzaro LA, Steinman RA, Croce CM, Huebner K, et al. Molecular cloning of cDNAs for the human granulocyte colony-stimulating factor receptor from HL-60 and mapping of the gene to chromosome region 1p32-34. Blood. 1992;79:1148-54.
9. Uzumaki H, Okabe T, Sasaki N, Hagiwara K, Takaku F, Tobita M, et al. Identification and characterization of receptors for granulocyte colony-stimulating factor on human placenta and trophoblastic cells. Proc Natl Acad Sci U S A. 1989;86:9323-6.
10. Giacomini G, Tabibzadeh SS, Satyaswaroop PG, Bonsi L, Vitale L, Bagnara GP, et al. Epithelial cells are the major source of biologically active granulocyte macrophage colony-stimulating factor in human endometrium. Hum Reprod. 1995;10:3259-63.
11. McCracken SA, Grant KE, MacKenzie IZ, Redman CW, Mardon HJ. Gestational regulation of granulocyte-colony stimulating factor receptor expression in the human placenta. Biol Reprod. 1999;60:790-6.
12. Novales JS, Salva AM, Modanlou HD, Kaplan DL, del Castillo J, Andersen J, et al. Maternal administration of granulocyte colony-stimulating factor improves neonatal rat survival after a lethal group B streptococcal infection. Blood. 1993;81:923-7.
13. Sugita K, Hayakawa S, Karasaki-Suzuki M, Hagiwara H, Chishima F, Aleemuzaman S, et al. Granulocyte colony stimulation factor (G-CSF) suppresses interleukin (IL)-12 and/or IL-2 induced interferon (IFN)-gamma production and cytotoxicity of decidual mononuclear cells. Am J Reprod Immunol. 2003;50:83-9.
14. Marino VJ, Roguin LP. The granulocyte colony stimulating factor (G-CSF) activates Jak/STAT and MAPK pathways in a trophoblastic cell line. J Cell Biochem. 2008;103:1512-23.
15. Ledee N, Lombroso R, Lombardelli L, Selva J, Dubanchet S, Chaouat G, et al. Cytokines and chemokines in follicular fluids and potential of the corresponding embryo: the role of granulocyte colony-stimulating factor. Hum Reprod. 2008;23:2001-9.
16. Schlaikjær Hartwig T, Ambye L, Gruhn JR, Petersen JF, Wrønding T, Amato L, et al.; COPL consortium. Cell-free fetal DNA for genetic evaluation in Copenhagen Pregnancy Loss Study (COPL): a prospective cohort study. Lancet. 2023;401(10378):762-71.
17. Zhu D, Wei X, Zhou XY, Deng LB, Xiong SY, Chen JP, et al. Chromosomal abnormalities in recurrent pregnancy loss and its association with clinical characteristics. J Assist Reprod Genet. 2023;40:1713-20.
18. Korkidakis A, Albert AY, Jiang I, et al. The Clinical Significance of Embryonic Chromosomal Errors in Recurrent Pregnancy Loss: an Analysis of 1107 Miscarriages. Reprod Sci. 2023;30:3019-26.
19. Li Y, Zhou R, Xia Z, Deng LB, Xiong SY, Chen JP, et al. Reproductive outcomes in couples with recurrent pregnancy loss after embryonic chromosomal microarray analysis. J Assist Reprod Genet. 2024;4:161-70.
20. Kornfield MS, Parker P, Rubin E, Garg B, O'Leary T, Amato P, et al. Patients with Recurrent Pregnancy Loss Have Similar Embryonic Preimplantation Genetic Testing Aneuploidy Rates and In Vitro Fertilization Outcomes to Infertility Patients. F S Rep. 2022;3(4):342-8.
21. Pantou A, Mitrakos A, Kokkali G, Petroutsou K, Tounta G, Lazaros L, et al. The impact of preimplantation genetic

testing for aneuploidies (PGT-A) on clinical outcomes in high risk patients. J Assist Reprod Genet. 2022;39(6):1341-9.
22. ESHRE Guideline Group on RPL; Bender Atik R, Christiansen OB, Elson J, Kolte AM, Lewis S, Middeldorp S, et al. ESHRE guideline: recurrent pregnancy loss: an update in 2022. Hum Reprod Open. 2023;2023(1):hoad002.
23. Practice Committee of the American Society for Reproductive Medicine. It replaces the document, "Definitions of Infertility and Recurrent Pregnancy Loss: a Committee Opinion," last published in 2013. Fertil Steril. 2020;113:533-5.
24. ESHRE Working Group on Recurrent Implantation Failure; Cimadomo D, de Los Santos MJ, Griesinger G, Lainas G, Le Clef N, McLernon DJ, et al. ESHRE good practice recommendations on recurrent implantation failure. Hum Reprod Open. 2023;2023(3):hoad023.
25. Carrington B, Sacks G, Regan L. Recurrent miscarriage: Pathophysiology and outcome. Curr Opin Obstet Gynecol. 2005;17(6):591-7.
26. Michimata T, Sakai M, Miyazaki S, Ogasawara MS, Suzumori K, Aoki K, et al. Decrease of T-helper 2 and T-cytotoxic 2 cells at implantation sites occurs in unexplained recurrent spontaneous abortion with normal chromosomal content. Hum Reprod. 2003;18:1523-8.
27. Porter TF, LaCoursiere Y, Scott JR. Immunotherapy for recurrent miscarriage. Cochrane Database Syst Rev. 2006;(2):CD000112.
28. Scarpellini F, Sbracia M. Use of granulocyte colony-stimulating factor for the treatment of unexplained recurrent miscarriage: a randomised controlled trial. Hum Reprod. 2009;24(11):2703-8.
29. Würfel W, Santjohanser C, Hirv K, Bühl M, Meri O, Laubert I, et al. High pregnancy rates with administration of granulocyte colony-stimulating factor in ART-patients with repetitive implantation failure and lacking killer-cell immunglobulin-like receptors. Hum Reprod 2010;25(8):2151-2.
30. Arefi S, Fazeli E, Esfahani M, Borhani N, Yamini N, Hosseini A, et al. Granulocyte-colony stimulating factor may improve pregnancy outcome in patients with history of unexplained recurrent implantation failure: An RCT. Int J Reprod Biomed (Yazd). 2018;16(5):299-304.
31. Busnelli A, Somigliana E, Cirillo F, Baggiani A, Levi-Setti PE. Efficacy of therapies and interventions for repeated embryo implantation failure: a systematic review and meta-analysis. Sci Rep. 2021;11(1):1747.
32. Gleicher N, Vidali A, Barad DH. Successful treatment of unresponsive thin endometrium. Fertil Steril. 2011;95(6):2123.e13-7.
33. Dale DC, Cottle TE, Fier CJ, Bolyard AA, Bonilla MA, Boxer LA, et al. Severe chronic neutropenia: treatment and follow-up of patients in the Severe Chronic Neutropenia International Registry. Am J Hematol. 2003;72(2):82-93.
34. Pessach I, Shimoni A, Nagler A. Granulocyte-colony stimulating factor for hematopoietic stem cell donation from healthy female donors during pregnancy and lactation: what do we know? Hum Reprod Update. 2013;19(3):259-67.
35. Boxer LA, Bolyard AA, Kelley ML, Marrero TM, Phan L, Bond JM, et al. Use of granulocyte colony stimulating factor during pregnancy in women with chronic neutropenia. Obstet Gynecol. 2015;125:197-203.
36. Condomines M, Quittet P, Lu ZY, Nadal L, Latry P, Lopez E, et al. Functional regulatory T cells are collected in stem cell autografts by mobilization with high dose cyclophosphamide and granulocyte colony-stimulating factor. J Immunol. 2006;176(11):6631-9.
37. Rossetti M, Gregori S, Roncarolo MG. Granulocyte-colony stimulating factor drives the in vitro differentiation of human dendritic cells that induce anergy in naive T cells. Eur J Immunol. 2010;40(11):3097-106.
38. Scarpellini F, Sbracia M. Modification of peripheric Treg andCD56^{brigh}NK levels in RIF women after egg donation, treated with GM-CSF or placebo. J Reprod Immunol. 2023;158:103983.
39. Scarpellini F, Klinger FG, Rossi G, Sbracia M. Immunohistochemical Study on the Expression of G-CSF, G-CSFR, VEGF, VEGFR-1, Foxp3 in First Trimester Trophoblast of Recurrent Pregnancy Loss in Pregnancies Treated with G-CSF and Controls. Int J Mol Sci. 2019;21(1):285.
40. Eapen A, Joing M, Kwon P, Tong J, Maneta E, De Santo C, et al. RESPONSE study group. Recombinant human granulocyte- colony stimulating factor in women with unexplained recurrent pregnancy losses: a randomized clinical trial. Hum Reprod. 2019;34(3):424-32.
41. Sbracia M, Scarpellini F, Stamenov G. G-CSFin RPL: what's new? Hum Reprod. 2020;35:1469-74.

CHAPTER 49

Role of Lymphocyte Immunotherapy

Mohan Raut, Mugdha Raut

ABSTRACT

Recurrent miscarriages are seen in 2–5% of women and 50% of these are labeled as unexplained as no underlying cause is found in them. Various studies have explained possible alloimmune basis in these couples. Lymphocyte immunization therapy (LIT) was the earliest immunomodulatory method suggested in these cases. Recent meta-analysis have shown that LIT is not only effective in the treatment of repeated miscarriages but it is also safe. Selection of subgroup of patients for LIT using immunological investigations is important. Large multicentric RCTs are required to further determine the efficiency of LIT.

Keywords: LIT, Lymphocyte immunotherapy, Repeated miscarriages, Alloimmune rejection, Lymphocyte crossmatch, TNF alpha, NK cells.

INTRODUCTION

Lymphocyte immunization therapy (LIT) is an active immunomodulatory treatment, used as a treatment for unexplained recurrent pregnancy loss (RPL), unexplained in vitro fertilization (IVF) failures, and unexplained infertility. It was the first immunomodulatory treatment recommended for unexplained repeated pregnancy loss.

Recurrent pregnancy loss can be a heterogeneous condition. This affects women of all ages and with a variety of conditions. As the cause of RPL is not always known, it is one of the most frustrating and challenging conditions in reproductive medicine. Also, the evidence for diagnostic and therapeutic methods is not always reliable. Many studies that examine the causes, management, and evaluation of RPL are flawed.[1] That is why, RPL treatment can often be frustrating.

American Society of Reproductive Medicine (ASRM) defines RPL as two or more miscarriages, while according to the European Society of Human Reproduction and Embryology (ESHRE), three or more miscarriages are required to label a case as RPL.[2] Recurrent miscarriages are seen in 2–5% of women. 50% of these patients do not have an underlying cause of repeated miscarriages.[3,4] Such patients are most likely to be benefited from LIT.

IMMUNOLOGY OF PREGNANCY: ROLE IN REPRODUCTIVE FAILURES

Fetus as Allograft

Pregnancy is nature's miracle, which is evident when you look at the immunological aspects of pregnancy.

A pregnancy has 50% genetic material from the father and 50% from the mother. The paternal part of the fetus carries with it the paternal antigens. These antigens are totally foreign to the mother's immunological system. So, logically speaking, the mother's immunological system should build an immunological response against the fetus, leading to the rejection of the fetus.[5] Thus, a fetus is a semiallograft in the immunologically active maternal immunological system.

The fetus survives and grows into a healthy baby, despite this. This is known as the "paradox in pregnancy."

The tolerance of the semiallogenic fetus requires an alteration in the maternal immune system so that the immune response to the fetus is changed. Thus, the paradox of pregnancy can be explained by the interplay between the inflammatory (Th1) and the anti-inflammatory (Th2) responses. This happens through alteration in the immune cells and cytokines at the fetomaternal interface. In this phenomenon, the uterine Natural Killer (NK) cells, T-reg cells, dendritic cells, and macrophages play an important role.[6,7]

Since immunomodulation in pregnancy is crucial, it has long been suspected that defects in this immune system can lead to fetal rejection causing pregnancy loss. It is in these cases that immunomodulatory treatment like LIT can be beneficial.

WHAT IS LIT?

Lymphocyte immunization therapy is the active immunomodulatory treatment that is used, to treat unexplained RM patients. As the name suggests, it involves the immunization of the prospective mother with allogeneic mononuclear cells, mainly lymphocytes.

Lymphocytes are the most important cells in the immune system. They play an important role both in cell-mediated immune responses and in humoral immune responses. They are the key players in rejection response against immunologically different substrates. Hence, the use of lymphocytes has been suggested to modulate the immune response against immunologically different fetuses in the mother's body (semiallograft).[8]

Lymphocyte immunization therapy is of two types:

1. *Paternal LIT*: In this, lymphocytes from the husband's blood are used to cause immunomodulation.
2. *Donor LIT*: In this, lymphocytes from the donor's blood are used to cause immunomodulation. It may involve a single donor or can use pooled donor lymphocytes.

HISTORY OF LYMPHOCYTE IMMUNIZATION THERAPY

The immunological basis of pregnancy was always considered by researchers, and various theories were put forward to explain the mechanisms that help in the maintenance of pregnancy. Once the alloimmune basis of pregnancy was established, various immunological treatments were put forward to treat complications of pregnancy, resulting from the disturbances in alloimmune imbalance. The possibility of immunization of paternally marked cells was explored to counter the immune response of the mother toward the fetus. One of the first modalities of immunomodulatory treatment that was tried and recommended was LIT.

History

It was Sir Peter Medawar, who first proposed that the maternal immune system has a big part to play in maintaining pregnancies that are immunologically different. He first put forward the question, "How does a pregnant mom sustain a fetus with antigenically foreign characteristics for several weeks and months? He suggested that whether it is due to physical separation by the placenta or by other means, the maternal immune response must be insensitive to the fetal presence in some way.[9]

Lymphocyte immunization was first described by Billingham et al.[10] Billingham RE et al. observed that skin transplants among fraternal twins were accepted, but not between nontwin siblings. They suggested that blood cells exchanged via the twin placentas continued and maintained an immunologic tolerance.

The first LIT was used by Taylor and Faulk. This study was based on the hypothesis that it should be possible to artificially stimulate protective factor production in the mother by infusing her with allogenic leukocytes, thereby, protecting the fertilized egg at implantation.[11]

Dr Beer suggested that paternal MHC-antigen sharing could be linked to adverse pregnancy consequences. According to him, insufficient maternal recognition of paternal antigens can lead to low tolerance for the pregnancy. Therefore, it was suggested that immunizations with paternal mononuclear cells could improve maternal recognition of paternal alloantigens and allow patients with spontaneous, recurrent abortions (or other forms) to continue a pregnancy to term.[12]

The first randomized controlled trial of LIT in unexplained, recurrent spontaneous abortions was conducted by Mowbrey, et al.[11] In this study, results showed that 17 out of 22 women (77.2%), who were given paternal cells were successful, while only 10 of 27 (37%) were successful in the control arm.

Later, a meta-analysis was conducted in 1994 by the Recurrent Miscarriages Immunotherapy Trialists Group (RMITG). It reported the efficacy of LIT in women with spontaneous primary abortions, who were negative for anti-paternal antibodies.[13]

In a subsequent meta-analysis, allogeneic lymphocyte transplantation was found to significantly increase the chance of live birth [odds ratio (OR): 1.94] in patients with primary recurrent miscarriage without anti-paternal antibodies.[14] Although studies from different parts of the world were yielding conflicting results, research in the field of LIT has continued.

MECHANISMS OF ACTION OF LYMPHOCYTE IMMUNIZATION THERAPY

Lymphocyte immunization therapy produces its protective immunomodulatory effect through different mechanisms **(Fig. 1)**:

- *Development of blocking antibodies (asymmetric antibodies)*: They are produced when allogenic lymphocytes are presented to the maternal immune system. These antibodies protect pregnancy.[15-17]

  Normally, antibodies have two antigen-binding fragments (Fab) regions. After LIT, the antibodies that are produced have post-translational high mannose glycosylations of one or both Fab chains, This makes the antibodies functionally univalent and is called asymmetrical antibodies. This asymmetric antibody is unable to form complexes, thus inhibiting complement fixation and phagocytosis. The other Fab fragment, being unmodified, has the antigen binding capacity and it competitively inhibits the unmodified symmetric antibody. Asymmetric antibody levels have also been shown to increase following LIT, as shown by Zenclussen et al.[17]
- *Increasing the number and distribution of T regulatory cells*: LIT could increase tolerance by increasing the number and distribution of T regulatory cells. When a sufficient number of lymphocytes are injected into the dermis, they interact with dendritic cells, macrophages, and mast cells. This can lead to an increased number of Treg cells, which may prove beneficial in maintaining pregnancy. It is reported that the Th17/Treg ratio significantly reduces after LIT,[18] and the Th1/Th2 cytokine ratio also decreases significantly after LIT, favoring the continuation of pregnancy.[19]
- *Role of dendritic cells:* The maintenance of immune tolerance could also be achieved by dendritic cells by turning on T regulatory cells that suppress immune responses to semi-allogenic pregnancy.[20]
- *Regulation of human leukocyte antigen-G (HLA-G):*[21] It maintains maternal-fetal immune tolerance at the maternal-fetal interface. It reduces inflammation and immune responses and strengthens transplantation tolerance.[22,23]
- *Role of CD200:* The immunomodulatory effect of LIT could also be mediated by the lymphocyte surface marker CD200.[24]

INDICATIONS AND CONTRAINDICATIONS FOR LYMPHOCYTE IMMUNIZATION THERAPY

- *Indications*:
  - Unexplained repeated pregnancy loss
  - Unexplained recurrent implantation failure (RIF)
  - Unexplained infertility

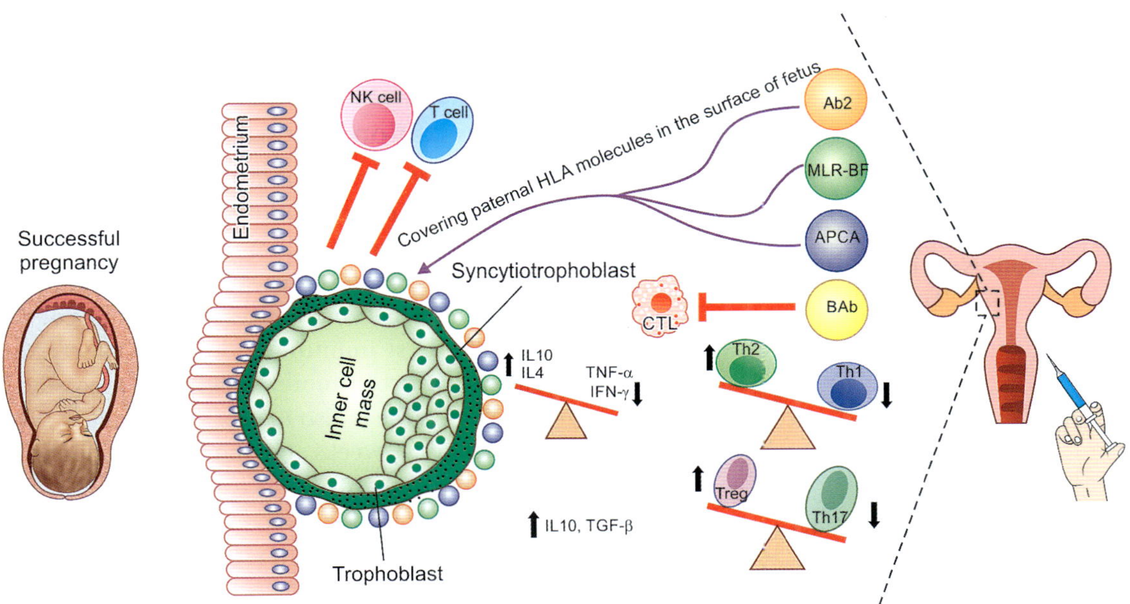

Fig. 1: Mechanisms of action of LIT.[50] (BAb: blocking antibodies; CTL: cytotoxic T-cell; IFN: interferon; IL: interleukin; MLR-BF: mixed lymphocyte reaction blocking factor; TGF: transforming growth factor)

- *Contraindications:*
  - Known factor for RPL/RIF
  - Selection criteria not fulfilled
  - Presence of infection in husband [human immunodeficiency virus (HIV), hepatitis C virus (HCV), venereal disease research laboratory test (VDRL), and hepatitis B surface antigen (HBsAg)—(donor lymphocytes can be used)]

SELECTION OF COUPLES FOR LYMPHOCYTE IMMUNIZATION THERAPY

Lymphocyte immunization therapy holds much potential as a safe and effective treatment approach for reproductive patients who have failed with less aggressive protocols when used correctly on a well-selected patient. The selection of a couple for LIT depends on many factors. Strict selection criteria should be followed.

Studies have suggested the need for laboratory criteria to identify couples who may benefit from LIT, as well as for the evaluation after LIT, before allowing the couple to attempt a new pregnancy. These tests are discussed further.

Lymphocyte Crossmatch

The crossmatch between the serum of the patient and the spouse's lymphocytes to detect anti-lymphocyte maternal antibodies is the most commonly used test to select a couple for the LIT procedure.[25]

Alloimmune recognition plays a very important role in this by the formation of Blocking Antibodies. Women suffering pregnancy loss have significantly lower levels of asymmetric antibodies than their healthy counterparts.[26]

Many studies confirm the association between recurrent abortions and parental similarity of HLA which induces hyporesponsiveness and inhibits the production of blocking antibodies as immunological regulators to maintain the pregnancy. These antibodies are considered as part of regulators that cover paternal HLA molecules on the surface of the fetus and make a barrier for the attacking maternal T cells and NK cells.[27]

Lymphocyte crossmatch or HLA crossmatch helps in the detection of antipaternal antibodies in the mother's blood.[28]

A negative lymphocyte crossmatch test in the presence of unexplained RPL or RIF indicates an alloimmune cause and that immunomodulation (LIT) will be beneficial in such a case.

Natural Killer Cells in Peripheral Blood

Increased concentration or proportion of NK cells and abnormal NK cell inhibition assay indicate the presence of the alloimmune factor. These cases benefit from immunotherapy.

Natural Killer Cells in Endometrium

Increased UNK cell CD56 or the presence of CD57 indicates a higher association with alloimmune causes for RPL.

Serum TNF-α

Elevated levels of serum TNF-α are associated with RM, RIF, or IVF failure. Even after treatment with immunotherapy, the success rates are limited in the presence of elevated serum TNF-α. Levels of TNF-α should be brought to normal with medications before planning a pregnancy or IVF cycle.

It has been shown by Wu et al. that in patients with unexplained RPL, immunotherapy (LIT) with paternal mononuclear cells leads to the secretion of the Treg-associated cytokine transforming growth factor beta (TGF-β), and Th2 cytokines, while the secretion of Th17-associated cytokine IL-17A and Th1 cytokine production was decreased. The Th1/Th2 cytokine ratio significantly decreased. The Th17/Treg ratio also significantly decreased. This Th2 and Treg bias was beneficial for pregnancy.[18]

Procedure of Lymphocyte Immunization Therapy

Lymphocyte immunization therapy involves the separation of paternal or donor lymphocytes and injecting them into the mother. Usually, intradermal injections are given. Some centers give subcutaneous and intravenous injections also. Lymphocytes from freshly collected blood have the best immunomodulatory effect. Most of the centers use two or more doses of LIT. A patented protocol of a single dose is also in use. The couple is asked to plan pregnancy 4–6 weeks after the LIT procedure.

SAFETY OF LYMPHOCYTE IMMUNIZATION THERAPY

The studies conducted to know the safety of LIT indicate that LIT is safe and well tolerated in most women and is not associated with increased incidence of acute allergic reactions, autoimmunity, graft versus host disease (GVHD), pregnancy complications, or neonatal thrombocytopenia.[29,30] However in 2006 King[31] reported local reactions like redness itching and blisters up to 2 weeks after LIT. In a prospective questionnaire after 2–3 years revealed that 4/1914 patients developed thromboembolism which was not due to antiphospholipid antibodies (APLA) syndrome.

Many studies have shown that LIT in the mother does not affect the health of the infant.[32,33] The incidence of congenital anomalies was not significantly different in the immunized and the nonimmunized mothers.[34] No appreciable difference in the rate of low-birth-weight babies and other complications has been seen either.[35]

CONTROVERSIES ABOUT LYMPHOCYTE IMMUNIZATION THERAPY

While there are a lot of success reports on LIT, there are equal numbers of reports that have not found beneficial effects of LIT. This has led to a lot of controversies and LIT has met with scepticism.

In 1999, a large multicentric study [REMIS (Recurrent miscarriage) Study] showed that LIT did not improve the chances of having a successful pregnancy in women with recurrent miscarriages.[34] However, this study met with a lot of criticism, as it did not take into account important factors like the concentration of paternal lymphocytes injected, storage of cells, the time between collection of blood and administration of immunizations, presence or absence of autoimmune disorders [antinuclear antibody (ANA) positive], different routes for immunotherapy, number of doses, etc.[24,37,38]

A series of Cochrane Reviews have also been published reporting the ineffectiveness of LIT.[39,40] However, the review also noted that the quality of evidence is quite low, and the results of the meta-analysis were skewed by the result of a single REMIS study which itself had issues with inclusion criteria. Not surprisingly, the Cochrane review itself has been criticized due to various flaws associated with it.[24]

In a systematic review and meta-analysis,[38] the results showed that there was no significant difference between the study and the control group in terms of clinical pregnancy rates.

RECENT EVIDENCE ABOUT THE EFFICACY OF LYMPHOCYTE IMMUNIZATION THERAPY

As more studies were published about LIT in reproductive failure, newer meta-analyses were available. In the latest systematic review and meta-analysis, 18 carefully selected randomized placebo-controlled clinical research studies were included. The overall results showed that there is a significant increase in live births after LIT with an OR of 4.02.[41]

In another meta-analysis of 20 publications of randomized clinical trials of LIT, the outcome showed that LIT was associated with an increased live birth rate with an odds ratio of 3.13.[42]

The systematic review and meta-analysis were recently updated by Cavalcante et al (2021).[43] This meta-analysis included all the studies reported in the two most relevant meta-analyses[41,42] together with the data from a large multicentric clinical trial published by Sarno et al.[42] This meta-analysis[43] revealed that women with LIT had an increased rate of live birth than the control arm with OR 3.22 **(Table1)**.

The odds ratios are for live births. The meta-analysis of all the studies shows an odds ratio of 3.22, which indicates that LIT is effective in the treatment of recurrent miscarriages.

However, it is of note that though most of the meta-analyses supporting the usefulness of LIT are quasi-experimental studies, there are a few randomized, double-blind studies.[49] Thus, now is the time to revisit LIT with more systematic and uniform multicentric randomized clinical trials (RCTs) to determine its clinical utility.

Review of Odds Ratios of Various Meta-Analyses of Lymphocyte Immunotherapy Studies in Recurrent Miscarriages

Table 2 summarizes the outcomes of various systematic-reviews and meta-analyses published on the efficiency of LIT in women with recurrent miscarriages. It is clear that as compared to earlier studies recent meta-analyses, with newer studies have shown a beneficial effect of LIT and the odds ratios for live birth rates are significantly high.

TABLE 1: Data derived from meta-analyses[41-43] of LIT for the treatment of RM.

	Odds ratio
Study or subgroup	*MH fixed 95% CI*
Mowbray 1985	5.78 (1.63, 20.51)
Cauchi 1991	0.51 (0.14, 1.83)
Clark 1991	4.38 (0.56, 33.95)
Ho 1991	1.95 (0.76, 5.00)
Gatenby 1993	2.60 (0.72, 9.36)
Christiansen 1994	2.69 (0.95, 7.64)
Illeni 1994	0.45 (0.09, 2.32)
Kilpatrick 1994	1.33 (0.23, 7.63)
Reznikoff 1994	1.62 (0.53, 4.95)
Scott 1994	2.10 (0.38, 11.59)
Stray–Pederson 1994	1.09 (0.37, 3.25)
Carp 1997	1.52 (0.37, 6.12)
Ober 1999	0.45 (0.22, 0.91)
Pandey 2002	24.00 (1.69, 340.99)
Hong 2003	18.00 (2.40, 134.83)
Pandey 2004	12.25 (2.92, 51.42)
Yanping 2011	4.48 (1.72, 11.68)
Lin 2012	5.39 (2.06, 14.09)
Aiwu 2013	7.06 (4.97, 10.03)
Bin 2013	5.33 (1.90, 14.97)
Sarno 2019	3.04 (2.33, 3.97)
Total (95% CI) 1573(LIT) 1434 (control)	*3.22 (2.74, 3.78)*

(CI: confidence interval; LIT: lymphocyte immunization therapy; MH: Mantel-Haenszel pooled odds ratio)

TABLE 2: Summary of the systematic reviews and meta-analyses on LIT for recurrent miscarriages and the associated odds ratio.[45]

Year	*Meta-analysis*	*Number of studies*	*Odds ratio*
2014	Cochrane (Paternal lymphocytes)	12	1.23
2014	Cochrane (Donor lymphocytes)	3	1.39
2014	Cochrane (Data by Ober et al. removed)	11	1.63
2016	Liu Z et al. (Data by Ober et al. and Stray–Pedersen removed)	18	4.02
2016	Cavalcante et al (Data by Ober et al. included)	20	3.13
2021	Cavalcante et al.	21	3.22

What could lead to such a difference in the outcomes of LIT in earlier studies as compared to the recent studies is a matter of speculation. Unlike the early studies, the protocol to prepare and store the lymphocytes has become more uniform. Further, the types of patients that will benefit from LIT are now clear and hence the inclusion criteria across studies are homogeneous. Above all, the dosage and timings for the administration of LIT and the time to pregnancy are now optimized. Also, recent studies have carried out adjustments for different variables that were not identified or reported in earlier studies. These could be possible reasons for the observed beneficial effects of LIT in recent studies.

The odds ratio is for the live births when the patients are treated with LIT. This analysis indicates that the recent meta-analyses show higher odds ratios favoring the efficacy of LIT positively in repeated miscarriages.

A recent systematic analysis also supports a beneficial effect of LIT therapy in RPL associated with alloimmunity.[46]

LYMPHOCYTE IMMUNIZATION THERAPY AND GUIDELINES

Considering the uncertainties associated with LIT many societies have released their guidelines for practicing clinicians. ESHRE (2017) guidelines recommend that LIT should not be used as a treatment for unexplained RPL as it has no significant effect and there may be serious adverse effects.[47]

Keeping in line with the ESHRE Guidelines, RCOG guidelines (Green-top guidelines 2011) recommend that Paternal cell immunization, third-party donor leukocytes, trophoblast membranes, and intravenous immunoglobulin in women with previous unexplained recurrent miscarriage do not improve the live birth rate.[48] and should not be considered as a first-line therapy for women with LIT. Similarly, ASRM Guidelines do not recommend immunomodulatory treatments (including LIT) in recurrent miscarriages or RIF.[49] Unfortunately, in the absence of any clinical data from Asian or African countries, there are no guidelines released by any of the Asian or African fertility-related organizations. It is time these countries generate new evidence with well-conducted multicentric randomized controlled trials to determine the benefits of LIT. This should definitely help the clinicians who deal with women with recurrent miscarriages.

FUTURE OF LYMPHOCYTE IMMUNIZATION THERAPY

The immunomodulation induced by allogeneic lymphocytes has been successful in overcoming the immune rejection seen in some women, thus preventing RPL/RIF/UI. Various studies have proved the efficacy of LIT. Various recent meta-analyses have underlined the success of LIT in these conditions.

The bigger challenge that we have faced about LIT is to know the underlying mechanism that leads to the success of LIT. The changes induced by LIT at the molecular and cellular levels need to be researched further. It is then possible to use the component or cytokine responsible for the immunomodulatory effect rather than injecting lymphocytes themselves.

It is important to identify which subgroups will benefit from LIT. For patients to be eligible for this treatment, it is very important to strictly decide the inclusion and exclusion criteria for LIT. To select couples for LIT, it is necessary to perform more precise diagnostic tests.

Lymphocyte immunization therapy can revolutionize the treatment of Infertility/RPL/recurrent IVF Failure in the future. As we know more and more about the intricacies of the immune system and the immune basis of different diseases, immunomodulation by LIT can play an important role in the fields of medicine other than reproductive immunology.

CONCLUSION

Lymphocyte immunization therapy is one of the earliest immunomodulatory methods suggested for women with recurrent miscarriages. With the plethora of knowledge and experience in the area, newly conducted clinical trials with improved patient selection criteria, and optimized dosage and route of demonstration, LIT has shown beneficial effects in terms of live birth rates. While the safety of LIT is unquestionable there is now mounting evidence that LIT may be beneficial for women experiencing repeated miscarriages with euploid embryos.

Large multicentric RCTs are however required to further determine their efficiency. However, LIT is a personalized therapy, and RCTs, especially double-blind in nature will be difficult to conduct. It is time we evolve new guidelines and develop standard operating protocols for the use of LIT in women with recurrent miscarriages.

REFERENCES

1. Christiansen OB, Nybo Andersen AM, Bosch E, Daya S, Delves PJ, Hviid TV, et al. Evidence-based investigations and treatments of recurrent pregnancy loss. Fertil Steril 2005;83(4):821-39.
2. American Society for Reproductive Medicine. Definitions of infertility and recurrent pregnancy loss. Fert Steril. 2008;90(Suppl 5):S60.
3. ESHRE Guideline Group on RPL; Bender Atik R, Christiansen OB, Elson J, Kolte AM, Lewis S, et al. ESHRE guideline: recurrent pregnancy loss. Hum Reprod Open. 2018;2018(2):hoy004.
4. Practice Committee of the American Society for Reproductive Medicine. Evaluation and treatment of recurrent pregnancy loss: a committee opinion. Fertil Steril. 2012;98(5):1103-1111.
5. Labarrere CA. Allogeneic recognition and rejection reactions in the placenta. Am J Reprod Immunol 1989; 21(3-4):94-9.
6. Mor G, Cardenas I. The Immune System in Pregnancy: A Unique Complexity. Am J Reprod Immunol. 2010;63(6): 425-33.
7. Murata H, Tanaka S, Okada H. Immune tolerance of the human decidua. J Clin Med. 2021; 10: 1-16.
8. Medawar PB. Some immunological and endocrinological problems are raised by the evolution of viviparity in vertebrates. Symp Soc Exp Biol. 1953;7:320-38.
9. Raut MK, Raut MM. Lymphocyte Immunization Therapy (LIT) in Reproductive Failures: New Horizons. Singapore: Springer, 57;2022. https://doi.org/10/1007/978-981-19-2960-1_6
10. Billingham RE, Brent L, Medawar PB. Actively acquired tolerance of foreign cells. 1953. J Immunol. 2010; 184(1):5-8.
11. Taylor C, Faulk WP. Prevention of recurrent abortion with leucocyte transfusions. Lancet. 1981;318(8237):68-70.
12. Beer AE, Semprini AE, Zhu XY, Quebbeman JF. Pregnancy outcome in human couples with recurrent spontaneous abortions: HLA antigen profiles; HLA antigen sharing; female serum MLR blocking factors; and paternal leukocyte immunization. Expm Clin Immunogenet. 1985;2(3):137-53.
13. Recurrent Miscarriages Immunotherapy Trialists Group (RTIMG). Worldwide collaborative observational study and meta-analysis on allogenic leukocyte immunotherapy for recurrent spontaneous abortion. Recurrent Miscarriage Immunotherapy Trialists Group. Am J Reprod Immunol. 1994;32(2):55-72.
14. Daya S, Gunby J. The effectiveness of allogeneic leukocyte immunization in unexplained primary recurrent spontaneous abortion. Recurrent Miscarriage Immunotherapy Trialists Group. Am J Reprod Immunol. 1994;32(4):294-302.
15. Margni RA, Perdigon G, Gentile T, Abatangelo C, Dokmetjian J. IgG precipitating and non-precipitating antibodies in rabbits repeatedly injected with soluble and particulate antigens. Vet Immunol Immunopathol. 1986;13(1-2):51-61.

16. Pandey MK, Agrawal S. Induction of MLR-Bf and protection of fetal loss: a current double blind randomized trial of paternal lymphocyte immunization for women with recurrent spontaneous abortion. Int Immunopharmacol. 2004;4(2):289-98.
17. Zenclussen AC, Gentile T, Kortebani G, Mazzolli A, Margni R. Asymmetric antibodies and pregnancy. Am J Reprod Immunol. 2001;45(5):289-94.
18. Wu LI, Luo LH, Zhang YX, Li Q, Xu B, Zhou GX, et al. Alteration of Th17 and Treg cells in patients with unexplained recurrent spontaneous abortion before and after lymphocyte immunization therapy. Reprod Biol Endocrinol. 2014;12:74.
19. Liu M, Zhen X, Song H, Chen J, Sun X, Li X, et al. Low-dose lymphocyte immunotherapy rebalances the peripheral blood Th1/Th2/Treg paradigm in patients with unexplained recurrent miscarriage, Reprod Biol Endocrinol. 2017;15(1):95.
20. Steinman RM1, Nussenzweig MC. Avoiding horror autotoxicus: the importance of dendritic cells in peripheral T cell tolerance. Proc Natl Acad Sci USA. 2002;99(1):351-8.
21. Rizzo R, Vercammen M, van de Velde H, Horn PA, Rebmann V. The importance of HLA-G expression in embryos, trophoblast cells, and embryonic stem cells. Cell Mol Life Sci. 2011;68(3):341-52.
22. Carosella ED, Rouas-Freiss N, Roux DT, Moreau P, LeMaoult J. HLA-G: An immune checkpoint molecule. Adv Immunol. 2015;127:33-144.
23. González A, Rebmann V, LeMaoult J, Horn PA, Carosella ED, Alegre E. The immunosuppressive molecule HLA-G and its clinical implications. Crit Rev Clin Lab Sci 49(3):63-84.
24. Clark DA, Chaouat G. Loss of surface CD200 on stored allogeneic leukocytes may impair anti-abortive effect in vivo. Am J Reprod Immunol. 2005;53(1):13-20.
25. Yu HL, Deng XH, Chao L, Chen C, Han YL. [Study on positive rate of blocking antibody in women with recurrent spontaneous abortion administered by route and frequency of paternal lymphocyte immunotherapy]. Zhonghua Fu Chan Ke Za Zhi. 2013;48(12):903-6.
26. Barrientos G, Fuchs D, Schrocksnadel K, Ruecke M, Garcia MG, Klapp BF, et al. Low levels of serum asymmetric antibodies as a marker of threatened pregnancy. J Reprod Immunol. 2009;79(2):201-10.
27. Higuchi K1, Aoki K, Kimbara T, Hosoi N, Yamamoto T, Okada H. Suppression of natural killer cell activity by monocytes following immunotherapy for recurrent spontaneous aborters. Am J Reprod Immunol. 1995;33(3):221-7.
28. Erard F, Wild MT, Garcia-Sanz JA, Le Gros G. Switch of CD8 T cells to noncytolytic CD8-CD4- cells that make TH2 cytokines and help B cells. Science. 1993;260(5115):1802-5.
29. Raut MK, Raut MM. Lymphocyte Immunization Therapy (LIT) in Reproductive Failures: New Horizons. Singapore: Springer, 95-98;2022. https://doi.org/10/1007/978-981-19-2960-1_11
30. Coulam CB, Clark DA, Collins J, Scott JR. Worldwide collaborative observational study and meta-analysis on allogenic leukocyte immunotherapy for recurrent spontaneous abortion. Am J Reprod Immunol. 1994; 32:55-72.
31. Kling C, Steinmann E, Westphal J, Magez D. Kabelitz Adverse Effects of Intradermal Allogeneic Lymphocyte Immunotherapy: Acute Reactions and Role of Autoimmunity. Hum Reprod. 2006;21(2):429-35.
32. Christansen OB, Mathiesen O, Husth M, Lauritsen JG, Grunnet N. Placebo-controlled trial of active immunization with third party leukocytes in recurrent miscarriage. Acta Obstet Gynecol Scand. 1994;73(3):261-8.
33. Cavalcante MB, Costa Fda S, Araujo Júnior E, Barini R. Risk Factors Associated With a New Pregnancy Loss and Perinatal Outcomes in Cases of Recurrent Miscarriage Treated With Lymphocyte Immunotherapy J Matern Fetal Neonatal Med. 2015;28(9):1082-6.
34. Carp HJ, Ben-Shlomo I, Toder V, Nebel L, Mashiach S. Congenital Malformations After Immunotherapy for Habitual Abortion: Is There an Increase? Gynecol Obstet Invest. 1993;36(4):198-201.
35. Nonaka C, Takahashi M, Nonaka C, Enomoto T, Takakuwa K. Studies on the infants born to the patients with Unexplained Recurrent Abortion who underwent immunotherapy using their husband's lymphocytes Austin J Obstet Gynecol. 2017;4(1):1067
36. Ober C, Karrison T, Odem RB, Barnes RB, Branch DW, Stephenson MD. Mononuclear-cell immunisation in prevention of recurrent miscarriages: a randomised trial. Lancet. 1999;354(9176):365-9.
37. Clark DA. 2009 Cell-surface CD200 may predict efficacy of paternal mononuclear leukocyte immunotherapy in treatment of human recurrent pregnancy loss. Am J Reprod Immunol. 2009;61(1):75-84.
38. Achilli C, Duran-Retamal M, Saab W, Serhal P, Seshadri S. The role of immunotherapy in in vitro fertilization and recurrent pregnancy loss: a systematic review and meta-analysis. Fertil Steril. 2018;110(6):1089-100.
39. Wong LF, Porter TF, Scott JR. Immunotherapy for recurrent miscarriage. Cochrane Database Syst Rev. 2014; 2014(10):CD000112.
40. Porter TF, La Coursiere Y, Scott JR. Immunotherapy for recurrent miscarriage. Cochrane Database Syst Rev. 2006;19(2):CD000112.
41. Liu Z, Xu H, Kang X, Wang T, He L, Zhao A. Allogenic lymphocyte immunotherapy for unexplained recurrent spontaneous abortion: a meta-analysis. Am J Reprod Immunol. 2016;76(6):443-53.
42. Cavalcante MB, Sarno M, Edward AJ, Costa FDS, Barini R. Lymphocyte immunotherapy for recurrent miscarriages: Predictors of therapeutic success. Arch Gynaecol Obstet. 2018;79(6):e12833.
43. Cavalcante MB, Sarno M, Barini R. Lymphocyte immunotherapy in recurrent miscarriage and recurrent implantation failure. Am J Reprod Immunol. 2021;85(4): e13408.

44. Sarno M, Cavalcante MB, Niag M, Pimentel K, Luz I, Figueiredo B, et al. Gestational and perinatal outcomes in recurrent miscarriages couples treated with lymphocyte immunotherapy. Eur J Obstet Gynecol Reprod Biol X. 2019; 3:100036.
45. Raut MK, Raut MM. Role of lymphocyte immunization therapy (LIT) in repeated miscarriages - A review. Am J Reprod Immunol. 2023;89(2):e13629.
46. Francisco PD, Tan-Lim CSC, Jesus MSLA. Efficacy of lymphocyte immunotherapy in the treatment of recurrent pregnancy loss from alloimmunity: a systematic review and meta-analysis. Am J Reprod Immunol. 2022;88(4): e13605.
47. www.eshre.eu. (2017). Recurrent Pregnancy Loss–ESHRE- Clinical practice guidelines. [Online] Available from https://www.eshre.eu/-/media/sitecore-files/Guidelines/Recurrent-pregnancy-loss/ESHRE-RPL-Guideline_27112017_FINAL_v2.pdf [Last accessed December, 2024].
48. Royal College of Obstetricians and Gynaecologists. Recurrent Miscarriage (Green-top Guideline No. 17). [Online] Available from https://www.rcog.org.uk/guidance/browse-all-guidance/green-top-guidelines/the-investigation-and-treatment-of-couples-with-recurrent-miscarriage-green-top-guideline-no-17/ [Last accessed December, 2024].
49. Khalife D, Ghazeeri G, Kutteh W. Review of current guidelines for recurrent pregnancy loss: new strategies for optimal evaluation of women who may be superfertile. Semin Perinatol. 2019;43(2):105-15.
50. Hajipour H, Nejabati HR, Latifi Z, Hamdi K, Bahrami-Asl Z, Fattahi A, et al. Lymphocytes immunotherapy for preserving pregnancy: Mechanisms and Challenges. Am J Reprod Immunol. 2018;80(3):e12853.

CHAPTER 50

Role of Micronutrients and Antioxidants

Kiran Kurtkoti

ABSTRACT

Pregnancy is a state of increased demand of both macro- and micronutients. Borderline micronutrient deficiencies during pre-pregnancy period will manifest during pregnancy. Deficiency of certain nutrients like folate, vitamins B_{12} and D is associated with poor pregnancy outcomes. Other micronutrients like selenium, thiamine, and vitamin E have not been adequately researched. Pregnancy is also a state of heightened oxidative stress due to trophoblast invasion. Build up of free radicals may lead to defective placentation and pregnancy damage. However, there is a paucity of research on antioxidant supplementation during pregnancy.

Keywords: Micronutrients RPL, Selenium, Antioxidants, Reactive oxygen species, Vitamin E.

INTRODUCTION

Pregnancy loss includes all losses from conception to 20–24 weeks gestation and is defined as the spontaneous termination of a pregnancy before the fetus has attained viability.[1] Fetal demand for both macro and micronutrients during pregnancy has to be fulfilled through the mother. Borderline deficient nutritional states of the mother will be uncovered during pregnancy. Pregnancy is also a state of free radical build up due to trophoblastic invasion of decidua. A robust maternal antioxidant system can handle it efficiently. Notably, the term "recurrent pregnancy loss" does not encompass ectopic or molar pregnancies.[1]

Although there are many different contributing variables to the etiology of RPL, such as genetic, hormonal, anatomical, immunological, and environmental ones, new studies have highlighted the possible roles that antioxidants and micronutrients may have in the treatment and prevention of RPL.

MICRONUTRIENTS

Due to changes in a woman's physiology and the needs of a developing baby, pregnancy is a time of heightened metabolic demands.[2,3] A condition of biological competition between the mother and the conceptus may result from inadequate intake of vital vitamins and minerals, which could be harmful to both parties' health.[4] Pregnancy-related trace element deficiencies are strongly linked to the newborn's morbidity and death.[5]

Deficits in particular antioxidant activities linked to the micronutrients such as manganese, copper, zinc, and selenium can lead to adverse pregnancy outcomes, such as preeclampsia,[7] fetal growth restriction,[6] and the corresponding elevated risk of adult diseases, such as type 2 diabetes and cardiovascular disease.[8-11]

Micronutrients, such as vitamins and minerals, are necessary for immunological response, hormone regulation, DNA synthesis, and cellular activity—all critical processes for a successful pregnancy. RPL is one of the unfavorable pregnancy outcomes that has been connected to deficiencies in specific micronutrients. Therefore, lowering the risk of RPL may require optimizing micronutrient status both before and during pregnancy.

Numerous studies have looked at the importance of macronutrients during pregnancy, particularly the consequences of maternal under- and overnutrition on the long-term health of the fetus.[12,13] Many theories have been put up to explain how nutrition from the mother influences the fetus and embryonic stages as well as how the offspring's cardiovascular and metabolic systems are programmed.[14,15] Studies have lately started to concentrate on the significance of necessary specific micronutrients, so named because they are an absolute requirement and are needed in very tiny amounts daily, in addition to the contribution of macro-nutrition to a successful pregnancy.[16]

ANTIOXIDANTS

In order to promote optimal embryonic and fetal growth, the expectant mother must prepare both her body for

Flowchart 1: The antioxidant pathway.

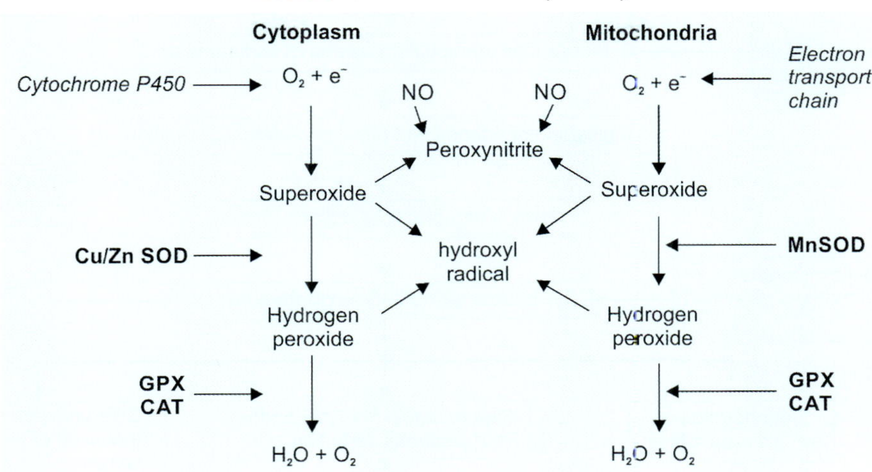

(CAT: catalase; Cu: copper; GPX: glutathione peroxidase; H_2O: water; MnSOD: manganese superoxide dismutase; NO: nitric oxide; O_2: oxygen; SOD: superoxide dismutase; Zn: zinc)

labor and delivery as well as the subsequent demands of nursing by providing a source of nutrition and gaseous exchange. Additionally, a delicate balance needs to be struck between allowing the semiallogenic conceptus to implant and survive and providing immunological surveillance to shield the mother against infection.[17,18] In order to successfully maintain the health of the mother and to allow the development of the embryo and growth of the fetus, the placenta and its circulatory system must develop and establish.

It is necessary for placental-derived extravillous trophoblast from anchoring cytotrophoblast columns to invade the mother's decidua and spiral arteries in order for the fetoplacental circulation to function. Trophoblast plugs in the spiral arteries, which are there to shield the embryonic DNA from oxidative stress, are released during the first 8 weeks of pregnancy, allowing placental circulation to begin.[19] Oxidative stress is produced when trophoblast plugs are released and blood flows into the intervillous gap.[20]

Antioxidants are substances that prevent oxidation, counteracting the negative effects of free radicals in the body. Numerous reproductive problems, including RPL, have been linked to oxidative stress, which is caused by an imbalance between the body's antioxidant defenses and the generation of free radicals. The proper balance of oxidative stress is essential for healthy embryo implantation, placental development, and fetal growth during pregnancy. Pregnancy loss can result from excessive oxidative stress that harms sperm, oocytes, embryos, and the uterine environment.

The placenta, however, is equipped with antioxidant defenses that guard against any injury to the placenta.[21-24] These defenses include the selenium-dependent glutathione peroxidases, thioredoxin reductases, selenoprotein P, and copper/zinc and manganese superoxide dismutases (Cu/Zn and MnSODs).

The process of physiological conversion, which is carried out by the extravillous trophoblast cells as they migrate through the spiral artery wall, increases the vessel lumen and maximizes blood flow to the intervillous space, allowing the placental syncytiotrophoblast to receive the maximum amount of nutrients and gases.

Deficient extravillous trophoblast invasion is the main abnormality causing preeclampsia,[25,26] fetal growth restriction,[27,28] and sporadic miscarriage.[29] It is linked to decreased spiral artery remodeling, which reduces blood flow and increases oxidative stress within the placenta. Reduced levels of antioxidant enzyme protection have also been linked to preeclampsia, which can worsen placental damage.[30-32]

Oxidative stress has been linked to the pathophysiology of several poor pregnancy outcomes, such as preeclampsia and fetal growth restriction,[33] as well as a number of neonatal outcomes.[34] Preeclampsia, also known as de novo proteinuric hypertension, is thought to affect roughly 3% of pregnancies and is a major contributor to maternal and perinatal mortality as well as morbidity in the West.[35,36] Preeclampsia, in conjunction with other hypertensive disorders of pregnancy, is estimated to be the cause of

Flowchart 2: Placental oxidative stress and pregnancy outcome.

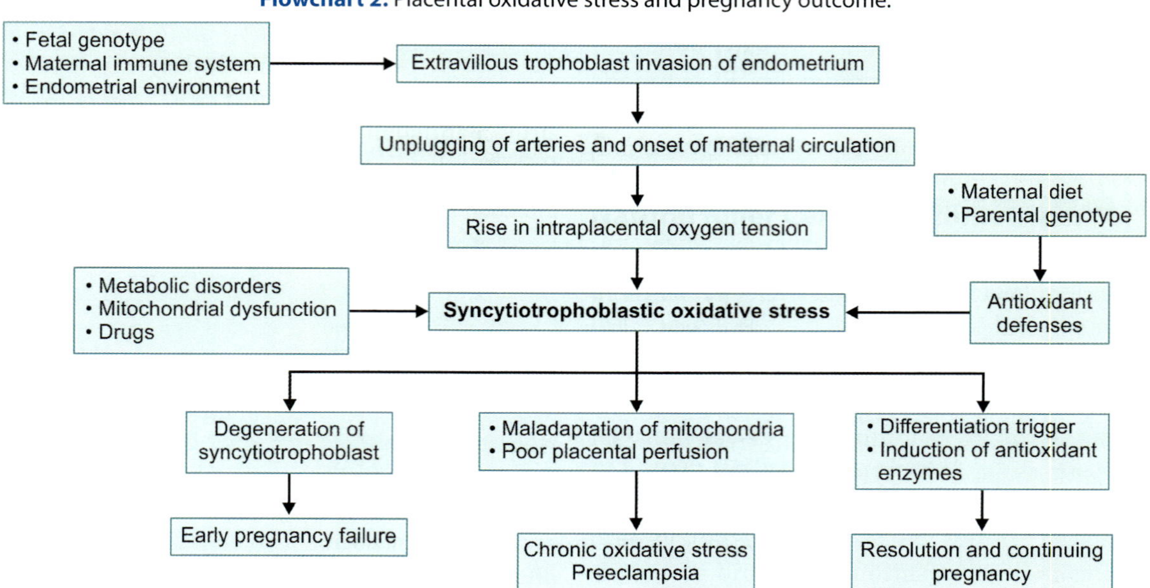

60,000 maternal deaths annually[37] and five times higher rates of perinatal mortality.[38]

The baby must frequently be delivered early in order to provide the best possible outcome for the mother and child, which increases the risk of preterm birth and low newborn birth weight. The syndrome includes maternal systemic oxidative stress and placental stress.[39,40] These factors also lead to a generalized activation of maternal systemic inflammation. Excessive generation of reactive oxygen species (ROS) has been linked to placental ischemia-reperfusion damage, which releases placental proteins that trigger inflammatory responses.[41]

CONCLUSION

Increased neonatal death and morbidity are linked to fetal growth limitation.[42] Placental ischemia/hypoxia is a likely contributing factor, though the exact mechanisms are still unknown.[43] It is believed that ischemia-reperfusion injury may contribute to oxidative stress and may release ROS into the mother's circulation, which may cause oxidative DNA damage and may be the reason behind the development of fetal growth restriction.[44] A recent review article[45] concluded that deficient antioxidant protection may be one of the mechanisms in unexplained RPL. There are however very few studies to elucidate the effect of antioxidant therapy during pregnancy. Currently both antioxidant supplementation and micronutrient therapy is not indicated during pregnancy but makes a good ground for research in high risk population.

REFERENCES

1. ESHRE Guideline Group on RPL; Bender Atik R, Christiansen OB, Elson J, Kolte AM, Lewis S, et al. ESHRE guideline: recurrent pregnancy loss. Hum Reprod Open. 2018;2018(2):hoy004.
2. Practice Committee of the American Society for Reproductive Medicine. Evaluation and treatment of recurrent pregnancy loss: a committee opinion. Fertil Steril. 2012;98(5):1103-11.
3. Broughton Pipkin F. Maternal physiology. In: Edmonds DK, (Ed). Dewhurst's Textbook of Obstetrics and Gynaecology. Oxford, UK: Blackwell Publishing; 2007.
4. Bader RA, Bader ME, Rose DF, Braunwald E. Hemodynamics at rest and during exercise in normal pregnancy as studies by cardiac catheterization. J Clin Invest. 1955;34(10):1524-36.
5. King JC. The risk of maternal nutritional depletion and poor outcomes increases in early or closely spaced pregnancies. J Nutr. 2003;133(5 Suppl 2):1732S-1736S.
6. Srivastava S, Mehrotra PK, Srivastava SP, Siddiqui MK. Some essential elements in maternal and cord blood in relation to birth weight and gestational age of the baby. Biol Trace Elem Res. 2002;86(2):97-105.
7. Fall CH, Yajnik CS, Rao S, Davies AA, Brown N, Farrant HJ. Micronutrients and fetal growth. J Nutr. 2003;133(5 Suppl 2):1747S-1756S.
8. Rumbold A, Duley L, Crowther CA, Haslam RR. Antioxidants for preventing pre-eclampsia. Cochrane Database Syst Rev. 2008;2008(1):CD004227.
9. Bellamy L, Casas JP, Hingorani AD, Williams DJ. Pre-eclampsia and risk of cardiovascular disease and cancer in later life: systematic review and meta-analysis. BMJ. 2007;335(7627):974.
10. Lykke JA, Langhoff-Roos J, Sibai BM, Funai EF, Triche EW, Paidas MJ. Hypertensive pregnancy disorders and

subsequent cardiovascular morbidity and type 2 diabetes mellitus in the mother. Hypertension. 2009;53(6):944-51.
11. Vikse BE, Irgens LM, Leivestad T, Skjaerven R, Iversen BM. Preeclampsia and the risk of end-stage renal disease. N Engl J Med. 2008;359(8):800-9.
12. Staff AC, Dechend R, Pijnenborg R. Learning from the placenta: acute atherosis and vascular remodeling in preeclampsia-novel aspects for atherosclerosis and future cardiovascular health. Hypertension. 2010;56(6):1026-34.
13. Armitage JA, Khan IY, Taylor PD, Nathanielsz PW, Poston L. Developmental programming of the metabolic syndrome by maternal nutritional imbalance: how strong is the evidence from experimental models in mammals? J Physiol. 2004;561(Pt 2):355-77.
14. Armitage JA, Taylor PD, Poston L. Experimental models of developmental programming: consequences of exposure to an energy rich diet during development. J Physiol. 2005;565(Pt 1):3-8.
15. Solomons NW. Developmental origins of health and disease: concepts, caveats, and consequences for public health nutrition. Nutr Rev. 2009;67(suppl 1):S12-S16.
16. Wells JC. The thrifty phenotype as an adaptive maternal effect. Biol Rev Cambridge Philos Soc. 2007;82(1):143-72.
17. Cetin I, Berti C, Calabrese S. Role of micronutrients in the periconceptional period. Hum Reprod Update. 2010;16(1):80-95.
18. Challis JR, Lockwood CJ, Myatt L, Norman JE, Strauss JF 3rd, Petraglia F. Inflammation and pregnancy. Reprod Sci. 2009;16(2):206-15.
19. Hanson LA, Silfverdal SA. The mother's immune system is a balanced threat to the foetus, turning to protection of the neonate. Acta Paediatr. 2009;98(2):221-8.
20. Ornoy A. Embryonic oxidative stress as a mechanism of teratogenesis with special emphasis on diabetic embryopathy. Reprod Toxicol. 2007;24(1):31-41.
21. Jauniaux E, Watson AL, Hempstock J, Bao YP, Skepper JN, Burton GJ. Onset of maternal arterial blood flow and placental oxidative stress. A possible factor in human early pregnancy failure. Am J Pathol. 2000;157(6):2111-22.
22. Wang Y, Walsh SW. Antioxidant activities and mRNA expression of superoxide dismutase, catalase, and glutathione peroxidase in normal and preeclamptic placentas. J Soc Gynecol Investig. 1996;3(4):179-84.
23. Vanderlelie J, Venardos K, Clifton VL, Gude NM, Clarke FM, Perkins AV. Increased biological oxidation and reduced anti-oxidant enzyme activity in pre-eclamptic placentae. Placenta. 2005;26(1):53-8.
24. Mistry HD, Kurlak LO, Williams PJ, Ramsay MM, Symonds ME, Broughton Pipkin F. Differential expression and distribution of placental glutathione peroxidases 1, 3 and 4 in normal and preeclamptic pregnancy. Placenta. 2010;31(5):401-8.
25. Rayman MP. Selenoproteins and human health: insights from epidemiological data. Biochim Biophys Acta. 2009;1790(11):1533-40.
26. Redman CW, Sargent IL. Placental debris, oxidative stress and pre-eclampsia. Placenta. 2000;21(7):597-602.
27. Burton GJ, Jauniaux E. Placental oxidative stress: from miscarriage to preeclampsia. J Soc Gynecol Investig. 2004;11(6):342-52.
28. Brosens I, Dixon HG, Robertson WB. Fetal growth retardation and the arteries of the placental bed. Br J Obstet Gynaecol. 1977;84(9):656-63.
29. Brosens IA, Robertson WB, Dixon HG. The role of the spiral arteries in the pathogenesis of preeclampsia. Obstet Gynecol Annu. 1972;1:177-91.
30. Gupta S, Agarwal A, Banerjee J, Alvarez JG. The role of oxidative stress in spontaneous abortion and recurrent pregnancy loss: a systematic review. Obstet Gynecol Surv. 2007;62(5):335-47; quiz 353-4.
31. Perkins AV. Endogenous anti-oxidants in pregnancy and preeclampsia. Aust N Z J Obstet Gynaecol. 2006;46(2):77-83.
32. Nakamura M, Sekizawa A, Purwosunu Y, Okazaki S, Farina A, Wibowo N, et al. Cellular mRNA expressions of anti-oxidant factors in the blood of preeclamptic women. Prenat Diagn. 2009;29(7):691-6.
33. Mistry HD, Wilson V, Ramsay MM, Symonds ME, Broughton Pipkin F. Reduced selenium concentrations and glutathione peroxidase activity in preeclamptic pregnancies. Hypertension. 2008;52(5):881-8.
34. Myatt L, Cui X. Oxidative stress in the placenta. Histochem Cell Biol. 2004;122(4):369-82.
35. Saugstad OD. Update on oxygen radical disease in neonatology. Curr Opin Obstet Gynecol. 2001;13(2):147-53.
36. Steegers EA, von Dadelszen P, Duvekot JJ, Pijnenborg R. Pre-eclampsia. Lancet. 2010;376(9741):631-44.
37. Sibai B, Dekker G, Kupferminc M. Pre-eclampsia. Lancet. 2005;365(9461):785-99.
38. Broughton Pipkin F. Risk factors for preeclampsia. N Engl J Med. 2001;344(12):925-6.
39. Roberts JM, Lain KY. Recent Insights into the pathogenesis of pre-eclampsia. Placenta. 2002;23(5):359-72.
40. Poston L. The role of oxidative stress. In: Critchley H, MacLean A, Poston L, and Walker J, (Eds). Pre-eclampsia. London, UK: RCOG Press; 2004.
41. Redman CW, Sargent IL. Pre-eclampsia, the placenta and the maternal systemic inflammatory response—a review. Placenta. 2003;24 Suppl A:S21-7.
42. Hung TH, Burton GJ. Hypoxia and reoxygenation: a possible mechanism for placental oxidative stress in preeclampsia. Taiwan J Obstet Gynecol. 2006;45(3):189-200.
43. Cetin I, Foidart JM, Miozzo M, Raun T, Jansson T, Tsatsaris V, et al. Fetal growth restriction: a workshop report. Placenta. 2004;25(8-9):753-7.
44. Biri A, Bozkurt N, Turp A, Kavutcu M, Himmetoglu O, Durak I. Role of oxidative stress in intrauterine growth restriction. Gynecol Obstet Invest. 2007;64(4):187-92.
45. Zejnullahu VA, Zejnullahu VA, Kosumi, E. The role of oxidative stress in patients with recurrent pregnancy loss: a review. Reprod Health. 2021;18(1):207. doi: 10.1186/s12978-021-01257-x.

CHAPTER 51

Role of Stem Cells for Ovarian Rejuvenation

Nayana Patel, Niket H Patel, Molina Patel, Harsha Bhadarka, Paresh Ghoghari, Piyush Chudasama, Kairavi Vyas

ABSTRACT

Ovarian rejuvenation techniques are emerging as innovative strategies to restore ovarian function and address infertility in menopausal women. Methods such as platelet-rich plasma (PRP) and stem cell therapy aim to enhance follicular activation, improve hormonal balance, and repair ovarian tissue. These approaches hold potential not only for improving reproductive outcomes but also for addressing broader health concerns associated with menopause. While promising, these therapies require further research to validate their safety, efficacy, and long-term benefits.

Keywords: Ovarian rejuvenation, Platelet-rich plasma (PRP), Stem cell therapy, Menopause, Infertility, Follicular activation, Hormonal balance, Ovarian function, Reproductive health, Menopausal symptoms.

INTRODUCTION

Ovarian rejuvenation, an emerging field in reproductive medicine, focuses on utilizing stem cells to enhance ovarian function and restore fertility in women facing age-related decline or premature ovarian insufficiency (POI).[1] This chapter aims to provide a comprehensive understanding of the significant role of stem cells in the ovarian rejuvenation procedure, exploring their therapeutic implications and future prospects.

- The identification, isolation, and establishment of ovarian stem cells challenge the long-held belief of a fixed primordial follicles pool, suggesting the potential for expanding this pool and enhancing ovarian function.
- Ovarian stem cells hold promise in postponing ovarian aging and delaying the decline in reproductive capability associated with aging.[2]
- The reduction of reproductive capability during ovarian aging is primarily attributed to the aging and disintegration of ovarian stem cell nests, rather than the senescence of germ cells themselves.[2]
- Recent research highlights the involvement of the immune and circulatory systems in the development and control of ovarian germline stem cell niches.[2]
- The proliferation and differentiation of ovarian stem cells are regulated by a combination of cellular and hormonal signals.[2]
- Improving the immune system and circulatory system can have a positive impact on ovarian function and potentially delay ovarian aging.[2]
- Stem cell therapy emerges as a promising avenue for the treatment of premature ovarian failure (POF) and infertility, offering new possibilities for addressing these conditions.[2]

FOLLICULOGENESIS

Folliculogenesis **(Fig. 1)** is a crucial process in the ovaries that produces oocytes for reproduction. It involves various genes and proteins that regulate follicular development, growth, ovulation, and atresia (follicle degeneration).[3] Key factors include growth factors such as follicle-stimulating hormone (FSH) and luteinizing hormone (LH), signaling pathways such as mTOR and PI3K, and hormones such as anti-Müllerian hormone (AMH) and estrogen. Imbalances in these processes can affect fertility. Understanding these mechanisms helps advance reproductive medicine for managing infertility and related conditions.[4]

OVARIAN STEM CELLS

Ovarian stem cells have emerged as a fascinating area of research, offering new insights into the regenerative potential of the ovary.[5] These specialized cells, found within the ovarian tissue, possess the unique ability to self-renew and differentiate into various cell types involved in

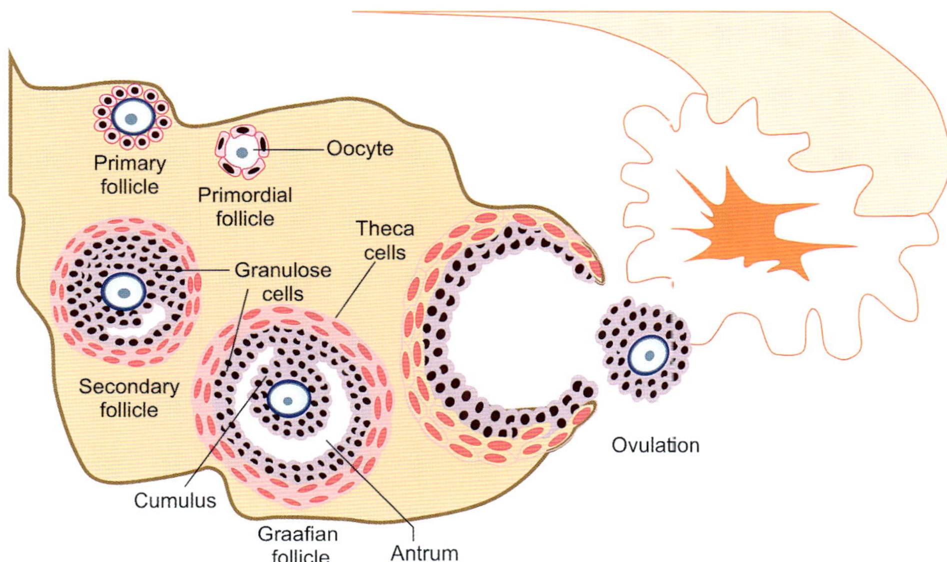

Fig. 1: Folliculogenesis. Granulosa and theca cells assist oocyte progression toward ovulation. Follicle development is shown in the figure.[4]

follicular development and oocyte production.[6] Unlike the fixed primordial follicle pool theory that previously dominated reproductive medicine, the discovery of ovarian stem cells challenges the traditional understanding of ovarian aging and opens up possibilities for rejuvenation.[7] By harnessing the regenerative capabilities of these stem cells, researchers aim to replenish the declining pool of follicles, promote the development of healthy oocytes, and potentially delay the onset of ovarian aging.[8] Understanding the properties and behavior of ovarian stem cells holds significant promise for advancing fertility treatments and providing hope to individuals facing infertility or premature ovarian failure.[9]

Ovarian Stem Cell Niche

The ovarian stem cell niche, also known as the stem microenvironment, was initially proposed by Schofield. It is composed of various components, including niche cells, extracellular matrix, and cytokines.[4] The niche plays a crucial role in the histogenesis of ovarian stem cells, providing a specialized microenvironment that supports their self-renewal and differentiation processes.[4] The niche cells, along with the extracellular matrix and cytokines, create a dynamic and interactive environment that regulates the behavior and fate of ovarian stem cells.[4] This intricate network of cellular and molecular interactions within the niche is essential for maintaining the balance between self-renewal and differentiation, ensuring the proper functioning and longevity of the ovarian stem cell population.[4]

Ovarian Stem Cell Nest

The ovarian stem cell nest is a complex structure composed of granulosa cells, vascular endothelial cells, immunologically relevant cells, and various molecules **(Fig. 2)**.[10] It serves as the microenvironment surrounding the ovarian reproductive stem cells, providing essential support and regulation for their functions.[10] Granulosa cells along with the other cell types present within the nest, contribute to the maintenance, and differentiation of ovarian stem cells. Vascular endothelial cells ensure proper blood supply and nutrient delivery to the stem cells, while immunologically relevant cells play a role in immune responses and cell signaling within the nest.[10] Additionally, the molecules present within the nest serve as key regulators of stem cell behavior and function.[10] The interactions and dynamics within the ovarian stem cell nest are crucial for maintaining the delicate balance required for normal ovarian function and fertility.[10]

AGE-RELATED OVARIAN DECLINE

Age-related ovarian decline is characterized by a decrease in both the quantity and quality of oocytes, leading to a decline in female fertility **(Fig. 3)**.[11] Factors such as

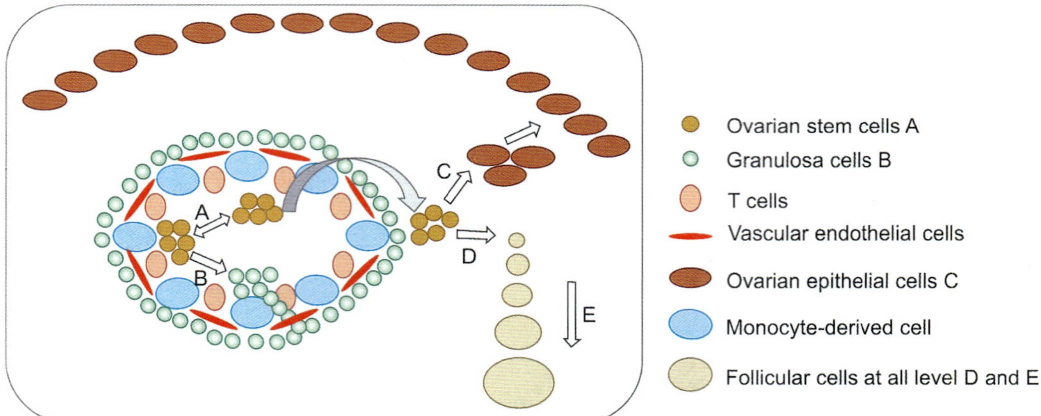

Fig. 2: The composition and function of ovarian stem cells nests.[10] A: Ovarian germ stem cells self-proliferation; B: Ovarian germ stem cells differentiate into granulosa cells; C: Ovarian germ stem cells differentiate into ovarian epithelial cells that can compensate for ovarian epithelial loss when ovulation; D: Ovarian germ stem cells differentiate into primordial follicles; E: Primordial follicular development to follicles at all levels.

increased risk of complications, changes in the ovulatory cycle, and potential decline in uterine health further contribute to this decline.[11]

Ovarian aging presents a substantial obstacle to fertility, demanding the exploration of innovative approaches to restore reproductive potential. Conventional treatments for ovarian aging have their limitations, prompting the need for alternative solutions.[11] Stem cell therapy has emerged as a promising avenue that has the potential to revolutionize the field of reproductive medicine.[11] By harnessing the regenerative capabilities of stem cells, this therapy aims to address the underlying causes of ovarian aging and restore fertility. This groundbreaking approach brings renewed hope and opens up new possibilities in the fight against ovarian aging, enabling women to pursue their reproductive aspirations with optimism.[11]

In individuals experiencing deficient ovarian sex hormones and decreased ovarian reserve, there is a significant impact on ovarian function, leading to an accelerated decline in reproductive capacity and an early onset of menopause.[11] The depletion of ovarian follicles occurs, rendering them unable to function normally as both reproductive and endocrine organs.[11] Consequently, this condition often results in subfertility or infertility, primarily due to hypoestrogenism, which manifests as menstrual irregularities and recurrent pregnancy failures.[11]

STEM CELLS AND REGENERATIVE HEALTH

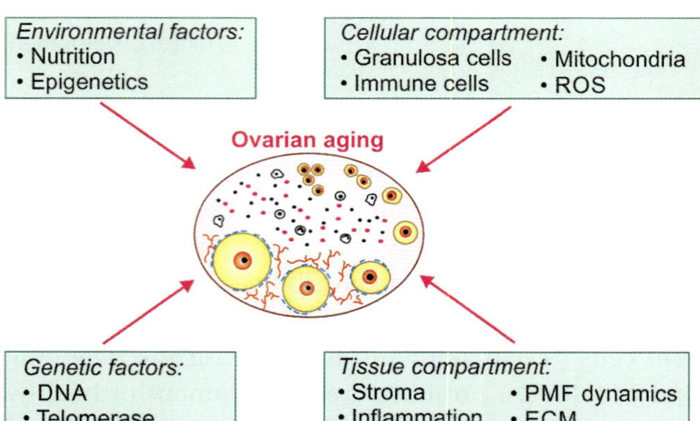

Fig. 3: Factors affecting ovarian aging.[11]
(ECM: extracellular matrix; PMF: primary myelofibrosis; ROS: reactive oxygen species)

- Stem cells, including embryonic stem cells (ESCs) and adult stem cells (ASCs), have the potential to differentiate into various cell types and play a crucial role in tissue maintenance, repair, and regeneration.[12]
- Regenerative health focuses on harnessing the regenerative properties of stem cells to develop innovative therapies and treatments.[12]
- *Tissue regeneration:* Stem cells show promise in regenerating damaged or diseased tissues such as bone, cartilage, heart muscle, and nerve cells, with the goal of repairing and regenerating these tissues.[13]
- *Organ transplantation:* Stem cells offer the potential to grow functional organs in the laboratory through organogenesis, addressing the shortage of donor organs for transplantation.[13]
- *Disease modeling and drug testing:* Stem cells serve as valuable tools for modeling diseases in the laboratory,

aiding in understanding disease mechanisms and testing potential drug therapies.[13]

- *Cellular therapies:* Stem cells can be transplanted into the body to replace damaged or dysfunctional cells, with hematopoietic stem cell (HSC) transplantation being a well-established treatment. Ongoing research aims to expand the use of stem cells for conditions such as diabetes, Parkinson's disease, and spinal cord injuries.[13]
- Ethical considerations and safety protocols are essential in stem cell research and regenerative health.
- Innovative therapies utilizing stem cells have the potential to revolutionize disease treatment and improve patients' quality of life.[13]

Sources of Various Stem Cells

Stem cells possess remarkable abilities for self-renewal and differentiation, making them pivotal in regenerative medicine and biomedical research.[14] This chapter explores different stem cell sources, their characteristics, and their implications in development, disease modeling, and potential therapies.

- *Embryonic stem cells:* Derived from the inner cell mass of blastocysts, ESCs exhibit pluripotency, differentiating into ectoderm, mesoderm, and endoderm. Valuable for studying human development, modeling diseases, and regenerative therapies; ethical concerns surround their use due to embryo destruction.[15]
- *Adult stem cells:* Also known as somatic or tissue-specific stem cells, ASCs are present in various organs, promoting tissue homeostasis and repair. Unlike ESCs, they have limited differentiation potential within specific tissues. They are easily accessible from sources such as bone marrow and adipose tissue; their utility may be restricted in certain therapeutic contexts.[16]
- *Induced pluripotent stem cells (iPSCs):* iPSCs are generated by reprogramming adult somatic cells, bypassing ethical concerns associated with embryonic sources. Similar to ESCs, they differentiate into multiple cell types and facilitate personalized medicine and disease modeling. Challenges include reprogramming and genomic instability.[17]
- *Perinatal stem cells:* Derived from tissues surrounding birth, perinatal stem cells include umbilical cord blood, amniotic fluid, and placenta. Ethically advantageous and readily available, they exhibit multipotency and have shown promise in regenerative therapies, particularly in hematopoietic disorders.[18]
- *Other sources of stem cells:* Diverse tissues harbor stem cells, expanding potential sources. Dental pulp stem cells, hair follicle stem cells, and intestinal stem cells contribute to odontoblasts, hair growth, and intestinal lining regeneration, respectively. Exploring these niche-specific stem cells reveals further regenerative potential.[19]

The understanding of various stem cell sources has advanced regenerative medicine, disease modeling, and personalized therapies. Each source presents unique advantages and limitations, driving ongoing research and optimization for future breakthroughs.

TYPES OF ADULT STEM CELLS

- Adult stem cells in various tissues are vital for tissue regeneration, offering potential in regenerative medicine.[20]
- Hematopoietic stem cells generate blood cells and are used in transplantation for hematological disorders and cancers.[20]
- Mesenchymal stem cells (MSCs) differentiate into various cell types and have immunomodulatory properties for treating conditions such as bone defects, cartilage damage, and autoimmune diseases.[20]

METHOD FOR ISOLATION OF STEM CELLS

- Stem cell isolation methods include manual methods [density gradient centrifugation, fluorescence-activated cell sorting (FACS), magnet-activated cell sorting (MACS)] and automated methods (microfluidics, robotic systems, and automated cell separators).
- In ovarian rejuvenation, stem cells differentiate into granulosa cells and oocytes, replenishing the follicular pool.
- Differentiation involves molecular signals and cellular interactions guided by specific factors and growth factors.
- Differentiated ovarian cells integrate into existing ovarian tissue, contribute to follicular development, and promote the development of healthy oocytes.
- Stem cells also release growth factors and cytokines that enhance the overall health and function of the ovarian environment.

- This breakthrough has the potential to revolutionize fertility treatment and provide new options for age-related infertility.

MECHANISMS OF ACTION

The differentiated ovarian cells integrate into the existing tissue, interact with surrounding cells, and participate in follicular development **(Fig. 4)**. This promotes the development of healthy, functional oocytes, crucial for successful fertility outcomes. Stem cells also release growth factors and cytokines that support the overall ovarian environment, offering new possibilities for age-related infertility.[4]

Controlled differentiation is vital in stem cell-based ovarian rejuvenation to ensure functionality and prevent tumorigenesis. Strict control over the differentiation process is necessary to replenish the follicular pool and promote proper oocyte development. Researchers employ techniques such as specific culture conditions, growth stimulants, and signaling molecules to direct stem cells toward the desired cell fate while minimizing the risk of uncontrolled proliferation.[4]

Characterization and quality control procedures are essential to maintain the phenotypic and functional characteristics of differentiated ovarian cells. These measures ensure the reliability and effectiveness of stem cell-based ovarian rejuvenation as a promising approach in fertility treatment.[4]

Indication: The treatment options available for ovarian aging **(Figs. 5A and B)** are not very robust.[21]

- *Diminished ovarian reserve (DOR):* Stem cell-based ovarian rejuvenation is considered for women with DOR, characterized by a reduced number of oocytes and impaired ovarian function.[21]
- *Premature ovarian insufficiency:* Women diagnosed with POI, which refers to the loss of ovarian function before the age of 40 years, may be potential candidates for ovarian rejuvenation using stem cells.[21]
- *Poor ovarian response:* Individuals who exhibit a poor response to ovarian stimulation during in vitro fertilization (IVF) treatment, with a limited number of retrieved oocytes, may benefit from ovarian rejuvenation with stem cells to enhance follicular development and improve IVF outcomes.[21]

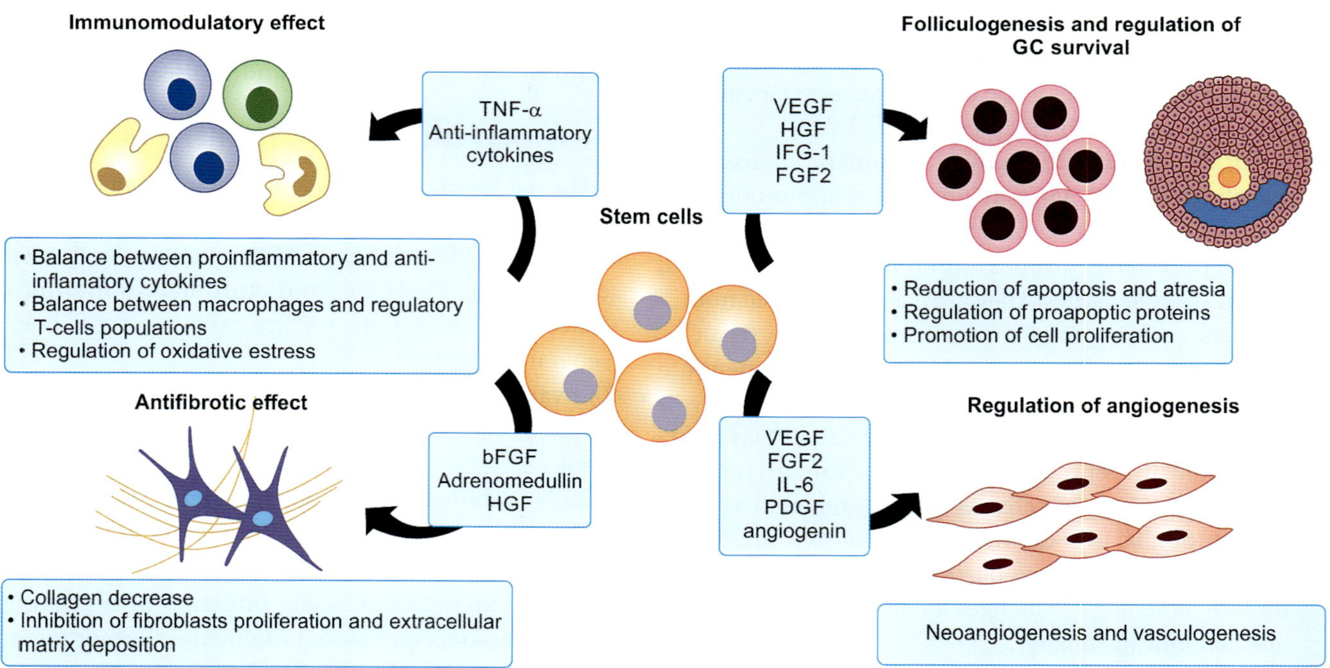

Fig. 4: Mechanism of stem cells.[4]

(bFGF: basic fibroblast growth factor FGF2: fibroblast growth factor-2; GC: granulosa cell; HGF: hepatocyte growth factor; IGF-1: insulin-like growth factor-1; IL-6: interleukin-6; PDGF: platelet-derived growth factor; TNF-α: tumor necrosis factor-α; VEGF: vascular endothelial growth factor)

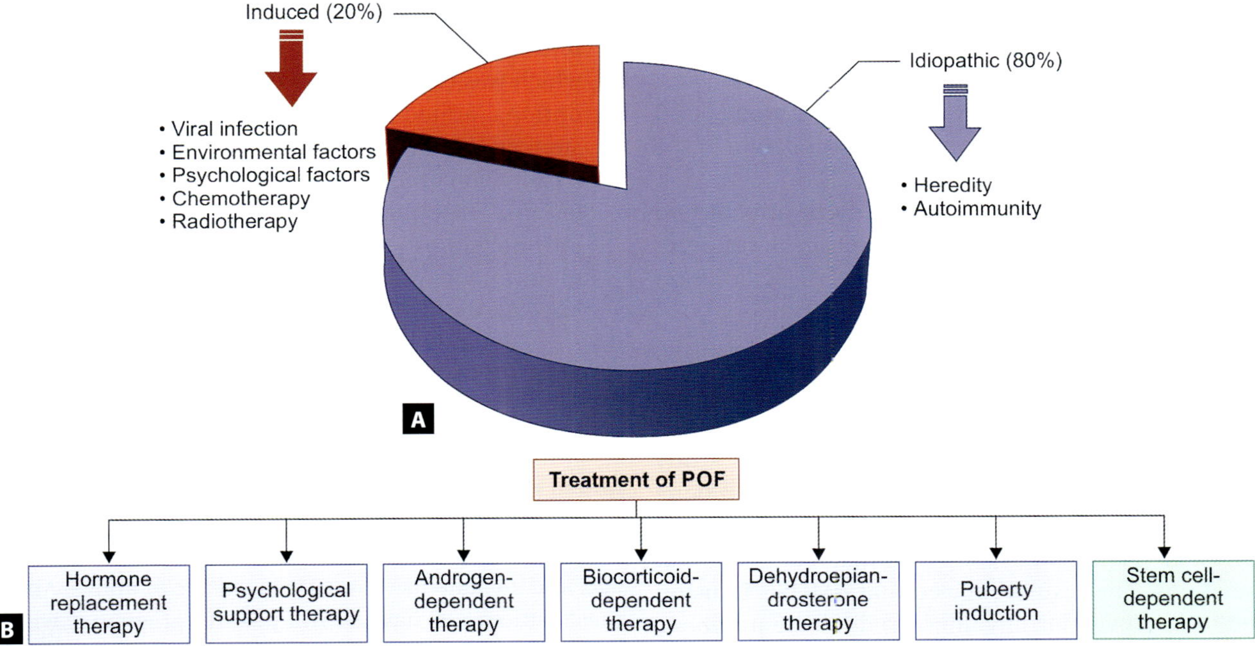

Figs. 5A and B: The pathogenic factors and treatment options of premature ovarian failure (POF).[21]

- *Age-related infertility:* Ovarian rejuvenation using stem cells is being explored as a potential solution for age-related infertility, with the goal of restoring the ovarian environment and improving oocyte quality.[21]
- *Reproductive aging:* Women experiencing the natural decline in ovarian function associated with aging may consider ovarian rejuvenation with stem cells as a means to potentially enhance fertility and reproductive outcomes.[21]

PROCEDURE

Transvaginal ovarian rejuvenation with stem cell therapy is a minimally invasive procedure performed by introducing stem cells directly into the ovaries through the vaginal route.[22] Using specialized instruments and guided by ultrasound imaging, a small needle is carefully inserted into the ovaries to deliver the stem cells.[22] This targeted approach aims to replenish the pool of follicles and promote the development of healthy oocytes, thereby restoring ovarian function and improving fertility outcomes.[23]

Laparoscopic ovarian rejuvenation with stem cell therapy involves a surgical approach where a small incision is made in the abdomen to access the ovaries.[22] Through laparoscopic instruments and visualization, the stem cells are precisely injected into the ovarian tissue.[22] This technique allows for a more comprehensive evaluation of the ovaries and enables the delivery of stem cells to specific areas of interest. The goal is to stimulate follicular growth and enhance the overall health and functionality of the ovaries.

Both transvaginal and laparoscopic approaches offer the potential benefits of stem cell therapy for ovarian rejuvenation.[24] The specific choice of procedure depends on various factors, including patient preferences, clinical indications, and the expertise of the healthcare team. It is important to consult with a qualified healthcare professional to determine the most suitable approach for individual cases.

Role of stem cells in polycystic ovary syndrome (PCOS) and endometriosis:

- Based on the analysis of follicular fluid lymphocytes, the Th1 response of PCOS patients was significantly higher when compared with the control group.[25]
- Human MSCs can suppress human Th1 response, which could influence the internal inflammatory environment in PCOS.[25]
- The ovarian function may recover after the cessation of autoimmune reaction and the regression of concurrent endocrine disease in accordance with these alterations.
- Human MSCs preserve the capacity to suppress human Th1 response that may influence the internal inflammatory environment of PCOS.[25]

- Endometriosis with its inflammatory response and increased release of cytokines could affect fertility via alteration of ovum formation, gamete transport through impairment of tubal movement, and endometrial development through modulation of the Wnt signaling pathway.[26]
- Recent experimental evidence in both animal and human models has documented promising results of stem cell-based therapy for the restoration of fertility in patients with endometriosis.

Several studies have investigated the role of stem cells in ovarian rejuvenation like:

- *Fertility rescue and ovarian follicle growth promotion by bone marrow stem cell infusion:*[27] This study aimed to assess whether the infusion of human bone marrow-derived stem cells (BMDSCs) could promote follicle development in patients with impaired ovarian functions. The results showed that BMDSC infusion led to improved fertility, increased follicle numbers, and enhanced ovarian vascularization. These findings suggest that promoting ovarian angiogenesis through BMDSC infusion could be a potential approach to improve follicular development in women with impaired ovarian function.[27]
- *Role of autologous BMDSC therapy for follicular recruitment in premature ovarian insufficiency:* Review of literature and a case report of World's first baby with ovarian autologous stem cell therapy in a perimenopausal woman of age 45 years.[28]
- *Autologous stem cell ovarian transplantation to increase reproductive potential in patients who are poor responders:*[29] Autologous stem cell ovarian transplant (ASCOT) was evaluated for its effects on ovarian reserve and IVF outcomes in poor responder women with a very poor prognosis. The study found that ASCOT led to a significant improvement in antral follicular count (AFC) and serum AMH levels. Ovarian function improved in 81.3% of women associated with the presence of fibroblast growth factor-2 and thrombospondin. ASCOT also increased the number of stimulable antral follicles and oocytes during controlled ovarian stimulation, although the embryo euploidy rate was low. Five pregnancies were achieved, indicating the potential of ASCOT to improve follicle and oocyte quantity for successful pregnancies in poor responders.
- *"Rejuvenation of premature ovarian failure with stem cells (ROSE-1)"*[30] was an ongoing clinical trial aimed at investigating the potential of stem cells for rejuvenating premature ovarian failure. The trial, which was conducted to explore innovative treatment options, aimed to assess the efficacy and safety of stem cell therapy in improving ovarian function and fertility outcomes in patients with premature ovarian failure. The study involved rigorous evaluation and monitoring of participants, with the ultimate goal of advancing medical knowledge and providing new hope for individuals facing this challenging condition.

OUR EXPERIENCE

Our hospital has been at the forefront of utilizing stem cells for ovarian rejuvenation treating a total of one hundred and fifteen patients until 2022. The age distribution of these patients was as follows: 54 patients were 35 years of age or below, 34 patients were between 36 and 39 years of age, and 28 patients were 40 years of age or above. Among these patients, 38 have shown positive pregnancy with 19 patients under the age of 35 years, 9 patients between 36 and 39 years of age, and 10 patients aged 40 years or above. However, we have also encountered challenges along the way, with 9 experiencing negative results and opted for donor egg. Majority of cases are done in 2022 which patient are still trying. Additionally, 14 patients were lost to follow-up, making it difficult to assess the long-term effectiveness of the treatment, and 53 others are still trying. Our dedication to advancing the role of stem cells in ovarian rejuvenation continues as we strive to improve the success rate and expand the benefits of this innovative treatment option (See Appendix 1 Case 11).

CONCLUSION

Rejuvenating the ovaries is a very new territory in menopause, lying between conventional treatment for infertility and regenerative therapies. Techniques like PRP and stem cell application can show some promise in reinitiating ovarian function and hormone balance. While preliminary outcomes are encouraging, further research, standardized protocols, and long-term studies are essential to establish efficacy and safety comprehensively. This field holds immense potential to redefine reproductive healthcare, offering hope to menopausal women seeking advanced therapeutic interventions.

REFERENCES

1. Martirosyan YO, Silachev DN, Nazarenko TA, Birukova AM, Vishnyakova PA, Sukhikh GT. Stem-cell-derived

extracellular vesicles: unlocking new possibilities for treating diminished ovarian reserve and premature ovarian insufficiency. Life. 2023;13(12):2247.
2. Ali I, Padhiar AA, Wang T, He L, Chen M, Wu S, et al. Stem cell-based therapeutic strategies for premature ovarian insufficiency and infertility: a focus on aging. Cells. 2022;11(23):3713.
3. Rimon-Dahari N, Yerushalmi-Heinemann L, Alyagor L, Dekel N. Ovarian Folliculogenesis. In: Piprek RP (Ed). Molecular Mechanisms of Cell Differentiation in Gonad Development. Cham: Springer International Publishing; 2016. pp. 167-90.
4. Polonio AM, García-Velasco JA, Herraiz S. Stem Cell Paracrine Signaling for Treatment of Premature Ovarian Insufficiency. Front Endocrinol (Lausanne). 2021;11: 626322.
5. Truman AM, Tilly JL, Woods DC. Ovarian regeneration: the potential for stem cell contribution in the postnatal ovary to sustained endocrine function. Molecular and cellular endocrinology. 2017;445:74-84.
6. Ng A, Barker N. Ovary and fimbrial stem cells: biology, niche and cancer origins. Nat Rev Mol Cell Biol. 2015;16(10): 625-38.
7. Hong W, Wang B, Zhu Y, Wu J, Qiu L, Ling S, et al. Female germline stem cells: aging and anti-aging. J Ovarian Res. 2022;15(1):79.
8. Qamar AY, Hussain T, Rafique MK, Bang S, Tanga BM, Seong G, et al. The role of stem cells and their derived extracellular vesicles in restoring female and male fertility. Cells. 2021;10(9):2460.
9. Sfakianoudis K, Rapani A, Grigoriadis S, Retsina D, Maziotis E, Tsioulou P, et al. Novel Approaches in Addressing Ovarian Insufficiency in 2019: Are We There Yet? Cell Transplant. 2020;29:963689720926154.
10. Ye H, Zheng T, Li W, Li X, Fu X, Huang Y, et al. Ovarian Stem Cell Nests in Reproduction and Ovarian Aging. Cell Physiol Biochem. 2017;43(5):1917-25.
11. Camaioni A, Ucci MA, Campagnolo L, De Felici M, Klinger FG; Italian Society of Embryology, Reproduction and Research (SIERR). The process of ovarian aging: it is not just about oocytes and granulosa cells. J Assist Reprod Genet. 2022;39(4):783-92.
12. Stocum DL. Stem cells in regenerative biology and medicine. Wound Repair Regeneration. 2001;9(6):429-42.
13. Bajada S, Mazakova I, Richardson JB, Ashammakhi N. Updates on stem cells and their applications in regenerative medicine. J Tissue Eng Regen Med. 2008;2(4):169-83.
14. Donnelly H, Salmeron-Sanchez M, Dalby MJ. Designing stem cell niches for differentiation and self-renewal. J R Soc Interface. 2018;15(145):20180388.
15. Wobus AM, Boheler KR. Embryonic Stem Cells: Prospects for Developmental Biology and Cell Therapy. Physiol Rev. 2005;85(2):635-78.
16. Ntege EH, Sunami H, Shimizu Y. Advances in regenerative therapy: A review of the literature and future directions. Regen Ther. 2020;14:136-53.
17. Aboul-Soud MA, Alzahrani AJ, Mahmoud A. Induced pluripotent stem cells (iPSCs)—roles in regenerative therapies, disease modelling and drug screening. Cells. 2021;10(9):2319.
18. Atala A, Cetrulo KJ, Taghizadeh RR, Cetrulo CL, Murphy S. Perinatal stem cells: research and therapy. London, UK: Academic Press; 2018
19. Fournier BPJ, Larjava H, Häkkinen L. Gingiva as a Source of Stem Cells with Therapeutic Potential. Stem Cells Dev. 2013;22(24):3157-77.
20. Mahla RS. Stem Cells Applications in Regenerative Medicine and Disease Therapeutics. Int J Cell Biol. 2016;2016:1-24.
21. Wang J, Liu W, Yu D, Yang Z, Li S, Sun X. Research Progress on the Treatment of Premature Ovarian Failure Using Mesenchymal Stem Cells: A Literature Review. Front Cell Dev Biol. 2021;9:749822.
22. Museridze N, Chokhonelidze A. Advances in Stem Cell Therapy for Reproductive Medicine: Applications, Techniques, and Potential Outcomes. Medical Times. 2024; 2(1):42-9.
23. Hu B, Wang R, Wu D, Long R, Ruan J, Jin L, et al. Prospects for fertility preservation: the ovarian organ function reconstruction techniques for oogenesis, growth and maturation in vitro. Front Physiol. 2023;14:1177443.
24. Kim HK, Kim TJ. Current Status and Future Prospects of Stem Cell Therapy for Infertile Patients with Premature Ovarian Insufficiency. Biomolecules. 2024;14(2):242.
25. Nasri F, Doroudchi M, Namavar Jahromi B, Gharesi-Fard B. T helper cells profile and CD4+ CD25+ Foxp3+ regulatory T cells in polycystic ovary syndrome. Iran J Immunol. 2018;15(3):175-85.
26. Saha S, Roy P, Corbitt C, Kakar SS. Application of stem cell therapy for infertility. Cells. 2021;10(7):1613.
27. Herraiz S, Buigues A, Díaz-García C, Romeu M, Martínez S, Gómez-Seguí I, et al. Fertility rescue and ovarian follicle growth promotion by bone marrow stem cell infusion. Fertil Steril. 2018;109(5):908-918.e2.
28. Gupta S, Lodha P, Karthick MS, Tandulwadkar SR. Role of Autologous Bone Marrow-Derived Stem Cell Therapy for Follicular Recruitment in Premature Ovarian Insufficiency: Review of Literature and a Case Report of World's First Baby with Ovarian Autologous Stem Cell Therapy in a Perimenopausal Woman of Age 45 Year. J Hum Reprod Sci. 2018;11(2):125.
29. Herraiz S, Romeu M, Buigues A, Martínez S, Díaz-García C, Gómez-Seguí I, et al. Autologous stem cell ovarian transplantation to increase reproductive potential in patients who are poor responders. Fertil Steril. 2018;110(3): 496-505.e1.
30. Igboeli PI, Gavilova-Jordan L, Brakta S, El Andaloussi A, Sportes C, Pantin J, et al. Rejuvenation of Premature Ovarian Failure with Stem Cells. In: Reproductive Sciences. Sage Thousand Oaks, CA USA: Publications Inc.; 2018. pp. 250A-250A.

CHAPTER 52

Role of Stem Cells for Endometrial Rejuvenation

Nayana Patel, Niket H Patel, Molina Patel, Paresh Ghoghari, Harsha Bhadarka, Piyush Chudasama, Kairavi Vyas

ABSTRACT

Irreversible endometrial damage can result in a thin nonreceptive endometrium resulting in implantation failure or early miscarriages. Stem cell therapy has been successfully tried in these cases. Autologous stem cells are harvested from the bone marrow and concentrated by either manual or automated methods. They are then injected with the intention of replacing endometrial progenitor mesenchymal stem cells (eMSC) and improving the quality of the endometrium. The routes of injecting stem cells can be intrauterine instillation, hysteroscopic injection in the basal endometrium or direct insertion into the uterine spiral arterioles via uterine artery catheterization. Further studies are required to formulate treatment protocols and indications for therapy.

Keywords: Endometrial stem cell niche, Bone marrow stem cells, Adipose stem cells, Hysteroscopic injection, Uterine artery catheterization, Ashermans syndrome, Intrauterine adhesions.

INTRODUCTION

The endometrium plays a critical role in the reproductive process, providing a favorable internal environment for embryo implantation and pregnancy maintenance.[1] Its thickness on the day of human chorionic gonadotropin (hCG) administration is a crucial factor affecting successful implantation, with thin endometrium defined as <7 mm.[2]

The basal layer of the endometrium, being the deepest layer, contains high levels of reactive oxygen species that can hinder implantation and embryo development.[3] Malfunctioning of endometrial stem/progenitor cells is linked to thin endometrium, lower implantation rates, and increased miscarriages.[4] The inadequate thickness affects embryo attachment and pregnancy support, leading to a decreased likelihood of successful implantation.[4]

Understanding the factors contributing to thin endometrium is essential for improving reproductive outcomes.[5] Identifying the underlying causes and developing strategies to address them can enhance endometrial receptivity and increase the chances of successful implantation and healthy pregnancies.[6]

IRREVERSIBLE ENDOMETRIAL DAMAGE

Irreversible endometrial damage can occur due to several factors and conditions, including multiple miscarriages, termination of pregnancy, repeated diagnostic curettage, postpartum dilatation and curettage, and intrauterine infections.[7] These factors can disrupt the structure and function of the endometrial lining, reducing its receptivity to future pregnancies.[8]

Such damage has significant implications for reproductive health, as it can pose challenges in achieving successful pregnancies and increase the risk of complications like infertility or recurrent miscarriage.[9]

The condition known as Asherman syndrome (AS) defines intrauterine adhesions (IUAs) and is characterized by infertility, recurrent miscarriage, hypomenorrhea, pelvic pain, and amenorrhea.[10]

Causes of thin endometrium are as follows:

- History of dilatation and curettage
- Postpartum and endometritis
- Septic miscarriage
- Myoma
- Radiation
- In uetero diethylstilbestrol exposure
- Hypothalamic hypogonadism
- Mullerian anomalies
- Premature ovarian insufficiency

Endometrium basalis: The permanent, deeper layer of the endometrium containing stem cells for regeneration.[11]

Endometrium functionalis: The superficial layer of the endometrium that undergoes cyclic changes and is shed during menstruation **(Fig. 1)**.[12]

Management of thin endometrium: Various treatment options are available for management of thin endometrium with varying results **(Flowchart 1)**.

REGENERATIVE MEDICINE

Regenerative therapy, a rapidly emerging field, offers the promise of repairing damaged tissues and organs. It encompasses various approaches to disease management, aiming to repair or regenerate human tissues, enhance the function of existing tissues or organs, and address infertility issues.[13] Platelet-rich plasma (PRP) and stem cell (SC) therapies have gained popularity as tools for tissue repair and rejuvenation in male and female infertility treatments.[14] PRP is derived from plasma and contains a high concentration of platelets rich in growth factors and enzymes, facilitating tissue repair and wound healing.[15] On the other hand, stem cells have the ability to self-renew and differentiate into various cell types, releasing growth factors and cytokines that accelerate the healing process at the site of tissue damage.[16] Despite the fact that both therapies' have similar functions, they differ in preparation procedures and functionality.

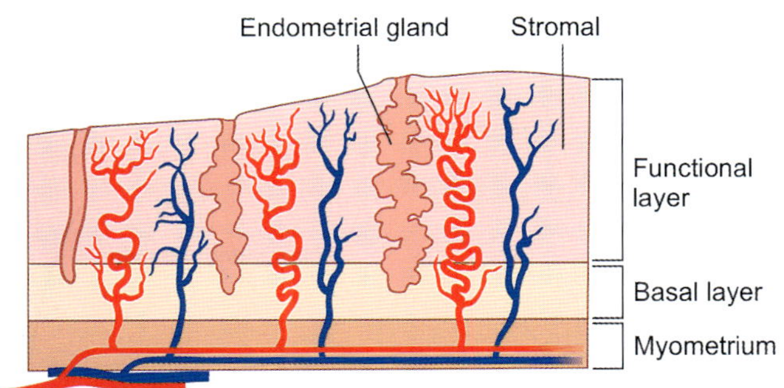

Fig. 1: Endometrium basal and functional layers.

Platelet-rich Plasma

Platelet-rich plasma is sourced from venous blood and is composed of growth factors and cytokines. Its mechanism of action involves anti-inflammatory and regenerative properties, making it effective in younger patients with minimal side effects.[17]

Stem Cell

Stem cells, originating from embryos, bone marrow, or other tissues, are undifferentiated and can differentiate into specific cell types, exhibiting immunosuppressive, anti-inflammatory properties, and aiding tissue regeneration. Stem cell therapy shows more promise than PRP treatments.[18]

Stem cells are classified into pluripotent and multipotent types based on their differentiation potential. Pluripotent stem cells, such as embryonic stem cells (ESCs), can differentiate into various cell types, but ethical concerns and cancer risks limit their frequent use. Induced pluripotent stem cells (iPSCs) and mesenchymal stem cells (MSCs) offer alternatives for research. iPSCs are reprogrammed specialized cells without ethical concerns, and MSCs, derived from the mesoderm, exhibit multipotent capabilities and low immunogenicity. MSCs are valuable for therapeutic applications, as they can be obtained from various sources like bone marrow and adipose tissue. However, their self-renewal potential might be constrained by donor age and invasive collection methods.

Flowchart 1: Management of thin endometrium.

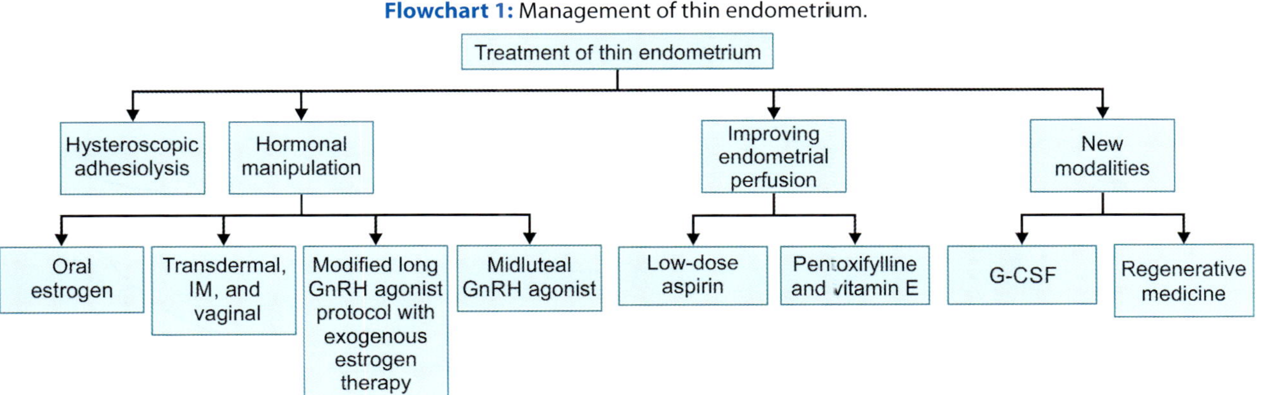

(G-CSF: granulocyte-colony stimulating factor; GnRH: gonadotropin-releasing hormone; IM: intramuscular)

Sources of Various Stem Cells

Stem cells have significantly transformed regenerative medicine and biomedical research due to their extraordinary abilities in self-renewal and differentiation. In this exploration, we delve into distinct stem cell origins, their traits, advantages, and constraints:

- *Embryonic stem cells:* Derived from the inner cell mass of a blastocyst, ESCs are pluripotent, capable of differentiating into cells from all germ layers. While they provide insights into human development, ethical concerns arise from embryo destruction during extraction.
- *Adult stem cells (ASCs):* Present in various tissues, ASCs play a pivotal role in tissue repair. They are multipotent or unipotent and offer ease of isolation. However, their differentiation capacity is more limited compared to ESCs.
- *Induced pluripotent stem cells (iPSCs):* Reprogrammed from adult somatic cells, iPSCs resemble ESCs, and enabling patient-specific cell lines without ethical dilemmas. Genomic instability poses challenges for clinical use.
- *Perinatal stem cells (PSC):* Obtained from tissues surrounding birth like umbilical cord blood, amniotic fluid, and placenta, PSCs hold ethical and logistical advantages. They exhibit multipotency and promising potential for regenerative therapies.
- *Other stem cell sources:* Stem cells have been discovered in diverse tissues such as dental pulp, hair follicles, adipose tissue, and the gastrointestinal tract. Unveiling these niche-specific stem cells broaden their potential applications **(Fig. 2)**.

Grasping the sources of stem cells deepens our understanding of regenerative medicine, disease

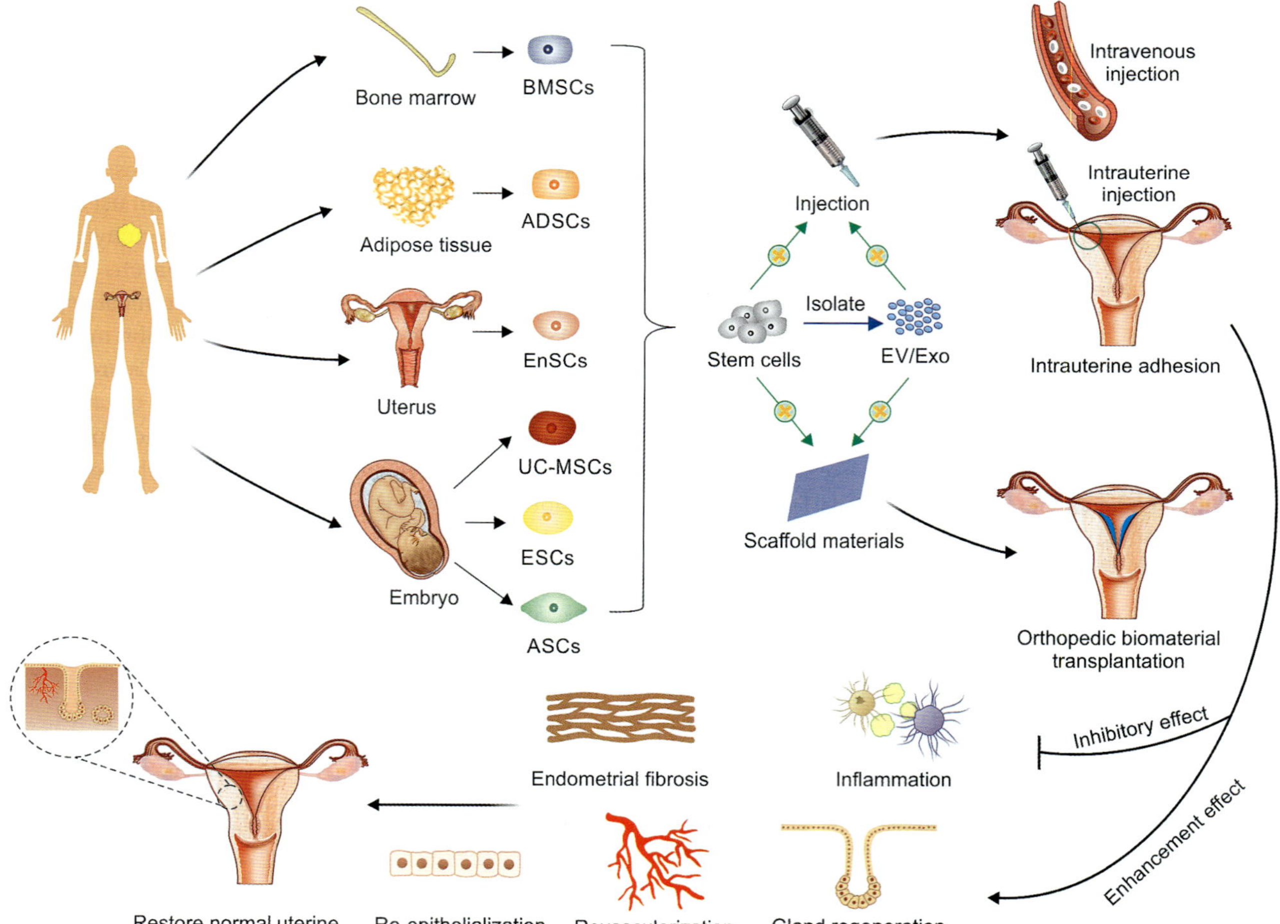

Fig. 2: Sources of stem cells.[19] (ADSCs: adipose-derived stem cells; ASCs: adult stem cells; BMSCs: bone marrow-derived mesenchymal stromal cells; EnSCs: endometrial stem cells; ESCs: embryonic stem cells; UC-MSCs: umbilical cord-mesenchymal stem cells)

modeling, and personalized treatments. Each source presents distinct merits and constraints, propelling continuous research for future break-through.[19]

Methods to Isolate Stem Cells

Categorized into two main approaches, stem cell isolation techniques can be broadly divided into manual and automated methods, each playing a pivotal role in stem cell research and therapeutic applications, offering distinct advantages and considerations.[20] Let us delve into these techniques further:

Manual methods:

- *Density gradient centrifugation:* This conventional technique involves layering a stem cell-containing sample onto a density gradient solution and centrifuging it. Stem cells move to specific density layers, enabling their separation from other cell types.[20]
- *Fluorescence-activated cell sorting (FACS):* FACS employs fluorescently labeled antibodies binding to stem cell markers on cell surfaces. Flow cytometers sort labeled cells based on fluorescence intensity, enabling the isolation of highly pure stem cells.[20]
- *Magnetic-activated cell sorting (MACS):* MACS employs magnetic beads coated with antibodies targeting specific stem cell markers. Passing the cell mixture through a magnetic field retains cells expressing the target marker, facilitating stem cell separation.[20]

Automated methods:

- *Microfluidics:* Microfluidics platforms use miniature channels and chambers to manipulate and sort cells based on physical or biochemical properties. Microfluidic devices isolate stem cells according to size, deformability, or specific surface markers.[20]
- *Robotic systems:* Equipped with specialized instruments and robotic arms, robotic systems precisely sort and isolate cells. They recognize specific stem cell markers or properties and automatically separate stem cells.[20]
- *Automated cell separators:* Similar to manual methods, automated cell separators use magnetic or fluorescent techniques. These separators process large sample volumes, ensuring high-throughput stem cell isolation.

The choice between manual and automated methods hinges on factors like research objectives, sample size, desired purity, and available resources. Manual methods offer flexibility and control but are time-intensive. Automated methods provide higher throughput and efficiency, often requiring specialized equipment and expertise. Researchers can combine different approaches to optimize stem cell isolation based on their specific requirements and research aims.[20]

Detection of Stem Cells

Detecting endometrial stem cells is a pivotal aspect of understanding their role in regenerative medicine and potential therapeutic applications. Various methods are employed to identify and isolate these specialized cells from the endometrial tissue.[11]

- Immunohistochemistry involves using specific antibodies that bind to surface markers characteristic of endometrial stem cells, allowing their visualization under a microscope.[11]

  Flow cytometry utilizes fluorescently labeled antibodies to sort and quantify stem cells based on their unique molecular profiles.[21]
- Gene expression analysis assesses the presence of specific genes associated with stem cell properties.[22] Techniques such as immunofluorescence and in situ hybridization provide visual insights into stem cell location within the endometrial tissue. These detection methods collectively contribute to unraveling the intricate characteristics of endometrial stem cells and their potential in regenerative therapies.[14]

Mode of Action

- *Bone marrow-derived stem cells:* Bone marrow-derived stem cells (BMDCs) have shown potential in regenerating endometrial damage, providing a promising therapeutic approach to address conditions such as thin endometrium and recurrent pregnancy loss. These stem cells have the ability to stimulate tissue repair and modulate the endometrial micro-environment, offering hope for improved fertility and reproductive outcomes in affected women.[19]
- *Umbilical cord stem cells:* Umbilical cord stem cells possess regenerative properties and can promote tissue repair in the endometrium. Their ability to modulate the microenvironment and stimulate cell growth holds potential for enhancing fertility and addressing endometrial issues, providing new hope for women facing reproductive challenges.[19]
- *Adipose tissue-derived stem cells:* Adipose tissue-derived stem cells have emerged as a potential tool for repairing endometrial damage. With their regenerative

capabilities and ability to secrete growth factors, these stem cells can promote tissue healing and regeneration in the endometrium. Utilizing these stem cells may offer new therapeutic avenues to improve fertility outcomes and address conditions such as thin endometrium and recurrent pregnancy loss.[19]

ENDOMETRIAL STEM CELLS

Endometrial stem cells, located in the basal layer of the endometrium, are crucial for the dynamic changes these undergo during the menstrual cycle to prepare for embryo implantation.[4] These progenitor cells have remarkable regenerative capabilities, rapidly replacing the functional layer of the endometrium each cycle. They exhibit high proliferation, continuously dividing to maintain a constant supply of cells for endometrial renewal. Additionally, endometrial stem cells can self-renew, generating identical daughter cells to preserve the stem cell population. Moreover, their multilineage differentiation potential allows them to form various endometrial tissue components, contributing to successful embryo implantation and pregnancy development.[11]

Understanding these stem cells is vital for comprehending the complexities of female reproductive health **(Fig. 3)**.[23]

Endometrial Stem Cell Niche

Endometrial stem cells play a crucial role in the regeneration and maintenance of the endometrial lining, which is essential for successful embryo implantation and pregnancy. The concept of the "stem cell niche," first proposed by Schofield in 1978 for hematopoietic stem cells, applies to endometrial stem cells as well. Stem cell niches are specialized microenvironments that support and regulate the self-renewal and differentiation of stem cells.[23]

Within the endometrium, stem cell niches are composed of various components that create a dynamic and finely tuned environment:

- *Cellular components:* Different types of cells, such as stromal cells, immune cells, and endothelial cells, interact with endometrial stem cells and provide important signals for their maintenance and differentiation.[23]
- *Secreted factors:* Growth factors, cytokines, and other signaling molecules are secreted by neighboring cells and create a signaling network that influences the behavior of endometrial stem cells.[23]
- *Extracellular matrix (ECM):* The ECM is a network of proteins and carbohydrates that provides structural support and biochemical cues to stem cells. It

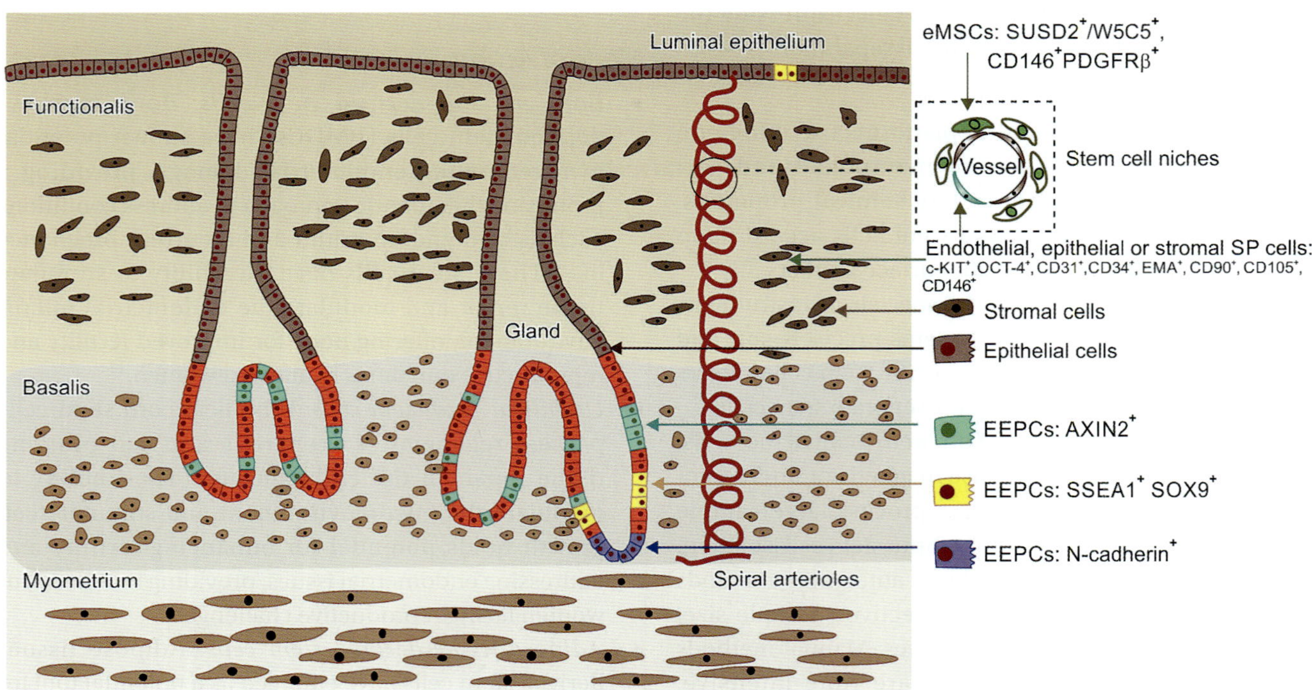

Fig. 3: Endometrial stem cells.[23]

helps regulate stem cell behavior and response to environmental signals.[23]

- *Physical parameters:* The mechanical properties of the stem cell niche, such as stiffness and elasticity, can influence stem cell behavior and fate.[23]
- *Environmental signals:* Environmental factors, such as oxygen levels and nutrient availability, can impact the function of endometrial stem cells and their ability to self-renew or differentiate.[23]

STEM CELL THERAPY

- The stem cell niche's bidirectional regulation means that stem cells also influence the surrounding microenvironment through their secreted factors and interactions with neighboring cells. This intricate crosstalk helps maintain the balance between self-renewal and differentiation of endometrial stem cells, ensuring the proper functioning of the endometrium during the menstrual cycle and pregnancy.
- Endometrial damage is a common cause of infertility, and traditional treatments have limited efficacy.
- Loss of plasticity of endometrial stem cells has been reported in cases of recurrent miscarriages.[5]
- Stem cell therapy is a promising new technology for treating endometrial damage, as stem cells have the ability to differentiate into various cell types and can promote tissue regeneration.
- Menstrual blood endometrial stem cells have been identified as a potential source of stem cells for endometrial repair, as they are easily accessible and have a high proliferation rate.
- However, there are still limitations to the clinical utility of stem cells, such as colonization rates, long-term efficacy, tumor formation, and storage and transportation.
- The mechanism by which stem cells repair endometrial damage is through replacement of damaged sites, paracrine effects, interaction with growth factors, and other new targets.
- Research is ongoing to solve these issues and optimize the clinical application of stem cells, including the development of functional bioscaffolds and multifunctional platforms to enhance stem cell colonization and differentiation.
- Overall, stem cell therapy shows great promise for the treatment of endometrial damage and infertility, but further research is needed to fully understand its potential and limitations.

Mechanism of Action

This mechanism includes four aspects **(Fig. 4)**:

- *Replacement of damaged sites:* Stem cells can differentiate into endometrial cells and replace the damaged tissue, promoting tissue regeneration.

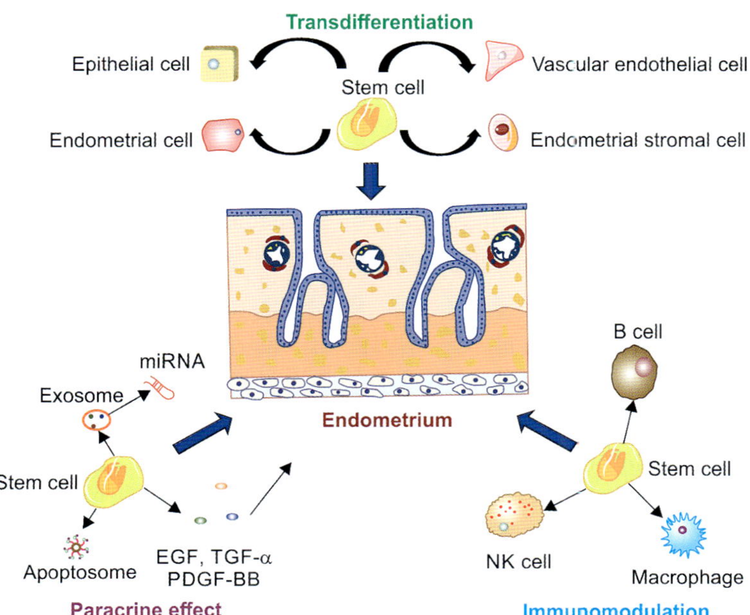

Fig. 4: Mechanism of action of stem cells.[4] (EGF: epidermal growth factor; PDGF-BB: platelet-derived growth factor-BB; TGF-α: transforming growth factor-α)

- *Paracrine effects:* Stem cells can secrete various growth factors, cytokines, and extracellular vesicles that can promote angiogenesis, reduce inflammation, and enhance tissue repair.
- *Interaction with growth factors:* Stem cells can interact with growth factors in the local microenvironment to promote tissue repair and regeneration.
- *Other new targets:* Stem cells can also interact with other cells in the local microenvironment, such as immune cells, to promote tissue repair.[4]

Routes of Therapy

- *Intrauterine instillation:* This medical procedure involves the direct injection of a small volume (0.5 mL) of bone marrow into the uterine cavity. It is performed 2–8 days before either an embryo transfer or an intra-uterine insemination (IUI) procedure. This procedure is used mostly to inject PRP.[24]
- *Hysteroscopic subendometrial injection:* Hysteroscopy involves the insertion of a thin hysteroscope into the uterine cavity to visualize the endometrial lining. During this procedure, a small injection is administered through an oocyte retrieval needle directly into the subendometrial space, i.e., 1 cm below the endometrial surface in the early follicular phase of the cycle.
- *Directly into uterine artery by spiral arterioles:* This innovative procedure involves the targeted instillation of BMDCs into the spiral arterioles of the uterine artery.[25] This is done by cannulating the uterine artery via the femoral artery under fluoroscopic control. This approach aims to replenish cellular components of the functional endometrial layer and holds promise for treating conditions such as AS and endometrial atrophy (EA). It ensures delivery into the basal layer of the endometrium.

DRUGS MODIFYING STEM CELL COLONIES IN THE ENDOMETRIUM

In patients with RPL, the endometrial progenitor mesenchymal stem cells (eMSC) population is decreased and there is excessive decidual senescence. Sitagliptin, an antidiabetic drug, has been shown to increase the eMSC population. In a randomized double-blind study, it decreases endometrial senescence thereby preventing miscarriage.[26]

CONCLUSION

In conclusion, the use of stem cells in the endometrium rejuvenation holds promising potential in addressing infertility and enhancing endometrial health. Despite the ongoing debate surrounding other treatment modalities, stem cells, with their regenerative capabilities, offer a fresh approach. Varieties of stem cells, such as endometrial mesenchymal stem cells (MSCs), eMSCs, bone marrow-derived mesenchymal stromal cells (BScs), and umbilical cord-mesenchymal stem cells (UC-MSCs), have shown positive impacts on restoring damaged endometrial tissue. This innovative therapy targets the endometrial niche, aiming to rejuvenate the functional layer and tackle conditions such as and EA. The regenerative power of endometrial stem cells opens doors to future possibilities in regenerative medicine, signifying a significant advancement in addressing various endometrial disorders. As the field progresses, ethical considerations and interdisciplinary cooperation will guide the integration of stem cell therapies, potentially reshaping the landscape of fertility treatments and bringing renewed hope to those seeking parenthood.

REFERENCES

1. Geller Sen B, Brosens JJ. Cyclic decidualization of the human endometrium in reproductive health and failure. Endor Rev. 2014;35(6):851-905.
2. Bu Z, Sun Y. The impact of endometrial thickness on the day of human chorionic gonadotrophin (chg.) administration on ongoing pregnancy rate in patients with different ovarian response. Plops One. 2015;10(12):e0145703.
3. Garcia-Velasco JA, Acevedo B, Alvarez C, Alvarez M, Beller J, Fontes J, et al. Strategies to manage refractory endometrium: state of the art in 2016. Repro'd Biomed Online. 2016;32(5):474-89.
4. Cen J, Zhang Y, Bai Y, Ma S, Zhang C, Jin L, et al. Research progress of stem cell therapy for endometrial injury. Mater Today Bio. 2022;16:100389.
5. Mahajan N, Sharma S. The endometrium in assisted reproductive technology: how thin is thin? J Hum Repro'd Sci. 2016;9(1):3-8.
6. Governini L, Luongo FP, Haxhiu A, Piomboni P, Luddi A. Main actors behind the endometrial receptivity and successful implantation. Tissue Cell. 2021;73:101656.
7. Santamaria X, Isaacson K, Simón C. Asherman's syndrome: it may not be all our fault. Hum Reprod. 2018;33(8):1374-80.
8. Neykova K, Tosto V, Giardina I, Tsibizova V, Vakrilov G. Endometrial receptivity and pregnancy outcome. J Matern Fetal Neonatal Med. 2022;35(13):2591-605.

9. Makker A, Singh MM. Endometrial receptivity: clinical assessment in relation to fertility, infertility, and antifertility. Med Res Rev. 2006;26(6):699-746.
10. Guerra ATBB. (2017). Asherman syndrome: current and future perspectives on treatment and prevention of recurrence. [online] Available from https://repositorio.ul.pt/handle/10451/30848 [Last accessed December, 2024].
11. Gargett CE, Nguyen HPT, Ye L. Endometrial regeneration and endometrial stem/progenitor cells. Rev Endocr Metab Disord. 2012;13(4):235-51.
12. Critchley HOD, Maybin JA, Armstrong GM, Williams ARW. Physiology of the Endometrium and Regulation of Menstruation. Physiol Rev. 2020;100(3):1149-79.
13. Upadhyay RK. Role of regeneration in tissue repairing and therapies. J Regen Med Tissue Eng. 2015;4(1):1.
14. Eguren AR. Regenerative Therapies to Treat Infertility of Endometrial Origin: From Basic to Clinics [PhD Thesis]. Universitat de Valencia (Spain); 2024; 31565208. [online] Available from https://search.proquest.com/openview/950f879c0d6aadba7b05d92b24e81f2e/1?pq-origsite=gscholar&cbl=2026366&diss=y [Last accessed December, 2024].
15. Lubkowska A, Dolegowska B, Banfi G. Growth factor content in PRP and their applicability in medicine. J Biol Regul Homeost Agents. 2012;26(2 Suppl 1):3S-22S.
16. Kanji S, Das H. Advances of Stem Cell Therapeutics in Cutaneous Wound Healing and Regeneration. Mediators Inflamm. 2017;2017:1-14.
17. Samy A, Abbas AM, Elmoursi A, Elsayed M, Hussein RS. Effect of autologous platelet-rich plasma transfusion in the treatment of infertile women with thin endometrium and its implications in IVF cycles: a literature review. Middle East Fertil Soc J. 2020;25(1):5.
18. Sarkar A, Saha S, Paul A, Maji A, Roy P, Maity TK. Understanding stem cells and its pivotal role in regenerative medicine. Life Sci. 2021;273:119270.
19. Song YT, Liu PC, Tan J, Zou CY, Li QJ, Li-Ling J, et al. Stem cell-based therapy for ameliorating intrauterine adhesion and endometrium injury. Stem Cell Res Ther. 2021;12(1): 556.
20. Mukherjee S, Malik P, Mukherjee TK. Isolation and purification of various mammalian cells: single cell isolation. In: Mukherjee TK, Malik P, Mukherjee S, (Eds). Practical Approach to Mammalian Cell and Organ Culture. Singapore: Springer Nature Singapore; 2023.
21. Pruszak J, Sonntag KC, Aung MH, Sanchez-Pernaute R, Isacson O. Markers and methods for cell sorting of human embryonic stem cell-derived neural cell populations. Stem Cells. 2007;25(9):2257-68.
22. Chin MH, Mason MJ, Xie W, Volinia S, Singer M, Peterson C, et al. Induced pluripotent stem cells and embryonic stem cells are distinguished by gene expression signatures. Cell Stem Cell. 2009;5(1):111-23.
23. Lv Q, Wang L, Luo X, Chen X. Adult stem cells in endometrial regeneration: Molecular insights and clinical applications. Mol Reprod Dev. 2021;88(6):379.
24. Kim JH, Park M, Paek JY, Lee WS, Song H, Lyu SW. Intrauterine infusion of human platelet-rich plasma improves endometrial regeneration and pregnancy outcomes in a murine model of Asherman's syndrome. Front Physiol. 2020;11:105.
25. Saad-Naguib MH, Kenfack Y, Sherman LS, Chafitz OB, Morelli SS. Impaired receptivity of thin endometrium: therapeutic potential of mesenchymal stem cells. Front Endocrinol. 2024;14:1268990.
26. Tewary S, Lucas ES, Fujihara R, Kimani PK, Polanco A, Brighton PJ, et al. Impact of sitagliptin on endometrial mesenchymal stem-like progenitor cells: a randomised, double-blind placebo-controlled feasibility trial. EBioMedicine. 2020;51:102597.

CHAPTER 53

Tender Loving Care and Reassurance Scans

Mala Arora, Pragati Oswal

ABSTRACT

Many studies confirm that pregnancy outcome in patients with unexplained recurrent pregnancy loss (RPL) can be positive with empathetic care without the need for any pharmacotherapy. This emphasizes the capacity of the body to heal itself and the role played by stress in pregnancy outcome. Stress has the capacity to alter the immune response and the endocrinal axis. Analyzing the consequences of stress in reproduction, a new field of psychoneuroimmunology has emerged. Stress relieving therapies like psychotherapy, empathetic care, and cognitive behavioral therapy are now a well recognized part of therapy in RPL.

Keywords: Tender loving care, CBT, RPL, Psychotherapy, Self-healing, Psychoneuroimmunology.

INTRODUCTION

It has been proven without doubt that in a patient with unexplained recurrent pregnancy loss (RPL), tender loving care (TLC) can give surprisingly positive outcomes. As early as 1991, Liddell et al., showed how supportive care for this group of women had successful results.[1] Most clinicians are aware of the need of supportive care for women with recurrent miscarriages. However, TLC is a very subjective and ambiguous concept and cannot be quantified in randomized control trials. It was defined very recently as "the care of mentally distressed patients by health professionals based on compassion and empathy, thereby reducing anxiety and improving mental wellbeing." A conceptual analysis of TLC was published in a journal of midwifery.[2]

HOW DOES TENDER LOVING CARE AFFECT RECURRENT PREGNANCY LOSS?

The limbic system of the brain is the seat of emotions. The limbic system mainly comprises the hippocampus and the amygdala. The thalamus and hypothalamus regulate hormones and many physiological systems of the body. A projection from the thalamus goes directly to the amygdala by passing the cerebral cortex. Hence, the emotional system acts independent from the cerebral cortex. Hence, emotional reactions may have no cortical participation at all.[3] The amygdala that stores memories will make us enact a response to an experience, without rationalizing because of the shortcut from the thalamus to the amygdala, something like a neural back lane, as opposed to the projection to the cortex which is the neural highway.

It has been shown that in the initial milliseconds of any experience, we will decide whether we like it or not.[4] Thus, the cognitive brain not only presents to us the awareness of what we experience, but also an opinion about it that is stored in the subconscious mind. It is possible then for emotions to have a mind of their own, one which can hold views quite independent of our rational mind.[5] This is precisely the reason why some experiences trigger stress emotions which are contrary to logical reasoning. One such event in a woman's life is a miscarriage.

Robert Ader,[6] a psychologist at University of Rochester, United States, discovered that the immune system, like the brain, could learn. His findings were a shock. The prevailing wisdom was that only the brain and the central nervous system could respond to an experience by changing how they behaved. Ader's findings led to the investigation of many ways in which the central nervous system and the immune system communicate. There are biological pathways not yet clearly defined, which make the mind, emotions, and physiological processes of the body intimately intertwined.

Immune system is the body's brain, so to say, defining the bodies' own sense of self and nonself. Immune cells permeate the entire body, making contact with every tissue. Those cells recognized as self are spared, but those they fail to recognize will be attacked and killed. This property of immune cells defends us against pathogens and cancer. Sometimes, this process may misidentify some "self-antigens" and create an autoimmune disease, and in the same light can mount an attack against the growing embryo to destroy it.

In a simple experiment that Ader conducted, he fed white rats a chemical that suppressed the disease fighting T-cells in the body. The chemical was fed to the rats in saccharin-flavored water. Later, the rats were fed plain saccharin water without the medication. This plain water also resulted in the depleting their T-cell count to the point of sickness and even death. Their immune system had learnt to suppress the T-cells in response to saccharin water. How was this possible?

Until recently, we believed that the central nervous system and the immune system functioned as two independent entities. There are no demonstrable anatomical pathways that connect the brain centers with the T cells. Ader's modest discovery has led to the new field of psychoneuroimmunology or PNI.[7,8] This field demonstrates close interaction between our immune system and the central nervous system.

David Felton[9] (a colleague of Ader) demonstrated that the autonomic nervous system (ANS) was in close contact with the immune system. He noted that emotions had a direct powerful effect on the ANS, which, in turn, regulated many physiological processes. Insulin secretion, blood pressure regulation and gut motility were all controlled by the ANS. Felton demonstrated that the ANS also influenced activity of lymphocytes and macrophages.[10] Electron microscopy shows synapses, where the ANS nerve endings are in close contact with immune cells in the lymph nodes, spleen, and thymus. The neurotransmitters released by the ANS regulate the activity of immune cells and the communication is bidirectional.

To test his discovery, Felton conducted an experiment in which he removed the nerves from the spleen and lymph nodes in animals. Then he challenged these animals with a virus. The immune response to the virus was suboptimal. Hence, the nervous system controls the proper functioning of the immune system.

Another key pathway linking emotions and pregnancy is the influence of hormones released by the hypothalamus. Under stress, it releases more catecholamines (adrenalin and noradrenalin), cortisol, and prolactin. Each of these impacts the immune system. This hormonal response also modifies the reproductive function. As an example, raised prolactin levels are luteolytic resulting in both infertility and miscarriage. It is nature's way of saying that if the mother is endangered, she need not be lumbered with a pregnancy.

A large multicentric study showed that people with chronic anxiety have a higher risk of asthma, arthritis, peptic ulcers, and heart disease.[11] This may also apply to miscarriages. In a cross-sectional study on RPL couples, there was a high degree of stress and anxiety in both the male and female partner.[12] In another prospective study, there was a high degree of posttraumatic stress disorder (PTSD) among women with miscarriage and ectopic pregnancy.[13]

HOW CAN WE PROVIDE TENDER LOVING CARE?

In a recent publication, it has been shown that *mirthful laughter* can affect natural killer (NK) cell activity which may change the outcome of pregnancy.[14] A recent publication re-enforced that laughter therapy is a nonpharmacological intervention that can be universally applied to reduce stress.[15]

In the field of *metaphysical healing*, it is thought that physical and mental disease has a deep root in the subconscious mind. Illness can be cured by pulling out its hidden roots by positive affirmations that are repeated by the conscious mind deeply and attentively till they permeate to the subconscious mind. Patience and attentive intelligent repetitions work wonders in arousing our healing powers. The power of positive thought is successfully exploited to heal the body of various chronic illnesses.[16]

Self-healing can also be accomplished at a metaphysical level. A prerequisite is to establish ones' sense of worth, independent of any external factors. The process involves a loving introspection of subjective sense of lack or loss (in this case a miscarriage) or other triggers that challenge one's sense of worth and accepting it.

The role of dispensing TLC alone in unexplained RPL has been recommended (Evidence level III—well-conducted case-control or cohort studies with risk of confounding bias).[17] It is estimated that supportive care alone, without any pharmacological intervention will also improve pregnancy outcome in unexplained RPL.[18]

Sigmund Freud, a contemporary of Alfred Ader, is considered the father of the "talking cure" now popularly

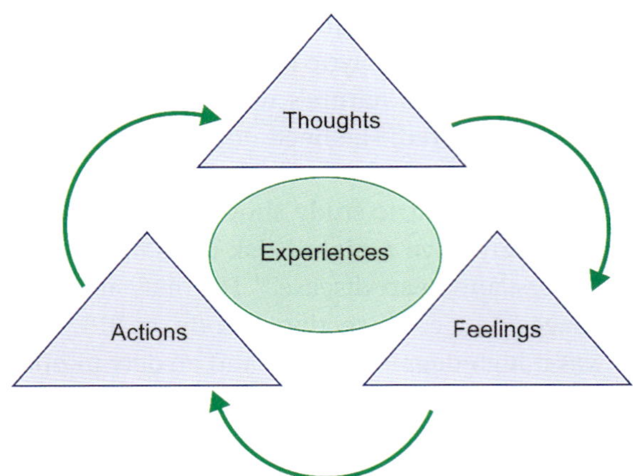

Fig. 1: Components of cognitive behavioral therapy (CBT).

known as psychotherapy.[19] He suggested that human behavior is affected by subconscious thoughts and memories. Talking about them can lead to catharsis. In the 1970s, the concept of cognitive behavioral therapy (CBT)[20] was introduced. CBT breaks down an experience into four components, viz., thoughts (cognition), feelings (emotions), behavior, and physiology or biological process **(Fig. 1)**. It then attempts to change the automatic negative thoughts that arise from the subconscious mind and lead to emotional problems. Identifying negative thoughts and replacing them with more objective positive ones can alleviate depression and anxiety. This has shown to have beneficial effect in patients with RPL.

VARIOUS TECHNIQUES OF COGNITIVE BEHAVIORAL THERAPY

- *Cognitive processing therapy (CPT)*—writing about the stressful event, and with help from the therapist, analyzing your emotions and reactions
- *Cognitive therapy (CT)* combatting over generalization of negative emotions and engaging in pleasurable activities
- *Dialectical behavior therapy (DBT)* educating people to interact with the experience in a less emotional way
- Rational emotive behavior therapy (REBT) allows you to identify and challenge irrational thoughts (e.g., if I have failed once I am bound to fail again) with more positive and productive thoughts (e.g., 80% of women that miscarry go on to have healthy babies)
- Mindfulness-based cognitive therapy (MBCT)[21]—to cultivate a nonjudgmental response to the event/living in the present only attitude
- Acceptance and commitment therapy (ACT)[22] that focusses on acceptance rather than modification of dysfunctional feelings toward an event.

HOW DOES PSYCHOTHERAPY HELP IN RECURRENT PREGNANCY LOSS?

Although psychotherapy has been beneficial in depression, anxiety, and other psychiatric disorders, its role in RPL is still in its infancy. It is now well established that emotions can affect the neuroendocrine-immune system.[23] Derangements in the endocrine system mediated through prolactin and the immune system mediated through T reg cells and NK cells will negatively affect embryo implantation thus leading to a miscarriage. Hence, a woman with one sporadic miscarriage may become prone to another miscarriage through high levels of anxiety.[24]

A triple arm randomized control trial assessed the effect of CBT, pharmacotherapy with sertraline and a control group with no intervention. CBT was clearly superior to pharmacotherapy in reducing stress and depression. The control group with no intervention had the highest stress and depression scores.[25]

OTHER INTERVENTIONS TO RELIEVE STRESS

- Having a separate early pregnancy clinic will provide privacy and shield patients from women that are full term.
- Having blogs/self-help groups where patients are able to interact with other couples undergoing similar experiences.
- Helpline to listen to patients and reassure them
- Frequent clinic visits for RPL patients preferably weekly appointments in the first trimester

REASSURANCE SCAN

Also known as comfort scans are early pregnancy scans in couples who had a previous miscarriage. The purpose of the scan is to demonstrate that the fetus is viable and growing. This provides reassurance to the couple that pregnancy is progressing well. Recent study suggested that after a miscarriage, you are never pregnant in the same way again, and need repeated reassurance that the pregnancy is progressing well. Performing extra scans in the first trimester becomes an integral part of pregnancy care in women that miscarry.[26]

- It dispels her doubts about the outcome of pregnancy and positively regulates the decidual environment for the growth of the embryo.

CONCLUSION

In simple language, negative emotions are toxic just like smoking and alcohol. There is a statistical link between stress and miscarriage. Clinical experience teaches us that couples may be emotionally distraught after an unexplained miscarriage. Some may treat it as emotionally disturbing as losing a child. Although vast majority of these couples will be able to fulfil their needs of parenthood.[27,28] Counseling and TLC or positive emotional support is required in the recovery phase. A current systematic review[29] and latest ESHRE guidlines[30] conclude that counseling is an important component of therapy. Some of the ways we can counsel positively are as follows:

- Encourage to practice selfcare post miscarriage, i.e., nutrition, light exercise, and sleep are important for mental healing.
- Acknowledge that a pregnancy existed and was lost as something was not quite right with the developing embryo.
- Avoid feelings of guilt and blame.
- Encourage to connect to a support group to share grief
- Consider memorializing the baby or giving the event a closure in a family/couple memorial.

REFERENCES

1. Liddell HS, Pattison NS, Zanderiqo A. Recurrent Miscarriage—outcome after supportive care in early pregnancy. Aust N Z J Obstet Gynecol. 1991;31(4):320-2.
2. Kido K, Mitani A, Uemura Y. Tender Loving Care: A Conceptual Analysis. Women, Midwives Midwifery. 2023;3(2):13-23.
3. Kunst-Wilson WR, Zajonc RB. Affective discrimination of stimuli that cannot be recognized. Science. 1980;207(4430):557-8.
4. Cahill L, Prins B, Weber M, McGaugh JL. Beta-adrenergic activation and memory for emotional events. Nature. 1994;371(6499):702-4.
5. Varela F. Immune system as the body's brain. The mind and life meeting proceedings. Dharamsala, India;1990.
6. Chemical messengers between brain and immune system. In: Ader R, Felten DL, Cohen N (Eds). Psychoneuroimmunology, 2nd edition. San Diego: Academic Press; 1990.
7. Besedovsky HO, Rev AD. Physiology of psychoneuro-immunology: a personal view. Brain Behav Immun. 2007;21(1):34-44.
8. Blalock JE, Smith EM. Conceptual development of the immune system as a sixth sense. Brain Behav Immun. 2007;21(1):23-33.
9. Felten DL, Felten SY, Carlson SL, Olschowka JA, Livnat S. Noradrenergic and peptidergic innervation of lymphoid tissue. J Immunol. 1985;135(2 Suppl):755s-765s.
10. Rabin BS, Cohen S, Ganguli R, Lysle DT, Cunnick JE. Bidirectional interaction between the central nervous system and the immune system. Crit Rev Immunol. 1989;9(4):279-312.
11. Friedman H, Boothby-Kewley S. The disease prone personality: a meta-analytic view. Am Psychol. 1987;42(6):539-55.
12. Voss P, Schick M, Langer L, Ainsworth A, Ditzen B, Strowitzki T, et al. Recurrent pregnancy loss: a shared stressor—couple-orientated psychological research findings. Fertil Steril. 2020;114(6):1288-96.
13. Farren J, Jalmbrant M, Ameye L, Joash K, Mitchell-Jones N, Tapp S, et al. Post-traumatic stress, anxiety and depression following miscarriage or ectopic pregnancy: a prospective cohort study. BMJ Open. 2016;6(11):e011864.
14. Bennett MP, Zeller JM, Rosenberg L, McCann J. The effect of mirthful laughter on stress and natural killer cell activity. Altern Ther Health Med. 2003;9(2):38-45.
15. Akimbekov NS, Razzaque MS. Laughter therapy: A humor-induced hormonal intervention to reduce stress and anxiety. Curr Res Physiol. 2021;4:135-8.
16. Sri Paramhansa Yogananda. Scientific Healing Affirmations. Kolkata: Yogoda Satsanga Society of India; 1917.
17. Jeve YB, Davies W. Evidence based management of recurrent miscarriages. J Hum Reprod Sci. 2014;7(3):159-69.
18. Clifford K, Rai R, Regan L. Future pregnancy outcome in unexplained recurrent first trimester miscarriage. Hum Reprod. 1997;12(2):387-9.
19. Cherry K. An Overview of Sigmund Freud's Theories. How the Father of Psychology Came to Be. 2024.
20. CBT https://www.nhs.uk/mental-health/talking-therapies
21. Patel A, Dinesh N, Sharma PSVN, Kumar P, Binu VS. Outcomes of Structured Psychotherapy for Emotional Adjustment in a Childless Couple diagnosed with Recurrent Pregnancy Loss: A Unique Investigation. J Hum Reprod Sci. 2018;11(2):202-7.
22. Salari N, Khazaie H, Hosseinian-Far A, Khaledi-Paveh B, Ghasemi H, Mohammadi M, Shohaimi S. The effect of acceptance and commitment therapy on insomnia and sleep quality: A systematic review. BMC Neurol. 2020;20(1):300.
23. González-Díaz SN, Arias-Cruz A, Elizondo-Villarreal B, Monge-Ortega OP. Psychoneuroimmunoendocrinology: clinical implications. World Allergy Organ J. 2017;10(1):19.
24. Sugiura-Ogasawara M, Furukawa TA, Nakano Y, Hori S, Aoki K, Kitamura T. Depression as a potential causal factor in subsequent miscarriage in recurrent spontaneous aborters. Hum Reprod. 2002;17(10):2580-84.
25. Basirat Z, Kheirkhah F, Faramarzi M, Esmaeilzadeh S, Khafri S, Tajali Z. Pharmacotherapy or Psychotherapy?

Selective Treatment Depression in The Infertile Women with Recurrent Pregnancy Loss: A Triple-Arm Randomized Controlled Trial. Int J Fertil Steril. 2022;16(3): 211-19.
26. Koert E, Hartwig TS, Hviid Malling GM, Schmidt L, Nielsen HS. 'You're never pregnant in the same way again': prior early pregnancy loss influences need for health care and support in subsequent pregnancy. Hum Reprod Open. 2023;2023(3):hoad032.
27. Ali S, Majid S, Niamat Ali M, Taing S, El-Serehy HA, Al-Misned FA. Evaluation of etiology and pregnancy outcome in recurrent miscarriage patients. Saudi J Biol Sci. 2020;27(10):2809-17.
28. El Hachem H, Crepaux V, May-Panloup P, Descamps P, Legendre G, Bouet PE. Recurrent pregnancy loss: current perspectives. Int J Womens Health. 2017;9:331-45.
29. Hennessy M, Dennehy R, Meaney S, Linehan L, Devane D, Rice R, et al. Clinical practice guidelines for recurrent miscarriage in high-income countries: a systematic review. Reprod Biomed Online. 2021;42(6):1146-71.
30. European Society of Reproduction and Embryology. (2023). ESHRE Early Pregnancy Guideline Development Group (GDG). Recurrent Pregnancy Loss. [online] Available from http://www.eshre.eu/en/Guidelines-and-Legal/Guidelines/Recurrent-pregnancy-loss [Last accessed December, 2024].

SECTION

10 Failed Pregnancy

CHAPTER

54 Hysteroscopic Evacuation of the Uterus

Oshri Barel, Moty Pansky

ABSTRACT

Hysteroscopic evacuation of the uterus offers certain advantages. It offers a chance to inspect the gestational sac and the embryo as in the technique of hystero-embryoscopy, and to take the embryo separately for accurate genetic evaluation. It minimizes chances of uterine perforation and allows us to see the site of implantation in the uterus which may be important for cornual or lower segment implantations. Finally, it allows us to check that the evacuation has been complete with no adherent remnants of retained products. The risk of adhesion formation is minimized. Challenges are poor visualization, lengthy procedure, and fluid overload.

Keywords: Hystroscopic evacuation of the uterus, Missed miscarriage, Intrauterine adhesions.

INTRODUCTION

Management of early miscarriage today is done either medically or surgically by dilatation and curettage (D&C). The optimal management necessitates complete evacuation of the uterus, with minimal endometrial damage (to conserve future fertility) and minimal need for future follow-up and intervention. D&C and aspiration curettage in the first trimester are safe procedures, with a small percentage of major complications (approximately 0.16%) or minor complications (approximately 1%).[1] However, these procedures are done blindly and rely mainly on the surgeon's experience. Some of the well-known complications of D&C include:

- Uterine perforation
- Retained products of conception (RPOC)
- Adhesion formation

The use of hysteroscopy in the treatment of failed pregnancies has some possible advantages that may assist in diagnosing the cause of miscarriage and preventing possible complications such as uterine perforation, RPOC, and intrauterine adhesions. Nevertheless, this method has a few disadvantages as well: These procedures are more expensive than standard D&C; they require specific equipment; and there is a learning curve related to performing the procedure successfully, mainly related to the learning curve of identifying the trophoblast and diagnosing embryonal malformations.

DIAGNOSTIC USES OF THE HYSTEROSCOPIC EVACUATION OF THE UTERUS

Embryoscopy and fetoscopy have been used increasingly in treating missed miscarriages in the last two decades. This procedure is done simply by transcervical hysteroscopy during pregnancy. The fact that we can directly view the embryo in the gestational sac allows us to document and describe the fetal morphology and to note different anatomical malformations **(Fig. 1)**. Philipp et al.[2] described in 2001 the use of embryoscopy prior to evacuation of the uterus in early missed miscarriages to

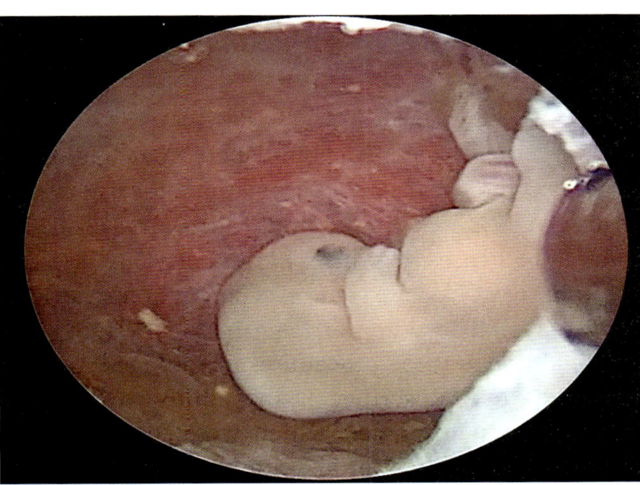

Fig. 1: Embryoscopy of a missed miscarriage of an 8-week embryo using a TruClear Elite 6-mm tissue removal device.

diagnose anatomical malformations and allow sampling of the fetal tissues for genetic testing. This group also demonstrated that patients with repeated pregnancy loss are more likely to have morphologically normal embryos and less aneuploidy in cytogenetic analysis.[3] Using fetal tissue obtained in embryoscopy allows for more accurate genetic testing and diagnosis and reduces the number of maternal cells in the specimen.[4,5] This procedure might also assist in diagnosing uterine malformations or structural abnormalities that might be related to the cause of the miscarriage.

REDUCING COMPLICATIONS

In a recent systematic review, the rate of intrauterine adhesions (IUAs) after D&C for miscarriages ranged between 16% and 21% and higher in cases of a repeat D&C. After more than one D&C, the risk of IUA is doubled.[6] The treatment of severe IUA and Asherman's syndrome is complex. These adhesions tend to recur and can result in secondary infertility and litigations.

Many options have been suggested to treat or prevent IUAs, including specific surgical techniques for different pathologies, specific surgical instruments, the use of antibiotics (prophylactic or postprocedures), and the use of intrauterine device (IUD) or intrauterine balloons. The use of estrogen to improve endometrial regeneration and the use of intrauterine antiadhesive gels or amnion grafts have also been implemented.[7-13] Hysteroscopic treatment might present a way to target the gestational sac without damage to uninvolved uterine walls, thus preventing possible adhesion formation.[14-17]

HYSTEROSCOPIC RESECTION OF MISCARRIAGES

A few studies have been published in recent years describing the use of hysteroscopy to treat early missed miscarriages. de Codt et al.[6] published a retrospective study of 358 cases, of which 173 underwent D&C and 185 underwent hysteroscopic evacuation of miscarriage. They reported less hemorrhage in the hysteroscopy group, although these procedures took longer. Another advantage they described is the ability to diagnose intrauterine pathologies, which were found in >5% of the cases. Meshaal et al.[7] compared hysteroscopic management of first-trimester pregnancy loss to surgical evacuation either blind or under ultrasound guidance. It included 315 patients, divided equally into three groups. All women were assessed for retained products, surgical complications, the need for further management, and pregnancy rates within 2 years of follow-up. The rate of RPOC and the need for further treatment were significantly higher in the group that underwent blind D&C compared to the other two groups. The conception rate within 2 years was also significantly lower in the group that underwent blind D&C.

According to the results of this study, women who underwent hysteroscopy for evacuation of the uterus following miscarriage needed a significantly shorter time to conceive.

Catena et al.[8] and Young et al.[9] have also published their experience with hysteroscopic treatment of miscarriages.

HYSTEROSCOPIC MORCELLATION OF MISSED MISCARRIAGE

Hysteroscopic morcellation has been used for intrauterine tissue extraction for over 20 years. Hysteroscopic morcellators have been shown to allow for rapid and complete resection of polyps, fibroids, uterine septa, and RPOC.[18] These instruments use a rotating blade and a suction system that allow for specimen removal under direct hysteroscopic visualization. Compared with standard resectoscopic techniques, hysteroscopic morcellators probably save time and allow complete specimen removal.[19]

The use of the hysteroscopic morcellator for resection of fetal tissue in early missed miscarriages has been gaining popularity in recent years. This technique was assessed in one case for a woman with previous Ashreman's syndrome and was found to be feasible. However, the authors state that visibility was poor while resecting the implantation site due to high vascularization.[20] A study by our group showed that this technique is feasible and safe.[21]

The technique we developed starts with hysteroscopic visualization of the uterine cavity and the location of the gestational sac. This is followed by creating a window in the gestational sac and performing an embryoscopy. Later it is followed by resection of the gestational sac and review of the uterine cavity and assessment for RPOC **(Videos 1 and 2)**. This procedure can sometimes be done (especially when learning the technique) using ultrasound guidance **(Video 3)**.

CHALLENGES AND MODIFICATIONS IN THE CURRENT TECHNIQUES

In most cases, as well as in our experience, there are a few challenges in the hysteroscopic management of missed miscarriages. This involves difficulty in visualization due to bleeding, difficulty in estimating complete uterus evacuation, fluid overload, and prolonged procedures.

A few modifications and methods have been used to overcome these challenges. The use of oxytocin, and sometimes vasopressin, can decrease blood loss, improve visibility, and decrease fluid overload. Also, the use of larger instruments allows for quicker procedures with less blood loss. The learning curve for adequately estimating an empty uterine cavity can be expedited using ultrasound assistance in the initial procedures until the hysteroscopic picture becomes clear.

HYSTEROSCOPIC-ASSISTED EVACUATION OF THE UTERUS FOLLOWING MISCARRIAGE

Unlike the previous techniques described, a few authors have suggested the use of hysteroscopic assistance prior to suction D&C; this includes hysteroscopy to target the location of the gestational sac and perform a uterine assessment and a morphological fetal assessment (embryoscopy), with or without obtaining an embryonic/fetal sample for genetic evaluation. A targeted D&C follows this to reduce the possibility of uterine damage. A lower level of hysteroscopic skill and expertise is necessary using this technique, and the learning curve is much shorter. Following the procedure, a hysteroscopy can be performed to ensure no RPOC were left behind.

VIDEO LEGENDS

Video 1: Hysteroscopic evacuation of a missed miscarriage at 6 weeks

Video 2: 9 weeks missed miscarriage with a gestational sac in anterior wall with fetus and an anembryonic gestational sac in posterior wall

Video 3: Ultrasound guided hysteroscopic evacuation of the uterus

REFERENCES

1. Upadhyay UD, Desai S, Zlidar V, Weitz TA, Grossman D, Anderson P, et al. Incidence of emergency department visits and complications after abortion. Obstet Gynecol. 2015;125:175-83.
2. Philipp T, Kalousek DK. Transcervical embryoscopy in missed abortion. J Assist Reprod Genet. 2001;18(5):285-90.
3. Feichtinger M, Wallner E, Hartmann B, Reiner A, Philipp T. Transcervical embryoscopic and cytogenetic findings reveal distinctive differences in primary and secondary recurrent pregnancy loss. Fertil Steril. 2017;107(1):144-9.
4. Campos-Galindo I1, García-Herrero S, Martínez-Conejero JA, Ferro J, Simón C, Rubio C. Molecular analysis of products of conception obtained by hysteroembryoscopy from infertile couples. J Assist Reprod Genet. 2015;32(5):839-48.
5. Hooker A, Fraenk D, Brölmann H, Huirne J. Prevalence of intrauterine adhesions after termination of pregnancy: a systematic review. Eur J Contracept Reprod Health Care. 2016;21(4):329-35.
6. de Codt M, Balza C, Jadoul P, Forget P, Squifflet J-L, Bernard P, et al. Hysteroscopic Resection for Missed Abortion: Feasibility, Operative Technique and Potential Benefit Compared to Curettage. Front Surg. 2020;7:64.
7. Meshaal H, Salah E, Fawzy E, Abdel-Rasheed M, Maged A, Saad H. Hysteroscopic management versus ultrasound-guided evacuation for women with first-trimester pregnancy loss, a randomised controlled trial. BMC Womens Health. 2022;22(1):190.
8. Catena U, D'Ippolito S, Campolo F, Dinoi G, Lanzone A, Scambia G. Hysteroembryoscopy and hysteroscopic uterine evacuation of early pregnancy loss: A feasible procedure in selected cases. Facts Views Vis Obgyn. 2022;14(2):193-7.
9. Young S, Miller CE. Hysteroscopic resection for management of early pregnancy loss: a case report and literature review. F S Rep. 2022;3(2):163-7.
10. Shazly SA, Laughlin-Tommaso SK, Breitkopf DM, Hopkins MR, Burnett TL, Green IC, et al. Hysteroscopic Morcellation Versus Resection for the Treatment of Uterine Cavitary Lesions: A Systematic Review and Meta-analysis. Minim Invasive Gynecol. 2016;23(6):867-77.
11. Harpham M, Abbott J. Use of a hysteroscopic morcellator to resect miscarriage in a woman with recurrent Asherman's syndrome. J Minim Invasive Gynecol. 2014;21(6):1118-20.
12. Weinberg S, Pansky M, Burshtein I, Beller U, Goldstein H, Barel O. A Pilot Study of Guided Conservative Hysteroscopic Evacuation of Early Miscarriage. J Minim Invasive Gynecol. 2021;28(11):1860-7.
13. Cholkeri-Singh A, Zamfirova I, Miller CE. Increased Fetal Chromosome Detection with the Use of Operative Hysteroscopy During Evacuation of Products of Conception for Diagnosed Miscarriage. J Minim Invasive Gynecol. 2020;27(1):160-5.
14. Deans R, Abbott J. Review of intrauterine adhesions. J Minim Invasive Gynecol. 2010;17:555-69.
15. Hooker AB, Lemmers M, Thurkow AL, Heymans MW, Opmeer BC, Brölmann HA, et al. Systematic review and meta-analysis of intrauterine adhesions after miscarriage:

prevalence, risk factors and long-term reproductive outcome. Hum Reprod Update. 2014;20(2):262-78.
16. Kodaman P, Arici A. Intrauterine adhesions and fertility outcome: how to optimize success? Curr Opin Obstet Gynecol. 2007;19:207-14.
17. Lee WL, Liu CH, Cheng M, Chang WH, Liu WM, Wang PH. Focus on the Primary Prevention of Intrauterine Adhesions: Current Concept and Vision. Int J Mol Sci. 2021;22(10): 5175.
18. Schenker JG, Margalioth EJ. Intrauterine adhesions: an updated appraisal. Fertil Steril. 1982;37:593-610.
19. Schenker JG. Etiology of a therapeutic approach to synechia uteri. Eur J Obstet Gynecol Reprod Biol. 1996;65:109.
20. Tam WH, Lau WC, Cheung LP, Yuen PM, Chung TK-H. Intrauterine adhesions after conservative and surgical management of spontaneous abortion. J Am Assoc Gynecol Laparosc. 2002;9:182-5.
21. van Dongen H, Emanuel MH, Wolterbeek R, Trimbos JB, Jansen FW. Hysteroscopic morcellator for removal of intrauterine polyps and myomas: a randomized controlled pilot study among residents in training. J Minim Invasive Gynecol. 2008;15(4):466-71.

CHAPTER

55

Placental Pathology

Sunil Jaiman

ABSTRACT

Histopathological study of placenta in cases of late fetal losses is highly recommended. Placental study will identify if there is chorionic villitis of unknown etiology, massive perivillous fibrin deposition, maternal vascular malperfusion, fetal vascular malperfusion and/or umbilical cord defects. This may help to identify which patients will benefit with antithrombotic therapy or control of placental inflammatory conditions.

Keywords: Placental pathology, Chronic histiocytic intervillositis, Multiple chorangioma syndrome, Maternal vascular malperfusion, Fetal vascular malperfusion.

INTRODUCTION

Miscarriage is defined as pregnancy loss before the 20th week of gestation.[1,2] It affects 50–70% of all gestations, while 15–20% of clinically recognized pregnancies can show miscarriage.[3-7] Additionally, the risk of miscarriage increases with the number of previous miscarriages.[8,9]

Recurrent pregnancy loss (RPL), on the other hand, as defined by the World Health Organization (WHO) is the loss of three or more consecutive pregnancies before the 20th week of gestation and it affects 1–5% of pregnancies.[6,7,10-12] After two pregnancy losses, the risk of miscarriage in a subsequent pregnancy is 30%, and it rises to 33% after three losses.[13] Therefore, the American Society for Reproductive Medicine has redefined RPL as two or more failed clinical pregnancies.[11,14] RPL carries significant demographic, social, psychological, and economic impact.[15]

Primary RPL can be defined as the absence of previous pregnancy at term or beyond the 24 weeks of gestation; while secondary RPL can be defined as the presence of two or more consecutive losses occurring in women with a previous child or whose previous pregnancy reached the 24 weeks of gestational age.[16]

Although examined in only a few studies, abnormalities of the umbilical cord, membranes, or placenta have been identified in >50% of pregnancy losses occurring before 20 weeks of gestation.[17] Studies on structurally normal stillbirths suggest that hypoxia resulting from placental dysfunction is the primary mechanism of fetal death in most cases, underscoring the critical importance of placental evaluation.[18,19] Moreover, the Stillbirth Collaborative Research Network study, focused on fetal deaths at or beyond 20 weeks, found that placental pathological examination was useful in identifying the cause of pregnancy loss in 64.6% of cases.[20] The American College of Obstetricians and Gynecologists Committee on Genetics recommends that placental examination should be a routine clinical tool in evaluating pregnancy loss.[21,22] This includes gross and microscopic examination of the placenta, membranes, and umbilical cord to identify potential causes of fetal death.[21] Placental pathology in cases of fetal death is now considered a research priority to better understand the causes and mechanisms of these occurrences.[19,22,23]

What are the placental lesions implicated in recurrent pregnancy loss?

Placental lesions with the propensity to show recurrence in the subsequent pregnancy include common and uncommon lesions. The common placental lesions include: (1) Villitis of unknown etiology (RR: 25–50%);[24] (2) Placenta accreta (RR: 10–25%);[25] (3) Maternal vascular malperfusion (RR: 10–25%);[26] (4) Preterm acute chorioamnionitis (RR: 10–25%);[27] (5) Placental abruption (RR: 4–5%).[28] The uncommon lesions include: (1) Chronic histiocytic intervillositis (RR: 75–90%);[29] (2) Massive perivillous fibrin/maternal floor infarction (RR: 30–60%);[30] (3) Multiple chorangioma syndrome (RR: 35–40%).[31] Patients at higher risk of recurrence typically exhibit advanced or extensive placental pathology.

Currently, there is no effective technology to identify important pathologic processes in the placenta, thereby making histologic evaluation essential for detecting these lesions.[32]

What is the classification of recurrent pregnancy loss placenta correlates?

Recurrent pregnancy loss is attributed to factors that persist throughout the reproductive life of the parents, compromising multiple pregnancies.[33] RPL can be classified into (1) previable and (2) postviable RPL.

- *Placental correlates in previable recurrent pregnancy loss:*

  The placental pathology in RPL is listed in **Table 1**.

  Abnormal uterine anatomy can cause recurrent inadequate embryonic implantation. For instance, large submucosal leiomyomas or uterine malformations (such as bicornuate uterus, which has a miscarriage rate of up to 60%) can contribute to RPL.[34]

  Although there are no specific embryo placental correlates with first trimester losses in these cases, maternal vascular malperfusion within affected placentas may manifest as inadequate fetal and/or placental growth in later gestation.

  Cervical incompetence can occur due to procedures like LEEP or cone biopsy and can result in recurrent mid-gestational previable delivery in up to 70% of patients, the risk of which drops significantly (to 5–30%) with cerclage.[35]

  Common obstetric syndromes in this context include preterm premature membrane rupture, amniotic fluid infection, and "inflammatory" abruption.[33] Histologic chorioamnionitis would be the embryo placental correlates in these cases.

  Chromosomal disorders such as parentally inherited aneuploidy, from unbalanced translocations or single-gene mutations, can lead to recurrent early pregnancy failure. The placental phenotype is correlated with the specific genetic abnormality. For example, maternally heritable autosomal dominant gestational trophoblastic disease causes recurrent molar pregnancies due to an NLRP7 gene imprinting mutation on chromosome 19q13. This phenotype evolves due to defective placenta-specific imprinting, resulting in the overexpression of paternally expressed transcripts.[36]

  Antiphospholipid antibodies can sometimes cause recurrent spontaneous abortion associated with early onset severe decidual arteriopathy. Decidual tissue fragments may demonstrate histologic features of maternal vascular malperfusion including arteriolar fibrinoid necrosis, and villous infarction.[37] Lupus anticoagulant and anticardiolipin antibodies are often implicated in these cases.[38]

  Immunomodulatory therapy (comprising aspirin, prednisone, heparin, and/or hydroxychloroquine) has been shown to reduce pregnancy loss from 76% in index pregnancies to 14% in subsequently treated gestations.[38]

- *Placental correlates in postviable recurrent pregnancy loss*:
  - *Chronic histiocytic intervillositis (CHI):* CHI also termed "chronic intervillositis of unknown etiology" (CIUE), is defined as an infiltrate of CD68+ mononuclear cells occupying ≥5% of the intervillous space "in the absence of clinical or histopathological signs of infection".[39] CHI is T-cell-driven maternal histiocytic infiltrate confined to the intervillous space, often with abundant fibrin.[29,39-43]

    CD68 positive mononuclear cells in the absence of clinical or histopathological signs of infection are what distinguishes CHI from the infectious causes of intervillositis, for example, *Plasmodium falciparum*, cytomegalovirus, dengue virus, Zika virus, parvovirus B19, SARS-CoV-2, *Chlamydia psittaci*, and *Listeria monocytogenes*. Moreover, the infection-induced intervillositis does not appear to recur.[44]

    This condition is associated with both early and late recurrent stillbirth as well as intrauterine growth restriction in live births. The recurrence risk, absent immunologic intervention, is very high (70–80%).[29,45]

TABLE 1: Placental pathology in RPL.

	Placental lesion	*Recurrence rate (Ref)*
1.	Villitis of unknown etiology	25–50%[24]
2.	Placenta accreta	10–25%[25]
3.	Maternal vascular malperfusion	10–25%[26]
4.	Preterm acute chorioamnionitis	10–25%[27]
5.	Placental abruption	4–5%[28]
6.	Chronic histiocytic intervillositis	75–90%[29]
7.	Massive perivillous fibrin/maternal floor infarction	30–60%[30]
8.	Multiple chorangioma syndrome	35–40%[31]

Women with recurrent CHI and their families have a predisposition to autoimmune diseases, suggesting an alloimmune pathology for CHI. This observation has led to attempts at preventing CHI with various maternal immunosuppression strategies.

Empirical administration of immunomodulatory agents, including low-molecular weight heparin, aspirin, and steroids, has proven effective in supporting 67% of pregnancies to live birth, though preterm deliveries occurred in about half of these cases (30% of all pregnancies).[45]

- *Chronic villitis of unknown etiology (VUE):* Chronic VUE is a destructive chronic inflammatory lesion of the chorionic villi characterized by a maternal T lymphocytes infiltrate along with elevated numbers of fetal macrophages (Hofbauer cells) in the villous stroma.[19,46,47] As with CHI, the diagnosis of VUE requires exclusion of an infectious cause. VUE can be low or high grade. Low-grade VUE shows presence of chronic inflammation affecting less than 10 contiguous villi in any one histologic focus; low-grade VUE can be focal (one slide, less than 10 villi) or multifocal (more than one histology slide). High-grade VUE shows presence of multiple foci, on more than one section, at least one of which shows inflammation affecting more than 10 contiguous villi; high-grade VUE can be patchy (multiple foci, with at least one focus with 10 or more contiguous villi) or diffuse (>30% of all distal villi are involved).[48]

  The antigenic stimuli (fetal/placental/environmental) that elicit this maternal host versus fetal graft reaction are unknown. VUE becomes more common as pregnancy progresses. However, severe early onset villitis is typically associated with fetal growth restriction and RPL. Conditions associated with VUE include fetal growth restriction, neurodisability in live births, and stillbirth. Diffuse high-grade chronic villitis, particularly with stem villous obliteration and/or extensive intervillous fibrin, is associated with adverse fetal/neonatal outcomes, including recurrent late fetal losses and recurrent complications in live births (e.g., FGR, abnormal neurological presentation).[49,50] The baseline rate of recurrent high-grade chronic villitis is reported at 60%.[49]

  Immunomodulatory agents like aspirin and corticosteroids have been reported to effectively reduce recurrent fetal morbidity and mortality.[51]

- *Massive perivillous fibrin deposition (MPFD)/maternal floor infarction (MFI):* MPFD/MFI defined by the presence of extensive deposition of fibrinoid material in the intervillous space encasing and suffocating the chorionic villi.[52] Three patterns of MPFD have been described: classic, borderline, and transmural.[52] *Classic MPFD or MFI* shows encasement of basal villi by fibrinoid along the presence of fibrinoid though the entire maternal floor which is ≥3 mm in thickness on at least one histology slide. *Borderline MPFD* shows involvement of 25–50% of villi on at least one histologic slide with transmural or nearly transmural distribution. *Transmural MPFD* shows transmural perivillous fibrinoid extension, with encasement of ≥50% of villi on at least one histology slide.[30,48,52]

  The MPFD/MFI involves immunologically mediated deposition of two types of fibrinoids: fibrin-type fibrinoid and matrix-type fibrinoids in the intervillous (MPFD) and basal (MFI) areas.[52] This fibrinoid forms a lattice that strangulates the chorionic villi, impairing fetomaternal gas exchange. This process is accompanied by areas of degenerative trophoblastic injury.[53]

  These conditions are associated with disorders such as antiphospholipid antibody syndrome, coagulation pathway mutations, and long-chain 3-hydroxyacyl-CoA dehydrogenase (LCHAD) deficiency. Reported stillbirth and recurrence rates can be as high as 30–50% and up to 80%, respectively.[30,54-56]

- *Maternal vascular malperfusion (MVM):* MVM diagnosis represents a constellation of findings involving the villous parenchyma and/or involving maternal decidual vasculature.[19,48,57-59] MVM lesions are categorized as villous or vascular depending upon the presence of pathology.
  - *Villous lesions include:*
    - *Villous infarct(s)* are dead villi in which the trophoblastic nuclei are clumped and necrotic with smudged partly dispersed DNA (recent infarct); or when there is collapse of intervillous space, with villous crowding and

complete disappearance of nuclear DNA (remote infarct).
  - *Increased syncytial knots*: When there are aggregates of syncytiotrophoblastic (ST) nuclei along proximal stem villi or the ST nuclei aggregate at one or more poles of distal villi.
  - *Villous agglutination*: It is adherence of distal villi agglutinated by fibrin and/or by bridging syncytial knots.
  - *Increased intervillous fibrin*: It is when abnormal amounts of intervillous fibrinoid coat either the proximal stem villi or get deposited to distal villi resulting in eccentric adherence.
  - *Distal villous hypoplasia*: It is paucity of terminal villi in relation to the surrounding stem villi. The villi are slender, elongated and with increased syncytial knots. These features are seen in the lower two-thirds of the placental parenchyma involving at least 30% of one full-thickness parenchymal histology slide.
- *Vascular lesions include:*
  - *Persistent muscularization of basal plate arteries*: It is the persistence of vascular smooth muscle cells in the walls of large spiral arteries at the basal plate.
  - *Mural hypertrophy of decidual arterioles*: It is the thickening of the muscular wall of extraplacental membranous arterioles.
  - *Acute atherosis of basal plate arteries and/ or decidual arterioles*: It is the eosinophilic fibrinoid necrosis of arterial smooth muscles along with the presence of subendothelial or medial foam cells (macrophages) in the basal maternal arteries.

  Maternal vascular malperfusion is rarely a cause of unexplained fetal demise in developed countries due to routine antenatal surveillance identifying at-risk fetuses. However, in under-resourced countries, MVM remains a primary cause of intrauterine demise.[33] Underlying maternal disorders are broadly classified into those mediated by hypertension and those mediated by maternal autoimmunity.[60,61] RPL occurs with unmodifiable or untreated disease or in resource-poor societies without the capacity for preterm intervention of high-risk pregnancies.[62]

- *Diabetes-associated pregnancy losses* can be recurrent if affected mothers have unstable glucose control ("brittle" disease), glucose-resistant disease, or reside in societies without the capacity for detection and intervention. Diabetes can lead to RPL[63] through mechanisms like MVM, fetal vascular malperfusion (FVM), fetal hypertrophic cardiomyopathy, and complications of fetal macrosomia.

  A recent study on women with RPL has shown that the risk of gestational diabetes mellitus (GDM) was higher in women with secondary RPL compared to those with primary RPL.[64] The authors speculate that it may be due to women with secondary RPL being more exposed to the diabetogenic effects of pregnancy, primarily during the second half, making them more susceptible to GDM in subsequent pregnancies. Recent observations suggest that higher numbers of pregnancies are an independent risk factor of GDM. Moreover, the association between number of pregnancies and GDM appears to be more prominent among women who were ≥30 years old or with a prepregnancy BMI <24 kg/m^2.[65]

  A recent study on nonhypertensive GDM found that placental histomorphology and its association with perinatal outcomes were observed more frequently in placentas of GDM pregnancies compared to the controls.[66]

  The histoarchitectural placental correlates include increased: (1) syncytial knots per villous; (2) maternal inflammatory response; (3) fetal inflammatory response; (4) chronic inflammation such as chronic villitis and chronic deciduitis; (5) MVM lesions including distal villous hypoplasia, decidual vasculopathy, villous infarction, and increased fibrin deposition; and (6) villous dysmaturity (delayed villous maturation).[66]
- *Abnormal uterine anatomy:* It can predispose to recurrent pregnancy complications, including RPL after gestational viability.[34] The etiologies include: (1) MVM related to implantation over large submucosal leiomyomas with limited arteriolar uteroplacental perfusion; (2) FVM due to space constraint-induced umbilical cord compression (e.g., bicornuate uterus with bilobate placentation within the uterine horns and velamentous cord insertion between the lobes); (3) placenta accreta/

percreta (e.g., due to C-section site implantation) complicated by uterine rupture, placental abruption, and/or fetal hemorrhage.

- *Fetal vascular malperfusion*: Fetal vascular malperfusion is a term applied to a group of placental lesions indicating reduced or absent perfusion of the villous parenchyma by the fetus.[19,48,58,59,67-69] Just as MVM lesions, FVM lesions are categorized as villous or vascular depending upon the presence of pathology.
  - *Villous lesions include:*
    - *Villous stromal-vascular karyorrhexis*: It is when three or more histologic foci show two or more terminal villi displaying karyorrhexis of nucleated erythrocytes, leukocytes, endothelial cells, and/or stromal cells albeit with preserved contiguous trophoblasts.
    - *High-grade FVM (severe)*: It is the finding of more than one focus of avascular villi (a cumulative assessment of ≥45 avascular villi over three histologic sections examined or an average of >15 villi per section) with or without thrombus; or finding two or more occlusive or nonocclusive thrombi in chorionic plate vessels or the vessels of major stem villi; or finding multiple nonocclusive thrombi.
    - *Avascular villi*: Small foci are the finding of three or more foci of two to four terminal villi show complete loss of villous capillaries along with bland hyaline fibrosis of the villous stroma; intermediate foci are when similar changes are observed in five to ten villi; and large foci are when ten or more villi show these changes.
  - *Vascular lesions include:*
    - *Thrombi large fetal vessels*: Organized blood clot, occlusive or nonocclusive, of any age (defined by 2 or more of the following: fibrin strands, glassy texture with slight hematoxylin blush, adherence to endothelium) compromising the lumen of fetal vessels in the chorionic plate or proximal origin of the villous tree.
    - *Intramural fibrin deposition (IFD)*: It is when the fibrin deposition is subendothelial or intramuscular, and thus intramural. These deposits by definition are nonocclusive. Recent IFD is depicted by fibrin or fibrinoid deposition either subendothelial or intramuscular, within the wall of large fetal vessels. While similar lesions with calcification indicate remote IFD.
    - *Stem vessel obliteration (synonymous with fibromuscular sclerosis)*: Show marked thickening of the vessel wall with resultant closure of the vascular. This results in loss of fetal circulation, loss of endothelial lining, and downstream avascular villi.
    - *Vascular ectasia*: It is characterized by the finding vessels that are four times the luminal diameter of the surrounding corresponding vessel.

  Fetal vascular malperfusion, though a common cause of late fetal demise, is almost always sporadic. When recurrent, the responsible mechanisms persist from one pregnancy to another. The recurrent causes may include: (1) maternal or fetal thrombophilia (maternal antiphospholipid antibodies, fetal protein C or S deficiency); (2) umbilical cord abnormalities recurring due to narrow cord, abnormal insertion, and oligohydramnios-induced cord compression; (3) diabetes-associated fetal thrombosis and/or delayed villous maturation; (4) cord compression due to abnormal uterine anatomy;[33] (5) recurrent umbilical cord hypercoiling or stricture perhaps due to maternal or genetic component influencing cord geometry.[70]

- *Multiple chorangioma syndrome:* Multiple chorangioma syndrome (placental chorioangiomatosis, diffuse placental chorioangiomatosis) is a very rare condition characterized by numerous chorangiomas ranging from a few millimeters to several centimeters and occupying up to 80% of the placental parenchymal volume.[31,71] Its genetic basis has not been established, although increased expression of angiogenic growth factors (e.g., angiopoietin) and decrease in several anti-angiogenic factors have been implicated.[72,73] Multiple chorangioma syndrome is associated with recurrent miscarriage and fetal coagulopathies including disseminated intravascular coagulation and cerebral thromboemboli.[74]

CONCLUSION

Study of placental pathology will help us identify the pathophysiology of RPL. Trained obstetric pathologist that specialize in placental study are required. Depending on the lesions identified in the placenta, preventive measures can then be instituted prior to/during the next pregnancy to avert a pregnancy loss.

REFERENCES

1. Dugas C, Slane VH. (2022). Miscarriage (Archived). [online] Available from https://www.ncbi.nlm.nih.gov/books/NBK532992/. [Last accessed December, 2024]
2. World Health Organization. WHO: recommended definitions, terminology and format for statistical tables related to the perinatal period and use of a new certificate for cause of perinatal deaths. Modifications recommended by FIGO as amended October 14, 1976. Acta Obstet Gynecol Scand. 1977;56(3):247-53.
3. Ammon Avalos L, Galindo C, Li DK. A systematic review to calculate background miscarriage rates using life table analysis. Birth Defects Res A Clin Mol Teratol. 2012;94(6):417-23.
4. Brezina PR, Kutteh WH. Classic and cutting-edge strategies for the management of early pregnancy loss. Obstet Gynecol Clin N Am. 2014;41(1):1-18.
5. Larsen EC, Christiansen OB, Kolte AM, Macklon N. New insights into mechanisms behind miscarriage. BMC Med. 2013;11:154.
6. Ford HB, Schust DJ. Recurrent pregnancy loss: etiology, diagnosis, and therapy. Rev Obstet Gynecol. 2009;2(2):76-83.
7. Rai R, Regan L. Recurrent miscarriage. Lancet (London, England). 2006;368(9535):601-11.
8. Knudsen UB, Hansen V, Juul S, Secher NJ. Prognosis of a new pregnancy following previous spontaneous abortions. Eur J Obstet Gynecol Reprod Biol. 1991;39(1):31-6.
9. Regan L, Braude PR, Trembath PL. Influence of past reproductive performance on risk of spontaneous abortion. BMJ. 1989;299(6698):541-5.
10. Clifford K, Rai R, Watson H, Regan L. An informative protocol for the investigation of recurrent miscarriage: preliminary experience of 500 consecutive cases. Hum Reprod. 1994; 9(7):1328-32.
11. Li TC, Makris M, Tomsu M, Tuckerman E, Laird S. Recurrent miscarriage: aetiology, management and prognosis. Hum Reprod Update. 2002;8(5):463-81.
12. Stirrat GM. Recurrent miscarriage. Lancet. 1990;336(8716):673-5.
13. American College of Obstetricians and Gynecologists. ACOG practice bulletin. Management of recurrent pregnancy loss. Number 24, February 2001. (Replaces Technical Bulletin Number 212, September 1995). American College of Obstetricians and Gynecologists. Int J Gynaecol Obstet. 2002;78(2):179-90.
14. Practice Committee of the American Society for Reproductive Medicine. Evaluation and treatment of recurrent pregnancy loss: a committee opinion. Fertil Steril. 2012;98(5):1103-11.
15. Murphy S, Cacciatore J. The psychological, social, and economic impact of stillbirth on families. Semin Fetal Neonatal Med. 2017;22(3):129-34.
16. Bender Atik R, Christiansen OB, Elson J, Kolte AM, Lewis S, Middeldorp S, et al. ESHRE guideline: recurrent pregnancy loss. Hum Reprod Open. 2018;2018(2):hoy004.
17. Man J, Hutchinson JC, Heazell AE, Ashworth M, Jeffrey I, Sebire NJ. Stillbirth and intrauterine fetal death: role of routine histopathological placental findings to determine cause of death. Ultrasound Obstet Gynecol. 2016;48(5):579-84.
18. Pacora P, Romero R, Jaiman S, Erez O, Bhatti G, Panaitescu B, et al. Mechanisms of death in structurally normal stillbirths. J Perinat Med. 2019;47(2):222-40.
19. Jaiman S, Romero R, Pacora P, Jung E, Bhatti G, Yeo L, et al. Disorders of placental villous maturation in fetal death. J Perinat Med. 2020. Online ahead of print.
20. Page JM, Christiansen-Lindquist L, Thorsten V, Parker CB, Reddy UM, Dudley DJ, et al. Diagnostic Tests for Evaluation of Stillbirth: Results From the Stillbirth Collaborative Research Network. Obstet Gynecol. 2017;129(4):699-706.
21. Committee on Genetics. ACOG Committee Opinion No. 383: Evaluation of stillbirths and neonatal deaths. Obstet Gynecol. 2007;110(4):963-6.
22. Pinar H, Koch MA, Hawkins H, Heim-Hall J, Shehata B, Thorsten VR, et al. The Stillbirth Collaborative Research Network (SCRN) placental and umbilical cord examination protocol. Am J Perinatol. 2011;28(10):781-92.
23. Flenady V, Wojcieszek AM, Middleton P, Ellwood D, Erwich JJ, Coory M, et al. Stillbirths: recall to action in high-income countries. Lancet. 2016;387(10019):691-702.
24. Freedman AA, Miller GE, Ernst LM. Chronic villitis: Refining the risk ratio of recurrence using a large placental pathology sample. Placenta. 2021;112:135-40.
25. Roeca C, Little SE, Carusi DA. Pathologically Diagnosed Placenta Accreta and Hemorrhagic Morbidity in a Subsequent Pregnancy. Obstet Gynecol. 2017;129(2):321-6.
26. Christians JK, Huicochea Munoz MF. Pregnancy complications recur independently of maternal vascular malperfusion lesions. PLoS One. 2020;15(2):e0228664.
27. Himes KP, Simhan HN. Risk of recurrent preterm birth and placental pathology. Obstet Gynecol. 2008;112(1):121-6.
28. Ananth CV, Cnattingius S. Influence of maternal smoking on placental abruption in successive pregnancies: a population-based prospective cohort study in Sweden. Am J Epidemiol. 2007;166(3):289-95.
29. Boyd TK, Redline RW. Chronic histiocytic intervillositis: a placental lesion associated with recurrent reproductive loss. Hum Pathol. 2000;31(11):1389-96.

30. Faye-Petersen OM, Ernst LM. Maternal Floor Infarction and Massive Perivillous Fibrin Deposition. Surg Pathol Clin. 2013;6(1):101-14.
31. Redline R, Bagby C, Ravishankar S. Multiple Chorangioma Syndrome. In: Khong TY ME, Nikkels PGJ, Morgan TK, Gordijn SJ (Eds). Pathology of the Placenta: A Practical Guide. Switzerland: Springer Nature; 2019. pp. 168-70.
32. Redline RW, Roberts DJ, Parast MM, Ernst LM, Morgan TK, Greene MF, et al. Placental pathology is necessary to understand common pregnancy complications and achieve an improved taxonomy of obstetrical disease. Am J Obstet Gynecol. 2023;228(2):187-202.
33. Boyd TK. Recurrent Pregnancy Loss. In: Redline RW, Boyd TK, Roberts DJ (Eds). Placental and Gestational Pathology. Diagnostic Pediatric Pathology. Cambridge: Cambridge University Press; 2017. pp. 327-30.
34. Żyła MM, Wilczyński J, Nowakowska-Głąb A, Maniecka-Bryła I, Nowakowska D. Pregnancy and Delivery in Women with Uterine Malformations. Adv Clin Exp Med. 2015;24(5):873-9.
35. Sneider K, Christiansen OB, Sundtoft IB, Langhoff-Roos J. Recurrence rates after abdominal and vaginal cerclages in women with cervical insufficiency: a validated cohort study. Arch Gynecol Obstet. 2017;295(4):859-66.
36. Sanchez-Delgado M, Martin-Trujillo A, Tayama C, Vidal E, Esteller M, Iglesias-Platas I, et al. Absence of Maternal Methylation in Biparental Hydatidiform Moles from Women with NLRP7 Maternal-Effect Mutations Reveals Widespread Placenta-Specific Imprinting. PLoS Genet. 2015;11(11):e1005644.
37. Nayar R, Lage JM. Placental changes in a first trimester missed abortion in maternal systemic lupus erythematosus with antiphospholipid syndrome; a case report and review of the literature. Hum Pathol. 1996;27(2):201-6.
38. Mekinian A, Alijotas-Reig J, Carrat F, Costedoat-Chalumeau N, Ruffatti A, Lazzaroni MG, et al. Refractory obstetrical antiphospholipid syndrome: Features, treatment and outcome in a European multicenter retrospective study. Autoimmun Rev. 2017;16(7):730-4.
39. Bos M, Nikkels PGJ, Cohen D, Schoones JW, Bloemenkamp KWM, Bruijn JA, et al. Towards standardized criteria for diagnosing chronic intervillositis of unknown etiology: A systematic review. Placenta. 2018;61:80-8.
40. Benachi A, Rabant M, Martinovic J, Bouchghoul H, Vivanti AJ, Leon J, et al. Chronic histiocytic intervillositis: manifestation of placental alloantibody-mediated rejection. Am J Obstet Gynecol. 2021;225(6):662.e1-e11.
41. Bendon RW, Coventry S, Thompson M, Rudzinski ER, Williams EM, Oron AP. Significance of C4d Immunostaining in Placental Chronic Intervillositis. Pediatr Dev Pathol. 2015;18(5): 362-8.
42. Labarrere CA, Hardin JW, Haas DM, Kassab GS. Chronic villitis of unknown etiology and massive chronic intervillositis have similar immune cell composition. Placenta. 2015;36(6):681-6.
43. Sato Y, Maekawa K, Aman M, Yamashita A, Kodama Y, Maki Y, et al. CD39 downregulation in chronic intervillositis of unknown etiology. Virchows Arch. 2019;475(3):357-64.
44. Cornish EF, McDonnell T, Williams DJ. Chronic Inflammatory Placental Disorders Associated With Recurrent Adverse Pregnancy Outcome. Front Immunol. 2022;13:825075.
45. Mekinian A, Costedoat-Chalumeau N, Masseau A, Botta A, Chudzinski A, Theulin A, et al. Chronic histiocytic intervillositis: outcome, associated diseases and treatment in a multicenter prospective study. Autoimmunity. 2015;48(1):40-5.
46. Russell P. Inflammatory lesions of the human placenta. III. The histopathology of villitis of unknown aetiology. Placenta. 1980;1(3):227-44.
47. Redline RW, Patterson P. Villitis of unknown etiology is associated with major infiltration of fetal tissue by maternal inflammatory cells. Am J Pathol. 1993;143(2):473-9.
48. Khong TY, Mooney EE, Ariel I, Balmus NC, Boyd TK, Brundler MA, et al. Sampling and Definitions of Placental Lesions: Amsterdam Placental Workshop Group Consensus Statement. Arch Pathol Lab Med. 2016;140(7):698-713.
49. Redline RW, Abramowsky CR. Clinical and pathologic aspects of recurrent placental villitis. Hum Pathol. 1985;16(7):727-31.
50. Tamblyn JA, Lissauer DM, Powell R, Cox P, Kilby MD. The immunological basis of villitis of unknown etiology—review. Placenta. 2013;34(10):846-55.
51. Boog G. Chronic villitis of unknown etiology. Eur J Obstet Gynecol Reprod Biol. 2008;136(1):9-15.
52. Katzman PJ, Genest DR. Maternal floor infarction and massive perivillous fibrin deposition: histological definitions, association with intrauterine fetal growth restriction, and risk of recurrence. Pediatr Dev Pathol. 2002;5(2):159-64.
53. Redline RW. Extending the Spectrum of Massive Perivillous Fibrin Deposition (Maternal Floor Infarction). Pediatr Dev Pathol. 2021;24(1):10-1.
54. Bane AL, Gillan JE. Massive perivillous fibrinoid causing recurrent placental failure. BJOG. 2003;110(3):292-5.
55. Andres RL, Kuyper W, Resnik R, Piacquadio KM, Benirschke K. The association of maternal floor infarction of the placenta with adverse perinatal outcome. Am J Obstet Gynecol. 1990;163(3):935-8.
56. Whitten AE, Romero R, Korzeniewski SJ, Tarca AL, Schwartz AG, Yeo L, et al. Evidence of an imbalance of angiogenic/antiangiogenic factors in massive perivillous fibrin deposition (maternal floor infarction): a placental lesion associated with recurrent miscarriage and fetal death. Am J Obstet Gynecol. 2013;208(4):310.e1-e11.
57. Baergen RN, Burton GJ, Kaplan CG. Benirschke's Pathology of the Human Placenta, 7th edition. Switzerland AG: Springer, Cham; 2022. p. XV, 939.

58. Khong TY, Mooney EE, Nikkels PGJ, Morgan TK, Gordijn SJ. Pathology of the placenta: a practical guide. Switzerland AG: Springer Cham; 2019. p. XVI, 395.
59. Redline RW, Boyd TK, Roberts DJ. Placental and Gestational Pathology. Cambridge: Cambridge University Press; 2018.
60. Smith GC, Yu CK, Papageorghiou AT, Cacho AM, Nicolaides KH. Maternal uterine artery Doppler flow velocimetry and the risk of stillbirth. Obstet Gynecol. 2007;109(1): 144-51.
61. Allen RE, Morlando M, Thilaganathan B, Zamora J, Khan KS, Thangaratinam S, et al. Predictive accuracy of second-trimester uterine artery Doppler indices for stillbirth: a systematic review and meta-analysis. Ultrasound Obstet Gynecol. 2016;47(1):22-7.
62. Reddy UM. Prediction and prevention of recurrent stillbirth. Obstet Gynecol. 2007;110(5):1151-64.
63. Moore LE. Recurrent risk of adverse pregnancy outcome. Obstet Gynecol Clin N Am. 2008; 35(3):459-71, ix.
64. Ticconi C, Pietropolli A, Specchia M, Nicastri E, Chiaramonte C, Piccione E, et al. Pregnancy-Related Complications in Women with Recurrent Pregnancy Loss: A Prospective Cohort Study. J Clin Med. 2020;9(9):2833.
65. Liu B, Song L, Zhang L, Wang L, Wu M, Xu S, et al. Higher Numbers of Pregnancies Associated With an Increased Prevalence of Gestational Diabetes Mellitus: Results From the Healthy Baby Cohort Study. J Epidemiol. 2020;30(5):208-12.
66. Lai YM, Tan GC, Shah SA, Abd Rahman R, Mohd Saleh MF, Mansor S, et al. Non-hypertensive gestational diabetes mellitus: Placental histomorphology and its association with perinatal outcomes. Placenta. 2024;147:21-7.
67. Redline RW, Ravishankar S. Fetal vascular malperfusion, an update. APMIS. 2018; 126(7):561-9.
68. Kraus FT. Fetal Thrombotic Vasculopathy: Perinatal Stroke, Growth Restriction, and Other Sequelae. Surg Pathol Clin. 2013;6(1):87-100.
69. Redline RW, Ariel I, Baergen RN, Desa DJ, Kraus FT, Roberts DJ, et al. Fetal vascular obstructive lesions: nosology and reproducibility of placental reaction patterns. Pediatr Dev Pathol. 2004;7(5):443-52.
70. Bakotic BW, Boyd T, Poppiti R, Pflueger S. Recurrent umbilical cord torsion leading to fetal death in 3 subsequent pregnancies: a case report and review of the literature. Arch Pathol Lab Med. 2000;124(9):1352-5.
71. Benirschke K. Recent trends in chorangiomas, especially those of multiple and recurrent chorangiomas. Pediatr Dev Pathol. 1999;2(3):264-9.
72. Guschmann M, Henrich W, Dudenhausen JW. Chorioangiomas—new insights into a well-known problem. II. An immuno-histochemical investigation of 136 cases. J Perinat Med. 2003;31(2):170-5.
73. Gallot D, Marceau G, Laurichesse-Delmas H, Vanlieferinghen P, Dechelotte PJ, Lemery D, et al. The changes in angiogenic gene expression in recurrent multiple chorioangiomas. Fetal Diag Ther. 2007;22(3):161-8.
74. Russell RT, Carlin A, Ashworth M, Welch CR. Diffuse placental chorioangiomatosis and fetal hydrops. Fetal Diag Ther. 2007;22(3):183-5.

CHAPTER 56

Grief Counseling

Kamini A Rao, Vyshnavi A Rao

ABSTRACT

Recurrent pregnancy loss leaves a deep psychological impact on the couples mental health. The loss of a pregnancy results in grief, guilt, anxiety, as well as post traumatic stress disorder. Creating awareness of these feelings and couple counseling will enable her to cope with these issues. This chapter deals with types of counseling required by couples and to identify the personnel in the care givers team who can provide these services.

Keywords: Pregnancy loss, Mental health, Counseling, Stress.

INTRODUCTION

Counseling is defined as a confidential interaction between a health professional and a client aimed at enabling the client to cope with stressful situations and take personal decisions related to problem areas. Recurrent pregnancy loss (RPL) poses a mental health challenge to a couple, be it a biochemical pregnancy, early first trimester loss or late second trimester loss. Early losses are often not perceived in this light by a busy obstetrician. This chapter will elaborate on the need for one on one counseling by the obstetric team and its benefits for the affected couple.

TYPES OF COUNSELING

The aim of counseling is to explore, understand, and resolve issues arising from RPL and its treatment and to clarify ways of dealing with the problem more effectively. In counseling, one should focus on the patient's emotional and psychosocial needs by:

- Understanding the situation of childlessness
- Implications of counseling
- Support counseling
- Therapeutic counseling.

A distinction is made in those aspects of care that are considered part of good clinical practice such as providing information, discussing options, and assessing implications, versus the more specialized psychological techniques for helping distressed people.

Grief Counseling

Grief counseling is a type of psychotherapy that is done to help people cope with physical, emotional, social, spiritual, and cognitive responses to loss of a particular person or a thing. It is a form of therapy needed when there is a loss of a loved one, or any kind of significant life-altering loss or losing a pregnancy.[1]

Grief counselors play a pivotal role in counseling. People have different ways of experiencing and expressing grief, which largely depends on family background, cultural values, intrinsic values, and types of personalities.[2]

Theories of Grief Counseling

Joanne Jozefowski in the year 1999 through "The Phoenix Phenomenon: Rising from the Ashes of Grief" summarizes five stages to rebuild a shattered life:

1. *Impact:* Shock, denial, anxiety, fear, and panic
2. *Chaos:* Confusion, disbelief, actions out of control, irrational thoughts and feelings, and agony from imagining their physical harm, and shattered beliefs
3. *Adapting:* Bringing order back into daily life while one continues to grieve—take care of basic needs (personal grooming, shopping, cooking, cleaning, and paying bills), learning to live without the loved one, accepting help, focusing on helping children cope, connecting with other grieving families for mutual support, taking control of grieving so that grief does not control oneself, slowly accepting the new reality.

4. *Equilibrium:* Attaining stability and routines—reestablishing a life that works alright, enjoying pleasant activities with family members and good times with friends, doing productive work, choosing a positive new direction in life while honoring the past, learning how to handle people who ask questions about what they have been through.
5. *Transformation:* Rethinking the purpose in life and the basis for identity; looking for meaning in tragic, senseless loss; allowing oneself to have both painful and positive feelings about the loss and choosing which feelings to focus on; allowing oneself to discover that the struggle has led them to develop a stronger, better version of oneself than expected; learning how to talk with others about heroic healing journey without exposing them to the pain; becoming supportive of others trying to deal with their losses.

There are number of losses experienced during the process of reproductive life:

- Loss of control of one's body
- Loss of a pregnancy during miscarriage
- Loss of ability to conceive a baby naturally
- Loss of identity within society
- Loss of experience of pregnancy, sexual identity, and confidence.

The losses are multiple, and one may move in and out of this grief model multiple times. Hence, the treatment process for infertility/pregnancy loss is described as a roller coaster.

Deep sadness, depressed mood, irritability, worry, anxiety, and changes in eating and sleeping patterns are considered part of a normal grief response.[3]

Although grief is a natural, nonpathological phenomenon, it can lead to complicated grief reactions, where symptoms are disruptive, long lasting than those of normal grief.[4] Complicated grief is a chronic impairing form of grief resulting from interference with the healing process.[5] This evokes exacerbated reactions whose symptoms affect the quality of life and can lead to substance abuse and increased risk of suicide.[6-11]

Grief Counseling in Pregnancy Loss

Repeated pregnancy losses are devastating experiences that can disrupt a couple's view of themselves and their future life together. Each reproductive cycle activates feelings of hope, helplessness, and uncertainty. The physical, psychological, and financial stress of repeated in vitro fertilization (IVF) attempts or repeated miscarriages can place some couples at risk of relationship breakdown. The loss of such a pregnancy may not be discussed or made known to others, and the couple may grieve alone and isolate themselves to avoid feelings of shame. They may try to manage the grief associated with their loss by embarking quickly on another pregnancy attempt without recognizing the difficulties in their relationships or related to their repeated experience of loss.

For parents making exciting and hopeful plans for the baby's future, a death incident occurring during pregnancy makes them lose their hopes and dreams. The death of a baby is one of the most painful experiences of patients and is difficult problem to handle.[12]

Patient-focused care is important in the treatment of patients in the immediate period after traumatic loss such as RPL stillbirth or neonatal death.

Health professionals medicalize the prenatal loss period from a medical perspective. They should understand the emotional status of the woman experiencing loss, provide appropriate support, and communicate empathetically. Therefore, training should be provided to improve their empathetic skills and abilities to provide appropriate and effective care services after a pregnancy loss.

Women experiencing loss require support of healthcare professionals and also support from social and religious-based institutions. So, perinatal mourning programs should be employed by educational institutions.

Male Partner Counseling

For both mother and father, pregnancy losses are considered to be significant emotional issues. The feeling of loss is real for both partners.[12] While much of the discussion on pregnancy loss is found around women, men also experience it. Father who experiences miscarriages realizes that there will not be a child to watch grow up, and their dreams of children are just as real and meaningful.

The typical male attitude in the events of crisis is to fix things. As miscarriage cannot be fixed, and it is the time that will heal the scar of the loss of embryonic life. In that sense, the father will feel powerless and hopeless to address his own feelings. But fathers may try to fix it by talking about other pregnancies, and the mother needs only a listening ear, sympathy, and reassurance of your love for her.

Many researchers suggest that up to 30% pregnancy losses are associated with significant emotional reaction. Of the 30%, 10% of women may display signs such as depression, anxiety, and post-traumatic stress disorder (PTSD).

DISPOSAL OF PRODUCTS OF CONCEPTION

Women's focus when undergoing miscarriages is on the state of being pregnant rather than disposal of the fetal tissue. The fetal tissue is different from other waste because of it being sensitive tissue and should be handled with care and dignity. It has to be separated from clinical waste. The method of disposal by incineration was generally acceptable to most women in comparison to ceremonial methods, which are considered inappropriate by most women.[13,14]

Women may experience curiosity after miscarriage as to what happened to the fetal tissue. So, availability of information on disposal was thought to be important but it should be a woman's choice whether and to what degree they can access it.

Studies have explored women's opinion regarding donation of fetal tissue for research purposes but found that women wanted reassurance that the fetus no longer existed in any material form.[15]

COUNSELING IN INFERTILITY

The continuum of patient-centered care, counseling, and psychotherapy in relation to infertility in patients with RPL is outlined in **Table 1**.

QUALIFICATIONS NEEDED TO OFFER COUNSELING

According to the American Society for Reproductive Medicine (ASRM), the counselor should have the following qualifications:

- Graduate degree in mental health profession (psychology, social work)
- A license to practice (registration/certification/chartered status)
- Training in medical and psychological aspects of infertility
- Minimum of 1 year for clinical experience
- Regular attendance at certified education programs.

Any patient can benefit from professional counseling, and all patients should be given the opportunity to avail the help they need. The following groups of people are identified as the ones needing or benefiting from counseling:

- Patients who use donated gametes, surrogacy or adoption to achieve parenthood.
- Patients who experience distress in the form of depression or anxiety or any other negative affective reaction. About 15–20% of patients taking infertility treatment are expected to experience this level of distress.

TABLE 1: Counseling in infertility.

Domain in the continuum	*Types of counseling*	*Focus areas*	*Delivered by*
Patient-centered care	• Information gathering and assessment • Implication and decision making	• Evaluation of medical and biological factors associated with infertility and eligibility for ART • Discussing the implications of infertility, options for treatment, and helping people in making decisions regarding their treatments	Medical and nursing staff of fertility clinic
Infertility counseling	• Supportive counseling • Crisis counseling	• Providing emotional support to patients in distress • Short-term support in crisis (e.g., acute grief) • Long-term support for people with multiple or long-term problems	Trained clinic counselor (medical or nursing staff or mental health professional such as a counselor, psychologist, and psychiatric social worker)
Psychotherapy	Therapeutic counseling	• Specific psychotherapeutic techniques such as problem solving, interpersonal therapy, and cognitive behavior therapy for longstanding problems	Qualified mental health professional (counselor, psychologist, psychotherapist, and psychiatrist)

(ART: assisted reproductive technology)

- Patients considered to be at risk because of their psychological history.
- Patients who require some form of genetic counseling as part of their fertility treatment (preimplantation genetic diagnosis).
- Patients with acute grief reactions following pregnancy loss and perinatal loss.
- Elderly primigravida, who may perceive RPL post ART to shatter their dreams of being a biological mother.

CONCLUSION

The negative psychosocial manifestations of response to grief are depression, despair or loss of hope, guilt, anger, anxiety, frustration, anguish, shock, suicidal thinking, and isolation. The most frequently reported positive manifestations are the hope of becoming pregnant and acceptance of infertility after attempting infertility treatment. Therefore, psychological support before, during, and after treatment is crucial for managing psychosocial aspects of responses to grief in infertile couples and patients with pregnancy loss, as women who seek alternatives to becoming pregnant strive for a future pregnancy as a resolution of their grief. Despite advances in assisted reproductive technologies (ARTs), the prenatal period still carries many mysteries. Counseling can help raise awareness of the area of grief among women with RPL and infertility and promote policy development for physical and mental health.

REFERENCES

1. Kneip R. Psychology of grief. GLPG.
2. Hoy WG. Bereavement Groups and the Role of Social Support: Integrating Theory, Research, and Practice, 1st edition. New York: Routledge/Taylor and Francis; 2016.
3. Koopmans L, Wilson T, Cacciatore J, Flendy V. Support for mothers, fathers and families after perinatal death. Cochrane Database Syst Rev. 2013;2013(6):CD000452.
4. Kersting A, Wagner B. Complicated grief after perinatal loss. Dialogues Clin Neurosci. 2012;14(2):187-94.
5. Shear MK. Grief and mourning gone awry: pathway and course of complicated grief. Dialogues Clin Neurosci. 2012;14(2):119-28.
6. American Psychiatric Association. (2022). Diagnostic and statistical manual of mental disorders (5th ed., text rev.). https://doi.org/10.1176/appi.books.9780890425787
7. Barreto P, de la Torre O, Pérez-Marín M. Detección de duelo complicado. Psicooncología. 2012;9(2-3):355.
8. Toedter LJ, Lasker JN, Janssen HJ. International comparison of studies using the perinatal grief scale: a decade of research on pregnancy loss. Death Stud. 2001;25(3):205-28.
9. Badenhorst W, Riches S, Turton P, Hughes P. The psychological effects of stillbirth and neonatal death on fathers: systematic review. J Psychosom Obstet Gynaecol. 2006;27(4):245-56.
10. Burden C, Bradley S, Storey C, Ellis A, Heazell AEP, Downe S, et al. From grief, guilt pain and stigma to hope and pride – a systematic review and meta-analysis of mixed-method research of the psychosocial impact of stillbirth. BMC Pregnancy Childbirth. 2016;16:9.
11. Obst KL, Due C, Oxlad M, Middleton P. Men's grief following pregnancy loss and neonatal loss: a systematic review and emerging theoretical model. BMC Pregnancy Childbirth. 2020;20(1):11.
12. Meaney S, Corcoran P, Spillane N, O'Donoghue K. Experience of miscarriage: an interpretative phenomenological analysis. BMJ Open. 2017;7(3):e011382.
13. Royal College of Nursing (RCN). Managing the Disposal of Pregnancy Remains: RCN Guidance for Nursing and Midwifery Practices. London: RCN; 2007.
14. The Institute of Cemetery and Crematorium Management (ICCM). The Sensitive Disposal of Fetal Remains: Policy and Guidance for Burial and Cremation Authorities and Companies. 2015. [online] Available from www.iccm-uk.com/iccm/wp-content/library/iccm_Fetal%20Remains%20Policy%20Updated%20Sept2015%20.pdf [Last accessed December, 2024].
15. Pfeffer N. What British women say matters to them about donating an aborted fetus to stem cell research: a focus group study. Soc Sci Med. 2008;66(12):2544-54.

CHAPTER 57

Medicolegal Implications

Usha Ahluwalia, Mala Arora

ABSTRACT

Women are likely to sue when unexpected and unwelcome events happen. Recurrent pregnancy loss (RPL) is one such event and medicolegal implications may ensue for not diligently identifying the cause of this mishap and also from ensuing complications like hemorrhage, retained products of conception, chronic endometritis or a uterine perforation, that may jeopardize her chances of a future pregnancy. If a medico legal case is filed, the court needs to prove medical negligence on the part of the practitioner. Hence, it is the duty of the gynecologists to maintain adequate records and to prove that no medical negligence was involved in any ensuing complication.

Keywords: RPL, Retained products of conception, Uterine perforation, Hemorrahge, Cervical incompetence, Chronic endometritis, Medical negligence, Vicarious liability.

INTRODUCTION

Like any other healthcare professional, gynecologists too have a legal obligation to adhere to a reasonable standard of care while acting in their professional capacity (the "duty of care"). A breach of this duty, whether due to an individual's actions such as poor clinical skill/inappropriate decision-making or administrative causes such as inadequate safety culture in the organization, could lead to litigation.

Women are likely to sue when unexpected and unwelcome events happen!

Complications that are most likely to lead to litigation while managing recurrent miscarriage cases may be:

- Early physical complications:
  - Hemorrhage
  - Retained products
  - Perforation/trauma
- Late complications:
  - Infertility
  - Cervical incompetence
  - Psychological trauma

These are less likely to lead to litigation because it may be hard to lay blame on the miscarriage, and the law may regard these complications as not being reasonably foreseeable.

Litigation arises because of inadequate counseling or insufficient explanation when complications do occur. Many complications involving litigation are nonspecific to actual process of having gone through miscarriage or an operative procedure itself, for example:

- Issue concerning consent
- Anesthetic mishap
- Retained swab
- Drug errors
- Equipment failure

First-trimester complications (incidence 0.3–0.5%) that may cause litigation include:

- Hemorrhage requiring transfusion
- Uterine perforation that may require laparotomy
- Infection
- Cervical injury
- Retained products

Second-trimester complications (incidence 4.1%) may be:

- Hemorrhage
- Pelvic infection
- Cervical injury

Failure to diagnose ectopic pregnancy has such serious consequences for the patient that a legal suite seems likely to follow, though presently with very sensitive beta human chorionic gonadotropin (hCG) assay and transvaginal scanning, it is highly unlikely that ectopic pregnancy may be missed. However, if any doubt, products of conception/

uterine contents must be sent for histological confirmation for presence of chorionic villi.

There may be heterotopic pregnancy—intrauterine and ectopic pregnancy being present simultaneously (incidence 1:5,000), in which case, missing an ectopic pregnancy will not amount to negligence. However, if any pelvic mass is suspected, an appropriate outpatient follow-up must be arranged.

Hemorrhage is usually associated with retained products or, more rarely, with damage such as cervical or uterine injury. Incidence of major hemorrhage (i.e., >500 mL) is approximately 2–2.5%. Patients are unlikely to sue for damage unless it is associated with retained products.

Retained products with or without infection and hemorrhage are the most common cause of legal problems. Much of the litigation deals with this problem even though actual number of patients who actually sue is quite small. Many of the complaints concern not so much the occurrence of a complication but incorrect or delayed management by the hospital staff and general practitioners. Re-evacuation is required in approximately 1.5–4.0%.

Various techniques that help us to ensure complete evacuation include:

- Use of oxytocic
- Performing evacuation under ultrasound guidance
- Evacuation under hysteroscopic guidance is also beneficial for collecting the embryo for genetic testing.
- Performing hysteroscopy postevacuation will identify retained products of conception and guide to their location.

If retained products are suspected, the patient should be kept in the hospital for observations and rescan as soon as possible to confirm/exclude retained products.

When the patient has returned to the hospital with retained products, she should be given antibiotics and repeat evacuation must be carried out by an experienced/senior doctor. It is prudent to inform the patient during and after the event about the inevitability of occasional complications, as a frank sympathetic discussion will often avoid litigation.

TRAUMA AND PERFORATION

- Cervical trauma
- Uterine perforation

Cervical Trauma

Cervical trauma may have:

- An immediate effect such as bleeding
- Long-term effect such as cervical incompetence

Immediate cervical trauma, usually in the form of tearing of the cervix, is produced by the vulsellum, whereas the latter is produced by forcible dilatation of the internal orifice of the uterus (os). The overall incidence is 1%. Such risks may be minimized by preoperative use of prostaglandins, such as misoprostol priming.

Cervical incompetence is a late complication and is a rare cause for litigation per se as it is very difficult to prove. Any litigation for this is therefore likely to flounder.

Uterine Perforation

Uterine perforation is dangerous and probably happens more often than is realized or even admitted. The introduction of instruments into the abdominal cavity, especially suction cannula, can lead to major hemorrhage, bowel injury, infection, and infertility, although perforation does not seem to significantly weaken the uterine wall in a subsequent pregnancy. Bowel injury is particularly likely to lead to litigation [*Bovenzi vs. Kettering Health Authority* (1991)]. A laparoscopy is mandatory if bowel injury is suspected during the course of evacuation.

The incidence of uterine perforation is 1%, mandating laparotomy in 0.1% of cases. When a small perforation (such as with sound or small dilator) is suspected and thought to have just happened, the patient is kept in the hospital for observation and put on antibiotics to avoid any subsequent infection. In case of a larger perforation with curette or suction cannula or where there is doubt about when and how it occurred, a laparoscopy must be performed to assess the extent of damage.

On laparoscopy, we should look for:

- Intra-abdominal bleeding
- Suspected bowel injury, which will warrant an immediate laparotomy

In the present litigious climate, it is wise to tell the patient even if there has been only a small perforation needing no further treatment. Unfortunately, words such as perforation or damage to the internal organs will suggest to the patient that something was done incorrectly even though there may not have been any negligence in law. When bowel injury occurs, the gynecologist should realize and anticipate the probability that this problem may reach the lawyers. It is therefore both prudent and in the patient's best interest to call an experienced general surgeon for help.

Swabs and Packs

Small swabs and/or packs are sometimes left in the vagina in an attempt to control excessive bleeding from cervical trauma or uterine atony. A swab inadvertently left in the vagina may lead to a serious infection, which further potentiates the legal consequences.

The surgeon is responsible for swabs and packs, which may get left behind in the body cavities. The nurse, if one scrubbed, is an assistant only and therefore not responsible. Medical staff must always:

- Do a loud swab count before and after the procedure
- Check the vagina after the procedure for any swab/ pack left behind.

There is usually no defense against a proven swab left inside the vagina or abdomen by a surgeon—*Dryden vs. Surrey County Council* (1936) and *Gardener vs. Morrell* (1963).

Rhesus Immunization

Rhesus immunization is another occurrence likely to lead to litigation. Anti-D immunoglobulin should always be given to rhesus negative women undergoing evacuation following miscarriage. The risk of sensitization is about:

- 2% at 8 weeks
- 9% at 12 weeks

Failure to give immunoglobulin is likely to lead to successful legal action even if the patient is not actually sensitized because of the worry and mental tension caused by the doctor's negligence. While the standard dose is 250 IU, it is probably wise to assess the amount of fetomaternal transfusion and decide the dose in the following cases:

- Mid-trimester miscarriage
- Major hemorrhage

Infection

Infection is usually associated with retained products and occasionally with other complications such as cervical trauma or uterine perforation. Routine use of antibiotics, therefore, is not advocated but they should certainly be used if complications likely to lead to infection occur. Acute infection may further increase the chances of:

- Chronic infections
- Ectopic pregnancy
- Infertility

While infection is unlikely to lead to litigation, secondary infertility may lead the patient to take action if she thinks postevacuation infection was incorrectly or inadequately treated.

Other possible causes of legal action by the patient following any miscarriage or related surgical procedure may be:

- Psychological problems
- Pelvic pain/discomfort

In any claim of negligence, once the facts are gathered, it is then necessary to seek an expert opinion as to the defensibility of the claim. Under English civil law, the claimant has only to prove her case on the "balance of probabilities" (unlike criminal cases where confirmation of negligence has to be "beyond reasonable doubt").

If a patient suffers damage as a result of medical practice, the civil action, which usually applies, is the action for negligence. Occasionally, there may be a possibility of an action for breach of contract, especially in a private set-up rather than in National Health Service (NHS) setting. If the action is taken for medical negligence, as is more likely, the claimant must satisfy three separate criteria:

1. That the defendant owed her a duty of care
2. That there was a breach of that duty
3. That the breach of duty caused the alleged damage, which must not be too "remote" in legal terms

Finally, if the claim succeeds, the amount of compensation to be awarded must be quantified (quantum of damage).

Negligence is the breach of legal duty of care owed by a defendant to a claimant, which results in damage caused by the defendant to the claimant. That such a legal duty of care is owed by a medical practitioner has long been recognized and established in common law *Pippin vs. Sheppard* (1822) and *Edgar vs. Lamont* (1914). This duty of care attaches to all those who hold themselves out as skilled in medical, nursing, and paramedical matters and arises independently of any contractual relationship. A litigant may therefore sue concurrently in contract and tort. The duty of care is imposed even when a practitioner acts gratuitously in voluntary capacity—*Goode vs. Nash* (1979).

Negligence is no more than a failure to come up to the standard of care, which is needed to be expected from colleagues with similar training skills and experience. A doctor is not negligent if they act in accordance with a practice accepted, at the time, properly by a responsible body of medical opinion, skilled in particular form of treatment; even though there is a body that might adopt a different technique. There are numerous authoritative cases in which the standard of professional judgment within medical profession has been ruled to be the criterion by which the conduct of doctors is to be judged—as in *Bolam vs. Friern Hospital Management Committee* (1957) 2 ALL ER 118 and reiterated in *Sidaway vs. Bethlem Royal Hospital* [1985] 1 ALL ER 643. The law imposes duty of care, but the standard of care is a matter of medical judgments. In *Bolitho vs. City* and Hackney Health Authority, the defending doctor was acquitted both at the original trial, in the Court of Appeal, and finally in the House of Lords. In his opinion, Lord Browne-Wilkinson accepted the principle that a judge would have to consider whether a body of medical opinion was logical, but decided that the opinion used by the defense in Bolitho was indeed logical.

Lord Scarman explained in *Maynard vs. West Midlands Area Health Authority* (1985) 1 All ER 635 "differences of opinion and practice exist, and will always exist, in the medical and the other professions. There is seldom one answer, exclusive of all others, to problems of professional judgment. A court may prefer one body of opinion to the other, but that is no basis for a conclusion of negligence."

The obstetrician can be held negligent only if the standards exhibited by him/her fall below the standards laid down by the peers/textbooks. This, in the eyes of law, can never be construed as negligence but is a pure "*misadventure*" that is not actionable, and hence no compensation becomes due and payable.

The *Supreme Court in Kusum Sharma & Others vs. Batra Hospital & Medical Research Centre & Others* holds:

- Medical science has conferred great benefits on mankind, but these benefits are attended by considerable risks. Every surgical operation is attended by risks. We cannot take the benefits without taking risks. Every advancement in technique is also attended by risks.
- In *Roe and Woolley vs. Minister of Health* (1954) 2 QB 66, Lord Justice Denning said: "It is so easy to be wise after the event and to condemn as negligence that which was only a misadventure. We ought to be on our guard against it, especially in cases against hospitals and doctors. Medical science has conferred great benefits on mankind but these benefits are attended by unavoidable risks. Every surgical operation is attended by risks. We cannot take the benefits without taking the risks. Every advance in technique is also attended by risks. Doctors, like the rest of us, have to learn by experience; and experience often teaches in a hard way." It was also observed in the same case that "We must not look at the 1947 accident with 1954 spectacles."

Occasionally, an expert opinion is not necessary because things are so obvious that it speaks for itself—res ipsa loquitur. The classic example is retained swabs or wrong patient operated—such cases are simply not defensible because care provided failed to reach the required standard and is unlikely that the matter will proceed to trial.

At last, the claimant must prove that he has suffered damage, which was caused by the defendant's negligence. If no damage is proved, there is no cause for action. Cases appearing to indicate gross failures on the part of practitioners, such as failing to attend a patient despite requests can often fail at this hurdle—*Barnett vs. Kensington Hospital Management Committee* (1969). In consent cases, the patient also has to establish that if the warning of the risk had been made clear, they would not have agreed to the treatment or operation.

EXPERT OPINIONS

While defending a case in the courts for alleged medical malpractice, it is not only wise but also prudent to base one's defense on expert opinions. Courts give a lot of credence to such expert opinions.

The *Supreme Court in Martin F. D'souza vs. Mohd. Ishfaq* holds:

- "The courts and Consumer Fora are not experts in medical science, and must not substitute their own views over that of specialists."
- *Guarantee and warranty with respect to the end results of treatment in cases of Recurrent Pregnancy Losses.* Law does not require any professional (this includes the lawyers as well) to give guarantee or warranty with respect to the end results of the services rendered by them. What law requires is that the services rendered must not be sub-standard or below par and the services rendered must be without any shortcomings.

The *Supreme Court in Jacob Mathew vs. State of Punjab & Anr.* holds:

- "He does not assure his client of the result. A lawyer does not tell his client that the client shall win the case in all circumstances. A physician would not assure the patient of full recovery in every case. A surgeon cannot and does not guarantee that the result of surgery would invariably be beneficial, much less to the extent of 100% for the person operated on. The only assurance which such a professional can give or can be understood to have given by implication is that he is possessed of the requisite skill in that branch of profession which he is practicing and while undertaking the performance of the task entrusted to him, he would be exercising his skill with reasonable competence. This is all what the person approaching the professional can expect."

WHEN THINGS GO WRONG, WHAT MAY I TELL THE PATIENT?

Surgeons have an obligation to inform patients of the benefits and potential harms of surgical treatment prior to undergoing a procedure. Although surgeons strive in daily practice to avoid harm (primum non nocere), adverse events and unfortunate outcomes occur. As complications arise, surgeons should strive to be transparent with patients about matters related to their care, in a manner that avoids confusion and self-incrimination. A natural tension exists between the surgeon's honest goals of explaining how errors may have occurred and empathizing with the patient and their families while avoiding legal hazards.

Surgeons have a duty to communicate complications that result from surgical procedures, but this puts them in a state of dilemma. On the one hand, he/she is encouraged to disclose adverse outcomes, and his/her human instinct is to empathize with the patient and their families, and on the other hand, they are warned that apologies and disclosures can be seen as inviting lawsuits and lessening the ability to defend oneself if sued. Silence and secrecy are increasingly considered ethically and legally unacceptable responses to medical injury.

Do not withhold the *"facts"* about the case from the patient but also do not discuss the *legal liability*, e.g., by commenting about or speculating on the known facts. Modern medical practice often involves team work and all the facts must be carefully established by proper inquiry from each member of the team (both medical and nonmedical) before speculating or admitting any legal liabilities to the patient.

In *Davis vs. Wooster Orthopaedics & Sports Medicine*, the court held, in a wrongful death action, that the surgeon's statements to the family directly after a surgical procedure resulting in the death of the patient were admissible as an admission of fault.

In *Strout vs. Central Maine Medical Center*, the court found that a statement in an otherwise redacted letter was admissible as evidence in a subsequent lawsuit filed by the patient for emotional distress. The letter was from the medical center to the patient in response to the patient's grievance regarding the surgeon's preemptive disclosure of a cancer diagnosis to the patient prior to the receipt of biopsy results.

WHAT DO THE DEFENSE ORGANIZATIONS/ INSURANCE AGENCIES THINK?

Despite the best efforts on part of the clinicians, accidents do still occur. The manner in which these are handled will usually determine whether they will result in litigation. The NHS Litigation Authority encourages the medical staff to render apology. Frequently, though not always, an explanation or an apology from the team will stave off the claim.

The essence of negligence is that the standard is one, which is set by the clinicians, rather than the lawyers. Although, the lawyers set the principles but it is the privilege of clinicians to define what comes up to the standard of a reasonable, responsible doctor at any given time. If the distinguished support is forthcoming to establish that the required standard has been maintained, the protection societies will be able to mount a defense to the claim.

National professional bodies, such as the Royal College (UK) or Federation of Obstetric and Gynaecological Societies of India (FOGSI), have clearly the most useful and important role to play in helping to delineate the boundaries of currently acceptable standards of clinical care.

PREVENTIVE MEASURES

Claims are like cancer, better prevented than cured!

It is impossible to emphasize too strongly the importance of good communications and the need for those human qualities of kindness, sympathy, tolerance, and understanding in dealing with patients. Communication is necessary for the busy practitioner to be seen to have time to listen and give the impression that the patient whom she/he is currently dealing with is of all-consuming interest and importance.

Communication also involves keeping up-to-date with current trends, research, and technological developments in the specialty and the need to be aware of the unwanted effects and interactions of highly potent therapeutic substances and adverse effects of medical interventions, which are part of the modern armamentarium of the clinicians.

There is also a need for communication with colleagues, junior staff, and the nursing staff so that there is clearest possible understanding as to how the individual cases are to be managed.

Strategies for preventing retained surgical items are directed at patient care processes and the work environment in the operating room. Unfortunately, no prevention strategy is entirely foolproof. Sponges should be separated, audibly counted, and concurrently viewed during the count procedure by two individuals, typically the scrub nurse and circulating nurse. If a discrepancy in any of the counts is identified, the entire surgical team is responsible for carrying out appropriate steps to locate the missing item.

The maintenance of an "optimal operation room/operation theater environment" should "allow focused performance of operative tasks" [American College of Surgeons (ACS)]. Distractions including interruptions, noise, conversation, and traffic in the operating room should be limited. When personnel changes occur during a procedure, complete and accurate transmission of relevant information about the surgical field and its contents needs to be conveyed. Focused time for these tasks, particularly the surgical count, should reduce errors.

Finally, one cannot overstress the importance of *good clinical contemporaneous records* and one has to remember that it is the consultant's responsibility to ensure that adequate notes are made in respect of those patients for whom she/he is ultimately responsible. Complaints and claims may not develop for years and only the documentation made at that time will prove to be the practitioner's best help against litigation. However, notes must be able to bear scrutiny in a court of law, and it is wise to make entries in case notes without sarcasm, wit, or subjective comment as one day the same wit may not seem quite so amusing when read in court.

CLINICAL MANAGEMENT

Among the main aims of managing patients with recurrent miscarriage is responding to the anxiety of the women (and her partner). *Uncertainty is the most important cause of anxiety and every effort must be made to determine her exact condition and as quickly as possible.* Anxiety is a state of mind which, in contrast to grief, serves little purpose. For that reason, every woman complaining of blood loss in first or second trimester should be seen on emergency basis, and proper diagnosis made without more delay than is reasonably necessary.

Several circumstances are perhaps not direct causes of recurrent miscarriage but increase the statistical risk of miscarriage, e.g., smoking, substance misuse, and certain occupational hazards. Obviously, in advising patients with recurrent miscarriage during prepregnancy counseling, one should try to make the circumstances for further pregnancy as favorable as possible. If a cause is not found, treatment is not always possible! When nothing positive has been discovered, the doctor should not resort to "empirical treatment options" but try to win the couple with a realistic view of the facts as they are known.

CONSENT FOR TREATMENT

Ethically, the requirement for patients to consent for treatment indicates respect for their autonomy. Consent has two purposes:

1. *Clinical:* It stems from the fact that in many instances the cooperation of the patient and the patient's faith or at least the confidence to the efficiency of the treatment is a major factor contributing to the treatment's success.

   Failure to obtain consent not only deprives the patient and the medical staff of the advantage but also will make it much more difficult to administer treatment.
2. *Legal:* The legal purpose is to provide those concerned with the treatment with a defense to a criminal charge of assault/battery or a civil claim for damages for trespass to the person. However, it does not provide them with a defense to negligently carried out treatment.

One of the two distinct actions is possible if consent is absent, and on the same occasion, both of these may be pleaded.

Only a competent adult is capable of giving a valid consent. An incompetent adult or a minor cannot give a valid consent as they have no legal capacity to do so. Failure to provide the amount of information, required by law for a valid consent, amounts to negligence. *Wells vs. Surrey Area Health Authority*, The Times, July 29, 1978, provides an illustration of operation of trespass to the person and negligence in relation to consent to treatment, where a woman gave consent for sterilization along with cesarean section, which was undertaken after long and difficult labor. She claimed that being Roman Catholic, she would have never consented to tubal ligation, and her consent was not held valid because she was in a weak and confused condition when she signed the form.

Negligence

In *Hatcher vs. Black*, Lord Denning explained the law on the subject of negligence against doctors and hospitals in the following words:

- Before I consider the individual facts, I ought to explain to you the law on this matter of negligence against doctors and hospitals. Mr. Marvan Evertt sought to liken the case against a hospital to a motor car accident or to an accident in a factory. That is the wrong approach. In the case of accident on the road, there ought not to be any accident if everyone used proper care; and the same applies in a factory; but in a hospital when a person who is ill goes in for treatment, there is always some risk, no matter what care is used. Every surgical operation involves risks. It would be wrong, and indeed bad law, to say that simply because a misadventure or mishap occurred, the hospital and the doctors are thereby liable. It would be disastrous to the community if it were so. It would mean that a doctor examining a patient or a surgeon operating at a table instead of getting on with his work, would be forever looking over shoulder to see if someone was coming up with a dagger; for an action for negligence against a doctor is for him like unto a dagger. His professional reputation is as dear to him as his body, perhaps more so, and an action for negligence can wound his reputation as severely as a dagger can his body. You must not, therefore, find him negligent simply because something happens to go wrong; if for instance, one of the risk inherent in an operation actually takes place or some complication ensues which lessens or takes away the benefits that were hoped for, or if in a matter of opinion he makes an error of judgment. You should only find him guilty of negligence when he falls short of the standard of a reasonably skilful medical man, in short, when he is deserving of censure for negligence a medical man is deserving of censure."

Vicarious Liability

Vicarious liability arises when the law holds one person or institution responsible for the tortuous actions of another, even though there is no misconduct or blame on that person or institution—employer being held liable for the negligence of an employee. A practitioner is obviously responsible in law for his own actions and will be liable personally if found to have caused damage by his negligence.

In suing the employer who is responsible for the acts of all the team, the patient can establish the negligence more easily rather than at an individual level.

Doctors need to be insured by Medical Defense Union (MDU) or Medical Protection Society (MPS) or another private insurance agency, but many paramedical practitioners and most nurses are not required to be insured. In United Kingdom, the current provision of so-called "Crown indemnity" (Clinical Negligence Scheme for Trusts), which came into force in respect of claims lodged on or after January 1, 1990, require health authorities to assume responsibility for medical negligence action arising out of acts of their employees including all staff—*R vs. North West Thames Regional Health Authority*, ex parte Daniels (1993). The argument that hospital authority has a personal nondelegable duty of care coupled with the doctrine of vicarious liability has been instrumental in establishing the main action in medical malpractice in an action of negligence. NHS litigation authority that deals with all litigation cases is now called "NHS Resolution".

CONCLUSION

What can clinicians do to avoid litigation associated with miscarriages/related surgical procedures?

- *Counseling:* The woman should be told about potential problems and possible prognosis including the possibility of probable operative procedures.
- Adequate explanation of complications of all the procedures she is about to undergo must be given prior to embarking upon them.
- Any complications encountered must be managed correctly and swiftly. Junior staff must call for timely senior help. *Ignorance* in *law* does not excuse.
- If the guidance in the judgment of Sideway case is applied, complications expected in excess of 1% have to be discussed with the patient.
- Junior staff should be adequately trained to perform the procedure before they are left without supervision.
- Any procedure, if required, should always be performed in centers, which has adequate equipment and sufficient staff. If the anesthetists, junior staff, or

consultants cannot cope with the workload, they should not be doing it—as being "too busy"/"overworked" is not an excuse in a court of law. Similarly, if the equipment is old or inefficient, the health authority should be informed about this, and the procedure should be canceled rather than performed with defective equipment.

- Good clinical records should not only have preoperative, operative, and postoperative details but should also record what has been told to the woman including the risks of any treatment offered and future implications to her.
- A follow-up appointment for all cases, either with the general practitioner or the hospital or the clinic, must be made. If the patient does not attend, a further appointment must be given, and a record is kept of the information.
- It is advisable to send products of conceptions for histology, especially where there is any doubt about diagnosis. It should also be sent for genetic analysis to be able to offer an explanation of the miscarriage to the couple.
- Early notification of the events to your defense organization (MDU/MPS) should be made, if there is likelihood of possible litigation.
- There should be clear and concise protocol to be followed for the management of recurrent miscarriages, including the plan of investigations to be carried out.
- It is a good practice to anticipate and discuss potential legal problems in your own departmental "clinical governance meetings" even if there has not been any complaint so as to improve future outcomes.

KEY PRINCIPLES

- *Always put the patient first:* Medicine exists to serve people, and as doctors, we must always act responsibly and where appropriate, engage openly and transparently with our patients and their relatives about their care and treatment, respecting their wishes at all times.
- *Zero harm and patient safety:* Provision of high-quality care that is safe, clinically effective, and enhances the experience of all patients should be foremost in our minds, which includes good multidisciplinary team working, following clinical standards and guidelines, and measuring outcomes.
- *Creating outstanding leadership and working together as teams of professionals:* Consultants have the responsibility to lead the profession, which includes challenging colleagues or employers when there is clear evidence of poor practice. As leaders, they must provide support and supervision to the trainees/juniors and work closely with other colleagues to offer safe and good-quality care through professional team working for the benefit of the women they serve.
- *Regulation, inspection, and accountability:* The colleges should have a role in accreditation and hospital visits to ensure that quality standards in education, training, and service provision are maintained.
- *Metrics and outcomes:* Both individual clinicians and hospitals must collate accurate and truthful data on patient care so as to monitor service quality and produce outcome metrics for quality assurance and revalidation purposes.

SUGGESTED READING

1. Alberman E, Dennis KJ. Late abortions in England and Wales. In: Report of a National Confidential Study. London: Royal College of Obstetricians and Gynaecologists; 1984.
2. Alberman E, Elliott M, Creasy M, Dhadial R. Previous reproductive history in mothers presenting with spontaneous abortions. Br J Obstet Gynaecol. 1975;82(5): 366-73.
3. American College of Surgeons (ACS) Committee on Perioperative Care. Revised statement on the prevention of unintentionally retained surgical items after surgery. Bull Am Coll Surg.2016;101(10):50-1.
4. Argent VP. Therapeutic miscarriage—clinical litigation. Obstet Gynaecol. 1985;118.
5. Chamberlain G. The risks of obstetrics and gynaecology in practice. Int J Risk Saf Med. 1991;2(2):129-32. doi: 10.3233/JRS-1991-22-308. PMID: 23511865
6. Clements RV. Litigation in obstetrics and gynaecology. Br J Obstet Gynaecol. 1991;98(5):423-6. doi: 10.1111/j.1471-0528.1991.tb10334.x. PMID: 2059586.
7. Edozein LC. Patient safety in operation theatre: an overview. Clin Risk. 2005;11(5):177-84.
8. Edozien LC. Risk management in gynaecology: principles and practice. Best Pract Res Clin Obstet Gynaecol. 2007; 21(4):713-25.
9. Freda VJ, Gorman JG, Galen RS, Treacy N. The threat of Rh immunisation from abortion. Lancet. 1970;2(7664):147-8.
10. Hatcher vs. Black (1954) Times, 2nd July.
11. Joint Study of the Royal College of General Practitioners and the Royal College of Obstetricians and Gynaecologists. Induced abortion operations and their early sequelae. J R Coll Gen Pract. 1985;35(273):175-80.
12. Martin F. D' Souza vs Mohd. Ishfaq on 17 February, 2009 Equivalent citations: AIR 2009 Supreme Court ... Appellate Jurisdiction Civil Appeal No. 3541 of 2002 Martin F. D'Souza

.. Appellant -versus- Mohd. Ishfaq .. Respondent Judgment Markandey Katju, J.
13. Negligence in Health: Clinical Claims and Risk. by Vivienne Harpwood | 1 May ... Legal Issues in Obstetrics (Medico-Legal Series). by Vivienne Harpwood. Amazon books
14. NHS Litigation Authority. (2017). [online] Available from http:// www.nhsla.com [Last accessed December, 2024].
15. Poland BJ, Miller JR, Jones DC, Trimble BK. Reproductive counseling in patients who have had a spontaneous abortion. Am J Obstet Gynecol. 1977;127(7):685-91.
16. RCOG Guidelines. (2018). [online] Available from https:// www. rcog.org.uk [Last accessed December, 2024].
17. Reginald PW, Beard RW, Chapple J, Forbes PB, Liddell HS, Mowbray JF, et al. Outcome of pregnancies progressing beyond 28 weeks gestation in women with a history of recurrent miscarriage. Br J Obstet Gynaecol. 1987;94(7):643-8.
18. Roth DB. The frequency of spontaneous abortion. Int J Fertil. 1963;8:431-4.
19. Sage WM, Gallagher TH, Armstrong S, Cohn JS, McDonald T, Gale J, et al. How policy makers can smooth the way for communication-and-resolution programs. Health Aff (Millwood). 2014;33(1):11-9.
20. Savage W, Paterson I. Abortion: methods and sequelae. Br J Hosp Med. 1982;28(4):364, 369-72 passim.
21. Sonne-Holm S, Heisterberg L, Hebjøorn S, Dyring-Anderson K, Anderson JT, Hejl BL. Prophylactic antibiotics in first-trimester abortions: a clinical, controlled trial. Am J Obstet Gynecol. 1981;139(6):693-6.
22. Supreme Court of India. Page 1 of 21. Case no.: Appeal (crl.) 144-145 of 2004. Petitioner: Jacob Mathew. Respondent: State of Punjab & Anr. Date of judgment: 05 /08/2005
23. Warburton D, Fraser FC. Spontaneous abortion risks in man: Data from reproductive histories collected in a medical genetics unit. Am J Hum Genet. 1964;16(1):1-25.
24. Warburton D, Strobino B. Recurrent spontaneous miscarriage. In: Bennett MJ, Edmonds DK (Eds). Spontaneous and Recurrent Miscarriages. Oxford: Blackwell Scientific Publications; 1987. pp. 193-213.
25. Zitter JM. Admissibility of evidence of medical defendant's apologetic statements or the like as evidence of negligence. Am Law Rep. 2014;97:519-2.

SECTION 11

The Future

CHAPTER 58

Resurgence of Statins in Recurrent Pregnancy Loss

Yona Grossman, Asher Bashiri

ABSTRACT

Statins were classed as category X drug by Food and Drug Administration (FDA). This posed a dilemma for physicians treating elderly patients with high cholesterol, triglyceride levels during pregnancy. Besides statins were found to be anti-inflammatory and hence were useful as adjuvant therapy in women with APLA syndrome. Recently FDA has issued a statement that statin use is safe during pregnancy, which will positively impact maternal health during pregnancy and may improve fetal outcomes as well.

Keywords: Statins, RPL, APLA syndrome, Preeclampsia, Pravastatin, FDA.

INTRODUCTION

Statins have become a mainstay of therapy and prophylaxis for cardiovascular disease worldwide.[1] Yet in obstetrics and gynecology, their use has been widely debated. Initially classified as teratogenic, statins were once contraindicated in pregnancy.[2] However, new data suggests that the teratogenicity risk is minimal,[3] with evidence only existing from older in vitro studies.[4] New research has shown the adjunct benefits of statins as an anti-inflammatory agent, which may have indication in recurrent pregnancy loss (RPL). This chapter will discuss the pharmacology of statins, their indications, the evolution of their use within pregnancy, and new research indicating their potential use in certain cases of RPL.

STATIN PHARMACOLOGY

Statin medications are the first-line therapy for hypercholesterolemia. Of all dyslipidemia medications, statins have shown the greatest reduction in cholesterol levels. They have also been proven to reduce mortality from ischemic heart disease and are thus prescribed as standard therapy post myocardial infarction (MI). The statin family is a class of drugs that inhibit cholesterol synthesis.[5] They competitively inhibit the hydroxymethylglutaryl-coenzyme A (HMG-CoA) reductase enzyme, thereby halting the conversion of HMG-CoA to mevalonate, the rate-limiting step in cholesterol synthesis.[5] By decreasing de novo cholesterol production, the body is forced to resorb the available cholesterol circulating through the bloodstream. The body thus upregulates its low-density lipoprotein (LDL) receptors so that LDL can migrate from the blood to the liver.[5] This LDL recycling effectively lowers cholesterol levels within the blood. Statins have an additional anticholesterol property as they limit the liver's production of Apolipoprotein B100 (ApoB100). Without ApoB100, LDL and very low-density lipoproteins (VLDL) cannot be secreted into the bloodstream.[5]

While the primary effect of statins lies in their cholesterol-lowering properties, statins also possess pleiotropic effects.[2] They have antioxidant, anti-inflammatory, immunomodulatory, and antithrombotic properties. Statins have been shown to decrease reactive oxygen species (ROS), thereby lowering oxidative stress within the body.[2] They increase the production and mobilization of hematopoietic stem cells and vascular endothelial growth factor (VEGF) promoting angiogenesis. Statins additionally modulate the effects of immunogenic mediators such as nuclear factor-kappa B (NF-κB), lowering proinflammatory cytokines reducing inflammation. Despite being independent of the lipid-lowering effects, all the pleiotropic effects of statins originate from the inhibition of HMG-CoA reductase. Mevalonate, the product of HMG-CoA reductase's conversion is critical to two pathways: the cholesterol pathway and the prenylated protein pathway. Statins' inhibition of this second prenylated protein pathway confer the downstream pleiotropic effects **(Flowchart 1)**.

Flowchart 1: HMG-CoA reductase pathways and the downstream effects of statins (an HMG-CoA reductase inhibitor).

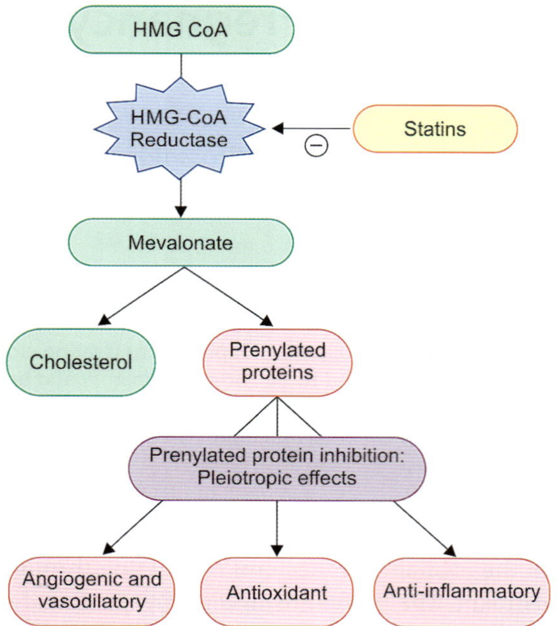

(HMG-CoA: hydroxymethylglutaryl-coenzyme A)

MEDICAL INDICATIONS FOR STATINS

Statins are the most widely prescribed medication worldwide.[2] They have many indications and are used for both treatment and prophylaxis for atherosclerosis and cardiovascular events.[5] They are indicated for treatment of hyperlipidemia, mixed dyslipidemia, hypertriglyceridemia, atherosclerosis, and primary prevention of atherosclerotic cardiovascular disease. They are even indicated for pediatric treatment of children with familial hypercholesterolemia. The guidelines set by the American Heart Association indicate that statins should be considered in any patient with a history of atherosclerotic cardiovascular disease, anyone with LDL ≥190 mg/dL, any diabetic patients between the ages of 40–75 years with LDL ≥70 mg/dL, or any patient aged 20–39 years with high risk of cardiovascular disease (LDL ≥160 mg/dL and family history of premature coronary artery disease).[5] The breadth of these statin guidelines results in a high proportion of the population receiving statins.

IMPORTANCE OF CHOLESTEROL, FATTY ACIDS, AND HYDROXYMETHYLGLUTARYL-COENZYME A REDUCTASE IN PREGNANCY

Pregnancy confers many physiological changes within the body to provide for the fetus and prepare for delivery. One such change includes a physiological hyperlipidemia, which occurs to assist with implantation, to provide nutrients to the growing fetus, and to facilitate fetal development. Cholesterol has a 25–50% increase during pregnancy while triglyceride levels increase two-to-fourfold.[2] Fatty acids and cholesterol are able to cross freely between maternal and fetal circulation via the placenta.[2] Increased triglycerides serve to provide the necessary free fatty acids that provide the fetus with sustenance and are critical to building fetal cells (i.e., the phospholipid bilayer).[2] Cholesterol is a crucial component of embryonic development as it stabilizes cell membranes and thus exists within all cells.[2] Additionally, cholesterol is the building block of steroid hormones, which are necessary to maintain pregnancy.[2] Cholesterol also activates signaling pathways that are fundamental to fetal development, such as Sonic the hedgehog (*SHH*) protein, which facilitates fetal brain and limb differentiation.[2] The importance of increased cholesterol levels during pregnancy garnered the initial suspicion that statin therapy, which serves to lower cholesterol and triglyceride levels, may confer high fetal risk and should thus be avoided during pregnancy.

CHANGING RESEARCH ON STATINS IN OBSTETRICS: REASSESSING TERATOGENICITY

The increase in both obesity rates and the average age of pregnant women has conferred a higher prevalence of pregnant women who should be receiving statin therapy. Therefore, it has recently become critical to reassess the effects of statins during pregnancy. In recent years, research on the risks of statin therapy during pregnancy has exploded, yielding fascinating findings. The following section will delineate the perceptions of statin therapy risk during pregnancy from early animal models to novel research insights.

Initial Claims Warning against Statin Use During Pregnancy

Until recently, statins were classified as teratogenic and thus assigned as class X by the Food and Drug Administration (FDA). This decision stemmed from early animal models testing the impacts of pravastatin on early pregnancy in rats and rabbits.[3] Two studies from 1987 noted the following teratogenic effects on progeny of rats and rabbits administered statin therapy: Gastroschisis and bone malformation in rats given 800 mg/kg/day of lovastatin and bone malformations only in rats given

6 mg/kg/day of fluvastatin.[2] Two additional studies conducted in 1990 and 1994 found no teratogenicity in animal models but a significant increase in first-trimester pregnancy losses.[6,7] In 2005, Kenis et al. opted to test the effect of statins on human placental tissue to assess deleterious effects.[4] This in vitro study compared first-trimester placental tissue grown on medium enriched with simvastatin to tissue grown on standard medium.[4] Results indicated that placental tissue exposed to simvastatin had significantly decreased progesterone secretion, increased cytotrophoblast cell apoptosis, and inhibited extra-villous trophoblast cell migration.[4] These studies have shown HMG-CoA reductase enzyme to be a critical component of successful placental development, leading to the FDA's contraindication of statin use during pregnancy.[2]

A New Wave of Clinical Studies Leads to Changes in Food and Drug Administration Guidelines

The increase in worldwide statin use combined with increasing maternal age has rendered more women of childbearing age utilizing statins. Furthermore, guidelines have highlighted the importance of statins for primary prophylaxis of cardiovascular events. Questions have thus arisen in recent years regarding the potential maternal risks of removing statin therapy during pregnancy planning periods. Debates on the potential risks and benefits of continuing statin use during conception have become commonplace. Thus, researchers have begun to reassess the risks of using statins in early pregnancy, despite the FDA's initial warning. Researchers noticed that most of the prior research was conducted in vitro and that the dosages of statins used in these trials were much higher than the doses prescribed clinically.

Two early clinical studies did show a significant increase in adverse pregnancy events and fetal malformations in women utilizing statins, but only when lipophilic statins were used (atorvastatin, simvastatin, and lovastatin).[8,9] Hydrophilic statins (i.e., pravastatin) conferred no difference in pregnancy outcomes.[8] One review of case reports published in *The New England Journal of Medicine* in 2004 found fetal malformations in 20 out of 52 included reports, but in all the cases, mothers utilized lipophilic statins.[8] None of the 14 cases of pravastatin use during pregnancy cited fetal malformation.[8] This study also noted that none of the earlier animal trials that indicated adverse fetal outcomes with statin use utilized hydrophilic statins.[8] The differences in pregnancy outcomes between hydrophilic and lipophilic statins is likely due to the unique ability of lipophilic statins to cross the placental barrier. Taguchi et al. conducted the first prospective clinical trial of statin use during pregnancy.[9] However, 46 out of 64 (72%) of women in this trial utilized atorvastatin, a lipophilic statin while only 9 out of 64 used a hydrophilic statin (pravastatin).[9] This trial did find a decrease in neonatal weight and gestational age among statin users, but it did not highlight significant differences in congenital malformations, miscarriages or spontaneous fetal demise between statin users and controls.[9]

With this novel insight regarding the potentially lower fetal risk of hydrophilic statins, more studies began to explore the risks of statins on pregnancy outcomes. The first systematic review and meta-analysis on statin use in pregnancy was published in 2012 that included a total of 13 human studies (5 cohort studies, 2 case series, and 6 case reports) and 11 animal trials (all experimental).[10] It found no significant difference in teratogenicity risk among statin users compared to controls in human trials, although the animal experiments did show some increased risk.[10] This study also highlighted that all animal trials used lipophilic statins at higher doses than those prescribed to humans.[10] Two more recent systematic reviews confirmed the results of this first meta-analysis: A systematic review of 16 human trials in 2016 by Karalis et al.,[3] and most recently, a systematic review and meta-analysis of cohort and case-control studies by Karadas[11] including 5 human trials in 2022. Both the 2016 and 2022 systematic reviews found no increased risk of congenital malformations among statin users relative to controls.[3,11] However, the meta-analysis from 2022 did indicate a significantly lower live birth rate and an increased risk of spontaneous abortion among statin users.[11] The results of these recent systematic reviews and meta-analyses highlighting no difference in teratogenicity risk between statin users and controls have led to a recent change in guidelines: In July 2021, the FDA removed its black box warning against the use of statins during pregnancy.[12] Instead, healthcare professionals are urged to consider the individual needs of their patients and to evaluate their patients' cardiovascular risks.[12] Additionally, the FDA has now deemed use of statins during the preconception period as safe.[12] However, once pregnant, statins should still be stopped for most patients (unless individual benefit outweighs the risk) until further research is done.

Statin Use in Preeclampsia

With this new guideline update regarding statin use in pregnancy, the use of statins may be useful to pregnant women not only for prevention of cardiovascular events but also for their pleiotropic benefits. Some of the pleiotropic effects conferred by statins may be useful for certain conditions during pregnancy, namely preeclampsia.[2,13] Preeclampsia is a disease of pregnancy characterized by hypertension, proteinuria, and/or end-organ damage.[14] Its exact pathophysiology is debated, but it includes the failure of spiral arteries to remodel and dilate, resulting in insufficient placental perfusion and ischemia.[14] Since spiral arteries do not widen as they should, there is increased turbulent flow and endothelial damage, causing a release of ROS that further harm the placental villi.[14] The injured villi release antiangiogenic molecules into the maternal circulation leading to the clinical sequelae that characterize the disease.[14] Two important mediators of preeclampsia include thromboxane, a vasoconstrictor, and soluble fms-like tyrosine kinase-1 (sFlt1), which acts to destabilize VEGF.[14] The effects of these two molecules may be neutralized by the pleiotropic effects of statins. One pleiotropic effect of statins is their upregulation of nitric oxide (NO) within the body.[2] NO is a potent vasodilator that can antagonize the vasoconstriction mediated by thromboxane. Statins modulate NO by increasing its bioavailability through their antioxidant properties by increasing endothelial nitric oxide synthase (eNOS) phosphorylation and stabilizing eNOS ribonucleic acid (RNA).[2] Furthermore, the antioxidant effects of statins may help neutralize the ROS released by damaged villi, leading to a more upstream effect whereby fewer antiangiogenic molecules are released into maternal circulation.[13] Finally, statins have shown to increase circulating levels of VEGF, which may be useful to counteract the destabilization of VEGF that occurs in preeclampsia.[2,13]

Numerous experimental models have shown the in vitro ability of statins to reduce the sequelae of preeclampsia via the aforementioned mechanisms. In 2010, Constantine et al. utilized a mouse model to highlight how pravastatin administration significantly lowered sFlt1 levels and reduced vascular contractility in the presence of procontractile molecules (i.e., phenylephrine), indicating its potential benefit in preeclampsia.[15] Fox et al. demonstrated that mice who were induced to preeclampsia conditions via transfection with sFlt1 had a significant increase in NO levels after pravastatin treatment.[16] Levels of NO after treatment were the same as control mice who were not induced to preeclampsia.[16] Ahmed et al. found that pravastatin's increase in VEGF restores the balance between pro- and antiangiogenic molecules, preventing glomerular injury and protecting the pregnancy in mice.[17]

Based on these findings that pravastatin lowers sFlt1 levels in mice, Ahmed et al. conducted a randomized control trial (RCT) of women in the United Kingdom with preeclampsia between 24 and 32 weeks of gestation to understand whether these findings are translated clinically.[18] They found no significant reduction in sFlt1 levels in the treatment group, nor any significant clinical changes to clinical preeclampsia course in women treated with pravastatin.[18] However, this RCT did strengthen the notion that pravastatin use is safe during pregnancy as there was no increase in adverse fetal outcomes in the treatment group.[18] There are numerous limitations to this study including slow recruitment and low-medication compliance among the treatment group.[19] A critical study limitation is that treatment was only started in the second trimester. Although the clinical features of preeclampsia set in late, the source of the disease (failure of spiral artery remodeling and resulting placental ischemia) begins far earlier. Thus, it is possible that clinical benefits of pravastatin would only be seen if it is started earlier in the pregnancy, to prevent the increase in antiangiogenic molecule release.[18] Perhaps the clinical course of preeclampsia, despite its late onset, is predetermined early on. RCTs analyzing the use of statins earlier in pregnancy as preeclampsia prophylaxis should thus be conducted.

STATINS IN RECURRENT PREGNANCY LOSS: WHEN MIGHT THEY BE USEFUL?

Several animal studies have highlighted the ability of statins to prevent recurrent miscarriage.[13,20] Redecha et al. postulated that pravastatin's reduction of tissue factor (TF) expression on trophoblasts protects against placental degradation and pregnancy loss in CBA/J × DBA/2 mice (a specific mice model that shares many features with human RPL).[20] However, a 2022 systematic review found that statin use during pregnancy increased rates of spontaneous miscarriage and decreased live birth rates, though this review included all statins, not just hydrophilic ones.[11] Any treatment showing increase in spontaneous miscarriage rates warrants caution when considering its use for treatment of RPL. Thus, current studies of statin use in RPL have focused on a subset of women in which increased TF is a known mediator of pregnancy loss e.g., Antiphospholipid syndrome (APS).[21] In APS, the increased inflammation leads to higher levels of complement C5a.[21] C5a activates TF in neutrophils, increasing the respiratory burst, leading to trophoblast injury and ultimately, pregnancy loss.[21]

The current recommendations for pregnant women with APS are treatment with aspirin (ASA) and low-molecular weight heparin (LMWH).[22] Numerous studies have demonstrated promising results that pravastatin may be a helpful adjunct therapy in APS. In 2016, Lefkou et al. conducted an observational study of 21 pregnant women with APS who received conventional therapy (ASA + LMWH) yet still developed either preeclampsia or intrauterine growth restriction (IUGR).[23] At the onset of complication, 11 women received 20 mg/day of pravastatin while ten women continued solely with standard treatment.[23] Women receiving pravastatin had significant improvement in their blood pressure and proteinuria, remained pregnant for longer and delivered closer to term.[23] Additionally, neonatal survival outcomes were greatly increased in the pravastatin group with a 100% survival rate relative to 45% in controls.[23] Lefkou et al. further studied the addition of pravastatin to standard ASA + LMWH treatment in 2020 to elucidate the mechanism of additional statin therapy.[24] They found that the addition of statins increased endothelial NO, reducing uteroplacental vessel resistance, and increasing placental health, thereby prolonging pregnancy.[24] One systematic review of 313 pregnancies published in 2021 evaluated the safety and efficacy of numerous second-line therapies [pravastatin, hydroxychloroquine, steroids, intravenous immunoglobulin (IVIG), plasma exchange, rituximab and tumor necrosis factor-alpha (TNF-α) inhibitors] for pregnancies complicated by APS that were refractory to conventional therapy (ASA + LMWH).[22] Of all second-line therapies, pravastatin was associated with the highest live birth rate (100%) and lowest number of severe pregnancy complications (8.3%). The use of pravastatin is thus currently under consideration to become a potential standard of therapy for APS refractory to conventional treatment.[25]

CONCLUSION

The use of statins during pregnancy has evolved from an absolute contraindication to relative safety. Updated clinical trials have not demonstrated the teratogenic outcomes that were originally established by in vitro animal models. Furthermore, pravastatin, a hydrophilic statin, does not cross the placental barrier and thus likely possesses an even lower risk of adverse fetal outcomes. This updated research has shifted the conception of the safety profile of statins during pregnancy, with FDA recommendations changing as a result. With the explosion of statin use worldwide, this update in guidelines has drastic implications on the increasing number of women who utilize statins and are pursuing pregnancy. This revitalized notion of statin safety during pregnancy has provided opportunities to research whether the antioxidant, angiogenic, and anti-inflammatory effects of statins could be employed within pregnancy disease states. Statins have subsequently been shown in animal models to reduce sequelae of preeclampsia and have been successful in human observational studies in improving pregnancy outcomes in refractory APS, a common cause of RPL. More robust clinical trials should be done to elucidate the ability of statins to improve pregnancy outcomes in preeclampsia, APS, and other causes of RPL.

REFERENCES

1. O'Malley PG, Arnold MJ, Kelley C, Spacek L, Buelt A, Natarajan S, et al. Management of dyslipidemia for cardiovascular disease risk reduction: synopsis of the 2020 updated U.S. Department of Veterans Affairs and U.S. Department of Defense Clinical Practice Guideline. Ann Intern Med. 2020;173(10):822-9.
2. Lecarpentier E, Morel O, Fournier T, Elefant E, Chavatte-Palmer P, Tsatsaris V. Statins and pregnancy: between supposed risks and theoretical benefits. Drugs. 2012; 72(6):773-88.
3. Karalis DG, Hill AN, Clifton S, Wild RA. The risks of statin use in pregnancy: a systematic review. J Clin Lipidol. 2016;10(5):1081-90.
4. Kenis I, Tartakover-Matalon S, Cherepnin N, Drucker L, Fishman A, Pomeranz M, et al. Simvastatin has deleterious effects on human first trimester placental explants. Hum Reprod. 2005;20(10):2866-72.
5. Sizar O, Khare S, Patel P, Talati R. Statin medications. StatPearls. Treasure Island: StatPearls Publishing; 2024.
6. Zapletalova K, Valenzuela I, Greyling M, Regin Y, Frigolett C, Krofta L, et al. The effects of prenatal pravastatin treatment in the rabbit fetal growth restriction model. Biomedicines. 2023;11(10):2685. PMID: 37893059.
7. Dostal LA, Schardein JL, Anderson JA. Developmental toxicity of the HMG-CoA reductase inhibitor, atorvastatin, in rats and rabbits. Teratology. 1994;50(6):387-94.

8. Edison RJ, Muenke M. Central nervous system and limb anomalies in case reports of first-trimester statin exposure. N Engl J Med. 2004;350(15):1579-82.
9. Taguchi N, Rubin ET, Hosokawa A, Choi J, Ying AY, Moretti ME, et al. Prenatal exposure to HMG-CoA reductase inhibitors: effects on fetal and neonatal outcomes. Reprod Toxicol. 2008;26(2):175-7.
10. Kusters DM, Lahsinoui HH, van de Post JAM, Wiegman A, Wijburg FA, Kastelein JJP, et al. Statin use during pregnancy: a systematic review and meta-analysis. Expert Rev Cardiovasc Ther. 2012;10(3):363-78.
11. Karadas B, Uysal N, Erol H, Acar S, Koc M, Kaya-Temiz T, et al. Pregnancy outcomes following maternal exposure to statins: a systematic review and meta-analysis. Br J Clin Pharmacol. 2022;88(9):3962-76.
12. Bittencourt MS. Statins and pregnancy - new FDA recommendations. Arq Bras Cardiol. 2022;119(1):1-2.
13. Girardi G. Can statins prevent pregnancy complications? J Reprod Immunol. 2014;101-102:161-7.
14. Chappell LC, Cluver CA, Kingdom J, Tong S. Pre-eclampsia. Lancet. 2021;398(10297):341-54.
15. Costantine MM, Tamayo E, Lu F, Bytautiene E, Longo M, Hankins GDV, et al. Using pravastatin to improve the vascular reactivity in a mouse model of soluble fms-like tyrosine kinase-1-induced preeclampsia. Obstet Gynecol. 2010;116(1):114-20.
16. Fox KA, Longo M, Tamayo E, Kechichian T, Bytautiene E, Hankins GDV, et al. Effects of pravastatin on mediators of vascular function in a mouse model of soluble Fms-like tyrosine kinase-1-induced preeclampsia. Am J Obstet Gynecol. 2011;205(4):366.e1-5.
17. Ahmed A, Singh J, Khan Y, Seshan SV, Girardi G. A new mouse model to explore therapies for preeclampsia. PLoS One. 2010;5(10):e13663.
18. Ahmed A, Williams DJ, Cheed V, Middleton LJ, Ahmad S, Wang K, et al. Pravastatin for early-onset pre-eclampsia: a randomised, blinded, placebo-controlled trial. BJOG. 2020;127(4):478-88.
19. Costantine MM. Pravastatin to ameliorate early-onset pre-eclampsia: promising but not there yet. BJOG. 2020;127(4):489.
20. Redecha P, van Rooijen N, Torry D, Girardi G. Pravastatin prevents miscarriages in mice: role of tissue factor in placental and fetal injury. Blood. 2009;113(17):4101-9.
21. Redecha P, Franzke CW, Ruf W, Mackman N, Girardi G. Neutrophil activation by the tissue factor/factor VIIa/PAR2 axis mediates fetal death in a mouse model of antiphospholipid syndrome. J Clin Invest. 2008; 118(10): 3453-61.
22. Ruffatti A, Tonello M, Favaro M, Ross TD, Calligaro A, Ruffatti AT, et al. The efficacy and safety of second-line treatments of refractory and/or high risk pregnant antiphospholipid syndrome patients. A systematic literature review analyzing 313 pregnancies. Semin Arthritis Rheum. 2021;51(1):28-35.
23. Lefkou E, Mamopoulos A, Dagklis T, Vosnakis C, Rousso D, Girardi G. Pravastatin improves pregnancy outcomes in obstetric antiphospholipid syndrome refractory to antithrombotic therapy. J Clin Invest. 2016;126(8):2933-40.
24. Lefkou E, Varoudi K, Pombo J, Jurisic A, Jurisic Z, Contento G, et al. Triple therapy with pravastatin, low molecular weight heparin and low dose aspirin improves placental haemodynamics and pregnancy outcomes in obstetric antiphospholipid syndrome in mice and women through a nitric oxide-dependent mechanism. Biochem Pharmacol. 2020;182:114217.
25. Kaneko K, Ozawa N, Murashima A. Obstetric antiphospholipid syndrome: from pathogenesis to treatment. Immunol Med. 2022;45(2):79-93.

CHAPTER 59

Role of Surrogacy

Asher Bashiri, Talya Kresch-Jaffe, Yuval Cherlow, Yona Grossman

ABSTRACT

Surrogacy can help couples with implantation issues that cannot be corrected with therapy. This is a small subset of recurrent pregnancy loss (RPL) patients nevertheless, this needs to be considered as part of management when all other therapies fail. Currently there are different surrogacy laws in different countries and this encourages surrogacy tourism. Having unified international guidelines to regulate surrogacy indications and safety put forth by professional bodies like ESHRE, ASRM, RCOG is the first step in urging governmental policy change.

Keywords: Surrogacy, RPL, Surrogacy tourism, Gestational surrogacy.

"Behold now, the Lord has restrained me from bearing; please come to my handmaid; perhaps I will be built up from her." (Genesis 16:2)

INTRODUCTION

From as early as biblical times, variations of surrogacy have been a documented method of producing offspring among women who could not conceive or maintain a pregnancy. The past few decades have exploded with medical advancement, affording greater understanding of the human body and the processes involved in conception and pregnancy. With the advent of assisted reproductive technology (ART), many women who once thought childbirth to be merely a dream are experiencing successful pregnancies. While many advancements have been made, there are still women who cannot successfully conceive and maintain a pregnancy and who unfortunately experience recurrent pregnancy loss (RPL). If numerous pregnancy attempts fail, many treatments including ART and preimplantation genetic testing (PGT) have already been tried, and the etiology of RPL is unknown, surrogacy can be a viable option.[1]

WHAT IS SURROGACY AND WHAT TYPES OF SURROGACIES EXIST?

Surrogacy is a consensual arrangement in which a woman agrees to carry and deliver a child for another couple or individual.[2] Prior to the advent of ART, surrogacy was defined as an arrangement in which the surrogate and a male intended parent (IP) are genetically related to the conceived child.[3] This arrangement is entitled traditional surrogacy (TS). New advancements have allowed for both IPs to be genetically related to the child. With the assistance of ART, eggs and sperm can be harvested from the IPs, which can then be used to grow successful embryos to be implanted in the uterus of the surrogate. This modern form of surrogacy is termed gestational surrogacy (GS).[3] Surrogacy arrangements can be further classified into altruistic and commercial surrogacies, where the former does not receive compensation other than pregnancy-related expenses, whereas the latter receives formal payment for her services.[4]

Gestational surrogacy has successfully been implemented worldwide and is proving to be invaluable for many individuals who were previously unable to conceive children. Thus, the number of surrogacy requests has increased dramatically in the last decade, with the United States indicating a two and a half-fold increase,[5] Israel citing a fourfold increase,[6] a fertility center in Canada experiencing a 10-fold increase,[7] and a Mexican center exhibiting a 23-fold increase.[8] The global success of GS has shown its positive effect as a medical intervention at providing tangible hope to individuals and couples who wish to build a family and have been previously unsuccessful.

WHO IS SURROGACY FOR?

The desire for surrogacy is multifaceted and complex with several factors leading to the decision to seek surrogacy.

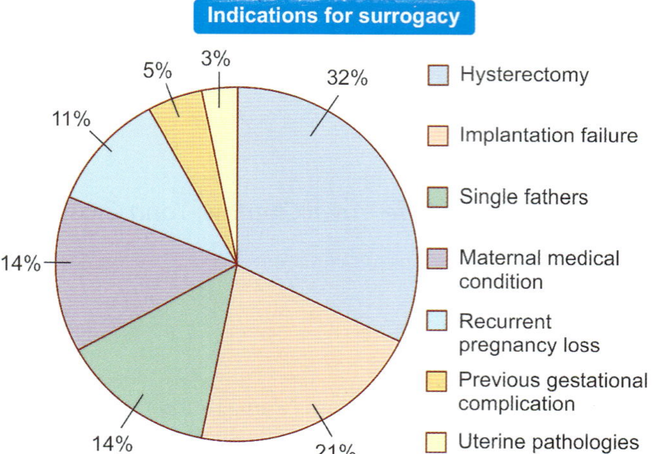

Fig. 1: Graphical representation outlining the percentage of surrogacy requests made by individuals among each indication category for gestational surrogacy.
Source: Cabra et al.[8]

The American Society for Reproductive Medicine (ASRM) has set broad indications for surrogacy including an inability to conceive or carry a child biologically (including same-sex couples and single parents), significant uterine anomalies, and medical or psychological contraindications to pregnancy.[9] RPL and recurrent implantation failure (RIF) are also relative indications for surrogacy[9] and are among the most commonly cited reasons for obtaining surrogacy.[7,8] Approximately 21% of all desired surrogacies were due to RIF and 11–14% were because of RPL[7,8] **(Fig. 1)**.

WHAT IS THE SURROGACY PROCESS?

The technological advancement facilitating GS has allowed for detachment of the surrogate from biological parentage. As such, surrogacy could theoretically be conducted transactionally between human beings, like any other contract providing goods and services. However, due to the sensitivity and ethical complexity of surrogacy, various legalities have been instated to regulate this process. Once an individual or couple decides to pursue surrogacy, they begin a long and complex journey. Helping them navigate this process is a multidisciplinary team comprised of physicians, fertility centers, lawyers, and psychosocial counselors.[10] There are six basic elements in the surrogacy process, each with their own set of potential roadblocks:

1. Finding a surrogate
2. Initial counseling including the medical and psychological assessments
3. Drafting a legal arrangement
4. The fertilization process
5. The pregnancy
6. Claiming parentage postdelivery.[10]

The following section will outline the process of surrogacy, according to chronological timeline of the process.

The first step to obtain surrogacy is finding a surrogate. Surrogates can be arranged by agencies, but one quarter of all surrogates are friends or relatives of the IPs. Rigorous guidelines have been set by both the European Society of Human Reproduction and Embryology (ESHRE)[11] (in 2005) and the ASRM[12] (in 2022) to ensure proper screening of gestational carriers (surrogates). The two guidelines are similar to each other with slight variations, with ASRM guidelines being more updated to the current practice of surrogacy. Both guidelines highlight the importance of screening surrogates for eligibility, including the age of the surrogate (maximum age limit of 45 years). Both guidelines also indicate that surrogates must have at least one child of their own. Additionally, both guidelines only recommend one embryo transfer at a time. While ESHRE guidelines only allow for altruistic surrogacies, ASRM believes that commercial surrogacy should be allowed. Additionally, ASRM recommends women to be surrogates only if they have a stable family life with ample support. A full list of surrogate criteria can be viewed in **Table 1**. Fertility centers and surrogacy agencies may have additional restrictions and criteria, such as requiring financial and criminal background checks and undergoing infectious disease screening.[4] While these guidelines may seem prohibitive, they exist to mitigate undesirable outcomes so that all parties experience the surrogacy process as optimally as possible. Understandably, even the first step of finding and selecting a surrogate can be fatiguing due to possible holdups or failed screenings.

Once a suitable surrogate has been obtained, legal proceedings begin to ensure a smooth surrogacy process and mitigate potential risks.[10] Guidelines recommend that the IPs and surrogates must be represented by separate counsel to protect the best interest of both parties.[12] The purpose of the agreement is to discuss about any potential conflicts or circumstances that could alter the surrogacy arrangement. Thus, articles in the contract often include issues of parentage, medical procedures, compensation, conditions for pregnancy termination, and divorce or death of IPs.[13] It is important to note that despite efforts to devise these legal agreements, it is often difficult to enforce

TABLE 1: ESHRE and ASRM guidelines to ensure surrogate eligibility.

Category	*ESHRE 2005*[11]	*ASRM 2022*[12]
Payment	Only altruistic surrogacy is acceptable	Compensation for surrogacy is allowed
Screening	The same precautions used for gamete donation should be used. Separate screening by independent specialists should be done	All FDA required screening guidelines for the use of donor gametes should be used. Additionally, psychologic counseling, genetic screening, medical evaluation, and legal consultation (independent legal counsel for each party) are recommended
Surrogate age	The surrogate should be <35 years of age for partial (traditional) surrogacy and <45 for full (gestational) surrogacy	The surrogate must be of legal age; preferably between 21 and 45
Prerequisites	The surrogate must have at least one child	History of at least one term uncomplicated pregnancy
Contraindications	Not mentioned	The GC should not have had >5 deliveries or >3 cesarean deliveries
Embryo transfer	Strongly recommends the transfer of only one embryo. Transfer of a maximum of 2 embryos may be considered with poor quality embryos, oocyte donor of >35 years of age or low number of fertilized embryos	Strongly recommends single embryo transfer. May consider multiple embryo transfer when oocyte provider is >38 years of age
Family environment	Not addressed	Stable family environment and ample support to handle the increased stress of pregnancy
Limits	Recommends a maximum of one act of surrogacy except in the case of the same commissioning parents	Not addressed
Surrogate rights	The surrogate has the legal right to make decisions about her pregnancy, regardless of the original agreement, and the intended parents should be informed of this	Not addressed
"Cooling off" period	All parties involved should take time to consider their decisions	Not addressed

(ASRM: American Society for Reproductive Medicine; ESHRE: European Society of Human Reproduction and Embryology; FDA: Food and Drug Administration; GC: gestational carrier)

the contracts, as countries often have limited protocols within the law regarding surrogacy.[10]

The physical surrogacy process begins identically to the traditional in vitro fertilization (IVF) process, as embryos need to be prepared prior to transfer to the surrogate. Either a short gonadotropin-releasing hormone (GnRH) antagonist or long GnRH agonist protocol may be used for egg retrieval from the IP.[7] Prior to transfer, the endometrium of the surrogate must be prepared: Oral estrogen, followed by progesterone is used to thicken the endometrial lining.[7] Embryos may be fresh or frozen when transferred, as determined by the contract. However, if a fresh embryo is used, efforts must be made to ensure hormonal synchronization between the IP/egg donor and the surrogate via oral contraceptive pills, progesterone pills, or progesterone injections.[4] Typically, only one embryo is utilized per cycle (unless extenuating circumstances exist, and multiple embryo transfer has been agreed upon in the aforementioned legal contract).[12] Once pregnancy has been achieved, a standard pregnancy follow-up protocol is used i.e., initial ultrasound (6–8 weeks), nuchal translucency (week 11–13.6 weeks), early (14–18 weeks), and late (20–22 weeks) anatomy scans and growth scans (28 and 34–36 weeks).[10] While this is the standard protocol, all medical arrangements including additional screenings and involvement of IPs in follow up should be stipulated in the contract.

One major limitation to surrogacy is the cost associated with each segment of the surrogacy process; even if the surrogate does not request compensation, there are still heavy attorney fees and medical bills associated with the fertilization and pregnancy process. In 2021, the median cost of surrogacy was cited to range between £25,000 in the United Kingdom to up to £50,000 in Israel[6,14] and £120,000 in the United States.[15]

HOW HAS SURROGACY CHANGED OUTCOMES FOR COUPLES DESIRING CHILDREN?

While the goal of surrogacy is to provide the opportunity for children, the sensitive nature of successfully having children and the complexity of the surrogacy process and relationship have many physical and psychological effects. It is thus critical to understand how surrogacy as a medical intervention changes the physical and psychological outcomes for both the IPs and the surrogate.

While the reasons individuals seek surrogacy are multifaceted **(Fig. 1)**, it is often due to a physical barrier to pregnancy, including same sex couples, inability to conceive, or RPL. For these individuals, GS, when successful, has an incredibly positive outcome in providing the IPs with the offspring they desired. However, other physical outcomes must be measured with respect to the surrogate, especially whether surrogacy has more complications or adverse pregnancy outcomes relative to nonsurrogate mothers. Several studies showed that pregnancy complications are similar in surrogates and nonsurrogates; Dar, et al. cited a complication rate of 9.8% among surrogates with 92.3% of those complications being relatively minor.[7] One study conducted in the United States examined the difference in pregnancies among surrogates compared to nonsurrogates undergoing IVF.[8] They found no significant difference between the two groups in the rate of miscarriage or preterm delivery. However, they found that surrogate mothers had a significantly higher rate of implantation [adjusted risk ratio (aRR) 1.22, 95% confidence interval (CI) 1.17–1.26], clinical pregnancies (aRR 1.14, 95% CI 1.10–1.19) and live birth rates, and a decreased level of low-birth-weight deliveries (aRR 1.17, 95% CI 1.12–1.21) relative to nonsurrogates.[8] These outcomes are unsurprising since surrogacy criteria indicate that surrogates must have had a prior live-birth pregnancy, whereas many women undergoing IVF are experiencing difficulty in conceiving or maintaining pregnancy.

The surrogacy process is incredibly vulnerable, with relationships forming between the IP and the fetus, the surrogate and the fetus, and the IPs with the surrogate. The surrogate and the IPs each go through unique psychological challenges while undergoing the surrogacy journey. The surrogate must contend with the many physical and psychological obstacles of pregnancy, while additionally fighting the inevitable emotional attachment that will form with the fetus that is not genetically related to them. Additionally, there is immense psychological burden postdelivery when the surrogate must give up the child to the IPs. One study found that 23% of the surrogates in the study experienced anxiety or depression postsurrogacy with 4% of surrogates experiencing long-term depression specifically attributed to the surrogacy process.[16] Another 2003 study by Jadva highlighted that many of the psychological struggles experienced by the surrogate occur shortly after relinquishing the child to the IPs but resolve within weeks.[17] While the psychological barriers to surrogacy are often universal among surrogates, some challenges faced by IPs depend on their reasons for seeking surrogacy. For example, couples who previously experienced RPL understand the pregnancy experience and may exhibit feelings of loss or even guilt during the surrogate's pregnancy, since they are so closely connected to the surrogate and her pregnancy. However, there are also several similar psychological challenges experienced by all IPs, including the financial burden of surrogacy, the tedious bureaucratic process for obtaining a surrogate, the ups and downs of experiencing the pregnancy along with the surrogate, and any other complications that occur.[3] An Iranian qualitative study highlights the psychological issues that arise due to the shame felt by requiring a surrogate; as a result, some couples do not disclose their use of a surrogate to family and friends, and thus, lack a support system throughout the process.[18] While psychological outcomes among surrogate mothers are well studied, few investigations have been done regarding the psychological outcomes of surrogacy on IPs, with no studies specifically measuring psychological outcomes of couples experiencing RPL.[3]

WHAT DO DIFFERENT RELIGIONS SAY ABOUT SURROGACY?

Views on surrogacy are often polarizing among different religions, with some religions embracing it and others completely rejecting the proposition.[19] Opinions can even vary within branches of the same religion. For example, while Catholicism bans surrogacy and any form of ART, claiming that the intrusion of a third party into marital affairs is immoral, the Church of Latter-Day Saints embraces IVF in married couples but is still wary of surrogacy.[19] Islam is of similar opinion in that it accepts ART as a means of assisting married couples in achieving pregnancy. However, views on surrogacy differ between Sunni and Shia Muslims. According to Sunni scholars, the interference of a surrogate into the couple's marriage is not permitted.[20] Many Shia scholars, however, accept surrogacy as a viable method of procreation.[20] Judaism takes a more liberal view of surrogacy, with most rabbis accepting the idea, but with much debate about how it should ethically and religiously be put into practice.[19] For example, there is polarization among rabbis as to who may serve as a surrogate, since Jewish lineage is passed through the mother and the question of maternal identity (whether the IP or the surrogate is the true mother) is controversial.[21] Additionally, some rabbis posit that surrogates should be unmarried in order to avoid the controversy of adultery laws, whereby a married woman cannot have the child of another man who is not her husband. However, most rabbis now hold a more liberal opinion, stating that married surrogates are acceptable,[22] and changing trends in Israel indicate that the majority of surrogates are married.[23] Highlighting Jewish support of surrogacy is Israel's 1996 Embryo Carrying Agreement Law, the world's first primary law permitting and regulating GS.[24] Both Hinduism and Buddhism fully accept surrogacy, especially since Buddhists view all pregnancy as reincarnating an old soul.[19] While many countries have separation of church and state, religious views on surrogacy are still largely implicated in the state policy on surrogacy.

WHAT ARE THE LEGAL AND ETHICAL CONSIDERATIONS REGARDING SURROGACY?

State law is often built upon historic, cultural, and religious practices of the country. Thus, surrogacy laws vary significantly worldwide. Some countries accept both commercial and altruistic surrogacy; others prohibit all surrogacy forms, and several lack any discussion of surrogacy. For example, Canada allows for altruistic but not commercial surrogacy (however, reimbursement for pregnancy-related expenses is permitted)[7]. Both the United States and Mexico have variance even between states: In Mexico, only 2 out of 31 states have surrogacy regulation.[8] Likewise, some states in the United States have complete surrogacy bans, while others, like New York, welcome surrogacy and will immediately name the IPs as birth parents without any further bureaucracy.[25] The paucity of worldwide regulation of this medical intervention poses numerous legal and ethical issues that will be discussed in this section.

Legal Enforceability of Surrogacy Contracts

The most basic problem of minimal surrogacy regulation surrounds enforceability of surrogacy contracts. The surrogacy agreement is in place to protect the individual rights of both the IPs and the surrogate. Surrogacy treatment involves some loss of autonomy, as both the IPs and the surrogate are considered patients, and they are thus inextricably interconnected.[10] The contract thus ensures that both parties have realistic expectations of the upcoming journey, minimizes unexpected outcomes, and prevents exploitation. Furthermore, an enforceable agreement streamlines the process for the IPs to assume parentage once the child is born, which in unregulated systems can often be difficult.[8,25] Finally, the contract prevents the IPs from changing their minds or abandoning the child with the surrogate.[10] While limited regulation and a lack of bureaucracy may initially appear ideal for obtaining surrogacy, as there are fewer roadblocks within the process, it is in the best interest of all parties to pursue surrogacy in a place where a legal framework exists.

Surrogacy Tourism: Issues of Exploitation

With such high variance in both state surrogacy regulation and surrogacy costs, many couples opt to pursue surrogacy in foreign countries with more optimal surrogacy conditions.[15] This phenomenon is known as "surrogacy tourism." Though often done with pure intention, surrogacy tourism has proven to be problematic, with numerous issues of exploitation arising. In 2002, India was the leading locale for surrogacy tourism, with a commercial industry of over 3,000 fertility clinics that was estimated to be worth $400 million.[4] Many women opted to become surrogates as they were compensated well; the surrogate wages were approximately three times greater than the monthly salary obtained by the primary earner in the surrogate's family.[4] The cost of surrogacy, however, was still far less than surrogacy expenses in other countries, like the United States.[15] While the early years of India's surrogacy tourism industry cited increased quality of life among surrogates, the increased demand heavily burdened surrogates to continually carry pregnancies, eventually leading to physical exhaustion and psychological decline.[4] This exploitation of surrogates prompted India to change its regulations, banning the foreign pursuit of surrogacy in 2014 and prohibiting all forms of commercial surrogacy in 2016.[4]

Issues of Autonomy and Other Ethical Considerations

While surrogate exploitation is one moral problem with cross-border surrogacy, an ethical question of autonomy is also relevant here. As previously mentioned, surrogacy agreements are put in place to ensure the best interests of the surrogate (and IPs) while also helping both parties maintain autonomy. This is a fine balance: When does protection come at a cost to autonomy? As evidenced above, it is easy for the practice of surrogacy to become exploitative. However, the surrogate should also be able to maintain her right to autonomy by accepting a surrogacy proposal that is financially beneficial for her.[10] The question thus arises, is all commercial surrogacy exploiting women, since it often preys on those who have little means of supporting themselves? How can we ensure that the surrogate is not merely commodified for her reproductive capabilities? English law does not view all commercial surrogacy as morally suspect, as long as it is conducted in a manner that treats the surrogate holistically in a manner that values her as a person and does not objectify her.[26] Other countries disagree and cite the exploitative nature of all commercial surrogacy as their reasons for solely permitting altruistic surrogacy arrangements.[26] Thus, the process of surrogacy poses an important ethical dilemma regarding the line between free market and exploitation as well as the question of autonomy versus security. Several other ethical dilemmas arise when pondering the question of surrogacy. Questions, such as: Who should be allowed to access surrogacy services? Should surrogacy be reserved for those requiring it as a medical intervention or should all couples, even those not experiencing infertility, be able to pursue surrogacy? How would allowing all couples to pursue surrogacy impact the availability and the cost to those who really need it? Physicians currently provide the service to all couples and do not interfere with such personal matters.

Claiming Parentage within State Law

Another important legal issue occurs once the surrogacy process is completed, and a child is born. Prior to GS, when the surrogate was genetically related to the child, issues of legal parentage were paramount. However, GS has not completely alleviated this issue. Even though both the IPs are genetically related to the child, not all countries are willing to accept them as parents, and they may not even recognize the child's birth certificate.[13] This is especially problematic in countries that forbid surrogacy. France, for example, prohibits surrogacy, and thus, refused to recognize a child's birth certificate or provide children French citizenship as a punishment for pursuing surrogacy in a foreign country.[27] However, in the 2014 landmark case of *Mennesson vs. France*, the European Court of Human Rights ruled that withholding citizenship from children born through surrogacy infringes on their personal rights to privacy and identity, and as such, citizenship must be granted.[28] While this case highlights the strides made in Europe regarding surrogacy law, other countries still have no legal framework to claiming parentage, leaving the IPs stuck in endless bureaucratic limbo.[13]

IS SURROGACY INTERNATIONALLY REGULATED?

As previously mentioned, currently there is no international or legal framework that standardizes surrogacy practice worldwide, neither in international human rights law, nor by the World Health Organization (WHO).[29] As such, countries are free to regulate surrogacy, according to their own practice.

England was among the first countries to create any form of legislation regarding surrogacy.[26] However, this law does not permit surrogacy within the country, but allows for couples pursuing surrogacy elsewhere to bring their children back to England. In 1985, as a response to the "babies for cash" crisis, the English court hastily ratified the Surrogacy Arrangements Act.[26] While it may have been one of the first modern surrogacy laws enacted, the speed in which it was put in place left many loose ends within the legislation. Furthermore, the law has not been updated for modern surrogacy, leading to additional complications. The law not only prohibits commercial surrogacy, but also deems any form of surrogacy as "unenforceable."[26] Many IPs thus commissioned surrogates internationally,[26] lending to the ethical issues of exploitation mentioned above. Interestingly, despite the restrictiveness of England's law, the actual practice of obtaining parentage from cross-border surrogacy is permissive.[26] The 1985 Report of the Committee of Inquiry into Human Fertilization and Embryology ("The Warnock Report") created a bill to assist parents undergoing IVF stating that parentage was granted to the couple who bore the child and not the gamete donor.[26,30] This proved to be problematic for couples undergoing GS, as according to this law, the gestational carrier would be the mother; parents, as a result, had to adopt their own children.[26] Thus, in 1998 a provision was added to the law granting IPs in a foreign surrogacy agreement parentage to children born from surrogates under certain conditions: The parents must live with the child in the United Kingdom; the parentage claim must be made within 6 months of the child's birth; and the surrogate must consent to the parenthood claim made by the IPs.[26] Finally, in 2008, the Human Fertilisation and Embryology Act was passed, allowing for altruistic surrogacy in England.[26]

While England had the first legislation regarding surrogacy, Israel had one of the earliest laws in supporting surrogacy. In 1996, Israel enacted a law allowing heterosexual couples to apply for surrogacy within Israel.[31] In 2018, the law was amended to allow for single women to obtain surrogacy, and was re-amended in 2022 to include single males or same-sex couples.[6] Additionally, new controversial legislation has increased surrogacy eligibility for women who cannot get pregnant due to psychiatric reasons. Notably, Israeli law only allows GS and prohibits TS. Surrogacy applications are reviewed by a committee composed of two obstetric/gynecological specialists, an internal medicine physician, a psychiatrist, a lawyer, and a clergy member of the IPs religion. However, 99.5% of surrogacy applications have been approved by this committee since the enactment of the law.[6] The surrogacy law enacted in Israel is highly specific, indicating who can act as a surrogate (including minimum and maximum age), maximal compensation allowed to the surrogate, and clauses that must be included in the surrogacy contract, such as ensuring proper medical care for the surrogate.[6] While this thorough surrogacy process, including the application and contracting processes, are in place to ensure greater protection and an optimal surrogacy process, it increases the bureaucratic hurdles needed to obtain surrogacy. Many couples, therefore, still choose to pursue surrogacy elsewhere, where surrogacy is less regulated.

Other countries vary across the spectrum of prohibiting all forms of surrogacy, including cross-border surrogacy, to permit any types of surrogacies including commercial surrogacy. Additionally, variation exists within the law regarding what parts of the surrogacy process should be regulated. As previously mentioned, all parts of the Israeli surrogacy process are highly regulated. Contrarily, though Canadian regulations allow for altruistic surrogacy, they do not interfere with the surrogacy contract and are not litigated.[7] This discrepancy enables the surrogacy tourism industry, as people will procure surrogacy arrangements in the country whose regulations suit them best. International human rights associations and the WHO should work together to enact global surrogacy regulations to help provide this important medical intervention in a safe and optimal way for all surrogates and IPs alike.

There is a dire need for surrogacy to be Internationally regulated.

CONCLUSION

Surrogacy is a critical medical intervention to individuals and couples who desire offspring and cannot achieve it for any reasons. ART has allowed for GS, allowing couples to have biological offspring in previously impossible conditions. Common reasons for pursuing surrogacy include single parenthood, same sex couples, uterine abnormalities, prior gestational complications, and RPL. With so many factors involved in maintaining the quality of the surrogacy process and the inherent interconnection between the IPs and the surrogate, obtaining surrogacy can be long and tedious, with numerous implications on mental and physical well-being of all parties involved. While surrogacy as a medical intervention has helped so many, it is not without complication. There are several legal and ethical issues that arise, especially regarding exploitation, autonomy, and obtaining parentage. The lack of international surrogacy regulation only exacerbates these roadblocks. With the advancement of surrogacy as an intervention, it is critical to instate global surrogacy laws to protect the rights of parents and women worldwide. As part of this global surrogacy initiative, we call on organizations, such as ESHRE, ASRM, and WHO to regulate surrogacy processes, and define parentage antenatally under one uniform standard that can be implemented worldwide.

REFERENCES

1. Shah K, Bhat P, Bhat R, Sultana R. An update on recurrent early pregnancy loss: causes, controversies and cure. J Clin Diagn Res. 2018;12(10):QE01-5.
2. Yale Medicine. (2022). Surrogacy. [online] Available from www.yalemedicine.org/conditions/gestational-surrogacy [Last accessed December, 2024].
3. Payne JG, Korolczuk E, Mezinska S. Surrogacy relationships: a critical interpretative review. Ups J Med Sci. 2020;125(2): 183-91.

4. Patel NH, Jadeja YD, Bhadarka HK, Patel MN, Patel NH, Sodagar NR. Insight into different aspects of surrogacy practices. J Hum Reprod Sci. 2018;11(3):212-8.
5. Perkins KM, Boulet SL, Jamieson DJ, Kissin DM, National Assisted Reproductive Technology Surveillance System (NASS) Group. Trends and outcomes of gestational surrogacy in the United States. Fertil Steril. 2016;106(2):435-42.e2.
6. State of Israel Ministry of Health. (2023). Surrogacy in Israel. [online] Available from www.gov.il/he/service/embryo-carrying [Last accessed December, 2024].
7. Dar S, Lazar T, Swanson S, Silverman J, Wasser C, Moskovtsev SI, et al. Assisted reproduction involving gestational surrogacy: an analysis of the medical, psychosocial and legal issues: experience from a large surrogacy program. Hum Reprod. 2015;30(2):345-52.
8. Cabra R, Alduncin A, Cabra JR, Ek LH, Briceño M, Mendoza PB. Gestational surrogacy. Medical, psychological and legal aspects: 9 years of experience in Mexico. Hum Reprod Open. 2018;2018(1):hox029.
9. Agius A, Cajella-Agius J. Infertility, repeated loss, and surrogacy. In: Xuereb RB, Jomeen J (Eds). Perspectives on Midwifery and Parenthood. Cham, Switzerland: Springer International Publishing; 2022. pp. 67-82.
10. Bashiri A, Cherlow Y, Kresch-Jaffe T. Surrogacy: an important pathway to parenthood. A call for international standardization. J Reprod Immunol. 2024;163:104247.
11. Shenfield F, Pennings G, Cohen J, Devroey P, de Wert G, Tarlatzis B, et al. ESHRE task force on ethics and law 10: surrogacy. Hum Reprod. 2005;20(10):2705-7.
12. Practice Committee of the American Society for Reproductive Medicine, Practice Committee of the Society for Assisted Reproductive Technology. Recommendations for practices using gestational carriers: a committee opinion. Fertil Steril. 2022;118(1):65-74.
13. Shakargy S. Choice of law for surrogacy agreements: in the in-between of status and contract. J Priv Int Law. 2020; 16(1):138-62.
14. World Center of Baby (WCOB). (2023). Surrogacy in Israel. Surrogacy in Israel: costs, legal status, and laws. How much does surrogacy cost in Israel? [online] Available from https://worldcenterofbaby.com/countries/israel/#:~:text=How%20Much%20Does%20Surrogacy%20Cost,is%20up%20to%20EUR%2070%2C000. [Last accessed December, 2024]
15. Jadva V, Prosser H, Gamble N. Cross-border and domestic surrogacy in the UK context: an exploration of practical and legal decision-making. Hum Fertil (Camb). 2021;24 (2):93-104.
16. Imrie S, Jadva V. The long-term experiences of surrogates: relationships and contact with surrogacy families in genetic and gestational surrogacy arrangements. Reprod Biomed Online. 2014;29(4):424-35.
17. Jadva V, Murray C, Lycett E, MacCallum F, Golombok S. Surrogacy: the experiences of surrogate mothers. Hum Reprod. 2003;18(10):2196-204.
18. Hadizadeh-Talasaz F, Roudsari RL, Simbar M. Decision for disclosure: the experiences of Iranian infertile couples undergoing assisted reproductive donation procedures. Human Fertil (Camb). 2015;18(4):265-75.
19. Donnenfeld SR, Mehta A. The urologist's guide to religion and male factor fertility treatment. Urology. 2022;167:128-31.
20. Ghodrati F. A comparative study of surrogacy rights in Iran and European countries, a review article. Ethics Med Pub Health. 2023;27:100880.
21. Cherlow Y. The Ethical Protection of the Surrogate UNESCO chair in Bioethics, 10th world Conference on Bioethics, Medical Ethics and Health Law Zefat Bioethics Forum Jerusalem Jan 2015 Book of Abstracts.
22. Deri RRY. (2024). Permission for married women to act as surrogates. [online] Available from https://daat.ac.il/daat/psk/psk.asp?id=5605 [Last accessed December, 2024].
23. Sherlow RY. (2024). Rabbi Yuval Sherlow claims that it is time to update surrogacy laws. The Question is How? [online] Available from https://healthy.walla.co.il/item/3662085 [Last accessed December, 2024].
24. Birenbaum-Carmeli D. Thirty-five years of assisted reproductive technologies in Israel. Reprod Biomed Soc Online. 2016;2:16-23.
25. Piersanti V, Consalvo F, Signore F, Del Rio A, Zaami S. Surrogacy and "procreative tourism". What does the future hold from the ethical and legal perspectives? Medicina (Kaunas). 2021;57(1):47.
26. Fenton-Glynn C. Outsourcing ethical dilemmas: regulating international surrogacy arrangements. Med L Rev. 2016; 24(1):59-74.
27. Dickenson D, van Beers B. Surrogacy: new challenges to law and ethics. New Bioeth. 2020;26(4):293-7.
28. Kulkarni R. Ethical dilemmas in surrogacy. Hektoen Int. 2015;7(1).
29. UNICEF. (2022). Key considerations: children's rights and surrogacy - briefing note. [online] Available from https://www.unicef.org/media/115331/file [Last accessed December, 2024].
30. Priest JA. The report of the Warnock committee on human fertilisation and embryology. Mod Law Rev. 1985; 48(1):73-85.
31. State of Israel Ministry of Health. (1996). Law on agreements for the carrying of fetuses (Confirmation of the agreement and the status of the newborn), 5556. [online] Available from https://www.gov.il/he/pages/poriut05 [Last accessed December, 2024].

CHAPTER 60

Role of Artificial Intelligence

Valentina Bruno, Martina Betti, Matteo Pallocca, Enrico Vizza, Adalgisa Pietropolli, Emilio Piccione

ABSTRACT

Given the diversity of diagnostic factors and cellular changes identified in recurrent pregnancy loss (RPL) patients, it will be wise to apply advanced machine learning tools to accurately interpret data and help to arrive at valid conclusions. The field of genomics, epigenomics, transcriptomics and metabolomics is playing an expanded role in RPL research. It will not be humanly possible to combine clinical characteristics, diagnostic results, genetic mutations, and omics data to link the pieces of the jigsaw puzzle of unexplained RPL. We now have the tools at our disposal and are sitting at the brink of solving the puzzle of unexplained RPL with the help of artificial intelligence (AI).

Keywords: Artificial intelligence, Machine learning, ML, RPL, Advanced neural network, ANN, Genomics, Epigenomics, Transcriptomics, Metabolomics.

INTRODUCTION

Recurrent pregnancy loss (RPL) is a much debated field for both clinical practice and research issues. No shared agreement has been reached in terms of definition, terminology, and etiological factors to be studied and therapeutical approach to be applied. The heterogeneity in approach across different research groups leads to a lack in RPL scientific research and represents a limitation in reaching an evidence-based level, which is required to translate evidence into strong recommendations for clinical practice.

In the era of reproducible, multicentric, and multiomics studies, the RPL field has lagged behind. From a bioinformatics point of view, most RPL experimental data is based on either signal-based omics (e.g., microarrays) or targeted phenotypic profiles (e.g., flow cytometry). This kind of data shows low reproducibility and can be summed up as a mere phenotypic description (such as the cytokinome), without reconstructing the entire cascades of biological mechanisms behind it. These limitations make available data less comparable because of biotechnological-intrinsic noise and batch effect as shown by many meta-analyses.

There is a need to look at this disease from new and innovative perspectives. Bioinformatics tools, machine learning (ML), and advanced neural network (ANN) methods have a high potential in extracting hidden and relevant relationships from multiomic data; however, these approaches are highly demanding in terms of data numerosity and data quality. Therefore, while bioinformatics tools and artificial intelligence (AI) could revolutionize RPL research in terms of etiology, pathogenesis, and therapeutic options, their application is currently unfeasible due to the nature of data produced in this field.

To summarize, the main limitations arise from the following:

- Quantitative/qualitative limitations of the cohorts
- Data format incompatibility with standard bioinformatics tools
- Lack of dedicated databases
- Lack of reproducibility (e.g., microarray dataset)
- Lack of comparable or aggregable dataset due to heterogeneity in RPL definition criteria, diagnostic workup to perform, and etiological factors.

PRINCIPLES OF ARTIFICIAL INTELLIGENCE SUITABLE DATA SETS

Artificial intelligence encompasses a range of technologies and methodologies that extend beyond traditional statistical analysis, offering unique advantages in handling complex datasets and predictive modeling. At its core, AI leverages algorithms to enable machines to learn from data, make decisions, and predict outcomes without explicit programming for each task. This is particularly evident in ML, a subset of AI, where systems learn patterns from data and improve over time. One principal advantage of AI over traditional statistics is its ability to manage and extract insights from high-dimensional data—datasets with many variables—more effectively. Traditional statistical methods often struggle with the "curse of dimensionality," where increased data dimensions lead to exponential growth in computational complexity. AI, particularly through deep learning models, can navigate these complexities by identifying intricate structures in large datasets, which would be infeasible with conventional approaches. AI also introduces automation and scalability in data analysis, enabling rapid processing of vast datasets with minimal human intervention. For ML models to function effectively, the quality and characteristics of the dataset used are crucial. Following are several mandatory requirements for a dataset to be suitable for ML applications:

- *Sufficient volume:* The dataset must be large enough to represent the complexities of the real world that the model is expected to handle. Insufficient data can lead to underfitting, where the model fails to capture important patterns. The required size of the dataset can vary depending on the complexity of the problem and the type of ML model being used.
- *Quality and accuracy:* The dataset should be free from errors, biases, and inconsistencies. Accurate data ensures that the model's predictions are based on correct and relevant information, which is critical for the model's performance and trustworthiness.
- *Relevance:* The data used must be relevant to the specific problem or decision-making process at hand. Irrelevant or extraneous features in the data can confuse the model and degrade its performance. Although not strictly a requirement of the dataset itself, effective feature engineering is crucial for enhancing model performance.
- *Labeling for supervised learning:* In supervised learning, where the model predicts an output based on input features, the dataset must include correct labels or outputs associated with each input. Properly labeled data is crucial for training the model to make accurate predictions.
- *Balance and representation:* The dataset should adequately represent all classes or outcomes in a balanced way, especially in classification tasks. Imbalanced datasets can lead to models that are biased toward the more frequent classes, resulting in poor generalization on less frequent classes.
- *Diversity:* Datasets should capture the diversity of scenarios that the model will encounter in actual use. This includes variations in data that mimic real-world changes and challenges, helping the model to be robust and perform well under different conditions.

Ensuring that these requirements are met not only enhances the performance of ML models but also contributes to their fairness, transparency, and acceptance in practical applications.

ARTIFICIAL INTELLIGENCE APPLICATION IN OMICS AND CLINICAL SETTING

Artificial intelligence in medicine encompasses the use of ML, deep learning, and other computational methods to analyze large datasets, make predictions, and assist in clinical decisions. AI applications range from image analysis in radiology and pathology to predictive analytics in patient monitoring.

Genomics

In genomics, AI is instrumental in analyzing vast amounts of deoxyribonucleic acid (DNA) sequencing data to identify genome-wide variations or single mutations that could be linked to diseases. AI models, particularly those based on deep learning, are adept at sifting through high-dimensional genomic data to find patterns that may escape traditional analysis. Key applications of AI in genomics are (1) variant interpretation, for which ML helps in interpreting genetic mutations and predicting their impact on diseases by integrating multiple annotation resources and different strategies of scoring and (2) genome wide associations, which is an intrinsically complex problem for which the employment of AI has been proven to be particularly useful.

Transcriptomics

Transcriptomics, the study of ribonucleic acid (RNA) transcripts produced by the genome, benefits immensely from AI. During the past 15 years, total RNA-sequencing (RNA-seq) approaches have led to great discoveries in terms of macroscopic profiling of diseases. However, the topic has been quickly exhausted and, nowadays, RNA-seq hardly provides sufficient information by itself, especially for novel biomarkers discovery. Since RNA-seq-derived results often present a great number of false positives, many downstream approaches can be used to effectively use RNA-seq data (e.g., epigenetic regulation mechanisms and proteomics). Whenever this is not feasible or desired, RNA-seq data can be improved by complex data structures and ML-aided approaches. Transcriptomic data can be injected with prior knowledge to derive more meaningful and interpretable information. For instance, the expression profile of specific immune cell types can be utilized to estimate immune cell abundances within a given tissue (e.g., CIBERSORTx, xCell) thanks to expectation maximization algorithms (EM models), dimensionality reduction techniques, and other types of supervised classification approaches. Transcriptomics data can also be represented through a more complex but efficient data structure, such as a graph, which can then either be explored in its topology, to gain a better representation of the expression profile clusters and interactions across sets of genes, or be classified through graph neural networks.

Other Omics

In the field of proteomics, ML has played and keeps playing an essential role in unraveling the high complexity and degree of freedom of protein 3D conformation and protein interaction prediction. In epigenomics, graph data structure, and specifically graph topology, is currently being tested as an efficient data representation strategy.

Clinical Setting

Lastly, ML can be applied to low-complexity settings, as in the case of outcome prediction models that uniquely rely on clinically annotated samples, with an order of features of 10–50 features. In the previous cases, ML and deep learning are essential to capture complex patterns from high-dimensionality data. In the latter cases ML algorithms serve as an integrative and weighted evaluation of the relevant parameters for a given disease to predict a clinical outcome of interest, possibly in a human-interpretable way. In this case, "lighter" models (lower number of trainable parameters) are preferred to favor interpretability and avoid overfitting.

ARTIFICIAL INTELLIGENCE APPLICATION IN RECURRENT PREGNANCY LOSS: OUTCOME PREDICTION MODELS AND OMICS BIOMARKERS

Omics Datasets and Biomarkers

Along with hormonal and metabolic factors, immunological dysregulation is a critical aspect to be considered for explaining RPL. The immune system must balance tolerance to the semiallogenic fetus while protecting against infections; therefore, alterations in this balance may compromise implantation. More specifically, literature has shown that across immunological factors, the cytokine profile and natural killer (NK) cells activity may play a crucial role.[1] To investigate these factors by using reproducible and robust approaches, the employment of omics data is essential. All studies regarding the attempt to use AI methods on omics, such as predictive ML models and/or bioinformatics tools, or even advanced statistical analysis, such as enrichment analysis of differentially expressed genes (DEGs), are limited by low numerical power and cohorts' numerosity.[2] For instance, very few datasets reach a minimum of 10 patients per group: RNA-seq on 10 RPL and 10 infertile (FASTQ available at SRP052612) and microarray gene expression from 24 RPL and 24 controls endometrial samples (series matrix GSE165004). Moreover, only one RPL dataset of single cell-RNA-seq exists, which provides the gene expression levels in the decidua of three RPL samples versus three control samples. The most useful dataset regarding RPL (series matrix GSE165004) comes from the Gene Expression Omnibus (GEO) database (https://www.ncbi.nlm.nih.gov/gds) of the National Center for Biotechnology Information, which provides comprehensive expression profiles for a wide range of diseases, enabling researchers to conduct diverse data analyses.

Through their analysis of the GEO dataset, Chen et al. identified *Atp6v1g3* as a key gene associated with recurrent spontaneous miscarriage;[3] while Yujia Luo, by using functional enrichment analysis on the screened DEGs, three ML techniques to generate the optimally characterized genes (OFGs), and CIBERSORTx analysis to examine the immune infiltration and investigate the correlation between OFGs and immune cells, revealed that *ZNF90*, *TPT1P8*, *FGF2*, and *FAM166B* are potential RPL biomarkers, offering new avenues for research into the molecular mechanisms of RPL immune modulation and early detection. Recently, Wei et al. showed that *WBP11*, *ACTR2*, and *NCSTN* were identified as diagnostic biomarkers of RPL and that there is an imbalance in immune cell infiltration in RPL, by using the same dataset with a subsequent validation cohort.[4] In this case, a wide combination of bioinformatics and ML approaches has been applied: Differential expression analysis enrichment, weighted coexpression network analysis (WGCNA), and

CMap for the bioinformatics part, and a set of different algorithms such as LASSO (least absolute shrinkage and selection operator) regression, support vector machine-recursive feature elimination (SVM-RFE), Random Forest, and neural networks.

Seven macrophage-related genes closely associated with recurrent miscarriage were screened and experimentally validated by Gustafsson et al. using single-cell sequencing technology combined with comprehensive bioinformatics analysis, which may have potential value in characterizing more specifically immune cells of the decidua.[5] In this case, the exploratory cohort used is too small to reach any significant conclusion.

Furthermore, a noninvasive source, such as menstrual blood, has been shown by Tsang et al.[6] to hold several opportunities to assess and monitor reproductive health by using ML algorithms. A combination of immune subsets (Ki67+CD8+ T cells, regulatory T cells, CD27+ B cells, NK bright cells, and CD24HiCD38Hi B cells) allows for robust identification of immune parameters with possible diagnostic value in RPL.

Omics and Artificial Intelligence

All studies that used omics and AI tools have reached different but promising results, especially in the investigation of etiological factors potentially involved in unexplained RPL cases, mostly including immunological features. However, none of these studies have seen a real-life application due to their low numerosity and the impossibility of validating such results on external cohorts.

Bruno et al. attempted to develop a decision support system tool that categorizes RPL patients into various risk categories through a diagnostic process.[7] This process aims to confirm its effectiveness for accurate prognosis and potential treatment strategies. The diagnostic workup they established includes more features than those in the ESHRE (European Society of Human Reproduction and Embryology) guidelines, achieving greater accuracy than the guidelines themselves. The predictive model from this study effectively assessed miscarriage risk in immune-abnormal pregnancies, outperforming the pregnancy risk management system and proving economically beneficial. Wu et al. have produced a model to effectively assess miscarriage risk in immune-abnormal pregnancies, outperforming the pregnancy risk management system and proving economically beneficial.[8] These and other studies have gathered large cohorts and shown promising outcomes, though they have included important clinical features while entirely overlooking the omics perspective, missing opportunities to shed light on unexplained RPL cases.

Studies are still being conducted to integrate the clinical factors and the omics feature through ML but those still rely on the same set of heterogeneous and scarce datasets.[9] Studies that use both AI and advanced bioinformatics tools have the highest potential in the investigation of etiological factors potentially involved in unexplained RPL cases, mostly including immunological features. However, none of these studies have seen a real-life application due to their low numerosity and the impossibility of validating such results on external cohorts.

Imaging and Artificial Intelligence

Several diagnostic techniques leverage imaging modalities, such as hysteroscopy, ultrasound, and flow cytometry.[10-13] These methods have progressively aligned with high-quality and standardized formats, making them highly suitable for ML research applications. The transition toward standardized imaging data has opened avenues for more robust and scalable ML models, which can be trained with a higher degree of accuracy and generalizability. In the context of endometrial health, significant progress has been made in utilizing imaging data for ML applications. Classifiers have been extensively trained and tested on datasets derived from radiology and hysteroscopy. This research has helped in the early detection and classification of various endometrial conditions, such as benign and malignant lesions or infertile status, enhancing the predictive capabilities of medical diagnostics.

However, in the domain of RPL, the integration of imaging-based ML approaches has been relatively focused. Additionally, ultrasound imaging has played a crucial role in monitoring the growth of the gestational sac, which is pivotal in the early stages of pregnancy. Through ML models trained on ultrasound datasets, researchers have been able to predict and monitor the viability of pregnancies.[14] Despite these advancements, the overall application of imaging in RPL research remains limited, with a notable lack of focus on hysteroscopic data. Given the potential of hysteroscopic imaging in enhancing our understanding and management of RPL, there is a compelling case for increased research in this area. By incorporating hysteroscopic and ultrasound data into ML models, researchers could unlock new diagnostic pathways and treatment options, ultimately improving outcomes for patients experiencing RPLs. Most notably, cytometry-based imaging has been employed to monitor systemic immunity—an essential factor in the etiology of RPL. Research in this area has leveraged flow cytometry to understand immune cell dynamics that could influence pregnancy outcomes.[15]

FURTHER PERSPECTIVES OF ARTIFICIAL INTELLIGENCE IN RECURRENT PREGNANCY LOSS

Although AI's potential in genomics and transcriptomics is immense, several challenges remain, which are as follows:

- *Data quality and quantity:* High-quality, annotated omics datasets are crucial, and their scarcity can limit AI's effectiveness.
- *Interpretability:* AI models, especially deep learning, often act as "black boxes," making clinical adoption challenging due to the lack of transparent decision-making processes. Results and advantages need to prove essential, otherwise their integration into the clinical practice will be unjustified.
- *Standardization of data sharing platforms:* The Cancer Genome Atlas and other similar consortia have reached astonishing results in cancer research by setting a standard for open data. Following this example, other conditions may be approached in a similar way to allow dataset aggregation and avoid clinical annotation heterogeneity.
- *Integrative omics approaches:* Combining genomics, transcriptomics, proteomics, and metabolomics to gain a comprehensive understanding of the biological pathways involved in RPL
- *Personalized medicine:* Tailoring treatments based on individual genetic backgrounds, such as using targeted therapies for specific genetic mutations or immunological treatments based on immune profiling.

CONCLUSION

Innovative research approaches and settings, by using high-dimensional data enabling the employment of advanced AI modeling techniques, could improve RPL research to reach a precision/personalized medicine level, as already experimented in the cancer field. Nevertheless, standardization in RPL research among all different groups—in terms of definition, terminology, etiological factors to be studied, and therapeutical approach to be applied—should be pursued to build proper RPL databases to be analyzed by all new methodological approaches. RPL research should aim to reach cancer research standards to be suitable for an extended AI methods application.

REFERENCES

1. Tilburgs T, Claas FHJ, Scherjon SA. Elsevier trophoblast research award lecture: unique properties of decidual T cells and their role in immune regulation during human pregnancy. Placenta. 2010;31:S82-6.
2. Betti M, Vizza E, Piccione E, Pietropolli A, Chiofalo B, Pallocca M, et al. Towards reproducible research in recurrent pregnancy loss immunology: learning from cancer microenvironment deconvolution. Front Immunol. 2023;14:1082087.
3. Gellersen B, Brosens IA, Brosens JJ. Decidualization of the human endometrium: mechanisms, functions, and clinical perspectives. Semin Reprod Med. 2007;25(6):445-53.
4. Wei C, Wei Y, Cheng J, Tan X, Zhou Z, Lin S, et al. Identification and verification of diagnostic biomarkers in recurrent pregnancy loss via machine learning algorithm and WGCNA. Front Immunol. 2023;14:1241816.
5. Gustafsson C, Mjösberg J, Matussek A, Geffers R, Matthiesen L, Berg G, et al. Gene expression profiling of human decidual macrophages: evidence for immunosuppressive phenotype. PLoS One. 2008;3(4):e2078.
6. Tsang HF, Cheung YS, Yu CA, Chan CS, Wong CT, Yim KA, et al. Menstrual blood as a diagnostic specimen for human papillomavirus genotyping and genital tract infection using next-generation sequencing as a novel diagnostic tool. Diagnostics (Basel). 2024;14(7):686.
7. Bruno V, D'Orazio M, Ticconi C, Abundo P, Riccio S, Martinelli E, et al. Machine learning (ML) based-method applied in recurrent pregnancy loss (RPL) patients diagnostic work-up: a potential innovation in common clinical practice. Sci Rep. 2020;10(1):7970.
8. Wu Y, Yu X, Li M, Zhu J, Yue J, Wang Y, et al. Risk prediction model based on machine learning for predicting miscarriage among pregnant patients with immune abnormalities. Front Pharmacol. 2024;15:1366529.
9. Luo Y, Zhou Y. Identification of novel biomarkers and immune infiltration features of recurrent pregnancy loss by machine learning. Sci Rep. 2023;13(1):10751.
10. Neofytou MS, Tanos V, Pattichis MS, Kyriacou EC, Pattichis CS, Schizas CN. Color multiscale texture classification of hysteroscopy images of the endometrium. Annu Int Conf IEEE Eng Med Biol Soc. 2008;2008:1226-9.
11. Kitaya K, Yasuo T, Yamaguchi T, Morita Y, Hamazaki A, Murayama S, et al. Construction of deep learning-based

convolutional neural network model for automatic detection of fluid hysteroscopic endometrial micropolyps in infertile women with chronic endometritis. Eur J Obstet Gynecol Reprod Biol. 2024;297:249-53.

12. Takahashi Y, Sone K, Noda K, Yoshida K, Toyohara Y, Kato K, et al. Automated system for diagnosing endometrial cancer by adopting deep-learning technology in hysteroscopy. PLoS One. 2021;16(3):e0248526.
13. Zhang Y, Wang Z, Zhang J, Wang C, Wang Y, Chen H, et al. Deep learning model for classifying endometrial lesions. J Transl Med. 2021;19(1):10.
14. Wang Y, Zhang Q, Yin C, Chen L, Yang Z, Jia S, et al. Automated prediction of early spontaneous miscarriage based on the analyzing ultrasonographic gestational sac imaging by the convolutional neural network: a case-control and cohort study. BMC Pregnancy Childbirth. 2022;22(1):621.
15. Benner M, Feyaerts D, Lopez-Rincon A, van der Heijden OWH, van der Hoorn ML, Joosten I, et al. A combination of immune cell types identified through ensemble machine learning strategy detects altered profile in recurrent pregnancy loss: a pilot study. F S Sci. 2022;3(2):166-73.

Appendices

APPENDIX 1

Recurrent Pregnancy Loss Cases

CASE 1: RECURRENT PREGNANCY LOSS WITH RESISTANT ANTIPHOSPHOLIPID SYNDROME AND SUCCESSFUL ADDITIONAL TREATMENT WITH HYDROXYCHLOROQUINE

Asher Bashiri, Judah Benjamin Smith, Israel David Gabay

A 34-year-old female presented with a history of three first-trimester pregnancy losses. Her medical background was unremarkable, with no other medical conditions, surgeries, medications, allergies, or known environmental exposures. The family history revealed that her mother had one miscarriage after two successful pregnancies, and her sister had a normal pregnancy.

The patient experienced menarche at the age of 12 and had a regular menstrual cycle of 4/28 days. Her pregnancy history included three losses: The first at 7 weeks treated with misoprostol, the second at 11 weeks treated with dilation and curettage (D&C), and the third at 13 weeks also treated with D&C. All three pregnancies resulted in fetal death without complications during the treatments.

On physical examination, the patient appeared well with normal vital signs (heart rate, blood pressure, and body temperature). She weighed 85 kg, had a height of 1.65 m, and had a body mass index (BMI) of 31, indicating obesity. An anatomical investigation showed a normal uterine cavity on 3D ultrasound. A full evaluation for recurrent pregnancy loss (RPL) was performed **(Box 1)**. Lupus anticoagulant (LAC) was abnormally elevated (1.4) in the first blood samples and was also elevated 12 weeks later (1.5) upon repeated tests.

The diagnosis for this patient was *antiphospholipid syndrome (APS)*, confirmed by two positive *LAC tests* 12 weeks apart. The management plan included daily low molecular weight heparin (LMWH) 40 mg from the first positive beta-human chorionic gonadotropin (β-hCG) until delivery, aspirin (ASA) 100 mg daily when planning a pregnancy or upon a positive β-hCG until delivery, dydrogesterone 10 mg twice daily from 2 to 3 days after ovulation or upon positive β-hCG until 20 weeks' gestation, *vitamin D supplementation* (1,000 IU/day), and folic acid supplementation (5 mg/day starting 3 months before a planned pregnancy), healthy lifestyle habits including regular physical activity, maintaining normal BMI, emotional support, and stress reduction were recommended before a new pregnancy.

BOX 1: Patient serum lab values.

Acquired thrombophilia:
- **Lupus anticoagulant (LAC)—1.4 (0.8–1.20 ratio). After 12 weeks—1.5**
- Anticardiolipin (ACL) antibodies IgM—0.6 U/mL (0–20 U/mL)
- Anticardiolipin antibodies IgA—0.7 U/mL (0–20 U/mL)
- Anticardiolipin antibodies IgG—normal 4 U/mL (0–20 U/mL)
- Anti-β2 glycoprotein 1 (aβ2GP1) IgG—normal 5 U/mL (0–20 U/mL)
- Anti-β2 glycoprotein 1 (aβ2GP1) IgM—2 U/mL (0–20 U/mL)

Hereditary thrombophilia:
- Factor V Leiden mutation—normal
- Prothrombin mutation—normal
- Antithrombin III—114% (80–120%)
- Protein S—74% (60–150%)
- Protein C—81% (70–150%)

Hormonal and metabolic:
- Thyroid-stimulating hormone (TSH)—1.9 mum/L—(0.2–2.5 mU/L)
- Antithyroglobulin—<20 IU/mL (10–40 IU/mL)
- Antithyroid peroxidase—negative >35 U/mL
- Vitamin D levels—*70 nmol/L* (recommended level 75–125 nmol/L)
- Fasting glucose—82 mg/dL (>95 mg/dL)
- HbA1c—5.2% (normal range <5.4%)
- Prolactin—18 ng/mL

Immunologic:
- Rheumatoid factor—13 IU/mL (0–30 IU/mL)
- Antinuclear antibody (ANA)—negative

Genetic:
- Paternal karyotype—46,XY
- Maternal karyotype—46,XX

Three months later the patient's fourth pregnancy had normal initial follow-up evaluations. However, at the 13-week ultrasound, no fetal heartbeat was detected. Genetic testing from the product of conception (POC) showed a normal karyotype (XX). Despite following the known treatment regimen for APS, the patient had another fourth pregnancy loss.

Since the fourth pregnancy was unsuccessful and the patient is considered to have *Refractory APS*, a decision was made to add hydroxychloroquine 400 mg daily. This treatment was started 3 months before the next planned pregnancy after normal ophthalmologic examination. The patient was placed under very close follow-up prenatal care including blood tests, nuchal translucency anatomy scans, triple test, amniocentesis, glucose challenge test, at 27 weeks immunization for pertussis, and fetal weight estimation at 32 weeks. All showed normal findings. She also had blood tests for anti-XA activity and LMWH dosage was increased to 60 mg accordingly at 24 weeks gestational age.

Induction of labor was performed at 38 weeks' gestation after stopping LMWH and ASA for 24 hours, resulting in a normal spontaneous vaginal delivery with a healthy baby girl weighing 3,100 g with an Apgar score of 9/10. The woman renewed the treatment medication with ASA and LMWH the day after the delivery during the 6 weeks of the puerperium.

DISCUSSION

This woman was diagnosed with antiphospholipid antibodies (APLA) syndrome due to her history of three consecutive pregnancy losses and a positive LAC test.

APS can be divided into three different criteria based on the Sydney criteria.[7]

1. Obstetric antiphospholipid syndrome (OAPS), obstetric morbidity APS (OMAPS), and noncriteria APS (NC-APS), each with specific clinical and laboratory requirements. OAPS is diagnosed when a patient meets the Sydney criteria.[1]
2. OMAPS is diagnosed when there is incomplete clinical data; it includes patients who have experienced obstetric complications suggestive of APS but do not meet the full clinical criteria. This category captures those with recurrent early miscarriages or severe preeclampsia occurring later in pregnancy, which may still be linked to antiphospholipid antibodies but lack sufficient laboratory confirmation.
3. NC-APS includes patients who present with clinical manifestations consistent with APS but have incomplete laboratory data. This can occur when only one antiphospholipid antibody test is positive when

BOX 2: Clinical and laboratory descriptions for OAPS and its variants OMAPS and NC-OAPS.[1]

OAPS

Clinical criteria:

- More than equal to three consecutive miscarriages before week 10 of gestation
- At least one fetal loss after week 10 of gestation
- At least one premature birth before week 34 of gestation due to PE/eclampsia or placental insufficiency

Laboratory criteria:

- Two LA positive tests at least 12 weeks apart
- Two IgG or IgM aCL positive tests at least 12 weeks apart
- Two egg or IgM aβ32GPI positive tests at least 12 weeks apart

OMAPS

Clinical criteria:

- Two consecutive unexplained miscarriages of well-formed embryos
- Three or more non-consecutive miscarriages of well-formed embryos
- PE/eclampsia after week 34 of gestation or at puerperium
- Placental abruption
- Late premature birth
- Premature rupture of membranes
- Unexplained recurrent implantation failure in in vitro fertilization*

Laboratory criteria: Fulfill the laboratory criteria described for OAPS

Clinical criteria: Fulfill the clinical criteria described for OAPS

NC-OAPS

Laboratory criteria:

- Positivity for LA, aCL or aβ2GPI only detected once
- Low positive IgG/IgM aCL or aβ2GPI titers
- Persistent positivity for non-criteria aPL, including IgA-aCL and aβ2GPI
- Resistance to Annexin A5 anticoagulant activity
- Thrombocytopenia

*Failure of at least three embryo transfers of good-quality embryos. (aCL: IgG/IgM anticardiolipin antibodies; aβ2GPI: IgG/IgM antiβ2-glycoprotein I antibodies; aPL: antiphospholipid antibodies; LA: lupus anticoagulant; OAPS: obstetric antiphospholipid syndrome; NC-OAPS: noncriteria obstetric antiphospholipid syndrome; OMAPS: obstetric morbidity antiphospholipid syndrome; PE: preeclampsia)

the antibody titers are low, or if there are nonstandard antibodies involved.

This classification helps identify and manage patients who are at risk but do not fulfill the classical diagnostic criteria.[1] Given the detailed history and investigations; this patient falls into the category of obstetric APS (OAPS) because she fulfilled the Sydney criteria without previous thrombotic events **(Box 2)**.

Hydroxychloroquine was considered because it has been documented to have been successful in the treatment of APS. A study conducted by Mekinian et al. has demonstrated the efficacy of hydroxychloroquine in preventing RPL in patients with refractory obstetrical anti-APS.[2] The study showed that the rate of pregnancy loss significantly decreased from 86% (12 out of 14 pregnancies) to 29% (four out of 14 pregnancies) among women with refractory obstetrical APS. It was also considered based on recommendations in the literature as a "potential add-on treatment for recurrent thrombosis despite therapeutic-dose anticoagulant therapy (See Chapter 26)."

REFERENCES

1. Alijotas-Reig J, Esteve-Valverde E, Anunciación-Llunell A, Marques-Soares J, Pardos-Gea J, Miró-Mur F. Pathogenesis, diagnosis and management of Obstetric Antiphospholipid Syndrome: A comprehensive review. J Clin Med. 2022; 11(3):675.
2. Mekinian A, Lazzaroni MG, Kuzenko A, Alijotas-Reig J, Ruffatti A, Levy P, et al. The efficacy of hydroxychloroquine for obstetrical outcome in anti-phospholipid syndrome: Data from a European Multicenter Retrospective Study. Autoimmun Revi. 2015;14(6):498-502.

CASE 2: MULTIPLE EARLY AND LATE MISCARRIAGES WITH MULTIPLE ETIOLOGICAL FACTORS

Mala Arora

A 31-year-old married for 11 years G8A6L1.

First pregnancy: 5 weeks—no cardiac activity—medically terminated.

Second pregnancy: 12 weeks—missed miscarriage—suction evacuation.

Third pregnancy 2007: 6 weeks—no cardiac activity—suction evacuation.

Fourth pregnancy: 26 weeks—preterm premature rupture of membranes—female fetus—neonatal death [was empirically on low-dose aspirin (LDA) and LMWH in this pregnancy].

Registered to our clinic after her fourth pregnancy loss.

Complete RPL workup done.

Diagnosed: Septate uterus on 3D ultrasound scan (USS).

Hysteroscopic resection of a Broad Fundal Septum was done.

She was APLA positive and had moderate hyper-homocysteinemia with activated protein C Resistance and a family history of thrombophilia.

Fifth pregnancy after septum resection—full term lower segment cesarean section (LSCS) for fetal growth restriction—female baby 2.2 kg A and W (was on LDA and therapeutic dose of LMWH)

Sixth pregnancy—12 weeks miscarriage while on LDA and therapeutic dose of LMWH.

Seventh pregnancy—14 weeks miscarriage while on LDA and therapeutic dose of LMWH.

A relook hysteroscopy was done 2 cm residual fundal septum was seen which was resected.

Eighth pregnancy—she was on a therapeutic dose of LMWH and LDA. At 14 weeks, after a normal nuchal scan, a cervical stitch was inserted in view of multiple previous late pregnancy losses and a short cervix of 2 cm on a nuchal scan. She delivered a healthy male baby at term weighing 2.6 kg.

This case highlights the following:

- Multiple thrombotic abnormalities require a full dose of LMWH and close follow-up.
- Multiple etiologies may be seen in the same patient. In this case, the early miscarriages (5–7 weeks) were due to thrombotic etiology whereas the second trimester miscarriages were due to uterocervical pathology (See Chapter 19).
- Multiple second-trimester losses may lead to cervical insufficiency.

CASE 3: HOMOZYGOUS *MTHFR* GENE MUTATION

Mala Arora

A 36-year-old, A3 early miscarriages. Three early miscarriages between 5 and 6 weeks. The gestational sac was documented once and raised beta-hCG was documented on all three occasions, but no fetal pole was seen in any pregnancy. All pregnancies were medically treated with no results for POC analysis available.

- *FSH:* 4.84 mIU/mL
- *LH:* 2.58 mIU/mL
- *Prolactin:* 11.47 ng/mL
- *Testosterone (total):* 19.79 ng/dL
- *Thyroid-stimulating hormone (TSH):* 1.967 µIU/mL
- *Anti-Müllerian hormone (AMH):* 1.87 ng/mL
- *APLA* negative
- Thyroid profile—normal
- *Fibrinogen:* 2.98 g/L (Normal 1.5–4.0 g/L)
- Antithrombin III activity—normal
- Protein C activity—normal
- Protein S antigen normal
- **Serum Homocysteine = 14.80 umol/L (Normal 3.70–13.90 umol/L)**

THROMBOSIS GENE ASSAY

- Factor II prothrombin gene mutation *not* present
- *Factor V Leiden c.1601G > A mutation:* Not present
- *MTHFR c.665 C >T variant*: Not present
- *MTHFR c.1286A >C variant: Present (homozygote)—abnormal*

Recurrent early pregnancy loss with a maternal age of 36 years. In view of very early pregnancy losses and normal fecundity, she was suggested to track her ovulation by urine hCG kit and start treatment on postovulation or soon after documented ovulation.

- Aspirin 150 mg continuously
- Enoxaparin 40 mg subcutaneously (SC) injections on postovulation
- Folic acid 5 mg daily continuously
- Tab *Homochek* 1 daily containing cyanocobalamin 400 µg pyridoxine hydrochloride 10 mg and folic acid 1 mg.

She was taking all of the above medications and on subsequent positive pregnancy test, she was started on dydrogesterone 10 mg BID, LMWH 40 mg SC daily in view of her hyperhomocysteinemia.

She is now 28 weeks pregnant with a normal fetal anatomy scan and a normal uterine artery Doppler.

DISCUSSION

There is no consensus on whether *MTHFR* gene mutations are associated with unexplained RPL. Some studies have found an increased frequency of *MTHFR* gene mutation in patients with RPL. However, there are no randomized control trials on this issue.

This case illustrates that certain *MTHFR* gene mutations may play a role in RPL. Two important mutations are the MTHFR c.1286A >C variant and the *MTHFR* c.665C >T variant. Homocysteine levels may be checked in women harboring these mutations. If homocysteine levels are abnormal it will warrant treatment with folic acid, vitamin B_6, B_{12}, and LMWH in view of endothelial dysfunction (See Chapter 34).

CASE 4: ARTERIOVENOUS MALFORMATION AFTER MISCARRIAGE

Neelanjana Mukhopadhaya

A 25-year-old lady in her first pregnancy had a normal antenatal booking with an obstetric nuchal USS which appeared to be normal. She declined the first-trimester screening and was booked for an anomaly scan at 20 weeks. She had a spontaneous miscarriage at 19 weeks and the fetus was diagnosed to have trisomy 21. Following this, she had very heavy bleeding suggesting that the placenta was retained. It was manually removed with polyp forceps and seemed adherent at the fundus. It appeared complete on examination. She underwent a scan 1 week later when only a small area of retained products measuring 17 × 16 mm was seen at the fundus and in view of the small size she was managed conservatively.

She continued to experience some bleeding off and on, and a scan 3 weeks later suggested that the area of retained products was still present however there was an area of vascularity at the fundus, suggestive of possible arteriovenous malformation (AVM)**(Figs. 1A to C)**. She underwent a magnetic resonance imaging (MRI) scan and multidisciplinary team (MDT) discussion which involved consultant gynecologists and consultant radiologists.

The plan was to consider uterine artery embolization but in view of her desire for fertility, it was decided to manage her conservatively. She had two admissions with very heavy bleeding and was given depot gonadotropin-releasing hormone (GnRH) agonist 11.25 mg with calcium supplements. After an extensive MDT discussion, she was also commenced on high-dose progesterone, norethisterone 5 mg three times a day. She subsequently had two further episodes of moderate bleeding which did not require admission. She was given tranexamic acid orally with an explanation about the risk of thrombosis and to use it sparingly. She was seen at regular intervals and given detailed explanations and counseling/support and the AVM was resolved after about 4 months.

She was advised to use contraception and prophylactic iron tablets for the next 6 months.

We still await to see her future obstetric performance.

DISCUSSION

Arteriovenous malformation is a rare consequence of midtrimester miscarriage. They may lead to torrential hemorrhage. Treatment modalities are as follows:

Management of uterine AVM should be individualized, considering the woman's desire for future fertility and the stability of her health at presentation. The options include:

- Transcatheter uterine arterial embolization is an excellent treatment option in selected cases. The uterine artery is embolized with microparticles, coil, glue, or alcohol, while the collateral supply maintains uterine perfusion, thus preserving fertility.
- The effect of gonadotropin-releasing hormone agonist (GnRHa) on uterine AVM is well known. It can be used for reduction in the size of AVM where uterine artery embolization is not suitable.
- Oral contraceptives.
- Intramuscular (IM) and subsequent oral high dose progesterone can cause regression of lesions as seen on USS.
- The standard mode of treatment for uterine AVM was a hysterectomy, which is indicated for life threatening hemorrhage in women who have completed their family (See Chapter 21).

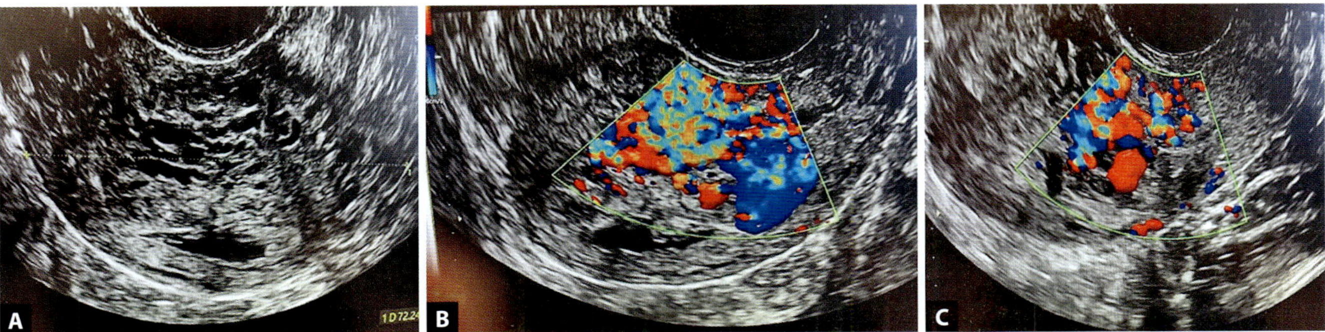

Figs. 1A to C: Arteriovenous malformation at the uterine fundus.

CASE 5: ADENOMYOSIS AND PELVIC ENDOMETRIOSIS WITH MULTIPLE COMORBIDITIES

T Ramanidevi

Mrs J, age 36 years G9P0L0A8

Married 2009

- *2011:* A1—missed miscarriage at 13 weeks—medically managed, check suction curettage done post spontaneous expulsion.
- *2012:* 2016—A2-A7—missed miscarriages between 5 and 10 weeks - Medical management
- *2017:* A8—placenta low-lying miscarried at 14 weeks after excessive bleeding per vaginum
- *2019:* G9—IUI conception

The couple had Rh incompatibility. Anti-D was administered post miscarriage from A3 onward.

After the third miscarriage, APLA testing was done and found to be positive. Since then, Aspirin 75 mg and LMWH 40 µg SC were administered in each pregnancy, fourth pregnancy onward.

The patient was diagnosed as:

- Type II diabetes mellitus (DM) post sixth miscarriage, controlled on oral hypoglycemic agents since 2015
- Hypothyroid since 2018 supplemented with thyroxine 50 µg. Thyroid antibodies negative.

Karyotyping of the couple was normal, which was done after five miscarriages.

Products of conception sent for karyotyping in the fifth miscarriage were inconclusive, due to failure of culture.

With eight pregnancy losses, she came under our care.

Problems diagnosed before reaching us:

- Rh incompatibility
- APLA syndrome
- Type II DM
- Hypothyroidism well controlled on supplementation
- Couple karyotyping—normal

Clinical examination revealed a normal BMI and general physical examination.

Diabetes mellitus was well controlled with metformin 750 mg twice daily, hypothyroidism was corrected on thyroid supplementation.

USG: Adenomyotic uterus, left ovary showed endometriotic cyst and right ovary was normal.

2019: Diagnostic hysterolaparoscopy done. Findings showed a bulky uterus with diffuse adenomyosis.

Left endometriotic cyst: 3 × 3 cm removed, the same side, and the left fimbrial cyst was also removed. The right ovary was normal.

Hysteroscopy showed simple endometrial (EM) hyperplasia without atypia. Histopathology of both removed specimens showed endometriosis.

Past history revealed hyperprolactinemia at the age of 33 years, treated with Cabergoline but currently, her prolactin level is normal.

Family history was positive for the presence of DM in both parents.

The malefactor was normal.

Treatment Given

In view of endometriosis/adenomyosis/EM hyperplasia, depot GnRH analogs, 3.75 mg IM was given, in three doses, 1 month apart. The patient was started on preconceptional folic acid. In view of advanced maternal age AMH was tested and reported as 1 ng/mL. Ovulation was induced with gonadotropins. She had two dominant follicles and IUI was done. Progesterone was supplemented in the luteal phase. She conceived and a scan showed a single live fetus. LDA, LMWH, insulin, thyroid supplementation, and intravenous immunoglobin were given once in 21 days for refractory APLA syndrome. Iron and calcium supplementation was given. The indirect Coombs test was negative and antenatal anti-D was given at 28 and 34 weeks. Ante natal period was uneventful, and growth scans showed normal growth of the fetus. Prophylactic steroids—dexamethasone was administered at 28 weeks in view of multiple comorbidities. The patient developed coronavirus disease 2019 (COVID-19) at 33 weeks of pregnancy. Her symptoms were mild and treated by home quarantine. She had a transient fall in AFI which recovered after COVID.

The growth profile was normal. The patient was posted for elective LSCS by 38 weeks. A 2.9 kg baby was delivered and was healthy. It did not need NICU care. The uterus was adenomyotic and adherent to the pelvis. The postoperative period was uneventful. LMWH continued for 2 weeks postpartum for thromboprophylaxis. The patient was inserted with LNG-IUS in the postnatal period and is on follow-up.

DISCUSSION

Multiple comorbidities were elicited which were well controlled. APLA syndrome refractory to Aspirin, LMWH, hence received intravenous immunoglobulin (IVIG) during this pregnancy.

Newer findings of endometriosis and adenomyosis were corrected by laparoscopic excision and prolonged GnRH suppression, preceding ovulation induction and intrauterine insemination, adequate luteal support and corrective treatment for refractory APLA syndrome helped in achieving a positive outcome (See Chapter 17).

CASE 6: UNDIAGNOSED DIABETES MELLITUS

BS Susheela Rani

- Patient 30-year-old, BMI 32
- Husband 32-year-old, BMI normal (not a smoker or alcoholic)
- First pregnancy spontaneous conception—biochemical pregnancy.
- Second pregnancy conceived after ovulation induction—6 weeks missed miscarriage, no fetal pole seen—evacuated with tablets
- Third pregnancy—conceived after IUI—6 weeks missed miscarriage; no fetal pole seen—evacuated with tablets.
- Point-of-care could not be checked as no fetal pole was seen.
- No significant family history

INVESTIGATIONS

- *CBC:* Normal
- *Liver function test (LFT) and renal function test (RFT):* Normal
- **Glycated hemoglobin (HbA1c): *7.7***
- **OGTT: Fasting 129 mg/dL, 2 hours—176 mg/dL**
- *Thyroid profile:* Normal. Anti-TPO antibodies—negative
- ANA—negative
- APLA—negative

The patient was started on tablet metformin 250 mg twice daily increased to 500 mg twice daily after 2 weeks.

She was advised to lose weight, exercise, and follow a diabetic diet.

She lost 4.5 kg in the next 4 months and conceived spontaneously.

Her sugars at 8 weeks despite metformin 500 mg twice daily were not controlled

Fasting was 110 mg/dL and post prandial 160 mg/dL.

She was started on insulin rapid-acting (Aspart) 6 units with meals and long-acting (Levemir) 4 units at bedtime.

Her insulin dose was increased during the course of pregnancy based on her glycemic profile.

She developed preeclampsia at 32 weeks.

An emergency lower segment cesarean section (LSCS) was done at 34 weeks for preterm premature rupture of membranes (PPROM). A healthy male baby of 2.2 kg was extracted which needed NICU care for 2 days.

Mother and baby were discharged in good condition on the sixth postnatal day.

COMMENTS

Repeated early pregnancy losses in this woman were possibly due to Hyperglycemia. Screening women by HbA1c levels is a good single-point screening strategy. Metformin with an incremental dosage of up to 2.5–3 g/day assists in normalizing her sugars. Exercise, a diabetic diet, and weight loss all helped her to conceive again spontaneously. Her diabetic status became very evident once she conceived. Insulin and metformin are ideal pharmacological agents to manage sugars in pregnancy and as in our case, they were responsible for a successful outcome (See Chapter 32).

CASE 7: RECURRENT FETAL ANEUPLOIDY WITH NORMAL PARENTAL KARYOTYPE

Seema Sharma

A 29-year-old housewife with her 31-year-old businessman husband, with whom she was married for 5 years, presented to our RPL clinic. The couple had of average BMI.

The first pregnancy was an intrauterine device (IUD) at 17 weeks. The fetus had ascites and hydrothorax on USS. The viral panel was normal, including parvovirus B19. A female fetus was expelled followed by a surgical suction evacuation. No genetic studies were done.

The second pregnancy ended in a missed miscarriage at 8 weeks and the POC were sent for examination. Double Trisomy of chromosomes 15 and 16 was reported.

The clinical examination of the mother was normal. Routine investigations were normal.

INVESTIGATIONS

- Blood group B positive
- *TSH/TPO antibody:* 3.3
- *HbA1c:* 5
- Thrombophilia:
  - LAC—negative
  - Anticardiolipin antibody—negative
  - B2 glycoprotein—normal
- Antinuclear antibody—negative
- **USG—3D bicornuate uterus with unequal horns**
- Karyotype of husband and wife—normal
- **POC testing—done in second abortus—trisomy 15 and trisomy 16**

DISCUSSION

This case poses the following problems:

- Structural abnormality of the uterus is not easy to correct surgically. One option to favor implantation in the larger horn to prevent a miscarriage is to insert an inert IUD in the smaller horn.[1]
- Recurrent fetal aneuploidy with normal parental karyotype will need genetic counseling and likely a more detailed genetic workup (See Chapters 2, 3, 4).

REFERENCE

1. Arora M, Basu H. Nonsurgical management of uterus didelphus. Saudi Medical Journal. 1989;10(1):141-2.

CASE 8: SECONDARY MISCARRIAGES WITH MULTIPLE COMORBIDITIES

Shobhna Mohandas

G6 P1 A4 nurse by profession, presented with 7 days missed period and positive urine pregnancy test.

- First pregnancy cesarean section at term, healthy baby girl, currently 11 years old.
- Four early first trimester miscarriages at 5-6 weeks, last miscarriage was 2 years ago. All pregnancies are medically terminated. No POC analysis was done as very early miscarriages.
- In her last pregnancy she was:
  - APLA positive
  - TSH was upper normal range and antithyroid antibodies were high.
  - Maturity onset DM controlled on metformin 750 mg twice daily.
  - Toxoplasma IgM titers were high for which she received treatment with a full course of spiramycin 1 g twice daily for 14 days.

She continued on levothyroxine (LT4) 75 µg/day. She was prescribed LMWH 40 mg daily, prednisolone 10 mg/three times daily for autoimmune thyroiditis, micronized progesterone 200 mg vaginally twice daily, and metformin 750 mg twice daily. She was also given hydroxychloroquine 400 mg twice daily and one dose of intralipid after a positive pregnancy test for refractory APLA syndrome. She had a healthy lifestyle and was also self-medicating with probiotics twice daily, vitamin C, and vitamin E.

The current pregnancy did not proceed beyond 6 weeks. Though a gestational sac was seen, subsequent scans failed to show a fetal pole and she miscarried a few days later.

DISCUSSION

After an uneventful first pregnancy, multiple early secondary miscarriages ensued. All known comorbidities were adequately addressed in this patient. She was also taking probiotics and antioxidants of her own accord. Yet we were unable to rectify the cause for recurrent early pregnancy losses.

CASE 9: RECURRENT BIOCHEMICAL PREGNANCY LOSSES

Seema Sharma

A 30-year-old female and 32-year-old male, married 3 years.

A1: Biochemical loss—overdue by 5 days—spontaneous bleeding the day urine pregnancy test came positive.

A2: 6 weeks 6 days missed miscarriage—suction evacuation done. POC normal comparative genomic hybridization microarray (CGH-MA) result.

A3: Beta-human chorionic gonadotropin grew till 380 then fell—spontaneous resolution of pregnancy.

A4: β-hCG rising slowly, growing by 10 units/day—maximum value was 180 IU/mL followed by spontaneous resolution.

MEDICAL HISTORY

- *MTFHR* gene mutation positive
- Anovulatory polycystic ovary syndrome (PCOS) positive
- The last two conceptions occurred after ovulation Induction with letrozole.
- *AMH:* 1.8
- TSH and antithyroid antibodies normal
- EM evaluation is normal
- Semen analysis is normal
- Sperm DNA fragmentation < 20

She has been advised to have the following tests prior to getting pregnant:

- Three-dimensional (3D) transvaginal scans to rule out the septate uterus
- Fasting serum homocysteine levels
- APLA profile
- Thrombophilia profile
- Testosterone panel to rule out hyperandrogenemia.
- Couple karyotyping
- HbA1c

DISCUSSION

This case illustrates that: Biochemical pregnancies should be a part of the definition of RPL. Recurrent biochemical pregnancies could be autoimmune or genetic. The *MTHFR* gene mutation as well as PCOS can also be present with this picture. Further evaluation of testosterone profile, fasting homocysteine levels, parental karyotyping, and autoimmune screening may need to be evaluated. POC are not always available for genetic testing in early losses. The debatable issue will be whether in vitro fertilization (IVF) and embryo testing for aneuploidy is warranted after the next pregnancy loss if all other factors have been evaluated and optimized (See Chapter 38).

CASE 10: AUTOIMMUNE THYROIDITIS

Asher Bashiri, Israel David Gabay, Liu Shuling

A 35-year-old lady was referred to the RPL clinic with four biochemical pregnancies before having a successful delivery of her son in 2014. It was a spontaneous planned pregnancy with an uneventful antenatal period and delivery of a healthy baby at 36 weeks weighing 2.4 kg.

She subsequently had another 16 pregnancy losses—11 biochemical pregnancies and four clinical pregnancy losses. She had a total of 21 pregnancies with one live birth.

She was diagnosed with hypothyroidism and was on thyroxine replacement of 700 μg/week (100 μg/day). She was a chronic smoker and smoked half a pack of cigarettes per day for the past 15 years. She did not have any other medical or surgical history of note.

Their family history included diabetes, autism, and colorectal cancer.

Physical examination was normal with a BMI of 18.4.

A 3D anatomical scan of the pelvis was normal.

Couple's karyotypes—normal

Tests for thrombophilia—normal

Tests for rheumatoid factor, antinuclear antibody (ANA) and antiphospholipid syndrome with LAC, anticardiolipin IgM and IgG antibodies, and anti-beta2 glycoprotein antibodies—all negative

Prolactin, vitamin D levels—normal

Blood sugars and HbA1C—normal

She had normal thyroid function at the delivery of her first child in 2014 and was only diagnosed with hypothyroidism in 2016, together with elevated thyroid peroxidase antibodies. She was on 700 μg thyroxine per week, i.e., 100 μg/day.

Her TSH fluctuated from 2.29 to 8.19 μU/mL.

Thyroid peroxidase antibodies were steadily rising from 2151 μIU/mL in 2016 to 9005 μIU/mL in 2018 **(Box 1)**. Her thyroglobulin antibodies were normal. Thyroid dysfunction with thyroid autoimmunity is a known factor for RPL and her thyroxine dose was increased by 30% in view of her suboptimal TSH level.

BOX 1: Results of recurrent pregnancy loss workup.

Acquired thrombophilia:
- Lupus anticoagulant (LAC)—1.1 (0.8–1.20 ratio)
- Anticardiolipin (ACL) antibodies IgM—2.4 U/mL (0–20 U/mL)
- Anticardiolipin antibodies IgA—3.6 U/mL (0–20 U/mL)
- Anticardiolipin antibodies IgG—6 U/mL (0–20 U/mL)
- Anti-β2 glycoprotein 1 (aβ2GP1) IgG—4 U/mL (0–20 U/mL)
- Anti-β2 glycoprotein 1 (aβ2GP1) IgM—6 U/mL (0–20 U/mL)

Hereditary thrombophilia:
- Factor V Leiden mutation—normal
- Prothrombin mutation—normal
- Antithrombin III—106% (80–120%)
- Protein S—84% (60–150%)
- Protein C—92% (70–150%)

Hormonal and metabolic:
- TSH **(Fig. 1)**
- Antithyroglobulin 47.8 IU/mL (10–40 IU/mL)
- Antithyroid peroxidase (TPO) **(Fig. 2)**
- Vitamin D—40 ng/mL (20–50 ng/mL)
- Fasting glucose—81 mg/dL (70–100 mg/dL)
- HbA1c—4.7% (<5.7%)
- Prolactin—24 ng/L (<25 ng/L)

Immunologic:
- Rheumatoid factor—normal
- Antinuclear antibody (ANA)—<1:80 ratio

Genetic:
- Paternal karyotype—46,XY
- Maternal karyotype—46,XX

Anatomical: 3D ultrasound of pelvis—normal uterine cavity

She was advised to be compliant with her thyroxine replacement and folic acid intake of 800 μg/day.

Healthy lifestyle habits were recommended to the couple including smoking cessation, reduction of stress, caffeine, and alcohol. An active lifestyle was also recommended to the couple. She was advised to attempt another pregnancy when her TSH level was below 2.5 μU/mL.

She managed to conceive naturally in 2020. The demand for thyroxine increases in pregnancy and therefore the weekly dosage of thyroxine was increased by 30% to 1,200 μg/week.

She was also given empirical prednisolone 10 mg/day and luteal support with dydrogesterone 10 mg three times per day till the 20th week of gestation. At 35 weeks and 5 days, she had preterm premature rupture of membrane, underwent a cesarean section, and delivered a healthy baby. A year later she had another successful pregnancy with the same management.

DISCUSSION

Thyroid dysfunction is a well-known cause of RPL. This is a special case illustrating the devastating effects of poorly controlled thyroid function on pregnancy outcomes in a patient with a history of 20 previous pregnancy loss. In patients with high antithyroid antibodies, thyroid replacement therapy may not be sufficient to prevent pregnancy loss (See Chapter 30).

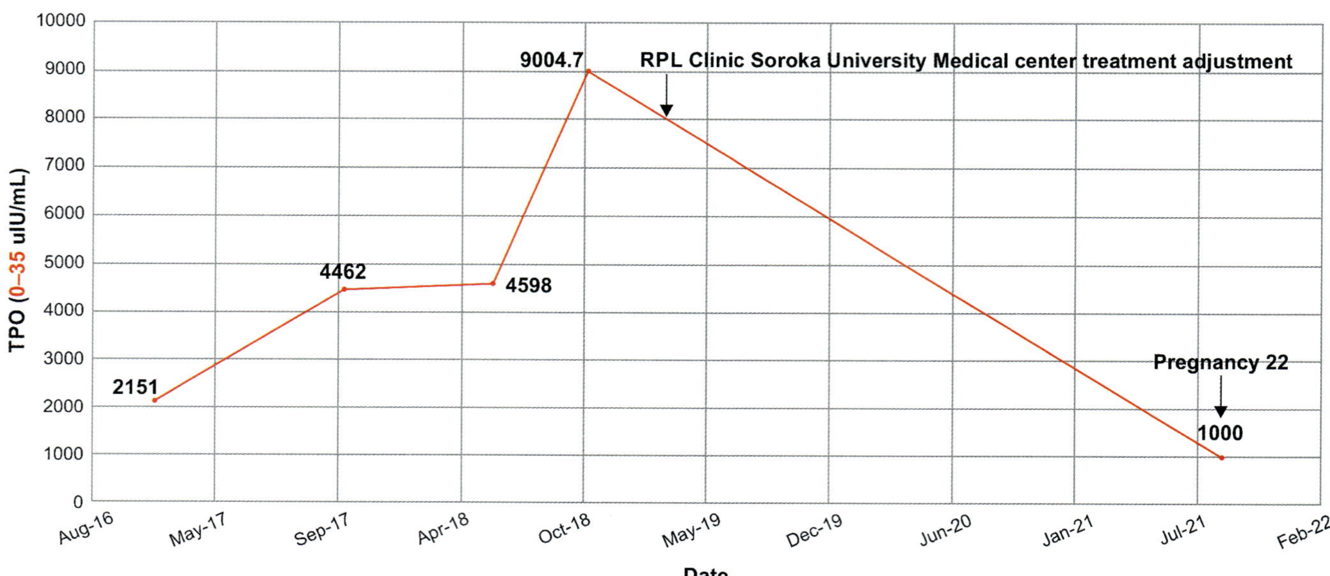

Fig. 1: Patient's thyroid peroxidase antibodies (TPOs) levels.

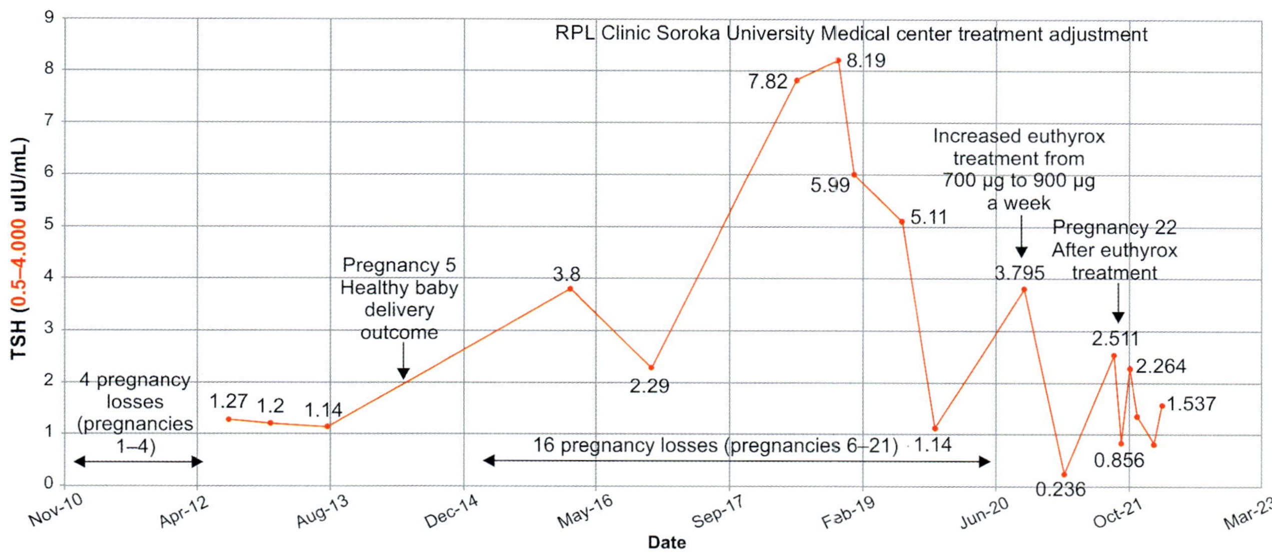

Fig. 2: Patient's thyroid-stimulating hormone (TSH) trend. (RPL: recurrent pregnancy loss)

CASE 11: ADVANCED MATERNAL AGE WITH AUTOIMMUNITY: STEM CELL OVARIAN REJUVENATION AND MULTIPLE DRUG THERAPY

Nayana Patel

A **46 years old**, married for 8 years. Regular menstrual cycle, duration 28–30 days with 4–5 days of flow.

HISTORY

- *Pregnancy losses:*
  - *First miscarriage:* October 2017 at 11 weeks.
  - *Second miscarriage:* July 2017 at 10 weeks (fetus had Down syndrome).
  - *Third miscarriage:* December 2017 at 8 weeks (missed abortion).
  - *Fourth miscarriage July 2020:* Conceived naturally but no heartbeat detected at 6 weeks.
- *Previous treatments:*
  - *May 2018:* One IVF cycle.
  - 13 follicles retrieved, 9 mature eggs, and two blastocysts formed, both with genetic abnormalities.

INVESTIGATIONS

- *Semen analysis:* Normal.
- *TVS:* Uterus anteverted with two small, 1–2 cm, anterior wall intramural fibroids, not indenting the EM cavity.
- *Immune cell investigations:*
  - **TNF-alpha: 133 high**
  - *Peripheral natural killer cells:* (CD16 + CD56): 2.3% (low)
  - **Anti-TPO: 115 high**
  - Antipaternal cytotoxic antibodies (APCAs) which is a lymphocyte crossmatch between husband and wife: Negative
  - **ANA: Strong positive 1:320**

TREATMENT

- Laparoscopy and hysteroscopy were done.
- Laparoscopy findings showed two small intramural myomas <2 cm. Bilateral intraovarian bone marrow-derived stem cell therapy, for in vitro activation (IVA) of ovaries to improve the quality of oocytes.
- *Hysteroscopy*: Normal findings. Sub-EM platelet-rich plasma (PRP) was injected to improve EM implantation.
- We treated her with lymphocyte immunotherapy (LIT) as APCA was negative. This will improve immune cell dysregulation and improve the maternal intolerance to the fetus.
- She continued thyroxine 50 µg daily.
- She received the following drugs for autoimmunity.

Tacrolimus 2 mg twice daily for 15 days, followed by 1.5 mg BD for 7 days, followed by 1 mg BD for 12 weeks (for high TNF alpha)

- Pentoxifylline 400 mg twice daily.
- Prednisolone 10 mg three times a day.
- Dydrogesterone 10 mg twice daily.

OUTCOMES

- Conceived naturally post-treatment.
- Genetic testing by NIPT confirmed the fetus was free of chromosomal abnormalities, including trisomies 13, 18, and 21.
- Delivered a healthy baby boy in July 2023.

DISCUSSION

This case illustrates that advanced maternal age (>40 years) is associated with a high percentage of embryos having genetic abnormalities.

Ovarian rejuvenation with stem cell therapy can result in spontaneous ovulation in women with advanced maternal age (See Chapter 51).

Pregnancy outcomes are poor with positive multiple autoimmune markers; hence she was administered steroids, tacrolimus, and pentoxyphylline. There is limited experience of the use of these drugs in pregnancy.

CASE 12: PREIMPLANTATION GENETIC TESTING

Aruna Ashok

HISTORY

The patient is a 29-year-old woman who has been married for 4 years as of June 2022. She has a history of secondary infertility, a BMI is 23, having failed to conceive in the past year despite efforts. The patient had three consecutive first-trimester miscarriages, each diagnosed as missed miscarriages, as here:

- *A1 (2018):* Missed miscarriage at 6 weeks
- *A2 (2020):* Missed miscarriage at 9 weeks
- *A3 (2021):* Missed miscarriage at 7 weeks

INVESTIGATIONS

- Uterine cavity—normal by 3D USS
- EB-CD138 count was negative
- Couple karyotyping—normal results
- Endocrine tests (75 g GTT, HbA1c, and TSH), showed normal results
- Autoimmune markers (ATA, APLA, ANA) all negative
- Hereditary thrombophilia normal profile
- MTHFR128C heterozygous positive nonsignificant
- The male partner had a sperm DNA fragmentation index (DFI) of 6.0%.
- Products of conception testing not done in previous miscarriages

She was advised ovulation induction and timed intercourse, but she had a *fourth missed miscarriage* at 8 weeks, despite treatment with aspirin 75 mg daily, dydrogesterone 10 mg BD, and a prophylactic dose of LMWH injections. During the last miscarriage (A4), chromosomal analysis of the POC revealed a pathogenic deletion on chromosome 11 (1.6Mb) and uncertain deletions on chromosomes 1 and 7. The pathogenic nature of the chromosome 11 deletion, which involved autosomal dominant mutations, suggested that the deletion was de novo, with a negligible recurrence risk.

After the fourth miscarriage, the patient was counseled regarding further treatment options, including ovulation induction (OI) with timed intercourse (TI) or IUI. She opted for IUI with hormonal support, injection LMWH, and LDA to aid implantation, resulting in a positive pregnancy test on June 20, 2022. However, this pregnancy also ended in a *fifth miscarriage*, at 6 weeks, confirmed by a serum beta-hCG drop and subsequent suction evacuation on July 16, 2022. Karyotyping of the POC from the fifth miscarriage revealed autosomal trisomy chromosome 16, which typically arises de novo due to meiotic nondisjunction during gametogenesis.

The overall rates of chromosomal abnormalities in groups with previous autosomal aneuploidy are significantly higher compared with the control group (67.8% for those whose previous aneuploidy arose after natural conception and 65.8% for those whose aneuploidy arose after Assisted reproduction, versus 34.0% in control).

TABLE 1: Results of preimplantation genetic testing for aneuploidy (PGT-A) and niPGT-A embryos.

Sample name	*Result*	*Mitoscore*	*Interpretation*
SV1	Monosomy of chromosome 21	NA	Aneuploid
SV2	Normal chromosome complement	0.0036	Euploid
SV3	Multiple chromosomal abnormalities	NA	Aneuploid
Sample name	*Result*	*Ploidy screening status*	
SV4	Normal chromosome complement	Euploid	

TREATMENT APPROACH AND PLAN

Given the pattern of RPL, the recurrent chromosomal abnormalities in the miscarried pregnancies, and the normal parental karyotyping, the decision was made to proceed with IVF, intracytoplasmic sperm injection (ICSI) combined with preimplantation genetic testing for aneuploidy (PGT-A). This strategy was aimed at selecting embryos with normal chromosomal content for transfer, reducing the risk of further miscarriages due to chromosomal aneuploidies.

Intracytoplasmic Sperm Injection and Preimplantation Genetic Testing for Aneuploidy

- 17 oocytes were retrieved, 12 fertilized, and four blastocysts on day 5.
- Three embryos underwent PGT-A and 1 noninvasive preimplantation genetic testing (NIPGT). A was done on culture media around blastocyst as trophectoderm (TE) grade C **Table 1**.
- *Day 6:* One embryo frozen grade C without biopsy after normal NIPGT-A result.

One euploid blastocyst was identified and frozen. One euploid embryo was transferred, with supportive medications. Ongoing pregnancy ensued with normal NIPT results. She is currently 20 weeks pregnant with normal anatomy scan results.

DISCUSSION

Recurrent pregnancy loss with a history of chromosomal abnormalities, showing trisomies and deletions, represents a challenging scenario in reproductive medicine. The risk of miscarriage in subsequent pregnancies after multiple RPLs due to chromosomal aneuploidy is significantly higher, with studies showing that 67.8% of patients who had previous aneuploidy are likely to experience similar events. In such cases, PGT-A has become an important tool in IVF to reduce the risk of miscarriage by selecting embryos with a normal chromosomal composition.

Preimplantation genetic testing aneuploidy offers a valuable diagnostic and therapeutic tool, especially in cases like this where previous miscarriages were attributed to chromosomal aneuploidies. While the pathogenic deletion on chromosome 11 is not detectable by PGT-A, its de novo nature and negligible recurrence risk provided reassurance. The inclusion of PGT-A in the treatment protocol will increase the likelihood of a successful pregnancy outcome by selecting embryos free of aneuploidies (See Chapter 10).

This case illustrates the complexities of managing RPL with chromosomal abnormalities and highlights the role of PGT-A in selecting viable embryos during IVF treatment. By utilizing ICSI with PGT-A, the patient can minimize the risk of further miscarriages and increase the likelihood of a successful pregnancy. Ongoing genetic counseling and appropriate supportive therapies will continue to play an essential role in ensuring the best possible outcome for this patient's future attempts at conception.

FUTURE CONSIDERATIONS

Continued research into improving the sensitivity of PGT-A for detecting a wider range of chromosomal abnormalities, including deletions.

APPENDIX

2 Further Reading

The guidelines pertaining to recurrent pregnancy loss (RPL) and related treatment modalities, published in the last two decades, are summarized below. A QR code is provided at the end of the appendix, for the reader to access the guidelines enumerated.

S. No	Society	Guidelines	Year	URL
1.	Indian Society of Assisted Reproduction (ISAR) and Indian Recurrent Pregnancy Loss Foundation (IRPLF)	Good clinical practice recommendations for RPL (upcoming)	2025 March	https://www.isarindia.net irplindia.org
2.	Australasian Position Paper	Recurrent pregnancy loss management Part 1	2024	https://obgyn.onlinelibrary.wiley.com/doi/full/10.1111/ajo.13821
3.	European Society of Human Reproduction and Embryology (ESHRE)	Recurrent pregnancy loss	2023	https://www.eshre.eu/Guidelines-and-Legal/Guidelines/Recurrent-pregnancy-loss
4.	Royal College of Obstetricians and Gynaecologist (RCOG) UK	Recurrent pregnancy loss green top guideline 17	2023	https://www.rcog.org.uk/guidance/browse-all-guidance/green-top-guidelines/recurrent-miscarriage-green-top-guideline-no-17/
5.	American College of Rheumatology (ACR) and European Alliance of Associations for Rheumatology (EULAR)	2023 ACR/EULAR antiphospholipid syndrome classification criteria	2023	https://ard.bmj.com/content/82/10/1258
6.	Queensland	Clinical prioritization criteria in infertility and RPL	2023	https://www.health.qld.gov.au/cpc/gynaecology/infertility
7.	FIGO Good Clinical Practice Recommendations (GCPR)	Progesterone use in recurrent pregnancy loss	2023	https://pubmed.ncbi.nlm.nih.gov/36958854/
8.	National Institute for Health & Clinical Excellence (NICE)	Threatened miscarriage	2022	https://pmc.ncbi.nlm.nih.gov/articles/PMC906694
9.	China	The association between 5, 10 – methylenetetrahydrofolate reductase and the risk of unexplained recurrent pregnancy loss in China	2021	https://pmc.ncbi.nlm.nih.gov/articles/PMC8084099/
10.	Clinical practice guidelines	Recurrent miscarriage in high-income countries: a systematic review	2021	https://pubmed.ncbi.nlm.nih.gov/33895080/
11.	Northern Ireland Public Health Agency	Recurrent pregnancy loss care pathway for Northern Ireland	2021	https://www.publichealth.hscni.net/sites/default/files/2020-02/RPL%20care%20pathway%201019.pdf

Contd...

Contd...

S. No	Society	Guidelines	Year	URL
12.	Israel Medical Association	Recurrent pregnancy loss: Causes, controversies, and treatment	2021	https://pubmed.ncbi.nlm.nih.gov/33443349
13.	European Society for Human Reproduction and Embryology (ESHRE)	ESHRE PGT Consortium good practice recommendations for the organization of PGT	2020	https://pubmed.ncbi.nlm.nih.gov/32524036/
14.	Am J Obstet Gynecol	Inherited susceptibility to miscarriage: A nested case-control study of 31,565 women from an intergenerational cohort	2020	https://pubmed.ncbi.nlm.nih.gov/31437424/
15.	Saudi guidelines	The role of progestogens in threatened and idiopathic recurrent miscarriage	2019	https://www.tandfonline.com/doi/full/10.2147/IJWH.S224159
16.	An Italian RPL Unit experience	What has to be pointed out in unexplained recurrent pregnancy loss research in the unsolved fields: Lessons from clinic	2019	https://art.torvergata.it/handle/2108/299330
17.	Review of Current Guidelines	Recurrent pregnancy loss: New strategies for optimal evaluation of women who may be superfertile	2019	https://www.sciencedirect.com/science/article/abs/pii/S0146000518301447
18.	Reprod Biomed Online	Comparison and appraisal of (inter)national recurrent pregnancy loss guidelines	2019	https://pubmed.ncbi.nlm.nih.gov/31182358/
19.	American College of Obstetrics and Gynecology (ACOG) Practice Bulletin No. 200	Early pregnancy loss	2018	https://pubmed.ncbi.nlm.nih.gov/30157093/
20.	Canadian Guideline	Joint CCMG-SOGC recommendations for the use of chromosomal microarray analysis for prenatal diagnosis and assessment of fetal loss in Canada	2018	https://jmg.bmj.com/content/55/4/215.abstract
21.	Australian Guideline	Recurrent pregnancy loss	2018	https://search.informit.org/doi/abs/10.3316/INFORMIT.708250628530903
22.	Recurrent Pregnancy Loss	Couples' perspectives on their need for treatment, support and follow up	2018	https://academic.oup.com/humrep/article/34/2/291/5248531
23.	ASRM	The use of preimplantation genetic testing for aneuploidy (PGT-A): A committee opinion	2018	https://pubmed.ncbi.nlm.nih.gov/29566854/
24.	Germen (DGGG), Austrian (OGGG) and Swiss (SGGG)	Recurrent miscarriage: Diagnostic and therapeutic procedures. Guideline of the DGGG, OEGGG and SGGG (S2k-Level, AWMF Registry Number 015/050)	2018	https://pmc.ncbi.nlm.nih.gov/articles/PMC5925690/
25.	The Society for Translational Medicine	Clinical practice guidelines for sperm DNA fragmentation testing in male infertility	2017	https://pmc.ncbi.nlm.nih.gov/articles/PMC5643607/
26.	2017 Guidelines of the American Thyroid Association	The diagnosis and management of thyroid disease during pregnancy and the postpartum	2017	https://pubmed.ncbi.nlm.nih.gov/28056690/
27.	South Africa	Medical conditions associated with recurrent miscarriage—Is BMI the tip of the iceberg?	2017	https://www.sciencedirect.com/science/article/abs/pii/S0301211517302282
28.	ASRM	Removal of myomas in asymptomatic patients to improve fertility and/or reduce miscarriage rate: a guideline	2017	https://www.sciencedirect.com/science/article/pii/S0015028217304934

Contd...

Contd...

S. No	Society	Guidelines	Year	URL
29.	Korean Society	Intravenous immunoglobulin G in women with reproductive failure: The Korean Society for Reproductive Immunology practice guidelines	2017	https://pubmed.ncbi.nlm.nih.gov/28428937/
30.	American Board of Internal Medicine	Practical work-up and management of recurrent pregnancy loss for the front-line clinician	2016	https://journals.lww.com/clinicalobgyn/abstract/2016/09000/practical_work_up_and_management_of_recurrent.10.aspx
31.	Utah, USA	The importance of an evidence-based workup for recurrent pregnancy loss	2016	https://journals.lww.com/clinicalobgyn/abstract/2016/09000/the_importance_of_an_evidence_based_workup_for.3.aspx
32.	National Standards for Bereavement Care	Following pregnancy Loss and perinatal death	2016	https://www.hse.ie/eng/services/list/3/maternity/bereavement-care/national-standards-for-bereavement-care-following-pregnancy-loss-and-perinatal-death.pdf
33.	French clinical practice guidelines	Pregnancy loss	2016	https://www.sciencedirect.com/science/article/abs/pii/S0301211516300513
34.	ASRM	Uterine septum: A guideline	2016	http://www.saegre.org.ar/biblioteca/reproduccion/Uterine%20septum%20A%20guideline%20%20ASRM.pdf
35.	RCOG	The Role of Natural Killer Cells in Human Fertility (Scientific Impact Paper No. 53)	2016	https://www.rcog.org.uk/guidance/browse-all-guidance/scientific-impact-papers/the-role-of-natural-killer-cells-in-human-fertility-scientific-impact-paper-no-53/
36.	IOWA, USA	Validating evidence and using standard outcomes for recurrent pregnancy loss tests and treatments	2016	https://pubmed.ncbi.nlm.nih.gov/27380206/
37.	Ireland, UK, NewZealand, Australia	Previous pregnancy loss has an adverse impact on distress and behavior in subsequent pregnancy	2015	https://obgyn.onlinelibrary.wiley.com/doi/abs/10.1111/1471-0528.13233
38.	NICE GUIDELINES	Hysteroscopic metroplasty of a uterine septum for recurrent miscarriage	2015	https://www.nice.org.uk/guidance/ipg510
39.	FOGSI Position statement on Progesterone use	Progesterone use in pregnancy	2015	https://www.fogsi.org/wp-content/uploads/2015/11/Progesterone-position-paper-Oct-2015.pdf
40.	ASRM	Subclinical hypothyroidism in the infertile female population: A guideline	2015	https://www.fertstert.org/article/S0015-0282(15)00379-9/fulltext
41.	Clinics of North America	Recurrent miscarriage clinics	2014	https://www.researchgate.net/publication/260090148_Recurrent_Miscarriage_Clinics
42.	American College of Medical Genetics (ACMG) Practice Guideline	Lack of evidence for MTHFR polymorphism testing	2013	https://www.sciencedirect.com/science/article/pii/S1098360021009163
43.	Hum Reprod (Netherland)	Recurrent miscarriage: do professionals adhere to their guidelines	2013	https://pubmed.ncbi.nlm.nih.gov/23970335/

Contd...

Contd...

S. No	Society	Guidelines	Year	URL
44.	American Association of Gyanecological Laparoscopist (AAGL) Practice Report	Practice guidelines for the diagnosis and management of submucous leiomyomas	2012	https://pubmed.ncbi.nlm.nih.gov/22381967/
45.	VTE, Thrombophilia, Antithrombotic Therapy, and Pregnancy	Antithrombotic Therapy and Prevention of Thrombosis, 9th ed: American College of Chest Physicians Evidence-Based Clinical Practice Guidelines	2012	https://www.sciencedirect.com/science/article/abs/pii/S0012369212601366
46.	Clinical Practice Guidelines for Hypothyroidism in Adults	Cosponsored by the American Association of Clinical Endocrinologists and the American Thyroid Association	2012	https://www.sciencedirect.com/science/article/pii/S1530891X20430307
47.	American Society of Reproductive Medicine (ASRM)	Evaluation and treatment of recurrent pregnancy loss: A committee opinion	2012	https://www.asrm.org/practice-guidance/practice-committee-documents/evaluation-and-treatment-of-recurrent-pregnancy-loss-a-committee-opinion-2012/
48.	Patients' perspectives	Supportive care for women with unexplained recurrent miscarriage	2011	https://academic.oup.com/humrep/article-abstract/26/4/873/628219
49.	Acta Obstet Gynecol Scand	Identification of barriers for good adherence to a guideline on recurrent miscarriage	2011	https://pubmed.ncbi.nlm.nih.gov/21241265/
50.	Appraisal of Guidelines for Research and Evaluation II (AGREE II)	Development, reporting and evaluation in health care	2010	https://www.cmaj.ca/content/182/18/E839.short
51.	Management of recurrent miscarriage	Evaluating the impact of a guideline	2007	https://academic.oup.com/humrep/article-abstract/22/5/1298/2914754
52.	Best Practice and Research Clinical Obstetrics and Gynaecology	Psychological morbidity following miscarriage	2007	https://www.sciencedirect.com/science/article/abs/pii/S1521693406001568
53.	The one-stop recurrent miscarriage clinic	Evaluation of its effectiveness and outcome	2004	https://academic.oup.com/humrep/article-abstract/19/12/2952/2356356
54.	DENMARK	Maternal age and fetal loss: Population based register linkage study	2000	https://pmc.ncbi.nlm.nih.gov/articles/PMC27416/

Index

Page numbers followed by *b* refer to box *f* refer to figure, *fc* refer to flowchart and *t* refer to table

D

E

F

P

Q

R

S

T

U

V

W

X

Y

Z